The Leeds Teaching Hospitals
NHS Trust **NHS**

The NHS Staff Library at the L.G.I.

Textbook of Peritoneal Dialysis

2nd Edition

Textbook of Peritoneal Dialysis

2ND EDITION

Edited by

R. Gokal
Manchester Royal Infirmary, Manchester, UK

R. Khanna
MA 436 Health Services Centre, Columbia, U.S.A.

R. Th. Krediet
Academisch Medisch Centrum, Amsterdam, The Netherlands

and

K. D. Nolph
University of Missouri, Columbia, MO, U.S.A.

Kluwer Academic Publishers

Dordrecht / Boston / London

A C.I.P. Catalogue record for this book is available from the Library of Congress

ISBN 0-7923-5967-4

Published by Kluwer Academic Publishers,
P.O. Box 17, 3300 AA Dordrecht, The Netherlands.

Sold and distributed in North, Central and South America
by Kluwer Academic Publishers,
101 Philip Drive, Norwell, MA 02061, U.S.A.

In all other countries, sold and distributed
by Kluwer Academic Publishers Group
P.O. Box 322, 3300 AH Dordrecht, The Netherlands

Printed on acid-free paper

Printed and bound in Great Britain by MPG Books, Bodmin, Cornwall

Table of contents

List of Principal Authors

G. Abraham
Department of Medicine
Sri Ramachandra Medical College and Research
  Institute
Deemed University
Porur
Chennai-600 116
India

T. Apostolou
108 A Sofokli Venizeioùs St.
16 342 Athens
Greece

J.M. Bargman
Department of Medicine
University of Toronto
Toronto General Hospital
200 Elizabeth Street
10EN-216
Toronto
Ontario M5G 2C4
Canada

P.G. Blake
Division of Nephrology and Optimal Dialysis
  Research Unit
London Health Sciences Centre
South Street
London
Ontario N6A 4G5
Canada

E.W. Boeschoten
Department of Internal Medicine
Division of Renal Medicine
Academic Medical Center F4-215
1105 AZ Amsterdam
The Netherlands

J.M. Burkart
Department of Internal Medicine
Wake Forest University School of Medicine
Medical Center Blvd
Winston-Salem
NC 27157-1053
USA

D.N. Churchill
Department of Medicine
McMaster University
St. Joseph's Hospital
50 Charleton St East
Hamilton
Ontario L8N 4A6
Canada

G.A. Coles
Institute of Nephrology
University of Wales College of Medicine
Heath Park
Cardiff
CF14 4XN
UK

M. Feriani
Department of Nephrology
St. Bortolo Hospital
I-36100 Vicenza
Italy

M.F. Flessner
Department of Medicine and Pharmacology and
  Physiology
601 Elmwood Avenue
Rochester
NY 14642
USA

L. Fried
Department of Medicine
Renal Electrolyte Division
University of Pittsburgh Medical Center
A919 Sciafe Hall
Terrace Street
Pittsburgh
PA 15261
USA

R. Gokal
Department of Renal Medicine
Manchester Royal Infirmary
Oxford Road
Manchester
M13 9WL
UK

L. Gotloib
Department of Nephrology and Hypertension
Kupat Holim
'Ha'emek' Medical Center
Afula 18101
Israel

A. Hutchison
Renal Dialysis and Transplant Unit
Manchester Road Infirmary
Oxford Road
Manchester
M13 9WL
UK

P. Kathuria
Department of Internal Medicine
The University of Oklahoma
Health Sciences Center
2808 South Sheridan Road
Tulsa
OK 74129-1077
USA

R. Khanna
Division of Nephrology
Department of Medicine
MA 436 Health Sciences Center
University of Missouri-Columbia
Columbia
MO 65212
USA

R.T. Krediet
University of Amsterdam
Department of Medicine
Division of Nephrology
Secretariat F4-215
PO Box 22700
1100 DE Amsterdam
The Netherlands

N. Lameire
Universiteit Gent
Nefrologie
Universitair Ziekenhuis
De Pintelaan 185
B-9000 Gent
Belgium

R.A. Mactier
Stobhill Hospital Renal Unit
Balornock Road
Glasgow
G21 3UW
UK

R. Maiorca
Divisione di Nefrologia
Spedali Civili di Brescia
Piazza Spedali Civili 1
25123 Brescia
Italy

R. Mehrotra
Peritoneal Dialysis Program
Division of Nephrology and Hypertension
Harbor-UCLA Medical Center
1000 W. Carson Street, Box 406
Torrance
CA 90509
USA

M. Misra
Department of Internal Medicine
Third-Year Nephrology Fellow
MA 436 Health Sciences Center
University of Missouri
Columbia
MO 65212
USA

S. Mujais
Renal Division
Baxter Healthcare Corporation
McGaw Park
Illinois
USA

K.D. Nolph
Department of Internal Medicine
MA 436 Health Sciences Center
University of Missouri-Columbia
Columbia
MO 65212
USA

D.G. Oreopoulos
Toronto Hospital Western Division
399 Bathurst Str.
E Wing, 6 Flr
Toronto
Ontario M5T 258
Canada

C.A. Pollock
Department of Medicine
The Royal North Shore Hospital
DX3332 St. Leonards
New South Wales
Australia

S.S. Prichard
Royal Victoria Hospital
Divison of Nephrology
687 Pine Avenue West, Room R2.38
Montreal
Quebec H3A 1A1
Canada

Z.J. Twardowski
Department of Internal Medicine
Division of Nephrology
MA 436 Health Sciences Center
University of Missouri
Colombia
MO 65212
USA

L. Uttley
Department of Renal Medicine
Manchester Royal Infirmary
Oxford Road
Manchester
M13 9WL
UK

B.A. Warady
Section of Nephrology
Children's Mercy Hospital
2401 Gilham Road
Kansas City
MS 64108
USA

R. White
Nephrology Section
VA Hospital
Mail Code 111 N
Shreveport
LA 71101
USA

Preface

The *Textbook of Peritoneal Dialysis*, in its 2nd edition, covers the advances made in the field over the past 25 years. In the past two decades, the time during which the therapy has been increasingly utilized, this book has been recognized as a major source of the discipline's base knowledge. The evolution of this text from its previous independent volumes parallels the growth of peritoneal dialysis from continuous ambulatory peritoneal dialysis in the eighties to the current therapies that encompass manual and automated therapies with full emphasis on adequacy of dialysis dose.

Peritoneal dialysis represents an intracorporeal technique for blood purification. This unique dialysis system represents one of man's several attempts to manipulate nature for sustenance of life. The past few years of advances have focused on further improvement of the technique. The areas that have fueled the interest of researchers include adequacy of dialysis doses, further improvement in catheter technology, automated techniques, further definition of indications and the ideal time to initiate dialysis. Newer insights into the host–defense mechanisms have also made the past decade of advances in the field more meaningful for the clinicians.

The second edition of the *Textbook of Peritoneal Dialysis* is in a way a compilation of all the explosive new knowledge in the field. It cites and describes in great detail all the new discoveries on a background of prior understanding of the subjects. These advances have made the therapy better in terms of diagnosis and management of patient care. The current group of Editors has worked with the experts in the field to attain balance between the new inventions and contentious issues. An attempt has been made to update bibliographies as recently as possible. To that end, the contributions of *Advances In Peritoneal Dialysis*, the annual publication of selected papers from the Annual Conference of Peritoneal Dialysis, and *Peritoneal Dialysis International*, the official publication of the International Society for Peritoneal Dialysis, have been enormous and can be judged by their frequent citation in the book.

As in the past edition, we have not edited the overlaps between chapters, since we feel the readers might benefit by exposure to different perspectives of complex material.

The Editors have tried in this text to sustain a balance between clinical and theoretical knowledge. We would like to credit our devoted authors for expending their busy time on writing and proofreading their respective chapters. We offer our heartfelt thanks to all the authors for their hard work, extraordinary contributions, and superb cooperation in editing this monumental work. To the many individuals at Kluwer Academic Publishers, we acknowledge their professionalism and intense labor. We appreciate the fine editorial assistance provided by Peggy Gray.

We hope that readers will find this text a useful resource for both clinical and research problems when dealing with patients on peritoneal dialysis.

The Editors
January 2000

1 | History of peritoneal dialysis

R. GOKAL

Introduction

Peritoneal dialysis (PD) has now become an established form of renal replacement therapy. Its use throughout the world is increasing and has provided a means of managing some patients who would otherwise have been denied treatment because haemodialysis was inappropriate, failed or unavailable. The current state of art has been a combination of painstaking efforts, dedication and ingenuity on the part of several innovative pioneers in this field over the past two centuries. This chapter describes these historical developments leading up to PD as it is practised today. This chapter also gives an overview of the state of the art of PD, details of most aspects being given in the relevant chapters that follow.

Historical review of peritoneal dialysis

Probably the first observers of the peritoneal cavity were the early morticians in Egypt, who delicately prepared the remains of influential Egyptians to ensure that the body would remain 'uncorrupted' for eternity [1]. Cunningham [2] reports that 'the Egyptians recorded in the Ebers papyrus, written about 3000 BC, the peritoneal cavity to be a definite entity in which the viscera were somehow suspended'. In conjunction with these anatomical studies these Egyptians also attempted to treat impaired renal function by inducing diarrhoea with the use of purgatives or forced diuresis, using beer. They were thus aware of oedema and understood the effects of diuresis. In Greek times Galan, a physician, made detailed descriptions of the abdomen whilst treating injuries of gladiators. He provided precise details of the peritoneal cavity and peritoneum [1]. Even though gradually, over the centuries, the peritoneal structure became more clearly

defined, its functioning and role better understood, it has remained an enigma and enchanted physiologists, surgeons and gynaecologists. More recently nephrologists joined this band of investigators.

Invention of peritoneal lavage (1744–5)

The concept of peritoneal lavage goes back over 150 years when it served a purpose totally different from that of removal of toxins. Christopher Warrick, a surgeon from Truro in England, presented his findings about a new – rather drastic – method of treating recurrent ascites [3]. He managed a female patient, aged 50, with severe ascites, by infusing a mixture of one-half Bristol water and one-half claret into the peritoneal cavity after draining the ascites. She miraculously recovered from the ensuing syncope and pain. He asked the lady if she thought herself capable of undergoing the procedure a second time! She answered 'in the affirmative'; he then prepared a stronger mixture of claret and water and injected the preparation as before. The patient complained of 'heavy pungent pain, darting through all the viscera' and Warwick became alarmed when her breathing became difficult, her pulse faltered, the syncope returned and the patient became speechless. He withdrew the cannula, ended the procedure and, much to his relief, the patient recovered! During a month of follow-up the ascites did not recur. It is interesting to note that Warrick felt that this was 'ascitic lymph' and was looking for a method whereby the 'ruptured lymphatics must close their mouths' – in his patient he felt that his manoeuvres had 'closed these mouths'.

The idea of peritoneal lavage came from a clergyman, Reverend Stephen Hales, who happened to be present at the presentation of Warrick at the Royal Society of Medicine. Reverend Hales felt pity for the old lady and wrote a letter to the Secretary of the Royal Society suggesting a more gentle modification of Warrick's methods [4]. His technique entailed

R. Gokal, R. Khanna, R.Th. Krediet and K.D. Nolph (eds.), Textbook of Peritoneal Dialysis, 2nd Edition, 1–17.
© 2000 *Kluwer Academic Publishers. Printed in Great Britain.*

introducing two trochars, one on each side of the abdomen, allowing the 'liquor' to flow in and out of the abdomen (Fig. 1).

This first description of peritoneal lavage was essentially identical to the continuous peritoneal lavage later to be used for the treatment of uraemia.

IV. *A Method of conveying* Liquors *into the* Abdomen *during the Operation of* Tapping; *proposed by the* Reverend Stephen Hales, *D. D. and F. R. S. on Occasion of the preceding Paper*; *communicated in a Letter to* Cromwell Mortimer, *M. D. Secr. R. S.*

S I R,   Feb. 22. 1743-4.

Read Feb. 23. IT occurred to me, on your reading,
1743-4.   *Thurfday* laft, before the Society, the Cafe of the Woman at *Truro* in *Cornwall*, who was cured of a Dropfy, by injecting into the *Abdomen Briftol* Water and *Cohore* Wine, after having drawn off a good Quantity of the dropfical *Lympha*; that, in cafe of further Trial, that, or any other Liquor, fhall be found effectual to the Purpofe, it might be more commodioufly injected in the following Manner; *viz.*

By having Two *Trochars* fixed at the fame time, one on each Side of the Belly; one of them having a Communication with a Veffel full of the medicinal Liquor by means of a fmall leathern Pipe: This Liquor might flow into the *Abdomen*, as faft as the dropfical *Lympha* paffed off through the other *Trochar*; whereby the dropfical *Lympha* might be conveyed off, to what Degree it fhall be thought proper; and that without any Danger of a *Syncope* from Inanition; becaufe the *Abdomen* would, through the whole Operation, continue diftended with Liquor, in fuch a Degree as fhall be found proper, by raifing or lowering the Veffel with the medicinal Liquor in it.

It is probable, that, if the Surface of the medicinal Liquor be about a Foot higher than the *Abdomen*, it may be fufficient for the Purpofe.

It were eafy to find the Force with which the *Abdomen* is diftended by the dropfical *Lympha*, by feeing to what Height it arofe in a Glafs Tube fixed to the *Trochar*; which Tube being taken away, it might, I fuppofe, be fufficient to have the medicinal Liquor flow in from a leffer perpendicular Height, than that to which the dropfical *Lympha* arofe in the Glafs Tube. I am,

S I R,

Your humble Servant,

Stephen Hales.

Figure 1. The Rev Stephen Hales' letter to the secretary of the Royal Society (from ref. 3).

Early studies of the peritoneum (1877–1922)

The peritoneum as a semi-permeable membrane

Not much is known of the fate of lavage in managing recurrent ascites. The next publication on experimental peritoneal lavage was published more than 130 years later in the late 19th century by Wegner, a German investigator [5], who in 1877 published the results of a series of animal experiments, perfusing the abdominal cavity of rabbits with cold saline solution, observing a decrease of the animals' body temperature. The results of other animal experiments were more important: he found that hypertonic solutions of sugar, salt or glycerine increased in volume when injected into the peritoneal cavity of animals. These findings were confirmed by a group of English physiologists, headed by Starling and Tubby, who in 1884 showed that hypertonic intraperitoneal solutions would increase whilst hypotonic solutions would decrease in volume [6]. They studied the absorption of such substances as indigo, carmine, and methylene blue from the peritoneal cavity, and concluded that the solute exchange was primarily between solutions and blood; the exchange with lymph was negligible. Cunningham in 1920 showed the complete absorption of a 10% dextrose solution from the rat peritoneal cavity in about 12 hours [7]. Similar results were obtained by Clark [8], who showed that, after introduction of a sodium chloride solution, first absorption occurs and later slower diffusible substances enter the peritoneal cavity from the blood. When dextrose was introduced, making the fluid hypertonic and preventing the absorption of the fluid, water and crystalloids entered the peritoneal fluid. He also further showed that absorption was temperature related; it increased by elevating the temperature of the solution or applying heat to the abdominal wall.

The permeability of the peritoneum

Many of the early investigations [6–8] and other experimental data [9, 10], provided convincing evidence that the peritoneal membrane is permeable in two directions. Starling and Tubby [6] also showed this bidirectional permeability of the peritoneum for larger solutes. When they injected methylene blue, indigo carmine or eosin into the peritoneal cavity, it appeared rapidly in the blood and subsequently in the urine; when these substances were injected intravenously, they appeared rapidly in the peritoneal fluid.

Spurred on by these interesting physiological studies and the report of Abel in 1913 on 'vivi' diffusion (haemodialysis) in animals [11], Putnam published his work in dogs, characterizing the peritoneum as a dialysing membrane [12]. His studies were extensive, looking at fluid removal (ultrafiltration) and exchange of various solutes and varying intervals of dwell time. He concluded that 'under certain circumstances, fluids in the peritoneal cavity can come into an apparently complete osmotic equilibrium with the plasma', and that the 'speed of diffusion of different molecules through the peritoneum appeared to vary with their respective sizes'. He also pointed out that 'changes in volume reflected the osmotic forces at work'.

This work, as well as that of others [7, 8], presented convincing evidence that the peritoneal membrane was permeable in two directions. The movement of water and crystalloids could be explained on the basis of the 'known physical laws of osmosis and diffusion', in a similar way to the pigs' bladder membrane or a membrane of non-biological material such as parchment *in vitro*, a phenomenon first described by Graham in 1861 who also coined the word dialysis [13]. These studies on transfer of colloids and crystalloids in a bidirectional manner across the peritoneal membrane were fundamental in establishing the principles of solute transport and ultrafiltration, which are still true to this day. These studies were further amplified by Engel, who showed that the clearance of solute was proportional to the molecular size and solution pH, and high flow rate maximized the transfer of solutes which also depended on peritoneal surface area and blood flow [14].

Further progress and practical application of this acquired knowledge was relatively slow, mainly because most work was undertaken by scientists. The clinical investigators had not appreciated the medical application so far. However, two paediatricians, Blackfan and Maxey, did utilize the peritoneal cavity for the administration of fluids to dehydrated children [15].

Early experiences of PD in uraemia (1923–45)

Ganter, a German clinical investigator, is traditionally credited with the first attempts to utilize PD in a human being [16]. Originally (in 1918) he removed a pleural effusion from a uraemic man, replacing the fluid with 0.75 L of a sodium chloride solution. He observed some improvement during the next 2 days. He also performed a series of experimental PD in rabbits and guinea pigs made uraemic by ureteric ligation. Injecting 40–60 ml of saline into the peritoneal cavity of a guinea pig, Ganter removed the remaining fluid after 2–4 h and then instilled fresh solution; the procedure was repeated every 3 h. There was almost complete equilibration of non-protein nitrogen in dialysate with that in the blood. There appeared to be some clinical improvement in the animals. What Ganter performed in his animals was later to become intermittent peritoneal dialysis.

Ganter used this technique to treat a uraemic woman suffering from obstructive uropathy from uterine cancer. He introduced 1.5 L of salt solution through a needle in the peritoneal cavity. There was transient improvement in symptoms when the solution was removed but the patient subsequently died. From his experience with the use of PD he was able to elicit several features upon which he based his recommendation. He advocated the use of 1–1.5 L per exchange with close monitoring of the equilibration time; the use of hypertonic solutions with an anaesthetic to minimize pain; and continuous lavage for cases of poisoning but a dwell phase between exchanges for uraemia. He postulated that with improvements this procedure could become an innovative and useful form of renal care.

In the years after World War I, several German investigators were active in the field of replacement of renal function, either with the still-experimental extracorporeal haemodialysis (the so-called 'external dialysis' [17, 18]), or with PD (the so-called 'internal dialysis'). Necheles was unable to reproduce the work of Ganter and Putman and wrote to Abel in 1924 saying that 'the clinical results are negative probably because the intervention is too drastic'.

A number of other reports subsequently confirmed the usefulness of PD in uraemia. Heusser and Werder [19] performed PD in three patients with acute renal failure from mercury poisoning. They modified Ganter's technique, inserting two catheters and perfusing the peritoneal cavity continuously. They noted that not only were nitrogenous substances extracted, but also mercury; they also noted some protein loss in the dialysis fluid. The patients died. Balazc and Rosenaks in 1934 [20] also dialysed patients with mercury poisoning without success. Wear *et al.* [21] were more successful in the treatment of five patients. Dialysing for longer, they noted a fall in serum creatinine and non-protein nitrogen. One patient improved enough to tolerate surgical removal of bladder stones – he recovered. This probably represents the first successful use of PD for acute renal failure. Rhodes [22] treated two uraemic patients with chronic renal failure with PD using for the first time intermittent methods as first described by Ganter in his experimental animals with a single catheter and a dwell period of about 15 min. The outcome was again unsuccessful. In most of these reports outcome was very poor related to poor removal of urea, with dialysis not being done for long enough periods.

During World War II, thousands of cases of acute renal failure caused by severe trauma harshly alerted the surgeons and physicians (no nephrologists then) to this grave problem. In this context, it is worth quoting the remark made by a Dr E D Churchill from Boston at a meeting of the American Surgical Association in April 1946 after Fine *et al.* [23] presented their classic paper on the treatment of acute renal failure by PD: 'despite all the optimistic reports on the successful management of shock in this war, renal shutdown was the stonewall against which we butted our heads many a times ... the surgeons caring for these patients tried many forms of treatment ... but they died of uraemia. Dr Fine's method represents one more procedure that may be applicable to men suffering from renal shutdown. I hope it will prove successful.'

Successful treatment of acute renal failure with PD (1946)

In March 1946 Fine *et al.* [23] reported a successful application of peritoneal irrigation in a patient with severe uraemia from sulphathiazol-induced anuria. The patient survived after 4 days of continuous peritoneal lavage. These investigations by the Boston team [24, 25] were the first in the field of peritoneal lavage to be based on sound scientific principles. This is indeed a landmark report in the history of treatment of uraemia. From then the tide turned.

The Boston investigators were convinced that the peritoneum was an efficient dialysis membrane. They made numerous studies in animals before turning to PD for the treatment of uraemic patients. Emphasizing the importance of a meticulous technique and observing a painstaking sterility, they adopted the continuous-flow technique. Their irrigation fluid, originally Ringer solution with dextrose, was later changed to Tyrode solution prepared in 5 gallon (19 L) Pyrex carboys.

Odel *et al.* [26] reviewed the literature between 1923 and 1948 and reported that 53 patients had received PD over this period. Of these 27 had reversible causes, 13 irreversible and in 13 the diagnosis was uncertain. There was recovery in 17 of the cases with reversible causes; death in the remaining cases

was predominantly related to uraemia, pulmonary oedema and peritonitis. Muehrcke [27], in the literature until 1948, found a total of 101 uraemic patients treated with PD; 63 were diagnosed as having acute renal failure, 32 had irreversible causes and six were related to poisoning. Of the acute group 32 survived. Derot *et al.* [28] reported the first successful experience in acute renal failure with nine out of 10 survivors. Following the work of Grollman *et al.* [29], who demonstrated the use of intermittent PD in nephrectomized dogs, Legrain and Merrill [30] used this form of dialysis in three patients. In one of them three procedures were performed in a 2-week period. They stressed frequent dialysis, dietary salt and protein restrictions and avoidance of infection.

In the early 1950s PD was still an experimental procedure, considered by many as a last resort in cases of terminal uraemia.

Methods, techniques and PD fluids

Over this period, up to 1950, the methods and techniques involved ingenious improvization. Catheters were made from tubings available on the ward and included gallbladder trochars [21], rubber catheters, whistle-tip catheters and stainless-steel sump drains [23]. In the early 1950s polyvinylchloride [28, 30] and polyethylene plastic tubes [29] were employed to gain peritoneal access but were troubled with kinking, leakage and blockage. Leakage was a common problem and a double-lumen catheter, with a flexible distal extension and a collar sewn in the subcutis, was designed to prevent this by Rosenak and Oppenheimer [31]. Maxwell *et al.* [32] described a nylon catheter with small perforations and a curved distal end. This catheter became commercially available and widely used subsequently. A major advance to this catheter was made by Weston and Roberts in 1965 [33]. They inserted a pointed stylet in the Maxwell catheter, thus eliminating the need for a trochar and sutures, considerably simplifying temporary peritoneal access.

The techniques varied from continuous flow (two catheters used) [23, 28, 30] to intermittent (one catheter with tip in pelvis) [32, 34, 35]. The former technique was bedevilled by fluid leakage and the risk of peritonitis was high.

The fluid composition varied considerably from normal saline to 5% dextrose. In retrospect the complications and undesirable side-effects were readily explained by the unsuitable composition of different dialysis fluids. Odel *et al.* [26], in their literature review, also assessed the electrolyte composition and found that hyperchloraemic metabolic acidosis was a frequently observed side-effect with the Lock–Ringer and modified Tyrode solutions and normal saline. High dialysis fluid sodium concentrations were used and Reid et al. [35], who performed the first PD in England in 1946, used twice normal saline. Peripheral and pulmonary oedema and hypertension often accompanied PD in the 1950s; soon a low dialysate sodium and appropriate amounts of bicarbonate (or acetate/lactate) were incorporated as a routine to avoid these complications. Bicarbonate in PD fluids ranged from 26 mmol/L [36] to 35–40 mmol/L [34]. The bicarbonate was soon replaced by lactate when commercial fluid became available in 1959. Since dextrose (up to 7 g/100 ml) was being used to induce ultrafiltration this created a problem during the sterilization process. Caramelization of glucose had to be avoided during the sterilization, and in addition solutions containing both calcium and bicarbonate could not be stored because of precipitation of calcium carbonate. In the late 1950s intermittent PD became a relatively safe and standardized procedure, in particular related to the work of Doolan et al. [37] and Maxwell and colleagues [32], who developed the hanging-bottle PD using commercially prepared rinsing fluids.

In the late 1950s and early 1960s, intermittent PD became a safe and standardized procedure. Kinetic studies looked at clearance (mainly equilibration of small solutes) as well as significance of dialysate flow rates. These changes and improvements, though important, did not allow the use of PD on a long-term basis for the management of patients in end-stage renal failure. Further advances were primarily related to catheter improvements which made long-term therapy possible.

Intermittent chronic PD (1960–76)

The successful application of intermittent PD to acute renal failure led to the use of repeated PD in patients with terminal end-stage renal failure at a time when a similar venture was being tried with intermittent haemodialysis.

The first such patient was treated in early 1960 by Rubin and Doolan at the US Naval Hospital in Oakland, California, by what later became known as 'periodic' PD. After the first PD through a Murphy–Doolan peritoneal catheter, she was diagnosed as having end-stage renal failure (bilaterally shrunken small kidneys). A second dialysis was done a week later when her clinical condition deteriorated. This initiated a pattern of dialysis on an outpatient basis every time the blood urea went above 20 mg/dl (1770 μmol/L). This patient survived for 6 months, after which she refused further treatment. This was the first chronic patient successfully treated with 'periodic' PD. The case report was never published; it was presented for publication but rejected [38]. Just from the single case experience it became obvious that the major problem lay with adequate and safe peritoneal access.

Repeated access to the peritoneal cavity

In the early 1960s various devices were tried to achieve easy and frequent access into the peritoneal cavity. In Seattle, Boen and colleagues tried the Seattle Teflon and silicone rubber tubes [39]. Merrill and colleagues [40] attempted repeated peritoneal irrigation in four patients with end-stage renal failure utilizing a plastic conduit for repeated insertion of the catheter. They had little success: a number of technical problems necessitated revision or removal of the conduits within 2 weeks to 4 months. Because of the bad results with implanted 'buttons' or other conduits, the Seattle group tried the so-called repeated puncture technique, introducing a catheter for each treatment and removing it at the end of each treatment. Tenckhoff et al. [41] carried this out in a patient for 3 years, entailing 380 catheter punctures with a low peritonitis rate. However, this procedure could not be used on a large scale as it was too time-consuming.

In the early 1960s, many centres attempted periodic PD for end-stage renal failure, using various implanted devices for repeated access to the peritoneal cavity. The reports, however, were discouraging [42]. The main problem was peritonitis from infection along the channel of the indwelling devices and from manually changing bottles. Repeated episodes of peritonitis were often followed by the development of adhesions with partial and more extensive obliteration of the peritoneal cavity, decreasing the dialysis efficiency. Most patients died within a few months.

The approach of the Seattle group was different. Boen and colleagues [43] developed the repeated puncture technique with automatic cycling machines. Initially 20-L Pyrex carboys were tried, to be replaced by even larger bottles with volumes of 45 L. The improved cycling machine facilitated uninterrupted cycling without breaking the continuity of the closed sterile fluid administration circuit. In addition the problem of nursing time was largely solved. It also enabled complete freedom between dialysis sessions. This technique, in addition, could be adapted for home use and was done in a woman patient, who was trained to do so in 1964. A doctor's visit was necessary once or twice a week to insert the peritoneal catheter. This was not practical; neither was the need to shift large amounts of fluid.

Overall, this early experience was indeed discouraging. PD was utilized as a 'holding procedure' for patients waiting for a place in a chronic haemodialysis programme or while waiting for vascular access to mature. In an editorial in the *Lancet* [44], it was stated that 'PD is obviously no silver bullet for renal failure but in suitable cases it is a good leaden bullet, which is more commonly fired'. PD lagged technically behind and remained the 'Cinderella' treatment for chronic renal failure. Long-term treatment was frequently associated with recurrent episodes of peritonitis, protein loss, malnutrition and progressive wasting.

In the late 1960s and early 1970s two technical developments changed this scene and gave some impetus to furthering the therapy. So far peritoneal access was the 'bottleneck' of long-term dialysis. One development was better access and the other was automation.

Indwelling catheters

A major advance was brought about in gaining peritoneal access by Palmer *et al.* [45] with further advances made by Gutch [46] and McDonald *et al.* [47], who all utilized silicone rubber catheters, which incorporated perforations at the distal end and a triflanged step or a Teflon velour skirt for seating the tube in the deep fascia and peritoneum. However, it was not until Tenckhoff's design of the indwelling silicone rubber catheter which had two dacron cuffs that intermittent PD became accepted as a long-term therapy for renal failure patients [48]. This catheter or its subsequent modifications became accepted as the only practical access device. The original Tenckhoff catheter was basically a modification of the curled Palmer catheter [45]; the curled section of the Palmer catheter was replaced by a straight intra-abdominal portion. It was inserted either surgically through a mini-laparotomy or with local anaesthesia and the aid of a special trochar at the bedside. Subsequent modifications have tried to minimize the various complications – dislocation, obstruction, fluid leaks and catheter

infections. Using automated machines and this catheter a large experience was built up in the Seattle area [49]. Tenckhoff and colleagues in this report related the experience of 12,000 PD sessions in 69 patients who were mostly at home.

Automatic cycling machines

Another major development, which made periodic PD much more dependable, was the introduction of automatic cycling machines by Boen and colleagues [42, 43]. Several models of 'cyclers' were described [50, 51] but basically, were relatively simple with timers set for inflow time, dwell period and outflow, freeing nurses from manual operations. Premixed, sterile dialysis fluid was supplied in carboys containing 19–45 L, and both machines and fluid were commercially available. There were problems to these cyclers. Sterility could not be guaranteed, because containers had to be changed, and bacterial filters did not seem very reliable and safe.

In 1969 a prototype of a proportioning PD system was constructed and described by Tenckhoff and colleagues [52]. Because of the necessity of a water still and a large water sterilization tank, it was bulky. An automatic system using reverse osmosis for tap-water purification and sterilization was designed 3 years later [53]. The purified sterile water was mixed with sterile concentrate in a ratio of 20 to 1. A commercial model of this system was available. These machines were expensive but the running costs relatively cheap. These machines had an important advantage in that the fluid factory and the peritoneal circuit formed a closed system, which was not broken during dialysis – the risk of bacterial contamination was minimal.

Further modifications were introduced in the early 1970s mainly to enhance efficiency. These modifications included reciprocating PD [54], fresh fluid, semi-continuous PD [55], and regeneration PD [56]. These developments were overshadowed by the introduction of continuous ambulatory PD (CAPD).

Outcomes

By 1977, in the Seattle area 161 patients had been on PD, many of them for over 4 years and a few for 8 years [57]. Similar experience was reported by Oreopoulous in 1975 [58] and subsequently by centres in Europe [59, 60]. Long-term therapy beyond 4 years was not often achieved with a cumulative technique survival of 27% for 3 years in the

Seattle group of patients [61]. Inadequate dialysis was one reason for conversion to haemodialysis, as was repeated peritonitis. Enhancement of PD efficiency was attempted in various ways; the influence of dialysis fluid flow and exchange volumes, effect of temperature, optimization of dwell time, increase of solute transfer by convection, and utilization of pharmacological methods were all tried without too much success [62]. For these reasons, haemodialysis remained the cornerstone of dialysis therapy and for PD to challenge this position a major rethink was necessary. This came about in the mid-1970s.

Continuous ambulatory PD (1976 onwards)

The concept of CAPD had its origin in Austin, Texas, USA, when in 1975 Dr R Popovich and Dr J Moncrief were discussing ways to dialyse a patient who could not receive haemodialysis or intermittent PD. This 'brainstorming' session induced Dr Popovich, a biomedical engineer with knowledge of membrane kinetics, to theorize the use of long dwell cycles to achieve adequate removal of uraemic waste products to sustain life. Based on mathematical calculations using several assumptions (70 kg male with no residual renal function, stable blood urea of 29 mmol/L, nitrogen generation rate of 5.7 mg/min, and dialysate/plasma ratio for urea of 1 = total equilibration) they arrived at five daily exchanges of 2 L, 7 days a week. With 2 L of ultrafiltrate this would give a total daily exchange of 12 L. Moncrief tried this in a patient and found that the results matched the theoretical ones. Ironically, the first description and account of the clinical experiences was not accepted for presentation at the American Society for Artifical Internal Organs (Fig. 2) [63].

It was initially called a 'portable/wearable equilibrium dialysis techniques'. This group described the theoretical mass transfer characteristics for this procedure. Popovich demonstrated that a double pool model is valid for a low dialysis clearance system, such as the equilibration dialysis he described. The accumulation of the metabolites in the body would be equal to the rate of generation minus the rate of residual renal clearance, minus the overall dialysate clearance (diffusive and convective). Popovich postulated that the accumulation term, being a time derivative of total mass of the metabolite in the

THE DEFINITION OF A NOVEL PORTABLE/WEARABLE EQUILIBRIUM PERITONEAL DIALYSIS TECHNIQUE. Robert P. Popovich, Jack W. Moncrief, Jonathan F. Decherd, John B. Bomar* and W. Keith Pyle.' Depts. Chem. Engr. and Biomed Engr., The Univ. of Texas and Austin Diag. Clin., Austin, Texas.

An analysis will be presented which predicts that acceptable blood metabolite levels will result if 10 liters of dialysate per day are allowed to continuously equilibrate with body fluids. Accordingly, a portable/wearable dialysis procedure based upon equilibrium-intermittent peritoneal dialysis has been defined. Two liters of standard hypertonic dialysate fluid are infused peritoneally via a Tenckhoff catheter and allowed to equilibrate 5 hours while the patient conducts his normal activities. The dialysate is then drained and replaced with the procedure being repeated five times per day.

In a preliminary clinical study metabolite equilibration between blood and dialysate was achieved for BUN and creatinine but not for vitamin B-12. Steady state metabolite levels for BUN and creatinine were 40 and 9.5 mg% respectively. The patient was maintained 5 months with the new procedure with excellent clinical results followed by a successful transplant.

It is concluded that a new portable/wearable dialysis procedure has been defined. The technique does not require blood access and results in steady, low blood metabolite levels: middle molecule removal greatly exceeds that of conventional techniques.

Figure 2. The abstract of the first description of CAPD by the pioneers Dr Popovich and Dr Moncrief as it appeared in the abstract book of the American Society of Artificial Organs meeting of 1976.

system, should equal zero if the dialysis treatment is continuous and the concentrations and volumes remain constant.

The concept of CAPD utilizes the smallest volume of dialysate, i.e. the lowest dialysate flow rate, to prevent uraemia. The significant reduction in dialysate volume allows 'portability' during the procedure. If 2 L of dialysate is allowed to totally equilibrate with the blood, the drained dialysate volume will then equal the urea clearance. If one assumes that adequate urea dialysis is achieved when blood urea nitrogen is maintained at 70 mg%, the dialysate drained volume, which is equilibrated with blood urea nitrogen, will have 700 mg of urea nitrogen per litre. Urea nitrogen generation in the average 70 kg man, who eats a diet containing 1 g/kg of body weight, will be 7000 mg/day. Working on this accepted urea generation rate [64] and a desired

steady-state BUN level (70–80 mg%), they estimated that over a 24 h day the daily clearance
requirements equalled about 10 L of dialysis fluid
exchanged. The theory therefore predicted that a
patient will maintain a steady BUN level of about
80 mg/dl, if 10 L of PD fluids are allowed to equilibrate with body fluids on a daily basis. This indeed
was borne out in the clinical experiences, described
in three patients [65]. The efficiency of CAPD was
also assessed in comparison to hemodialysis and
intermittent PD (Table 1). This shows that the
CAPD system is more efficient at removing larger
molecular weight substances (creatinine) than urea.
As the molecular weight of the substance under consideration increases, so there is greater removal with
long dwells. They also calculated the removal rates
of water using glucose as an osmotic agent.

A major cooperative study was begun in 1977
supported by the National Institutes of Health.
These included clinical studies at the Austin Diagnostic clinic, Texas (Dr Moncrief), at the University
of Missouri (Dr K Nolph), with the biomedical engineering support of the University of Texas (Dr
Popovich). This joint experience in nine patients
(duration of CAPD 5–26 weeks) was described in
1978 [66] and the name of the technique was
changed to continuous ambulatory peritoneal dialysis (CAPD).

The main advantages of this new technique
(Table 2) were good steady-state biochemical control, more liberal dietary and fluid intakes than
haemodialysis, improvement in anaemia and well-
being of the patients and freedom from machines,
which allowed patients to travel long distances.
However, these studies utilized PD solutions in bottles. Connections and disconnections of tubing and
bottles to the Tenckhoff catheter were required with
each exchange, and chances of contamination were
high. Hence, not only was the technique cumbersome and time-consuming, but it was complicated
by a high incidence of peritonitis (one episode/10
patient-weeks).

Table 2. Advantages and disadvantages of CAPD as compared to haemodialysis as perceived and later documented
in the early days after the introduction of the technique

Advantages	Disadvantages
Well-being	Peritonitis
Easier diet and fluid management	Catheter related problems
Steady-state biochemistry	Hernias
Improved anaemia	Patient dislikes, fatigue
Less hypertension	Obesity
Better for children, diabetics and elderly	Hyperlipidaemia
Lower cost	Loss of ultrafiltration

In September 1977 Dr Oreopoulos started his first
patient on CAPD using a novel modification of the
above technique with PD fluid in polyvinylchloride
(PVC) bags. Following instillation of the fluid, the
plastic bag, still connected to the administration set,
was rolled up and carried under clothing without
much difficulty. After a dwell period of 4–8 h the
fluid was allowed to drain into the same bag under
the 'force of gravity' without disconnecting the tube
from the Tenckhoff catheter [67]. The technique
details were first presented in January 1978, at the
11th Annual Contractors Conference of the Artifical
Kidney Programme, Institutes of Arthritis, Metabolism, Digestive Disease in Bethesda, USA. The Oreopoulos modification made CAPD easier to perform
and decreased (but did not eliminate) the rather high
incidence of peritonitis when using bottled PD fluid
(one episode/10 patient-weeks, to one episode/eight
patient-months). This represented a major advance
and the use of CAPD increased in an explosive way.
By June 1980, 115 patients were managed on CAPD
at the Toronto Western Hospital [68].

In September 1978 the Food and Drug Administration approved sale of PD solution in plastic
bags in the United States; this led to many centres
developing CAPD Programmes [69]. Another
major step in the growth of CAPD in the USA was
the announcement by the Health Care Financing

Table 1. Clearances (L/week) for different solutes by varying dialysis techniques. IPD – intermittent peritoneal dialysis; CCPD – continuous cyclic peritoneal dialysis; CAPD – continuous ambulatory peritoneal dialysis

	Haemodialysis 15 h/week	IPD 40 h/week	CAPD continuous	Nocturnal	CCPD diurnal	Total	Normal kidney
Urea (60 daltons)	135	60	76–84	54	12.7	66.7	604
Creatinine (113 daltons)	90	28	58	46.2	12.5	58.7	1200
B12 (1350 daltons)	30	15–16	50	34.8	10.1	44.9	1200
Indulin (5200 daltons)	5	12	30	–	–	–	1200

Administration (Medicare), in October 1979, that CAPD was reimbursable and an accepted alternative to chronic haemodialysis. The growth, therefore, has been exponential. By July 1980 over 1700 patients were treated in 190 centres [70].

Growth of CAPD worldwide

The growth in the United States was mirrored in other leading Western Nations with rapid increase in numbers in Canada [68], Europe [71–75] and Australia [76]. All these reports related to certain advantages of CAPD over IPD and haemodialysis (Table 2), but the technique was still compromised by the high rate of peritonitis and catheter-related problems. These reviews were substantiated by individual centre experiences in the UK and Canada [77, 78] and proved beyond any doubt that maintenance of good dialysis and well-being could be achieved over several years on CAPD treatment.

Over the ensuing years there has been a steady increase in the number of patient on PD worldwide and industrial sources reported that this number worldwide was 76,000 patients at the end of 1992 (see Fig. 1 in Chapter 2). Also over the years the percentage increase of patients on an annual basis has been much higher on PD as compared to haemodialysis, and for the years 1991/92 this was a 16% increase for PD as compared to a 9% increase for haemodialysis.

Evolution of CAPD technique

The CAPD technique, as eventually proposed by Popovich and Moncrief, entailed four exchanges of 2 L volumes, using a combination of three 1.36% glucose and one 3.8% glucose to produce a 10 L dialysate volume over a 24 h period. This necessitated a 4–8 h dwell period adjusted to fit into the patient's daily routine. The initial use of glass bottles

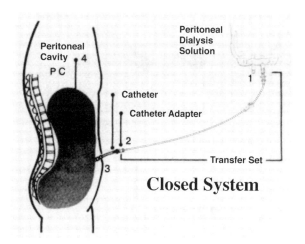

Figure 3. The CAPD System. 1 – connection between transfer set and PD fluid bag. This connection is broken three or four times a day to effect exchanges. 2 – connection between Tenckhoff catheter and transfer set, incorporating the titanium connector. This connection is undone every 6 months for transfer set changes. 3 – exit site. 4 – peritoneal cavity.

resulted in an unacceptable peritonitis rate [66] but with the introduction of the PVC bags there was a dramatic improvement [67].

The basic CAPD system, which to this day remains unchanged, consists of the PVC bag containing 0.5–3 L of PD fluid, a transfer set and a Tenckhoff catheter (Fig. 3). The connection between the bag and transfer set is broken four times a day, and the exchange procedure transferring the set from the spent bag to the new bag has to be performed using a strict non-touch technique. Various devices (connectors) were developed to minimize the risk of contamination and this gave rise to the science of 'connectology'. However, this site remains the major source of contamination and peritonitis [80]. 'Initially spike' connectors, at Sites 1 and 2 (Fig. 3), led to accidental catheter and bag disconnections. In addition, bag leaks and fluid leaks from defective materials used in the manufacture of connectors [81] plagued the procedure and maintained a high peritonitis rate. The connection between Tenckhoff catheter and transfer set (Site 2) was improved substantially by the introduction of a luer-locking titanium peritoneal catheter adaptor in 1979 [69]. This led to a further reduction in the peritonitis rate. From the initially weekly transfer set changes advocated by Oreopoulos [67], monthly set changes were introduced in 1979 [82]. Improvements in transfer set material have led to set changes being performed at roughly 6-monthly intervals.

Table 3. Number of patients in individual countries on CAPD by 1980, also expressed as a percentage of total dialysis population

Country	No. CAPD patients	Percentage of dialysis population	Reference
Australia	102	—	76
Belgium	99	12	71
France	254	3.2	72
Italy	240	2	73
UK	230	10	74
USA	2500	13	79

An inherent problem with this technique is that, having made a connection of transfer set to a new bag, fluid is instilled into the peritoneal cavity. If the exchange procedure has led to a contamination of the connector, the microorganisms will pass with the fluid into the peritoneal cavity. The Italian Y set connector system, utilizing the closed double bag, overcomes this inherent problem [83, 84]. Buoncristiani and colleagues [83] were the first to use this system, which includes two bags, one containing the PD fluid while the other is empty. They are connected by Y tubing with a sterile capped needle. After the connections are made the dialysate from the peritoneal cavity is drained into the empty bag followed by drainage of fresh fluid from the other bag into the peritoneal cavity. The two-bag system is then disconnected and the Y piece is filled with chlorhexidine. This system had two major advantages: any contamination at the time of the connection was 'washed out' and in addition it enabled the patient to be bag-free at all times, between the exchanges. This is the principle of 'flush before fill' (Fig. 4). Use of the system has resulted in low peritonitis rates, and in a controlled randomized trial peritonitis rates were halved as compared to the standard system [85] (Fig. 5). Initially, other than

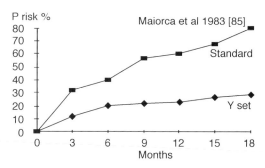

Figure 5. The first randomized prospective trial of the disconnect versus standard systems. This shows a dramatic reduction in the risk of developing peritonitis in the Y-set group [85].

in Italy, the use of the system was limited but in the late 1980s there has been a dramatic increase in its use and now there is a whole range of disconnect systems that are available [86], which have substantially reduced the peritonitis rate. Thus disconnect/Y systems are now accepted as the normal and the use is increasing [87]. The effects of all these technical changes with the introduction of the new systems and connector devices has, over the years, had a dramatic impact on the peritonitis rate. It is now generally accepted that with the use of disconnect systems a peritonitis rate of an episode every 2 years should be possible, and this has been verified in several individual centre reports. In addition the impact of the disconnect system on CAPD results is also significant [88, 89].

The development of techniques of CAPD has brought with it the realization that, though CAPD is simple, the procedure does require motivation, discipline, compliance and a certain degree of technical skill. The early literature emphasized the need to have an organized programme for training and an adequate nursing staff to fulfil the teaching aims [90, 91]. This of course still applies today, and where this has not been possible (as in some countries such as the UK) where the use of CAPD has expanded rapidly the high dropout and peritonitis rates may be related to limited facilities and staff, especially in the early 1980s [92].

Early results and subsequent developments

It was fairly evident after a few years of the introduction of CAPD that the therapy worked and produced good biochemical control. Because of its continuous nature it provided steady-state values for electrolytes and nitrogenous waste products. Control of sodium, potassium was reportedly easier

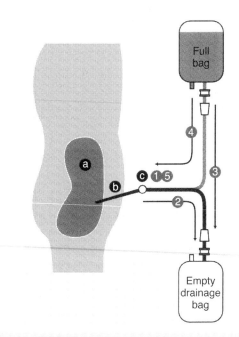

Figure 4. CAPD disconnect system. Steps in the exchange procedure are: **1** Connect Y system (double bag) to Tenckhoff catheter. **2** Drain out from patient. **3** Flush line before fill. **4** Drain in. **5** Disconnect. **a** = Peritoneal cavity; **b** = Tenckhoff catheter; **c** = point of connection/disconnection between Y sytem and catheter.

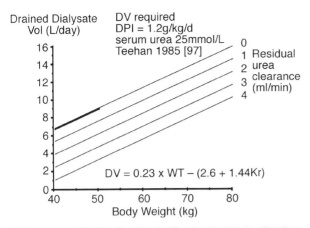

Figure 6. Theoretical evaluation of the dialysate volume (DV) required to maintain a steady-state urea level on a dietary protein intake (DPI) of 1.2 g/kg, based on body weight and residual urea clearance [95].

[69], and a mild chronic acidosis [93] was easily corrected by an increase in the dialysate lactate concentration [94]. This was also the forerunner of changes in fluid composition to improve 'biocompatibility' of PD solutions.

The levels of BUN and creatinine no longer reflected the level of uraemia, but instead a combination of factors, including the dietary intake, muscle mass, residual renal function and amount of dialysis. The amount of solute clearance started to assume greater importance, and this was the prelude to the concepts of 'adequacy' and 'prescription'.

Ten years after the introduction of CAPD, Teehan et al. [95], theorized that the dialysate volume required to maintain a steady-state BUN, on a requisite protein intake, was heavily dependent on the body weight and the level of residual renal function (Fig. 6). In spite of this there appeared to be limited attempts at varying the prescription to take these variables into account. Furthermore, early work on the 'permeability' of the peritoneum [96], eventually leading to the peritoneal equilibration test (PET) [97], suggested that this parameter was also important in setting a prescription. Yet most patients were on a set daily prescription of 4×2 L exchanges. No account was taken of declining residual renal function, changes in weight or permeability. This changed in the late 1980s.

Permeability, peritoneal fibrosis and loss of ultrafiltration (UP)

Early ultrastructural studies of the peritoneum after CAPD were reported as early as 1981 by Dobbie et al. [98]. They found that the mesothelial cells,

Table 4. European experience of loss of UF in CAPD

Reference	No. of patients affected	Time to loss of UF (months)	Buffer
Faller and Marichal [101]	27/27	18	Acetate
Slingeneyer et al. [102]	13/66	18	Acetate
Rottembourg et al. [103]	26/101	12	Acetate
Wideroe et al. [104]	5/9	—	Lactate
Bazzato et al. [105]	7/55	18	Acetate

exposed to PD solutions, showed intracellular oedema with disruption of cytoplasmic structures. There was also disruption of collagen bundles in the sub-mesothelium and an increase in fibroblasts and mast cells. After several months of CAPD there was an increase in the distance between the mesothelium and capillaries to 20–40 μm. Changes related to peritonitis were also described by Verger et al. [99]. In severe episodes of peritonitis there was total disappearance of the mesothelium and fibrous reaction of the sub-mesothelial layers.

It soon became apparent that in some patients it was proving difficult to maintain adequate fluid status because of loss of UF [100]. Peritonitis and PD solutions were thought to be responsible for this. In Europe the incidence was high related to the use of acetate-buffered dialysate (Table 4). The incidence of this in North America was much less [106], but the analysis found a significant correlation between incidence of peritonitis and late (>18 months CAPD) onset loss of UF. This raised the question of how long the peritoneal membrane would last to support CAPD [107].

The alarm raised by these studies resulted in an International Cooperative cross-sectional study of UF in 29 participating centres worldwide [108]. Significant correlations were noted with use of acetate-buffered dialysate and time on CAPD. There was a strong negative correlation between glucose absorption and UF. Various other causative factors were incriminated in the pathogenesis of loss of UF – glucose metabolites [109], chlorhexidine [110] and dialysate particulate matter [111]. In an attempt to propose a final common pathway to account for all the causes and loss of UF, Shaldon et al. developed the interleukin-1 hypothesis [112]. They suggested that in CAPD the peritoneal macrophage was in a state of over-stimulation with increased production of IL-1. This stimulates production of collagen from fibroblasts and prostacyclin from endothelial cells; this hypothesis would account for both loss of UF and development of sclerosing peritonitis – the end-result of several factors discussed above.

The changes in the peritoneum leading to UF loss were not entirely clear, but Verger *et al.* were able to delineate two types of peritoneal permeability in these patients [97, 113]. They assessed 'permeability' on the basis of dialysate/plasma equilibration curves derived from hourly measurements of urea and glucose over a 6-h dwell. They proposed a number of types of 'permeability' changes (Table 5). Type I loss of UF corresponded to a hyperpermeable membrane which corresponded histologically with loss of mesothelial microvilli and increased cell separation. Type II loss of UF is associated with low permeability and, histologically, adhesions or sclerosing peritonitis [114]. Type I changes were regarded as reversible.

The complication of loss of UF became even more alarming when French investigators described the syndrome of progressive sclerosing encapsulating peritonitis (SEP) in their CAPD patients [115]. The sclerosis took the form of marked thickening of the peritoneal membrane, encasing all the bowel loops like a cocoon. Most patients died of intestinal obstruction and malnutrition. Factors implicated in the pathogenesis were the same as for loss of UF. There were various other reports, including morphology [110, 116, 117]. An international survey by Slingeneyer revealed the problem to be fairly widespread [118].

Early outcome results

The early results in the first 5–8 years after the introduction of CAPD in 1976 were poor. Mortality was high, as was 'drop-out' to HD. The main reasons were those related to the inherent problems of the CAPD technique – access, peritonitis, inadequate dialysis and patient fatigue. This was a period when some countries utilized CAPD to increase their take-on rates because of limited HD facilities (e.g. the UK). The initial data from Europe were indeed

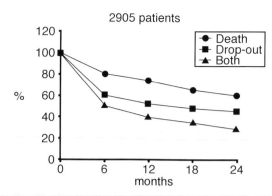

Figure 7. Outcome of patients undergoing CAPD in 1982 from the EDTA registry [119].

poor (Fig. 7) [119], with <30% being on therapy after 2 years of CAPD. Shaldon *et al.* [120] regarded this therapy as a 'second class treatment, for second class patients, by second class doctors' – a comment that aroused high feelings, but may have been a major stimulus to the subsequent improvements.

Automated PD (APD)

Whilst the growth of CAPD in the 1980s was dramatic, the use of intermittent modes of PD lagged behind considerably. Intermittent dialysis therapy in 1986 provided dialysis for only 700 out of 90,000 end-stage renal disease patients. In the United States the percentage was 0.7% [121]. The major disadvantages compared to haemodialysis were the inadequacy of dialysis, minimal adequate clearances and symptoms of thirst, sodium and water imbalance and blood pressure control. CAPD compared more favourably to hemodialysis in terms of clearances, symptomatology and also pyschosocial adjustments.

However, there was a resurgence of interest in APD with the introduction of continuous cyclic PD (CCPD) described by Nakayawa *et al.* in 1981 [122]. CCPD was based on the concept of continuous equilibration dialysis initially proposed by

Table 5. Peritoneal permeability alterations and types of loss of ultrafiltration [113]

Type	Dialysate glucose equilibration	Dialysate urea equilibration	Volume drained	Dialysate Na decrease	Reason
I	Rapid	Rapid	Low	No	Hyperpermeable – reversible mesothelial alterations
II	Slow	Normal or slow	Low	No	Hypopermeable – adhesions or sclerosing peritonitis
III	Normal	Normal	Low	No	Early adhesions or sclerosis
IV	Normal	Normal	Low	Yes	Leakage
Normal	Normal	Normal	Normal	Yes	Normal

Moncrief and Popovich but incorporated the automation provided by a cycler [123]. CCPD uses multiple short (usually three), nocturnal exchanges, while the patient is connected to the cycler, and a long diurnal exchange with the patient ambulatory. Thus, it is a virtual reversal of the CAPD schedule. The primary objective of CCPD was to provide automated, continuous PD in a convenient manner, freeing the daytime hours from all procedures. The secondary goal was to reduce the rate of peritonitis. Within the first decade of experience of CCPD it was felt that the original goals were fulfilled.

CCPD has been of particular benefit to those patients in need of assistance with the procedure due to their poor muscular coordination, blindness and generalized weakness and patients who are unable to perform manual dialysis exchanges. Thus, the use of CCPD for the very young, the elderly, and the diabetic patient has been substantial. Growth of CCPD has been moderate, with about 10% of the dialysis population undertaking this treatment in the mid-1980s.

Another variant of intermittent dialysis therapy was the development of nightly intermittent peritoneal dialysis (NIPD). This is performed every night and may be considered as CCPD without long-dwell daytime exchanges, but performed with an intermittent flow technique of rapid exchanges, and was utilized to a small extent by Twardowski [121]. It was used mainly in patients with recurrent abdominal leaks and hernias, bladder prolapse, rapid glucose absorption resulting in poor ultrafiltration on CAPD, abdominal discomfort, chronic hypertension and patient preference. In 1985 Scribner postulated 'some form of nightly peritoneal dialysis (NPD), may prove as the best compromise of all forms of PD' [124]. However, because of reduced dialysis time compared to CAPD or CCPD, the main problem was to achieve adequate clearances. The efficiency of PD is dependent upon peritoneal transport characteristics in individual patients and the measurement of this was established in a simplified procedure – the peritoneal equilibration test (PET) [97]. The curves that were obtained over a 4 h dwell of 2.27% glucose solution discriminated patients into four categories of low, low average, high average and high peritoneal transport rates based on measurements of glucose and creatinine in dialysate and bloods. Using this test one could prognosticate and prescribe the preferred dialysis regime. This ability to tailor dialysis has certainly popularized APD, which is now the fastest-growing PD modality.

Other intermittent dialysis techniques have been introduced to try to maximize the efficiency of the dialysis. One such technique is tidal PD (TPD). Here, after an initial flow into the peritoneal cavity, only a portion of the dialysate is drained and replaced by fresh dialysis fluid, leaving the majority of dialysate in constant contact with the peritoneal membrane until the end of the dialysis session when the fluid is drained as completely as possible [121]. TPD is approximately 20% more efficient than NIPD with a dialysis flow of 3.5 L/h.

The introduction of APD meant that patients on PD could be maintained longer on this technique. It also meant that psychosocial factors and patient preference could be more readily accommodated such that therapy could be adjusted depending upon clinical situations, changes in peritoneal membrane characteristics, and loss of residual renal function. In spite of this knowledge prescriptions remained fairly standard.

Patient selection

The availability of PD makes a renal centre more flexible in managing a patient in end-stage renal failure. In the early years of experience with CAPD no 'profile' of a perfect CAPD patient emerged. Selection, therefore, became a process of assessing a multitude of factors, some of which are listed in Table 6.

For new patients, essential factors were, and still are, motivation, physical and mental capabilities of carrying out the procedure, and some insight into symptoms of uraemia. They needed low-key scientific knowledge of dialysis for renal failure. A desire to be independent and attain home dialysis was important. Certain categories of patients may have major difficulties in undergoing other types of dialysis. These were the 'high-risk' patient population such as diabetics and those with severe cerebro- and cardiovascular

Table 6. Factors influencing choice of CAPD in new patients starting dialysis

Medical factors	Psychosocial factors
Age	Patient preference
Ischaemic heart disease	Motivation
Diabetes mellitus	Compliance
Ease of transplantation	Family support
Extensive abdominal surgery	Distance from centre
Blindness	Occupation
Severe pulmonary disease	Concern with body image
Peripheral vascular disease	Travel
Lumbar disc problems	
Extensive diverticulitis	

disease, in whom there was little option but to treat on CAPD as HD was contraindicated.

Indications for CAPD

For patients already on haemodialysis or IPD, CAPD is indicated for problems such as vascular access, excessive weight gain between dialyses, severe hypertension, postdialysis disequilibration and severe anaemia. It may also be indicated for those in certain (hospital) dialysis patients showing a desire to undertake home dialysis.

For new patients, about to commence dialysis therapy, the factors in Table 6 need to be assessed carefully. However, certain diseases may be preferentially managed by CAPD. Diabetics may be a group in whom CAPD may be an absolute indication, as would those in whom HD would be hazardous. Patients awaiting a kidney transplant can be safely maintained on CAPD and this is even more important for children in whom CAPD would be preferred therapy prior to transplantation.

Contraindications

An inappropriate peritoneal cavity from adhesions, secondary to previous operations or systemic inflammatory disease, is the only absolute contraindication to CAPD. This in the early years was assessed, according to Moncrief and Popovich, by instilling 2 L of PD fluid via an acute catheter and measuring the creatinine concentration in the dialysate and blood after 6 h [125]. If this ratio was <40%, failure of CAPD was likely. Adhesions may also lead to poor inflow and drainage. In general, previous abdominal surgery is not a contraindication to CAPD.

Other relative contraindications

1. Recurrent chronic backache with pre-existing disc disease. This may be aggravated by the exaggerated lordosis associated with the constant presence of fluid in the peritoneal cavity.
2. Abdominal hernias. These may well have to be repaired before CAPD is started.
3. The presence of colostomy, ileostomy, nephrostomy and ileal conduit may increase the risk of peritonitis; unless absolutely necessary these patients are better managed on HD.
4. Progressive neurological diseases, movement disorders and severe arthritis make CAPD impossible to perform. In such cases a spouse or relative may be able to carry out the exchanges.

5. Severe psychological and social problems. A cooperative and compliant patient is essential for independent home dialysis. Patients who are psychotic, belligerent, or uncooperative are unlikely to succeed in this form of therapy and may be better managed on hospital/in-centre HD.
6. Chronic obstructive airways disease patients may not be able to tolerate 2 L of fluid because of an impaired vital capacity; this is however relatively uncommon.
7. Severe diverticular disease of the colon in the elderly may be associated with repeated Gram-negative peritonitis or perforation, which has a high mortality.
8. Hepatitis B antigenaemia (HBsAg). For units that do not routinely dialyse these patients this may be an absolute contraindication because of the risk to staff and other patients within the unit. However, CAPD may be carried out in designated hepatitis units where the staff have been vaccinated or in departments or a hospital for infectious diseases. It is important to remember that the dialysate is HBsAg positive and needs to be treated with 1% hypochlorite before discarding.

It became apparent soon after the introduction of CAPD that it was an integral part of the renal replacement programme. However, there appeared to be obvious bias against CAPD and this was not helped by the initial poor results. Patient selection remained a problem where the various treatment modalities were not integrated. This remains so to this day; renal units should be able to provide all the therapies and be prepared to adjust treatment according to the patients' needs or justified desire. The development of CAPD and its various modifications brought with it the realization that, even though the exchange procedure was simple, it required motivation, discipline, compliance and a degree of technical skill. The early literature emphasized the need to have an organized programme for training, and an adequate nursing staff to fulfil the teaching aims [126, 127].

Conclusion

The historical development of PD provides a fascinating study in ingenuity, resourcefulness, and enterprise by the many pioneers and dedicated scientists. The fruits of their endeavours are clear to see for all, in what has developed into the modern PD, as will be portrayed in the following pages. We salute these pioneers who made possible the success of this therapy.

References

1. McBride P. Taking the first steps in the development of peritoneal dialysis. Perit Dial Bull 1982; 100–2.
2. Cunningham RS. The physiology of the serous membranes. Physiol Rev 1926; 6: 242–56.
3. Warrick C. An improvement of the practice of tapping, whereby that operation instead of relief of symptoms, becomes an absolute cure for ascites, exemplified in the case of Jane Roman. Phil Trans R Soc 1744; 43: 12–9.
4. Hale SA. Method of conveying liquors into the abdomen during the operation of tapping. Phil Trans R Soc 1744; 43: 20–1.
5. Chirurgische Bemerkungen uber die Peritonealhohle, mit besonderer Berucksichtigung der ovariotome. Arch Klin Chir 1877; 20: 51–4.
6. Starling EH, Tubby AH. The influence of mechanical factors on lymph production. J Physiol 1894; 16: 140–8.
7. Cunningham RS. The effect of dextrose upon the peritoneal mesothelium. Am J Physiol 1920; 53: 458–88.
8. Clark AJ. Absorption from the peritoneal cavity. J Pharmacol Exp Ther 1921; 16: 415–22.
9. Klapp R. Uber Bauchfelresorption (On resorption by the peritoneum). Mitt Grenzeb Med Chir 1902; 10: 254.
10. Hertzler AE. The Peritoneum structure and function in relation to principles of abdominal surgery. St Louis: CV Mosby, 1919, vol. 1.
11. Abel JJ, Rowntree LG, Turner BB. Removal of diffusible substances from the circulating blood of living animals by dialysis. J Exp Ther 1913; 5: 275–316.
12. Putnam J. The living peritoneum as a dialysing membrane. Am J Physiol 1923; 63: 548–65.
13. Graham T. Liquid diffusion applied to analysis. Philos Trans R Soc 1861; 151: 183.
14. Engel D. Beitrage permeabilitas problem: Entgeft ungsstudien mettils des Lebendin peritoneums als 'Dialysator'. Z Gesarite Ex Med 1927; 55: 544–601.
15. Blackfan KD, Maxey KF. The intraperitoneal injection of saline solution. Am J Dis Child 1918; 21: 257–65.
16. Ganter G. Uber die Beseitgung giftiger Stoffe aus dem Blute durch Dialse. Muench Med Wochenschr 1923; 70: 1478–80.
17. Necheles H. Uber dialysieren des stromenden Blutes am Lebenden (On dialysis of the circulating blood *in vivo*). Klin Wochenschr 1923; 2: 1257–65.
18. Haas G. Dialysieren des stromenden Blutes am Lebenden (Dialysing the circulating blood). Klin Wochenschr 1925; 4: 13–19.
19. Heusser H, Werder H. Untersuchungen uber Peritonealdialyse. Bruns Beitr Klin Chir 1927; 141: 384–9.
20. Balazc J, Rosenaks S. Zur behandlung der sublimatanurie durch Peritoneal Dialse. Wein Klin Wochenschr 1934; 47: 851–4.
21. Wear JB, Sisk IR, Trinkle AJ. Peritoneal lavage in the treatment of uraemia. J Urol 1938; 39: 53–62.
22. Rhoads JE. Peritoneal lavage in the treatment of renal insufficiency. Am J Med Sc 1938; 39: 53–62.
23. Fine JH, Frank HA, Seligman AM. The treatment of acute renal failure by peritoneal irrigation. Ann Surg 1946; 124: 857–75.
24. Frank HA, Seligman AM, Fine JH. Treatment of uraemia after acute renal failure by peritoneal irrigation. JAMA 1946; 130: 703–12.
25. Fine JH, Frank HA, Seligman AM. Further experiences with peritoneal irrigation for acute renal failure. Ann Surg 1948; 128: 561–9.
26. Odel HM, Ferris DO, Power H. Peritoneal lavage as an effective means of extra-renal excretion. Am J Med 1950; 9: 63–77.
27. Muehrcke RC. Acute Renal Failure. St Louis: CV Mosby, 1969.
28. Derot M, Tanzet P, Roussillion J, Bernier JJ. La dialyse peritoneal dans le traitment de l'ureme aigue. J Urol 1949; 55: 113–21.
29. Grollman A, Turner LB, McLean JA. Intermittent peritoneal lavage in nephrectomised dogs and its application to the human being. Arch Intern Med 1951; 87: 379–90.
30. Legrain M, Merrill JP. Short term continuous trans peritoneal dialysis. N Engl J Med 1953; 248: 125–9.
31. Rosenak SS, Oppenheimer GD. An improved drain for peritoneal lavage. Surgery 1948; 23: 832–7.
32. Maxwell MH, Rockney RE, Kleman CR, Twiss MR. Peritoneal dialysis. JAMA 1959; 170: 917–24.
33. Weston RE, Roberts M. Clinical use of stylet catheter for PD. Arch Intern Med 1965; 15: 659–64.
34. Boen ST. Kinetics of peritoneal dialysis. Medicine 1961; 40: 243–87.
35. Reid R, Penfold JB, Jones RN. Anuria treated by renal encapsulation and peritoneal dialysis. Lancet 1946; 2: 749–51.
36. Abbot WE, Shea P. The treatment of temporary renal insufficiency by peritoneal lavage. Am J Med Sci 1946; 211: 312–9.
37. Doolan PD, Murphy WP, Wiggins RA *et al*. An evaluation of intermittent peritoneal lavage. Am J Med 1959; 268: 314–8.
38. Drukker W. History of peritoneal dialysis. In: Maher JF, ed. Replacement of Renal Function by Dialysis. Dordrecht: Kluwer, 1989, pp. 476–515.
39. Boen ST, Milman AS, Dillard DH, Scribner BH. Periodic peritoneal dialysis in the management of chronic uremia. Trans Am Soc Artif Intern Organs 1962; 8: 256–62.
40. Merrill JP, Sabbaga E, Henderson L, Welzant W, Crane C. The use of an inlying plastic conduit for chronic peritoneal irrigation. Trans Am Soc Artif Intern Organs 1962; 8: 252–6.
41. Tenckhoff H, Shillipetar G, Boen ST. One year's experience with home peritoneal dialysis. Trans Am Soc Artif Intern Organs 1965; 11: 11–4.
42. Boen ST, Curtis FK, Tenckhoff H, Scribner BH. Chronic hemodialysis and peritoneal dialysis. Proc Eur Dial Transplant Assoc 1964; 1: 221–3.
43. Boen ST, Mion C, Curtis F, Shilipetar G. Periodic PD using the repeated puncture technique and an automatic cycling machine. Trans Am Soc Artif Intern Organs 1964; 10: 409–13.
44. Anonymous. Intermittent peritoneal lavage. Lancet 1959; 2: 551–2.
45. Palmer RA, Quinton WE, Gray JF. Prolonged PD for chronic renal failure. Lancet 1964; 1: 700–2.
46. Gutch CF. Peritoneal dialysis. Trans Am Soc Artif Intern Organs 1964; 10: 406–7.
47. McDonald HP, Gerber N, Mishra D, Woln L, Peng B, Waterhouse K. Subcutaneous Dacron and Teflon cloth adjuncts for silastic AV shunts and peritoneal dialysis catheters. Trans Am Soc Artif Intern Organs 1968; 14: 176–80.
48. Tenckhoff H, Schechter HA. Bacteriologically safe peritoneal access device. Trans Am Soc Artif Intern Organs 1973; 19: 363–70.
49. Tenckhoff H, Blagg C, Curtis HF, Hickman RO. Chronic peritoneal dialysis. Proc EDTA 1973; 10: 363–70.
50. Jarrel B, Lasker N, Roberts M. A simple system of automated peritoneal dialysis. Dial Transplant 1974; 3: 36–9.
51. Vercellone A, Piccoli G, Cavalli PL, Ragni R, Alloatte S. A new automatic peritoneal dialysis system. Proc Eur Dial Transplant Assoc 1968; 5: 344–9.
52. Tenckhoff H, Shilipetar G, van Paasschen WH, Swanson E. A home peritoneal dialysate delivery system. Trans Am Soc Artif Intern Organs 1969; 15: 103–7.
53. Tenckhoff H, Meston B, Shilipetar G. A simplified automatic peritoneal dialysis system. Trans Am Soc Artif Intern Organs 1972; 18: 436–9

54. Stephen RL. Reciprocating peritoneal dialysis with a subcutaneous peritoneal catheter. Dial Transplant 1978; 7: 834–8.
55. Di Paolo N. Semicontinuous peritoneal dialysis. Dial Transplant 1978; 7: 839–42.
56. Gordan A, Greenbaum M, Maxwell MH. Sorbent regeneration of peritoneal dialysate. Trans Am Soc Artif Intern Organs 1974; 20A: 130.
57. Tenckhoff H. Advantages and shortcomings of peritoneal dialysis. Seminar Uro Nephrol Hopital Pitie 1977; 10: 71–8.
58. Oreopoulos DG. Home peritoneal dialysis. Proc EDTA 1975; 12; 139–42.
59. Buoncristiani U. Clinical results of long term peritoneal dialysis. Proc EDTA 1975; 12: 145–8.
60. Heal MR, England AG, Goldsmith HJ. Four years experience with indwelling silastic cannulae for long term peritoneal dialysis. Br Med J 1975; 2: 596–600.
61. Ahmed S, Gallagher N, Shen F. Intermittent peritoneal dialysis: status reassessed. Trans Am Soc Artif Intern Organs 1979; 25; 86–8.
62. Gutman RA. Towards enhancement of peritoneal clearances. Dial Transplant 1979; 8: 107–26.
63. Popovich RP, Moncrief JW, Decherd JF, Bomar JB, Pyle WK. The definition of a novel portable/wearable equilibrium dialysis technique. Abstct. Trans Am Soc Artif Intern Organs 1976; 5: 64.
64. Gotch FA, Sargeant JA, Keen M, Lam M, Prowitt M, Grasy M. Solute kinetics in intermittent dialysis therapy. 9th Annual Contractors Conference. Artificial Kidney Chronic Uremia Prog 1976; 9: 98–101.
65. Popovich RP, Moncrief JW, Dechert JF, Pyle WK, Morris S, Lindley JD. Clinical developments of the low dialysis clearance hypothesis via equilibium peritoneal dialysis. Proc Annual Contractors Conf. Artif Kidney-Chronic Uremia Prog (NIAMDO) 1977; 10: 123–5.
66. Popovich RP, Moncrief JW, Nolph KD, Ghods AJ, Twardowski Z, Pyle WK. Continuous ambulatory peritoneal dialysis. Ann Intern Med 1978; 88: 449–56.
67. Oreopoulos DG, Robson M, Izatt S, Clayton S, de Veber GA. A simple and safe technique for CAPD. Trans Am Soc Artif Intern Organs 1978; 24: 484–9.
68. Oreopoulos DG, Khanna R, Williams P, Dombros N, Carmichael D. Efficacy of and clinical experience with CAPD in Canada. In: Aktins R, Thomson N, Farrell PC, eds. Peritoneal Dialysis. Edinburgh: Churchill Livingstone, 1981, pp. 114–25.
69. Nolph KD. Continuous ambulatory peritoneal dialysis. Am J Nephrol 1981; 1: 1–10.
70. Moncrief JW, Popovich PR. Efficiency and clinical experience with CAPD in the USA. In: Aktins R, Thomson N, Farrell PC, eds. Peritoneal Dialysis. Edinburgh: Churchill Livingstone, 1981, pp. 165–70.
71. Lamiere N, De Paepe M, Van Holder R, Verbanck J, Ringoir S. Experience with CAPD in Belgium. In: Aktins R, Thomson N, Farrell PC, eds. Peritoneal Dialysis. Edinburgh: Churchill Livingstone, 1981, pp. 104–13.
72. Mion C, Slingeneyer A, Canard B. CAPD in France: results of a national survey and two years experience at one centre. In: Aktins R, Thomson N, Farrell PC, eds. Peritoneal Dialysis. Edinburgh: Churchill Livingstone, 1981, pp. 126–35.
73. La Greca G, Biasioli S, Chiaramonte S, Fabris A, Feriani M, Pisani E, Ronco C. Italian clinical experience of CAPD. In: Aktins R, Thomson N, Farrell PC, eds. Peritoneal Dialysis. Edinburgh: Churchill Livingstone, 1981, pp. 136–8.
74. Gokal R, Ward MK. Clinical experience with CAPD in the United Kingdom. In: Aktins R, Thomson N, Farrell PC, eds. Peritoneal Dialysis. Edinburgh: Churchill Livingstone, 1981, pp. 162–4.
75. Lindholm B, Alverstrand A, Furst P, Trandeus A, Bergstrom J. Efficiency and clinical experience of CAPD – Stockholm, Sweden. In: Aktins R, Thomson N, Farrell PC, eds. Peritoneal Dialysis. Edinburgh: Churchill Livingstone, 1981, pp. 147–61.
76. Thomson N, Atkins R, Hooke D, Maydom B, Scott D. Long term clinical experience with CAPD in Australia. In: Aktins R, Thomson N, Farrell PC, eds. Peritoneal Dialysis. Edinburgh: Churchill Livingstone, 1981, pp. 93–103.
77. Gokal R, McHugh M, Fryer R, Ward MK, Kerr DNS. CAPD: one year's experience in a UK dialysis unit. Br Med J 1980; 281: 474–7.
78. Fenton SSA, Cattram DC, Allen AF et al. Initial experience with CAPD. Artif Organ 1979; 3: 206–9.
79. Mocrief JW, Popovich R. Continuous ambulatory peritoneal dialysis. In: Nolph KD, ed. Peritoneal Dialysis. Dordrecht: Martinus Nijhoff, 1985, pp. 209–46.
80. Gokal R. Peritonitis in CAPD. Antimicrob Chemother 1982; 9: 417–22.
81. Gokal R, Manos J, Mallick NP. Defects in CAPD equipment. Lancet 1982; 2: 382 and 671.
82. Oreopoulos DG, Khanna R, Williams P, Vas SI. Continuous ambulatory peritoneal dialysis. Nephron 1982; 30: 292–303.
83. Buoncristiani U, Bianchi P, Cozzari M. A new safe simple connection system for CAPD. Int J Nephrol Urol Androl 1980; 1: 50–3.
84. Bazzato G, Coli U, Landini S. CAPD without wearing a bag: complete freedom of patient and significant reduction of peritonitis. Proc EDTA 1980; 17: 266–75.
85. Maiorca R, Cantaluppi A, Cancarini GC et al. Prospective controlled trial of a Y-connector and disinfectant to prevent peritonitis in CAPD. Lancet 1983; 2: 642–4.
86. Viglino G, Cantaluppi A, Gandolfo C, Peluso F, Cavalli PL. Y-set evolution. In: La Greca G, Ronco C, Feriani M, Chiaramonte S, Conz P, eds. Peritoneal Dialysis. Milan: 1991, pp. 281–93.
87. Buoncristiani V. The Y-set with disinfectant is here to stay. Perit Dial Int 1989; 9: 149–50.
88. Maiorca R, Cancarini GC, Comerini C, Monili L. Morbidity and mortality of CAPD and haemodialysis. Kidney Int 1993; 43 (suppl. 40): S4–S15.
89. Maiorca R, Cancarini GC, Comerini C, Monili L, Brunori G. The impact of the Y-system and low peritonitis rate on CAPD results. In: Hatano M, ed. Nephrology. Tokyo: Springer Verlag, 1991, pp. 1592–601.
90. Clayton S, Finer C, Quinton C et al. Training patients for CAPD at Toronto Western Hospital. In: Legrain M, ed. Continuous Ambulatory Peritoneal Dialysis. Amsterdam: Excerpta Medica, 1980, pp. 162–6.
91. Oreopoulos DG. Requirements for the organisation of a CAPD programme. Nephron 1979; 24: 261–3.
92. Gokal R, Marsh FP. Survey of CAPD in the United Kingdom, 1982. Perit Dial Bull 1984; 4: 261–3.
93. Teehan BP, Schleifer CR, Reichard CA, Cupit MC, Sigler MH, Haff AC. Acid–base studies in CAPD. In: Moncrief J, Popovich R, eds. CAPD Update. Masson, 1982, pp. 95–102.
94. Nolph KD, Prowant B, Serkes KD et al. Multi-centre evaluation of a new peritoneal dialysis solution with a high lactate and a low magnesium concentration. Perit Dial Bull 1983; 3: 63–5.
95. Teehan B, Schleifer C, Sigler M, Gilgore G. A quantitative approach to CAPD prescription. Perit Dial Bull 1985; 5; 152–6.
96. Verger C, Brunschvicg O, Le Charpentier Y, Lavergne A, Vantelon J. Structural and ultrastructural peritoneal membrane changes and permeability alterations during CAPD. Proc EDTA 1981; 18; 199–203.
97. Twardowski Z, Nolph KD, Khanna R et al. Peritoneal equilibration test. Perit Dial Bull 1987; 7: 138–47.
98. Dobbie J, Zaki M, Wilson M. Ultrastructural studies on the peritoneum with reference to CAPD. Scot Med J 1981; 26: 213–23.
99. Verger C, Luger A, Moore LH, Nolph KD. Acute changes in peritoneal morphology and transport properties with infectious peritonitis and mechanical injury. Kidney Int 1983; 23: 823–31.
100. Faller B, Marichal JF. Loss of ultrafiltration in CAPD. In: Gahl GM et al. eds, Advances in Peritoneal Dialysis. Amsterdam: Excerpta Medica, 1981, pp. 227–32.

101. Faller B, Marichal JF. Loss of ultrafiltration in CAPD: a role for acetate. Perit Dial Bull 1984; 4: 10–14.
102. Slingeneyer A, Canaud B, Mion C. Permanent loss of ultrafiltration capacity of the peritoneum in long term peritoneal dialysis: an epidemiological study. Nephron 1983; 33: 133–8.
103. Rottembourg J, Issad B, Langlois P et al. Loss of ultrafiltration and sclerosing peritonitis during CAPD: evaluation of the potential risk factors. Proc V Nat Conf CAPD 1985, pp. 109–17.
104. Wideroe TE, Smeby LC, Mjaland S et al. Long term changes in transperitoneal water transport during CAPD. Nephron 1984; 38: 238–47.
105. Bazzato G, Coli U, Landini S et al. Restoration of ultrafiltration capacity of peritoneal membrane in patients on CAPD. Int J Artif Organs 1984; 7: 93–6.
106. Manuel FA. Failure of ultrafiltration in patients on CAPD. Perit Dial Bull 1983; 3: S38–40.
107. Oreopoulos DG, Gotloib L, Calderaro V, Khanna R. For how long can peritoneal dialysis be continued? Can Med Assoc J 1981; 124: 12–13.
108. Nolph KD, Legrain M, Rottembourg, J et al. A survey of ultrafiltration in CAPD. Perit Dial Bull 1984; 4: 137–42.
109. Henderson IS, Couper IA, Lumsden A. The effects of shelf life of peritoneal dialysis fluid on ultrafiltration in CAPD. In: La Greca G, Ronco C, eds. Second International Course in Peritoneal Dialysis. Milan: Wichtig Editore, 1986, pp. 85–6.
110. Junor BJR, Briggs JD, Forewell M, Dobbie J, Henderson I. Sclerosing peritonitis – the contribution of chlorhexidine in alcohol. Perit Dial Bull 1985; 5: 101–4.
111. Lasker N, Burke JF, Patchefsky A, Haughey E. Peritoneal reactions to particulate matter in peritoneal dialysis solutions. Trans Am Soc Artif Intern Organs 1975; 21: 342–4.
112. Shaldon S, Koch KM, Quellhorst E, Dinarello CA. Pathogenesis of sclerosing peritonitis in CAPD. Trans Am Soc Artif Intern Organs 1984; 30: 193–4.
113. Verger C. Clinical significance of ultrafiltration alterations in CAPD. In: La Greca G, Ronco C, eds. Second International Course in Peritoneal Dialysis. Milan: Wichtig Editore, 1986, pp. 91–4.
114. Verger C, Celicont B. Peritoneal permeability and encapsulating peritonitis. Lancet 1985; I: 986–7.
115. Slingeneyer A, Canaud B, Maurad B et al. Sclerosing peritonitis: late and severe complication of long term home peritoneal dialysis. Trans Am Soc Artif Intern Organs 1983; 29: 633–8.
116. Gandhi VC, Humayan HM, Ing TS et al. Sclerotic thickening of the peritoneal membrane in maintenance peritoneal dialysis patients. Arch Intern Med 1980; 140: 1201–3.
117. Dobbie J, Henderson I, Wilson L. New evidence on the pathogenesis of sclerosing encapsulating peritonitis obtained from serial biopsies. Adv Perit Dial 1987; 7: 138–42.
118. Slingeneyer A. Preliminary report on a cooperative international study on sclerosing encapsulating peritonitis. Contrib Nephrol 1987; 57: 239–47.
119. Wing AJ, Broyer M, Brunner FB et al. Combined report on regular dialysis and transplantation in Europe, XIII, 1982. Proc EDTA 1983; 20: 2–75.
120. Shaldon S, Koch KM, Quellhorst E, Lonnemann G, Dinarello CA. CAPD is a second class treatment. Contrib Nephrol 1985; 44: 163–72.
121. Twardowski ZJ. New approaches to intermittent peritoneal dialysis therapies. In: Nolph KD, ed. Peritoneal Dialysis. Dordrecht: Kluwer Academic Publishers, 1989, pp. 133–51.
122. Nakayawa D, Price C, Stinebraugh B, Suki W. Continuous cyclic peritoneal dialysis: a viable option in the treatment of chronic renal failure. Trans Am Soc Artif Intern Organs 1981; 2: 755–7.
123. Diaz-Buxo JA, Walker PJ, Farmer CD. Continuous cyclic peritoneal dialysis – a preliminary report. Artif Organs 1981; 5: 157–62.
124. Scriber BH. Foreword. In: Neph KD, ed. Peritoneal Dialysis. 2nd edn. Dordrecht: Kluwer, 1985, pp. xi–xii.
125. Moncrief J, Popovich R. CAPD worldwide experience. In: Nolph KD, ed. Peritoneal Dialysis. The Hague: Martinus Nijhoff, 1981, pp. 178–212.
126. Prowant B, Fruto LV. Inpatient home training for CAPD. In: Legrain M, ed. Continuous Ambulatory Peritoneal Dialysis. Amsterdam: Excerpta Medica, 1980, pp. 158–161.
127. Clayton S, Finer C, Quinton C et al. Training patients for CAPD at the Toronto Western Hospital. In: Legrain M, ed. Continuous Ambulatory Peritoneal Dialysis. Amsterdam: Excerpta Medica, 1980, pp. 162–66.

2 | Current status of peritoneal dialysis

R. Mehrotra and K. D. Nolph

Introduction

It was in 1923 that Ganter performed the first peritoneal dialysis (PD) in a woman with renal failure [1]. However, the early experience with intermittent peritoneal dialysis was discouraging and led to the belief that PD was not an appropriate renal replacement therapy for patients with end-stage renal disease (ESRD) [2]. The introduction of the concept of continuous ambulatory peritoneal dialysis (CAPD) by Popovich et al. [3] was initially met with scepticism but the successful clinical experience in nine patients at two centres in the United States [4] convinced sceptics about the potential of the technique as a viable alternative to haemodialysis. Over the last two decades PD has grown worldwide to become the third most common modality for renal replacement therapy.

Epidemiology

Patient numbers on PD

During the 1980s there occurred a rapid growth in the utilization of chronic PD. This rapid growth continued into the first half of this decade, with annual global growth rates reaching 15% for the period 1991–94 [5]. However, since then there has occurred a slowing in the global growth rate: the worldwide PD population grew at 7.3% from 1993 to 1997 (Fig. 1). The reasons for this slow-down are unclear and are possibly multi-factorial. At the end of 1997 the chronic PD population worldwide was an estimated 115,000, representing 14% of global dialysis patients [6]. The vast majority of these patients are concentrated in North America, Latin America, Europe and Japan (Fig. 2).

There are wide variations in the utilization of PD in different countries. The proportion of patients on dialysis treated with PD varies from over 80% in Mexico and Hong Kong to less than 5% in Argentina, Romania and Chile (Fig. 3) [7–14]. Even within the same country there are wide variations in the use of PD. In the United States the point prevalence of PD, in the period 1994–96, ranged from 10.3% in Texas to 20.5% in Network 12 (Iowa, Nebraska, Missouri and Kansas) [7]. Similarly, at the end of 1996, only 13% of patients in the Northern Territory in Australia were treated with PD as against 47% in the state of Tasmania [8]. In Italy the disparity in use of PD, among regions, has increased, varying from 0% to 55% [9]. Finally, in France, there are large differences in the use of PD and the percentage of patients treated with PD can vary from 0% to 22% between different towns in the same region [15]. The reasons for these differences are multiple and complex and are discussed in a subsequent section.

Growth of automated PD (APD)

While in the 1980s and the early 1990s, the growth in PD was almost entirely due to the expansion of CAPD programmes, it is the growth in automated PD that is sustaining the ongoing increase in the number of patients on PD (Fig. 4). There has been a 10-fold increase in the number of patients on APD in the United States and Canada over the past decade [7, 10] and over the past 5 years the numbers of patients on APD in Australia and New Zealand have increased 5- and 7-fold respectively [16]. In both the United States and Canada, in the period 1994–96, there has been a 14% decrease in the absolute number of patients on CAPD [7, 10]. In the same time-period the number of patients on APD has more than doubled [7, 10], accounting for the small overall increase in the number of patients on PD. The growth of APD has been spurred by an increasing emphasis on adequacy and the simplified automated machines address the concerns of some patients about lifestyle issues [17]. It is anticipated

R. Gokal, R. Khanna, R.Th. Krediet and K.D. Nolph (eds.), Textbook of Peritoneal Dialysis, 2nd Edition, 19–35.

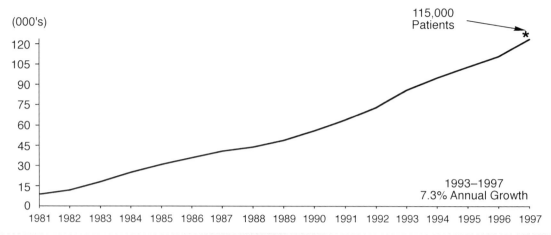

Figure 1. Growth of global PD patients, 1981–97. Source: 1997 Baxter Health Care Report [6].

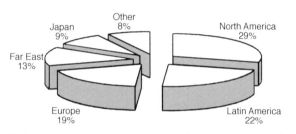

Figure 2. Geographical distribution of the 115,000 patients on PD. Source: 1997 Baxter Health Care [6].

that the use of APD will continue to expand and will sustain the growth of PD.

Factors affecting the choice of PD

The disparity in the use of PD in different countries and different parts of the same country has stimulated tremendous interest in elucidating the factors that determine the choice of PD as the modality for renal replacement. A large number of factors impact

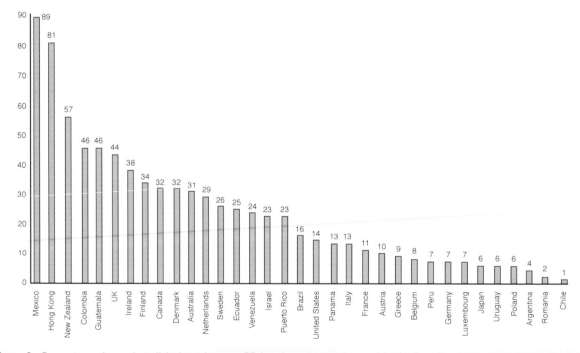

Figure 3. Percentage of prevalent dialysis patients on PD in selected countries worldwide. Data for all countries, except Australia, Canada, New Zealand and United States are for prevalent patients in 1995. For Canada and the United States the data are for prevalent patients on 31 December 1996, and for Australia and New Zealand the data are for prevalent patients in March 1998 [7–14].

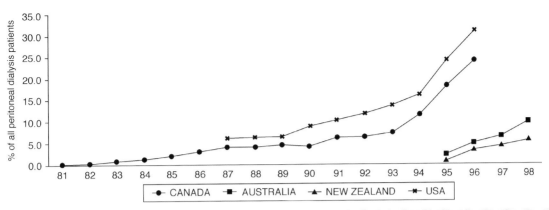

Figure 4. Growth of proportion of PD patients on APD in United States, Canada, Australia and New Zealand [7, 8, 10].

upon this choice (Table 1); non-medical factors, however, are primary in the decision-making process [9, 15, 18–20].

It appears that the greater the involvement of the 'public' (as opposed to 'private') facilities in the provision of dialysis care, the larger the proportion of dialysis patients on chronic PD (Fig. 5) [9, 15, 19, 21]. Within the same country a similar difference exists in the utilization of PD between public and private dialysis facilities (Fig. 6) [6, 15]. The reason for this is obvious: when the annual healthcare budget is fixed, PD, because of its lower cost, is highly utilized [9]. Physician reimbursement is significantly influenced by the health care system and has been identified as the most important determinant of the choice of PD by some [9, 15, 19] but not others [20]. Moreover, when the facility reimbursement is paid at a flat rate, the proportion of patients on PD declines as higher fixed cost for PD reduces the margin of profit [15].

Table 1. Factors determining the choice of peritoneal dialysis

Economic factors
   Health care system
   Physician/facility reimbursement
   Resource availability

Psychosocial factors
   Physician bias
   Educational deficits (physician/patient)
   Time of referral
   Patient preference/lifestyle attributes

Medical factors
   Age
   ? Diabetes
   Cardiovascular instability
   Availability of vascular access
   Abdominal pathology

Physician bias is second only to the aforementioned economic factors in the utilization of PD [9, 15, 19, 22]. The nature of patient education is dependent on the physician bias, and in non-urgent situations the decisions of patients depend mostly on the information provided by their doctors [15, 20, 22]. In the Dialysis Morbidity and Mortality Study (DMMS), Wave 2, only 25% of the patients who chose HD reported that PD was discussed with them, whereas 68% of the patients who chose PD reported that HD was discussed with them [22]. Time of referral is another important determinant: patients who are referred late are more likely to be initiated on HD and are likely to stay on it [19, 21–24]. Once all the psychosocial factors are eliminated, it is the patient preference that finally determines the choice of therapy. Patient factors include their psychological profile, family environment, type of housing, distance from the HD unit, and the desire to be independent and/or continue working [15, 25, 26]. On balance it is the patients who are willing to take an important role in their care who choose PD. In fact, 84% of the PD patients and only 47% of the HD patients enrolled in the DMMS Wave 2 study appeared to contribute substantially to the decision [22].

PD is the dialysis modality of choice in children. However, medical reasons play a role in the selection of the dialysis modality in only a minority of adult patients [20]. Of 150 consecutive adult patients started on dialysis at a single Canadian centre, only 15% were referred to one of the two modalities for medical reasons (cardiovascular instability and inability to obtain a vascular access for choosing PD or an unusable abdomen for choosing HD) [20]. It has been claimed that PD is the best method for treating patients with diabetes [27] but current evidence does not support its preferential use in these patients [28].

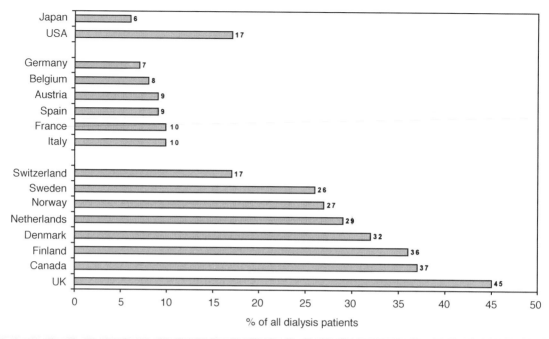

Figure 5. Use of PD as a modality for dialysis in various countries, based upon the funding of the dialysis provider. The top panel (Japan, USA) are with predominantly private dialysis providers; the middle panel (Germany, Belgium, Austria, Spain, France, Italy) are with mixture of public and private providers, and the bottom panel (Switzerland, Sweden, Norway, Netherlands, Denmark, Finland, Canada, UK) are with predominantly public providers [21].

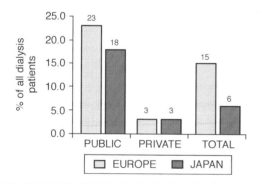

Figure 6. Proportion of all dialysis patients on PD in public and private dialysis units in Europe and Japan. Source: 1997 Baxter Health Care [6].

Technique survival

When PD was initially introduced in clinical practice it was anticipated that a quarter of all patients on chronic dialysis would be on PD [29]. In the United States, even though about 20% of incident ESRD patients are initiated on PD, it accounts for only 14% of the prevalent population [7]. A lower technique survival rate seemingly accounts for this disparity. Technique failure usually implies departure from PD due to death or transfer; transplantation is usually censored.

There are differences in the proportion of patients stopping PD per year between different countries [7, 30, 31]; these national differences are in large part due to the differences in the rate of transplantation. However, there is clearly a tremendous variability in the technique survival between various centres [32–34]. The difference in technique success between CAPD and HD is greatest in the youngest patients and progressively diminishes in the other age groups [35]. Furthermore, some racial groups may have a lower short-term technique survival than others [36] and patients who are referred late are more likely to be transferred to HD than those who are referred early [23]. With improvements in patient selection, training and aggressive management of complications, it is possible to obtain technique survival in excess of 80% [37, 38].

The early modifications in the technique of PD led to significant increases in the technique survival. The declining rates of peritonitis in the second half of the 1980s led to continuing improvements in the technique success [30]. However, over the past decade the improvement has been more modest. In the United States the 36% overall 2-year survival rate in the period 1981–88 [39] increased to 36–40% for the period 1988–90 [40] and further to 40–44% for the period 1991–93 [7].

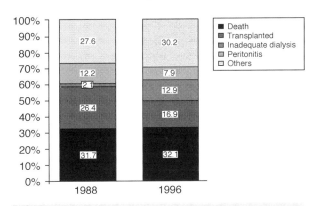

Figure 7. Change in the aetiology of stopping PD in Canada, 1988–96. Source: CORR report, 1998 [11].

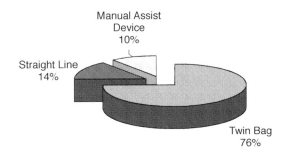

Figure 8. Frequency of use of different connection techniques worldwide, 1997. Source: 1997 Baxter Health Care [6].

If death and transplantation are excluded, infectious complications have been the most common reason for transfer-out from PD [39, 41–43]. However, with refinements in technology there has been a significant reduction in the rates of infectious complications. This has been paralleled by an increasing recognition of the importance of adequacy, both in terms of small solute clearance and ultrafiltration capacity. This change is clearly reflected in the trends in the aetiology of technique failure in Canada (Fig. 7) [10]. The proportion of patients transferring out of PD secondary to peritonitis declined from 12.2% in 1988 to 7.9% in 1996. This was paralleled by an increase in the number of patients transferring out because of inadequate dialysis from 2.1% in 1988 to 12.9% in 1996.

These data are very compelling, and call for similar studies in other countries; it is likely that similar trends will be noticeable in other parts of the world.

PD: the technique

A major innovation early on was the introduction of sterile plastic bags for dialysate [44]. Since then, the basic PD system consists of a PVC bag containing 0.5–3 L of PD fluid, a transfer set and a catheter access to the peritoneal cavity. Significant advances in the technique of PD have occurred over the past two decades.

Trends in connectology

The initial bag-and-spike system was recognized to result in an unacceptably high incidence of peritonitis from touch contamination. In Italy a double-bag Y-set device was developed that used a disconnect system with a flush before fill technique [45]. The early success in Italy was confirmed in centres in Europe [46] and North America [47, 48] and is now the system of choice for PD (Fig. 8). Over 90% of all patients in North America, Europe, Australia and New Zealand now use these disconnect devices [5, 8]. The increased monetary cost of the twin-bag system is more than offset by the reduction in the time to first peritonitis and the number of episodes of peritonitis [49].

Trends in catheter design

Tenckhoff's design of the indwelling silicone rubber catheter with two dacron cuffs was instrumental in making IPD a viable long-term therapy for renal replacement [50]. To date the Tenckhoff catheter remains the most widely used catheter worldwide [30, 51]. Several variations in the catheter design have been introduced and include the number of cuffs (single vs. double), design of the subcutaneous pathway (permanently bent or 'swan-neck' vs. straight) and the intra-abdominal portion (straight vs. coiled) [52]. Double-cuff catheters are associated with a lower incidence of both peritonitis [51, 53, 54] and exit-site infections [55, 56]. Similarly, a downward-directed exit site results in a reduction in the incidence of exit-site infections and peritonitis [43, 53]. However, the benefit of the swan-neck design was demonstrable in the USRDS study only after adjusting for possible centre effects [51]. No convincing evidence exists for the superiority of the coiled design of the intraperitoneal portion of the catheter [52].

Consistent with these studies, the proportion of patients in the United States with double-cuff catheters has increased from 72% in 1989 to 89% in 1996 [22, 51]. The use of other catheter designs remains uncertain. The innovations in connectology and catheter design have resulted in a 1-year catheter survival of over 80% [43].

Patient outcome: morbidity

Peritonitis

Prevention

Infectious complications, particularly peritonitis, have long been the proverbial 'Achilles heel' of PD and have long accounted for technique failure [39, 41–43] and catheter loss [43, 57, 58]. Based on the source of infection, episodes of peritonitis can be classified into one of four categories (Table 2) [59].

Refinements in connectology and use of the twin-bag systems have led to significant declines in the rates of peritonitis from touch contamination. The number of episodes of peritonitis has declined from about 1.4 episodes per patient-year to 0.5 episodes per patient-year in most centres [39, 59]. Touch contamination, however, still remains the most common aetiology of peritonitis.

Rates of exit-site and tunnel infections, on the other hand, have remained relatively stable. The use of double-cuffed catheters and a downward-pointing tunnel lead to reductions in catheter-related infections. Over the past few years, several other strategies have been tested. Nasal carriage of *Staphylococcus aureus* has been identified as an important risk factor for this complication and several recent studies have demonstrated that the risk of *S. aureus* peritonitis can be reduced by prophylaxis for nasal carriage [60–64]. This can be achieved either by intra-nasal application of mupirocin [61, 63] or cyclical rifampin [60] or the daily application of mupirocin to the exit site [62, 64]. Widespread application of these strategies is likely to result in a further decline in peritonitis rates.

Another strategy that is being tested to reduce the incidence of catheter-related infections is the use of silver-impregnated catheters or silver ring devices at the exit site. Animal studies have reported that silver-coated catheters enhance healing of exit sites [65] and lead to a reduction in infectious complications [66, 67]. However, a prospective trial of humans with silver-coated PD catheters had to be discontinued because of complications from the improper

Table 2. Sources of infection of the peritoneal cavity in patients on peritoneal dialysis

Touch contamination
Catheter-related infections (exit-site/tunnel infections)
Enteric
Iatrogenic (enteric, bacteremic, gynecologic)

manufacture of the catheter [68]. Recently, a preliminary evaluation of the silver ring device showed a significant reduction of exit-site infections [69]. However, a larger randomized, multi-centre trial from Germany has been unable to demonstrate any benefit in the prevention of either exit-site or tunnel infections or rates of peritonitis [70].

It is believed that aggressive treatment of constipation may reduce the incidence of enteric peritonitis, and iatrogenic (or procedure-related) peritonitis can be decreased by use of antibiotic prophylaxis for procedures such as extensive dental work, colonoscopy or endometrial biopsies [59].

It is anticipated that incorporation of these advances in clinical practice and ongoing research in this area will lead to further declines in rates of peritonitis.

Treatment

The emergence of vancomycin-resistant enterococci has forced us to re-evaluate the empiric regimen for treatment of PD-related peritonitis. The ad hoc treatment guidelines of 1996 recommended the use of a first-generation cephalosporin, in combination with gentamicin, as first-line therapy [71]. While one study has provided support for this change [72], others have found significant under-treatment [73, 74], leading to a call for centre-specific treatment guidelines [74].

Nutritional status

Malnutrition at the time of initiation of dialysis, and subsequently, has emerged as an important surrogate marker of an adverse patient outcome. This observation makes the assessment of nutritional status and prevention of malnutrition an important clinical priority.

Trends

Malnutrition is widely prevalent in the PD population [75–77]. In the three multi-centre studies that have looked at this issue, estimates of severe malnutrition range from 4% to 8% [75, 76] and mild to moderate malnutrition from 33% to 55% [75–78]. There is evidence to suggest that the protein malnutrition is more widely prevalent than energy malnutrition in patients on PD [79–81]. This information is useful as it helps us direct our efforts in the direction of improvement of protein stores.

Strategies to improve nutritional status in PD patients

Significant progress has been made in this field over the past 5 years. The various interventions that have been tested are listed in Table 3. It is unclear, however, if improvement in nutritional status will result in a reduction in morbidity or mortality of our patients.

Residual renal function. There has been an increasing recognition of the importance of residual renal function in maintaining the nutritional status of patients on chronic dialysis [75, 76, 82]. Loss of residual renal function correlated with muscle wasting, and contributed to anorexia and the symptoms of severe malnutrition in patients studied in an international study [75]. Likewise, in the Canadian–USA (CANUSA) multicentre study, after 6 months of initiation of PD there was a progressive decline in nutritional parameters with declining residual renal function [76]. Hence, preserving residual renal function should be an important goal.

Adequacy of dialysis. Several cross-sectional studies have shown a relationship between the dose of PD and the dietary protein intake and the nutritional status of patients. However, this has not been widely accepted. The results of the CANUSA study should put this controversy to rest. In this study, during the first 6 months of CAPD, the addition of dialysis clearance to the residual renal function resulted in a marked increase in solute clearances. This was associated with significant improvements in several estimates of nutritional status (subjective global assessment, protein catabolic rate and lean body mass) and these changes were significantly correlated with both the estimates of the dose of dialysis [83].

Correction of metabolic acidosis. The adverse impact of chronic metabolic acidosis on nutritional status has long been recognized. Recently, both short-term [84] and long-term [85] correction of acidosis have been shown to be beneficial. In the latter study an improvement in plasma bicarbonate from 25 to 30 mmol/L was associated with an increase in body weight, triceps skinfold thickness and mid-arm circumference over a 12-month treatment period.

Use of intraperitoneal amino acid (IAA) solutions. Earlier studies with amino-acid solutions enrolled small numbers of patients, were uncontrolled, and used solutions not available commercially. However, three recent well-conducted trials support the use of these solutions. In a 35-day, inpatient study of 19 malnourished CAPD patients, one exchange a day of IAA induced a positive nitrogen balance, improved plasma amino-acid profile and increased serum albumin and transferrin levels [86]. In an outpatient study of 15 CAPD patients from France, there was a progressive increase in serum albumin and transferrin levels over a period of 6 months in patients with or without malnutrition [87]. Finally, a large multicentre, prospective, randomized, open-label study confirmed the nutritional benefits of 1.1% amino-acid solutions in malnourished CAPD patients [88]. The beneficial effect of the solution may have been partially offset by induction of acidosis in almost 50% of patients with a decrease in mean CO_2 level by 2–4 mEq/L [88]. Hence, more aggressive control of acidosis may be necessary to obtain the maximal benefit of these solutions.

Patient outcome: mortality

The current practice of care of the ESRD patient is based on the premise that haemodialysis and PD are equivalent therapies. Several recent studies have put this issue on the centre stage.

Comparisons of mortality in USA and Canada

The premise of equivalent patient outcomes on PD and HD has recently been challenged by Bloembergen: in the cohort of prevalent patients in the United States from 1987 to 1989, using the Poisson regression model, they showed that the relative risk of death was 1.19 in prevalent CAPD patients compared with prevalent HD patients [89]. The risk was relatively strong in females and in diabetics. These results caused considerable consternation in the PD community. Vonesh and Moran followed up their study with an identical analysis of death risk in four subsequent cohorts (1988–90, 1989–91, 1990–92, 1991–93) [90]. Based on the same model, there was no difference in the average death risk between PD and HD patients, both overall and by

Table 3. Recommended interventions to improve nutritional status in PD patients

Preservation of residual renal function
Adequacy of dialysis
Correction of metabolic acidosis
Use of intra-peritoneal amino acid solutions

gender. These differences may be explained, in part, by the inclusion of incident patients in the USRDS report since the 1989–91 cohort. Subgroup analysis of these data indicates that, except among older diabetics, especially female diabetics, patients treated with PD have similar (non-diabetics) or better (younger diabetics) survival than patients treated with HD [91]. Finally, Wolfe compared the 1-year mortality between the PD and HD patients, in the 65–74-year age group, initiating dialysis in 1994 in the United States. Adjusting for age, race, sex, diabetes and pre-ESRD Medicare costs (as an index of co-morbidity), the relative risk of mortality was significantly lower among PD patients than among HD patients ($RR = 0.809$, $p = 0.01$) [92].

The results from Canada have been different in several respects. Fenton and co-workers enrolled 11,970 incident patients who initiated dialysis between January 1990 and December 1994 [93]. Adjusting for age, primary renal diagnosis, centre size, and pre-dialysis co-morbid conditions, the relative risk of mortality, as estimated by Poisson regression, was significantly lower among PD patients ($RR = 0.73$, 95% CI 0.68–0.78). The increased mortality for HD was concentrated in the first 2 years of follow-up. Censoring patients at transplantation had little impact; the lower mortality was not altered when patients were censored at the time of the first modality switch and the relative risk of death was unchanged when deaths occurred within 30, 60 and 90 days of a treatment switch attributable to a previous modality.

Limitations of mortality comparisons between modalities

As illustrated above, modality comparisons are very sensitive to the method of analysis. While there are many reasons for the difference in the results of the studies, some of the potential reasons are summarized in Table 4.

Failure to include all co-morbid conditions can result in different outcomes. In a recent study, different risk-stratification methods applied to the same cohort of patients yielded significant variation

Table 4. Limitations of modality comparisons

Failure to include all co-morbid conditions
Failure to grade all co-morbid conditions
Failure to account for adequacy of dialysis
Failure to account for compliance
Failure to adjust for differences in residual renal function

in the proportion of patients in each risk group and survival in each group varied depending on the method of risk stratification used [94]. Failure to grade the severity of the identified co-morbid conditions is an obvious limitation of the current methods of analysis [95] and is the likely reason for the significantly higher mortality of PD patients in US, as compared to Canada in the CANUSA study. The emphasis on improving the adequacy of dialysis for PD came significantly after that for HD. At this present time, under-dialysis is more widely prevalent among PD patients. The 1998 Core-Indicators study from the United States reported that only 45% of CAPD patients met the DOQI guidelines for adequacy based on Kt/V [96] as against 72% of HD who met the Dialysis Outcome Quality Initiative (DOQI) guidelines of adequacy based on urea reduction ratio (URR) [97]. It is likely that the magnitude of under-dialysis was significantly greater during the period of the studies mentioned in the previous section. Unpublished results of Keshaviah compared CANUSA high-dose PD with Minnesota high-dose HD and found high but similar survival rates for both therapies. Finally, self-reported non-compliance among CAPD patients is higher than among HD patients [22] and recent studies suggest that the actual non-compliance with therapy may actually be higher than the self-reported non-compliance [98].

Hence, current comparisons of the two therapies are flawed. There is little reason to believe that one modality of therapy is superior over the other, though it is likely that PD may have an advantage early on.

Adequacy of PD

In the early years of PD it was commonly accepted that subjective clinical judgement was enough for determining that a patient was well dialysed [99]. Even though the concept of urea kinetic modelling was first extended to PD in the mid-1980s [100], it was not until recently that the importance of adequate dialysis has been recognized. Several studies over the past few years suggest that the concept of adequacy should be extended to include ultrafiltration capacity.

Adequacy: small solute clearances

Several indices for small solute clearances have been used to assess the adequacy of PD but weekly $Kt/$

V_{urea} and creatinine clearance (litres/week/1.73 m^2) are now accepted as independent estimates of dialysis dose that complement each other.

Small solute clearances and patient outcome

Some small, single-centre studies were initially conducted that demonstrated the dependence of patient morbidity and mortality on small solute clearances [101–105]. This led to the multi-centre CANUSA study, the results of which were published in 1996 [76]. This showed that both weekly Kt/V_{urea} and creatinine clearance were strong predictors of patient survival, and survival improved continuously with increasing small solute clearance, without an apparent threshold. Higher dialysis dose, including residual renal function, was also associated with better technique survival and less hospitalization. This study has clearly documented the importance of adequate small solute clearances in improving patient outcome. However, this study was unable to address the importance of peritoneal clearances: while both total weekly Kt/V_{urea} and creatinine clearance and residual renal function correlated with patient survival, peritoneal Kt/V_{urea} and creatinine clearance were not predictive at all. This probably reflects the lack of sufficient variation in these indices due to the uniformity of prescriptions, and does not undermine the importance of peritoneal clearances.

Targets for adequacy

Shortly after the publication of the landmark CANUSA study, the landmark report of the Peritoneal Dialysis Adequacy Workgroup of the Dialysis Outcome Quality Initiative (DOQI) of the National Kidney Foundation was published [106]. These recommendations are likely to become the standard of care in many parts of the world.

The current targets for adequacy for CAPD are a weekly Kt/V_{urea} of 2.0 and a creatinine clearance of 60 L/week/1.73 m^2; for CCPD, a weekly Kt/V_{urea} of 2.1 and a creatinine clearance of 63 L/week/1.73 m^2 and for NIPD, a weekly Kt/V_{urea} of 2.2 and a creatinine clearance of 66 L/week/1.73 m^2.

Trends in PD prescription/small solute clearances

There has been a trend towards an increase in the use of exchange volume and number of exchanges per day in patients maintained on PD in the United States (Fig. 9) [22, 51], Australia and New Zealand (Fig. 10) [8] and Canada [10]. In the United States the number of patients in whom adequacy was mea-

sured at least once has increased from 66% in 1995 to 81% in 1998 [96]. There was an increase in the mean weekly Kt/V_{urea} and creatinine clearance for the prevalent CAPD and continuous cycler PD (CCPD) population in the United States from 1995 to 1997 [107]. The proportion of CAPD patients meeting the DOQI guideline for adequacy based on Kt/V_{urea} has increased from 36% in 1997 to 45% in 1998 and based on creatinine clearance has increased from 34% to 41% in the same time period [96, 108]. Similarly, 46% of CCPD patients met the Kt/V_{urea} guideline and 35% met the creatinine clearance guideline in 1998 [96]. For patients on nocturnal intermittent PD (NIPD), only 35% of the patients achieved the Kt/V_{urea} guideline and only 27% met the creatinine clearance guideline [96]. These trends reflect the increasing emphasis on adequacy, and it is likely that similar changes are occurring in the practice of PD in other parts of the world. This should translate into improved patient outcome. However, this reinforces the fact that under-dialysis is widely prevalent and a major focus of our efforts should be directed at improving adequacy of therapy.

Strategies to improve small solute clearances

The standard CAPD prescription will need to be modified to achieve the adequacy targets. The most efficient way of increasing small solute clearances is to increase the volume, rather than the number, of exchanges. Using the assumption that a patient uses 4 exchanges/day, all of the same instillation volume, the d/p urea is always 0.95 and the drainage volume is equal to the instillation volume plus 1.5 L of ultrafiltration. If a patient uses 2, 2.5 or 3 L exchanges, the body weights above which weekly Kt/V_{urea} target would not be achieved in functionally anephric patients are 52 kg, 63 kg and 74 kg respectively [5]. In heavier patients, or those who are unable to increase the dialysate volumes, based on the peritoneal transport, available resources and patient preference, either CCPD or tidal PD [109] or PD-plus [110] can often be used successfully to achieve the adequacy targets.

Adequacy: ultrafiltration

There is increasing evidence that peritoneal function, as assessed by the PET, can influence outcome. High transporters have a higher relative risk of death or technique failure than those with high-average or low-average transporters despite similar levels of small solute clearances [111–115]. These patients

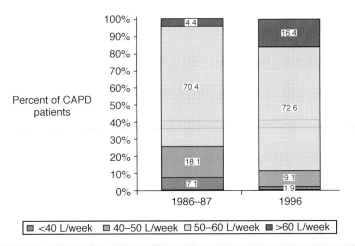

Figure 9. Change in the CAPD prescription in the United States over the past 10 years. Source: USRDS 1992 and USRDS 1997 annual reports [22, 51].

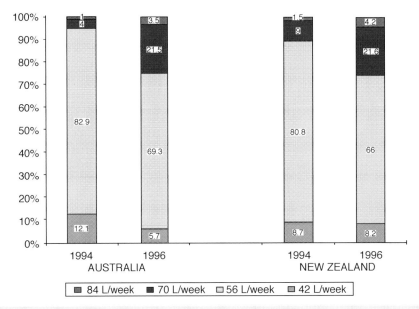

Figure 10. Change in the CAPD prescription in Australia and New Zealand. Source: ANZDATA, 1998 [8].

also have a higher morbidity while on dialysis [116]. These data are compelling enough for us to add ultrafiltration as another dimension of adequacy of PD. It is likely that the adverse impact of loss of residual renal function may be a result of both loss of small solute clearances and loss of ultrafiltration and, to compensate for this loss, enhancement of ultrafiltration has also to be ensured. In fact, high transporters may do better on automated PD or use alternative osmotic agents to ensure adequate ultrafiltration.

New solutions

The limitations of the currently available glucose-based solutions are increasingly being recognized. The long-term use of bio-incompatible solutions may be responsible for some of the complications of PD (Fig. 11). The areas of concern are the unphysiological pH and buffer combinations, hypertonicity and the role of glucose in the non-enzymatic glycation, formation of advanced glycosylation end-products (AGE) and glucose degradation products

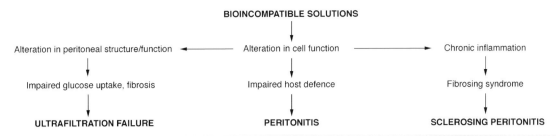

Figure 11. Consequences of long-term use of bio-incompatible PD solutions.

Table 5. Clinical role of the new peritoneal dialysis solutions

Improved ultrafiltration
Prolonged technique survival
Improved membrane viability
Nutritional management
Reduced glucose load

Table 6. Biocompatibility of the new peritoneal dialysis solutions

	Bicarbonate/ lactate	Amino acid	Icodextrin
Improved pH	√	√	
Bicarbonate buffer	√		
Iso-osmolar			√
Reduced GDPs	√	√	
Reduced AGE formation	√	√	√
Reduced glucose level		√	√

(GDP). To overcome these and other concerns, alternative solutions have been designed, each targeted to achieve a clinical goal (Table 5). These solutions, in addition, meet some or all of the concerns with the present solutions (Table 6).

Improved ultrafiltration

Icodextrin is a glucose polymer which has undergone clinical trials since the early 1990s. As it has a large particle size, unlike glucose, it is able to maintain an osmotic gradient for longer periods of time. The use of 7.5% icodextrin for an overnight exchange in patients with CAPD can generate 3.5 times greater ultrafiltration at 8 h than the 1.5% dextrose solution and similar to the 4.25% dextrose solution [117]. The amount of ultrafiltration with icodextrin can be further augmented by adding nitroprusside and this is associated with an increase in urea and creatinine clearances [118]. When used instead of standard glucose solutions for the long daytime dwell in patients on CCPD, it generates significantly greater ultrafiltration and this is associated with increases in 24-h creatinine clearances [119]. No clinical adverse effect has been noticed in the short-term clinical studies although serum maltose levels increased in both CAPD and CCPD patients [117, 120]. There was no increase in the episodes of peritonitis, and during such episodes no further increase in maltose concentration occurred [121]. These encouraging results, coupled with the recognition of the importance of ultrafiltration in determining patient outcome, will lead to a greater use of these solutions in clinical practice.

Prolonged technique survival

The ability of icodextrin to maintain an osmotic gradient during the period of dwell has been exploited in patients with ultrafiltration failure and impending technique failure. Two retrospective studies have demonstrated the ability of glucose polymer solutions to sustain ultrafiltration and increased technique survival [122, 123].

Improved membrane viability

The use of more biocompatible solutions is expected to lead to improved viability of the peritoneal membrane. However, this has not been tested formally in clinical trials.

Nutritional management

The role of intraperitoneal amino acid solutions in the nutritional management of CAPD patients has been discussed earlier.

Future directions

Over the past two decades PD has established a niche for itself in the therapy of end-stage renal disease. Indications are that it will continue to grow and its role is likely to evolve further in the years to come.

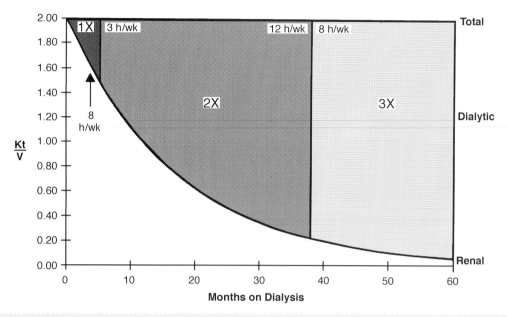

Figure 12. Results of kinetic modelling for HD as therapy for incremental dialysis [143]. Reproduced with permission.

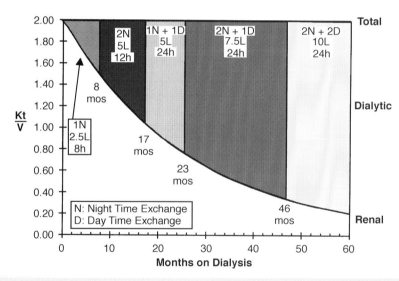

Figure 13. Results of kinetic modelling for PD as therapy for incremental dialysis [143]. Reproduced with permission.

PD and capitation

As discussed earlier, non-medical factors are the most important determinant of choice of PD, and it is anticipated that these factors will continue to influence the use of this therapy. In the United States, changes in Medicare policy will result in increased managed-care oversight and Medicare itself will move from the traditional fee for service to capitated payment. This will lead to an increased emphasis on managing the total cost of care for dialysis patients. In a capitated environment, poten-

tial for returns will be based on our ability to provide high-quality, cost-effective therapy [124]. At least two recent studies suggest that the cost of PD at some centres is lower than that for HD [125, 126]. Medicare payments for patients on CAPD/CCPD are significantly lower than for patients on HD in all age groups [7]. All this suggests an advantage of PD over HD in a capitated environment. It is likely that similar pressures related to cost-containment will soon be felt in other parts of the world, also, if not already so.

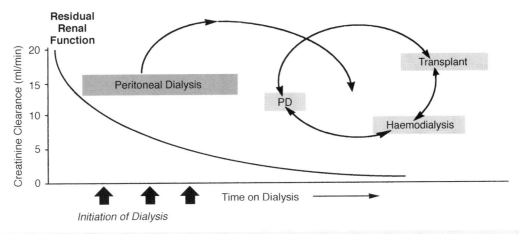

Figure 14. A model of integrated ESRD care. Source: 1997 Baxter Health Care [6].

'Healthy' start of dialysis and incremental dialysis

Even though targets have been set for small solute clearance clearances on dialysis, patients with chronic renal failure are allowed to dwindle to clearances far below the adequacy target before dialysis is initiated [22, 76, 127–130]. This practice is unacceptable as progressive renal failure leads to nutritional decline [131, 132] and the lower the small solute clearances [127,133,134] and the worse the nutritional status [51, 76, 83, 135–140] at the time of initiation of dialysis, the worse is the patient outcome. As the relationship between dietary protein intake and small solute clearances in pre-dialysis patients is similar to that in patients on CAPD [141], adequacy targets for CAPD have been recommended as targets for initiation of chronic dialysis [106]. The PD subcommittee of the NKF-DOQI recommends that chronic dialysis should be initiated in an incremental fashion once the renal weekly Kt/V_{urea} declines to below 2.0. The conditions that may indicate that dialysis is not yet necessary (even though renal weekly Kt/V_{urea} is <2.0) are a stable or increased oedema-free weight, the dietary protein intake, as estimated by urea kinetics, is equal to or greater than 0.8 gm/kg per day and there is complete absence of signs or symptoms attributable to uraemia [106]. The dose of dialysis should be gradually increased such that the sum of the renal and dialytic weekly Kt/V_{urea} should remain near 2.0 at all times. Even though scientific evidence for this approach is lacking, given the importance of small solute clearances in affecting patient outcome, this approach seems rational.

At least two nomograms have been constructed to guide physicians in prescribing incremental dialy-sis, using either haemodialysis peritoneal dialysis [106, 142, 143]. These two approaches are summarized in Figs 12 and 13. As is apparent, for the patient on HD, once-weekly haemodialysis is adequate only for 5 months and, even during this period, the duration of dialysis has to keep increasing to keep pace with declining renal function. Moreover, given the short-term viability of once-weekly HD and the wide swings of BUN and other small molecular weight indicators, it is recommended that the patient be directly initiated with twice-weekly HD with a switch to thrice-weekly at the appropriate point in time [143]. On the other hand, for the patient on PD, only nocturnal exchanges are required up to 18 months from initiation, thus allowing the patient freedom to pursue daytime activities [143]. Incremental exchanges can be added to the dialysis regimen without need for significant retraining. Timely initiation and incremental dialysis may therefore be easier with PD than with HD. Once all residual renal function has been lost, and it is not possible to achieve an adequate Kt/V, a switch from PD to HD should be considered (Fig. 14). Other advantages of PD include better preservation of residual renal function [144–149], delaying the use of blood access sites, continued liberalization of diet to ensure nutritional rehabilitation and lower overall cost [6].

References

1. Ganter G. Uber die Beseitgung giftiger Stoffe aus dem Blute durch Dialse. Muench Med Wochenschr 1923; 70: 1478–80.
2. Ahmad S, Gallagher N, Shen F. Intermittent peritoneal dialysis: status re-assessed. Trans Am Soc Artif Intern Organs 1979; 25: 86–9.
3. Popovich RP, Moncrief JW, Decherd JF, Bomar JB, Pyle WK. The definition of a novel portable/wearable equilibrium

dialysis technique (Abstract). Trans Am Soc Artif Intern Organs 1976; 5: 64.

4. Popovich RP, Moncrief JW, Nolph KD, Ghods AJ, Twardowski ZJ, Pyle WK. Continuous ambulatory peritoneal dialysis. Ann Intern Med 1978; 88: 449–56.

5. Nolph KD. Has peritoneal dialysis peaked? The impact of the CANUSA study. ASAIO J 1996; 42: 136–8.

6. Annual Baxter World-wide Survey, February 1998. Baxter Healthcare Corporation, Deerfield, Illinois.

7. US Renal Data System: USRDS 1998 Annual Data Report. The National Institutes of Health, National Institute of Diabetes and Digestive and Kidney Diseases, Bethesda, MD, 1998.

8. Disney APS (ed.) ANZDATA Report 1997. Adelaide, South Australia, Australia and New Zealand Dialysis and Transplant Registry, 1998.

9. Nissenson AR, Prichard SS, Cheng IKP et al. ESRD modality selection into the 21st century: the importance of non-medical factors. ASAIO J 1997; 43: 143–50.

10. Annual Report 1998, Volume 1: Dialysis and Renal Transplantation, Canadian Organ Replacement Register, Canadian Institute for Health Information, Ottawa, Ontario, June 1998.

11. European Dialysis and Transplant Association: Report on Management of Renal Failure in Europe, XXVI, 1995. Nephrol Dial Transplant 1996; 11: 1–32.

12. The Italian Registry of Dialysis and Transplantation (Salomone M: personal communication).

13. Rutkowski B, Puka J, Lao M et al. Renal replacement therapy in an era of socio-economic changes – report from the Polish registry. Nephrol Dial Transplant 1997; 12: 1105–8.

14. Ursea N, Mircescu G, Constantinovici N, Verzan C. Nephrology and renal replacement therapy in Romania. Nephrol Dial Transplant 1997; 12: 684–90.

15. Mignon F, Michel C, Viron B. Why so much disparity of PD in Europe? Nephrol Dial Transplant 1998; 13: 1114–17.

16. ANZDATA. Australia and New Zealand Dialysis and Transplant Registry. (Disney APS: personal communication).

17. Oreopoulos DG. Peritoneal Dialysis – Year 2010. Perit Dial Int 1996; 16: 109–12.

18. Friedman EA. Rationing of uremia therapy. Artif Organs 1992; 16: 90–7.

19. Nissenson A, Prichard SS, Cheng IKP et al. Non-medical factors that impact on ESRD modality selection. Kidney Int 1993; 43 (suppl. 40): S120–7.

20. Prichard SS. Treatment modality selection in 150 consecutive patients starting ESRD therapy. Perit Dial Int 1996; 16: 69–72.

21. Van Biesen W, Wiedemann M, Lameire N. End-stage renal disease treatment: a European perspective. J Am Soc Nephrol 1998; 9: S55–62.

22. US Renal Data System: USRDS 1997 Annual Data Report. The National Institutes of Health, National Institute of Diabetes and Digestive and Kidney Diseases, Bethesda, MD, 1997.

23. Slingeneyer A, De Vecchi A, Faller B et al., European GFR Group. Multicenter study on patient referral to dialysis. J Am Soc Nephrol 1998; 9: 226A.

24. Lameire N, Van Biessen W, et al. The referral pattern of patients with ESRD is a determinant in the choice of dialysis modality. Perit Dial Int 1997; 17: S161–6.

25. Groome PA, Hutchinson TA, Prichard SS. ESRD treatment modality selection: which factors are important in the decision? Adv Perit Dial 1991; 7: 54–6.

26. Hamburger R, Schreiber MJ, Sorkin M et al. A dialysis modality selection guide on the experience of six dialysis centres. Dial Transplant 1990; 19: 66–70.

27. Friedman EA. Dialytic therapy for the diabetic ESRD patient: comprehensive care essentials. Semin Dial 1997; 10: 193–202.

28. Finkelstein FO, Smith JD. Peritoneal dialysis for patients with diabetes and end-stage renal disease. Sorting out the biases? ASAIO J 1996; 42: 1–3.

29. Tenckhoff H. Peritoneal dialysis today: a new look. Nephron 1974; 12: 420–36.

30. Lupo A, Tarchini R, Cancarini G et al. Long-term outcome in continuous ambulatory peritoneal dialysis: a 10-year survey by the Italian Cooperative Peritoneal Dialysis Study Group. Am J Kidney Dis 1994; 24: 826–37.

31. Kawaguchi Y, Hasegawa T, Nakayama M, Kubo H, Shigematu T. Issues affecting longevity of the continuous peritoneal dialysis therapy. Kidney Int 1997; 52 (suppl. 62): S105–7.

32. Maiorca R, Vonesh EF, Cavalli PL et al. A multicentre selection-adjusted comparison of patient and technique survivals on CAPD and hemodialysis. Perit Dial Int 1991; 11: 118–27.

33. Gentil MA, Carriazzo A, Pavon MI et al. Comparison of survival in continuous ambulatory peritoneal dialysis and hospital hemodialysis: a multicentre study. Nephrol Dial Transplant 1991; 6: 444–51.

34. Geerlings W, Tufveson G, Ehrich JHH et al. Combined report on regular dialysis and transplantation in Europe, XXI, 1990. Nephrol Dial Transplant 1991; 6 (suppl. 4): 5–29.

35. Maiorca R, Cancarini GC, Zubani R et al.CAPD viability: a long-term comparison with hemodialysis. Perit Dial Int 1996; 16: 276–87.

36. Shih D, Cline KN, Firanek CA, Vonesh EF, Korbet SM. Racial differences in survival in an urban peritoneal dialysis program. J Am Soc Nephrol 1998; 9: 226A.

37. Jindal KK, Hirsch DJ. Excellent technique survival on home peritoneal dialysis: results of a regional program. Perit Dial Int 1994; 14: 324–6.

38. Bistrup C, Holm-Nielsen A, Pedersen RS. Technique survival and complication rates in a newly started CAPD centre (five years of experience). Perit Dial Int 1996; 16: 90–1.

39. Continuous ambulatory peritoneal dialysis in the USA. In: Lindblad AS, Novak JW, Nolph KD, eds. Final report of the National CAPD registry 1981–1988. Dordrecht: Kluwer, 1989.

40. US Renal Data System, USRDS 1995 Annual Data Report, The National Institutes of Health, National Institute of Diabetes and Digestive and Kidney Diseases, Bethesda, MD, 1995.

41. Burkart JM. Significance, epidemiology, and prevention of peritoneal dialysis catheter infections. Perit Dial Int 1996; 16: S340–6.

42. Woodrow G, Turney JH, Bownjohn M. Technique failure in peritoneal dialysis and its impact on patient survival. Perit Dial Int 1997; 17: 360–4.

43. Golper TA, Brier ME, Bunke M et al. Risk factors for peritonitis in long-term peritoneal dialysis: the Network 9 peritonitis and catheter survival study. Academic Subcommittee of the Steering Committee of the Network 9 Peritonitis and catheter survival studies. Am J Kidney Dis 1996; 28: 428–36.

44. Oreopoulos DG, Robson M, Izatt S, deVeber GA. A simple and safe technique for continuous ambulatory peritoneal dialysis. Trans Am Soc Artif Intern Organs 1978; 24: 484–9.

45. Buonocristiani U, Bianchi P, Gorazzi M et al. A new, safe disconnection system for CAPD. Int J Nephrol Urol Androl 1980; 1: 50–3.

46. Maiorca R, Cantaluppi A, Cancarini GC et al. Prospective controlled trial of a Y-connector and disinfectant to prevent peritonitis in CAPD. Lancet 1983; 2: 642–4.

47. Canadian CAPD Clinical Trials Group. Peritonitis in continuous ambulatory peritoneal dialysis (CAPD): A multicenter randomized clinical trial comparing the Y-connector disinfectant systems to standard systems. Perit Dial Int 1989; 9: 159–63.

48. Port FK, Held PJ, Nolph KD, Turenne MN, Wolfe RA. Peritonitis rates and risk assessment in CAPD patients: a national study. Kidney Int 1992; 42: 967–74.

49. Harris DC, Yuill EJ, Byth K, Chapman JR, Hunt C. Twin-versus single-bag disconnect systems: infection rates and cost of continuous ambulatory peritoneal dialysis. J Am Soc Nephrol 1996; 7: 2392–8.

50. Tenckhoff H, Schechter H. A bacteriologically safe peritoneal access device. Trans Am Soc Artif Intern Organs 1973; 10: 181–7.

51. US Renal Data System: USRDS 1992 Annual Data Report. The National Institutes of Health, National Institute of Diabetes and Digestive and Kidney Diseases, Bethesda, MD, 1992.

52. Gokal R, Alexander S, Ash S et al.Peritoneal catheters and exit-site practices toward optimum peritoneal access: 1998 update. Perit Dial Int 1998; 18: 11–33.

53. Waraday BA, Sullivan EK, Alexander SR. Lessons from the peritoneal dialysis database: a report of the North American Pediatric Renal Transplant Cooperative Study. Kidney Int 1996; 49 (suppl. 53): S68–71.

54. Honda M, Iitaka K, Kawaguchi H et al. The Japanese National Registry Data in Pediatric CAPD patients: a ten-year experience. A report of the study group of the pediatric conference. Perit Dial Int 1996; 16: 269–75.

55. Lindblad AS, Hamilton RW, Nolph KD, Novak JW. A retrospective analysis of catheter configuration and cuff type: a National CAPD registry report. Perit Dial Int 1988; 8: 129–33.

56. Favazza A, Petri R, Montanaro D, Boscutti G, Bresadola F, Mioni G. Insertion of a straight peritoneal catheter in an arcutae subcutaneous tunnel by a tunneler: long term experience. Perit Dial Int 1995; 15: 357–62.

57. Eklund BH, Honkanen EO, Kala AR, Kyllonen LE. Peritoneal dialysis access: prospective randomized comparison of the swan neck and Tenckhoff catheters. Perit Dial Int 1995; 15: 353–6.

58. Weber J, Mettang T, Hubel E, Kiefer T, Kuhlmann U. Survival of 138 surgically placed straight double cuff Tenckhoff catheters in patients on continuous ambulatory peritoneal dialysis. Perit Dial Int 1993; 13: 234–7.

59. Piraino B. Peritonitis as a complication of peritoneal dialysis. J Am Soc Nephrol 1998; 9: 1956–64.

60. Zimmerman SW, Ahrens E, Johnson CA et al. Randomized controlled trial of prophylactic rifampin for peritoneal dialysis-related infections. Am J Kidney Dis 1991; 18: 225–31.

61. Perez-Fontan M, Garcia-Falcon T, Rosales M et al. Treatment of *Staphylococcus aureus* nasal carriers in continuous ambulatory peritoneal dialysis with mupirocin: Long term results. Am J Kidney Dis 1993; 22: 708–12.

62. Bernardini J, Piraino B, Holley J, Johnston JR, Lutes R. A randomized trial of *Staphylococcus aureus* prophylaxis in peritoneal dialysis patients: Mupirocin calcium ointment 2% applied to exit site versus oral rifampin. Am J Kidney Dis 1996; 27: 695–700.

63. Mupirocin Study Group. Nasal mupirocin prevents *Staphylococcus aureus* exit site infection during peritoneal dialysis. J Am Soc Nephrol 1996; 11: 2403–8.

64. Thodis E, Bhaskaran S, Pasadakis P, Bargman JM, Vas SI, Oreopoulos DG. Decrease in *Staphylococcus aureus* exit-site infections and peritonitis in CAPD patients by local application of mupirocin ointment at the catheter exit site. Perit Dial Int 1998; 18: 261–70.

65. Kathuria P, Moore HL, Mehrotra R, Prowant BF, Khanna R, Twardowski ZJ. Evaluation of healing and external tunnel histology of silver-coated peritoneal catheters in rats. Adv Perit Dial 1996; 12: 203–8.

66. Dasgupta MK. Autochthonous bacterial spread from catheter exit site is reduced by silver catheters. Perit Dial Int 1995; 15: S49 (abstract).

67. Fung LC, Khoury AE, Vas ST, Smith C, Oreopoulos DG, Mittelman MW. Biocompatibility of silver-coated peritoneal dialysis catheter in a porcine model. Perit Dial Int 1996; 16: 398–405.

68. Vas S. Randomized clinical trial with silver coated PD catheter. Perit Dial Int 1996; 16: S56.

69. Kahl AA, Grosse-Siestrup C, Kahl KA et al. Reduction of exit site infections in peritoneal dialysis by local application of metallic silver: a preliminary report. Perit Dial Int 1994; 14: 177–80.

70. Pommer W, Brauner M, Westphale HJ et al. Effect of a silver device in preventing catheter related infections in peritoneal dialysis patients: silver ring prophylaxis at the catheter exit study. Am J Kidney Dis 1998; 32: 752–60.

71. Keane WF, Alexander SR, Bailie GR et al. Peritoneal dialysis-related peritonitis treatment recommendations. 1996 update. Perit Dial Int 1996; 16: 557–73.

72. Lai MN, Kao MT, Chen CC, Cheung SY, Chung WK. Intraperitoneal once-daily use of cefazolin and gentamicin for treating CAPD peritonitis. Perit Dial Int 1997; 17: 87–9.

73. Vas S, Bargman J, Oreopoulos DG. Treatment in PD patients of peritonitis caused by gram-positive organisms with single daily dose of antibiotics. Perit Dial Int 1997; 17: 91–4.

74. Van Biesen W, Vanholder R, Vogelaers D et al. The need for a center-tailored treatment protocol for peritonitis. Perit Dial Int 1998; 18: 274–81.

75. Young GA, Kopple JD, Lindholm B et al. Nutritional assessment of continuous ambulatory peritoneal dialysis patients: an international study. Am J Kidney Dis 1991; 17: 462–71.

76. Canada-USA (CANUSA) Peritoneal Dialysis Study Group: Adequacy of dialysis and nutrition in continuous peritoneal dialysis: association with clinical outcomes. J Am Soc Nephrol 1996; 7: 198–207.

77. Cianciaruso B, Brunori G, Kopple JD et al. Cross-sectional comparison of malnutrition in continuous ambulatory peritoneal dialysis and hemodialysis patients. Am J Kidney Dis 1995; 26: 475–86.

78. Flanigan M, Rocco MV, Frankensfield D et al.for the PD-CIS Workgroup. 1997 ESRD core indicators study for peritoneal dialysis (PD-CIS); nutritional indicators. J Am Soc Nephrol 1998; 9: 233A.

79. Kopple JD. Effect of nutrition on morbidity and mortality on maintenance dialysis patients. Am J Kidney Dis 1994; 24: 1002–9.

80. Wolfson M. Nutritional management of the continuous ambulatory peritoneal dialysis patient. Am J Kidney Dis 1996; 27: 744–9.

81. Flanigan MJ, Bailie GR, Frankenfield DL, Frederick PR, Prowant BF, Rocco MV. 1996 Peritoneal Dialysis Core Indicators Study: Report on Nutritional Indicators. Perit Dial Int 1998; 18: 489–96.

82. Keshaviah PR, Nolph KD. Protein catabolic rate calculations in CAPD patients. ASAIO Trans 1991; 37: M400–2.

83. McCusker FX, Teehan BP, Thorpe KE, Keshaviah PR, Churchill DN for the Canada-USA (CANUSA) Peritoneal Dialysis Study Group. How much peritoneal dialysis is required for maintaining a good nutritional state? Kidney Int 1996; 50 (suppl. 56): S56–61.

84. Graham KA, Reaich D, Channon SM et al.Correction of acidosis in CAPD decreases whole body protein degradation. Kidney Int 1996; 49: 1396–400.

85. Stein A, Moorhouse J, Iles-Smith H et al. Role of an improvement in acid–base status and nutrition in CAPD patients. Kidney Int 1997; 52: 1089–95.

86. Kopple JD, Bernard D, Messana J et al. Treatment of malnourished CAPD patients with an amino acid based dialysate. Kidney Int 1995; 47: 1148–57.

87. Faller B, Aparicio M, Faict D et al.Clinical evaluation of an optimized 1.1% amino-acid solution for peritoneal dialysis. Nephrol Dial Transplant 1995; 10: 1432–7.

88. Jones M, Hagen T, Boyle CA et al. Treatment of malnutrition with 1.1% amino acid peritoneal dialysis solution: results of a multicenter outpatient study. Am J Kidney Dis 1998; 32: 761–9.

89. Bloembergen WE, Port FK, Mauger A, Wolfe RA. A comparison of mortality between patients treated with hemodialysis and peritoneal dialysis. J Am Soc Nephrol 1995; 6: 177–83.

90. Vonesh E, Moran J. Mortality in end-stage renal disease: a reassessment of the differences between patients treated with

hemodialysis and peritoneal dialysis. J Am Soc Nephrol 1999; 10: 354–65.

91. Vonesh E, Moran J. Subgroup comparisons of mortality between hemodialysis and peritoneal dialysis. J Am Soc Nephrol 1998; 9: 229A.

92. Wolfe RA, Hirth RA, Port FK *et al.* Mortality and costs in the first year of dialysis: a comparison between hemodialysis and peritoneal dialysis controlling for costs prior to ESRD. J Am Soc Nephrol 1998; 9: 241A.

93. Fenton SS, Schaubel DE, Desmeules M *et al.* Hemodialysis versus peritoneal dialysis: a comparison of adjusted mortality rates. Am J Kidney Dis 1997; 30: 334–42.

94. Khan IH, Campbell MK, Cantarovich D *et al.* Comparing outcomes in renal replacement therapy: how should we correct for case-mix? Am J Kidney Dis 1998; 31: 473–8.

95. Nolph KD. Why are reported relative mortality risks for CAPD and HD so variable? (Inadequacies of the Cox proportional hazards model). Perit Dial Int 1996; 16: 15–18.

96. Health Care Financing Administration. Highlights from the 1998 ESRD Core Indicators Project for Peritoneal Dialysis patients. Retrieved from the World Wide Web http://www.hcfa.gov/quality/qlty-3.htm

97. Health Care Financing Administration. Highlights from the 1998 ESRD Core Indicators Project for Hemodialysis patients. Retrieved from the World Wide Web http://www.hcfa.gov/quality/qlty-3.htm

98. Bernardini J, Piraino B. Compliance in CAPD and CCPD patients as measured by supply inventories during home visits. Am J Kidney Dis 1998; 31: 101–7.

99. Twardowski ZJ, Nolph KD. How much peritoneal dialysis is enough? Semin Dial 1988; 1: 75–6.

100. Teehan BP, Schleifer CR, Sigler MH *et al.* A quantitative approach to the peritoneal dialysis prescription. Perit Dial Bull 1985; 5: 152–6.

101. Teehan BP, Schleifer CR, Brown JM, Sigler MH, Raimondo J. Urea kinetic analysis and clinical outcome on CAPD. A five year longitudinal study. Adv Perit Dial 1990; 6: 181–5.

102. Blake PG. Balaskas E, Blake R, Oreopoulos DG. Urea kinetics has limited relevance in assessing adequacy of dialysis in CAPD. Adv Perit Dial 1992; 8: 65–70.

103. Lameire NH, Vanholder R, Veyt D, Lambert MC, Ringoir S. A longitudinal, five year survey of urea kinetic parameters in CAPD patients. Kidney Int 1992; 42: 426–32.

104. Brandes JC, Piering WF, Beres JA, Blumenthal SS, Fritsche C. Clinical outcome of continuous ambulatory peritoneal dialysis by urea and creatinine kinetics. J Am Soc Nephrol 1992; 2: 1430–5.

105. Teehan BP, Schleifer CR, Brown J. Urea kinetic modeling is an appropriate assessment of adequacy. Semin Dial 1992; 5: 189–92.

106. NKF-DOQI Clinical practice guidelines for peritoneal dialysis adequacy. Am J Kidney Dis 1997; 30 (3; suppl. 2): S69–133.

107. Rocco M, Frankenfield D, Frederick P, Flanigan M, Prowant B, Bailie G, for the HCFA Core Indicators Work-Group. Trends in clinical indicators of care for adult peritoneal dialysis patients in the U.S. from 1995 to 1997. Health Care Financing Administration (HCFA) ESRD peritoneal dialysis core indicators study (PD-CIS). J Am Soc Nephrol 1998; 9: 301A.

108. Health Care Financing Administration. 1997 Annual Report, End Stage Renal Disease Core Indicators Project. Department of Health and Human Services, Health Care Financing Administration, Office of Clinical Standards and Quality, Baltimore, Maryland, December, 1997.

109. Twardowski ZJ, Nolph KD. Is peritoneal dialysis feasible once a large muscular patient becomes anuric? Perit Dial Int 1996; 16: 20–3.

110. Diaz-Buxo JA. Enhancement of peritoneal dialysis: the PD Plus concept. Am J Kidney Dis 1996; 27: 92–8.

111. Wu CH, Huang CC, Huang JY, Wu MS, Leu ML. High flux peritoneal membrane is a risk factor in survival of CAPD treatment. Adv Perit Dial 1996; 12: 105–9.

112. Fried LF. PET test and survival. Perit Dial Int 1997; 17: S60.

113. Churchill DN, Thorpe KE, Nolph KD, Keshaviah PR, Oreopoulos DG, Page D. Increased peritoneal membrane transport is associated with decreased patient and technique survival for continuous peritoneal dialysis patients. J Am Soc Nephrol 1998; 1285–92.

114. Davies SJ, Phillips L, Russell GI. Peritoneal solute transport predicts survival on CAPD independently of residual renal function. Nephrol Dial Transplant 1998; 13: 962–8.

115. Wang T, Heimburger O, Waniewski J, Bergstrom J, Lindholm B. Increased peritoneal permeability is associated with decreased fluid and small solute removal and higher mortality. Nephrol Dial Transplant 1998; 13: 1242–9.

116. Heaf J. CAPD adequacy and dialysis morbidity. detrimental effect of a high peritoneal equilibration rate. Renal Failure 1995; 17: 575–87.

117. Mistry CD, Gokal R, Peers E. A randomized multicenter clinical trial comparing isosmolar icodextrin with hyperosmolar glucose solution in CAPD. Multicenter investigation of Icodextrin in Ambulatory Peritoneal Dialysis. Kidney Int 1994; 46: 496–503.

118. Douma CE, Hiralall JK, de Waart DR, Struijk DG, Krediet RT. Icodextrin with nitroprusside increases ultrafiltration and peritoneal transport during long CAPD dwells. Kidney Int 1998; 53: 1014–21.

119. Posthuma N, ter Wee PM, Verbrugh HA, Oe PL, Peers E, Sayers J, Donker AJ. Icodextrin instead of glucose during the daytime dwell in CCPD increases ultrafiltration and 24-h dialysate creatinine clearance. Nephrol Dial Transplant 1997; 12: 550–3.

120. Posthuma N, Ter Wee PM, Donker AJ, Oe LP, Verbrugh HA, Peers E. Disaccharide ('total maltose') levels in CCPD patients using icodextrin. J Am Soc Nephrol; 1995; 6: 513.

121. Gokal R, Mistry CD, Peers EM. Peritonitis occurrence in a multicenter study of icodextrin and glucose in CAPD. MIDAS Study Group. Multicenter Investigation of Icodextrin in Ambulatory Peritoneal Dialysis. Perit Dial Int 1995; 15: 226–30.

122. Peers EM, Scrimgeour AC. Icodextrin can prolong technique survival in CAPD patients with ultrafiltration failure. J Am Soc Nephrol 1995; 6: 513.

123. Wilkie ME, Plant MJ, Edwards L, Brown CB. Icodextrin 7.5% dialysate solution (glucose polymer) in patients with ultrafiltration failure: extension of CAPD technique survival. Perit Dial Int 1997; 17: 84–7.

124. Rubin RJ, Gaylin DS, Shapiro JR. Introduction: end-stage renal disease, managed care, and capitation: implications for the renal community. Adv Ren Replace Ther 1997; 4: 306–13.

125. McMurray SD, Miller J. Impact of capitation on freestanding dialysis facilities: can you survive? Am J Kidney Dis 1997; 30: 542–8.

126. Bruns FJ, Seddon P, Saul M, Zeidel ML. The cost of caring for end-stage kidney disease patients: an analysis based on hospital financial transaction records. J Am Soc Nephrol 1998; 9: 884–90.

127. Tattersall J, Greenwood R, Farrington K. Urea kinetics and when to commence dialysis. Am J Nephrol 1995; 15: 283–9.

128. Obrador GT, Ruthazer R, Arora P, Pereira BJG, Levey AS. What is the level of GFR in the U.S. ESRD population? J Am Soc Nephrol 1998; 9: 156A.

129. Jansen MAM, Korevaar JC, Dekker FW, Boeschoten EW, Krediet RT and the NECOSAD study group. Residual renal function and nutritional status at the start of chronic dialysis treatment. J Am Soc Nephrol 1998; 9: 212A.

130. Mehrotra R, Elivera H, Lee J, Ahmed Z. Renal function at initiation of dialysis: how far are we from DOQI guidelines? J Am Soc Nephrol 1998; 9: 220A.

131. Kopple JD, Berg R, Houser H, Steinman TI, Teschan P. For Modification of Diet in Renal Disease (MDRD) Study

Group. Nutritional status of patients with different levels of chronic renal insufficiency. Kidney Int 1989; 36 (suppl. 27): S184–94.

132. Ikizler TA, Greene JH, Wingard RL, Parker RA, Hakim RM. Spontaneous dietary protein intake during progression of chronic renal failure. J Am Soc Nephrol 1995: 6: 1386–91.

133. Bonomini V, Feletti C, Scolari MP, Stefoni S. Benefits of early initiation of dialysis. Kidney Int 1985; 28 (suppl. 17): S57–9.

134. Churchill DN. An evidence-based approach to earlier initiation of dialysis. Am J Kidney Dis 1997; 30: 899–906.

135. Churchill DN, Taylor DW, Cook RJ et al. Canadian hemodialysis morbidity study. Am J Kidney Dis 1992; 19: 214–34.

136. Gamba G, Mejia JL, Saldivar S, Pena JC, Correa-Rotter R. Death risk in CAPD patients. The predictive value of the initial clinical and laboratory variables. Nephron 1993; 65: 23–7.

137. Khan IH, Catto GRD, Edward N, MacLeod AM. Death risk during the first 90 days of dialysis: a case control study. Am J Kidney Dis 1995; 25: 276–80.

138. Iseki K, Uehara H, Nishime K et al. Impact of the initial levels of laboratory variables on survival in chronic dialysis patients. Am J Kidney Dis 1996; 28: 541–8.

139. Sesso R, Belasco AG. Late diagnosis of chronic renal failure and mortality in maintenance dialysis. Nephrol Dial Transplant 1996; 11: 2417–20.

140. Barrett BJ, Parfrey PS, Morgan J et al. Prediction of early death in end-stage renal disease patients starting dialysis. Am J Kidney Dis 1997; 29: 214–22.

141. Mehrotra R, Saran R, Moore HL et al. Towards targets for initiation of chronic dialysis. Perit Dial Int 1997; 17: 497–508.

142. Mehrotra R, Nolph KD, Gotch F. Early initiation of chronic dialysis: role of incremental dialysis. Perit Dial Int 1997; 17: 426–30.

143. Keshaviah PR, Emerson PF, Nolph KD. Timely initiation of dialysis: a urea kinetic approach. Am J Kidney Dis (in press).

144. Rottembourg J, Issad B, Gallego J et al. Evolution of residual renal function in patients undergoing maintenance hemodialysis or continuous peritoneal dialysis. Proc Eur Dial Transplant Assoc 1992; 19: 397–402.

145. Cancarini GC, Brunori G, Camerini C, Brasa S, Manili L, Maiorca R. Renal function recovery and maintenance of residual diuresis in CAPD and hemodialysis. Perit Dial Bull 1986; 6: 77–9.

146. Lysaght MJ, Vonesh EF, Gotch F et al. The influence of dialysis treatment modality on the decline of remaining renal function. ASAIO Trans 1991; 37: 598–604.

147. Hallett M, Owen J, Becker G, Stewart J, Farrell PC. Maintenance of residual renal function: CAPD vs. HD (abstract). Perit Dial Int 1992; 12 (suppl. 2): S46.

148. Lutes R, Perlmutter J, Holley JL, Bernardini J, Piraino B. Loss of residual renal function in patients on peritoneal dialysis. Adv Perit Dial 1993; 9: 165–8.

149. Feber J, Scharer K, Schaefer F, Mikova M, Janda J. Residual renal function in children in hemodialysis and peritoneal dialysis therapy. Pediatr Nephrol 1994; 8: 579–83.

3 | Functional structure of the peritoneum as a dialysing membrane

L. GOTLOIB, A. SHOSTAK AND V. WAJSBROT

... conduire ... par ordre mes pensées, en commençant par les objects les plus simples et les plus aisés à connaître, pour monter peu a peu, comme par degrés, jusque à la connaissance des plus composés ...

(René Descartes, in: *Discours de la mèthode*, 1637)

Introduction

More than 90 years ago Robinson [1], after summarizing more than two centuries of research, defined the diverse natural functions of the peritoneum as follows: (a) to regulate fluid for nutrient and mechanical purposes; (b) to facilitate motion; (c) to minimize friction, and (d) to conduct vessels and nerves to the viscera.

Several medical and scientific developments which occurred during the twentieth century originated a new approach for the peritoneum being used as a dialysing membrane for long-term life support [2–6]. These same developments created the need for a deeper understanding of peritoneal structure and function.

The peritoneum is a serous membrane embryologically derived from mesenchyma and composed of thin layers of the connective tissue covered by a sheet of mesothelium [7]. When the membrane is folded, forming the omentum and the mesentery, both luminal surfaces are covered by mesothelium.

The peritoneal surface area for the human adult is considered to range between 2.08 [8] and 1.72 m^2 [9], with a ratio of area/body weight of 0.284. The intestinal mesothelium, together with that of mesentery, makes up 49% of the total mesothelial area [10]. For infants having a body weight of 2700–2900 g, the total peritoneal surface was found to oscillate between 0.106 [10] and 0.151 m^2 [8], with an area to body weight ratio that fluctuates between 0.383 [10] and 0.522. In infants the contribution of intestine and mesentery to the total surface area is 67.5% [10].

Peritoneal thickness is not uniform and varies according to the area examined. Measurements are quite problematic in parietal and diaphragmatic peritoneum due to the considerable amount of connective tissue, and at times fat, intervening between the peritoneum itself and the underlying tissue (Fig. 1). The submesothelial connective tissue layer of visceral peritoneum is firmly bound to the fibrous tissue of the viscus. Therefore the mesentery, having mesothelial lining on both surfaces and including its trabecular connective framework, appears to be the most appropriate peritoneal portion for estimation of membrane thickness which, in the rabbit, ranges between 30 and 38 μm [11, 12] (Figs 2 and 3).

Normal mesothelium

Electron microscopic studies performed on mouse embryo disclosed that the mesothelium is derived from mesenchymal cells which become flattened, form their own basement membrane, and develop intercellular junctions, mostly desmosomes [13] (Fig. 4, inset). Both pinocytotic vesicles and rough endoplasmic reticulum were present. Yolk sac of human embryos at the 5th–7th week of gestation also exhibit flattened mesothelial cells lying on a hyaline, homogeneous basement membrane [14, 15].

The cell plasmalemma, when stained specifically, shows the typical trilaminar structure observed in all biological cell membranes [16]. The normal mesothelium occasionally shows macrophages implanted on the luminal peritoneal surface instead of mesothelial cells (Fig. 5).

The luminal aspect of the mesothelial cell plasmalemma has numerous cytoplasmic extensions: the microvilli (Figs 2, 3 and 4), whose existence was originally reported by Kolossov [17] and many

R. Gokal, R. Khanna, R.Th. Krediet and K.D. Nolph (eds.), Textbook of Peritoneal Dialysis, 2nd Edition, 37–106.
© 2000 *Kluwer Academic Publishers. Printed in Great Britain.*

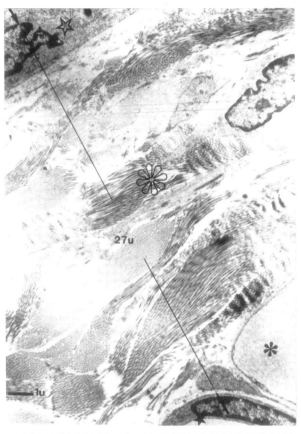

Figure 1. Sample of diaphragmatic rabbit peritoneum. The distance (straight line) between the peritoneal space (upper arrow) and the lumen of the blood capillary (black star) is around 27 μm. The actual pathway through the collagen fibres (open asterisk) is longer (open star: mesothelial cell; black asterisk: fenestrated capillary (×14 250).

years later confirmed by electron microscopy on the serosa covering the rat oviduct [18, 19]. Even though microvilli are more frequently observed in visceral than in parietal peritoneum [20, 21], their distribution is variable and fluctuates from very numerous to completely absent [21, 22]. It should be taken into account, however, that microvilli are extremely sensitive to minor injury or even to dryness, and can therefore be lost from the cell surface if removal and handling of samples are not done with extremely careful techniques. On the other hand, loss of microvilli, as described in CAPD patients [23] (Fig. 6), represent an early sign of impending apoptosis [24–26] that can be easily identified in mesothelial cell imprints (Fig. 7).

Light microscopy applied to the observation of resting mesothelium imprints [27] shows a continuous monolayer made up mostly of polygonal mononuclear cells (Fig. 8), showing, in mice visceral peritoneum, a density of about 300 000 cells/cm^2 [28]. The number of mesothelial cells per unit area seems higher on the visceral than on the parietal peritoneal surface. Of those cells 1–2% are binucleated (Fig. 8, lower left inset), whereas cells showing three nuclei can be observed (Fig. 8).

Under normal circumstances the cell population of the monolayer is not stained by vital dyes such as Trypan Blue (Fig. 9). This is an indication of their viability. In perpendicular cuts observed under light microscopy, the resting normal mesothelium appears as a continuous layer formed by flattened cells, that are apparently elongated, as a result of the angle of section (Fig. 10). The mesothelial sheet lies on a layer of connective interstitial tissue (Fig. 10), the thickness of which varies in the different portions of the peritoneum (Figs 1 and 3). The relevance of this point on peritoneal permeability will be discussed later.

Thickness of mesothelial cells in the rabbit ranges between 0.6 and 2 μm [11, 12] (Fig. 11).

The human omentum has not yet been studied in great depth. However, some ultrastructural investigations performed in mice and rats [19, 29] seem to indicate that there is little variation between species [30] and that, in mice, omental mesothelial cells can transiently increase their population of microvilli up to seven-fold, suggesting that their concentration in any given area could reflect functional adaptation rather than static structural variation [31].

The presence of pinocytotic vesicles in microvilli has been both reported [18, 20, 32], and denied [31].

Experimental studies done in mice and rats [32–34] using cationic tracers such as ruthenium-red (MW 551 da) and cationized ferritin (MW 445 da) revealed the existence of anionic fixed charges on the luminal surface of the microvilli cytoplasmic membrane (Fig. 12, inset). This cell membrane coating, or glycocalyx, composed of fine fibres that are continuous with the membrane itself [35], furnishes the microvilli surface with electronegative charge which most probably plays a significant role in the transperitoneal transfer of anionic macromolecules such as plasma proteins [33, 36], as well as in that of charged small molecules, as suggested by Curry and Michel [37] in their fibre matrix model of capillary permeability. This surface charge is substantially reduced in cells undergoing apoptosis [38]. The relevance of these charges upon peritoneal permeability will be discussed later.

Length of microvilli in rodents ranges between 0.42 and 2.7 μm, and their average diameter is 0.1 μm

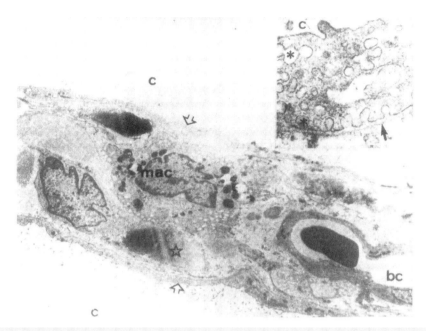

Figure 2. Section of normal rabbit mesentery showing the mesothelial layer (open arrows) covering both aspects of the mesenteric surface area facing the abdominal cavity (c). The interstitium contains a continuous blood capillaty (bc), bundles of collagen (open star), as well as a macrophage (mac). Numerous microvilli can be seen at the lower mesothelial surface (original magnification ×4750).
   Upper right inset. Parietal peritoneum of normal mice. Note the presence of numerous pinocytotic vesicles (*) which, on the left side of the electron micrograph, form a chain between the luminal aspect of the mesothelial cell facing the abdominal cavity (c) and the abluminal one, lying on the continuous basement membrane (arrow) (×41 500).

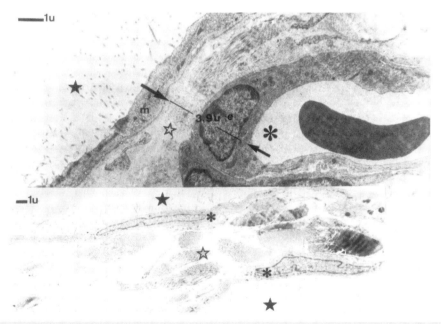

Figure 3. The main photograph shows a sample of rabbit mesenteric peritoneum where the distance (straight line) between the peritoneal space (upper black star) and the microvascular lumen (*) is 3.9 μm (open star: interstitial connective tissue) (×14 250).
   Lower inset. Section of a 42.1 μm length avascular rabbit mesenteric peritoneum sample (black star: peritoneal space; asterisk: mesothelial cell; open star: interstitial connective tissue) (×4750).

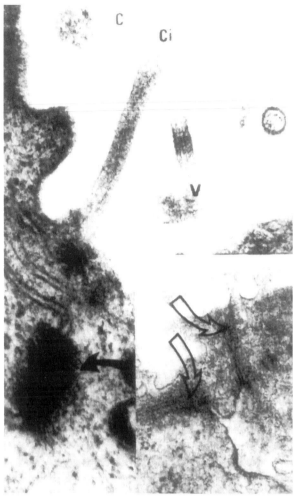

Figure 4. Biopsy of parietal peritoneum taken from a chronic uraemic patient on maintenance peritoneal dialysis. Note the presence of an oligocilium (Ci) showing the deviated axial microtubule (open arrow) and the attached basal body (black arrow). Their function is unknown (C: abdominal cavity; V: microvilli) (× 42 900).

Inset. (Lower right). Rabbit mesentery: the open arrows show tight junctions between adjoining mesothelial cells (× 62 500).

[11, 18, 20, 29). We have observed a similar range in adult humans. However, mesothelial cells of human embryos (5th–7th week of gestation) showed microvilli up to 3.5 μm long [14].

It has been estimated that microvilli present in the striated border of intestinal epithelium increase the surface area of the intestine by a factor of 20 [39]. Consequently, it has been speculated that mesothelial microvilli could increase the actual peritoneal surface up to 40 m² [40].

Plasmalemma of mesothelial cells, like that of microvilli, shows electronegatively charged glycocalyx (Fig. 12) [32–34, 41].

Plasmalemmal vesicles, or caveolae, originally described by Lewis [42] in macrophages of rat omentum, are conspicuously present in mesothelial cells at both the basal and luminal borders, as well as in the paranuclear cytoplasm [18–20, 29, 43–45] (Fig. 2, inset). Their average diameter is approximately 0.717 μm [11]. At times, pinocytotic vesicles appear clustered together and communicating with each other (Fig. 2, inset). Occasionally they appear forming transcellular channels similar to those described in endothelial cells of blood capillaries [46, 47] (Fig. 13, inset), apparently communicating both aspects, luminal and abluminal, of the mesothelial cell. These channels can be formed by a chain of several vesicles (Fig. 13, inset) or just by two adjoining vesicles (Fig. 14, inset). Often pinocytotic vesicles appear to open through the plasma membrane into the luminal or abluminal aspect of the cell (Fig. 2, inset; Fig. 12), as well as into the intercellular space (Fig. 12); exhibiting a neck and a mouth whose respective average diameters are 0.176 and 0.028 μm [11]. With respect to the density distribution of these caveolae, it has been suggested that the parietal mesothelium is less well endowed than the visceral [44].

Palade [48] first proposed that a large part of the macromolecular transport across capillary walls could be attributed to exchange of pinocytotic vesicles between the internal and external surfaces of endothelial cells. This concept was repeatedly applied to the mesothelium. Several electron-dense tracers such as native ferritin [45], iron dextran [11, 29] and melanin [19] were found randomly distributed within pinocytotic vesicles of mesothelial cells after being injected intraperitoneally. Casley-Smith and Chin [44] calculated that the median transit time of vesicles through mesothelial cells ranges between 3 and 5 s, and that approximately 40% of the released vesicles reach the cytoplasmic membrane on the opposite side of the cell. It was even observed that metabolic inhibitors such as dinitrophenol, poisons (cyanide) or slow cooling to 0°C did not completely preclude the uptake of electron-dense macromolecules by pinocytosis [45, 49]. This information, supporting Palade's prediction [48] that vesicles could be the structural equivalent of the large pore theory [50], was challenged by stereological analysis of plasmalemmal vesicles. This study apparently showed that vesicles represent merely invaginations of the plasmalemma from both sides of the capillary wall in frog mesentery [51]. It was suggested that this organization of the vesicular system is incompatible with the concept that macro-

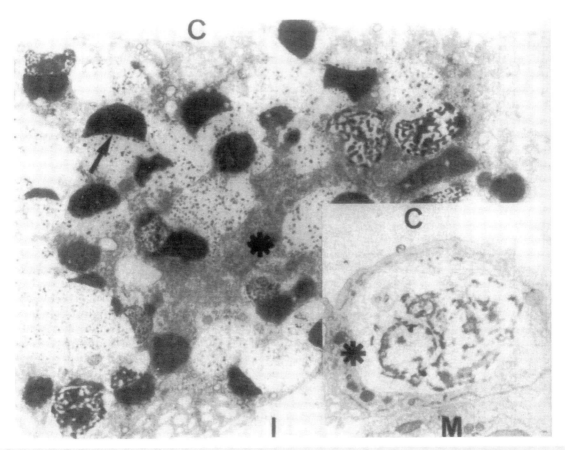

Figure 5. Mesentery of normal rabbit. A macrophage (*) is covering a denuded area of peritoneum (C: abdominal cavity; black arrow: lysosome; I: interstitium). Original magnification ×27 500.
   Inset. (Lower right). Mouse mesenteric mesothelium: a signet-ring macrophage (*) is covering a recently implanted mesothelial cell (M) (original magnification ×15 400).

molecules could be transferred across cells by vesicular transport. The methodology followed in this study has been reviewed and criticized, and its conclusions have been refuted [52].

Furthermore, a huge body of scientifically based evidence indicates that endocytosis, transcytosis, as well as potocytosis (an endocytic pathway that utilizes phosphatylinositol anchored membrane proteins and plasmalemmal vesicles or caveolae to concentrate and internalize small molecules) are basic mechanisms used by cells to carry in, out and through the cytoplasm a variety of substances [53]. The following part of our description applies to both mesothelium and endothelium.

Work done basically during the past decade shed new light on the intimal structure of pinocytotic vesicles. Even though their morphometric parameters are more or less homogeneous, differences in nature, function and biochemical structure identified at least two kinds of vesicles showing distinctive characteristics.

Caveolae or plasmalemmal vesicles are membrane domains that represent a subcompartment of the plasma membrane [54], characteristic of all vascular endothelium [55]. In capillary endothelial cells, morphological studies indicate that caveolae are effectors of transcytosis of certain macromolecules across the microvascular endothelium: native as well as modified albumins [56–64) LDL [65–68], protein hormones [69, 70], AGE [71], as well as orosomucoid [72], a 41 kDa glycoprotein that qualifies as a probe for the postulated small pore [73–75]. Furthermore, endocytosis and transcytosis of albumin–gold complexes have been observed in mice peritoneal mesothelium [76] (Fig. 15, inset; Fig. 16, inset).

Schnitzer has demonstrated that transendothelial transport of native albumin through caveolae in both experimental situations (*in vivo* as well as in the *in vitro* set-up) is dependent on the interactions of the probe with the endothelial cell surface protein albondin, a 60 kDa albumin binding protein for-

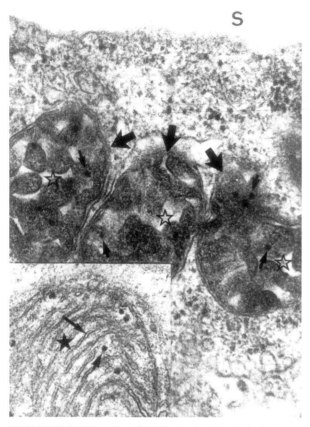

S

Figure 6. Section of a mesothelial cell seen in a biopsy of parietal peritoneum taken from a patient on CAPD. Mitochondria (open stars) assumed a condensed configuration with increased density of the matrix, blurring of cristae as well as fusions and adhesions of the inner membrane (thick arrows). The matrical granules are still visible (short arrows). These signs of cell injury, in addition to the absence of microvilli, are early signs of impending apoptosis (S: peritoneal space) (×54 600).

Inset. Intact mitochondrion (short star) showing normal cristae (long arrow) and matrical granules (short arrow) (×64 550).

merly called gp60 [60]. Other binding proteins, gp30 and gp18, appear to mediate the attachment, endocytosis and degradation of modified albumin. These vesicular carriers require key intracellular components that are sensitive to alkylation with N-ethylmaleimide. Indeed, this substance has been shown to substantially inhibit native albumin (MW: 67 kDa, $r = 36$ Å) and ferritin (MW ~ 500 kDa, $r = 100–110$ Å) uptake, both transcytosed by caveolae [77]. Additional experiments have shown that transcytosis and capillary permeability of insulin and albumin are selectively inhibited by filipin, a complex of polyene antibiotics obtained from *Streptomyces filipenensis,* but does not affect endocytosis mediated by the clathrin-coated vesicles [78]. This concept

that identifies two different vesicular pathways is completed with the recent discovery of caveolin, the major structural caveolar protein [79]. This substance is a 22 kDa integral protein that represents a subcompartment of the plasma membrane [54, 80]. Basically, it is a component of the coating covering the luminal aspect of caveolae [81] that, when specifically stained by immunocytochemical methods, serves as a useful marker to draw the diagnostic line between caveolae and other pinocytotic related structures, e.g. coated vesicles [82–84].

Coated pits and coated vesicles (Fig. 15, left and right insets) remain the most extensively characterized transport vesicles. They are involved in the intracellular transport of membrane proteins between a variety of membrane components, mediate endocytosis of transmembrane receptors and transport newly synthesized lysosomal hydrolases from the trans-Golgi network to lysosomes [85]. The luminal coat contains at least six polypeptides, in addition to the above-mentioned 180 kDa polypeptide clathrin [86, 87]. This type of vesicle is also involved in receptor-mediated endocytosis. Cell surface mediators operate endocytosis clusters into clathrin-coated pits, which pinch off to form vesicles that transport the receptors and their ligand [88]. The complex process of invagination, constriction and budding of clathrin-coated vesicles employs the coordinated actions of several proteins. The best-characterized of them is the expanding family of dynamin guanosine triphosphate phosphatases (GTPase), essential for receptor-mediated endocytosis [89, 90]. This enzyme appears to be assembled around the necks of clathrin-coated pits, and assists in pinching vesicles from the plasma membrane [90]. Recently published information suggests that dynamins mediate both clathrin-dependent endocytosis and the internalization of caveolae in microvascular endothelial cells [91, 92].

Some 60 years ago [93], it was suggested that junctions between capillary endothelial cells should be considered the main pathway for exchanges across the microvascular wall. This concept was later extended to the peritoneal blood microvessels and mesothelium, and extensively analysed within the frame of the two [74, 75], and lately, the three [94] pore size model of capillary and/or peritoneal permeability. (Assumed pores size: large pore: >150 Å; small pore: up to 40–45 Å; ultra-small pore: 2–5 Å.) To date, physiological studies and mathematical models have failed to convincingly identify the morphological equivalents of the hypothetical cylindrical water-filled pores [73]. On the other hand, however,

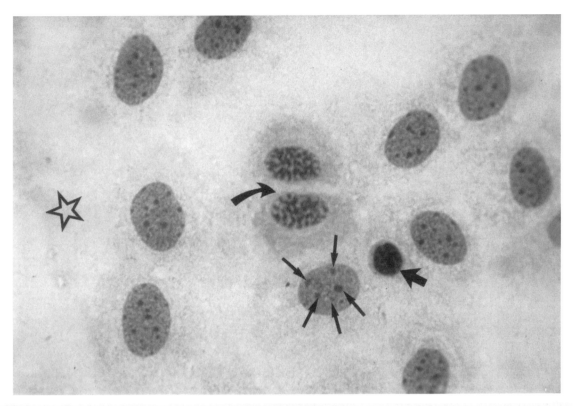

Figure 7. Sample from a mouse injected for 30 consecutive days with 4.25% glucose-enriched dialysis solution. The material was taken 7 days after interruption of the exposure to the dialysis solution (7 days of recovery). This photograph shows the two most critical moments in the life cycle of a mesothelial cell: mitosis (curved arrow), and apoptosis (short thick arrow). Open star shows an area of peritoneum where the mesothelial monolayer is absent (desertic peritoneum). Note the substantially reduced density distribution of cells (small arrows: nucleoli) (haematoxylin–eosin; ×1000).

this short review of the topic testifies that, at least for protein traffic, the vesicular carried hypothesis has been largely proven and accepted in the last few years [77].

Basically, that caveolae and transcellular channels function as a continuous operating conveyor belt, fusing with each other [46, 47, 95, 96], and moving through the cell [95, 96]. The source of energy fuelling vesicular movement remains one of the many questions still open [95–101].

Additionally, recently published evidence demonstrated not only the presence of aquaporin channels in mesothelial cells, but also that their expression can be modulated by both osmotic and non-osmotic stimulation [102]. The relevance of these channels for peritoneal permeability will be analysed in the section dealing with peritoneal microvasculature. Their presence in mesothelial cells is one more indication giving support to Henle's prediction that the essential anatomy and physiology of the peritoneum are located in its 'endothelia' [103].

Simionescu *et al.* [104] showed the existence of differentiated microdomains on the luminal surface of capillary endothelium where they found a distinct and preferential distribution of electronegative fixed charges, also called anionic sites. Cationic tracers, which did not bind to caveolae or to transcellular channels, decorated the luminal glycocalyx, coated pits and coated vesicles [95, 100, 104]. Recent studies applying cationic tracers such as ruthenium red and cationized ferritin in rat and mouse peritoneum, also showed a preferential distribution of negative charges at the level of the mesothelial cells luminal surface [33, 34, 41] (Figs 12 and 17). Density of these surface plasmalemmal charges is substantially reduced in cells undergoing apoptosis [38].

Mesothelial cell boundaries are tortuous, with adjacent cells often tending to overlap (Fig. 4, inset; Fig. 12). Tight junctions close the luminal side of the intercellular boundaries [11, 18, 29] (Figs 4 and 12). When studied in the horizontal plane by

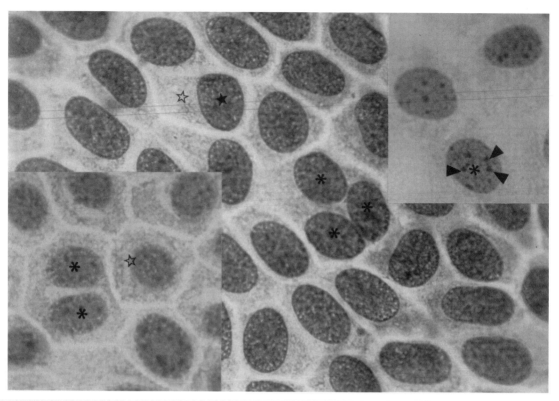

Figure 8. Normal density distribution of mesothelial cells observed in intact, unexposed animals. Asterisks indicate nuclei of a trinucleated cell, rarely seen in normal mesothelium (open star: cytoplasm of mesothelial cell; black star: nucleus). haematoxylin–eosin ×1000.

Lower left inset. Binucleated cells (asterisks) are seldom observed in intact, unexposed mesothelium. Note the polygonal shape of the cell (open star) (haematoxylin–eosin; ×1000).

Upper right inset. Arrow heads point at nucleoli of mesothelial cell nucleus (*) (haematoxylin–eosin; ×1000).

using the freeze–fracture technique these junctional contact areas were defined as cell extensions and finger-like processes, overlapping into the adjacent cell body. Cell processes were wedge-shaped and numerous, and the cell periphery appeared serrated [105]. Desmosomes have also been observed near the cellular luminal front [11, 20, 22, 29] (Fig. 18) and so have gap junctions [22]. The abluminal portions of cell interfaces usually show an open intercellular infundibulum (Fig. 18). Completely open intercellular interphases have not been observed in normal, resting mesothelium [11, 18, 29]. Even desquamated mesothelial cells showing severe degenerative changes can keep their junctional system almost intact (Fig. 19). These junctional morphological features are, however, different from those observed between mesothelial cells covering the diaphragmatic lymphatic lacunae, which are more cuboidal and prominent than mesothelial cells observed in other areas of the peritoneal surface.

The existence of stomata (open intermesothelial communications between the abdominal cavity and the submesothelial diaphragmatic lymphatics), predicted by William Hewson [1] 100 years before being discovered by Von Recklinghausen [106], have been the subject of a long and rich controversy along the years. Accepted by some [107–109] and denied by others [110–112], it was not until the advent of electron microscopy that their existence was demonstrated [41, 113, 114]. Scanning electron microscopy disclosed the patent intermesothelial junctions forming gaps whose average diameter ranged between 4 and 12 μm [113, 114] and circumscribed by cuboidal mesothelial cells. These gaps open into submesothelial lymphatics [41] and have not been observed in diaphragmatic mesothelium covering non-lacunar areas [114]. Additional studies have shown the passage of particles from the abdominal cavity into the submesothelial diaphragmatic lymphatics [115, 116]. These studies also con-

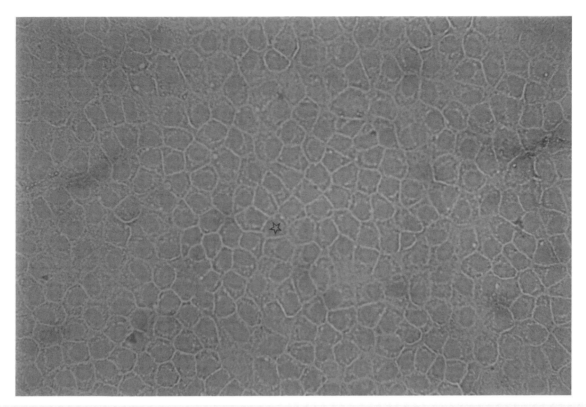

Figure 9. Cell viability evaluated on visceral mesothelium by Trypan-blue exclusion in an intact unexposed mouse. The stain did not permeate the cell membrane (open star: mesothelial cell) (× 400).

firm the results of experiments performed by Allen [117], who demonstrated the passage of frog erythrocytes through stomata of the mouse diaphragmatic peritoneum, and their appearance within submesothelial lymphatics. This pathway paved the way for intraperitoneal blood transfusions that have been successfully performed in fetuses [118, 119], human adults [120], rats, mice, dogs and lambs [121, 122]. On the other hand, intraperitoneal malignant cells [123] and bacteria [124] also leave the abdominal cavity on their way to the central venous circulation, through diaphragmatic stomata. The same pathway applies for absorption of albumin–gold complexes injected into the peritoneal cavity (Fig. 16) [76]. These structures can be found only between mesothelial cells overlying lacunae.

At the sites of stomata and their channels, mesothelial and lymphatic endothelial cells contain actin-like filaments [125] assumed to induce cell contraction, opening the stomatal pathway for the passage of macromolecules and cells. Cationized ferritin has been observed decorating the glycocalyx of mesothelial and lymphatic endothelial cells located along the stomata, as well as the coated pits and

coated vesicles of both types of cells [41, 126]. It should be noted that the presence of stomata has been recently detected in mouse mesenteric mesothelium [127], in omental, ovaric and pelvic peritoneum, as well as in that covering the anterior liver surface and the anterior abdominal wall [128, 129]. Therefore, it may be assumed that all these extradiaphragmatic openings contribute to the absorptive capacity of the entire peritoneal membrane. Albumin–gold complexes appear to be absorbed also from the peritoneal space through stomata [76] (Fig. 16), even though the capability of this pathway for the uptake of the probe did not seem to be much higher than that shown by non-stomatal mesothelial infundibular junctions that contained only 1% of the injected tracer.

Stomata have been ascribed the role of a preferential pathway for the output of fluids, cells, particles and bacteria from the abdominal cavity [130]. However, the luminal surface of mesothelial cells (which limits the gaps), after staining with cationized ferritin, displayed dense labelling of their cytoplasmic plasmalemma as well as coated pits and coated vesicles. The same cationic tracer also decorated the

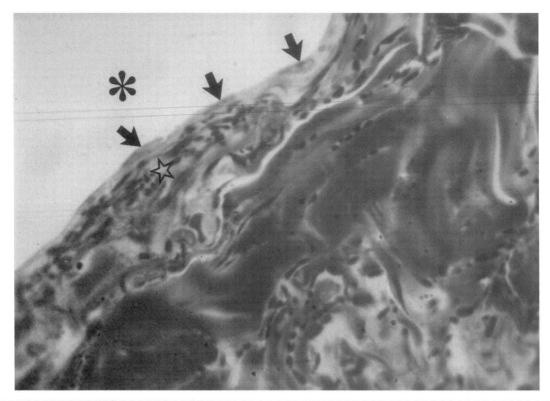

Figure 10. Biopsy of parietal peritoneum taken from a uraemic patient at the time of implanting the first dialysis catheter. Arrows point at nuclei of mesothelial cells. Open star was placed on the submesothelial interstitial tissue, the thickness of which ranges between 37 and 62 μm (*: peritoneal cavity) (toluidin blue; × 400).

lymphatic endothelial plasmalemma, which circumscribed the stomatal openings [41]. If this is so, the passage of solutes through stomata is most likely dependent not only on molecular weight, size and shape, but also on electric charge [41].

Studies in rat and mouse perfused with ruthenium red revealed that intermesothelial cell junctions were, in general, stained just at the level of their infundibulum, even though the dye now and then decorated the junctional complex, staining approximately 50% of its length [34] (Fig. 12).

Nuclei are generally located in the central region of mesothelial cells, showing an elongated, oval or reniform appearance with occasional irregularities in their outlines and sometimes protrusions and identations (Fig. 11). The chromatin is fine, evenly distributed and forms a dense rim around the nuclear membrane (Fig. 11). In normal unexposed mesothelium, around 2% of cells are binucleated [28] (Fig. 8, left lower inset; Fig. 20). Nucleoli have been reported both as present and absent [18, 29]. However, studies performed in imprints [28] showed that they are present and that their number ranges between 6 and 8 (Fig. 7). Rough endoplasmic

reticulum and ribosomes are dispersed in the cytoplasm. Mitochondria and the Golgi complex are evident mainly in perinuclear areas (Figs 6 and 11). Although seldom observed, isolated cilia may emerge from the luminal aspect of mesothelial cells, showing in their cytoplasmic part the axial microtubule as well as the attached basal body (Fig. 4). More frequently observed in splenic mesothelium [131], their functional significance is still unknown [132].

The submesothelial basement membrane, originally described by Todd and Bowman [133], and later reported as hyaline, homogeneous, one-layered and continuous [107, 134], with an average thickness of approximately 40 nm for mouse and rabbit peritoneum [11, 19], normally appears lying under the mesothelial layer of visceral, parietal and diaphragmatic peritoneum [135] (Figs 11 and 18). As an exception, the functional significance of which is still unknown, the omental mesothelium of mice and humans lacks basement membrane [19, 136].

Submesothelial basement membrane of visceral, parietal and diaphragmatic peritoneum of rat and mouse, perfused with the cationic tracer ruthenium

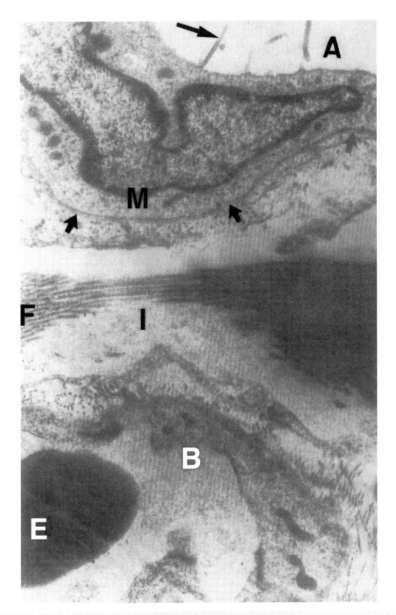

Figure 11. Rabbit mesentery: normal resting mesothelial cell (M) lying on a continuous basement membrane (short arrows) (A: abdominal cavity; long arrow: microvilli; I: interstitium; F: collagen fibres; B: blood capillary; E: erythrocyte) (original magnification ×27 500).

red, consistently showed anionic charges periodically distributed along the lamina rara externa and interna, most of the time, forming double rows [33, 34] (Fig. 12).

The reported average diameter of ruthenium red-stained particles in the basement membrane was 2.7 nm, whereas the average distance measured between the one-row oriented basal lamina dye particles ranged between 65 and 90 nm, not far from the interval value of 60 nm observed using the same

tracer in rats [137] and human kidney glomeruli [138].

The fact that these charges are, as stated above, distributed along both aspects of the basement membrane implies that the charge-free interval is actually smaller than the mean distance calculated for each membrane layer. The electric field of each particle of ruthenium is around 8–10 nm, and charge discrimination for negative tracers is effective for substances with a molecular radius around 1 nm,

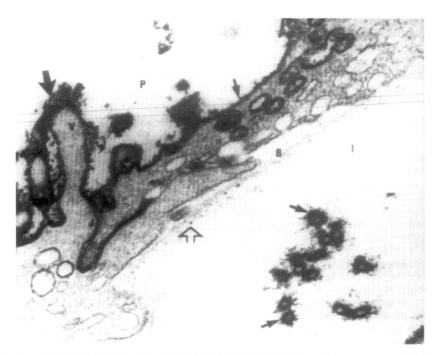

Figure 12. Section of rat mesentery showing microvilli (V) with heavily ruthenium-red decorated glycocalyx (large arrow), also evident on the mesothelial cell plasmalemma (small arrow). The cationic dye also stains a long portion of the intercellular junction (J). The basement membrane (B) shows quite regularly distributed anionic sites (open arrow) (P: abdominal cavity; I: interstitium). Original magnification ×50 720.

Inset. Rat mesentery: transversal section of microvilli showing the fibrilar ruthenium red-stained glycocalyx (arrows) (×50 720).

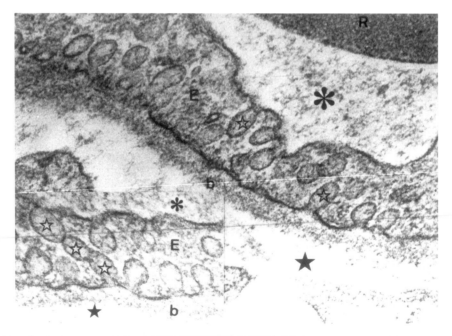

Figure 13. Continuous blood capillary of rat mesenteric peritoneum. Plasmalemmal vesicles (open stars) are open to both aspects of the endothelial cell (E) (R: red blood cell; *: microvascular lumen; b: subendothelial basement membrane; black star: interstitial space) (×87 000).

Inset. Another capillary from the same sample, showing a transcellular channel made up by a chain of three plasmalemmal vesicles (open stars), connecting both aspects of the endothelial cell (E) (*: microvascular lumen; b: subendothelial basement membrane; black star: subendothelial interstitial space) (×87 000).

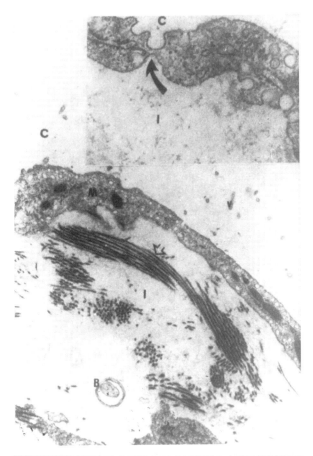

Figure 14. Sample of rat mesentery obtained after 13 intra-peritoneal injections of 0.2% furfural, performed on a daily basis. Microvilli (V) are present. The elongated mesothelial cell (M) is lying directly on the connective tissue. The basement membrane is absent. Note the intensity of interstitial edema (I), which is evident even between the collagen fibres (open arrow) (B: myelinoid body; C: abdominal space) (original magnification × 15 400).
Upper right inset. A different area of the same sample showing a transmesothelial channel (black arrow) formed by two vesicles. Notice the lack of submesothelial basement membrane (I: edematous interstitium; C: abdominal cavity) (original magnification × 41 500).

corresponding approximately to a globular molecule showing a molecular weight of 2 kDa [139]. In this sense it should be taken into account that the radius of macromolecular anionic albumin is 3.6 nm, whereas its molecular weight is 67 kDa.

It should be noted that the density distribution of these anionic fixed charges of the basement membrane almost disappears during the acute inflammatory reaction secondary to septic peritonitis [140] (Fig. 21), and is substantially reduced in rats, soon after 4 months of streptozotocin-induced, uncontrolled diabetes [141] (Fig. 17).

The relevance of the electronegative charge of the mesothelial monolayer upon the peritoneal permeability to anionic plasma proteins will be discussed in the section dealing with microvascular permeability.

Reduplicated submesothelial basement membrane has been observed in diabetic and non-diabetic chronic uraemic patients treated by maintenance peritoneal dialysis [142, 143] (Fig. 22). It has been shown that perivascular basement membrane thickness increases with age [144, 145] as well as in the direction of head to foot [145, 146]. This same ultrastructural alteration has been observed in diabetics [145, 147]. It has been suggested that diabetes alone is not responsible for excessive accumulation of basement membrane associated with ageing [148]. Therefore, it could be claimed that the reduplication of basement membrane observed in human mesothelium is a by-product of cell renewal regardless of the cause of cell death that triggers the process of repopulation [142, 149]. However, the fact that this phenomenon was also detected in the submesothelial basement membrane of diabetic rats suggests that a high glucose content in the extracellular fluid appears to be related to the mechanism(s) leading to these changes [141].

Interstitium

Connective tissue, which originates from mesenchyma, is composed of cells and fibres embedded in an amorphous substance. The main connective tissue cell is the fibroblast and the main fibre is collagen [150].

The submesothelial connective tissue normally has a low cell population surrounded by high molecular weight intercellular material. Fibroblasts, mast cells in the proximity of blood microvessels (Fig. 23), occasional monocytes and macrophages (Fig. 2) are frequently observed.

Substantial amounts of quite compact bundles of collagen are usually interposed between the blood microvessels and the mesothelial layer (Figs 1, 2 and 3). The collagen density distribution in the different regions of visceral peritoneum is quite variable [144].

The macromolecular common denomination of connective tissues is a broad molecular class of polyanions: the tissue polyaccharides. They form a gel-like structure with the collagen fibres [151] which, when stained with ruthenium red, shows the presence of anionic fixed charges [34].

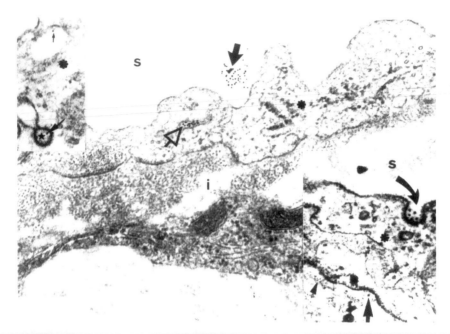

Figure 15. Diaphragmatic peritoneum of a mouse taken 10 min after intra-arterial perfusion with gold-labelled albumin. Some particles (black arrow) can be seen in the peritoneal space (s). The mesothelial cell (*) shows a multivesicular body (open arrow) containing particles of the tracer (I: interstitial space) (×41 500).
Upper left inset. Cytoplasmic compartment of a mesothelial cell (*) showing albumin–gold complexes decorating the membrane luminal aspect of a pynocytotic vesicle (small arrow), as well as that of coated vesicle (big arrow) (×64 550).
Lower left inset. Particles of the tracer decorating the luminal glycocalyx of a coated pit (curved arrow) of a mesothelial cell (*), seen in the same sample. The tracer is also present in the abluminal aspect of the mesothelial cell (straight arrow), between the plasmalemma and the submesothelial basement membrane (arrowhead) (×64 550).

Thickness of the interstitial layer is extremely variable in the different portions of the peritoneum. This heterogeneity can also be applied to the distances separating the submesothelial blood vessels from the peritoneal cavity, ranging between 1–2 μm to ⩾ 30 μm (Fig. 1). It should be noted that restriction of molecular movement through the interstitial tissue and its progression from or to the microvasculature is affected not only by their molecular weight, shape and electric charge, but also by the length of the pathway. According to Fick's law of diffusion, it is the difference in concentration per unit of distance (the concentration gradient) which determines the rate of movement of the solute. If we double the distance over which the same concentration difference occurred, the gradient and, therefore, the rate of transfer, would be cut in half. Therefore, the relevance of the interstitial compartment thickness in the transperitoneal transfer of solutes may well be critical [75, 152], and diffusion of solutes coming out from capillaries far from the abdominal cavity could be rendered useful only in long-dwell exchanges, like those performed in CAPD.

The question of the interstitium in terms of plasma to lymph traffic of macromolecules has been basi-cally investigated in lung interstitial tissue [153], which, at physiological pH, has the properties of a negatively charged membrane [154]. Therefore, the polyanionic glycosaminoglycans (mainly hyaluronan) and glycoproteins located in the interstitial ground substance have the capability of influencing the interstitial distribution volumes of plasma proteins coming out from the intravascular compartment, according to their molecular charge [155]. It has been suggested that these glycosaminoglycans restrict free diffusion through the interstitium [156] and can both reduce the interstitial distribution volume of anionic plasma proteins, and retard the plasma-lymph traffic of cationic macromolecules [153]. Anyway, the effect of protein charge on the interstitial hydraulic conductivity has been only partly clarified.

The extremely low and, at times, negative interstitial pressure (0 to −4 mmHg) [157–159] represents, together with the capillary permselectivity and the lymphatic drainage, one of the three key factors modulating the plasma-to-lymph fluid traffic, therefore, preventing the formation of interstitial oedema [160, 161]. Specifically, during peritoneal dialysis, studies by Flessner [162] have shown that transfer

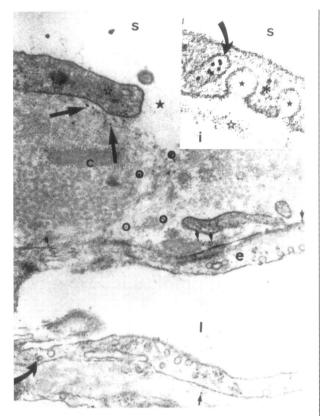

Figure 16. Diaphragmatic peritoneum of a mouse, taken 10 min after intraperitoneal injection of albumin–gold complexes. The black star points at stomata communicating the peritoneal space(s), and the submesothelial connective tissue (c). Albumin–gold complexes (large straight arrow) are present immediately under the mesothelial cell (open star), between collagen fibres (open circles), as well as in the submesothelial interstitial space, near the lymphatic lacuna (short straight arrows). The curved arrow points at a particle of the tracer included in an endothelial pinocytotic vesicle (l: lymphatic lacuna; c: interstitial space) ($\times 30\,740$).

Inset. Mouse diaphragmatic mesothelium taken 10 min after intraperitoneal injection of albumin–gold complexes. Arrow indicates an endosome containing particles of the tracer (S: peritoneal space; *: mesothelial cell cytoplasm; black star: plasmalemmal vesicles; open star: submesothelial basement membrane; l: interstitial space) ($\times 64\,550$).

Used with permission from *Kidney International*, **47**: 1274–84, 1995.

of small solutes through the tortuous interstitial pathways is primarily by diffusion, and that convection may contribute to overall transport in parietal tissue. As stated above, in normal conditions the interstitium has hydrostatic pressure near 0 [157, 162]. During clinical peritoneal dialysis the intra-abdominal pressure ranges between 4 and 10 cm H_2O [163, 164], thus creating a pressure gradient that drives fluid as well as solutes out of the

peritoneal cavity to the interstitium. Thus, fluid loss from the abdominal cavity to the periperitoneal interstitial space is directly proportional to intra-abdominal pressures higher than 2 cm H_2O [164].

Blood microvessels

Capillaries of human and rodent parietal [165] and visceral peritoneum [40, 166] have been reported to be of the continuous type (Figs 1, 3, 24, 25 and 26), according to the classification of Majno [167]. However, the existence of fenestrated capillaries in human parietal and rabbit diaphragmatic peritoneum (Figs 1 and 27), as well as in mouse mesentery [168–170] has been reported. The incidence of fenestrated capillaries in human parietal peritoneum appears to be low (1.7% of the total number of capillaries) [170]. The reported density of fenestrated microvessels in mouse mesentery and rabbit diaphragmatic peritoneum ranged between 26% and 29% of the observed capillaries, whereas their presence in parietal peritoneum of non-dialysed uraemic patients was only 1.7%. It should be noted, however, that the anterior abdominal wall of humans comprises less than 4% of the peritoneal surface area [10]. Diameter of fenestrae, which ranged between 60 and 90 nm, is well within the range of fenestrae observed in other capillary beds: 40–70 nm in renal peritubular capillaries [171], glomerular capillaries [167], and rabbit submandibular gland [172]. The reported density of fenestrae counted along the capillary circumference of mice mesenteric microvessels is 3.4 fenestrae/micron [173]. This value is quite close to that of 3 fenestrae/micron of capillary circumference observed in renal glomerular capillaries [167]. Density of fenestrae per square micron of endothelial surface is 45–60/μm^2 in renal peritubular capillaries [174] and 20/μm^2 in renal glomerular capillaries [167], whereas their frequency in mouse mesenteric capillaries is approximately 12/μm^2 [169].

The density distribution of submesothelial microvessels along the different portions of the peritoneum is variable. In the rabbit the mesentery appears to be the most vascularized peritoneal segment (contributing 71.1% of the total number of observed capillaries). The reported diaphragmatic and parietal contributions to the total microvascular bed examined were 17.9% and 10.9% respectively [175].

In rabbit mesentery the main population of continuous blood microvessels is represented by:

1. True capillaries (without perithelial cells), the mean luminal diameter of which is 7.2 μm and

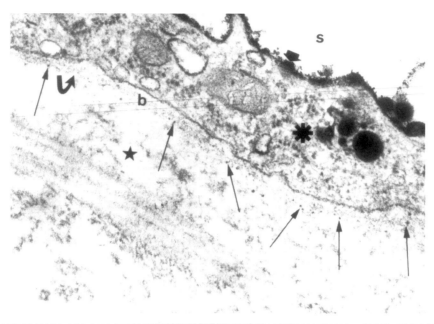

Figure 17. Mesenteric mesothelial cell of a diabetic rat (*). The animal was perfused with ruthenium-red 6 months after induction of the disease, with streptozotocin (glucose blood levels were higher than 500 mg/dl; glycated haemoglobin: $16.38 \pm 0.57\%$). Glycocalyx covering the cavitary aspect of the mesothelial cell is heavily decorated by the cationic tracer (thick arrow). The submesothelial basement membrane (b) shows few dispersed anionic sites (long arrows), as well as areas where they are completely absent (curved arrow) (s: peritoneal cavity; black star: interstitial space) ($\times 41\,500$).

whose mean wall thickness is 0.4 µm (Figs 11, 24, 25 and 26).

2. Venous capillaries usually formed by the confluence of two or three capillaries. These show a thin endothelial layer, occasional peripheral perithelial cells, and have a mean luminal diameter of 9.2 µm.

3. Postcapillary venules whose luminal diameter ranges between 9.4 and 20.6 µm [40].

With increasing luminal diameter there is a proportional increase in wall thickness due to the presence of more perithelial cells encircling the endothelial layer [176] (Fig. 25). The average ratio of luminal diameter to wall thickness is approximately 10/1 [176]. All aforementioned exchange vessels present at their luminal aspect a limiting area that separates the endothelial cell from the circulating blood and is formed by the plasmalemma with its trilaminar structure [16] (Fig. 26) and the glycocalyx (Fig. 26). The latter, originally described by Luft [35] in other vascular beds, has also been observed at the luminal aspect of peritoneal microvessels [36, 177] The presence of sialoconjugates, proteoglycans and acidic glycoproteins organized as a fibrous network provides the plasmalemmal glycocalyx with electronegative charge [178] (Fig. 28).

There is evidence that anionic plasma proteins (albumin and IgG) are adsorbed to the glycocalyx of microvascular endothelial cells [179]. The fibre-matrix model of capillary permeability envisages the glycocalyx as a meshwork of glycoprotein fibres which, after adsorbing circulating proteins, would tighten its mesh, thereby rendering the underlying endothelium less accessible to water and other water-soluble molecules [37]. Furthermore, it has been shown that the adsorption of circulating anionic plasma proteins to the glycocalyx renders the underlying endothelium relatively impermeable to large, electron-dense, anionic tracers such as native ferritin (MW ~ 450 kDa) [179].

The mean endothelial cell width of rabbit mesenteric capillaries is 0.4 µm, unless the cytoplasm bulges up to more than 1 µm at the site of the nucleus (compare Figs 3 and 24 with Fig. 26). The cytoplasm includes the usual cell organelles: mitochondria, rough endoplasmic reticulum and free ribosomes [11, 167].

The mitochondrial content of vascular endothelial cells in frog mesentery decreases gradually from arterioles towards venous capillaries and subsequently increases toward venules [180].

The Golgi complex displays variable degrees of development in biopsies taken from different

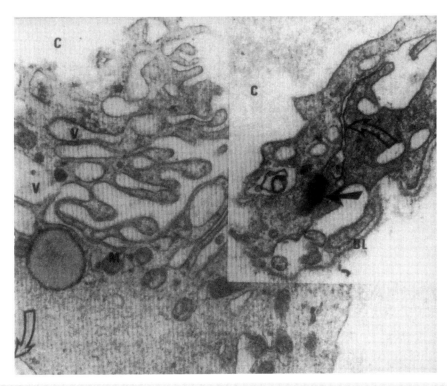

Figure 18. Biopsy of parietal peritoneum taken from a 67-years-old chronic uraemic patient, who was on IPD for a period of almost 2 years. A young mesothelial cell shows numerous vacuoles (V) giving a worm-like appearance, which is why this structure is called micropinocytosis vermiformis. The abluminal aspect of the mesothelial cell is lying on a hyaline basement membrane (open arrow) (C: abdominal cavity; M: mitochondrion) (× 26 000).
   Upper right inset. Another area of the same biopsy. This electron micrograph shows the vacuolized cytoplasm of two adjacent mesothelial cells developing a new intercellular junction (open arrow). Note the presence of a typical desmosome (black arrow). The basement membrane (BL) is still discontinuous (original magnification × 30 740).

patients. This same variability was observed when comparing different peritoneal microvascular endothelial cells present in a single sample.

The cytoplasmic matrix of endothelial cells shows long filaments, parallel to the longitudinal cellular axis. Their diameter ranges between 20 and 100 Å [167], and at times they appear in bundles. These intermediate-size filaments seem to be a common component of the cytoplasmic matrix of vascular endothelial cells showing, however, a lower density distribution than that observed in other cell types [132].

Nuclei are generally oval, elongated (Fig. 24) or occasionally kidney-shaped with focal surface irregularities (Fig. 11). Their mean short-axis width in rabbit mesentery is 0.957 ± 0.417 μm [11].

Plasmalemmal vesicles, which can be found in most cell types, are particularly common in capillary endothelia [181], where they occupy approximately 7% of the cell volume [98] (Fig. 25). Their outer diameter is approximately 700 Å (it ranges between 500 and 900 Å) [11, 33, 47] and they have a round

or oval shape surrounded by a three-layered membrane of 80 Å thickness (Fig. 26, inset).

According to their location in the cytoplasmic matrix, vesicles can be classified into three groups: (a) vesicles attached to the plasmalemma limiting the blood front of the endothelial cell; (b) free vesicles within the cytoplasmic matrix; (c) attached vesicles, but this time to the tissue front of the endothelial cell plasmalemma [47] (Fig. 25). The density population of plasmalemmal vesicles varies considerably from one vascular segment to another, even within the same microvascular territory [46, 47]. In the mouse diaphragm, arterioles show 200 vesicles/μm², true capillaries 900 μm², venular segments of capillaries 1200 μm² and postcapillary venules 600 μm² [46].

Most vesicles that open to the extracellular medium have necks whose diameter can be as small as 100 Å [47]. Transendothelial channels formed by a chain of vesicles opening simultaneously on both fronts of the endothelium have been described in capillaries of mouse diaphragmatic muscle [46] as

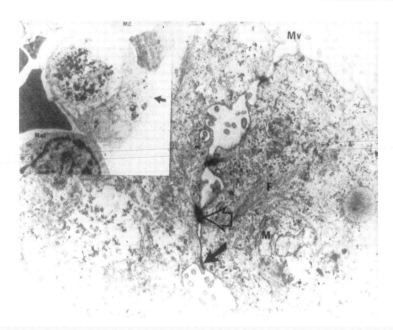

Figure 19. Effluent dialysate obtained from a non-infected patient on peritoneal dialysis. Two desquamated mesothelial cells show severe degenerative changes: swollen mitochondria (M) with broken membranes, sheaves of filaments (F), and swollen cytoplasm. Part of the tight junction is still present (black arrow), as well as a desmosome (open arrow) (M: microvilli) (original magnification ×15 400).
Upper left inset. Effluent dialysate obtained from the same patient. Note the presence of a signet-ring macrophage (arrow), as well as part of two floating mesothelial cells (Mc) (mac: macrophage) (original magnification ×8600).

well as in postcapillary venules of rabbit and rat mesentery (Figs 25 and 29) [11]. The relative frequency of transendothelial channels has been found to be higher in true capillaries than in arterioles and venules, with the highest density in the venular segment of capillaries [100]. Microvessels of frog mesentery showed a density distribution of three transendothelial channels for every 400 vascular profiles examined [180]. Just as in observations made on mesothelial cells, plasmalemmal vesicles and transendothelial channels do not bind cationic electron-dense tracers which, on the other hand, decorate the luminal aspect of coated pits and coated vesicles [95, 104] in the peritoneal microvasculature [34].

The functional significance of plasmalemmal vesicles or caveolae vesicles, transendothelial channels, coated pits and coated vesicles was discussed in the section on normal epithelium.

As stated above, in fenestrated capillaries, endothelial cells are pierced by fenestrae closed by a diaphram [182] (Fig. 24, inset; Figs 27 and 30). Fenestrae are not static structures. It has been shown that their prevalence can be increased under the effect of vitamin A metabolites [183], the influence of sexual hormones [166], thrombocytopenia [184], and by the acute inflammatory reaction

[167]. In this sense a microvascular bed (capillaries and postcapillary venules), supplied with a continuous endothelium, can rapidly develop endothelial fenestrations under the influence of vascular endothelial growth factor (VEGF), a 34–42 kDa cytokine, released by different cell types (eosinophils, neutrophils, and others) during the acute inflammatory reaction [185–188]. This effect has been demonstrated *in vivo* [189, 190], after acute and chronic exposure of different microvascular beds.

High concentrations of negative fixed charges (heparin and heparan sulphate) have been found on the blood front of fenestral diaphragms in several microvascular beds [95, 104, 182, 191–194]. They are expected to discriminate against anionic macromolecules, essentially anionic plasma protein. Similarly, mesenteric fenestrated capillaries of mice perfused with the cationic tracer ferritin showed densely packed anionic fixed charges on the endothelial cell glycocalyx, on the luminal aspect of fenestral diaphragms, as well as along both sides of the subendothelial basement membrane [173] (Fig. 27).

What is the role of fenestrae and intercellular junctions in the still ill-defined mechanisms related to capillary permeability? For more than 25 years the fenestral pathway was ascribed a major role in the permeability capabilities of fenestrated capillar-

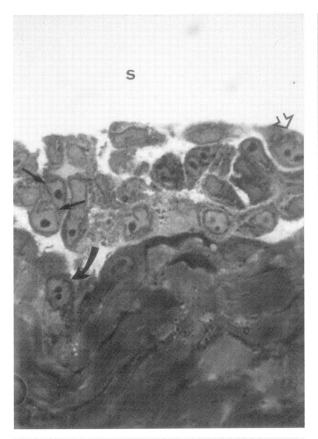

Figure 20. Peritoneal biopsy taken from a patient on CAPD (parietal peritoneum). Desquamating mesothelial cells (small arrows), one of them binucleated (open arrow). Curved arrow points at a binucleated mesothelial cell still forming part of the monolayer (s: peritoneal space) (haematoxylin–eosin; original magnification ×400).

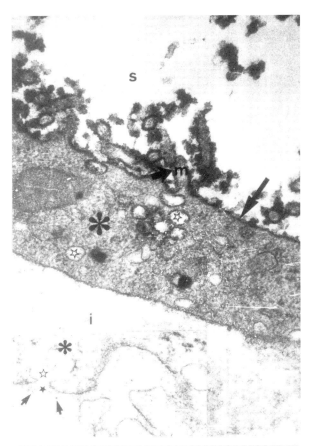

Figure 21. Rat mesenteric mesothelium. The animal was perfused with ruthenium-red, 24 h after experimental induction of *E. coli* peritonitis. Plasmalemmal vesicles or caveolae (open stars) can be seen in the cytoplasm of the mesothelial cell (*). The submesothelial basement membrane is absent, as well as the normally present anionic sites. The luminal aspect of microvilli (m) and that of the cellular membrane are decorated by the cationic tracer (short and long arrows respectively) (S: peritoneal space; I: oedematous interstitial space) (×41 500).

Inset. Another mesothelial cell (*) seen in the same tissue sample. Very few anionic sites (arrows) can be seen sporadically distributed along parts of the submesothelial basement membrane (black star). Open star: plasmalemmal vesicle or caveola, showing an open neck facing the abluminal aspect of the cell cytoplasm (I: interstitial space) (×84 530).

ies [195]. Some investigators suggested that, while open fenestrae could represent the ultrastructural equivalent of the large pore [74], fenestrae, closed by diaphragms (Fig. 27), could also provide a diffusive pathway for water- and lipid-soluble substances [196]. However, fenestral openings of 60–90 nm diameter are too large to be considered the structural equivalent of the hypothetical large pores, the radii of which range between 11 and 35 nm [74, 197]. Furthermore, the density of these pores, estimated at one every 20 μm^2 [47], is substantially lower than the density of fenestrae per square micron observed in microvascular beds.

At least from a theoretical point of view, the presence of anionic fixed charges at the level of fenestral diaphragms, as well as in the subendothelial basement membrane (Fig. 27), is a strong argument against the transfenestral passage of macromolecular anionic proteins [137, 198]. Indeed, previously reported physiological studies have demonstrated the selectivity and restriction of the fenestrated microvascular wall to the passage of electronegatively charged macromolecules [199–201]. Moreover, the permeability of fenestrated capillaries to anionic macromolecules is not higher than that of capillaries of the continuous type [202]. In this context Fig. 30 offers a descriptive account of the problem, observed in our laboratory [Shostak and Gotloib, unpublished observations]. Rat mesentery was perfused (*in vivo*) through the arterial tree with

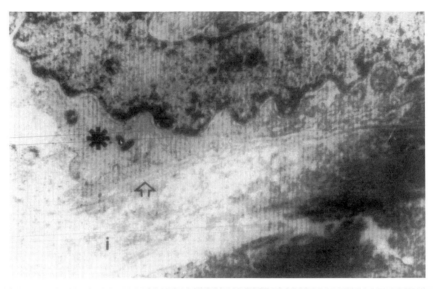

Figure 22. Parietal peritoneum taken from a 67-year-old patient on IPD. The open arrow shows the reduplicated submesothelial basement membrane (*: mesothelial cell; I: submesothelial interstitium) (original magnification ×24 600).

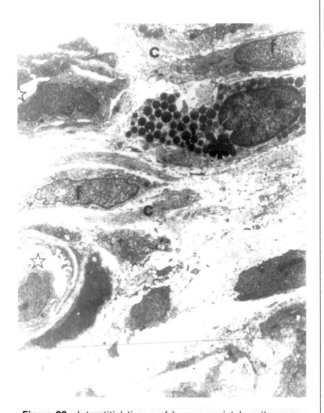

Figure 23. Interstitial tissue of human parietal peritoneum. Bundles of collagen (c) and fibroblasts (f) are interposed between the blood microvessels (open stars) and the mesothelial cells (not included in the electron micrograph). Mast cells (*) are frequently observed near blood microvessels (original magnification 42 900).

negatively charged albumin–gold complexes for a period of 30 min. As can be seen, substantial amounts of albumin–gold particles appear contacting the luminal aspect of the endothelial cell plasmalemma, as well as free into the capillary lumen. Particles of the tracer can be observed in close apposition to the luminal front of fenestral diaphragms. However, albumin–gold particles were not seen in the subendothelial space, even after 30 min perfusion. These observations support the hypothesis that fenestrae are not permeable to anionic plasma proteins. Consequently, it appears that fenestral openings are unrelated to the theoretically predicted large pore system [195, 198, 202, 203]. On the other hand, fenestrated endothelia have higher hydraulic conductivity, and are more permeable to small ions and molecules than continuous endothelia [204].

Capillary endothelial cells are linked to each other by tight junctions (zonula occludens), originally described by Farquhar and Palade [205–207] (Fig. 31). Communicating or gap junctions have been observed in arteriolar endothelium [206]. Postcapillary venules have loosely organized junctions with discontinuous ridges and grooves of which 25–30% appear to be open with a gap of 20–60 Å [47]. They also sometimes show gap junctions [11].

Cytoplasmic plasmalemma bordering both sides of junctions also shows anionic fixed charges [34]. Their functional significance in relation to the passage of charged molecules will be discussed later.

Research performed during the past 5–6 years revealed that interendothelial tight junctions appear

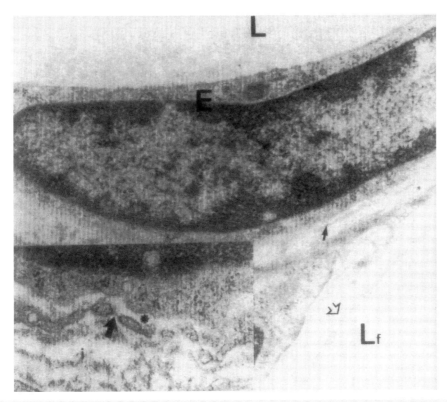

Figure 24. Continuous capillary of a blood mesenteric rabbit capillary whose endothelial layer (E) is lying on the basement membrane (black arrow). The lower right part of this electron micrograph shows a fenestrated capillary (open arrow) (L: lumen of continuous capillary; Lf: lumen of fenestrated capillary) (original magnification ×47 400).
    Lower left inset. Fenestrated capillary of human parietal peritoneum. The arrow points to a fenestral diaphragm (I: interstitium; *: lumen of fenestrated capillary) (original magnification ×42 900).

as a set of long, parallel, linear fibrils that circumscribe the cell, with short fibrillar fragments interconnecting the main parallel array. The number of fibres correlates with junctional permeability: the more densely packed the fibrillar mesh, the lower the junctional permeability [208]. Therefore, the tight junction is not a simple fusion between the outer plasmalemmal leaflets of neighbouring cells [209]; rather, it consists of protein molecules such as occludins and cadherins in tight junctions, desmoleins and desmocolins in desmosomes, and connexins in gap juctions [210, 211].

Occludin is an integral membrane protein, exclusively localized at tight junctions in both epithelial and endothelial cells [210], and is directly involved in sealing the cleft, creating the primary barrier to the diffusion of solutes through the paracellular pathway as well as regulating, according to the modulation of occludin expression, the permeability properties of different microvascular beds [212]. Occludin is bound on the endothelial cytoplasmic surface to ZO-1, a 220 kDa membrane-associated

protein likely to have both structural and signalling roles [213, 214].

Vascular endothelial cadherin, in turn, is an endothelial-specific cadherin that regulates cell to cell junction organization in this cell type, and provides strength and cohesion to the junction [215]. Cadherins are also implicated in junctional permeability, basically under the effect of inflammatory mediators such as tumour necrosis factor and histamine, which have been shown to induce a redistribution of these adhesion molecules to non-junctional regions and junctional disassembly [216, 217].

The role of tight junctions in the permeability capabilities of the microvasculature, during the situation of normal physiology, has been a topic for intensive research and controversy through the years. Whereas some groups considered the intercellular cleft as the main pathway for water, as well as for small and large solutes and electrolytes [218, 219], other groups developed the concept that tight junctions create a regulated paracellular barrier to the movement of water, solutes and immune cells

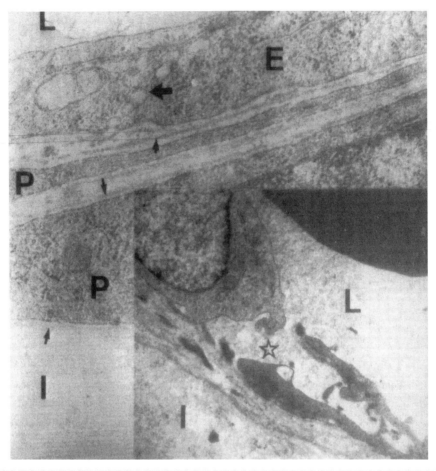

Figure 25. Postcapillary venule of rabbit mesentery. The large arrow shows a transcellular channel (L: microvascular lumen; E: endothelial cell; short arrow: subendothelial basement membrane; P: pericyte; small arrows: subperithelial basement membrane; I: interstitium) (×62 500).
    Lower right inset. Human parietal peritoneum taken from a 21-year-old patient with *E. coli* peritonitis. The star shows an open interendothelial junction of a blood capillary. Note part of an erythrocyte in the upper right quadrant (L: capillary lumen; I: interstitium) (original magnification ×41 500).

between the microvascular compartment and the interstitial space, enabling the endothelial monolayer to create compositionally different fluid compartments [208, 220–222]. Recent progress indicates that the presence of tight junctions does not imply a foolproof seal of the intercellular cleft. Instead, this structure contains discrete ion-selective pathways through the extracellular portion of the junction, regulated, at least in part, by the activity of the cytoskeleton [208, 223]. As stated above, the transmembrane protein occludin is an excellent candidate for the sealing protein. Understanding the mechanisms involved in junction permeability will require both a more detailed molecular characterization of tight junction proteins and the regulation by the endothelial cells of their attachment to the perijunctional cytoskeleton [220]. As stated by Renkin

[202] in 1977, identification of the tight junction with the diffusional pathway for macromolecular plasma proteins, in a situation of normal physiology, still remains questionable. Their role in capillary permeability is still debated.

As for blood cells, recent investigations showed that neutrophils preferentially migrate by crossing at tricellular corners, rather than passing through tight junctions that lie between two adjacent endothelial cells [224].

The basement membrane of true capillaries is normally a thin sheet at the interface between the abluminal aspect of the endothelial cell and the connective tissue (Figs 13 and 24). In postcapillary venules it is interposed between the endothelial and the perithelial cell (Fig. 25). Generally uniform for a given structure, its thickness varies among the

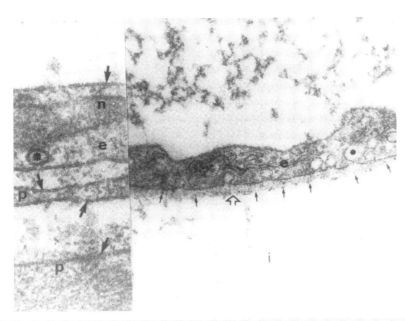

Figure 26. The right part of the figure shows part of a blood capillary wall observed in a sample of diaphragmatic peritoneum obtained from a normal rat. The luminal aspect (upper cell border) of the endothelial cell (e) shows a fine reticular glycocalyx stained by ruthenium red which, on the other hand, does not decorate pynocytotic vesicles (*). The subendothelial basement membrane (open arrow) is continuous and shows quite regularly distributed ruthenium-red stained anionic sites (small arrows) along both the lamina rara externa and the lamina rara interna (original magnification ×50 720).

Inset. Left part of the figure. Part of a postcapillary venule observed in mesentery of rat, 5 days after induction of peritonitis. The trilaminar structure of the endothelial (e) and perithelial cell plasmalemma is clearly observed (arrows), as well as that of the limiting membrane of the pinocytotic vesicle (*). Glycocalyx, basement membrane and anionic sites are absent (n: nucleus of endothelial cell) (original magnification ×84 530).

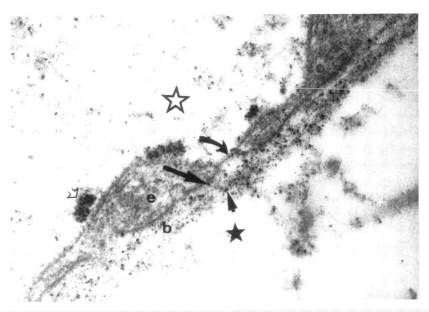

Figure 27. Fenestrated capillary of mouse mesenteric peritoneum. The animal was perfused with cationized ferritin. Particles of the tracer decorate the luminal (long straight arrow) and the abluminal (short black arrow) aspects of the basement membrane (b) laying under the endothelial cells (e). A fenestral diaphragm is also decorated on its luminal aspect by particles of cationized ferritin (curved arrow). Clumps of the tracer appear located on the luminal endothelial cell plasmalemma (open arrow) (open star: microvascular lumen; black star: subendothelial interstitial space) (×41 500).

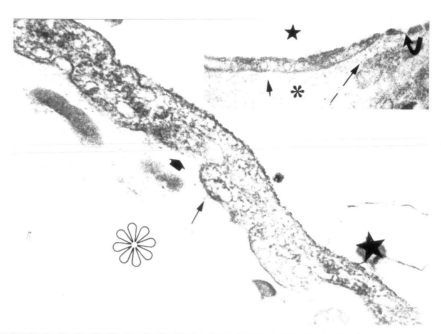

Figure 28. Continuous capillary of rat mesentery. The sample of tissue was recovered 24 h after induction of abdominal sepsis. Distribution of subendothelial anionic sites is irregular; at times they are totally absent (thick arrow), whereas in other portions of the basement membrane they can be seen, but showing an extremely low density (small thin arrow). The luminal aspect of the endothelial cell shows a black rim decorated by ruthenium red, indicating the still-present negative charges of the endothelial glycocalyx (star: microvascular lumen; *: edematous interstitial tissue) (ruthenium red; ×41 500).

Inset. Mesenteric fenestrated capillary taken from the same animal. Occasional anionic sites (long arrow) can be seen along the basement membrane. Most of its length is free from ruthenium-red decorated negative charges (short arrow) (*: structureless interstitial space; star: capillary lumen; curved arrow: fenestra) (ruthenium-red; ×30 740).

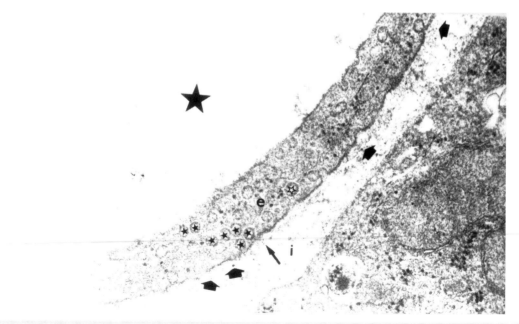

Figure 29. Mesenteric capillary of a rat 6 months after induction of diabetes with streptozotocin (glucose blood levels were higher than 500 mg/dl; glycated haemoglobin $16.38 \pm 0.57\%$). The animal was perfused with ruthenium red. The basement membrane (long arrow), lying under the endothelial cell (e), shows few and occasional anionic sites (thick arrows) (large black arrow: capillary lumen; open star: pinocytotic vesicle; small black stars: transendothelial channel; i: interstitial space) (×41 500).

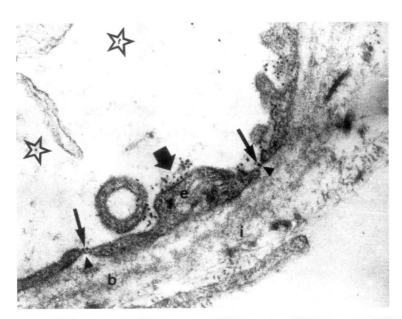

Figure 30. Fenestrated capillary of mouse mesentery taken 30 min after intra-arterial perfusion of the tissue with albumin–gold complexes. Particles of the tracer can be seen in the microvascular lumen (open stars), on the glycocalyx of the endothelial plasmalemma (short thick arrow), as well as on the luminal aspect (long arrows) of fenestral diaphragms (arrowheads). The tracer did not reach the subendothelial interstitial space (i) (b: subendothelial basement membrane) (× 50 720).

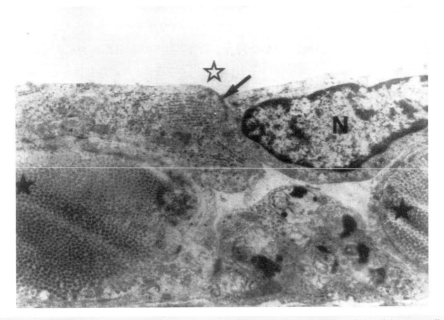

Figure 31. Blood capillary of rabbit mesentery. The black arrow points at a tight junction formed by two adjoining endothelial cells. A macrophage can be observed lying under the endothelial cells interposed between two bundles of collagen (black stars) (open star: capillary lumen; N: nucleus of endothelial cell) (original magnification × 85 000).

different parts of the body. True capillaries of normal rabbit mesentery have a mean basal membrane thickness of 0.234 ± 0.095 μm [11]. As described for the submesothelial basement membrane, that of human capillaries also exhibits a significantly increasing thickness in the direction of head to foot [145]. It has been suggested that these regional variations are secondary to differences in venous hydrostatic pressure effective on the capillary bed [145]. Diabetic and non-diabetic patients on long-term peritoneal dialysis, showing reduplicated submesothelial basement membrane, had similar alterations on the capillary basement membrane of parietal peritoneum [142]. These changes were also observed in postcapillary venules and small arterioles of parietal peritoneum taken from diabetic uraemics on CAPD (Figs 32 and 33), as well as in skin capillaries (Fig. 34). Additionally, reduplication of mesenteric subendothelial capillary basement membrane has been recently reported in streptozotocin-induced diabetic rats, as early as after 4 months of uncontrolled hyperglycaemia [141], whereas thickening was seen in the same animals 6 months after induction of the disease. These structural alterations of diabetic basement membranes seem to be derived from a substantial increased presence of collagen IV [147, 225–229] which, according to *in-vitro* studies, appears to derive from extended exposure of cells to high concentrations of glucose [230, 231].

In rats, both thickening and layering of microvascular basement membrane can also develop as a consequence of ageing [149, 232], but not before completing the first year of life [232].

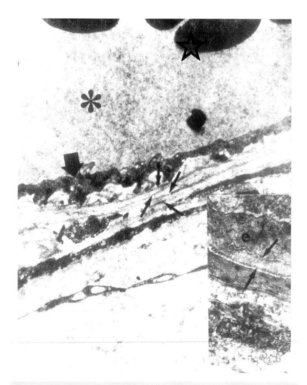

Figure 32. Subendothelial reduplicated basement membrane (small arrows) observed in a small venule of parietal peritoneum taken from a diabetic patient on CAPD (open star: red blood cells; *: vascular lumen; thick arrow: endothelial cell) (× 15 400).
   Inset. One arteriole from the same biopsy shows splitting of the subendothelial basement membrane (arrows) (e: endothelial cell) (× 12 600).

So far it may be speculated that reduplication or layering of submesothelial and peritoneal microvascular basement membranes in non-diabetics on CAPD could result from their continuous and long exposure to high glucose concentrations.

Subendothelial basement membranes of both continuous and fenestrated capillaries (Figs 26 and 27), have regularly distributed anionic fixed charges along both aspects of the membrane [36, 173]. Their density distribution in continuous capillaries ranges between 31 and 34 µm of basement membrane [36, 141]. These values, shown in the section devoted to the mesothelial basement membrane, are not far from those detected in other microvascular basement membranes.

The chemical composition of the fixed electronegative charges linked to the subendothelial basement membrane has been explored in several microvascular beds. Studies have shown that their main structural components are glycosaminoglycans such as heparan sulphate and chondroitin sulphate [104, 233–235]. This is at variance with the biochemical and histochemical observations made on the glycocalyx cell surface charges, the main component of which is sialic acid and sialo conjugate. This pattern has been detected in microvascular endothelium [236–240], pleural, pericardial and peritoneal mesothelial cells [241], as well as in macrophages [242], erythrocytes [243] and platelets [244].

What is the functional significance of these electronegative charges? A strong body of literature supports the concept that the permselectivity of capillary walls to anionic macromolecules is basically dependent on molecular charge, besides size and shape [137, 139, 165, 203, 234, 245–251]. Investigations performed in *in-vivo,* whole organ studies [153], in isolated perfused frog capillaries [252] and in isolated rat hindquarters [246] have demonstrated their presence evaluating permeability of different endogenous proteins in a variety of microvascular beds. Indeed, similar results were observed in patients on CAPD comparing dialysate to plasma concentrations of amino acids, having almost the same molecular weight but quite different charge [253], as well as in rat peritoneum, using charged dextrans [254]. The fact that endogenous proteins of graded size are hetereogeneous with respect to their molecular charge [255] lead to some conflicting results [256]. The key to this problem was found investigating clinical and experimental situations, where the permselectivity was substantially reduced or neutralized, enabling the observer to evaluate changes in permeability, derived from the absence

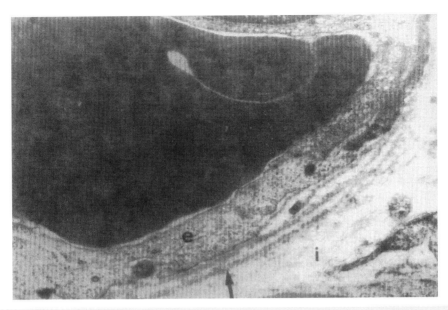

Figure 33. Blood capillary of parietal peritoneum taken from a 69-year-old uraemic patient on IPD for almost 3 years. The endothelial cell (e) is lying on a reduplicated basement membrane (arrow) (I: interstitium ($\times$24 600).

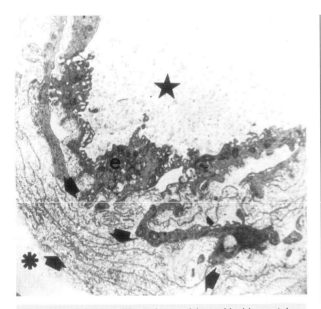

Figure 34. Blood capillary observed in a skin biopsy taken from the same diabetic chronic uraemic patient, whose parietal peritoneum was shown in Fig. 32. Arrows point at the multiple layers of basement membrane (star: microvascular lumen; e: endothelial cell; *: interstitial space) ($\times$5850).

of the normally present fixed electronegative charges. In the clinical set-up, type I diabetes [257], congenital [258, 259], and acquired nephrotic syndrome [260, 261] have been shown to expose the association of depleted glomerular negative charges and loss of the permselectivity of the capillary wall, leading to massive proteinuria. Experimental interventions performed in laboratory animals confirmed, in turn, the aforementioned findings. Enzymatic removal of sulphated (heparan sulphate) or non-sulphated (hyaluronic acid) glycosaminoglycans from the glomerular basement membrane resulted in a substantially increased permeability to bovine serum albumin [262]. Rats with streptozotocin-induced diabetic nephropathy showed reduced glycosaminoglycan contents in the glomerular basement membrane [263], decreased presence of their heparan sulphate-associated anionic sites [264], as well as significantly increased proteinuria [141]. Further observations made in the streptozotocin diabetic rat have shown a substantial reduction in the submesothelial and capillary subendothelial density distribution of anionic fixed charges (from 31 ± 2 to 12 ± 2 ruthenium red-decorated anionic sites/μm of basement membrane) and, at the same time, a significant increase of albumin losses in the peritoneal dialysis effluent, indicating a marked decrease of the permselective capabilities of the charged components of the peritoneal membrane (Fig. 17) [141]. Similar observations were made in intact rats after neutralization of the peritoneal negative charges with protamine sulphate [265].

The acute inflammatory reaction is the most spectacular experimental set-up to demonstrate the permeability changes derived from an acute reduction of the microvascular negative charge. This situation has been classically defined by the development of acute low hydrostatic pressure, high capillary permeability, and albumin-rich interstitial oedema [161, 266]. In this sense the generalized acute inflammatory reaction derived from abdominal sepsis promotes a major erosion of the density distribution of the anionic fixed charges in several microvascular beds, diaphragmatic and mesenteric peritoneum (showing values as low as six anionic sites/micron of basement membrane) [267], myocardium [268], skeletal muscle, pancreas, renal peritubular capillaries [269], as well as in the submesothelial basement membrane of rat diaphragmatic and mesenteric peritoneum [140] (Figs 21 and 28). Additional studies in the same experimental model of abdominal sepsis in rats demonstrated abnormally increased albumin content in mesenteric, diaphragmatic and pancreatic interstitial fluid [270]. This drastic loss of the permselectivity of the capillary wall derives from a massive liberation and reduced inactivation of a host of mediators of inflammation triggered by acute inflammation [271–273], including tumour necrosis factor alpha, inlerleukins, platelet-activating factor, leukotrienes, thromboxane A2, activators of the complement cascade, kinins, transforming growth factor B, vascular endothelial growth factor, as well as many others already known, or still waiting to be identified [183, 274–277].

The role of intercellular junctions in macromolecular leakage during acute inflammation is still controversial. Some groups pointed to the endothelial tight junction as the main pathway for extravasation of macromolecular plasma protein. It was postulated that inflammatory mediators such as histamine, serotonin, bradykinin and leukotriene E4 induced junctional openings (Fig. 25, inset), by means of endothelial cells contraction [278–281] or by a loss of occludin and cadherin from the junctional complex [282, 283]. Unpublished observations from our laboratory (Shostak and Gotloib) made in intact rats, as well as in rats with *E. coli* peritonitis, by means of intra-arterial injection of albumin–gold complexes, showed that most particles of the tracer cross the endothelial barrier transcellularly, via plasmalemmal vesicles. In both experimental situations, intact and infected rats, the tracer was not seen beyond the junctional infundibulum (Figs 35 and 36); just the opposite: the tracer was present in plasmalemmal vesicles (Fig. 36, inset), and reached the subendothelial space in areas far from intercellular junctions (Figs 35 and 36). This concept of transcellular transport of albumin through the capillary wall, also during acute inflammation, is supported by recently published evidence postulating a significant role for plasmalemmal vesicles and even for fenes-

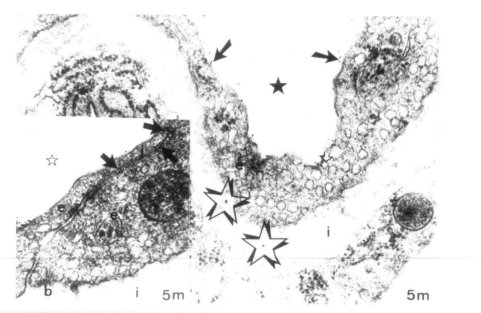

Figure 35. Blood continuous capillary of mouse diaphragmatic peritoneum. The material was taken 5 min after intra-arterial perfusion of the tissue with albumin–gold. Particles of the tracer decorate the luminal aspect (black arrows) of the endothelial cell, as well as that of pynocytotic vesicles (open arrows). Note the presence of albumin–gold complexes (open stars) in the subendothelial interstitial space (i), in an area free of intercellular junctions (×41 500).

Inset. Another aspect of the same sample shows particles of the tracer (arrows) in the luminal side of the intercellular junction (j), whereas the interstitial space (i) is devoid of albumin–gold complexes (open star: microvascular lumen; b: subendothelial basement membrane; e and e′: adjacent endothelial cells) (×41 500).

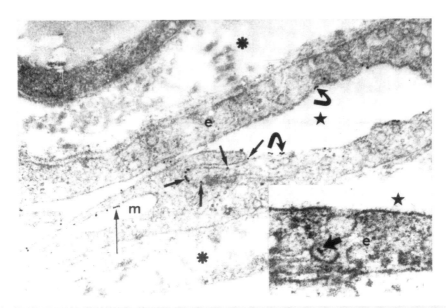

Figure 36. Mesenteric capillary of a rat with experimentally induced *E. coli* peritonitis. Intraarterial perfusion with albumin–gold was performed 24 h after provoking the disease. Particles of the tracer can be seen adsorbed to the luminal aspect of the endothelial cell membrane (curved arrows), as well as within the infundibulum of the interendothelial cell junction (short arrows). Some particles of the tracer (long thin arrow) are also present in a cytoplasmic multivesicular body (m) (*: interstitial space; e: endothelial cell; black star: capillary lumen) ($\times$ 41 500).

Inset: Another aspect of the sample taken from the same animal. Albumin–gold complexes are also present in a pinocytotic vesicle (arrow) (star: capillary lumen; e: endothelial cell) ($\times$ 84 530).

trations induced by vascular endothelial growth factor [284–286].

Water transport across endothelium of continuous capillaries was classically thought to occur almost completely via the paracellular pathway through intercellular junctions. Transcellular transport was considered to be nil.

However, the relevance of the transcellular pathway also for water has recently been brought to the forefront by the immunohistochemical identification of aquaporin-1 channels in peritoneal microvascular endothelium [287, 288], as well as in rat peritoneal mesothelium [102]. Expression of this transmembrane water channel protein in the endothelial cell surface of continuous capillaries appeared to be basically localized in plasmalemmal vesicles, and its concentration is quantitatively comparable to that seen in erythrocyte plasma membrane [289]. The presence of aquaporin–1 in microvascular endothelium provides a molecular explanation for the water permeability of some capillary beds [290], as well as a low-energy cost pathway [291] for almost 70% of the transmembrane transport of water [287]. Furthermore, this evidence confirms the predicted concept that, also during peritoneal dialysis, not less than 50% of the transperitoneal water flow occurs through ultra-small transcellular pores [94].

Summarizing the information obtained from ultrastructural and physiological studies, it can be stated that the microvascular endothelial cell should be considered a highly active structure, serving not only as a permeability barrier and an effective thromboresistant surface, but also as the location of important synthetic and other metabolic activities [180, 207].

Continuous capillaries are more permeable to larger molecules than are fenestrated capillaries [197]. Coated pits and coated vesicles are involved in receptor-mediated endocytosis, whereas the uncharged pinocytotic vesicles and transcellular channels are involved in the transfer of proteins and fluid-phase pinocytosis. The transcellular pathway plays a relevant role in the transmembrane transport of water and macromolecular plasma proteins. Additionally, all the resistances described by Nolph [75] along the pathway leading from the microvascular lumen to the abdominal cavity, are negatively charged [34, 36].

Lymphatics

The lymphatic system serves to drain, from the interstitial compartment, a range of materials such as water, proteins, colloid materials and cells [292], all elements included in the interstitial fluid. Under normal conditions fluid crosses the microvascular endothelial membrane at a rate whose magnitude depends on the Starling forces acting at each aspect of the capillary membrane, as well as on the permeability properties of the endothelial microvascular monolayer. The local autoregulation of interstitial volume is provided by automatic adjustment of the transcapillary Starling forces and lymphatic drainage [159]. Therefore, an alteration in the aforementioned forces results in interstitial accumulation of fluid which will eventually be removed by the lymphatic flow that, in situations of high capillary permeability oedema occurring during acute inflammation, can increase by a factor of ten [293]. In the abdominal cavity, lymphatics have a relevant role in the prevention of ascites [294].

Work during the last 20 years has revealed relevant evidence characterizing lymphatic structure and organization. The first stage of lymph collection occurs through a system of interstitial non-endothelial channels, or low-resistance pathways known as pre-initial lymphatics [295, 296], which have been seen in the cat and the rabbit mesentery [297].

This most peripheral part of the lymph vessel system is a completely open net of tissue channels which drain, at least in the cat mesentery, mainly along the paravascular area of the venous microvasculature, into a network of 0.5 mm long, irregularly shaped endothelial tubes, approximately 20–30 µm width [298]. By the time these tubes are completely filled they can reach a maximal diameter of up to 75 µm [299]. A single endothelial layer (Fig. 37, inset) forms these endothelial tubes defined as initial lymphatics or lymphatic capillaries [297, 299, 300].

The subendothelial area is most of the time devoid from basement membrane, as well as from a smooth muscle layer present in larger lymphatic collectors [301]. The sporadically observed patches of basement membrane have, as in blood capillaries, anionic fixed charges that can be decorated by cationic tracers [302]. Due to the absence of muscular layer, lymphatic capillaries lack the capability for spontaneous contractility [303]. However, the fact that lymphatic endothelial cells contain an abundant supply of fine actin-like filaments, 40–60 Å in diameter, arranged in bundles parallel to the long axis of the cell, led some investigators to postulate that these filaments could function as a contractile element of the lymphatic capillary wall [304, 305].

Anchoring filaments, having histochemical and ultrastructural characteristics similar to those observed in elastin-associated microfibrils, form a uniform population of fibrous elements, leading to the development of structural and functional continuity between the abluminal aspect of the lymphatic capillary endothelial cell and the elastic network of

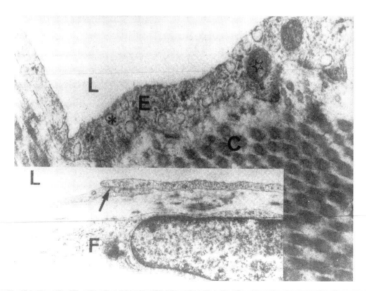

Figure 37. Partial view of a lymphatic lacuna observed in a sample of rabbit diaphragmatic peritoneum. The thin endothelial cell (E) shows numerous pinocytotic vesicles (*) and occasional mitochondria (star). Note the absence of subendothelial basement membrane (L: lacunar lumen; C: collagen fibres) (original magnification ×85 000).

Lower left inset. Lymphatic capillary of rabbit diaphragmatic peritoneum. Two adjoining endothelial cells, forming a tight junction (arrow), appear lying on the interstitial tissue. Basement membrane, as well as anchoring filaments, are not observed (L: capillary lumen; F: fibroblasts) (original magnification ×62 500).

the adjacent connective tissue [306]. The main role of these anchoring filaments is the prevention of capillary collapse, when the interstitial pressure gains strength as a consequence of expanded fluid content of the interstitial compartment [307]. This simple element enables the lymphatic system to launch a mechanism of fluid drainage that accounts for 25% of the safety factors that can prevent formation of interstitial oedema [307]. In this context it has been proposed that initial lymphatics directly sense and regulate the interstitial fluid volume [308].

The total surface area of pre-initial and initial lymphatics seems to be smaller than the total exchange area of blood microvessels [196]. Other studies on cat and rabbit mesentery showed the additional presence of flat, blind saccular structures up to 40 μm wide, with a wall made up of a simple layer of thin endothelial cells, devoid of basement membrane [196, 298].

Lymphatic endothelial cells are flat and elongated, showing an average thickness of 0.3 μm in non-nuclear areas [43, 304]. The luminal aspect of lymphatic endothelium, when exposed to cationic tracers such as cationized ferritin or ruthenium red, shows a high density of anionic fixed charges that, at times, can also be detected labelling the luminal aspect of the intercellular cleft (Fig. 38) [305, 309]. These charges prevent the adhesion of electronegatively charged blood cells to the endothelial luminal surface and may play a significant role in the movement of charged solutes from the interstitial compartment to the capillary lumen [309]. Furthermore, the absence of subendothelial and negatively charged basement membrane (Fig. 38) points at the asymmetry of the lymphatic capillary wall, that is at variance with the electric symmetry characteristic of blood capillaries.

Nuclei of endothelial cells are flattened and, on electron microscopy, appear elongated. Their irregular outline shows a thin peripheral rim of dense chromatin. Plasmalemmal vesicles [43, 310] and transendothelial channels, similar to those described for blood microvessels, are commonly observed [305]. Plasmalemmal vesicles have been shown to participate in the transcellular movement of albumin–gold complexes, from the submesothelial interstitial space to the lumen of capillary lymphatics [76] (Fig. 39). Furthermore, the endocytotic pathway has been shown up by the presence of the same tracer into cytoplasmic endosomes (Fig. 40).

Several types of interendothelial junctions have been described. Approximately 2% of the whole

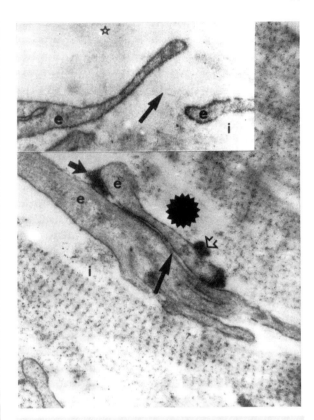

Figure 38. Mesenteric lymphatic capillary of a mouse perfused with cationized ferritin. The long arrow points at the intercellular junction formed by two adjacent endothelial cells (e). The short black arrow indicates the presence of the electropositive tracer on the luminal aspect of the intercellular junction, whereas the open arrow shows particles of ferritin decorating the endothelial luminal plasmalemma. Note the absence of subendothelial basement membrane (*: microvascular lumen. i: subendothelial interstitial space) (×41 500).

Inset. Mesenteric lymphatic capillary of an intact mouse. The arrow points at an open intercellular cleft formed by two adjacent endothelial cells (e). The junction serves as a valvular structure sensitive to the hydrostatic gradient between the interstitial space (i) and the microvascular lumen (open star) (×41 500).

junctional system consists of open junctions, showing gaps up to 100 nm width, that can, at times, be as wide as 1000 nm [305, 311]. These openings serve as a way in for macromolecular solutes such as gold-labelled albumin (Fig. 40) or cationized ferritin (Fig. 41). At times two adjoining endothelial cells overlap each other, forming a kind of valvular junction that can be easily opened by an eventual increase of interstitial pressure (Fig. 38, inset). Junctional infundibuli show anionic fixed charges similar to those observed in the luminal endothelial glycocalyx (Fig. 38). Around 10% of junctions are zonula

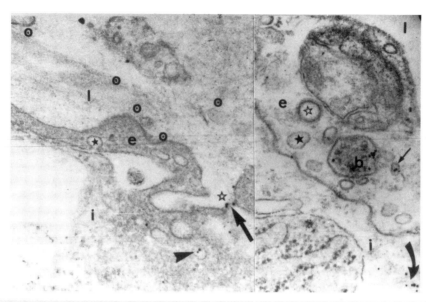

Figure 39. Diaphragmatic submesothelial lymphatic capillary taken from a mouse 10 min after intraperitoneal injection of albumin–gold complexes.
   Left inset. Albumin–gold complexes (long arrow) can be observed in their pathway through an open interendothelial cell junction (open star). More particles of the tracer are seen (open circles) within the luminal space (l) of the microvessel. Arrowhead points at albumin–gold included into a pinocytotic vesicle (i: subendothelial interstitial space; black star: plasmalemmal vesicle) (×41 500).
   Right inset. Lymphatic capillary endothelial cell (e). Albumin–gold complexes appear in an endosome (b) as well as in a pinocytotic vesicle (straight arrow). Curved arrow points at albumin–gold complexes present in the interstitium (i). Notice the absence of subendothelial basement membrane (black star: plasmalemmal vesicle; open star: coated vesicle) (×64 450).

Used with permission from *Kidney International,* **47**: 1274–84, 1995.

adherens, whereas the rest are tight junctions [299, 312]. It has been proposed that, in addition to the organized prelymphatic system [313], a small percentage of open junctions (1–6%) can account for a substantial proportion of the lymphatic pathway for fluid and small and large molecule drainage [299].

The diaphragmatic lymphatic capillary net is organized as a plexus along the submesothelial surface [314], which drains, through an intercommunicating microvascular system, into a plexus on the pleural side of the diaphragm [130]. The distribution of the whole diaphragmatic network is irregular, and varies in different species.

A prominent feature of diaphragmatic lymphatics is the presence of flattened, elongated cisternae or lacunae, approximately 0.3–0.6 cm length, with a long axis that is parallel to the long axis of the muscle fibres [314–316] (Fig. 42). The monolayer endothelial lining of the lymphatic lacunae is thin and shows no tight junctions. Adjacent cells usually overlap, forming valve-like processes, leaving an open interface that can be as wide as 12 µm. The cytoplasm of endothelial cells, basement membrane, and anchoring filaments of lymphatic lacunae are similar to those structures described for lymphatic capillaries. While anionic sites have not been observed, the glycocalyx of cisternal endothelium, when exposed to ferritin, is heavily decorated by the cationized tracer, which also appears along the open intercellular clefts [41, 317].

Diaphragmatic lymphatic lacunae, regularly connected by transverse anastomosis [115], and capillaries from the whole peritoneal lymphatic network, including the rich omental plexus [318], drain into a system of precollector, small-calibre lymph vessels that have a poorly developed smooth muscle layer underlying the endothelium. These vessels, which have semilunar valves [1, 319], drain, in turn, into the larger collecting vessels, whose diameter ranges between 40 and 200 µm [320]. The luminal aspect of the endothelial layer shows a sequence of valvular segments, with a semilunar bicuspidal valve at the distal end of each [130, 320]. The smooth muscle layer underlying the subendothelial basement membrane shows a spiral arrangement around the endo-

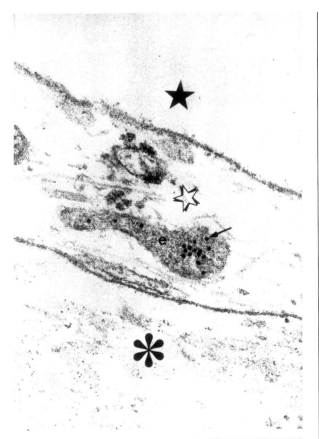

Figure 40. Diaphragmatic lymphatic capillary of a rat. The sample was taken 15 min after starting intraarterial perfusion with albumin–gold complexes. Endosome (e) present in the cytoplasm of the endothelial cell (open star) shows particles of the tracer. This may well represent the endocytotic pathway for degradation of the complex. Note the absence of subendothelial basement membrane (black star: microvascular lumen; *: interstitial tissue) (×87 000).

thelial tube that becomes more pronounced towards the downstream end of the intervalvular segment [303, 321, 322]. Distances between adjacent valves range between 0.1 and 0.6 mm [322]. Thereby, the anatomical and functional unit (lymphangion) is established, consisting of one valve and the following intervalvular segment, which measures 2–3 mm in length [323]. This collecting segment, limited by two-one way valves and an intrinsic smooth muscle layer, compresses the lymphatic lumen driving the intravascular fluid centrally into the next compartment, making up an escalated system of drainage which has, in the proximal part of each lymphangion, a valve which prevents retrograde flow [303]. The presence of valves also enables this part of the system to reach differential intraluminal pressures around 1–2 cm of water [324].

Capillary lymph that flows from the interstitium slowly moves downstream (average velocity for particles with diameter up to 5 μm = 1 μm/min) [301], drains into large collecting channels (40–200 μm diameter), and proceeds in the direction of the central venous circulation, propelled by peristaltic and rhythmic contractions of consecutive lymphangions [290, 301, 320, 325], with frequencies ranging between four and 12 contractions/minute [320, 325]. Within each lymphangion, hydrostatic pressure increases to a threshold of approximately 12 cm of water, after which the proximal valve is closed, and the downstream valve is opened. The cycle is repeated in the following segment. Contractility of lymphangions is modulated by a pacemaker site of spontaneous activity, apparently located, at least in bovine mesenteric lymphatics, in the vessel wall near the inlet valve of the unit. Activity propagates at a speed of 4 mm/s, and the ejection fraction was evaluated at 45–65% [326].

Contractions are generated by myogenic stimuli (hydrostatic pressure of 5–7 cm water) [326], and influenced by activation of α and β adrenoreceptors [327–329], histamine, leukotriene C4 and D4, platelet-activating factor [330, 331], PGF2 alpha, PGA2, PGB2 [332], bradykinin [333], and vasoactive intestinal peptide [334]. It should be noted that all the aforementioned vasoactive substances are mediators of inflammation present in high concentrations in blood and tissues during the localized or the generalized acute defense reaction [274].

Lymph flows from collectors to the thoracic duct and the right lymph duct, and finally drains into the subclavian veins. Lymphangions join larger collecting lymphatic vessels, forming a dichotomous tree that drains entire tissue regions. This arrangement has been described in the diaphragm as well as in mesentery [303, 324, 335].

Innervation of lymph vessels has been studied in the dog and cat mesentery, by means of silver stains [319]. It was shown that large lymphatic collectors have myelinated nerves that remain on the adventitial area, and non-myelinated nerve fibres that penetrate into the region of valve attachment and are considered to be the motor supply to the smooth muscle. Bovine mesenteric lymphatics show adrenergic nerve fibres in the media, as well as in the adventitia. Human mesenteric lymph collector neurotransmitters are both adrenergic and cholinergic, the former being prevalent. Lymphatic capillaries are devoid of innervation [336].

Since Starling [337, 338], it has been accepted that, besides the removal of excess interstitial tissue,

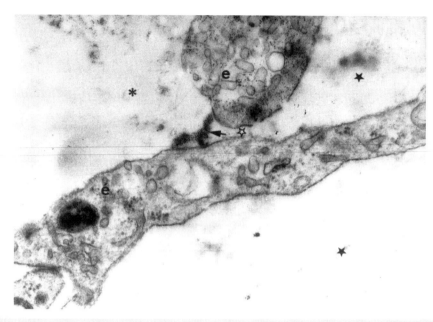

Figure 41. Mesenteric lymphatic capillary obtained from a mouse intraperitoneally injected with cationized ferritin. Particles of the tracer (arrow) can be seen entering the microvascular lumen (*) through the open interendothelial cell junction (open star). Again, note the absence of subendothelial basement membrane and anionic sites (e and e': lymphatic endothelial cells; black stars: interstitial space) (× 41 500).

the lymphatic system has the special function of absorbing protein. Normally, blood capillaries leak protein, which will not re-enter the blood vessels unless delivered by the lymphatic system [339]. It is generally accepted that the rate of lymph formation is equal to the net capillary efflux under normal physiological conditions, in order for the interstitial fluid volume to remain constant [308]. However, the mechanisms involved in the formation of lymph, at the level of the most peripheral part of the lymphatic system, are still controversial. According to Allen [340], who formulated the hydraulic theory, lymph formation is the end-result of hydraulic forces acting across initial lymphatics. Assuming that the interstitial hydrostatic pressure is zero, or even negative [157, 341], any rise will also increase the initial lymphatic flow, and oedema will eventually develop if and when the lymphatic drainage capabilities are exceeded [342–344]. This concept of increased hydrostatic pressure as the main factor in the process of lymph formation was extrapolated to the lymphatic absorption from the peritoneal cavity [345, 346]. In this context it was postulated that, during peritoneal dialysis, the intra-abdominal pressures [347, 348] modulated lymphatic drainage from the abdominal cavity well within the range of values observed in dialysed patients [163, 349]. This concept has been substantially challenged by a series

of elegant studies performed by Flessner *et al.* [164, 350], who showed that a significant proportion of the intra-abdominal fluid is lost to the abdominal wall, the rate of which is also dependent on the intra-abdominal pressure. This fluid, after being incorporated to the tissues surrounding the abdominal cavity, will be drained through the lymphatic circulation [351]. The eventual influence of the intrathoracic negative pressure upon the lymphatic downstream circulation [352] may well be an additional component of the hydrostatic forces involved in lymph progression to the venous-blood compartment.

The osmotic theory of lymph formation [353] postulates the existence of a protein-concentrating mechanism at the level of the initial lymphatics, the main result of which would be that only 10–40% of the fluid initially entering within the lymphatic network would flow downstream, back to the blood compartment, and the remaining fluid would be filtered out from the lymphatics as a protein-free solution. This process would eventually cause a high protein concentration, and an oncotic gradient between the contents of the initial lymphatics and the surrounding interstitial fluid. Other investigators have proposed a vesicular theory of lymph formation, which holds that plasmalemmal vesicles provide the major route for transendothelial transport

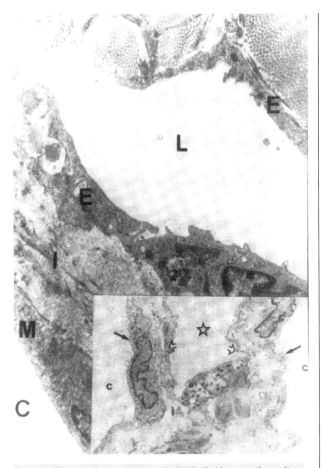

Figure 42. Lymphatic lacuna of rabbit diaphragmatic peritoneum. The wide lacunar lumen (L) is surrounded by the
lymphatic endothelium (E). Connective tissue (I) is
interposed between the lacuna and the mesothelial cell layer
(M) (G: abdominal cavity) (original magnification ×17 750).
Lower right inset. Lymphatic lacuna of rabbit mesentery.
The open star shows the lacunar lumen surrounded by a
thin endothelial layer (open arrows). Mesothelial cells (black
arrows) are covering both aspects of the mesenteric peritoneal surface (I: interstitium. C: abdominal cavity) (original
magnification ×4750).

each one could vary in different areas of the initial
lymphatic network [357].

The relevance of peritoneal lymphatics, as well as
their impact upon ultrafiltration during peritoneal
dialysis, is addressed in Chapter 6.

Peritoneal innervation

The first report announcing the presence of nerves
in the peritoneal interstitium was made by Haller in
1751 [358] and confirmed during the nineteenth
century by Ranvier and Robin who, using osmic
acid and silver nitrate, described nerve trunks,
branches and nerve endings accompanying arteries
and veins. Robinson [1] described the peritoneum
as being richly supplied with myelinated and non-
myelinated nerves (Fig. 43).

In rat mesentery, networks of adrenergic axons
innervate the principal and small arteries and arterioles. Precapillary arterioles, collecting venules and
small veins are not innervated, and are most likely
under the influence of humoral vasoactive substances [359]. Lymphatic innervation was described
in the previous section.

In 1741 Vater observed that the submesothelial
connective tissue of cat mesentery contained oval
corpuscles with a diameter of approximately
1–2 mm. In 1830 Paccini rediscovered and gave a
systemic description of this corpuscle, known as the
Vater–Paccini corpuscle [1]; it takes the form of a
non-myelinated nerve ending which, in transverse
section, appears as a sliced onion. In humans it has
been observed in the peritoneum of mesentery and
visceral ligaments, functioning as the main receptor
for perception of pressure.

Cytology of the peritoneal fluid

The peritoneal fluid of laboratory animals has classically been a favoured site for experiments dealing
with the inflammatory response [360], as well as
for those designed to analyse the biological reaction
to infection [361].

More than 50 years ago Josey and Webb realized
that fluid shifts into and out of the peritoneal cavity
could change the concentration of cells without
affecting their absolute number [362–365]. The
methodological answer to this question was given
by Seeley and colleagues, who weighed peritoneal
fluid and measured the cellular concentrations, and
so were able to estimate the absolute number of cells
[366]. Padawer and Gordon [364], after analysing

of protein, thereby creating the oncotic gradient
needed for further fluid flow between adjacent cells
or through transendothelial channels [354, 355].
This hypothesis is supported by recent studies that
have shown active transendothelial transport of
albumin in plasmalemmal vesicles [57, 356].
Figure 39 shows gold-labelled albumin transported
by plasmalemmal vesicles of a mouse diaphragmatic
lymphatic capillary.

On the other hand, it has been suggested that the
postulated mechanisms may not necessarily be
exclusive in the sense that some or all could function
simultaneously. However, the relative influence of

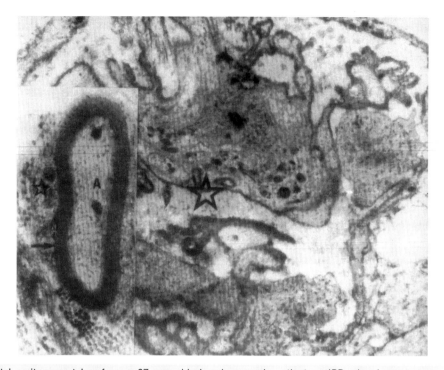

Figure 43. Parietal peritoneum taken from a 67-year-old chronic uraemic patient on IPD, showing a transversal section of an unmyelinated nerve (star) ($\times$ 12 600).
    Inset. Rabbit mesentery showing a myelinated nerve fibre (star: Schwann cell cytoplasma; arrow: myelin; A: axon) (original magnification $\times$ 47 400).

the cellular elements present in peritoneal fluid of eight different normal mammals, concluded that the most frequently observed cells were eosinophils, mast cells and mononuclears (including lymphocytic and macrophagic elements). Total cell numbers, as well as percentages of the different cells, varied greatly among the species examined. Neutrophils were never observed in normal animals. Total absolute counts were higher for females than for males, as well as for older animals compared with younger ones. In the individual animal, under normal conditions, the number of cells present within the abdominal cavity was constant [364].

Observation of peritoneal fluid obtained from healthy women showed that macrophages and mesothelial cells contributed more than 70% of the whole cell population, whereas lymphocytes and polymorphonuclears contributed to a lesser extent (18% and 7% respectively) [367]. Other investigators observed that at the midphase of the menstrual cycle, macrophages, which comprised 82–98% of the peritoneal cells, showed morphological as well as biochemical heterogeneity and were seen to be involved in phagocytosis of erythrocytes [368] (Fig. 44). However, other studies showed up to four different

types of cytological patterns in peritoneal fluid of women during the course of the menstrual cycle, in all of which mesothelial cells contributed substantially to the total cell counts. The paramenstrual type was in most cases haemorrhagic and highly cellular [369]. Ciliocytophtoria, anucleated remnants of ciliated mesothelial cells, can be occasionally observed in effluent dialysate, basically in young women. Inability to identify these structures can mislead the laboratory team as well as the physician to search for parasitic or fungal contamination [370].

The apparently puzzling effect of intraperitoneal saline inducing substantial influx of neutrophils into the abdominal cavity, which was observed long ago [361], was not confirmed when the experiments were carried out using sterile techniques. Bacterial lipopolysaccharides proved to be very effective in producing intraperitoneal exudate rich in cells [365]. This phenomenon was inhibited by prior intraperitoneal injection of cortisone [371].

In humans, sterile inflammatory effusions are characterized by a rich cellular content including neutrophils, lymphocytes, macrophages, mesothelial cells, eosinophils and basophils; usually in that order

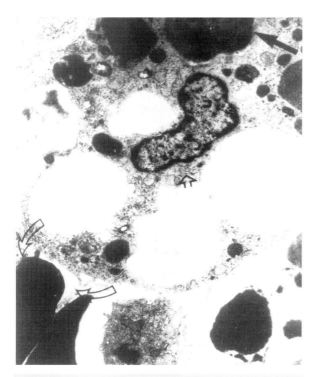

Figure 44. Peritoneal effluent obtained from a chronic urae-mic patient on peritoneal dialysis. The macrophages depicted in the figure show phagolysosomes digesting erythrocytes (black arrow). Note the presence of rough endoplasmic retic-ulum (short open arrow) near the nucleus (n). The former normally appears in macrophages when the cells are involved in phagocytic activity. The curved open arrows are pointing to cell processes engulfing red blood cells (× 8600).

of frequency [372]. The presence of macrophages, mesothelial cells, lymphocytes, eosinophils and even plasma cells has been confirmed by electron micro-scope studies [373–375].

Peritoneal eosinophilia (eosinophils > 10–50%) has been experimentally induced by intraperitoneal injection of iodine, chalk, nucleic acids, pilocarpine, haemoglobin or red blood cells, egg albumin, gold salts, mineral and vegetable oils, hydatidic fluid, and saline [372, 376]. On the other hand, intraperitoneal injection of bacteria and/or bacterial endotoxins induces a massive migration of neutrophils and monocytes into the peritoneal cavity [364, 377, 378].

The information presented above suggests that the cell content of effluent peritoneal dialysate is likely to be modified by so many factors that a concise description of a standardized cytological pattern becomes extremely difficult. There are, how-ever, a few aspects of peritoneal effluent dialysate which have been defined: (a) patients on CAPD have total cell counts up to 50 cells/ml [379]. (b) The

population of resident peritoneal cells observed in patients on long-term peritoneal dialysis is basically made up by macrophages (around 50% of the popula-tion), and lower prevalence of lymphocytes, mast cells and mesothelial cells [379–382]. (c) During infection there is a substantial increase in total cell number [383], as well as in the proportion of neu-trophils [379–382]. (d) Fluid eosinophilia is a basic component of the still ill-defined eosinophilic perito-nitis [384–386].

Ultrastructure of peritoneal fluid cells

Free-floating mesothelial cells are round or oval in shape and show a central, round nucleus (Fig. 45). Occasionally, binucleated mesothelial cells can be observed (Fig. 46). Nuclear chromatin is quite evenly distributed (Fig. 47, inset) and a small nucleolus may be observed. Numerous slender and sometimes branching microvilli emerge from the cytoplasmic membrane [373, 375, 387–389]. Branching microvilli, similar to those observed in human embryos [14], can be quite crowded in some cells, whereas in others they are scarce [375] (Fig. 47, inset). The glycocalyx covering the luminal aspect of the plasmalemma is endowed with electro-negative fixed charges as shown in preparations exposed to the cationic tracer ruthenium red (Fig. 48). Mitochondria, numerous cisternae of rough endoplasmic reticulum and free ribosomes are mainly located in the outer part of the cytoplasm, and so are pinocytotic vesicles [373, 389]. The pres-ence of intermediate-size filaments, perinuclear or irregularly scattered along the cytoplasm, has been documented in young free-floating mesothelial cells [372, 374], as well as in those recently implanted on the peritoneal surface (Fig. 49). These free-floating mesothelial cells should be distinguished from des-quamated, degenerating mesothelial cells wandering in the peritoneal fluid (Fig. 46) [390]. Free-floating mesothelial cells in culture undergo mitotic activity [155].

Macrophages, which can be observed in large numbers, usually show an irregular and, at times, kidney-shaped nucleus with distorted masses of chromatin concentrated along the nuclear mem-brane (Figs 44 and 45). The cytoplasmic outline of macrophages is irregular, with thin processes of vari-able length which, at times, engulf degenerated cells (Fig. 44) or take the form of signet-ring macrophages (Fig. 5, inset). Mitochondria, a small Golgi complex and phagolysosomes are more evident when the cell is involved in phagocytic activity (Fig. 44).

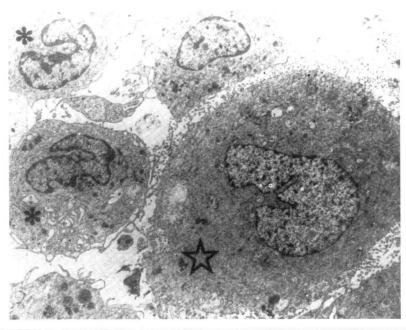

Figure 45. Effluent dialysate obtained from a non-infected uraemic patient, showing a floating mesothelial cell (star), as well as macrophages (*) (×6900).

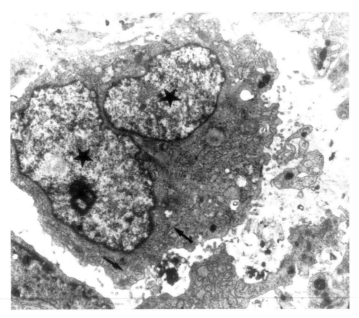

Figure 46. Binucleated mesothelial cell observed in effluent fluid from a patient on CAPD. Note the abundance of rough endoplasmic reticulum (arrows) (stars: nuclei of mesothelial cell) (×8600).

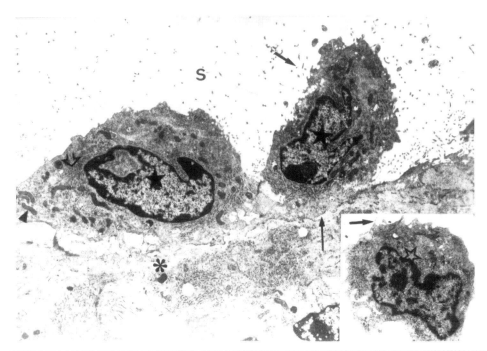

Figure 47. Sample taken from the parietal peritoneum of a patient on CAPD. Two recently implanted young and active mesothelial cells (black stars), showing numerous mitochondria (arrowhead), rough endoplasmic reticulum (open arrow) and microvilli (short arrow). The cell on the right is forming its own basement membrane (long arrow) (*: submesothelial connective tissue; S: peritoneal space) (× 6900).
Inset. Free-floating mesothelial cell (open star), seen in effluent dialysate of a CAPD patient (arrow: microvilli) (× 5600).

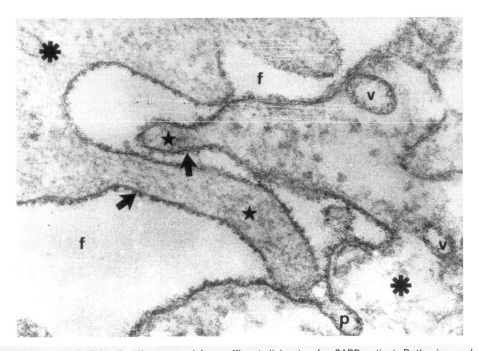

Figure 48. Wandering mesothelial cells (*) recovered from effluent dialysate of a CAPD patient. Ruthenium red decorates the electronegative plasmalemmal glycocalyx of microvilli (thick arrows), as well as that covering the internal aspect of a coated pit (p) and a pinocytotic vesicle (v) (f: peritoneal fluid) (× 87 000).

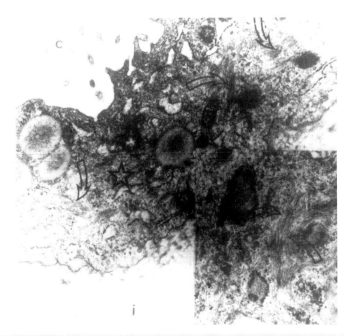

Figure 49. Biopsy of parietal peritoneum taken from a chronic uraemic patient 16 h after interruption of peritoneal dialysis. This recently implanted ($\sim$4–5 days) mesothelial cell (star) shows microvilli on its luminal aspect facing the abdominal cavity (c). The open arrows point to intermediate-size filaments. The basement membrane is still lacking (i: interstitium) ($\times$15 400).
Lower right inset. Intermediate-size filaments at higher magnification (open arrows) ($\times$24 600).

The ultrastructural aspect of inflammatory cells that eventually appear in the peritoneal fluid is similar to that classically described for other tissues.

Peritoneal ultrastructural changes during long-term peritoneal dialysis

Mesothelial cells are extremely sensitive to minor injury. Mild drying or wetting of rat caecal peritoneum for 5 min induced mesothelial cell degeneration and detachment, and severe interstitial oedema [391, 392]. Biopsies taken from CAPD patients also showed detachment of mesothelial cells (Fig. 20) and similar severe degenerative changes: widened intercellular spaces (Fig. 50) between mesothelial cells [393] and variable degrees of interstitial oedema (Figs 51, 52 and 53) [393, 394, 395].

In one of the deepest analyses of this topic, Di Paolo and colleagues described the (at that time) unexplained focal absence of microvilli, intercalated with areas where the other cells show a normal prevalence of these cytoplasmic prolongations (Figs 6 and 54) [23, 393]. This change is an early manifestation of impending apoptosis [25, 396–398], the prevalence of which has been shown to be increased

in mesothelial cells exposed *in vitro* [399] as well as *in vivo* (Fig. 7) to glucose-enriched dialysis solutions.

Cell organelles are also affected by the dialysis solutions. Mitochondria frequently show a condensed appearance with increased material density, blurring of cristae and fusions of the inner membrane (Fig. 6), rating as stage III in the classification of Trump describing mitochondrial profiles following cell injury [400]. This situation of cell injury is still compatible with cell survival [401], even though it indicates impaired ability for ATP synthesis. Mitochondrial stage III can be observed in cells undergoing either necrosis or apoptosis [402]. Lamellar bodies (Fig. 55, right inset) described in human mesothelium not exposed to dialysis solutions [403], as well as lipid droplets (Fig. 46) are frequently observed in the mesothelial cytoplasm of patients treated by CAPD, and in that of animals exposed to high glucose concentration fluids (Fig. 56).

Substantial hypertrophy of the rough endoplasmic reticulum (Fig. 57, left inset) is an additional pattern commonly seen in samples of mesothelium taken from CAPD patients. This same material observed under electron and light microscopy revealed the presence of large binucleated cells in the mesothelial monolayer (Fig. 20; Fig. 57, right inset), some of

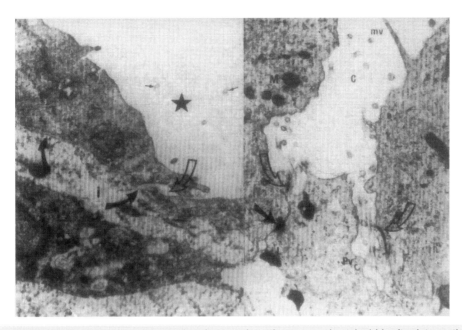

Figure 50. *Left.* Parietal peritoneum taken from a chronic uraemic patient, approximately 14 h after interruption of peritoneal dialysis. A few transversally sectioned microvilli (small arrows) can be seen in the peritoneal cavity (star). Two young adjacent mesothelial cells are separated by an open intercellular junction (open arrow). The basement membrane (black arrows) is, at times, interrupted (i: interstitium) (original magnification ×16 250).
Right. Another area of the same biopsy. The general appearance of the tissue is quite close to that observed in normals and to that reported by Ryan and Majno in rats, 7 days after injury. Note the presence of microvilli (mv), tight junctions (open arrows) and a desmosome (black arrow) (Pv: pinocytotic vesicles; M: mitochondria: L: lysosome; C: abdominal cavity) (original magnification ×16 250).

them exfoliating at times from the peritoneal luminal aspect (Fig. 20).

Furthermore, studies in rats treated for 6 weeks with daily intraperitoneal injections of a high-glucose-concentration dialysis solution showed a substantially increased mesothelial cell thickness [404]. These morphological alterations were interpreted as a reaction of the exposed cells to the continuous and long-term contact with unphysiological dialysis solutions. This concept was supported by evidence indicating that cultured mesothelial cells acutely [405–409] or chronically [410] exposed to dialysis solutions showed evidence of substantial functional and structural damage.

New challenges appeared after the early years of CAPD: biocompatibility of the dialysis solutions [411–416], the role of mesothelial cells in the defense mechanisms of the peritoneal cavity [417–419], and the eventual relevance of the mesothelial monolayer in the mechanisms of peritoneal permeability. On the other hand, research based only on ultrastructural observation of the mesothelium (electron microscopy) and light microscopy performed in biopsies taken from patients, carries some limitations. In patients, sequential observations

(biopsies) cannot be performed, the population of patients will be characterized by a substantial heterogeneity, and the circumstances and timing prevailing when the biopsy is obtained will also make difficult the evaluation and classification of data. In this sense the obtained information will deal mainly with reactions of the entire peritoneum as an organ in response to the detrimental effects of the dialysis solution, and the effects of infection and other complications inherent in the therapeutic procedure. Furthermore, electron microscopy provides information on a limited number of cells. On the other hand, studies on cultures examine specific reactions of cells that are exposed for minutes, or a few hours, to experimental solutions, the physicochemical composition of which remains constant. This situation is much different from the continuously changing steady-state characteristic of peritoneal dialysis [420]. Therefore, having the feeling that a complementary approach was to be found, we developed the experimental method of population analysis of mice mesothelium, based on the method of imprints originally designed by Efskind [27], and later refined by Raftery and Whitaker [421, 422]. This experimental model, in which animals receive daily

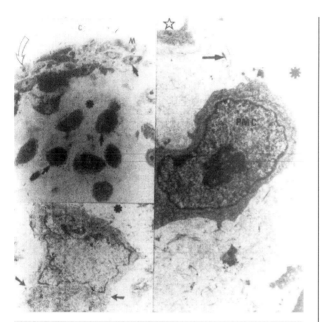

Figure 51. Biopsy taken from a chronic uraemic patient, 14 h after interruption of peritoneal dialysis.

Upper left. Mesothelial cell precursors (black arrows) appear to be progressing towards the peritoneal surface facing the abdominal cavity (C). One of these cells (open arrows) is already implanted on the luminal surface of the peritoneum. The elongated mesothelial cell (M) shows a nucleus quite similar to that of the precursors. The interstitium (*) is oedematous. This situation is similar to that observed by Ryan and Majno 3 days after experimentally induced severe mesothelial injury (original magnification × 400).

Lower left. This submesothelial interstitial cell (arrows) is interpreted as a mesothelial cell precursor. The cytoplasm shows protrusions and indentations. The irregularly shaped nucleus (N) shows fine and evenly distributed chromatin with a dense rim along the nuclear membrane. The presence of numerous cisternae of rough endoplasmic reticulum (R) indicates the high metabolic activity of this cell. The Golgi complex (G) is poorly developed as is usually observed in stem cells and fast-growing cells (*: interstitium) (original magnification × 10 450).

Right. This cell is interpreted as a primitive mesenchymal cell (PMC). The nucleus is oval, with some irregularities and shows a granular and even distribution of chromatin. A fine chromatin rim underlines the nuclear membrane. The nucleolus is prominent. These cells are usually arranged along interstitial blood capillaries (star). Note collagen fibres (arrow) between the cell and the blood capillary (*: interstitium) (× 4400).

intraperitoneal injections of a dialysis solution, provides the possibility of *in-vivo* exposure and practically *in-situ* observation of the mesothelial monolayer at any given time, during the period of exposure and that of recovery [28]. Studies using this experimental set-up concluded that mesothelium exposed to glucose-enriched dialysis solutions devel-

ops a hypertrophic phenotype, characterized by increased enzymatic activity at the level of the cell membrane: Na,K,ATP-ase (Fig. 58), alkaline phosphatase and 5-nucleotidase, and cytoplasmic enzymes such as acid phosphatase, cytochrome oxidase (Fig. 59) and glucose-6-phosphatase (Figs 60 and 61) [423]. Additional parameters indicating the hypertrophic change were reduced density distribution of the mesothelial cell population derived from increased mean cell and cytoplasmic surface area, and the substantially high prevalence of large (up to three times) multinucleated cells (up to seven nuclei) (Fig. 62) [28, 276, 424]. This pattern of increased mean cellular surface, in addition to the fact that Slater *et al.* [404] reported an increased mean cell thickness in mesothelium of mice exposed for 6 weeks to daily intraperitoneal injections of 4.25% glucose lactated fluid, suggests that after long-term exposure to this dialysis solution cells had a substantially higher volume. Large multinucleated cells have been also described in effluent fluid of rabbits dialysed with high glucose concentration solutions [425]. These hypertrophic changes showed a dose-dependent relationship with the concentration of glucose: the higher the concentration of the aforementioned osmotic agent, the more marked the manifestations of cell hypertrophy [28, 276]. These changes bore no relationship to the pH [28, 276], or with the osmotic pressure of the solution, since they were not observed in mesothelial cells of mice exposed to dialysis fluid, having mannitol in iso-osmolar concentration the same as the osmotic agent [426]. Furthermore, exposure of the mesothelial monolayer to a glucose-free, lactated dialysis fluid, using the same experimental set-up, failed to induce any of the hypertrophic changes observed during exposure to glucose-enriched solutions [427].

The mitotic rate observed in intact mice (0.33%) was not far from the 0.25% prevalence previously reported by another laboratory using a different methodological approach [428]. However, in one of our early studies [28], we detected a substantial increase in the prevalence of mitosis only after a short (2 h) exposure to high glucose concentration (4.25%) dialysis solution (Figs 63 and 64), whereas at the end of the following period the mitotic rate was nil. This intriguing development was further investigated using the same experimental model of population analysis, injecting a high glucose concentration fluid (4.25%) for 30 consecutive days [429]. Samples were taken before and 2 h after one daily intraperitoneal injection of the high glucose concentration (4.25%) lactated-experimental solution. As

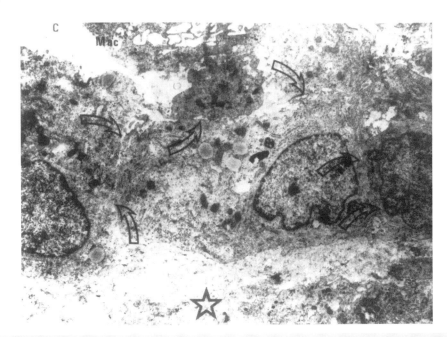

Figure 52. Biopsy of parietal peritoneum taken from a chronic uraemic patient 13 h after interruption of peritoneal dialysis. Note adjacent recently implanted mesothelial cells touching one another (open arrows), forming new intercellular junctions. There is no evidence of basement membrane. This situation is similar to that experimentally observed by Ryan and Majno 3–4 days after severe mesothelial injury (C: abdominal cavity; Mac: macrophage; star: interstitium) (original magnification ×5600).

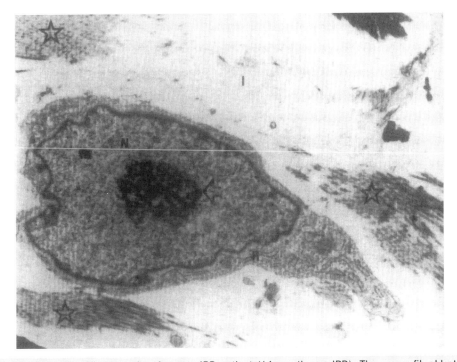

Figure 53. Biopsy of parietal peritoneum taken from an IPD patient (14 months on IPD). The young fibroblast depicted in the figure shows irregular cytoplasmic outline. The nucleus (N) is large, irregular with faint, widely distributed chromatin, which is concentrated at the nuclear periphery, forming a thin rim. Note a large, granular and central nucleolus (open arrow). The interstitium shows bundles of collagen fibres (open stars) as well as large areas of oedema (I) (R: endoplasmic reticulum) (×8600).

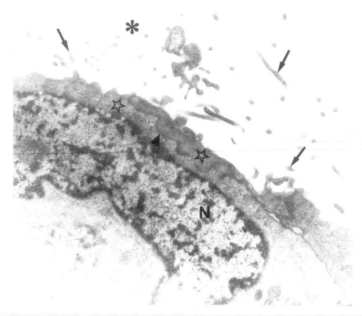

Figure 54. Parietal peritoneum of a patient on CAPD. Two adjacent mesothelial cells (open stars) show the normal presence of microvilli (arrows) (*: peritoneal space; arrowhead: intercellular junction; N: nucleus of mesothelial cell) ($\times$ 15 400).

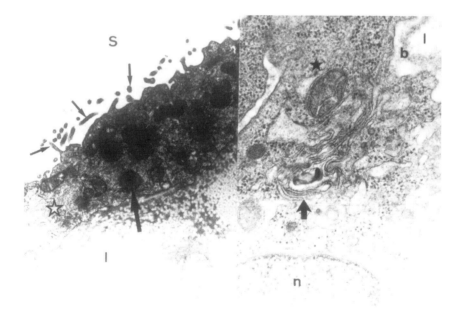

Figure 55. *Left.* Mesothelial cell (open star) observed in a biopsy of parietal peritoneum taken from a patient on CAPD. Note the presence of lipid droplets (long arrow) in the cytoplasm (S: peritoneal space; small arrows: microvilli; I: submesothelial interstitial space) ($\times$ 24 600).
Right. Lamellar body (arrow) in the cytoplasm (star) of a mesothelial cell seen in parietal peritoneum of another CAPD patient (n: nucleus of mesothelial cell; b: submesothelial basement membrane; I: interstitial space) ($\times$ 35 000).

shown in Fig. 65, this early acceleration of the cell cycle was maintained only during the first 3 days of exposure, reaching a prevalence of mitosis near zero on the 4th day (eight per 10 000 cells). This low prevalence lasted during the rest of the follow-up period (30 days). Additionally, mice exposed to lac-tate-free, high glucose concentration showed the same hypertrophic changes observed in animals treated with the commercially available high glucose solutions. This hypertrophied appearance, coupled to an extremely low mitotic activity observed *in vivo* as well as *in vitro* after long-term exposure [410],

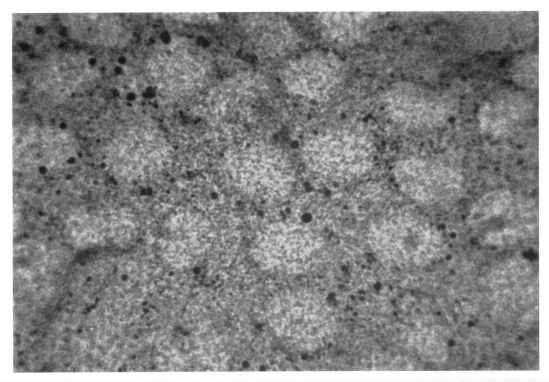

Figure 56. Mesothelial imprint taken from a mouse treated for 30 days with one daily intraperitoneal injection of high glucose (4.25%) dialysis fluid. The black dots are lipid droplets (Sudan black; ×1000).

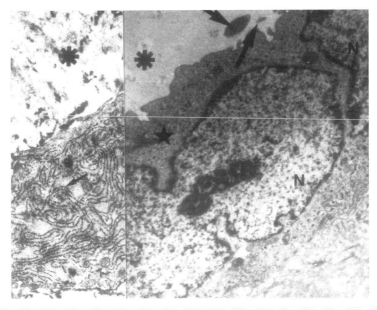

Figure 57. *Right.* Large binucleated mesothelial cell seen in parietal peritoneum of a CAPD patient (N and N′: nuclei of mesothelial cell; star: cytoplasm; arrows: microvilli; *: peritoneal space) (×24 600).
Left. Another mesothelial cell from the same biopsy. The arrow points at hypertrophic endoplasmic reticulum (*: peritoneal space) (×24 600).

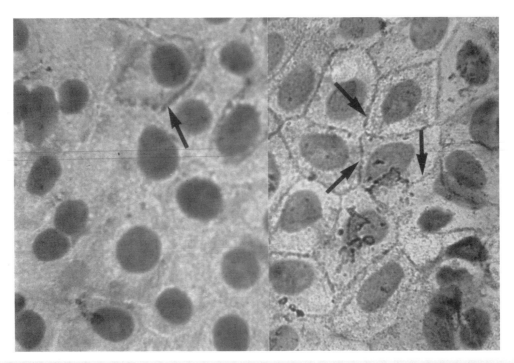

Figure 58. *Left.* Imprint taken from an intact mouse. Arrow points at the cell membrane of one mesothelial cell, showing positive staining for Na,K,ATPase.
Right. This sample was taken from a mouse exposed to 4.25% glucose-enriched dialysis fluid for 30 consecutive days. Note the substantial increased enzymatic activity (arrows) (Guth and Albers staining; ×1000).

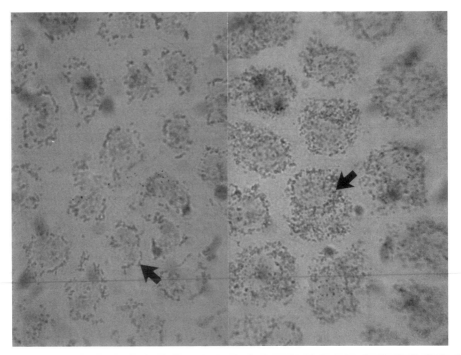

Figure 59. *Left.* Cytochrome-oxidase cytoplasmic activity (arrow points at granules) in a mesothelial cell imprint taken from an intact unexposed mouse (anterior liver surface) (DAB method of Seligman *et al.*; ×1000).
Right. This imprint was recovered from a mouse exposed to 4.25% glucose-enriched dialysis fluid for 30 consecutive days. Note the substantial increase of both the enzymatic activity (arrow) and the size of the cytoplasmic compartment (same staining and magnification).

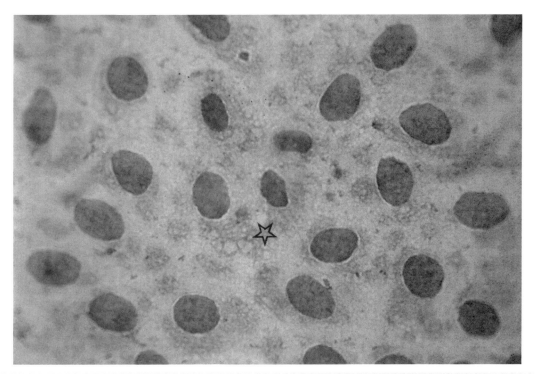

Figure 60. Visceral mesothelium of an intact mouse. Open star indicates staining of cytoplasmic glucose-6-phosphatase (lead method of Wachstein and Meisel; ×1000).

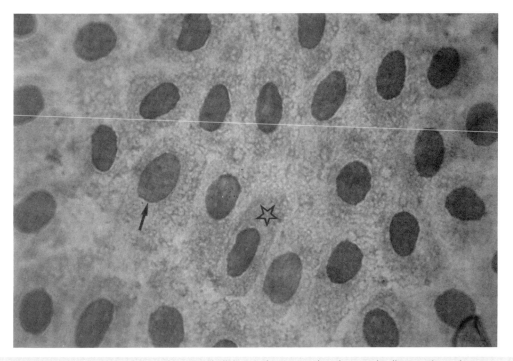

Figure 61. This material was obtained from the mesothelial monolayer covering the anterior liver surface of a mouse treated for 30 days with intraperitoneal injections of 4.25% glucose-enriched dialysis solution. Note the increased activity of the cytoplasmic glucose-6-phosphatase (open star pointing to the granules) (arrow: nucleus of mesothelial cell) (lead staining method of Wachstein and Meisel; ×1000).

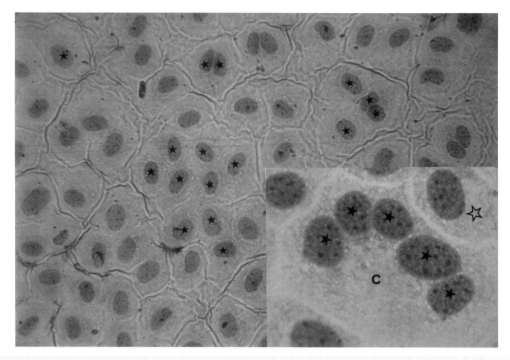

Figure 62. Mice exposed to high glucose concentration (4.25%) dialysis fluids for long periods of time (at least 30 days) can show as much as 50% of multinucleated cells (one star: mononuclear cell; two stars: binucleated cell; three stars: trinucleated cell; four stars: cell with four nuclei; six stars: cell showing six nuclei) (haematoxylin–eosin; ×400).

Inset. Imprint taken from the same mouse. Huge mesothelial cell (c) showing five nuclei. Compare with the normal size of a mononuclear cell (open star) (haematoxylin–eosin; ×1000).

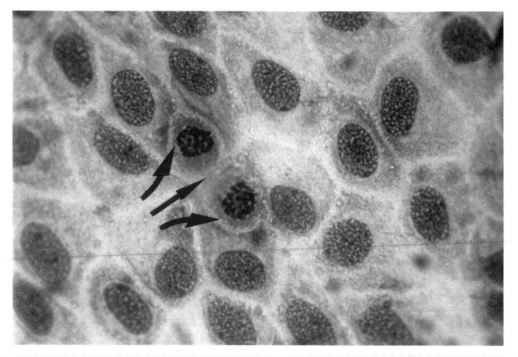

Figure 63. Normal, unexposed and unstimulated mesothelium shows a very low proportion of cells in mitosis at any given time. This photograph shows a mitotic cell at the time of cytokinesis (arrows) (haematoxylin–eosin; 1000).

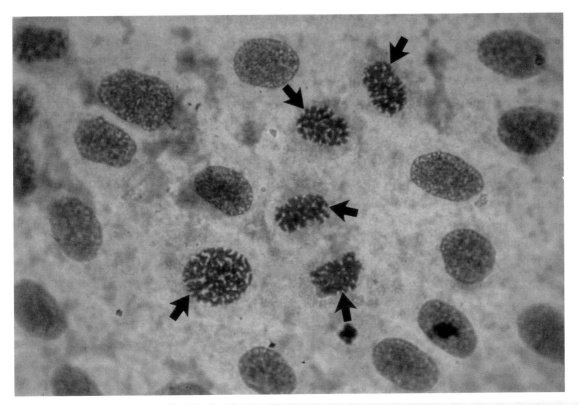

Figure 64. Sample of visceral mesothelium recovered from a mouse 2 h after one intraperitoneal injection of 4.25% glucose-enriched dialysis fluid. The photograph shows a substantial increase in the prevalence of cells in mitosis (arrows) (haematoxylin–eosin; ×1000).

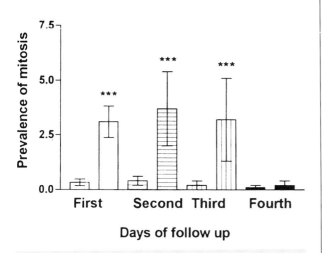

Figure 65. Bars at each time interval show prevalence of mitosis on each group of 10 mice, before and 2 h after the once-a-day intraperitoneal injection of the high glucose concentration (4.25%) lactate-free dialysis solution. The early acceleration of cell growth lasted only 3 days, after which the prevalence of mitosis remained of nil during the rest of the follow-up period (30 days).

indicates that glucose, in high concentration, induces in the exposed mesothelial monolayer the development of an hypertrophic phenotype of multinucleated (derived from defective cytokinesis) senescent cells, with low regenerative capabilities. This substantial change in the cell cycle of the mesothelial cell population was not related to the low pH, the presence of lactate, or to the high osmolality of the dialysis solution, but appeared specifically connected to the high concentration of glucose in the dialysis solution [28, 276, 426, 427]. Additionally, use of high glucose concentration in dialysis solutions is associated with a significant reduction of mesothelial cell viability (Figs 9 and 66).

What could be the link of high glucose concentration to these substantial changes of the cell cycle? Several reports have shown evidence indicating that different cell types, exposed to hydrogen peroxide, display a reduced rate of proliferation, increased multinucleation, expanded cell size, higher protein content indicating cellular hypertrophy, premature senescence, as well as higher prevalence of apoptosis

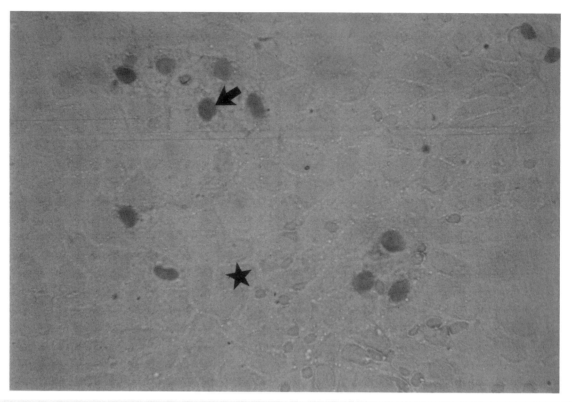

Figure 66. Trypan-blue exclusion performed in a sample of visceral mesothelium (anterior liver surface) recovered from a mouse after being injected for 30 consecutive days with high glucose (4.25%) dialysis fluid. The prevalence of non-viable cells (arrow) is higher than that seen in controls. Compare with Fig. 9 (star: viable cell) (× 400).

[430–432]. Additional studies have shown the existence of a dose-related effect. Indeed, low levels of oxidants potentiate cell growth signals and enhance proliferation, whereas higher oxidant concentrations can block cell proliferation which, in turn, results in premature senescence and the consequent activation of the mechanisms leading to apoptotic cell death [433–435].

High glucose concentration (20 mmol/L), and the subsequent increased generation of oxygen-reactive species derived from glucose auto-oxidation, has been shown to induce a delayed replication of human endothelial cells in culture [436]. In this sense, the fact that mesothelial cells in culture significantly increased the generation of hydrogen peroxide when exposed to high glucose concentration (24 mmol/L), coupled to the observation that 24–27 mmol/L concentration of D-glucose (432–480 mg/100 ml), and not equimolar concentrations of L-glucose or raffinose, induced a substantial impairment of hydrogen peroxide degradation by human endothelial and mesothelial cells [437, 438], are further arguments pointing at the D-glucose-specific metabolism, and the subsequent

increased generation of reactive oxygen species, as being the more suitable candidates to be blamed for the altered mesothelial cell cycle observed in our experimental animals. Therefore, it may be hypothesized that the D-glucose-dependent cell damage is a function of both the reduced production of scavengers, and the increased generation of reactive oxygen species [439], not only by the mesothelial cells, but also by the peritoneal phagocytes [440]. The fact that Amadori and AGE products are a source of H_2O_2 formation *in vitro* [441], and that glycation of peritoneal tissues is rapidly increased after 2 h of exposure to a 2.5% glucose dialysis fluid [442], suggests that these substances may well be an additional source of oxidative stress, acting on the exposed mesothelium.

All these elements, premature senescence due to accelerated cycle of the cell population, in addition to reduced viability, can be at the origin of areas of the peritoneal surface devoid from the normally present mesothelial monolayer observed in CAPD patients [443], as well as in experimental animals (Fig. 67). It may well be that a failure of the regenerative capabilities of the mesothelium can lead to

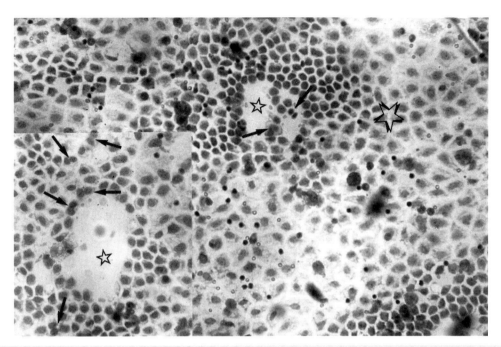

Figure 67. Imprint taken from a mouse after 7 days of recovery. The peritoneal cavity was exposed for 30 days to a high glucose (4.25%) dialysis solution. Open small star was placed in an area of the sample devoid of mesothelium. Arrows point at mitotic cells. Compare the higher density distribution of small cells in the mesothelial surface surrounding the area free from mesothelium, with the lower density observed in other part of the sample (double large star) (haematoxylin–eosin; × 160).

Inset. Another part of the same preparation. Several mitotic cells can be seen surrounding the area free from mesothelium (arrows) (haematoxylin–eosin; × 160).

repair the desertic peritoneal area, by means of fibrous tissue [444, 445]. This complication covers a wide range of morphological alterations starting from peritoneal opacification, passing through the tanned peritoneum syndrome, and finally reaching replacement of the serosal layer by fibrous tissue. This situation develops, in some patients, in the fearful syndrome of sclerosing encapsulating peritonitis (Fig. 68) [446, 447], in which a thickened, fibrous sheet of tissue envelops the small intestine. Fibrous bands may be present compromising spleen, liver and stomach, as well as pelvic organs. Light microscopy in both situations reveals serosal fibrosis and its worst consequence, sclerosing peritonitis, total absence of the mesothelial monolayer, replaced by a thick layer of connective fibrous tissue. Sclerosing peritonitis has been reported as idiopathic [448], associated with the use of some β-blockers such as practolol [449], propranolol [450], or timolol [451], as well as to metroprolol [452], and intraperitoneally administered antibiotics such as tetracycline [453]. In CAPD patients the origin of this complication is still ill-defined. Many possible factors have been invoked (acetate, hyperosmolarity, recurrent peritonitis, glucose, antiseptics, intraperitoneal antibiotics, bacterial endotoxins), even though there is

no available evidence clearly demonstrating specific relevance for any of them [444, 454]. Experimental studies have suggested that a substantial decrease in the mesothelial fibrinolytic activity could be the most likely initiating mechanism [455–457]. Increased thickness of the submesothelial collagenous layer, apparently leading to a decreased peritoneal ultrafiltration potential, has also been reported [395].

Some researchers have reported small plastic particles [393, 395] as well as cytoplasmic inclusions of crystals (Fig. 69), both probably resulting from the use of contaminated dialysis solutions or defective lines and/or bags.

It has been shown that the mesothelium has powerful regenerative capabilities [391, 392]. Comparison of experimental observations with those obtained from patients on maintenance peritoneal dialysis suggests that most of the observed peritoneal ultrastructural changes are the end-results of two processes occurring simultaneously: mesothelial injury and regeneration [458].

Biopsies taken from IPD patients approximately 14–16 h after completion of peritoneal dialysis showed peritoneal areas denuded of mesothelium and covered only by smooth muscle cells. Round,

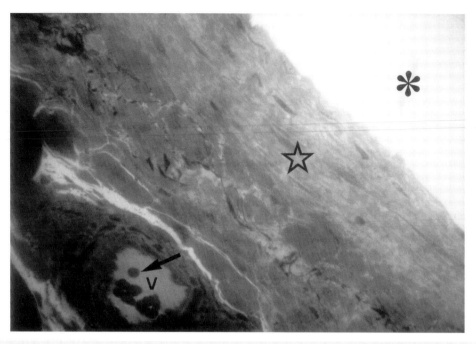

Figure 68. Biopsy of parietal peritoneum. The patient developed total membrane failure after being treated with CAPD for 39 months, at the time the biopsy was taken. Note the absence of mesothelium on the peritoneal surface facing the abdominal cavity (*). Huge amounts of fibrous tissue replaced the missing monolayer (open star). Thickness of the repair tissue ranges between 163 and 175 µm. Distance between the peritoneal cavity and the venule (v) is around 190 µm. With the diagnosis of peritoneal sclerosis the patient was referred to haemodialysis (compare with Fig. 10) (haematoxylin–eosin; × 400).

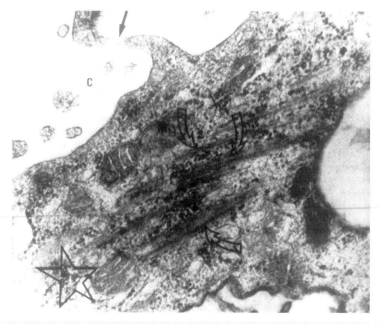

Figure 69. Biopsy of parietal peritoneum taken from a chronic uraemic patient, 10 days after interruption of peritoneal dialysis. This patient was on peritoneal dialysis for 7 months. The mesothelial cell (star) depicted in the figure shows crystalline inclusions (open arrows), mitochondria (M), smooth endoplasmic reticulum (framed by the open star), as well as microvilli (black arrow) (C: abdominal cavity) (× 50 720).

mononuclear, wandering mesothelial cells coming up from the peritoneum and, at times, macrophages were observed settling at the injured areas (Fig. 5; Fig. 70, inset). These findings resemble those made by Ryan *et al.* [391] 24 h after experimental mesothelial injury. Other areas of the same biopsies showed recently implanted young mesothelial cells (Figs 47 and 70). Both the mesothelial basement membrane and microvilli were absent. Adjoining mesothelial cells occasionally appeared forming new intercellular junctions which were still more or less open (Fig. 50, left; Fig. 70). The submesothelial interstitium was grossly oedematous (Figs 52 and 53). Similar ultrastructural features were observed experimentally 3 days after mesothelial injury [391, 392].

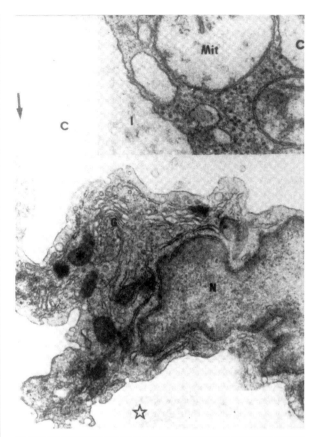

Figure 71. Mesentery of rat. The animal was sacrificed after 14 consecutive intraperitoneal injections of 0.2% furfural, on a daily basis. The young mesothelial cell appearing in this electron micrograph shows some microvilli (black arrow), an irregularly shaped nucleus (N), hypertrophic Golgi complex (G), and mitochondria (*). The normally observed submesothelial membrane is absent. The interstitial space (I) is grossly oedematous. A few collagen fibres (star) can be seen at the bottom (original magnification × 24 600).

Upper right inset. A different mesothelial cell of the same sample showing marked mitochondrial swelling (Mit) as well as absence of basement membrane (C: abdominal cavity; I: interstitium) (original magnification × 50 720).

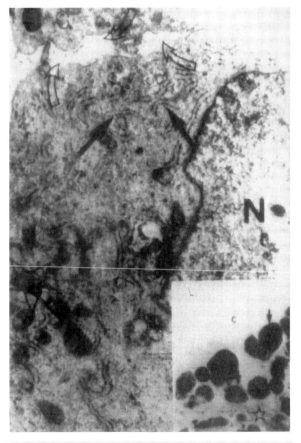

Figure 70. Parietal peritoneum of a patient on IPD. The biopsy was taken 13 h after peritoneal dialysis was interrupted. This electron micrograph shows two recently implanted new mesothelial cells, still separated by a wide intercellular space (open arrows). The cytoplasm is rich in rough endoplasmic reticulum (black arrows) and mitochondria (open star) (N: nucleus) (× 19 200).

Lower right inset. Wandering mesothelial cells (arrows) coming from the peritoneal space (c) are repopulating the denuded peritoneal surface. The smaller round cells are macrophages (original magnification × 400).

Other specimens, taken from patients approximately 14–16 h after peritoneal dialysis, showed young mesothelial cells building a new basement membrane (Figs 18 and 50), as well as new microvilli which sometimes took on the worm-like appearance of micropinocytosis vermiformis (Fig. 18). These were reminiscent of the branching microvilli observed in mesothelial cells of human embryos in the 5th–6th week of gestation [14]. This sequence of mesothelial regeneration is compatible with that observed 4–5 days after experimental mesothelial injury [391]. Biopsies taken 10 or more days after the last peritoneal dialysis had a normal mesothelial lining which, in one case, showed intracytoplasmic crystalline inclusions (Fig. 69).

In summary, studies performed on PD patients disclosed that different blocks taken from one biopsy of parietal peritoneum showed each of the above-mentioned steps of mesothelial regeneration taking place simultaneously in different areas of the perito-neal surface [458]. From these observations it can be inferred that the currently used peritoneal dialysis solutions induce a situation of continuous mesothe-lial injury, which is restored by a continuous process of regeneration and/or repair. Similar ultrastructural changes were experimentally induced by intraperito-neal injections of furfural, one of the many sub-stances resulting from the non-enzymatic degrad-ation of glucose (Fig. 14) [459].

The detrimental effects of the dialysis fluids do not spare the peritoneal microvasculature. Small venules show specifically fibrosis and hyalinization of the media. Immunofluorescence microscopy revealed extensive deposition of type IV collagen and laminin in the microvascular wall, whereas electron microscope observation detected substan-tially increased presence of collagen fibres and degenerative changes of smooth muscle cells [460].

Interstitial oedema (Figs 49 and 51) results from the inflammatory reaction after injury. The presence of wide-open intercellular channels (Fig. 50) occur-ring after mesothelial injury would reflect a specific stage in the process of building new junctions by the new mesothelial cells [388, 392, 461, 462] (Figs 50 and 52). Ultrastructural studies on mouse embryo [13] revealed that mesothelial cells directly derived from mesenchymal cells showed increasing numbers of microvilli according to the extent of the differen-tiation. Therefore, the aforementioned lack or scar-city of microvilli in recently implanted cells could also denote the presence of less mature, regenerating mesothelial cells at the peritoneal luminal surface [22].

The origin of the new mesothelial cells

It has been experimentally shown that small and large mesothelial wounds heal at the same rate within 7–10 days after injury [463]. The basal, nor-mally observed mitotic rate of mesothelial cells, as measured in the rat by ^{3}H-thymidine incorporation, is approximately 1%/day. This rate is significantly increased during peritonitis, reaching maximal values of up to 19% between 1 and 3 days after injury, and returning to the basal activity on the 4th or 5th day [464]. It should be noted, however, that

proliferations of fibroblasts, as well as mesothelial cell regeneration, are substantially inhibited in experimental uraemic animals [464–466].

The origin of the new mesothelial cells repopulat-ing denuded areas of injury is still controversial. Four different hypotheses have been proposed:

1. The repopulating cells originate from the bone marrow [99]. Other experimental studies showed, however, that whole-body irradiation sufficient to depress peripheral white blood cell count as well as cell replacement by the bone marrow did not prevent mesothelial healing [467]. Therefore, the existence of a circulating mesothelial precursor originating from the bone marrow seems unlikely.
2. Mature mesothelial cells from adjacent and/or opposed areas proliferate, exfoliate and migrate to repopulate the affected surface [462, 463, 468]. Other investigators [465, 469, 470] have not accepted this hypothesis.
3. Other studies [387, 465, 471] suggested the sequence of a two-stage process; during the first 24 h, macrophages forming the first line of defence [472] and coming from the peritoneal fluid repopulate the wound surface (Fig. 5, inset; Fig. 72). Later, during the second stage, new mesothelial cells, arising from metaplasia of mes-enchymal precursors located in the interstitial tissue well below the site of injury, migrate to the surface and differentiate into mature mesothelial cells (Fig. 51). This hypothesis has not been uni-versally accepted [22, 391, 392, 461, 463]. It has also been suggested that the early implanted macrophages are gradually transformed into mesothelial cells [461]. However, Raftery [473], after labelling peritoneal macrophages with poly-styrene spheres, presented strong evidence against the hypothesis that peritoneal macrophages could be transformed into mesothelial cells.

Primitive mesenchymal cells which have been observed deep in the interstitial tissue [474] (Fig. 51, right) are multipotential and can give rise to a wide variety of cells, including mesothe-lium [469, 475].

Mesothelial cell precursors coming up from the submesothelial connective tissue were also observed under the damaged areas. The nuclear and cytoplasmic aspects of these cells were iden-tical to that shown by new mesothelial cells already implanted on the peritoneal surface (Fig. 51, upper left). This approach is supported by observations made in imprints taken from

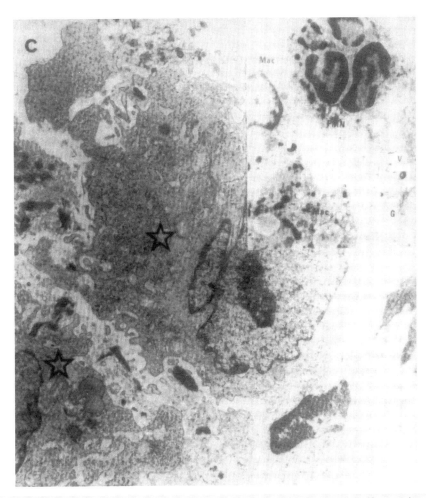

Figure 72. Biopsy of parietal peritoneum, taken during an episode of peritonitis, from a chronic uraemic patient on peritoneal dialysis. Recently implanted (1–2 days) mesothelial cells (stars), apparently coming from the abdominal cavity (C), are repopulating the denuded peritoneal surface (original magnification ×8400).
   Upper right inset. A different area of the same biopsy showing a recently implanted mesothelial cell with caveolae (V), rough endoplasmic reticulum (R) and hypertrophic Golgi complex (G). Notice the presence of macrophages (Mac) and polymorphonuclears (PMN) (original magnification ×12600).

intact unexposed mice that showed a prevalence of mitosis around 0.33% [28] (Fig. 7) and a substantial increase after a 2 h exposure to a high glucose concentration fluid (Fig. 64). Additional still-unpublished histochemical studies (Shostak, Wajsbrot and Gotloib) have detected in the unexposed mouse, passage of mesothelial cells through the G1 checking point, demonstrated by immunohistochemical assessment of PCNA (proliferative cell nuclear antigen) (Fig. 73). Furthermore, unexposed mesothelial cells enter S phase as indicated by their capability to incorporate tritiated thymidine, as shown by observations made using autoradiography (Figs 74 and 75). As observed with mitosis, this activity is substantially stimulated by

a 2 h *in-vivo* and *in-situ* exposure to a high glucose concentration solution (Fig. 76). In addition, mitotic cells can be observed surrounding areas devoid of mesothelium (Fig. 67), indicating the relevance of the local regenerative capabilities of the injured mesothelial monolayer [476].

4. Free-floating cells of the serosal cavity settle on the injured areas and gradually differentiate into new mesothelial cells [391, 392, 428, 469] (Figs 47 and 50). It should be noted that desquamated, mature mesothelial cells show degenerative changes which, as previously stated, are absent in the young, free-floating mesothelial cells. The relevance of this mechanism is attested by experiments showing the feasibility of autologous

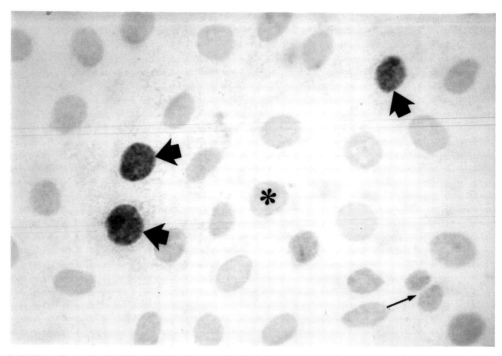

Figure 73. Imprint taken from an intact, unexposed control mouse. Arrows point at mesothelial cells passing through the G1 checkpoint (thick arrows) (*: cells before the G1 checkpoint; thin arrow: binucleated mesothelial cell) (PCNA staining; streptavidin–biotin system; ×400).

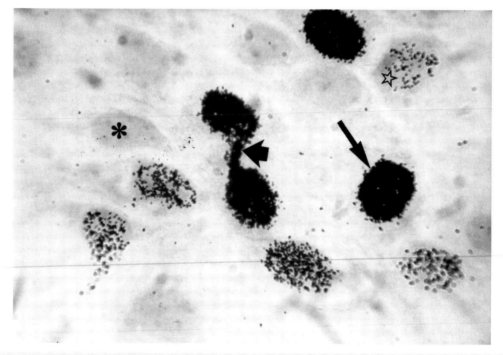

Figure 74. This photograph of a mesothelial cell imprint was taken from the anterior liver surface of a mouse. It shows, using the technique of autoradiography, the incorporation of tritiated thymidine within mesothelial cells, as well as different moments of the cell cycle. Asterisk indicates a cell in G1. Open star directs attention to a cell at the beginning of S phase. Long arrow indicates another cell at the end of S phase, or probably in G2. Short black arrow points at one cell processed at the time of cariokinesis (haematoxylin–eosin; ×1000).

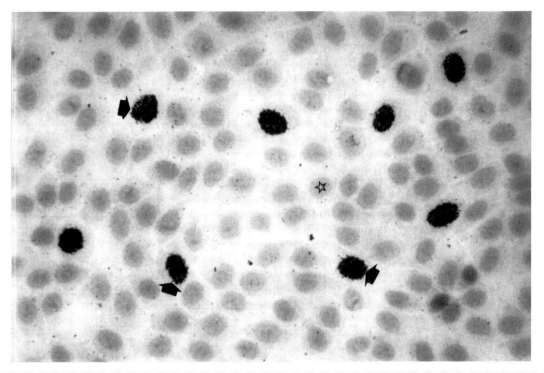

Figure 75. Thymidine incorporation seen in an imprint obtained from an intact, unexposed control animal (arrows: cells incorporating thymidine; open star: cells in G1) (autoradiography and haematoxylin–eosin; ×400).

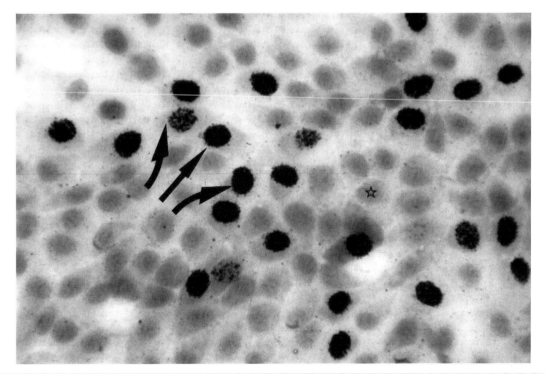

Figure 76. Mesothelial cell imprint obtained from a mice 2 h after intraperitoneal injection of a 4.25% glucose-enriched fluid for peritoneal dialysis. Note the substantial increase of cells incorporating thymidine (arrows); compare with previous figure (open arrow: cell in G1) (autoradiography and haematoxylin–eosin; ×400).

mesothelial cell implants in both experimental animals and human patients' [407].

All this evidence suggests that, most likely, mesothelial cell regeneration takes place through three different processes occurring simultaneously: implantation of young wandering mesothelial cells, migration of mesothelial cell precursors coming from the underlying connective tissue, and mitosis of young cells bordering the injured area.

Structural changes during septic peritonitis

This condition results in acute inflammatory changes affecting all the peritoneal structures. The density distribution of mesothelial cells is substantially reduced, and the presence of microorganisms can be detected in the denuded peritoneal surface as well as within mesothelial cells (Fig. 77). Mesothelial cells, necrotic or showing severe degenerative changes, exfoliate. The submesothelial basement membrane disappears (Fig. 21), together with the

normally present anionic fixed charges (Figs 21 and 78).

Experimental studies have shown that the anionic fixed charges of mesothelial glycocalyx and microvilli, which were still present 24 h after induction of peritonitis, were not observed 5 days later, and partially reappeared 13 days after the onset of the experiment [177].

The interstitium becomes grossly oedematous (Fig. 21), as well as infiltrated by acute inflammatory cells. The microvessels occasionally show wide-open intercellular junctions (Fig. 25, inset), as well as a sharp decrease in the subendothelial density distribution of anionic fixed charges (Fig. 25, left; Fig. 28) [177]. Endothelial mitochondria show signs of severe injury [Fig. 79).

Almost simultaneously, macrophages and young mesothelial cells start to repopulate the denuded luminal peritoneal surface (Fig. 70). Polymorphonuclears (Fig. 70, inset; Fig. 79) and monocytes are usually present at the luminal surface, as well as in

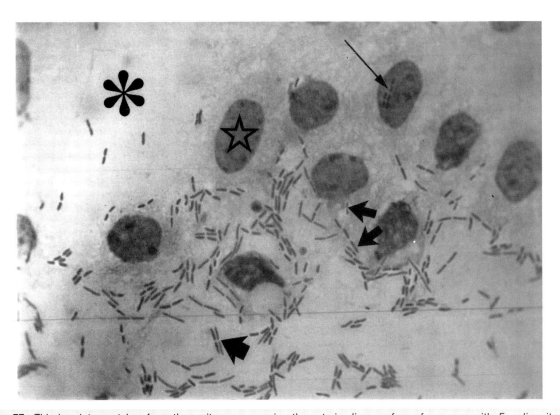

Figure 77. This imprint was taken from the peritoneum covering the anterior liver surface of a mouse with *E. coli* peritonitis. Bacterial rods (thick arrow) can be seen in areas devoid of mesothelial dressing, as well as within the cell cytoplasmic compartment (small arrows), and even into the nuclei (long thin arrow). Note the low-density distribution of mesothelial cells. (Open star: nucleus of mesothelial cell) and the presence of large peritoneal areas deprived of the monolayer (*) (haematoxylin–eosin; blue filter; × 1000).

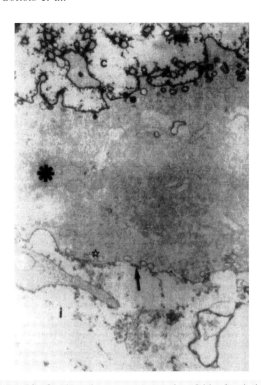

Figure 78. Section of rat mesentery taken 24 h after induction of *E. coli* peritonitis. The glycocalyx of mesothelial cell plasmalemma (short black arrow), as well as that of microvilli (open arrow) are still present. The mesothelial cell (*) is lying on an interrupted and disorganized basement membrane (long black arrow). Note the absence of submesothelial anionic sites as well as the intensity of the interstitial oedema (i) (star: uncoated pinocytotic vesicles; C: abdominal cavity) (original magnification × 24 600).

the submesothelial connective tissue. Light and electron microscopic studies have demonstrated that omental milky spots are the major route through which leukocytes migrate into the peritoneal cavity [477–479], as well as the main providers of peritoneal macrophages in situations where their increased presence is required [480].

Complete morphological and functional return to normality may be expected to occur approximately 2 weeks after recovery from the infectious episode.

Final remarks

It was not the purpose of the authors merely to deliver a cold and tedious description of anatomical structures. On the contrary, our goal has been to offer the reader a comprehensive and balanced analytical approach of structure and function covering, at least in part, their interactions. It is evident that the function of the peritoneum as a dialysis membrane cannot be evaluated only within the frame of passive diffusion through water-filled, cylindrical pores [202] and/or mathematical models [481], based on assumptions that, at times, lose sight of the formidable barrier of the living cell membrane as well as the structural organization of the tissues.

Research during the past 15 years provided enough evidence to characterize the peritoneum not as an inert dialysing sheet, but as a living and reusable membrane for dialysis [269], as predicted 20 years ago [482].

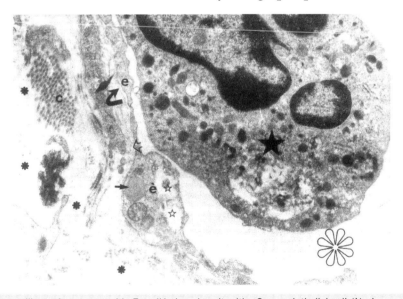

Figure 79. Mesenteric capillary of a mouse with *E. coli*-induced peritonitis. One endothelial cell (è) shows signs of severe injury, mitochondrion with inner compartment swelling (short arrow) and vascuolization of the cytoplasm (open stars). The subendothelial basement membrane (curved arrow) is, at times, absent (open arrow). The interstitial tissue is oedematous (black asterisks) (black star: polymorphonuclear cell; open asterisk: capillary lumen) (× 12 600).

In addition, it becomes evident that the mesothelial monolayer continuously exposed to dialysis solutions *in vivo* is structurally and functionally different, at least from the histochemical point of view, from that observed in unexposed–intact cells, or in those growing in the *in-vitro* set-up of culture and later exposed to experimental incubation [420]. Therefore, we have the feeling that a good deal of creative thinking is required to integrate data obtained during 40 years of physiological studies and mathematical models, with the realities of tissue structure and cell biology.

We do hope that this chapter offers the message we promised to ourselves during the preparation of the manuscript, and serves as a catalytic element for further research.

References

1. Robinson B. The Peritoneum. Chicago, IL: WT Keener, 1897, p. 13.
2. Ganter G. Uber die Beseitigung giftiger Stoffe aus dem Blute durch dialyse. Munchen Med Wochenschr 1923; 70: 1478–80.
3. Boen ST. Peritoneal dialysis in clinical medicine. Springfield, IL: Charles C. Thomas, 1964.
4. Tenckhoff H. Schechter H. A bacteriologically safe peritoneal access device for repeated dialysis. Trans Am Soc Artif Intern Organs 1968; 14: 181–7.
5. Popovich RP, Moncrief JW, Decherd JF, Bomar JB, Pyle WK. Preliminary verification of the low dialysis clearance hypothesis via a novel equilibrium peritoneal dialysis technique. Abst Am Soc Artif Intern Organs 1976; 5: 64.
6. Nolph KD, Sorkin M, Rubin J, Arfania D, Prowant B, Fruto L, Kennedy D. Continuous ambulatory peritoneal dialysis: three-year experience at one center. Ann Intern Med 1980; 92: 609–13.
7. Luschka H. Die Structure der serosen haute des menschen. Tubingen, 1851.
8. Putiloff PV. Materials for the study of the laws of growth of the human body in relation to the surface areas of different systems: the trial on Russian subjects of planigraphic anatomy as a mean of exact anthropometry. Presented at the Siberian branch of the Russian Geographic Society, Omsk, 1886.
9. Wegner G. Chirurgische bemerkingen uber die peritoneal Hole, mit Besonderer Berucksichtigung der ovariotomie. Arch Klin Chir 1877; 20: 51–9.
10. Esperanca MJ, Collins DL. Peritoneal dialysis efficiency in relation to body weight. J Pediatr Surg 1966; 1: 162–9.
11. Gotloib L, Digenis GE, Rabinovich S, Medline A, Oreopolous DG. Ultrastructure of normal rabbit mesentery. Nephron 1983; 34: 248–55.
12. Gosselin RE, Berndt WO. Diffusional transport of solutes through mesentery and peritoneum. J Theor Biol 1962; 3: 487.
13. Haar JL, Ackerman GA. A phase and electron microscopic study of vasculogenesis and erythropoiesis in the yolk sac of the mouse. Anat Rec 1971; 170: 199–224.
14. Ukeshima A, Hayashi Y, Fujimore T. Surface morphology of the human yolk sac: endoderm and mesothelium 1986; 49: 483–94.
15. Puulmala RM. Morphologic comparison of parietal and visceral peritoneal epithelium in fetus and adult. Anat Rec 1937; 68: 327–30.
16. Robertson JD. Molecular structure of biological membranes. In: Lima de Faria, A., ed. Handbook of Molecular Cytology. Amsterdam: North Holland, 1969, p. 1404.
17. Kolossow A. Weber die struktur des endothels der pleuroperitoneal hole der blut und lymphgefasse. Biol Centralbl Bd 1892; 12: S87–94.
18. Odor L. Observations of the rat mesothelium with the electron and phase microscopes. Am J Anat 1954; 95: 433–65.
19. Felix DM, Dalton AJ. A comparison of mesothelial cells and macrophages in mice after the intraperitoneal inoculation of melanine granules. J Biophys Biochem Cytol 1956; 2 (suppl. part 2): 109–17.
20. Baradi AF, Hope J. Observations on ultrastructure of rabbit mesothelium. Exp Cell Res 1964; 34: 33–4.
21. Baradi AF, Crae SN. A scanning electron microscope study of mouse peritoneal mesothelium. Tissue Cell 1976; 8: 159.
22. Whitaker D, Papadimitriou JM, Walters MNI. The mesothelium and its reactions: a review. CRC Crit Rev Toxicol 1982; 10: 81–144.
23. Di Paolo N, Sacchi G, De-Mia M et al. Morphology of the peritoneal membrane during continuous ambulatory peritoneal dialysis. Nephron 1986; 44: 204–11.
24. Kondo T, Takeuchi K, Doi Y, Yonemura S, Nagata S, Tsukita S. ERM (ezrin–radixin/moesin)-based molecular mechanism of microvillar breakdown at an early stage of apoptosis. J Cell Biol 1997; 139: 749–58.
25. Bonelli G, Sacchi MC, Barbiero G et al. Apoptosis of L929 cells by etoposide: a quantitative and kinetic approach. Exp Cell Res 1996; 228: 292–305.
26. Boe R, Gjertsen BT, Doskeland SO, Vintermyr OK. 8-Chloro-cAMP induces apoptotic cell death in a human mammary carcinoma cell (MCF–7) line. Br J Cancer 1995; 72: 1151–9.
27. Efskind L. Experimentelle Untersuchungen uber die Biologie des Peritoneums. 1. Die morphologische reaktion des peritoneums auf riexze. Oslo: Det Norske Videnk aps Academii, 1940.
28. Gotloib L, Wajsbrut V, Shostak A, Kushnier R. Acute and long-term changes observed in imprints of mouse mesothelium exposed to glucose-enriched, lactated, buffered dialysis solutions. Nephron 1995; 70: 466–77.
29. Fukata H. Electron microscopic study on normal rat peritoneal mesothelium and its changes in adsorption of particulate iron dextran complex. Acta Pathol Jpn 1963; 13: 309–25.
30. Lieberman-Meffet D, White H. The greater omentum: anatomy, physiology, pathology, surgery with an historical survey. Berlin: Springer-Verlag, 1983, p. 6.
31. Madison LD, Bergstrom MU, Porter B, Torres R, Shelton E. Regulation of surface topography of mouse peritoneal cells. J Cell Biol 1979; 82: 783.
32. Gotloib L, Shostak A. Ultrastructural morphology of the peritoneum: new findings and speculations on transfer of solutes and water during peritoneal dialysis. Perit Dial Bull 1987; 7: 119–29.
33. Gotloib L. Anatomical basis for peritoneal permeability. In: La Greca G, Chiaramonte S, Fabris A, Feriani M, Ronco G, eds. Peritoneal Dialysis. Milan: Wichtig Ed, 1986, pp. 3–10.
34. Gotloib L, Shostak A, Jaichenko J. Ruthenium red stained anionic charges of rat and mice mesothelial cells and basal lamina: the peritoneum is a negatively charged dialyzing membrane. Nephron 1988; 48, 65–70.
35. Luft JH. Fine structure of capillary and endocapillary layer as revealed by ruthenium red. Fed Proc 1966; 25: 1173–83.
36. Gotloib L, Bar-Sella P, Jaichenko J, Shostak A. Ruthenium red stained polyanionic fixed charges in peritoneal microvessels. Nephron 1987; 47: 22–8.
37. Curry FE, Michel CC. A fiber matrix model of capillary permeability. Microvasc Res 1980; 20: 96–9.
38. Morris RG, Hargreaves AD, Duvall E, Wyllie AH. Hormone-induced cell death. 2. Surface changes in thymocytes undergoing apoptosis. Am J Pathol 1984; 115: 426–36.
39. Moog F. The lining of the small intestine. Sci Am 1981; 2455: 116–25.

40. Gotloib L. Anatomy of the peritoneal membrane. In: La Greca G, Biasoli G, Ronco G, eds. Milan: Wichtig Ed., 1982, pp. 17–30.

41. Leak LV. Distribution of cell surface charges on mesothelium and lymphatic endothelium. Microvasc Res 1986; 31: 18–30.

42. Lewis WH. Pinocytosis. Bull Johns Hopkins Hosp 1931; 49: 17–23.

43. Casley-Smith JR. The dimensions and numbers of small vesicles in cells, endothelial and mesothelial and the significance of these for endothelial permeability. J Microsc 1969; 90: 251–69.

44. Casley-Smith JR, Chin JC. The passage of cytoplasmic vesicles across endothelial and mesothelial cells. J Microsc 1971; 93: 167–89.

45. Fedorko ME, Hirsch JG, Fried B. Studies on transport of macromolecules and small particles across mesothelial cells of the mouse omentum. Exp Cell Res 1971; 63: 313–23.

46. Simionescu N, Simionescu M, Palade GE. Structural basis of permeability in sequential segments of the microvasculature. II. Pathways followed by microperoxidase across the endothelium. Microvasc Res 1978; 15: 17–36.

47. Palade GE, Simionescu M, Simionescu N. Structural aspects of the permeability of the microvascular endothelium. Acta Physiol Scand Suppl 1979; 463: 11–32.

48. Palade GE. Fine structure of blood capillaries. J Appl Phys 1953; 24: 1424.

49. Florey HW. The transport of materials across the capillary wall. Q J Exp Physiol 1964; 49: 117–28.

50. Pappenheimer JR, Renkin EM, Borrero LM. Filtration, diffusion and molecular sieving through peripheral capillary membranes. A contribution to the pore theory of capillary permeability. Am J Physiol 1951; 167: 13–46.

51. Frokjaer-Jensen J. The plasmalemmal vesicular system in capillary endothelium. Prog Appl Microcirc 1983; 1: 17–34.

52. Wagner RC, Robinson CS. High voltage electron microscopy of capillary endothelial vesicles. Microvasc Res 1984; 28: 197–205.

53. Smart EJ, Foster DC, Ying YS, Kamen BA, Anderson RGW. Protein kinase G activators inhibit receptor-mediated potocytosis by preventing internalization of caveolae. J Cell Biol 1994; 124: 307–13.

54. Lisanti MP, Scherer PE, Vidugiriene J et al. Characterization of caveolin-rich membrane domains isolated from an endothelial-rich source: implications for human disease. J Cell Biol 1994; 126: 111–26.

55. Moldovan NI, Heltianu G, Simionescu N, Simionescu M. Ultrastructural evidence of differential solubility in Triton X–100 of endothelial vesicles and plasma membrane. Exp Cell Res 1995; 219: 309–13.

56. Shasby DM, Roberts RL. Transendothelial transfer of macromolecules *in vivo*. Fed Proc 1987; 46: 2506–10.

57. Shasby DM, Shasby SS. Active transendothelial transport of albumin. Interstitium to lumen. Circ Res.1985; 57: 903–8.

58. Milici AJ, Watrous NE, Stukenbrok M, Palade GE. Transcytosis of albumin in capillary endothelium. J Cell Biol 1987; 105: 2603–12.

59. Ghitescu L, Bendayan M. Transendothelial transport of serum albumin: a quantitative immunocytochemical study. J Cell Biol 1992; 17: 747–55.

60. Schnitzer JE, Oh P. Albondin-mediated capillary permeability to albumin. Differential role of receptors in endothelial transcytosis and endocytosis of native and modified albumins. J Biol Chem 1994; 269: 6072–82.

61. Ghitescu L, Galis Z, Simionescu M, Simionescu N. Differentiated uptake and transcytosis of albumin in successive vascular segments. J Submicrosc Cytol Pathol 1988; 20: 657–69.

62. Williams SK, Devenny JJ, Bitensky MW. Micropinocytic ingestion of glycosylated albumin by isolated microvessels: possible role in pathogenesis of diabetic microangiopathy. Proc Natl Acad Sci USA 1981; 78: 2393–7.

63. Ghitescu L, Fixman A, Simionescu M, Simionescu N. Specific binding sites for albumin restricted to plasmalemmal vesicles of continuous capillary endothelium: receptor-mediated transcytosis. J Cell Biol 1986; 102: 1304–11.

64. Predescu D, Simionescu M, Simionescu N, Palade GE. Binding and transcytosis of glycoalbumin by the microvascular endothelium of the murine myocardium: evidence that glycoalbumin behaves as a bifunctional ligand. J Cell Biol 1988; 107: 1729–38.

65. Dehouck B, Fenart L, Dehouck MP, Pierce A, Torpier G, Cecchelli R. A new function for the LDL receptor: transcytosis of LDL across the blood–brain barrier. J Cell Biol 1997; 138: 877–89.

66. Simionescu N, Simionescu M. Interactions of endogenous lipoproteins with capillary endothelium in spontaneously hyperlipoproteinemic rats. Microvasc Res. 1985; 30: 314–32.

67. Snelting-Havinga I, Mommaas M, Van-Hinsbergh VW, Daha MR, Daems WT, Vermeer BJ. Immunoelectron microscopic visualization of the transcytosis of low density lipoproteins in perfused rat arteries. Eur J Cell Biol 1989; 48: 27–36.

68. Vasile E, Simionescu M, Simionescu N. Visualization of the binding, endocytosis, and transcytosis of low-density lipoprotein in the arterial endothelium *in situ*. J Cell Biol 1983; 96: 1677–89.

69. Ghinea N, Hai MTV, Groyer-Picard MT, Milgrom E. How protein hormones reach their target cells. Receptor mediated transcytosis of hCG through endothelial cells. J Cell Biol 1994; 125: 87–97.

70. Bendayan M, Rasio EA. Transport of insulin and albumin by the microvascular endothelium of the rete mirabile. J Cell Sci 1996; 109: 1857–64.

71. Schmidt AM, Vianna M, Gerlach M et al. Isolation and characterization of two binding proteins for advanced glycosylation end products from bovine lung which are present on the endothelial cell surface. J Biol Chem 1992; 267: 14987–97.

72. Predescu D, Predescu S, McQuistan T, Palade GE. Transcytosis of alpha 1-acidic glycoprotein in the continuous microvascular endothelium. Proc Natl Acad Sci USA 1998; 95: 6175–80.

73. Pappenheimer JR. Passage of molecules through capillary walls. Physiol Rev 1953; 33: 387–423.

74. Grotte G. Passage of dextran molecules across the blood–lymph barrier. Acta Chir Scand 1956; Suppl. 211: 1–84.

75. Nolph KD. The peritoneal dialysis system. Contrib Nephrol 1979; 17: 44–9.

76. Gotloib L, Shostak A. Endocytosis and transcytosis of albumin–gold through mice peritoneal mesothelium. Kidney Int 1995; 47: 1274–84.

77. Schnitzer JE, Allard J, Oh P. NEM inhibits transcytosis, endocytosis and capillary permeability: implication of caveolae fusion in endothelia. Am J Physiol 1995; 168: H48–55.

78. Schnitzer JE, Oh P, Pinney E, Allard J. Filipin-sensitive caveolae-mediated transport in endothelium: reduced transcytosis, scavenger endocytosis, and capillary permeability of select macromolecules. J Cell Biol 1994; 127: 1217–32.

79. Tiruppathi G, Song W, Bergenfeldt M, Sass P, Malik AB. Gp60 activation mediates albumin transcytosis in endothelial cells by tyrosine kinase-dependent pathway. J Biol Chem 1997; 272: 25968–75.

80. Schnitzer JE, Oh P, Jacobson BS, Dvorak AM. Caveolae from luminal plasmalemma of rat lung endothelium: microdomains enriched in caveolin, Ca (2+)-ATPase, and inositol triphosphate receptor. Proc Natl Acad Sci USA 1995; 92: 1759–63.

81. Glenney JR, Soppet D. Sequence and expression of caveolin, a protein component of caveolae plasma membrane domains phosphorylated on tyrosine in Rous sarcoma virus-transformed fibroblasts. Proc Natl Acad Sci USA 1992; 89: 10517–21.

82. Bush KT, Stuart RO, Li SH et al. Epithelial inositol 1,4,5-triphosphate receptors. Multiplicity of localization, solubility, and isoforms. J Biol Chem 1994; 269: 23694–9.

83. Brown D, Lydon J, McLaughlin M, Stuart-Tilley A, Tyszkowski R, Alper S. Antigen retrieval in cryostat tissue sections and cultured cells by treatment with sodium dodecyl sulfate (SDS). Histochem Cell Biol 1996; 105: 261–7.

84. Breton S, Lisante MP, Tyszkowski R, McLaughlin M, Brown D. Basolateral distribution of caveolin-1 in the kidney. Absence from ATPase-coated endocytic vesicles in intercalated cells. J Histochem Cytochem 1998; 46: 205–14.

85. Schmid SL. Clathrin-coated vesicle formation and protein sorting: an integrated process. Annu Rev Biochem 1997; 66: 511–48.

86. Pfeffer SR, Drubin DG, Kelly RB. Identification of three coated vesicle components as alpha- and beta-tubulin linked to a phosphorylated 50,000-dalton polypeptide. J Cell Biol 1983; 97: 40–7.

87. Pearse BMF. Clathrin: a unique protein associated with intracellular transfer of membrane by coated vesicles. Proc Natl Acad Sci USA 1976; 73: 1255–9.

88. Lin HC, Duncan JA, Kozasa T, Gilman AG. Sequestration of the G protein beta gamma subunit complex inhibits receptor-mediated endocytosis. Proc Natl Acad Sci USA 1998; 95: 5057–60.

89. Damke H. Dynamin and receptor-mediated endocytosis. FEBS Lett 1996; 389: 48–51.

90. Sweitzer SM, Hinshaw JE. Dynamin undergoes a GTP dependent conformational change causing vesiculation. Cell 1998; 93: 1021–9.

91. Henley JR, Krueger EW, Oswald BJ, McNiven MA. Dynamin-mediated internalization of caveolae. J Cell Biol 1998; 141: 85–99.

92. Oh P, McIntosh DP, Schnitzer JE. Dynamin at the neck of caveolae mediates their budding to form transport vesicles by GTP-driven fission from the plasma membrane of endothelium. J Cell Biol 1998; 141: 101–14.

93. Chambers R, Zweifach BW. Capillary cement in relation to permeability. J Cell Comp Physiol 1940; 15: 255–72.

94. Rippe B. A three-pore model of peritoneal transport. Perit Dial Int 1993; 13 (suppl. 2): S35–8.

95. Simionescu N, Simionescu M, Palade GE. Differentiated microdomains on the luminal surface of capillary endothelium. I. Preferential distribution of anionic sites. J Cell Biol 1981; 90: 605–13.

96. Steinman RM, Mellman IS, Muller WA, Cohn ZA. Endocytosis and the recycling of plasma membrane. J Cell Biol 1983; 96: 1–27.

97. Shea SM, Karnovsky MJ. Brownian motion: a theoretical explanation for the movement of vesicles across the endothelium. Nature, Lond 1966; 212: 353–4.

98. Simionescu M, Simionescu N, Palade GE. Morphometric data on the endothelium of blood capillaries. J Cell Biol 1974; 60: 128–52.

99. Wagner JC, Johnson NF, Brown DG, Wagner MMF. Histology and ultrastructure of serially transplanted rat mesotheliomas. Br J Cancer 1982; 46: 294–9.

100. Petersen OW, Van Deurs B. Serial section analysis of coated pits and vesicles involved in adsorptive pinocytosis in cultured fibroblasts. J Cell Biol 1983; 96: 277–81.

101. Peters KR, Carley WW, Palade GE. Endothelial plasmalemmal vesicles have a characteristic stripped bipolar surface structure. J Cell Biol 1985; 101: 2233–8.

102. Takahashi H, Hasegawa H, Kamijo T *et al.* Regulation and localization of peritoneal water channels in rats. Perit Dial Int 1998; 18 (suppl. 2): S70.

103. Henle FGH. Splacnologie. Vol. II, p. 175, 1875.

104. Simionescu M, Simionescu N, Silbert J, Palade GE. Differentiated microdomains on the luminal surface of the capillary endothelium. II. Partial characterization of their anionic sites. J Cell Biol 1981; 90: 614–21.

105. Simionescu M, Simionescu N. Organization of cell junctions in the peritoneal mesothelium. J Cell Biol 1977; 74: 98.

106. Von Recklinghausen FD. Zur Fettresorption. Arch Pathol Anat Physiol 1863; Bd 26: S172–208.

107. Bizzozero G, Salvioli G. Sulla suttura della membrana serosa e particolarmente del peritoneo diaphragmatico. Giorn R Acad Med Torino 1876; 19: 466–70.

108. Allen L. The peritoneal stomata. Anat Rec 1937; 67: 89–103.

109. French JE, Florey HW, Morris B. The adsorption of particles by the lymphatics of the diaphragm. Q J Exp Physiol 1959; 45: 88–102.

110. Tourneux F, Herman G. Recherches sur quelques epitheliums plats dans la serie animale (Deuxieme partie). J Anat Physiol 1876; 12: 386–424.

111. Kolossow A. Uber die struktur des pleuroperitoneal und gefassepithels (endothels). Arch Mikr Anat 1893; 42: 318–83.

112. Simer PM. The passage of particulate matter from the peritoneal cavity into the lymph vessels of the diaphragm. Anat Rec 1948; 101: 333–51.

113. Leak LW, Just EE. Permeability of peritoneal mesothelium. J Cell Biol 1976; 70: 423a.

114. Tsilibarry EC, Wissig SL. Absorption from the peritoneal surface of the muscular portion of the diaphragm. Am J Anat 1977; 149: 127–33.

115. French JE, Florey HW, Morris B. The absorption of particles by the lymphatics of the diaphragm. Q J Exp Physiol 1959; 45: 88–102.

116. Abu-Hijleh MF, Scothorne RJ. Studies on haemolymph nodes. IV. Comparison of the route of entry of carbon particles into parathymic nodes after intravenous and intraperitoneal injection. J Anat 1996; 188: 565–73.

117. Allen L. The peritoneal stomata. Anat Rec 1937; 67: 89–103.

118. Hashimoto B, Filly RA, Callen PW, Parer JT. Absorption of fetal intraperitoneal blood after intrauterine transfusion. J Ultrasound Med 1987; 6: 421–3.

119. Smedsrood B, Aminoff D. Studies on the sequestration of chemically and enzymatically modified erythrocytes. Am J Hematol 1983; 15: 123–33.

120. Fowler JM, Knight R, Patel KM. Intraperitoneal blood transfusion in African adults with hookworm anaemia. Br Med J 1968; 3: 200–1.

121. Chandler K, Fitzpatrik J, Mellor D, Milne M, Fishwick G. Intraperitoneal administration of whole blood as a treatment for anaemia in lambs. Vet Rec 1998; 142: 175–6.

122. Aba MA, Pissani AA, Alzola RH, Videla-Dorna I, Ghezzi MS, Marcilese NA. Evaluation of intraperitoneal route for the transfusion of erythrocytes using rats and dogs. Acta Physiol Pharmacol Ther Latinoam 1991; 41: 387–95.

123. Remmele W, Richter IE, Wildenhof H. Experimental investigations on cell resorption from the peritoneal cavity by use of the scanning electron microscope. Klin Wochenschr 1975; 53: 913–22.

124. Dumont AE, Maas WK, Iliescu H, Shin RD. Increased survival from peritonitis after blockade of transdiaphragmatic absorption of bacteria. Surg Gynecol Obstet 1986; 162: 248–52.

125. Leak LV. Permeability of peritoneal mesothelium: a TEM and SEM study. J Cell Biol 1976; 70: 423–33.

126. Leak LV. Polycationic ferritin binding to diaphragmatic mesothelial and lymphatic endothelial cells. J Cell Biol 1982; 95: 103–11.

127. Ettarh RR, Carr KE. Ultrastructural observations on the peritoneum in the mouse. J Anat 1996; 188: 211–5.

128. Wassilev M, Wedel T, Michailova K, Kuhnel W. A scanning electron microscopy study of peritoneal stomata in different peritoneal regions. Anat Anz 1998; 180: 137–43.

129. Li J, Zhou J, Gao Y. The ultrastructure and computer imaging of the lymphatic stomata in the human pelvic peritoneum. Anat Anz 1997; 179: 215–20.

130. Yoffey JM, Courtice FC. Lymphatics, Lymph and Lymphoid Tissue. London: Edward Arnold, 1956, p. 176.

131. Andrews PM, Porter KR. The ultrastructural morphology and possible functional significance of mesothelial microvilli. Anat Rec 1973; 177: 409–14.

132. Ghadially FN. Ultrastructural Pathology of the Cell. London: Butterworths, 1978, p. 403.

133. Todd RB, Bowman W. The Physiological Anatomy and Physiology of Man, Vols I and II. London, 1845 and 1846.

134. Muscatello G. Uber den Bau und das Aufsaugunsvermogen des Peritanaums. Virchows Archiv Path Anat 1895; Bd 142: 327–59.

135. Baron MA. Structure of the intestinal peritoneum in man. Am J Anat 1941; 69: 439–96.

136. Maximow A. Bindgewebe und blutbildende gewebe. Handbuch der mikroskopischen Anatomie des menschen. von Mollendorf, 1927; Bd 2 T 1: S232–583.

137. Kanwar YS, Farquhar MG. Anionic sites in the glomerular basement membrane. *In vivo* and *in vitro* localization to the laminae rarae by cationic probes. J Cell Biol 1979; 81: 137–53.

138. Rohrbach R. Reduced content and abnormal distribution of anionic sites (acid proteoglycans) in the diabetic glomerular basement membrane. Virchows Arch B Cell Pathol Incl Mol Pathol 1986; 51: 127–35.

139. Ghinea N, Simionescu N. Anionized and cationized hemeundecapeptides as probes for cell surface charge and permeability studies: differentiated labeling of endothelial plasmalemmal vesicles. J Cell Biol 1985; 100: 606–12.

140. Gotloib L, Shostak A, Jaichenko J. Loss of mesothelial electronegative fixed charges during murine septic peritonitis. Nephron 1989; 51: 77–83.

141. Shostak A, Gotloib L. Increased peritoneal permeability to albumin in streptozotocin diabetic rats. Kidney Int 1996; 49: 705–14.

142. Gotloib L, Shostak A, Bar-Sella P, Eiali V. Reduplicated skin and peritoneal blood capillaries and mesothelial basement membrane in aged non-diabetic chronic uremic patients. Perit Dial Bull 1984; 4: S28.

143. Di Paolo N, Sacchi G. Peritoneal vascular changes in continuous ambulatory peritoneal dialysis (CAPD): an *in-vivo* model for the study of diabetic microangiopathy. Perit Dial Int 1989; 9: 41–5.

144. Gersh I, Catchpole HR. The organization of ground substances and basement membrane and its significance in tissue injury, disease and growth. Am J Anat 1949; 85: 457–522.

145. Williamson JT, Vogler NJ, Kilo CH. Regional variations in the width of the basement membrane of muscle capillaries in man and giraffe. Am J Pathol 1971; 63: 359–67.

146. Vracko R. Skeletal muscle capillaries in non-diabetics. A quantitative analysis. Circulation 1970; 16: 285–97.

147. Parthasarathy N, Spiro RG. Effect of diabetes on the glycosaminoglycan component of the human glomerular basement membrane. Diabetes 1982; 31: 738–41.

148. Vracko R. Basal lamina scaffold – anatomy and significance for maintenance of orderly tissue structure. A review. Am J Pathol 1974; 77: 313–46.

149. Vracko R, Pecoraro RE, Carter WB. Basal lamina of epidermis, muscle fibers, muscle capillaries, and renal tubules: changes with aging and diabetes mellitus. Ultrastruct Pathol 1980; 1, 559–74.

150. Hruza Z. Connective tissue. In: Kaley G, Altura BM, eds. Microcirculation. Baltimore, MD: University Park Press, 1977, Vol. I, pp. 167–183.

151. Comper WD, Laurent TC. Physiological function of connective tissue polysaccharides. Physiol Rev 1978; 58: 255–315.

152. Flessner MF. The importance of the interstitium in peritoneal transport. Perit Dial Int 1996; 16 (suppl. 1): S76–9.

153. Parker JC, Gilchrist S, Cartledge JT. Plasma–lymph exchange and interstitial distribution volumes of charged macromolecules in the lung. J Appl Physiol 1985; 59: 1128–36.

154. Lai-Fook SJ, Brown LV. Effects of electric charge on hydraulic conductivity of pulmonary interstitium. J Appl Physiol 1991; 70: 1928–32.

155. Gilchrist SA, Parker JC. Exclusion of charged macromolecules in the pulmonary interstitium. Microvasc Res 1985; 30: 88–98.

156. Haljamae H. Anatomy of the interstitial tissue. Lymphology 1978; 11: 128–32.

157. Guyton AC. A concept of negative interstitial pressure based on pressures in implanted perforated capsules. Circ Res 963; 12: 399–414.

158. Scholander PF, Hargens AR, Miller SL. Negative pressure in the interstitial fluid of animals. Fluid tensions are spectacular in plants; in animals they are elusively small, but just as vital. Science 1968; 161: 321–8.

159. Aukland K, Reed PK. Interstitial–lymphatic mechanisms in the control of extracellular fluid volume. Physiol Rev 1993; 73: 1–78.

160. Rutili G, Arfors KE. Protein concentration in interstitial and lymphatic fluids from the subcutaneous tissue. Acta Physiol Scand 1977; 99: 1–8.

161. Rutili G, Kvietys P, Martin D, Parker JC, Taylor AE. Increased pulmonary microvascular permeability induced by alpha-naphthylthiourea. J Appl Physiol 1982; 52: 1316–23.

162. Flessner MF. Peritoneal transport physiology: insights from basic research. J Am Soc Nephrol 1991; 2: 122–35.

163. Gotloib L, Mines M, Garmizo AL, Varka I. Hemodynamic effects of increasing intra-abdominal pressure in peritoneal dialysis. Perit Dial Bull 1981; 1: 41–2.

164. Flessner MF, Schwab A. Pressure threshold for fluid loss from the peritoneal cavity. Am J Physiol 1996; 270: F377–90.

165. Simionescu N. Cellular aspects of transcapillary exchange. Physiol Rev 983; 63: 1536–79.

166. Wolff JR. Ultrastructure of the terminal vascular bed as related to function. In: Kaley G, Altura BM, eds. Microcirculation. Baltimore, MD: University Park Press, 1977, Vol. I, pp. 95–130.

167. Majno G. Ultrastructure of the vascular membrane. Handbook of Physiology. Section II – Circulation, vol. III. Washington, DC: Am Physiol Soc, 1965, pp. 2293–375.

168. Gotloib L, Shostak A, Jaichenko J. Fenestrated capillaries in mice submesothelial mesenteric microvasculature. Int J Artif Organs 1989; 12: 20–4.

169. Gotloib L, Shostak A. In search of a role for submesothelial fenestrated capillaries. Perit Dial Int 1993; 13: 98–102.

170. Gotloib L, Shostak A, Bar-Sella P, Eiali V. Fenestrated capillaries in human parietal and rabbit diaphragmatic peritoneum. Nephron 1985; 41: 200–2.

171. Friederici HHR. The tridimensional ultrastructure of fenestrated capillaries. J Ultrastruct Res 1968; 23: 444–56.

172. Clough G, Smaje LH. Exchange area and surface properties of the microvasculature of the rabbit submandibular gland following duct ligation. J Physiol 1984; 354: 445–56.

173. Gotloib L, Shostak A, Jaichenko J, Galdi P, Fudin R. Anionic fixed charges in the fenestrated capillaries of the mouse mesentery. Nephron 1990; 55: 419–22.

174. Rhodin JAG. The diaphragm of capillary endothelial fenestrations. J Ultrastruc Res 1962; 6: 171–85.

175. Gotloib L, Shostak A, Bar-Sella P, Eiali V. Heterogeneous density and ultrastructure of rabbit's peritoneal microvasculature. Int J Artif Organs 1984; 7: 123–5.

176. Rhodin YAG. Ultrastructure of mammalian venous capillaries, venules and small collecting veins. J Ultrastruct Res 1968; 25: 452–500.

177. Gotloib L, Shostak A, Jaichenko J. Loss of mesothelial and microvascular fixed anionic charges during murine experimentally induced septic peritonitis. In: Avram M and Giordano G, eds. Ambulatory Peritoneal Dialysis. New York: Plenum, 1990, pp. 63–6.

178. Simionescu M, Simionescu N, Palade GE. Differentiated microdomains on the luminal surface of capillary endothelium: distribution of lectin receptors. J Cell Biol 1982 94, 406–13.

179. Schneeberger EE, Hamelin M. Interactions of serum proteins with lung endothelial glycocalyx: its effect on endothelial permeability. Am J Physiol 1984; 247: H206–17.

180. Bundgaard M, Frokjaer-Jensen J. Functional aspects of the ultrastructure of terminal blood vessels: a quantitative study

on consecutive segments of the frog mesenteric microvasculature. Microvasc Res 1982; 23: 1–30.

181. Palade GE. Transport in quanta across the endothelium of blood capillaries. Anat Rec 1960; 116: 254.

182. Milici AJ, L'Hernault N, Palade GE. Surface densities of diaphragmed fenestrae and transendothelial channels in different murine capillary beds. Circ Res 1985; 56, 709–17.

183. Lombardi T, Montesano R, Furie MB, Silverstein SC, Orci L. *In-vitro* modulation of endothelial fenestrae: opposing effects of retinoic acid and transforming growth factor beta. J Cell Sci 1988; 91: 313–8.

184. Kitchens CS, Weiss L. Ultrastructural changes of endothelium associated with thrombocytopenia. Blood 1975; 46: 567–78.

185. Horiuchi T, Weller PF. Expression of vascular endothelial growth factor by human eosinophils: upregulation by granulocyte macrophage colony-stimulating factor and interleukin-5. Am J Respir Cell Mol Biol 1997; 17: 70–7.

186. Collins PD, Connolly DT, Williams TJ. Characterization of the increase in vascular permeability induced by vascular permeability factor *in vivo*. Br J Pharmacol 1993; 109: 195–9.

187. Yeo KT, Wang HH, Nagy JA, Sioussat TM *et al.* Vascular permeability factor (vascular endothelial growth factor) in guinea pig and human tumor inflammatory effusions. Cancer Res 1993; 53: 2912–18.

188. Taichman NS, Young S, Cruchley AT, Taylor P, Paleolog E. Human neutrophils secrete vascular endothelial growth factor. J Leukoc Biol 1997; 62: 397–400.

189. Roberts WG, Palade GE. Increased microvascular permeability and endothelial fenestration induced by vascular endothelial growth factor: J Cell Sci 1995; 108: 2369–70.

190. Roberts WG, Palade GE. Neovasculature induced by vascular endothelial growth factor is fenestrated. Cancer Res 1997; 57: 765–72.

191. Simionescu M, Simionescu N, Palade GE. Sulfated glycosaminoglycans are major components of the anionic sites of fenestral diaphragms in capillary endothelium. J Cell Biol 1979; 83: 78a.

192. Milici AJ, L'Hernault N. Variation in the number of fenestrations and channels between fenestrated capillary beds. J Cell Biol 1983; 97: 336.

193. Peters KR, Milici AJ. High resolution scanning electron microscopy of the luminal surface of a fenestrated capillary endothelium. J Cell Biol 1983; 97: 336a.

194. Bankston PW, Milici AJ. A survey of the binding of polycationic ferritin in several fenestrated capillary beds: indication of heterogeneity in the luminal glycocalyx of fenestral diaphragms. Microvasc Res 1983; 26: 36–49.

195. Levick JR, Smaje LH. An analysis of the permeability of a fenestra. Microvasc Res 1987; 33: 233–56.

196. Wayland H, Silberberg A. Blood to lymph transport. Microvasc Res 1978; 15: 367–74.

197. Bearer EL, Orci L. Endothelial fenestral diaphragms: a quick freeze, deep-etch study. J Cell Biol 1985; 100: 418–28.

198. Simionescu M, Simionescu N, Palade GE. Preferential distribution of anionic sites on the basement membrane and the abluminal aspect of the endothelium in fenestrated capillaries. J Cell Biol 1982; 95: 425–34.

199. Deen WN, Satvat B. Determinants of the glomerular filtration of proteins. Am J Physiol 1981; 241: F162–70.

200. Deen WM, Bohrer MP, Robertson CR, Brenner BM. Determinants of the transglomerular passage of macromolecules. Fed Proc 1977; 36: 2614–8.

201. Kanwar YS, Linker A, Farquhar MG. Characterization of anionic sites in the glomerular basement membrane: *in vitro* and *in vivo* localization to the lamina rarae by cationic probes. J Cell Biol 1980; 86: 688–93.

202. Renkin EM. Multiple pathways of capillary permeability. Circ Res 1977; 41: 735–43.

203. Charonis AS, Wissig SL. Anionic sites in basement membranes. Differences in their electrostatic properties in continuous and fenestrated capillaries. Microvasc Res 1983; 25: 265–85.

204. Renkin EM. Cellular and intercellular transport pathways in exchange vessels. Am Rev Respir Dis 1992; 146: S28–31.

205. Farquhar MG, Palade GE. Junctional complexes in various epithelia. J Cell Biol 1963; 17: 375–442.

206. Simionescu M, Simionescu N, Palade GE.: Segmental differentiations of cell junctions in the vascular endothelium. J Cell Biol 1975; 67: 863–85.

207. Thorgeirsson G, Robertson AL Jr. The vascular endothelium. Pathobiologic significance. Am J Pathol 198; 95: 801–48.

208. Gumbiner B. Breaking through the tight junction barrier. J Cell Biol 1993; 123: 1631–3.

209. Gumbiner B. Structure, biochemistry, and assembly of epithelial tight junctions. Am J Physiol 1987; 253: C749–58.

210. Furuse M, Hirase T, Itoh M *et al.* Occludin: a novel integral membrane protein localized at tight junctions. J Cell Biol 1993; 123: 1777–88.

211. Furuse M, Itoh M, Hirase T *et al.* Direct association of occludin with ZO-1 and its possible involvement in the localization of occludin at tight junctions. J Cell Biol 1994; 127: 1617–26.

212. Hirase T, Staddon JM, Saitou M *et al.* Occludin as a possible determinant of tight junction permeability in endothelial cells. J Cell Sci 1997; 110: 1603–13.

213. Balda MS, Anderson JM. Two classes of tight junctions are revealed by ZO-1 isoforms. Am J Physiol 1993; 264: C918–24.

214. Mitic LL, Anderson JM. Molecular architecture of tight junctions. Annu Rev Physiol 1998; 60: 121–42.

215. Navarro P, Caveda L, Breviario F, Mandoteanu I, Lampugnani MG, Dejana E. Catenin-dependent and independent functions of vascular endothelial cadherin. J Biol Chem 1995; 270: 30965–72.

216. Leach L, Firth JA. Structure and permeability of human placental microvasculature. Microsci Res Tech 1997; 38: 137–44.

217. Alexander JS, Blaschuk OW, Haselton FR. An N-cadherin-like protein contributes to solute barrier maintenance in cultured endothelium. J Cell Physiol 1993; 156: 610–8.

218. Bundgaard M. The three dimensional organization of tight junctions in capillary endothelium revealed by serial-section electron microscopy. J Ultrastruct Res 1984; 88: 1–17.

219. Zand T, Underwood JM, Nunnari JJ, Majno G, Joris I. Endothelium and 'silver lines'. An electron microscopic study. Virchows Arch Pathol Anat 1982; 395: 133–44.

220. Anderson JM, Van-Itallie CM. Tight junctions and the molecular basis for regulation of paracellular permeability. Am J Physiol 1995; 269: G467–75.

221. Robinson PJ, Rapoport SI. Size selectivity of blood–brain barrier permeability at various times after osmotic opening. Am J Physiol 1987; 253: R459–66.

222. Blum MS, Toninelli E, Anderson JM *et al.* Cytoskeletal rearrangement mediates human microvascular endothelial tight junction modulation by cytokines. Am J Physiol 1997; 273: H286–94.

223. Schneeberger EE, Lynch RD. Structure, function and regulation of cellular tight junctions. Am J Physiol 1992; 262: L647–61.

224. Burns AR, Walker DC, Brown ES *et al.* Neutrophil transendothelial migration is independent of tight junctions and occurs preferentially at tricellular corners. J Immunol 1997; 159: 2893–903.

225. Rohrbach DH, Hassell JR, Klechman HK, Martin GR. Alterations in basement membrane (heparan sulfate) proteoglycan in diabetic mice. Diabetes 1982; 31: 185–8.

226. Chakrabarti S, Ma N, Sima AAF. Anionic sites in diabetic basement membranes and their possible role in diffusion barrier abnormalities in the BB-rat. Diabetologia 1991; 34: 301–6.

227. Shimomura H, Spiro RG. Studies on macromolecular components of human glomerular basement membrane and alterations in diabetes. Decreased levels of heparan sulfate, proteoglycan and laminin. Diabetes 1987; 36: 374–81.

228. Abrahamson DR. Recent studies on the structure and pathology of basement membranes. J Pathol 1986; 149: 257–78.

229. Hasslacher G, Reichenbacher R, Getcher F, Timpl R. Glomerular basement membrane synthesis and serum concentration of type IV collagen in streptozotocin-diabetic rats. Diabetologia 984; 26: 150–4.

230. Li W, Shen S, Khatami M, Rockey JH. Stimulation of retinal capillary pericyte protein and collagen synthesis in culture by high glucose concentration. Diabetes 1984; 33: 785–9.

231. Cagliero E, Maiello M, Boeri D, Roy S, Lorenzi M. Increased expression of basement membrane components in human endothelial cells cultured in high glucose. J Clin Invest 1988; 82: 735–8.

232. Ashworth CT, Erdmann RR, Arnold NJ. Age changes in the renal basement membrane of rats. Am J Pathol 1960; 36: 165–79.

233. Pino RM, Essner E, Pino LC. Location and chemical composition of anionic sites in Bruch's membrane of the rat. J Histochem Cytochem 1982; 30: 245–52.

234. Kanwar YS, Rosenzweig LJ, Kerjaschki DI. Glycosaminoglycans of the glomerular basement membrane in normal and nephrotic states. Ren Physiol 1981; 4: 121–30.

235. Kitano Y, Yoshikawa N, Nakamura H. Glomerular anionic sites in minimal change nephrotic syndrome and focal segmental glomerulosclerosis. Clin Nephrol 1993; 40: 199–204.

236. Torihara K, Suganuma T, Ide S, Morimitsu T. Anionic sites in blood capillaries of the mouse cochlear duct. Hear Res 1994; 77: 69–74.

237. Lawrenson JG, Reid AR, Allt G. Molecular characterization of anionic sites on the luminal front of endoneural capillaries in sciatic nerve. J Neurocytol 1994; 23: 29–37.

238. Lawrenson JG, Reid AR, Allt G. Molecular characteristics of pial microvessels of the rat optic nerve. Can pial microvessels be used as a model for the blood–brain barrier? Cell Tissue Res 1997; 288: 259–65.

239. Vorbrodt AW. Ultracytochemical characterization of anionic sites in the wall of brain capillaries. J Neurocytol 1989; 18: 359–68.

240. Dos-Santos WL, Rahman J, Klein N, Male DK. Distribution and analysis of surface charge on brain endothelium in vitro and in situ. Acta Neuropathol Berl 1995; 90: 305–11.

241. Ohtsuka A, Yamana S, Murakami T. Localization of membrane associated sialomucin on the free surface of mesothelial cells of the pleura, pericardium, and peritoneum. Histochem Cell Biol 1997; 107: 441–7.

242. Meirelles MN, Souto-Padron T, De-Souza W. Participation of cell surface anionic sites in the interaction between Trypanosoma cruzi and macrophages. J Submicrosc Cytol 1984; 16: 533–45.

243. Danon D, Marikovsky Y. The aging of the red blood cell. A multifactor process. Blood Cells 1988; 14: 7–18.

244. Lupu G, Calb M. Changes in the platelet surface charge in rabbits with experimental hypercholesterolemia. Artherosclerosis 1988; 72: 77–82.

245. Curry FE. Determinants of capillary permeability: a review of mechanisms based on single capillary studies in the frog. Circ Res 1986; 59: 367–80.

246. Haraldsson B. Physiological studies of macromolecular transport across capillary walls. Acta Physiol Scand 1986; 128 (suppl. 553): 1–40.

247. Hardebo JE, Kahrstrom J. Endothelial negative surface charge areas and blood–brain barrier function. Acta Physiol Scand 1985; 125: 495–9.

248. Brenner BM, Hostetter TH, Humes HD. Glomerular permeability: barrier function based on discrimination of molecular size and charge. Am J Physiol 1978; 234: F455–60.

249. Bray J, Robinson GB. Influence of charge on filtration across renal basement membrane films in vitro. Kidney Int 1984; 25: 527–33.

250. Skutelsky E, Danon D. Redistribution of surface anionic sites on the luminal front of blood vessel endothelium after interaction with polycationic ligand. J Cell Biol 1976; 71: 232–41.

251. Reeves WH, Kanwar YS, Farquhar MG. Assembly of the glomerular filtration surface. Differentiation of anionic sites in glomerular capillaries of newborn rat kidney. J Cell Biol 1980 85: 735–53.

252. Adamson RH, Huxley VH, Curry FE. Single capillary permeability to proteins having similar size but different charge. Am J Physiol 1988; 254: H304–12.

253. Nakao T, Ogura M, Takahashi H, Okada T. Charge-affected transperitoneal movement of amino acids in CAPD. Perit Dial Int 1996; 16 (suppl. 1): S88–90.

254. Leypoldt JK, Henderson LW. Molecular charge influences transperitoneal macromolecule transport. Kidney Int 1933; 43: 837–44.

255. Myers BD, Guasch A. Selectivity of the glomerular filtration barrier in healthy and nephrotic humans. Am J Nephrol 1993; 13: 311–7.

256. Krediet RT, Koomen GC, Koopman MG et al. The peritoneal transport of serum proteins and neutral dextran in CAPD patients. Kidney Int 1989; 35: 1064–72.

257. Vernier RL, Steffes MW, Sisson-Ross S, Mauer SM. Heparan sulfate proteoglycan in the glomerular basement membrane in type 1 diabetes mellitus. Kidney Int 1992; 41: 1070–80.

258. Vernier RL, Klein DJ, Sisson SP, Mahan JD, Oegema TR, Brown DM. Heparan sulfate-rich anionic sites in the human glomerular basement membrane. N Engl J Med 1983; 309: 1001–9.

259. Van-den-Heuvel LP, Van-den-Born J, Jalanko H et al. The glycosaminoglycan content of renal basement membranes in the congenital nephrotic syndrome of the Finnish type. Pediatr Nephrol 1992; 6: 10–15.

260. Washizawa K, Kasai S, Mori T, Komiyama A, Shigematsu H. Ultrastructural alteration of glomerular anionic sites in nephrotic patients. Pediatr Nephrol 1993; 7: 1–5.

261. Ramjee G, Coovadia HM, Adhikari M. Direct and indirect tests of pore size and charge selectivity in nephrotic syndrome. J Lab Clin Med 1996; 127: 195–9.

262. Rosenzweig LJ, Kanwar YS. Removal of sulfated (heparan sulfate) or nonsulfated (hyaluronic acid) glycosaminoglycans results in increased permeability of the glomerular basement membrane to ^{125}I–bovine serum albumin. Lab Invest 1982; 47: 177–84.

263. Wu VY, Wilson B, Cohen MP. Disturbances in glomerular basement membrane glycosaminoglycans in experimental diabetes. Diabetes 1987; 36: 679–83.

264. Van-den-Born J, Van-Kraats AA, Bakker MA et al. Reduction of heparan sulphate-associated anionic sites in the glomerular basement membrane of rats with streptozotocin-induced diabetic nephropathy. Diabetologia 1995; 38: 1169–75.

265. Galdi P, Shostak A, Jaichenko J, Fudin R, Gotloib L. Protamine sulfate induces enhanced peritoneal permeability to proteins. Nephron 1991; 57: 45–51.

266. Arfors KE, Rutili G, Svensjo E. Microvascular transport of macromolecules in normal and inflammatory conditions. Acta Physiol Scand Suppl 1979; 463: 93–103.

267. Gotloib L, Shostak A, Jaichenko J, Galdi P. Decreased density distribution of mesenteric and diaphragmatic microvascular anionic charges during murine abdominal sepsis. Resuscitation 1988; 16: 179–92.

268. Gotloib L, Shostak A, Galdi P, Jaichenko J, Fudin R. Loss of microvascular negative charges accompanied by interstitial edema in septic rats' heart. Circ Shock 1992; 36: 45–6.

269. Gotloib L, Shostak A. Lessons from peritoneal ultra-structure: from an inert dialyzing sheet to a living membrane. Contrib Nephrol 1992; 100: 207–35.

270. Shostak A, Gotloib L. Increased mesenteric, diaphragmatic, and pancreatic interstitial albumin content in rats with acute abdominal sepsis. Shock 1998; 9: 135–7.

271. Gotloib L, Barzilay E, Shostak A, Lev A. Sequential hemofiltration in monoliguric high capillary permeability pulmonary edema of severe sepsis: preliminary report. Crit Care Med 1984; 12: 997–1000.

272. Gotloib L, Barzilay E, Shostak A, Wais Z, Jaichenko J, Lev A. Hemofiltration in septic ARDS. The artificial kidney as an artificial endocrine lung. Resuscitation 1986; 13: 123–32.

273. Klein NJ, Shennan GI, Heyderman RS, Levin M. Alteration in glycosaminoglycan metabolism and surface charge on human umbilical vein endothelial cells induced by cytokines, endotoxin and neutrophils. J Cell Sci 1992; 102: 821–32.

274. Bone RC. The pathogenesis of sepsis. Ann Intern Med 1991; 115: 457–69.

275. Bone RS. Immunologic dissonance: a continuing evolution in our understanding of the systemic inflammatory response syndrome (SIRS) and the multiple organ dysfunction syndrome (MODS). Ann Intern Med 1996; 125: 680–87.

276. Gotloib L, Wajsbrot V, Shostak A, Kushnier R. Population analysis of mesothelium *in situ* and *in vivo* exposed to bicarbonate-buffered peritoneal dialysis fluid. Nephron 1996; 73: 219–27.

277. Sirois MG, Edelman ER. VEGF effect on vascular permeability is mediated by synthesis of platelet-activating factor. Am J Physiol 1997; 272: H2746–56.

278. Ryan GB, Grobety J, Majno G. Mesothelial injury and recovery. Am J Pathol 1973; 71: 93–112.

279. Gabbiani G, Badonnel MC, Majno G. Intra-arterial injections of histamine, serotonin, or bradykinin: a topographic study of vascular leakage. Proc Soc Exp Biol Med 1970; 135: 447–52.

280. Ryan GB, Majno G. Acute inflammation. A review. Am J Pathol 1977; 86: 183–276.

281. Joris I, Majno G, Corey EJ, Lewis RA. The mechanism of vascular leakage induced by leukotriene E4. Endothelial contraction. Am J Pathol 1987; 126: 19–24.

282. Gardner TW, Lesher T, Khin S, Vu G, Barber AJ, Brennan WA Jr. Histamine reduces ZO-1 tight-junction protein expression in cultured retinal microvascular endothelial cells. Biochem J 1996; 320: 717–21.

283. Kevil CG, Payne DK, Mire E, Alexander JS. Vascular permeability factor/vascular endothelial cell growth factor-mediated permeability occurs through disorganization of endothelial junctional proteins. J Biol Chem 1998; 273: 15099–103.

284. Predescu D, Palade GE. Plasmalemmal vesicles represent the large pore system of continuous microvascular endothelium. Am J Physiol 1993; 265: H725–33.

285. Esser S, Wolburg K, Wolburg H, Breier G, Kurzchalia T, Risau W. Vascular endothelial growth factor induces endothelial fenestrations *in vitro*. J Cell Biol 1998; 140: 947–59.

286. Feng D, Nagy JA, Hipp J, Pyne K, Dvorak AM. Reinterpretation of endothelial cell gaps induced by vasoactive mediators in guinea-pig, mouse and rat: many are transcellular pores. J Physiol Lond 1997; 504: 747–61.

287. Carlsson O, Nielsen S, Zakaria-el R, Rippe B. *In vivo* inhibition of transcellular water channels (aquaporin-1) during acute peritoneal dialysis in rats. Am J Physiol 1996; 271: H2254–62.

288. Panekeet MM, Mulder JB, Weening JJ, Struijk DG, Zweers MM, Krediet RT. Demonstration of aquaporin-CHIP in peritoneal tissue of uremic and CAPD patients. Perit Dial Int 1996; 16 (suppl. 1): S54–7.

289. Schnitzer JE, Oh P. Aquaporin-1 in plasma membrane and caveolae provides mercury-sensitive water channels across lung endothelium. Am J Physiol 1996; 270: H416–22.

290. Nielsen S, Smith BL, Christensen EI, Agre P. Distribution of the aquaporin CHIP in secretory and resorptive epithelia and capillary endothelia. Proc Natl Acad Sci USA 1993; 90: 7275–79.

291. Wintour EM. Water channels and urea transporters. Clin Exp Pharmacol Physiol 1997; 24: 1–9.

292. Ikomi F, Hunt J, Hanna G, Schmid-Schonbein GW. Interstitial fluid, plasma protein, colloid, and leukocyte uptake into initial lymphatics. J Appl Physiol 1996; 81: 2060–7.

293. Rutili G, Parker JC, Taylor AE. Fluid balance in ANTU-injured lungs during crystalloid and colloid infusions. J Appl Physiol 1984; 56: 993–8.

294. Drake RE, Gabel JC. Abdominal lymph flow response to intraperitoneal fluid in awake sheep. Lymphology 1991; 24: 77–81.

295. Ottaviani G, Azzali G. Ultrastructure of lymphatic vessels in some functional conditions. In: Comel M, Laszt L, eds. Morphology and Histochemistry of the Vascular Wall. Basel: Karger, 1966, pp. 325.

296. Foldi M, Csanda E, Simon M et al. Lymphogenic haemangiopathy. 'Prelymphatic' pathways in the wall of cerebral and cervical blood vessels. Angiologica 1968; 5: 250–62.

297. Hauck G. The connective tissue space in view of the lymphology. Experientia 1982; 38: 1121–2.

298. Crone G. Exchange of molecules between plasma, interstitial tissue and lymph. Pflugers Arch Suppl 1972: 65–79.

299. Casley-Smith JR. Lymph and lymphatics. In: Kaley G, Altura BM, eds. Microcirculation, vol. 4. Baltimore, MD: University Park Press, 1981, pp. 423.

300. Schmid-Schonbein GW. Mechanisms causing initial lymphatics to expand and compress to promote lymph flow. Arch Histol Cytol 1990; 53 (suppl. 1): 107–14.

301. Rhodin JA, Sue SL. Combined intravital microscopy and electron microscopy of the blind beginnings of the mesenteric lymphatic capillaries of the rat mesentery. A preliminary report. Acta Physiol Scand Suppl 1979; 463: 51–8.

302. Jones WR, O'Morchoe CC, Jarosz HM, O'Morchoe PJ. Distribution of charged sites on lymphatic endothelium. Lymphology 1986; 19: 5–14.

303. Schmid-Schonbein GW. Microlymphatics and lymph flow. Physiological Rev 1990; 70: 987–1028.

304. Leak LV, Burke JF. Fine structure of the lymphatic capillary and the adjoining connective tissue area. Am J Anat 1966; 118: 785–809.

305. Leak LV, Burke JF. Electron microscopic study of lymphatic capillaries in the removal of connective tissue fluids and particulate substances. Lymphology 1968; 1: 39–52.

306. Gerli R, Ibba L, Fruschelli G. Ultrastructural cytochemistry of anchoring filaments of human lymphatic capillaries and their relation to elastic fibers. Lymphology 1991; 24: 105–12.

307. Taylor AE. The lymphatic edema safety factor: the role of edema dependent lymphatic factors (EDLF). Lymphology 190; 23: 111–23.

308. Hogan RD, Unthank JL. The initial lymphatics as sensors of interstitial fluid volume. Microvasc Res 1986 31: 317–24.

309. Leak LV. Distribution of cell surface charges on mesothelium and lymphatic endothelium. Microvasc Res 986; 31: 18–30.

310. Leak V. Electron microscopic observations on lymphatic capillaries and the structural components of the connective tissue–lymph interface. Microvasc Res 1970; 2: 361–91.

311. Leak LV. The structure of lymphatic capillaries in lymph formation. Fed Proc 1976 35: 1863–71.

312. Shinohara H, Nakatani T, Matsuda T. Postnatal development of the ovarian bursa of the golden hamster *(Mesocricetus auratus)*: its complete closure and morphogenesis of lymphatic stomata. Am J Anat 1987; 179: 385–402.

313. Hauck G. Capillary permeability and micro-lymph drainage. Vasa 1994; 23: 93–7.

314. McCallum WG. On the mechanisms of absorption of granular material from the peritoneum. Bull Johns Hopkins Hosp 1903; 14, 105–15.

315. Tsilibary EC, Wissig SL. Absorption from the peritoneal cavity. SEM study of the mesothelium covering the peritoneal surface of the muscular portion of the diaphragm. Am J Anat 1977; 149: 127–33.

316. Leak LV, Rahil K. Permeability of the diaphragmatic mesothelium. The ultrastructural basis for stomata. Am J Anat 1978; 151: 557–92.

317. Leak LV. Lymphatic endothelial–interstitial interface. Lymphology 187; 20: 196–204.

318. Simer PM. Omental lymphatics in man. Anat Rec 1935; 63: 253–62.

319. Vajda J. Innervation of lymph vessels. Acta Morphol Acad Sci Hung 1966; 14: 197–208.

320. Hargens AR, Zweifach BW. Contractile stimuli in collecting lymph vessels. Am J Physiol 1977; 233: H57–65.

321. Gnepp DR, Green FH. Scanning electron microscopic study of canine lymphatic vessels and their valves. Lymphology 1980; 13: 91–9.

322. Ohtani O. Structure of lymphatics in rat cecum with special reference to submucosal collecting lymphatics endowed with smooth muscle cells and valves. I. A scanning electron microscopic study. Arch Hist Cytol 1992; 55: 429–36.

323. Moller R. Arrangement and fine structure of lymphatic vessels in the human spermatic cord. Andrologia 1980; 12: 564–76.

324. Zweifach BW, Prather JW. Micromanipulation of pressure in terminal lymphatics in the mesentery. Am J Physiol 1975; 228: 1326–35.

325. Horstmann E. Anatomie und Physiologie des lymphgefa B systems im bauchraum. In: Bartelheimer H, Heising N, eds. Actuelle Gastroenterologie. Stuttgart: Verh, Thieme, 1968, p. 1.

326. Ohhashi T, Azuma T, Sakaguchi M. Active and passive mechanical characteristics of bovine mesenteric lymphatics. Am J Physiol 1980; 239: H88–95.

327. Watanabe N, Kawai Y, Ohhashi T. Demonstration of both B1 and B2 adrenoreceptors mediating negative chronotropic effects on spontaneous activity in isolated bovine mesenteric lymphatics. Microvasc Res 1990; 39: 50–9.

328. Ohhashi T, Azuma T. Sympathetic effects on spontaneous activity in bovine mesenteric lymphatics (retracted by Ohhashi T, Azuma T. In: Am J Physiol 1986; 251: H226). Am J Physiol 1984; 247: H610–15.

329. Ohhashi T, Azuma T Pre and postjunctional alpha-adrenoceptors at the sympathetic neuroeffector junction in bovine mesenteric lymphatics. Microvac Res 1986; 31: 31–40.

330. Watanabe N, Kawai Y, Ohhashi T. Dual effects of histamine on spontaneous activity in isolated bovine mesenteric lymphatics. Microvasc Res 1988; 36: 239–49.

331. Ferguson MK, Shahinian HK, Michelassi F. Lymphatic smooth muscle responses to leukotrienes, histamine and platelet activating factor. J Surg Res 1988; 44: 172–7.

332. Ohhashi T, Kawai Y, Azuma T. The response of lymphatic smooth muscles to vasoactive substances. Pflugers Arch 1978; 375: 183–8.

333. Azuma T, Ohhashi T, Roddie IC. Bradykinin-induced contractions of bovine mesenteric lymphatics. J Physiol Lond 1983; 342: 217–27.

334. Ohhashi T, Olschowka JA, Jacobowitz DM. Vasoactive intestinal peptide inhibitory innervation in bovine mesenteric lymphatics. A histochemical and pharmacological study. Circ Res 1983; 53: 535–8.

335. Abu-Hijleh MF, Habbai OA, Moqattash ST. The role of the diaphragm in lymphatic absorption from the peritoneal cavity. J Anat 1995; 186: 453–67.

336. Fruschelli G, Gerli R, Alessandrini G, Sacchi G. Il controllo neurohumorale dalla contratilita dei vasi linfatici. In: Atti dalla Societa Italiana di Anatomia. 39th Convegno Nazaionale, 19/21 September. Firenze: I Sedicesimo, 1983, p. 2.

337. Starling EH, Tubby A. On absorption from and secretion into the serous cavities. J Physiol (Lond) 1894; 16: 140–55.

338. Starling EH. On the absorption of fluid from the connective tissue spaces. J Physiol (Lond) 1896; 19: 312–21.

339. Drinker CF, Field ME. The protein of mammalian lymph and the relation of lymph to tissue fluid. Am J Physiol 1931; 97: 32–45.

340. Allen L, Vogt E. Mechanisms of lymphatic absorption from serous cavities. Am J Physiol 1937; 119: 776–82.

341. Brace RA, Guyton AC. Interstitial fluid pressure: capsule, free fluid, gel fluid and gel absorption pressure in subcutaneous tissue. Microvasc Res 1979; 18: 217–28.

342. Guyton AC, Granger HJ, Taylor AE. Interstitial fluid pressure. Physiol Rev 1971; 51: 527–63.

343. Guyton AC, Taylor AE, Granger HJ, Gibson WH. Regulation of interstitial fluid volume and pressure. Adv Exp Med Biol 1972; 33: 111–8.

344. Guyton AC, Taylor AE, Brace RA. A synthesis of interstitial fluid regulation and lymph formation. Fed Proc 976; 35: 1881–5.

345. Zink J, Greenway CV. Intraperitoneal pressure in formation and reabsorption of ascites in cats. Am J Physiol 1977; 233: H185–90.

346. Zink J, Greenway CV. Control of ascites absorption in anesthetized cats: effects of intraperitoneal pressure, protein, and furosemide diuresis. Gastroenterology 1977; 73: 119–24.

347. Imholz AL, Koomen GC, Struijk DG, Arisz L, Krediet RT. Effect of an increased intraperitoneal pressure on fluid and solute transport during CAPD. Kidney Int 1993; 44: 1078–85.

348. Durand PY, Chanliau J, Gamberoni J, Hestin D, Kessler M. Intraperitoneal pressure, peritoneal permeability and volume of ultrafiltration in CAPD. Adv Perit Dial 1992; 8: 22–5.

349. Gotloib L, Garmizo AL, Varka I, Mines M. Reduction of vital capacity due to increased intra-abdominal pressure during peritoneal dialysis. Perit Dial Bull 1981; 1: 63–4.

350. Flessner MF. Net ultrafiltration in peritoneal dialysis: role of direct fluid absorption into peritoneal tissue. Blood Purif 1992; 10: 136–47.

351. Flessner MF, Parker RJ, Sieber SM. Peritoneal lymphatic uptake of fibrinogen and erythrocytes in the rat. Am J Physiol 1983; 244: H89–96.

352. Silk YN, Goumas WM, Douglass HO Jr, Huben RP. Chylous ascites and lymphocyst management by peritoneovenous shunt. Surgery 1991; 110: 561–5.

353. Casley Smith JR. A fine structural study of variations in protein concentration in lacteals during compression and relaxation. Lymphology 1979; 12: 59–65.

354. O'Morchoe CC, Jones WR 3d, Jarosz HM, O'Morchoe PJ, Fox LM. Temperature dependence of protein transport across lymphatic endothelium *in vitro*. J Cell Biol 1984; 98: 629–40.

355. Dobbins WO, Rollins EL Intestinal mucosal lymphatic permeability: an electron microscopic study of endothelial vesicles and cell junctions. J Ultrastruct Res 1970; 33: 29–59.

356. Shasby DM, Peterson MW. Effects of albumin concentration on endothelial albumin transport *in vitro*. Am J Physiol 1987; 253: H654–61.

357. Albertini KH, O'Morchoe CC. Renal lymphatic ultrastructure and translymphatic transport. Microvasc Res 1980; 19: 338–51.

358. Haller A. Primae linae physiologiae in usum Praelectionum Academicarum avetae et emendato. Gottingae, Capit 25, 1751, p. 41.

359. Furness JB. Arrangement of blood vessels and their relation with adrenergic nerves in the rat mesentery. J Anat 1973; 115: 347–64.

360. Beattie JM. The cells of inflammatory exudations: an experimental research as to their function and density, and also as to the origin of the mononucleated cells. J Pathol Bacteriol 1903; 8: 130–77.

361. Durham HE. The mechanism of reaction to peritoneal infection. J Pathol Bacteriol 1897; 4: 338–82.

362. Josey AL. Studies in the physiology of the eosinophil. V. The role of the eosinophil in inflammation. Folia Haematol 1934; 51: 80–95.

363. Webb RL. Changes in the number of cells within the peritoneal fluid of the white rat, between birth and sexual maturity. Folia Haematol 1934; 51: 445–51.

364. Padawer J, Gordon AS. Cellular elements in the peritoneal fluid of some mammals. Anat Rec 1956; 124: 209–22.

365. Fruhman GJ. Neutrophil mobilization into peritoneal fluid. Blood 1960; 16: 1753–61.

366. Seeley SF, Higgins GM, Mann FC. The cytologic response of the peritoneal fluid to certain substances. Surgery 1937; 2: 862–76.

367. Bercovici B, Gallily R. The cytology of the human peritoneal fluid. Cytology 1978; 22: 124.

368. Becker S, Halme J, Haskill S. Heterogeneity of human peritoneal macrophages: cytochemical and flow cytometric studies. J Reticuloendothel Soc 1983; (ES) 33: 127–38.

369. De Brux JA, Dupre-Froment J, Mintz M.: Cytology of the peritoneal fluids sampled by coelioscopy or by cul de sac puncture. Its value in gynecology. Acta Cytol 1968; 12: 395–403.

370. Mahoney CA, Sherwood N, Yap EH, Singleton TP, Whitney DJ, Cornbleet PJ. Ciliated cell remnants in peritoneal dialysis fluid. Arch Pathol Lab Med 1993; 117: 211–3.

371. Fruhmann GJ. Adrenal steroids and neutrophil mobilization. Blood 1962; 20: 335–63.

372. Spriggs AI, Boddington MM. The Cytology of Effusions, 2nd edn. New York: Grune & Straton, 1968, pp. 5–17.

373. Domagala W, Woyke S. Transmission and scanning electron microscopic studies of cells in effusions. Acta Cytol 1975; 19: 214–24.

374. Efrati P, Nir E. Morphological and cytochemical investigation of human mesothelial cells from pleural and peritoneal effusions. A light and electron microscopy study. Israel J Med Sci 976; 12: 662–73.

375. Bewtra Ch, Greer KP. Ultrastructural studies of cells in body cavity effusions. Acta Cytol 1985 29: 226–38.

376. Chapman JS, Reynolds RC. Eosinophilic response to intraperitoneal blood. J Lab Clin Med 1958; 51: 516–20.

377. Northover BJ. The effect of various anti-inflammatory drugs on the accumulation of leucocytes in the peritoneal cavity of mice. J Pathol Bacteriol 1964; 88: 332–5.

378. Hurley JV, Ryan GB, Friedman A. The mononuclear response to intrapleural injection in the rat. J Pathol Bact 1966; 91: 575–87.

379. Rubin J, Rogers WA, Taylor HM. *et al.* Peritonitis during continuous ambulatory peritoneal dialysis. Ann Intern Med 1980; 92: 7–13.

380. Cichoki T, Hanicki Z, Sulowicz W, Smolenski O, Kopec J, Zembala M. Output of peritoneal cells into peritoneal dialysate. Cytochemical and functional studies. Nephron 1983; 35: 175–82.

381. Strippoli P, Coviello F, Orbello G *et al.* First exchange neutrophilia is not always an index of peritonitis during CAPD. Adv Perit Dial 1989; 4: 121–3.

382. Kubicka U, Olszewski WL, Maldyk J, Wierzbicki Z, Orkiszewska A. Normal human immune peritoneal cells: phenotypic characteristics. Immunobiology 1989; 180: 80–92.

383. Gotloib L, Mines M, Garmizo AL, Rodoy Y. Peritoneal dialysis using the subcutaneous intraperitoneal prosthesis. Dial Transplant 1979; 8: 217–20.

384. Hoeltermann W, Schlotmann-Hoelledr E, Winkelmann M, Pfitzer P. Lavage fluid from continuous ambulatory peritoneal dialysis. A model for mesothelial cell changes. Acta Cytol 1989; 33: 591–4.

385. Chan MK, Chow L, Lam SS, Jones B. Peritoneal eosinophilia in patients on continuous ambulatory peritoneal dialysis: a prospective study. Am J Kidney Dis 1988; 11: 180–3..

386. Gokal R, Ramos JM, Ward MK, Kerr DN. 'Eosinophilic' peritonitis in continuous ambulatory peritoneal dialysis (CAPD). Clin Nephrol 1981; 15: 328–30.

387. Leak LV. Interaction of mesothelium to intraperitoneal stimulation. Lab Invest 1983; 48: 479–90.

388. Raftery AT. Regeneration of parietal and visceral peritoneum: an electron microscopical study. J Anat 1973; 115: 375–92.

389. Raftery AT. Mesothelial cells in peritoneal fluid. J Anat 1973; 115: 237–53.

390. Koss LG. Diagnostic Cytology and its Histopathologic Bases, 3rd edn. Philadelphia, PA: Lippincot, 1979, chs 16–25.

391. Ryan GB, Grobety J, Majno G. Postoperative peritoneal adhesions: a study of the mechanisms. Am J Pathol 1971; 65: 117–48.

392. Ryan GB, Grobety J, Majno G. Mesothelial injury and recovery. Am J Pathol 1973; 71: 93–112.

393. Di Paolo N, Sacchi G, De Mia M *et al.* Does dialysis modify the peritoneal structure? In: La Greca G, Chiaramonte S, Fabris A, Feriani M, Ronco G, eds. Peritoneal Dialysis, Milan: Wichtig Ed., 1956, pp. 11–24.

394. Dobbie JW, Zaki M, Wilson L. Ultrastructural studies on the peritoneum with special reference to chronic ambulatory peritoneal dialysis. Scot Med J 1981; 26: 213–23.

395. Verger G, Brunschvicg O, Le Charpentier Y, Lavergne A, Vantelon J. Structural and ultrastructural peritoneal membrane changes and permeability alterations during continuous ambulatory peritoneal dialysis. Proc EDTA 1981; 18: 199–205.

396. Susuki S, Enosawa S, Kakefuda T *et al.* A novel immunosuppressant, FTY720, with a unique mechanism of action, induces long-term graft acceptance in rat and dog allotransplantation. Transplantation 1996; 61: 200–5.

397. Nagata S. Fas-mediated apoptosis. Adv Exp Med Biol 1996; 406: 119–24.

398. Laster SM, Mackenzie JM Jr. Bleb formation and F-actin distribution during mitosis and tumor necrosis factor-induced apoptosis. Microsci Res Tech 1996; 34: 272–80.

399. Yang AH, Chen JY, Lin YP, Huang TP, Wu CW. Peritoneal dialysis solution induces apoptosis of mesothelial cells. Kidney Int 1997; 51: 1280–8.

400. Laiho KU, Trump BF. Mitochondria of Ehrlich ascites tumor cells. Lab Invest 1975; 32: 163–82.

401. Pentilla A, Trump BF. Studies on the modification of the cellular response to injury. III. Electron microscopic studies on the protective effect of acidosis on p-chloromercuribenzene sulfonic acid (PCMBS) induced injury of Ehrlich ascites tumor cells. Virchows Arch B Cell Pathol 1975; 18: 17–34.

402. Trump BF, Berezesky IK, Chang SH, Phelps PC. The pathways of cell death: oncosis, apoptosis, and necrosis. Toxicol Pathol 1997; 25: 82–8.

403. Dobbie JW, Anderson JD. Ultrastructure, distribution, and density of lamellar bodies in human peritoneum. Perit Dial Int 1996; 16: 488–96.

404. Slater ND, Cope GH, Raftery AT. Mesothelial hyperplasia in response to peritoneal dialysis fluid: a morphometric study in the rat. Nephron 1991; 58: 466–71.

405. Witowski J, Jorres A, Coles GA, Williams JD, Topley N. Superinduction of IL-6 synthesis in human peritoneal mesothelial cells is related to the induction and stabilization of IL-6 mRNA. Kidney Int 1996; 50: 1212–23.

406. Topley N, Williams JD. Effect of peritoneal dialysis on cytokine production by peritoneal cells. Blood Purif 1996; 14: 188–97.

407. Di Paolo N, Garosi G, Traversari L, Di Paolo M. Mesothelial biocompatibility of peritoneal dialysis solutions. Perit Dial Int 1993; 13 (suppl. 2): S109–12.

408. Breborowicz A, Rodela H, Oreopoulos DG. Toxicity of osmotic solutes on human mesothelial cells *in vitro*. Kidney Int 1992; 41: 1280–5.

409. Jorres A, Gahl GM, Topley N *et al. In vitro* biocompatibility of alternative CAPD fluids: comparison of bicarbonate-buffered and glucose-polymer-based solutions. Nephrol Dial Transplant 1994; 9: 785–90.

410. Shostak A, Pivnik K, Gotloib L. Daily short exposure of cultured mesothelial cells to lactated, high-glucose, low pH peritoneal dialysis fluid induces a low-profile regenerative steady state. Nephrol Dial Transplant 1996; 11: 608–13.

411. Topley N, Kaur D, Petersen MM *et al. In vitro* effects of bicarbonate and bicarbonate-lactate buffered peritoneal dialysis solutions on mesothelial and neutrophil function. J Am Soc Nephrol 1996; 7: 128–224.

412. Breborowicz A, Rodela H, Karon J, Martis L, Oreopoulos DG. *In vitro* stimulation of the effect of peritoneal dialysis solution on mesothelial cells. Am J Kidney Dis 1997; 29: 404–9.

413. Topley N. *In vitro* biocompatibility of bicarbonate-based peritoneal dialysis solutions. Perit Dial Int 1997; 17: 42–7.

414. Jorres A, Williams JD, Topley N. Peritoneal dialysis solution biocompatibility: inhibitory mechanisms and recent studies with bicarbonate-buffered solutions. Perit Dial Int 1997; 17 (suppl. 2): S42–6.

415. Di Paolo N, Garosi G, Monaci G, Brardi S. Biocompatibility of peritoneal dialysis treatment. Nephrol Dial Transplant 1997; 12 (suppl. 1): 78–83.

416. Holmes CJ. Peritoneal host defense mechanisms. Perit Dial Int 1996; 16 (suppl. 1): S124–5.

417. Zemel D, Krediet RT. Cytokine patterns in the effluent of continuous ambulatory peritoneal dialysis. Relationship to peritoneal permeability. Blood Purif 1996; 14: 198–216.

418. Topley N, Petersen MM, Mackenzie R *et al.* Human peritoneal mesothelial cell prostaglandin synthesis: induction of cyclooxygenase mRNA by peritoneal macrophage-derived cytokines. Kidney Int 1994; 46: 900–9.

419. Shostak A, Pivnik E, Gotloib L. Cultured rat mesothelial cells generate hydrogen peroxide: a new player in peritoneal defense? J Am Soc Nephrol 1996; 7: 2371–78.

420. Gotloib L. Large mesothelial cells in peritoneal dialysis: a sign of degeneration or adaptation? Perit Dial Int 1996; 16: 118–20.

421. Raftery AT. An enzyme histochemical study of mesothelial cells in rodents. J Anat 1973; 115: 365–73.

422. Whitaker D, Papadimitriou JM, Walters MN. The mesothelium; techniques for investigating the origin, nature and behaviour of mesothelial cells. J Pathol 1980; 132, 263–71.

423. Gotloib L, Shostak A, Wajsbrot V, Kushnier R. The cytochemical profile of visceral mesothelium under the influence of lactated-hyperosmolar peritoneal dialysis solutions. Nephron 1995; 69: 466–71.

424. Gotloib L, Wajsbrot V, Shostak A, Kushnier R. Morphology of the peritoneum: effect of peritoneal dialysis. Perit Dial Int 1995; 15 (suppl.): S9–11.

425. Di Paolo N, Garosi G, Petrini G, Monaci G. Morphological and morphometric changes in mesothelial cells during peritoneal dialysis in the rabbit. Nephron 1996; 74: 594–9.

426. Gotloib L, Wajsbrot V, Shostak A, Kushnier R. Effect of hyperosmolality upon the mesothelial monolayer exposed *in-vivo* and *in-situ* to a mannitol enriched dialysis solution. Nephron 1999; 81: 301–9.

427. Wajsbrot V, Shostak A, Gotloib L, Kushnier R. Biocompatibility of a glucose-free, acidic lactated solution for peritoneal dialysis evaluated by population analysis of mesothelium. Nephron 1998; 79, 322–32.

428. Walters WB, Buck RC. Mitotic activity of peritoneum in contact with a regenerative area of peritoneum. Virchows Arch B Zellpathol 1973; 13, 48–52.

429. Gotloib L, Shostak A, Wajsbrot V, Kushnier R. High glucose induces an hypertrophic, senescent mesothelial cell phenotype after long, *in vivo* exposure. Nephron 1999; 82: 164–7.

430. Vincent F, Brun H, Clain E, Ronot X, Adolphe M. Effects of oxygen free radicals on proliferation kinetics of cultured rabbit articular chondrocytes. J Cell Physiol 1989; 141: 262–6.

431. De Bono DP, Yang WD. Exposure to low concentrations of hydrogen peroxide causes delayed endothelial cell death and inhibits proliferation of surviving cells. Atherosclerosis 1995; 114: 235–45.

432. Bladier G, Wolvetang EJ, Hutchinson P, De Haan JB, Kola I. Response of a primary human fibroblast cell line to H_2O_2: senescence-like growth arrest or apoptosis? Cell Growth Difer 1997; 8: 589–98.

433. Nicotera P, Dypbukt JM, Rossi AD, Manzo L, Orrenius S. Thiol modification and cell signalling in chemical toxicity. Toxicol Lett 1992; 64–5 (Spec No.): 563–7.

434. Dypbukt JM, Ankarcrona M, Burkitt M *et al.* Different pro-oxidant levels stimulate growth, trigger apoptosis, or produce necrosis of insulin-secreting RINm5F cells. The role of intracellular polyamines. J Biol Chem 1994; 269: 30553–60.

435. Orrenius S, Burkitt MJ, Kass GE, Dypbukt JM, Nicotera P. Calcium ions and oxidative cell injury. Ann Neurol 1992; 32 (suppl.): S33–42.

436. Curcio F, Ceriello A. Decreased cultured endothelial cell proliferation in high glucose medium is reversed by antioxidants: new insights on the pathophysiological mechanisms of diabetic vascular complications *in Vitro*. Cell Dev Biol 1992; 28A: 787–90.

437. Kashiwagi A, Asahina T, Ikebuchi M *et al.* Abnormal glutathione metabolism and increased cytotoxicity caused by H_2O_2 in human umbilical vein endothelial cells cultured in high glucose medium. Diabetologia 1994; 37: 264–9.

438. Breborowicz A, Witowski J, Wieczorowska K, Martis L, Serkes KD, Oreopoulos DG. Toxicity of free radicals to mesothelial cells and peritoneal membrane. Nephron 1993; 65: 62–6.

439. Donnini D, Zambito AM, Perrella G, Ambesi-Impiombato FS, Curcio F. Glucose may induce cell death through a free radical-mediated mechanism. Biochem Biophys Res Commun 1996; 219: 412–7.

440. Kashwem A, Nomoto Y, Tanabe R *et al.* The effect of dialysate glucose on phagocyte superoxide generation in CAPD patients. Perit Dial Int 1998; 18: 52–9.

441. Elgawish A, Glomb M, Friedlander M, Monnier VM. Involvement of hydrogen peroxide in collagen cross-linking by high glucose *in vitro* and *in vivo*. J Biol Chem 1996; 272: 12964–71.

442. Friedlander MA, Wu YC, Elgawish A, Monnier VM. Early and advanced glycosylation end products. Kinetics of formation and clearance in peritoneal dialysis. J Clin Invest 1996; 97: 728–35.

443. Dobbie JW, Anderson JD, Hind G. Long-term effects on peritoneal dialysis on peritoneal morphology. Perit Dial Int 1994; 14 (suppl. 3): S14–20.

444. Dobbie JW: Pathogenesis of peritoneal fibrosing syndromes (sclerosing peritonitis) in peritoneal dialysis. Perit Dial Int 1992; 12: 14–27.

445. Verger G, Celicout B, Larpent L, Goupil A. Encapsulating peritonitis during continuous ambulatory peritoneal dialysis. A physiopathologic hypothesis. Presse Med 1986; 15: 1311–4.

446. Gandhi VC, Humayun HM, Ing TS *et al.* Sclerotic thickening of the peritoneal membrane in maintenance peritoneal dialysis patients. Arch Intern Med 1980; 140: 1201–3.

447. Slingeneyer A, Mion G, Mourad G, Canaud B, Faller B, Beraud JJ. Progressive sclerosing peritonitis: a late and severe complication of maintenance peritoneal dialysis. Trans Am Soc Artif Intern Organs 1983; 29: 633–40.

448. Foo KT, Ng-Kc, Rauff A, Foong WC, Sinniah R. Unusual small intestinal obstruction in adolescent girls: the abdominal cocoon. Br J Surg 1978; 65: 427–30.

449. Lee RE, Baddeley H, Marshall AJ, Read AE. Practolol peritonitis. Clin Radiol 1977; 28: 119–28.

450. Harty RF. Sclerosing peritonitis and propranolol. Arch Intern Med. 1978; 138: 1424–6.

451. Baxter-Smith DC, Monypenny IJ, Dorricott NJ. Sclerosing peritonitis in patient on timolol. Lancet 1978; 2: 149.

452. Clarck CV, Terris R. Sclerosing peritonitis associated with metoprolol. Lancet 1983; 1: 937.

453. Phillips RK, Dudley HA. The effect of tetracycline lavage and trauma on visceral and parietal peritoneal ultrastructure and adhesion formation. Br J Surg 1984; 71: 537–9.

454. Di Paolo N, Di Paolo M, Tanganelli P, Brardi S, Bruci A. Technique nefrologiche e dialitici. Perugia: Bios Editore, 1988, p. 5.

455. Myhre-Jensen O, Bergmann Larsen S, Astrup T. Fibrinolytic activity in serosal and synovial membranes. Rats, guinea pigs and rabbits. Arch Pathol 1969; 88: 623–30.

456. Gervin AS, Puckett ChL, Silver D. Serosal hypofibrinolysis. A cause of postoperative adhesions. Am J Surg 1973; 1225: 80–8.

457. Buckman RF, Woods M, Sargent L, Gervin AS. A unifying pathogenetic mechanism in the etiology of intraperitoneal adhesions. J Surg Res 1976; 20: 1–5.

458. Gotloib L, Shostak A, Bar-Sella P, Cohen R. Continuous mesothelial injury and regeneration during long term peritoneal dialysis. Perit Dial Bull 1987; 7: 148–55.

459. Gotloib L, Wajsbrot V, Shostak A, Kushnier R. Experimental approach to peritoneal morphology. Perit Dial Int 1994; 14 (suppl. 3): S6–11.

460. Honda K, Nitta K, Horita S, Yumura W, Nihei H. Morphological changes in the peritoneal vasculature of patients on CAPD with ultrafiltration failure. Nephron 1996; 72: 171–6.

461. Eskeland G, Kjaerheim A. Regeneration of parietal peritoneum in rats. 2. An electron microscopical study. Acta Pathol Microbiol Scand 1966; 68, 379–95.

462. Watters WB, Buck RC. Scanning electron microscopy of mesothelial regeneration in the rat. Lab Invest 1972; 26: 604–9.

463. Whitaker D, Papadimitriou J. Mesothelial healing: morphological and kinetic investigations. J Pathol Bac 1957; 73: 1–10.

464. Renvall SY. Peritoneal metabolism and intrabdominal adhesion formation during experimental peritonitis. Acta Chirurg Scand Suppl 1980; 503: 1–48.

465. Ellis H, Harrison W, Hugh TB. The healing of peritoneum under normal and pathological conditions. Br J Surg 1965; 52: 471–6.

466. Ellis H. The cause and prevention of postoperative intraperitoneal adhesions. Surg Gynecol Obstet 1971; 133: 497–511.

467. Whitaker D, Papadimitriou J. Mesothelial healing: morphological and kinetic investigations. J Pathol 1985; 145: 159–75.

468. Cameron GR, Hassan SM, De SN. Repair of Glisson's capsule after tangential wounds on the liver. J Pathol Bacteriol 1957; 73: 1–10.

469. Johnson FR, Whitting HW. Repair of parietal peritoneum. Br J Surg 1962; 49, 653–60.

470. Eskeland G. Regeneration of parietal peritoneum in rats. A light microscopical study. Acta Pathol Microbiol Scand 1966; 68: 355–78.

471. Williams DC. The peritoneum. A plea for a change in attitude towards this membrane. Br J Surg 42: 1955; 401–5.

472. Shaldon S. Peritoneal macrophage: the first line of defense. In: La Greca G, Chiaramonte S, Fabris A, Feriani M, Ronco G, eds. Peritoneal Dialysis. Milan: Wichtig. Ed., 1986, p. 201.

473. Raftery AT. Regeneration of parietal and visceral peritoneum. A light microscopical study. Brit J Surgery 1973; 60: 293–9.

474. Maximow AA, Bloom W. A Textbook of Histology. Philadelphia, PA: Saunders, 1942, pp. 63–66.

475. Gonzales S, Friemann J, Muller KM, Pott F. Ultrastructure of mesothelial regeneration after intraperitoneal injection of asbestos fibres on rat omentum. Pathol Res Pract 1991; 187: 931–5.

476. Watters WB, Buck RC. Mitotic activity of peritoneum in contact with a regenerating area of peritoneum. Virchows Arch B Cell Pathol 1973; 13: 48–54.

477. Mironov VA, Gusev SA, Baradi AF. Mesothelial stomata overlying omental milky spots: scanning electron microscopic study. Cell Tissue Res 1979; 201, 327–30.

478. Doherty NS, Griffiths RJ, Hakkinen JP, Scampoli DN, Milici AJ. Post-capillary venules in the 'milky spots' of the greater omentum are the major site of plasma protein and leukocyte extravasation in rodent models of peritonitis. Inflamm Res 1995; 44: 169–77.

479. Fukatsu K, Saito H, Han I. et al. The greater omentum is the primary site of neutrophil exudation in peritonitis. J Am Coll Surg 1996; 183: 450–6.

480. Krist LF, Eestermans IL, Steenbergen JJ. Cellular composition of milky spots in the human greater omentum: an immunochemical and ultrastructural study. Anat Rec 1995; 241: 163–74.

481. Leypoldt JK. Evaluation of peritoneal membrane pore models. Blood Purif 1992; 10: 227–38.

482. Gotloib L, Oreopoulos DG. Transfer across the peritoneum: passive or active? Nephron 1981; 29: 201–2.

4 The peritoneal microcirculation in peritoneal dialysis

R. WHITE AND D. N. GRANGER

Introduction

The peritoneal microcirculation is an intricate microvascular network through which physiological interactions occur between the systemic vasculature and the peritoneal cavity. In peritoneal dialysis these dynamic interactions are of paramount importance in maintaining effective dialysis. The peritoneal microcirculation participates in numerous physiological functions including solute transfer and exchange, regulation of fluid dynamics and ultrafiltration, delivery of nutrients and hormones, delivery of leukocytes to areas of inflammation and distribution of drugs. Physiological and pathophysiological changes, as well as the process of peritoneal dialysis, may affect many of these microvascular functions. The emphasis of this chapter will be to review available information regarding the peritoneal microcirculation and to integrate this information into a general functional knowledge as it relates to peritoneal dialysis. The chapter will examine: (1) the functional anatomy and blood supply of the peritoneum, (2) components of the peritoneal microvascular network, (3) peritoneal microvascular haemodynamics and the effects of vasoactive agents on the microcirculation and (4) inflammation in the peritoneal microcirculation with emphasis on leukocyte–endothelial interactions.

Overview of the functional anatomy and blood supply of the peritoneum

Functional anatomy of the parietal and visceral peritoneum

The peritoneum is a large, intricately arranged serous membrane which lines the abdominal wall (parietal peritoneum) and visceral organs of the abdominal cavity (visceral peritoneum). The peritoneal cavity is the potential space between the parietal and visceral layers of peritoneum [1]. The primary purpose of the peritoneum is to provide a smooth surface over which the abdominal viscera may easily move [2]. Normally, the peritoneal cavity contains less than 100 ml of fluid but can accommodate a 20-fold increase without patient discomfort. In peritoneal dialysis, intraperitoneal solution volumes of greater than 2 L are successfully used [3]. The peritoneal cavity is lined by a layer of mesothelial cells on a connective tissue base which is perfused with circulatory and lymphatic vessels. Specialized regions of peritoneum, the omenta and mesenteries, are double-layer folds of peritoneum which connect certain viscera to the posterior abdominal wall or to each other. For example, the greater omentum extends from the greater curvature of the stomach to attach to the transverse colon. Specific double-layered peritoneal folds attach solid viscera to the abdominal wall (e.g. the falciform ligament of the liver). The total surface area of the peritoneum in adults approximates the surface area of skin ($1–2 m^2$) [4]. However, the effective surface of the peritoneal membrane may be below $1 m^2$, and can be further reduced as a result of adhesions or prior abdominal surgery [5, 6]. The visceral peritoneum accounts for the majority of the total peritoneal membrane surface area [7, 8]. Considering that most of the surface area is composed of visceral peritoneum, one might intuitively suspect that the contribution of the visceral peritoneum to total peritoneal membrane exchange would predominate over that contribution made by the parietal peritoneum. However, animal studies have suggested that the contribution of the visceral peritoneum to peritoneal exchange is less than would be predicted from the relative anatomical surface area. For example, eviscerated rats exhibit only slight reductions in peritoneal absorption rates for urea, creatinine, glucose and inulin relative to control animals [9]. Studies

R. Gokal, R. Khanna, R.Th. Krediet and K.D. Nolph (eds.), Textbook of Peritoneal Dialysis, 2nd Edition, 107–133.
© 2000 *Kluwer Academic Publishers. Printed in Great Britain.*

in other evisceration animal models have shown similar findings with reductions in peritoneal mass transport of small solutes by only 10–30% [10–14]. In these eviscerated animal models, contact between the dialysate and the parietal peritoneal membrane may be improved, thus contributing to these findings. With regard to the visceral peritoneum, there are conditions in which transport across the visceral peritoneum may be improved. Animal studies reveal that small solute mass transfer is significantly enhanced with vibration in the intact rat (i.e. with the visceral peritoneum intact), but only marginally improved in the eviscerated animal. With vibration, improved dialysate to visceral membrane contact is thought to occur. Based on these animal studies it has been proposed that the parietal peritoneum can significantly contribute to small solute transport, and that visceral peritoneal transport may be improved when contact is enhanced between visceral peritoneal surfaces and dialysis solutions [15]. The correlation of these animal findings to clinical peritoneal dialysis currently remains speculative, but these results suggest that the relative contribution of the visceral and parietal peritoneum to small solute mass transport may not necessarily correlate to anatomical surface area.

Blood supply to the peritoneum

The vascular and lymphatic systems supplying the peritoneal membrane and intraperitoneal organs constitute a complex and efficient system for fluid and solute delivery to the peritoneum. The arterial blood supply to the visceral peritoneum and intraperitoneal organs arises from the coeliac, superior mesenteric and inferior mesenteric arteries. The arterial blood supply to the parietal peritoneum and underlying musculature arises from the circumflex, iliac, lumbar, intercostal, and epigastric arteries. The veins draining the visceral peritoneum and intraperitoneal organs empty into the portal vein, while the venous system of the parietal peritoneum empties into the systemic veins. A potentially important consequence of this venous vascular arrangement is that drugs and other solutes which are absorbed across the visceral peritoneum are subject to hepatic metabolism. Pharmacological studies have shown intraperitoneal administration of compounds such as atropine, caffeine, glucose, glycine and progesterone and some intraperitoneally administered vasoactive drugs are subject to metabolism by the liver [16, 17]. Another important example is insulin, which may be absorbed through the portal circulation and a

significant portion degraded through first-pass metabolism by the liver [18, 19]. Thus, the pharmacokinetic effects of hepatic first-pass metabolism may play an important role in the systemic availability of some intraperitoneally administered substances.

Summary

In summary, animal studies suggest that the contribution of the visceral and parietal peritoneal membrane to total solute transport may not necessary correlate to anatomical surface area. The importance of contact between peritoneal tissue and dialysis solutions was suggested both in the eviscerated animal model and in studies of the effect of vibration on solute transport in the intact animal model. The general vascular supply to the peritoneum was reviewed and the potential importance of the portal venous drainage was presented.

The peritoneal microvascular network

Peritoneal microvascular architecture

The large vessels supplying blood to the visceral peritoneum function primarily as conduits to supply blood to the visceral organs. As the large vessels course through the mesentery they divide and reflect over the bowel surface forming capillary beds which can presumably participate in transperitoneal solute and fluid exchange. Over 50 years ago, Chambers and Zweifach described the topography of the mesenteric microcirculation [20]. The typical capillary network consists of arterioles, terminal arterioles, precapillary sphincters, arteriovenous anastomoses, throughfare channels, capillaries, postcapillary venules, and venules (Fig. 1) [21]. Blood flows into the capillary system through arterioles and exits through venules. Arterioles and throughfare channels modulate blood flow into the network, while precapillary sphincters regulate blood flow to single capillaries. Arteriovenous anastomoses can divert blood flow from arterioles directly into venules, thereby bypassing capillary networks. The flow through a capillary network can be extremely variable with individual capillary flow starting, stopping, and sometimes reversing direction [22, 23]. Capillary recruitment may occur to meet metabolic demands or as a result of certain vasoactive agents. Capillary recruitment increases perfused capillary density and increases surface area for potential exchange processes. The

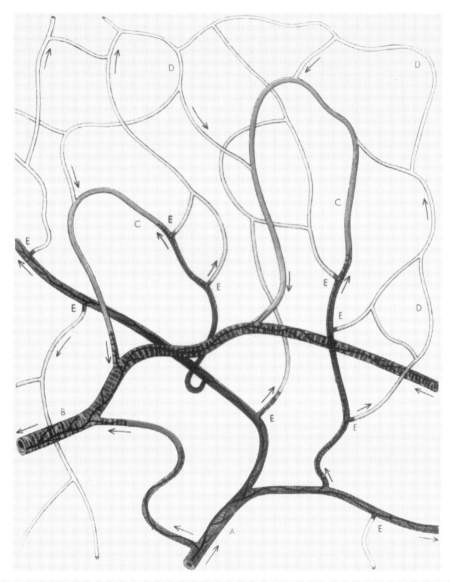

Figure 1. Structural elements of a typical mesenteric microcirculatory bed. A = arteriole, B = venule, C = thoroughfare channel, D = capillary, E = capillary sphincter (BW Zweifach: The microcirculation of the blood. Sci Am, 1959, January, pp. 54–60).

architecture of the peritoneal microvasculature in animal models has been previously reviewed by Miller [24]. The visceral microvasculature may be visualized on the mesenteric surface and includes abundant arterial and venular arcades that may function to equalize flow during periods of bowel compression. The parietal microvasculature may be represented by the vascular supply to the cremaster muscle, since this muscle extends from the abdominal wall musculature. Features of the cremaster microcirculation include the absence of short artery to vein anastomoses and the formation of arteriolar and venular arcades from which capillaries may arise [24–26].

Arterioles

The arterioles are the major site of microvascular resistance and regulate flow to capillary beds. Arterioles are lined by endothelial cells resting on a basal lamina surrounded by a layer of smooth muscle cells. Terminal arterioles may participate in the exchange process as they have a discontinuous muscle layer and portions of these vessels are lined only by endothelium and basement membrane. However, the relative contribution to overall peritoneal transport is minimal since the surface area and permeability of these vessels are much less than in capillaries and postcapillary venules. The distal smooth muscle layer of an arteriole may extend to form a ring around the site of capillary origin. This area is termed a precapillary sphincter and regulates flow to single capillaries. Marked arteriolar vasoconstriction can completely close the vascular lumen, resulting in no flow to its capillary distribution [27]. Figure 2 illustrates the haemodynamic pressure profiles and demonstrates that the greatest slope for microvascular pressure change occurs in arterioles 8 to 40 µm in diameter [28]. This figure also illustrates the pressure changes associated with vasoconstriction and vasodilation and the typical microvessel size gradations for arterioles, capillaries and venules.

Capillaries

In the peritoneal microvascular network capillaries are the principal sites for solute and fluid exchange [29, 30]. The wall of the capillary is composed of an endothelium and a basal lamina. Capillary size is approximately 5–8 µm, which is large enough to

let red blood cells (average diameter 7.5 µm) through, usually one at a time and with some deformity [27]. The capillaries have no smooth muscle and do not vasoactively participate in blood flow regulation. There are three types of capillary endothelium present in the mesenteric area: (1) continuous endothelium as in the peritoneal vessels, (2) fenestrated endothelium as in the intestinal villi and (3) discontinuous endothelium as found in the liver sinusoids [24]. Krediet will review the properties of peritoneal capillary transport in the following chapter. Some generalizations of peritoneal capillary structure as related to transport will now be briefly reviewed.

Permeability of the mesenteric microcirculation has been measured using estimates of the osmotic reflection coefficient (σ). The osmotic reflection coefficient describes the degree of macromolecular selectivity exhibited by the microvascular barrier and determines the effectiveness of an oncotic pressure gradient across the capillary membrane for a particular solute. An osmotic reflection coefficient of

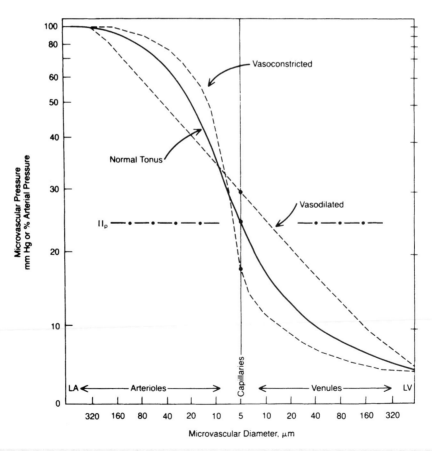

Figure 2. Microvascular pressure profiles as related to microvascular diameter. The dotted lines represent changes in microvascular pressure which occur with vasoconstriction and vasodilation (Renkin EM: Microcirculation and exchange. In: Patton HD, Fuchs AF, Hille B, Scher AM, Steiner R, eds. Textbook of Physiology. Philadelphia, PA: WB Saunders, 1989, pp. 860–78).

zero would imply a freely permeable membrane, while an osmotic reflection coefficient of one would indicate that the solute is impermeable and would generate 100% of its potential osmotic pressure [31]. Studies of osmotic reflection coefficients in the peritoneum indicate that the σ values of the peritoneum are similar to those reported for the continuous capillary beds of other organs [30–34]. The reflection coefficients for sodium chloride (MW 58), urea (MW 61), sucrose (MW 342), raffinose (MW 504), and vitamin B12 (MW 1354) range between 0.02 and 0.20 in the frog mesentery and rabbit, cat, and human peritoneum [35–41]. The reflection coefficients for myoglobin (21 Å radius), albumin (36 Å radius), Dextran 118 (61 Å radius) and Dextran 242 (90 Å radius) are 0.35, 0.82, 0.99 and 1.00 respectively [38, 40]. These studies indicate that there is a strong correlation between σ and molecular size. Thus, the peritoneal capillary barrier is not freely permeable to solutes but is a highly selective barrier with restrictive properties similar to those reported for other continuous capillary beds.

In animal models, intravital fluorescence microscopic observations of mesenteric capillaries have demonstrated the rapid passage of small solutes (MW 389–3400) along the entire length of most capillaries and the passage of larger molecular solutes (MW 19 000) in the venous capillaries and venules [42]. These types of observations suggest that peritoneal capillaries contain populations of small and large pores that regulate solute transport. Rippe, Stelin, Krediet and colleagues have developed and proposed a three-pore model of permselectivity which provides an ultrastructural framework to explain the restrictive properties and functional characteristics of transport in peritoneal capillaries [43–45]. In this model there are three population of pores: (1) a large number of transcellular, ultrasmall pores 2–5 Å radius; (2) a large number of small pores 40–55 Å radius; and (3) a small number of large pores 150–250 Å radius [43–46]. This theory predicts that nearly one-half of ultrafiltration would occur through ultrasmall pores and would be driven primarily by osmotic pressure differentials from the large glucose gradient across the peritoneal membrane. Recently, a family of membrane water channels known as the aquaporins (AQP) have been identified [47, 48]. AQP-1 is the pore type present in most continuous endothelium and is now thought to be the molecular correlate for the ultrasmall pore. Immunocytochemistry and immunoelectronmicroscopy have demonstrated AQP-1 labeling in the capillary and postcapillary venule endothelium of peritoneal tissue. In human peritoneal tissue, AQP-1, 3 and 4 have been shown to be present, with AQ-1 > 1 > 3 > 4. In addition, the sediment of dialysate contains the mRNA of AQP-1 and AQP-3 [49]. AQP-1 can be inhibited by mercurials, and Carlsson and colleagues have demonstrated in animal studies that $HgCl_2$ can inhibit transcellular water channels during acute peritoneal dialysis [50]. In this study $HgCl_2$ decreased water flow and inhibited sodium sieving without significant changes in microvascular permeability. Thus, aquaporins are thought to play a vital role in transendothelial water transport driven by osmotic gradients during peritoneal dialysis.

Postcapillary venules

The postcapillary venules participate in fluid and solute exchange, are an important site for microvascular leukocyte adhesion, and may demonstrate dramatic changes in permeability during inflammatory conditions. Small venules which are located just distal to the capillaries are often termed postcapillary venules. Postcapillary venules are generally 10–40 μm in diameter and are composed of endothelial cells resting on a basal lamina surrounded by pericytes with larger venules enclosed by muscular media [51].

Significant changes in microvascular permeability can occur in postcapillary venules. Numerous vasoactive agents, cytokines and drugs may induce changes in permeability. Histamine, bradykinin, platelet-activating factor, vascular permeability factor (vascular endothelial growth factor), certain components of the complement cascade, and drugs such as nitroprusside are examples of agents which can affect mesenteric microvascular permeability [52–59]. For example, Fig. 3 demonstrates the effects of vascular permeability factor on albumin permeability in a mesenteric postcapillary venule.

Intravital microscopic studies have demonstrated that the attachment and migration of leukocytes from the vascular space to the extravascular space is localized primarily to postcapillary venules [60–63]. A number of leukocyte adhesion molecules such as intracellular adhesion molecules (ICAM) and certain selectins (P-selectin and E-selectin) are located on the postcapillary endothelium. Selectin interactions are responsible for leukocyte rolling along the microvascular endothelium while ICAM interactions result in firm leukocyte adhesion to the endothelium [64–71]. In conditions such as peritoneal dialysis-associated peritonitis, these leukocyte–

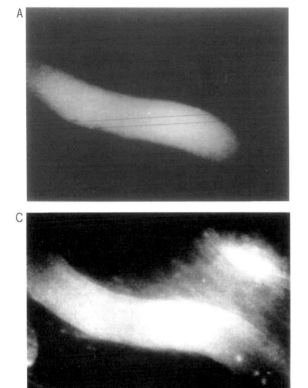
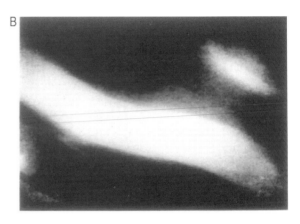

Figure 3. Fluorescence photomicrograph of the mesenteric microcirculation demonstrating the effects of vascular permeability factor (VPF) on permeability in the rat mesentery. **A**: No significant leakage of FITC-labelled albumin during basal conditions. **B**: Superfusion of VPF (660 pm) induces albumin leakage from the microcirculation after only 10 min of exposure to VPF. **C**: Albumin leakage into the interstitium continues to progress after 20 min of exposure to VPF. *In-vitro* studies by Kevil *et al.* of VPF on endothelial monolayers have demonstrated that VPF promotes changes in permeability through disorganization of endothelial junctional adhesion proteins [113]. (Photomicrograph courtesy of N. Yount, S. Ram and R. White).

endothelial interactions are critical for intraperitoneal leukocyte migration. The presence of adherent/emigrating leukocytes and inflammatory agents can also promote changes in permeability. These microvascular inflammatory interactions will be discussed in detail later in this chapter.

Endothelium

The microvascular endothelium is increasingly being recognized as having important regulatory roles in microvascular physiology [72–74]. Endothelial-derived substances can regulate microvascular haemodynamics, thrombogenesis, fibrinolysis, and leukocyte adhesion. Endothelial-derived vasoactive factors play a major role in the control of microvascular haemodynamics with the production of both relaxing and constricting factors. The endothelium-derived relaxing factor (EDRF) has been identified as nitric oxide (NO). NO is a diffusible, labile gas with a short biological half-life (seconds) [72, 75].

NO is synthesized from L-arginine by a family of enzymes known as nitric oxide synthases (NOS). Several isoforms of NOS have been identified and are broadly classified into constitutive and inducible isoforms. The endothelial-associated NOS is a constitutive, calcium–calmodulin dependent enzyme [75–77]. Once NO is produced in the endothelium it diffuses to the smooth muscle cells and produces smooth muscle relaxation via a cGMP-dependent mechanism [78]. NO production can be inhibited by several exogenous L-arginine analogues such as N^G-monomethyl-L-argine (L-NMMA), N^G-nitro-L-arginine methyl ester (L-NAME) and endogenous arginine analogues such as N^G,N^G-dimethylarginine (ADMA or asymmetrical dimethylarginine) [79–81]. Inhibition of NO synthesis produces mesenteric arteriolar vasoconstriction (Fig. 4) [82, 83]. This demonstrates that basal levels of NO are important in maintaining normal microvascular tone in the mesenteric microcirculation. Mesenteric post-capillary venules appear to be relatively spared from

Arteriole

Interstitium

Doppler
Velocimeter

Video Caliper

16 μm

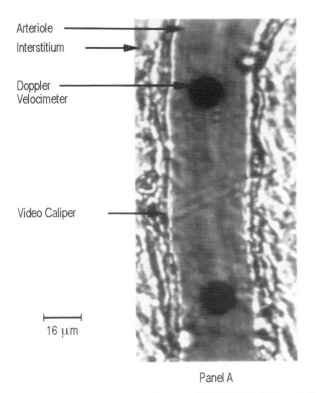
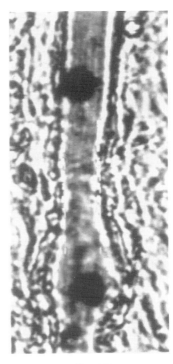

Panel A   Panel B

Figure 4. Haemodynamic effect of a nitric oxide synthesis inhibitor (ADMA) on an arteriole in the mesenteric microcirculation in the rat. **A**: The arteriole during basal conditions with superfusion of a buffer solution. **B**: ADMA (100 μm) added to the buffer solution induces marked arteriolar vasoconstriction. This demonstrates that basal levels of NO are important in maintaining normal microvascular tone in the mesenteric microcirculation (White R, Barefield D, Ram S, Work J. Peritoneal dialysis solutions reverse the hemodynamic effects of nitric oxide synthesis inhibitors. Kidney Int 1995; 48: 1986–93).

the vasoconstrictive effects of a decrease in basal NO production.

An important constricting factor produced by the endothelium is the potent vasoconstrictor endothelin. The endothelins (ET) are a family of amino acid peptides with diverse and overlapping biological activity. Four isoforms exist: ET-1, ET-2, ET-3, and ET-β [84–86]. Two human ET receptors have been cloned: ET_A and ET_B. ET_A receptors bind ET-1 > ET-2 > ET-3, whereas ET_B receptors bind these three ET with approximate equal affinity [87–89]. ET-1 is the most potent vasoconstrictor produced by the endothelium and induces sustained, intense vasoconstriction. Intravital microscopic observations of mesenteric arterioles have shown that ET-1 can completely arrest blood flow in the microcirculation. ET-1 has a short circulating half-life, but the effects may be sustained due to the slow dissociation of the bound peptide from its receptor [86]. In general, ET activates phospholipase C and increases the production of inositol trisphosphate which mobilizes calcium from the endoplasmic reticulum. ET can also activate calcium channels which

allow for the influx of calcium into the cytosol [90]. ET-1 produces vasoconstriction in both mesenteric arterioles and venules [91, 92]. ET-1 in small concentrations attached to ET_B may produce mild vasodilation through the release of NO and prostacyclin from endothelial cells, thus forming a potential feedback mechanism [72, 93].

NO and ET are not the only vasoactive substances produced by endothelial cells. Some other vasoactive mediators released from the endothelium include thromboxane A_2, superoxide, prostaglandin H_2, prostaglandin I_2, and endothelial-derived hyperpolarizing factor [72]. Despite the numerous vasoactive agents that have been catalogued, it appears that under usual circumstances the basal release of NO is the predominant endothelial factor influencing vascular tone [74]. Interestingly, ADMA and other guanidino compounds which inhibit NO production have been shown to accumulate in renal failure [80]. Levels of ET have been shown to be elevated in ESRD, and ET-1 is present in the peritoneal dialysis effluent of CAPD patients [94]. The relevance of some of these findings as it relates to peritoneal dialysis will be discussed in the next section.

NO and ET also have effects in modulating inflammatory processes. Inhibition of NO production is proinflammatory, as evidenced by an increase in the number of adherent leukocytes in postcapillary venules [95]. ET–1 is a proinflammatory cytokine and in cell culture ET-1 stimulates neutrophil adhesion to endothelial cell monolayers [96]. ET-1 increases the *in-vitro* endothelial expression of E-selectin [97]. *In-vivo* observations in the mesenteric microcirculation have shown that ET-1 increases leukocyte rolling in postcapillary venules [98].

The endothelium produces both growth promoters and growth inhibitors. An intact endothelium protects the microvascular wall from processes such as intimal hyperplasia which can occur when the endothelium is disrupted and smooth muscle growth factors are released. NO, heparin sulphates, and transforming growth factor β_1 are inhibitors of vascular smooth muscle proliferation; while angiotensin II, epidermal growth factor and platelet-derived growth factor contribute to smooth muscle proliferation [72]. ET-1 may also be considered an endothelial-derived growth factor. In the presence of certain cytokines (PDGF, TGF-α, EGF), ET-1 produces synergetic proliferative effects on rat vascular smooth muscle [86].

The biology of the endothelium is complex with cellular production of numerous haemodynamic, inflammatory and growth factors. Many intriguing questions remain to be answered concerning the process of peritoneal dialysis and endothelial function.

Junctional adhesion proteins

A developing area of endothelial cell biology is the architecture and physiological control of the intercellular tight junction. The tight junction forms an apical intercellular semipermeable diffusion barrier between cells in the endothelium [99, 100]. A number of proteins have been described which participate in the formation of the tight junction. Zonula occludens-1 (ZO-1) was the first tight junction protein described and is a peripheral membrane protein located near the plasma membrane [99, 101]. Occludin is another important junctional protein and is transmembrane in location at membrane–membrane sites [102–105]. Occludin appears to be bound near the cytoplasmic membrane to ZO-1. A possible molecular model has ZO-1 bound to

spectrin which is bound to actin [101]. Regulation of occludin has been suggested as a possible mechanism for controlling paracellular permeability [106]. Occludin is more concentrated in arterial junctions than in venous junctions. Kevil and colleagues have shown that arterial endothelial cells express 18-fold more occludin protein than venous endothelial cells. These authors suggest that the arterial and venous endothelial barriers reflect the level of expression of different junctional molecules [107].

In addition to ZO-1 and occludin, many other junctional proteins have been identified. Another cell-to-cell junctional structure is the adherens junction. Adherens junctions are formed by the transmembrane cadherins bound intercellularly to catenins anchored to actin [108–111]. For example, VE-cadherin is a junctional protein localized to the borders between endothelial cells [112]. Kevil *et al.* have shown vascular permeability factor increases permeability in endothelial monolayers through disorganization of endothelial junctional proteins. The increase in permeability has been related to the rearrangement of endothelial junctional proteins occludin and VE-cadherin. The mechanism involves a protein kinase signal transduction pathway [113]. Alexander *et al.* demonstrated that, in the presence of low extracellular calcium, endothelial monolayers have increased permeability. Treatment of endothelial monolayers with 0.12 mmol/L calcium resulted in the endocytosis of cadherins. This effect was attenuated by treatment with a protein kinase C inhibitor. These results suggest the possibility that regulation of the *in-vivo* endothelial barrier may involve a protein kinase C-dependent endocytosis of cadherins [114]. The potential role of junctional adhesion proteins in peritoneal dialysis remains to be investigated.

Basement membrane

The basement membrane functions as a substratum which acts as a solid support to anchor cells and limits the domain of connective tissue, thus producing distinct cellular compartments [115]. With the exception of large molecules such as plasma proteins, the basement membrane appears to be freely permeable to most solutes [116–120]. This concept is supported by the fact that the restrictive properties of the intestinal capillaries to endogenous macromolecules are similar to the capillaries found in the mesentery, skin and skeletal muscle, despite the fact that numerous large fenestrations are present in the intestinal capillary endothelium [121]. It has also been shown that colloidal carbon penetrates the intercellular clefts of continuous capillaries after exposure to histamine, but the transport of the colloidal carbon into the interstitial space is impeded at the basement membrane [122, 123]. These observations imply that the basement membrane may constitute a component of the barrier in the blood to lymph transport of large macromolecules. In addition, the proteoglycans in the basement membrane and interstitial gel matrix create an electrostatic barrier that retards the movement of anionic solutes [124]. These findings suggest that, although the basement membrane is permeable to small solutes, it may provide a significant transport barrier for large macromolecules under conditions of endothelial contraction and/or injury.

The peritoneal microvasculature in transport models

The peritoneal microcirculation plays an important role in peritoneal transport models. Peritoneal transport may be modelled through a variety of conceptualizations, all of which describe the transport of solutes and water between the microcirculation and the peritoneal cavity. These models include a combination of descriptive and mathematical conceptualizations. Understanding the details of these models can be challenging, and the reader is referred to the following chapter for an excellent discussion of the physiology of transport. For the purposes of this discussion an overview of the basic concepts involving the microcirculation in certain transport models will be summarized.

Barrier model

Nolph and colleagues describe the peritoneal transport process as occurring across several physiological and anatomical barriers (Fig. 5A) [125]. These barriers include:

R_1: a stagnant fluid layer within the peritoneal capillary
R_2: the capillary endothelium
R_3: the capillary basement membrane
R_4: the interstitium
R_5: the mesothelium
R_6: the stagnant fluid films within the peritoneal cavity.

According to this model, three of the major resistance barriers reside at the level of the capillary wall (i.e. R_1–R_3). Vasoactive agents alter R_2 primarily by modulating perfused capillary density, thus increasing or decreasing the total surface area available for exchange. Inflammatory and vasoactive agents may also affect R_2 through changes in permeability. R_1 is thought to have only minor effects. The characteristics of the basement membrane, R_3, were described above. An important aspect of this model is the compartmentalization of the process of transport as related to certain anatomical areas. This model is not a mathematically or statistically descriptive model, and thus will not quantitatively estimate transport properties. However, the model does provide an important visual, qualitative conceptualization of the transport process across tissue 'barriers'.

Distributive model

Flessner *et al.* have developed a quantitative descriptive model of peritoneal transport [126–128]. According to this model, capillaries are uniformly distributed in the tissue space surrounding the peritoneal cavity but are separated by varying distances from the dialysate (Fig. 5B). This model allows for the prediction of solute concentration gradients within the tissue space in relation to the peritoneal capillary distribution. It emphasizes that solute concentration profiles allow for a quantitative measure of the depth of tissue involved in transport and for the differentiation of the dominant transport process occurring based on tissue type. For example, this model predicts that the predominant mode of small solute transport in the viscera is diffusion to a depth of 400–600 μm from the serosal surface. Mathematical modelling of small solute transport suggests that the mechanisms of transport are identical in both directions. Thus, the distributed model defines a theoretic spatial arrangement of the microcirculation in a particular tissue. Using this model, estimates of tissue-specific transport properties can be calculated and refined based on experimental and peritoneal anatomical data. In peritoneal dialysis the relative contribution of a tissue to total transport must take into account the actual tissue surface area available for dialysis solution contact and solute exchange.

Pore model

Kinetic modelling using the concept of pores located in the microcirculation has given great insight into the dynamics of solute and fluid transport. As noted in the discussion of capillaries, a three-pore model has been proposed with: (1) a large number of transcellular, ultrasmall pores; (2) a large number of small pores; and (3) a small number of large pores (Fig. 5C).

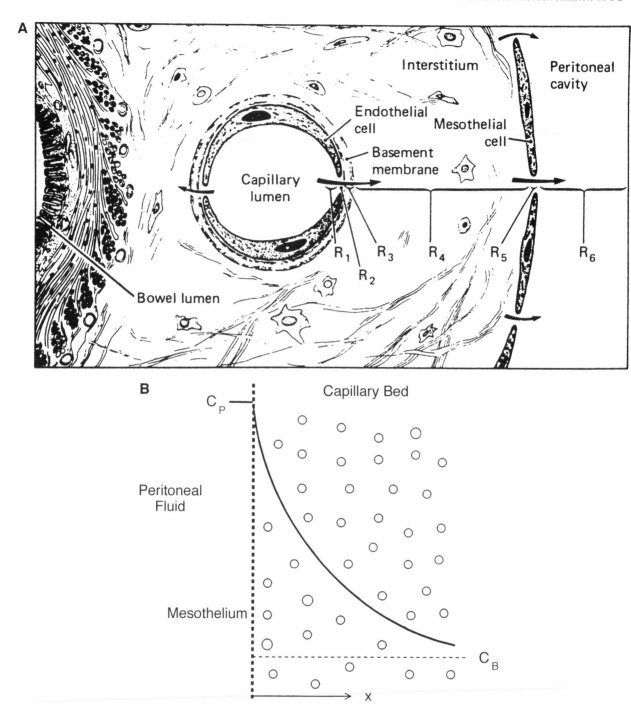

Figure 5. The peritoneal microcirculation in transport models. **A**: Diagrammatic representation of resistance to solute passage from peritoneal capillaries to dialysate (Nolph KD, Miller F, Rubin J, Popovich R. New directions in peritoneal dialysis concepts and applications. Kidney Int 1980; 18: S111–16). **B**: Distributed model concept in which transport in the peritoneal cavity-to-blood direction occurs as diffusion and convection across the mesothelium, through tissue space, and into blood capillaries which are distributed throughout the tissue space; 'x' is the distance into the tissue from the peritoneal surface. The small circles represent capillaries in the tissue space. C_P is the concentration of a substance in the peritoneal cavity. C_B is the concentration of a substance in the blood (Flessner MF. Peritoneal transport physiology: insights from basic research. J Am Soc Nephrol 1991; 2: 122–35). **C**: Hypothetical three-pore capillary membrane which illustrates the governing forces across each pore. The pore radius is given under each pore name. The forces are: P = hydrostatic pressure; Π = osmotic pressure. Large circles represent protein; small circles represent small solutes (Flessner MF. Peritoneal transport physiology: insights from basic research. J Am Soc Nephrol 1991; 2: 122–35).

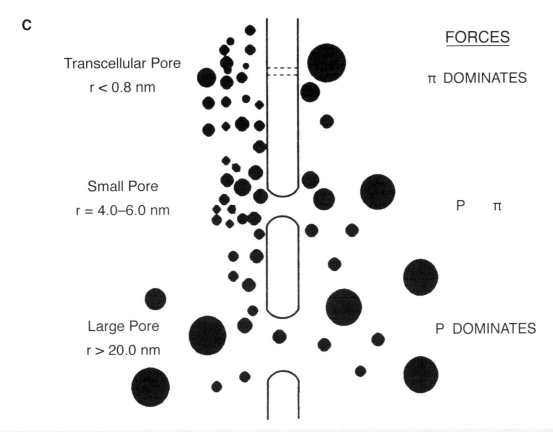

Figure 5c.

The physiological correlates to these pores are thought to be the aquaporins for the ultrasmall pores, interendothelial clefts for the small pores and venular endothelial gaps for the large pores [129]. With this model, pore size, pore distribution, and the effects of diffusion and convection on solute transport through pores can be mathematically modelled. The effects of diffusion and convection in relation to the pore variables can be correlated to measured solute clearances. As an example, application of the pore model has been performed with certain vasodilators such as nitroprusside. Intraperitoneal administration of nitroprusside has been correlated to an increase in pore radius of both small and large pores, with the large pores being affected to a greater degree [129]. This model helps explain the physiological effects of vasoactive agents such as nitroprusside in increasing clearances of both small and large solutes and changes in microvascular permeability.

The microcirculation and the peritoneal 'membrane'

Using concepts from these models Flessner has estimated transport characteristics of the peritoneal membrane. The peritoneal membrane is not one uniform tissue but a collection of different tissue areas which contribute to total 'membrane' transport. The contribution of different individual peritoneal 'tissues' (liver, hollow viscera, abdominal wall, and diaphragm) towards total mass transport can be estimated [130]. For example, theoretical calculations of specific tissue mass transport suggested that the liver could have significantly greater transport capabilities when compared to the other 'membrane' tissues. However, experimental evidence demonstrated only small differences in the mass transfer coefficient for mannitol across the surface of the liver as compared to the caecum, stomach and abdominal wall [131]. In peritoneal dialysis, estimates of mass transport of a substance in a 'tissue' must also take into account the actual surface area of tissue in contact with dialysis solutions. Since the liver has only a small portion of its total surface area in contact with peritoneal dialysis solution, the effective transport properties of the liver appear similar to the other peritoneal tissues. Thus, the physiological contribution of the liver to actual total transport is less than was theoretically predicted.

These results are interesting in reference to the earlier discussion of the eviscerated animal models, in which contributions of the visceral and parietal peritoneum to total transport may be partially explained by the increased contact of dialysate to tissue. In the eviscerated animal, improved dialysate contact to parietal surface area preserves transport capabilities, while in the non-eviscerated model vibration probably improves anatomical contact with visceral peritoneum enhancing visceral solute transport. Dialysate to tissue contact and the actual tissue surface area available for exchange are critical parameters in the transport process. Experimental findings have demonstrated the difficulty of modelling transport in a heterogenous peritoneal 'membrane'. Modelling numerous variables such as tissue-specific transport properties, the distribution and characteristics of the exchange vessels, and the actual tissue surface area available for dialysis contact is proving to be both intriguing and challenging.

Summary

The general architecture of the microvascular network and some important physiological processes occurring in arterioles, capillaries and postcapillary venules have been reviewed. Arterioles are the major site of microvascular resistance and regulate blood flow to the capillaries. Capillaries are the principal location for solute and fluid exchange. Postcapillary venules are important sites for leukocyte adherence and may show marked changes in permeability under inflammatory conditions. The endothelium is active in the physiological regulation of numerous microvascular processes including microvascular haemodynamics, leukocyte adhesion and production of growth factors and growth inhibitors. Endothelial adhesion molecules have been described and appear to have important roles in maintenance of tight junctions. The basement membrane appears to be freely permeable to small solutes, but restricts the transport of macromolecules. Finally, the role of the microcirculation in various transport models was introduced.

Peritoneal microvascular haemodynamics

In this section we will first consider the collective effect of peritoneal microvascular blood flow as it relates to solute clearance and ultrafiltration. The effect of vasoactive agents on the peritoneal microcirculation will then be considered. Finally, the effect

of peritoneal dialysis solutions and certain agents with elevated concentrations in renal failure on the microcirculation will be examined.

Effective peritoneal blood flow and clearance

Approximately 25% of cardiac output is directed to the splanchnic vascular bed in normal, resting individuals [132]. Excluding the parietal peritoneum, the total abdominal splanchnic blood flow usually exceeds 1200 ml/min at rest [133]. Granger *et al.* have measured superior mesenteric and peritoneal blood flow during intraperitoneal administration of a commercial dialysis solution in anaesthetized cats. The dialysis solution significantly increased blood flow to the mesentery, omentum, intestinal serosa and parietal peritoneum [134]. When considering the overall effective capillary blood flow in the peritoneum, an important question arises. Is the effective blood flow adequate to deliver solutes and fluid such that solute clearance is not primarily blood flow limited?

Due to the heterogeneous nature of peritoneal tissue and its vasculature it is difficult to precisely measure the effective blood flow in the peritoneal capillary bed. Indirect measures of effective peritoneal blood flow have been made using inert gas (H_2, Xe) washout techniques. Estimates of peritoneal blood flow range between 2.5 ml and 6.2 ml/min per kg body weight in rabbits to 7.5 ml/min per 100 g body weight in rats [135, 136]. Despite the difficulties in direct measurement of effective blood flow, Nolph *et al.* have presented indirect evidence that maximum clearance is not primarily blood flow limited [137]. This evidence relies on the interpretation of urea clearance data under conditions of decreased mesenteric blood flow as well as data derived from kinetic modelling. Maximum urea clearances obtained with rapid cycling and predicted clearances at infinite dialysis flow are in the range of 30–40 ml/min. If urea clearances were blood flow limited a severe restriction in mesenteric blood flow would be expected to reduce urea clearance. However, the results of studies in dogs subjected to circulatory shock have shown that urea clearances remain at 74% of control values despite a 38% reduction in mean arterial pressure [138]. In rabbits, urea clearances are affected when blood flow is reduced to 20% of normal [135, 139]. These findings demonstrate that, despite marked reductions in mesenteric blood flow, only modest decreases in urea clearance occur, suggesting that urea clearance is not primarily blood flow limited. Estimates of effective capillary blood flow have been made using gas diffusion techniques and range between 68 and 82 ml/min. Peritoneal clearances of carbon dioxide are approximately two to three times the maximum urea clearance. Using the ratio of urea clearance to peritoneal blood flow, Aune predicted that a doubling in blood flow would produce less than a 10% increase in urea clearance [135]. However, results obtained using gas diffusion techniques should be viewed with caution since they are based on the assumption that peritoneal gas clearance is equal to effective blood flow. Further studies using intraperitoneal vasodilators and kinetic modelling have also suggested clearance is not blood flow limited [124, 137, 140–145]. However, some authors have suggested that blood flow may be a limiting factor with rapid peritoneal exchanges such as with high flux automated peritoneal dialysis [146].

Kim and colleagues have performed recent experiments using diffusion chambers attached to the serosal side of the abdominal wall, stomach, caecum and liver in conjunction with laser Doppler flowmetry to directly evaluate the effect of decreased blood flow on mass transfer of solutes [147, 148]. In these experiments local blood flow beneath a diffusion chamber was monitored by Doppler flowmetry with simultaneous measurements of the disappearance of a tracer during conditions of baseline control blood flow, 30% of control and zero blood flow. No significant difference in the rate of mass transfer for mannitol or urea was demonstrated between control blood flow and 30% of control in the abdominal wall. There was a significant reduction in rates of mass transfer with no blood flow. In similar experiments involving the stomach, caecum and liver there was no difference in the urea mass transfer coefficient for the stomach and caecum when blood flow was reduced to 30% of control. There was a significant decrease in the urea mass transfer coefficient in the liver with reduction of flow to 30% of control. Significant reductions in mass transfer were again demonstrated with zero blood flow. These data demonstrate that reductions of blood flow by approximately 70% do not significantly reduce mass transfer in the parietal and visceral peritoneal areas tested, except in the liver. As noted previously, the relative contribution of a tissue to total transport must take into account the actual tissue surface area available for dialysis solution contact. Since the liver has only a relatively small effective exchange area available, total solute transport in peritoneal dialysis should not be greatly affected during conditions of decreased blood flow. Thus, with the exception of the liver, animal models suggest that solute clearance in the peritoneum does not appear to be blood flow limited as long as flow is greater than 30% of normal.

Effective peritoneal blood flow and ultrafiltration

Ultrafiltration occurs in peritoneal dialysis when there is net fluid filtration into the peritoneum. For osmotically driven ultrafiltration to occur, a physiological semipermeable membrane must separate two physiological compartments with one of the compartments having an effective osmolality to induce fluid shifts. The increased osmolality of hypertonic glucose containing peritoneal dialysis solutions produces an osmotic gradient which favours fluid movement from the vascular compartment to the peritoneal cavity [149, 150]. The capillary membrane has physiological characteristics of a semipermeable membrane. As noted previously, the peritoneal capillary barrier is not freely permeable to solutes but is a highly selective barrier with restrictive properties. The peritoneal microcirculation at the peritoneal surface would be directly exposed to the hyperosmotic effects of peritoneal dialysis solutions. The peritoneal blood flow would continuously present water for ultrafiltration between the vascular compartment and the intraperitoneal compartment. In animal models, dialysis solutions with a 1.5% glucose concentration produce an ultrafiltration rate of 3.0 ml/min per m^2 and the rate increases by approximately 1.7 ml/min per m^2 for each 1.0% increase in glucose concentration [151, 152]. In peritoneal dialysis the intraperitoneal glucose concentration decreases with time, resulting in decreased osmolality and reduced ultrafiltration. Eventually, osmotic equilibrium is obtained and at this point it would seem reasonable to assume intraperitoneal volume would be maximized. However, peak intraperitoneal volume does not necessarily coincide with osmotic equilibrium as peritoneal lymphatic absorption and intraperitoneal hydrostatic pressure can influence ultrafiltration [153–155]. The mechanisms for ultrafiltration in peritoneal dialysis will be discussed in other chapters of this book, but it is clear that the microcirculation plays a central role in the process.

Considering these concepts it is important to ascertain whether or not ultrafiltration is blood flow limited. To evaluate whether ultrafiltration may be limited by effective peritoneal blood flow, Grzegorzewska *et al.* studied the effects of ultrafiltration and effective peritoneal blood flow during peritoneal dialysis in the rat [156]. When maximum net ultrafiltration rate was obtained with hypertonic solutions, effective peritoneal blood flow was approximately five times greater than net ultrafiltration rate; and under isosmotic conditions effective peritoneal blood flow exceeded net ultrafiltration rate by 57 times. Since there is a great difference between effective peritoneal blood flow and net ultrafiltration rate, it is unlikely that normal peritoneal blood flow significantly limits ultrafiltration during peritoneal dialysis.

The effects of vasoactive agents on the peritoneal microcirculation

Numerous endogenous and exogenous vasoactive agents have been shown to modify blood flow in the peritoneal microcirculation. A wide variety of drugs, hormones, neurotransmitters and mediators of inflammation alter mesenteric vascular resistance. Peritoneal dialysis solutions also exhibit vasoactive properties. In addition to altering blood flow, many of these agents can also simultaneously affect perfused capillary density and microvascular permeability. The effects a particular vasoactive agent has on capillary blood flow, perfused capillary density and capillary permeability combine to determine physiological effect. In general, vasodilators in the splanchnic circulation enhance peritoneal clearances and increase capillary filtration coefficients while vasoconstrictors decrease peritoneal clearances and reduce capillary filtration coefficients (alterations in capillary filtration coefficients may reflect changes in perfused capillary density and permeability) [31, 124, 134, 140, 143]. While no broad generalization regarding the relationship between vasoactive agents and permeability may be made, it should be noted that many vasodilators also act to increase microvascular permeability [31]. For example, bradykinin, glucagon, and histamine increase both blood flow and permeability [157–159]. Secretin and cholecystokinin infusions increase blood flow but do not alter microvascular permeability to macromolecules [160]. This example demonstrates the lack of an absolute relationship between blood flow and alterations in vascular permeability [31]. Despite the lack of effect of secretin and cholecystokinin on macromolecular permeability, these agents increase the capillary filtration coefficient. The latter observation suggests that changes in capillary surface area secondary to capillary recruitment primar-

ily account for the ability of these agents to increase peritoneal clearances.

With regard to the various factors that modify peritoneal exchange in the clinical setting, perhaps the most important parameter is clearance. Table 1 catalogues many substances that may affect clearance in peritoneal dialysis. Nitroprusside and isoproterenol are among the most effec-

Table 1. Drugs and hormones which modify peritoneal clearance (modified from ref. 134)

Agents that may increase clearance

Albumin [161–164]
Aminoproprionate [165]
Anthranilic acid [166, 167]
Arachidonic acid [168]
Bradykinin [169]
Calcium channel blockers [170, 171]
Cetyl trimethyl NH_4Cl [172]
Cholecystokinin [173]
Cytochalasin D [174]
Desferrioxamine [175–177]
Dialysate alkalinization [178, 179]
Diazoxide [180]
Dioctyl sodium sulphosuccinate [181, 182]
Dipyridamole [183]
Dopamine [184, 185]
Edetate calcium disodium [186]
Ethacrynic acid [187]
Furosemide [187, 188]
Glucagon [189–192]
Histamine [193, 194]
Hydralazine [195]
Hypertonic glucose [196, 197]
Indomethacin [195]
Insulin [198]
Isoproterenol [144, 199–201]
Lipid in dialysate [202]
Nitroprusside [17, 124, 198, 203–205]
N-myristyl alanine [166]
Procaine hydrochloride [207]
Prostaglandin A1 [208, 209]
Prostaglandin E1 [208, 209]
Prostaglandin E2 [208, 209]
Phentolamine [210]
Protamine [211]
Puromycin [212]
Salicylate [184, 195]
Secretin [208]
Serotonin [184]
Streptokinase [184]
Tris hydroxymethyl aminomethane (THAM) [190, 195]

Agents that may decrease clearance

Calcium [190]
Dopamine [213]
Norepinephrine [214]
Prostaglandin F2 [208]
Vasopressin [184, 185]

tive agents which augment clearances in peritoneal dialysis [17, 129, 196, 203–205, 215]. Nitroprusside increases the clearance of urea, creatinine, inulin, and protein in a dose-dependent fashion. Small solute clearance appears to be most affected at lower doses, while large solute clearances are significantly increased at higher doses [216]. The maximum effect of intraperitoneally administered nitroprusside appears to occur after three to five consecutive exchanges with the drug, and the effects of nitroprusside are reversed when the drug is removed from the dialysis solution. With nitroprusside, mass transfer coefficients increase proportionately more for inulin than for urea, suggesting that alterations in permeability occur with exposure to the drug [17]. Nitroprusside also enhances the leakage of fluorescein-tagged albumin across the mesenteric microvessels [24, 58].

Studies of the effects of vasodilators and peritoneal dialysis solutions on small arteries (70 μm) and small veins (140 μm) in the rat caecum demonstrate that peritoneal dialysis solutions dilate both arteries and veins. Addition of nitroprusside to peritoneal dialysis solutions produced no further arterial vasodilation [140]. This suggests that, in peritoneal dialysis, the effects of nitroprusside on clearance are not secondary to increased blood flow via arteriolar vasodilation. Studies by Grzegorzewska et al. using gas diffusion techniques in patients receiving intermittent peritoneal dialysis showed that the intraperitoneal administration of nitroprusside produced no significant differences in the peritoneal transfer of CO_2 [217]. Nitroprusside did enhance the removal of certain solutes such as urea and total protein. Thus, the effect of nitroprusside on solute clearance did not appear to be attributable to changes in effective peritoneal blood flow. Studies by Douma et al. in CAPD patients also demonstrated that the mass area transfer coefficient of CO_2 was not significantly different after the intraperitoneal administration of nitroprusside in a glucose dialysate [129]. Since nitroprusside appears to have no significant effects on effective peritoneal blood flow in the setting of peritoneal dialysis (based on gas diffusion of CO_2), the effects of nitroprusside on other parameters such as capillary permeability and perfused capillary density need to be defined in order to explain the increase in solute clearance.

In the same study of CAPD patients, Douma et al. demonstrated that nitroprusside increased the mass transfer area coefficient of low molecular weight solutes and serum proteins. Using kinetic modelling and concepts of the pore theory, they related the effects of nitroprusside to an increase in the radius of both large and small pores and an increase in the effective peritoneal surface area. An increase in the number of perfused capillaries would increase the total number of pores available for exchange but theoretically should not alter the distribution of the sizes of the pores. Nitroprusside had a greater relative increase in the clearance of larger molecular proteins, suggesting a greater relative effect on the large pore radius. In this study the dialysate to plasma concentration of cGMP was greater with the addition of nitroprusside, suggesting a local generation of NO produced by nitroprusside. There was no difference in the dialysate concentrations of PGE_2, 6-keto-$PGF_2\alpha$, or thromboxane B_2 with the addition of nitroprusside. These workers also demonstrated that the ultrafiltration rate was increased with nitroprusside during the initial phase of dwell but the effect on net ultrafiltration was not significantly different for nitroprusside and control after 4 h. This information suggests that the effect of nitroprusside in improving clearance in the setting of peritoneal dialysis is not due to arteriolar vasodilation, but to changes in perfused capillary density and alterations in microvascular pore diameter.

Isoproterenol administered intraperitoneally increases peritoneal transport. The route of administration is important in determining isoproterenol's effects on clearance. Intravenous isoproterenol increases superior mesenteric blood flow by 88%, but does not alter peritoneal clearances of creatinine and inulin. In contrast, intraperitoneally administered isoproterenol increases superior mesenteric blood flow and increases solute clearance [200]. In animal studies it has been suggested that the vasoactive effects of isoproterenol increase capillary surface area through the recruitment of capillaries. Isoproterenol increases the mass transfer area coefficients of small solutes, especially in the early phases of the dialysis dwell [218].

A possible major disadvantage for clinical use of nitroprusside is the potential for systemic vasodilation. Some studies indicate the peripheral vasodilatory effects may be limited with appropriate intraperitoneal dosing [205]. In the study of CAPD patients by Douma et al. no marked blood pressure decreases were noted [129]. Intraperitoneal isoproterenol has been used in certain clinical situations [218]. Patients with vascular diseases such as scleroderma may experience decreased clearances during peritoneal dialysis. In a patient with scleroderma, addition of isoproterenol to the dialysis fluid appeared to improve clearance [219]. However, the clinical use of isoproterenol is hindered by its potential cardiac stimulatory actions [200].

The effects of peritoneal dialysis solutions on the peritoneal microcirculation

Routine peritoneal dialysis can markedly affect the mesenteric microcirculation. Topical application of dialysis fluid to arterioles in the rat caecum or cremaster muscle produces a transient vasoconstriction lasting 1–4 min, followed by a sustained vasodilation [24, 83, 141, 219–221]. Standard glucose-containing peritoneal dialysis solutions have a high osmolality as a result of elevated glucose concentration, a low pH, and contain an acetate or lactate buffer system. It is reasonable to postulate that alterations in osmolality, pH or the buffer may contribute to the vasoactive properties of peritoneal dialysis solutions. Indeed, superfusion of mesentery with a hypertonic solution containing glucose produces submaximal arteriolar vasodilation. Isomolar acetate or lactate solutions also produce submaximal arteriolar vasodilation. The combination of hyperosmolality and acetate or lactate produces maximal arteriolar vasodilation. Although maximal arteriolar vasodilation is achieved with peritoneal dialysis solutions, maximum mesenteric venular vasodilation does not occur. In the presence of peritoneal dialysis solutions the addition of nitroprusside produces significant increases in venular diameter [219]. It is unlikely that the low pH of peritoneal dialysis solutions accounts for their vasoactive properties, since adjustment of the pH to 7.0–7.4 does not alter the vasodilator response in the rat cremaster muscle [141].

It has been previously demonstrated that hyperosmolar sodium solutions perfused into intestinal lymph produced vasodilation of submucosal intestinal arterioles through a mechanism partly mediated by NO [222]. Could hyperosmolar peritoneal dialysis solutions vasodilate through a NO-dependent pathway? As previously noted, inhibition of NO synthesis produces mesenteric arteriolar vasoconstriction and several inhibitors of NO synthesis are present in renal failure. Asymmetrical dimethylarginine (N^G,N^G-dimethylarginine or ADMA), methylguanidine and aminoguanidine are endogenous guanidino compounds which accumulate in renal failure and inhibit NO production. ADMA is reported to accumulate in renal failure to plasma concentrations of approximately 5 µmol/L, while other investigators have reported ADMA concentrations in CAPD patients to be significantly less (0.70 µmol/L), [80, 81, 223, 224]. In animal models intravital microscopic studies of mesenteric arterioles have revealed that inhibition of basal NO synthesis with ADMA (100 µmol/L) and L-NAME (100 µmol/L) (N^G-nitro-L-arginine methyl ester) produces vasoconstriction of arterioles to 68% and 74% of baseline diameter respectively. This suggests that basal levels of NO are important in maintaining normal vascular tone and blood flow in the mesenteric microcirculation. Superfusion of a hyperosmolar peritoneal dialysis solution (1.5% and 4.25% solution) rapidly reverses the vasoconstrictive effects of these NO synthesis inhibitors [83]. When L-NAME and a 4.25% solution are simultaneously superfused the arteriole remained significantly vasodilated throughout a 1 h superfusion period. Thus, peritoneal dialysis solutions remain vasoactive despite arteriolar exposure to NO synthesis inhibitors, suggesting these glucose dialysis solutions possess vasoactive properties largely through a NO-independent mechanism.

It is important to note that although hypertonic, glucose-containing peritoneal dialysis solutions may acutely overcome the arteriolar vasconstrictive effects of NO synthesis inhibitors such as ADMA, the effect NO synthesis inhibitors may have on intraperitoneal production of NO, perfused capillary density and pore radius remain to be fully investigated. Breborowicz *et al.* have performed animal studies in which L-NAME was added to peritoneal dialysis solutions [225]. They found that the transperitoneal transport of larger solutes such as total protein was reduced in the presence of L-NAME (5 mg/ml). When intraperitoneal inflammation was induced with LPS, L-NAME also decreased the total protein transport when compared to LPS alone. These results suggest that NO is important in modulating microvascular permeability in peritoneal dialysis in both the basal state and during inflammation. In these studies, addition of L-NAME to the dialysis fluid also produced a dose-dependent increase in net ultrafiltration.

In studies of CAPD patients using amino acid-based peritoneal dialysis solutions, amino acid solutions increased estimated peritoneal blood flow. Based on nitrate and cGMP mass transfer area coefficients, this effect was not attributable to NO [226]. The exact mechanism through which peritoneal dialysis solutions are vasoactive remains imprecisely defined, but currently it does not appear to be primarily attributable to NO.

Summary

Animal studies and other evidence suggest that peritoneal clearance is not blood flow limited as long as effective peritoneal blood flow is greater than 30% of normal (with the exception of the liver). Ultrafiltration does not appear to be significantly limited by blood flow under usual conditions. Numerous vasoactive agents can affect peritoneal clearance and one of the most studied vasoactive agents is nitroprusside. In the setting of peritoneal dialysis, the effects of nitroprusside are not primarily related to arteriolar vasodilation, but to increases in perfused capillary density and alterations in microvascular pore radius. This demonstrates that the effect a particular vasoactive agent has on clearance is not solely dependent on haemodynamic changes (such as arteriolar vasodilation), but must take into account effects on perfused capillary density and changes in capillary/venular permeability. Peritoneal dialysis solutions are vasoactive and have primarily vasodilatory effects in the mesenteric microcirculation. In the presence of a peritoneal dialysis solution, the effects a particular vasoactive agent have on effective blood flow, perfused capillary density and capillary permeability combine to determine final physiological effect. Since peritoneal clearance does not under usual circumstances appear to be primarily blood flow limited, determining the effect a 'vasodilator' has on perfused capillary density and permeability may be the most important parameters to define.

The peritoneal microcirculation in inflammation

A fascinating area of investigation with relevance to the field of peritoneal dialysis is the role of the microcirculation in inflammation. The microcirculation plays a critical role in inflammatory responses associated with peritoneal dialysis. An important aspect of this response is the interaction of leukocytes with the vascular endothelium during inflammation. In pathophysiological states such as peritonitis the intraperitoneal leukocyte cell count may rapidly increase from a few cells to thousands of cells per mm^3. This rapid rise in the number of peritoneal leukocytes is dependent on factors that govern adhesive interactions between leukocytes and the microvascular endothelium. This section will focus on the microvascular physiological interactions involved in leukocyte adherence and in the microcirculation.

General principles of leukocyte–endothelial interactions

The attachment and subsequent migration of leukocytes from the vascular to the extravascular compartment involves numerous steps which occur in a sequential fashion. Leukocyte adhesion is localized primarily to postcapillary venules [60–63]. In order for a leukocyte to establish an adhesive interaction with the endothelium it must first be displaced from the centre stream to the vessel wall. This appears to be related to microvascular network topography and radial dispersive forces. As the blood vessel diameter increases from the capillary to the postcapillary venules, the more flexible erythrocytes begin to pass the leukocytes and deflect them towards the vessel wall [227]. Once displaced to the vessel wall, the leukocyte can begin to adhere. Adhesion begins as a rolling movement along the postcapillary endothelium. As the inflammatory process proceeds, the number of rolling neutrophils increases and the velocity of the rolling decreases. This exposes the leukocyte to low concentrations of chemotactic agents released from parenchymal cells and/or the endothelium. Leukocyte activation allows the establishment of firm (stationary) adhesive interactions. The firmly adherent leukocyte may then migrate across the endothelial barrier and enter the interstitium (Fig. 6) [65].

The adhesive interaction between the leukocyte and the endothelium is mediated by a complex, highly coordinated, dynamic interplay between adhesion glycoproteins expressed on the surface of both the leukocyte and the endothelium. Each of these glycoproteins belongs to one of three main families: the integrins, superimmunoglobulins, and selectins. The integrins are heterodimers composed of a common beta subunit (CD18) and a specific alpha subunit (CD11a, CD11b or CD11c). These subunits combine to form the integrins CD11a/CD18, CD11b/CD18 and CD11c/CD18. The superimmunoglobulin family is represented by intercellular adhesion molecules known as ICAM. The selectins are represented by L-selectin, E-selectin, and P-selectin. The integrins and L-selectin are expressed on the surface of neutrophils. ICAM-1 is present on endothelial cells and its expression may be increased by endotoxin and cytokines such as interleukin-1 and tumour necrosis factor (IL–1 and TNF). Cytokines can also activate endothelial cells to express E-selectin. P-selectin is present on platelets and vascular endothelial cells [65–71].

The sequence of events involved in neutrophil adherence and migration to sites of inflammation requires

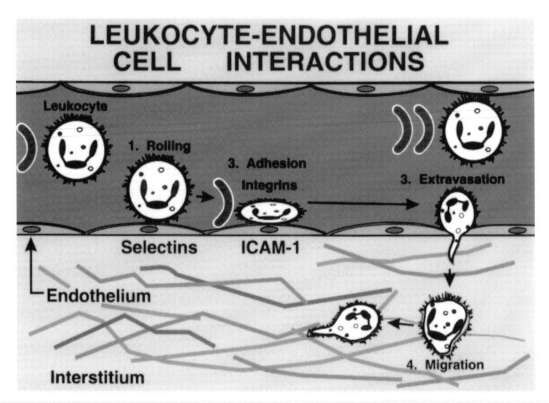

Figure 6. The sequence of events involved in leukocyte adherence and migration to sites of inflammation requires coordination of the adhesive interaction between the leukocyte and vascular endothelium. (1) The initial leukocyte rolling appears to involve interaction between L-selectin on the neutrophil and E-selectin and P-selectin on the vascular endothelium. (2) This interaction allows for the up-regulation of the leukocyte integrin CD11b/CD18 which can bind to ICAM-1 and strengthen neutrophil adhesion. (3) The firmly adherent leukocyte may then extravasate by a process that is dependent on CD11a/CD18, CD11b/CD18, and ICAM-1. (4) The leukocyte may then migrate into the interstitial tissue. (Figure courtesy of Kristine Bienvenu.)

coordination of the adhesive interactions between the neutrophil and vascular endothelium. The initial leukocyte rolling appears to involve interactions between L-selectin which is constitutively expressed on the surface of leukocytes and E-selectin and P-selectin which are located on the vascular endothelium. This interaction allows for the up-regulation of CD11b/CD18 which can bind to ICAM-1 and strengthen neutrophil adhesion (Fig. 7). L-selectin is then down-regulated (shed) from the cell surface. The firmly adherent neutrophil may then migrate across the vessel wall by a process that is dependent on CD11a/CD18, CD11b/CD18, and ICAM-1.

Inflammatory mediators and the microcirculation

The physiological interaction between leukocytes and the endothelium may be influenced by several factors. Intravital videomicroscopic approaches have provided a wealth of information regarding the influence of intravascular hydrodynamic dispersal forces [60, 228, 229], leukocyte capillary plugging [230–232], electrostatic charge [233], and chemical mediators on leukocyte–endothelial cell interactions during inflammation. Table 2 lists several agents which affect leukocyte rolling and adherence in post-capillary venules.

As examples, platelet-activating factor (PAF), leukotriene B_4 (LTB$_4$) and nitric oxide synthesis inhibitors (such as L-NAME and ADMA) and superoxide have been shown to increase microvascular leukocyte adherence. The presence of adherent leukocytes and inflammatory agents may also promote changes in permeability. As an example, adherent leukocytes mediate PAF-induced vascular leakage. Pretreatment with monoclonal antibodies directed against the common beta subunit of the leukocyte integrin CD11/CD18 largely prevents the increased vascular protein leakage caused by infusion of PAF [266]. In the cat mesentery, local intra-arterial infusion of either LTB$_4$ or PAF promotes leukocyte adherence, but only PAF alters microvascular permeability. This indicates that leukocyte

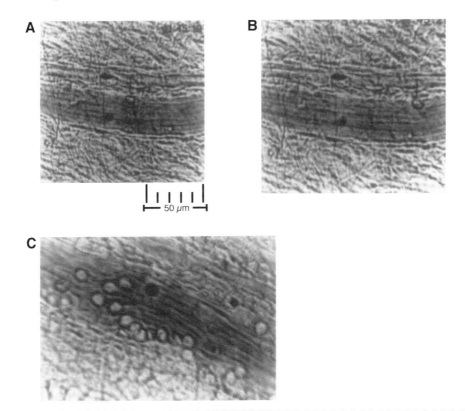

Figure 7. A: A mesenteric venule with a leukocyte (arrow) rolling along the length of the venule. **B**: This micrograph was taken 2 s after the micrograph depicted in **A** to demonstrate that the leukocyte moved approximately 40 μm downstream in the venule. **C**: A mesenteric venule during 2 ng/min platelet-activating factor (PAF) infusion. Note the numerous white blood cells adhering to the endothelial wall after PAF infusion (Kubes P, Suzuki M, Granger DN. Modulation of PAF-induced leukocyte adherence and increased microvascular permeability. Am J Physiol 1990; 259: G858–64).

adhesion alone does not always result in increased microvascular permeability. When LTB$_4$ and PAF are infused simultaneously, LTB$_4$ causes a further increase in microvascular permeability than is observed with PAF alone. While PAF *per se* may increase microvascular permeability in the presence of adherent leukocytes, it may also serve as a 'priming agent' that sensitizes neutrophils and/or the endothelium to other stimuli such as LTB$_4$ [246]. Reactive oxygen metabolites such as superoxide and hydrogen peroxide may be produced by neutrophils and endothelial cells [267–269]. Hydrogen peroxide appears to promote leukocyte adhesion to vascular endothelium by a PAF-mediated up-regulation or activation of CD11/CD18. Superoxide-induced increases in leukocyte adherence may be related to inactivation of nitric oxide by superoxide [270]. The inhibition of nitric oxide production by the vascular endothelium can produce an increase in microvascular protein efflux that is mediated in part by leukocyte-dependent mechanisms in the mesentery [271].

Thus, several agents promote leukocyte rolling and adherence in mesenteric postcapillary venules. Leukocyte adherence in the presence of an appropriate chemical stimulus may affect microvascular permeability. Since leukocyte adhesion has been associated with changes in permeability, the question arises as to whether leukocyte adhesion could modify endothelial junctional elements. Recent *in-vitro* studies have shown that PMN adhesion to endothelial cells activated by tumour necrosis factor results in VE-cadherin/catenin disorganization [272]. This effect could be blocked by an anti-integrin beta 2 antibody. PMN adhesion also resulted in increased endothelial cell permeability. *In-vivo* animal studies have shown that a monoclonal antibody against VE-cadherin increases vascular permeability and accelerates the entry of neutrophils into inflamed mouse peritoneum [273]. Thus, it appears that some agents which promote leukocyte adhesion may affect microvascular permeability through modulation of some junctional adhesion proteins.

Table 2. Substances or conditions that affect leukoctye adherence to postcapillary venules (modified from ref. 64)

A. Stimulants for leukocyte rolling

Superoxide [234–236]
Histamine [237]
Interleukin-1 [238]
Hydrogen peroxide [239]
Indomethacin [240]
Ischaemia–reperfusion [241]
Endothelin [98]

Stimulants for adherence

C5a [242]
PAF [55, 243, 244]
Leukotriene B4 [56, 245, 246]
N-formylmethionyl-leucyl-phenylalanine [229, 247]
Hydrogen peroxide [248]
Indomethacin [240, 249]
Nitric oxide synthesis inhibitors [95, 250]
Ischemia–reperfusion [251]
Endotoxin [57]
Superoxide [267–270]

Substances which reduce leukocyte adherence

Adenosine [254, 255]
PGI_2 [249, 256]
Iloprost (PGI_2 analogue) [257]
NO donors [234, 258]
8-Bromo-cGMP (cGMP analogue) [259]
Superoxide dismutase [61, 260]
Catalase [261]
Quinacrine (phosopholipase A_2 inhibitor) [262]
WEB2086 (PAF antagonist) [248]
Misoprostol (PGE_2 analogue) [249, 263]
Colchicine [264]
Methotrexate [255, 264]
Cromolyn (mast cell stabilizer) [265]
Salicylate [256]

The effect of peritoneal dialysis solutions on microvascular leukocyte adhesion

Peritoneal dialysis solutions can also affect leukocyte adhesion in the microcirculation. Intravital microscopic studies have shown that glucose-containing peritoneal dialysis solutions decrease leukocyte rolling and adherence in mesenteric postcapillary venules [274]. In studies by Jonasson *et al.*, superfusion of heat-sterilized glucose-containing peritoneal dialysis solutions decreased the concentration of rolling leukocytes and increased flow velocity when compared to buffer and filtered sterilized peritoneal dialysis solutions [275]. Since the heat-sterilized peritoneal dialysis solution decreased leukocyte rolling, it was hypothesized there is a disturbance in the presentation or binding capacity of selectins.

As previously noted, superfusion of L-NAME on the mesenteric microcirculation produces microvascular inflammation through increasing the number of firmly adherent leukocytes to postcapillary venules. A glucose-containing peritoneal dialysis solution (4.25% solution) attenuates L-NAME-induced leukocyte adhesion, returning leukocyte adhesion back to basal conditions [276]. This suggests a possible effect on either the integrins or ICAM. *In-vitro* studies have demonstrated that hyperosmolar solutions affect integrin expression. Kaupke and colleagues have demonstrated that incubation of blood with glucose-containing peritoneal dialysis solutions results in depressed basal neutrophil expression of CD11b and CD18 and monocyte expression of CD14 [277]. In addition, the glucose-containing peritoneal dialysis solutions decrease the LPS up-regulation of CD11b and CD18. Peritoneal dialysis solutions in which sodium chloride was substituted for glucose to obtain similar osmolalities as the glucose-based peritoneal dialysis solutions also show a reduction in basal and LPS-stimulated expression of CD11b. The decreased leukocyte adhesion molecule expression was shown to be primarily an osmolality-related event and pH independent. In other animal models there is experimental evidence to suggest that hyperosmolar solutions attenuate leukocyte adherence in the microcirculation. In the rat haemorrhagic model of ischaemia–reperfusion, muscle reperfusion injury is significantly attenuated when animals are treated with hypertonic saline [278]. *In-vivo* animal studies of the mesenteric microcirculation have also suggested that hyperosmolar non-glucose-containing buffer solutions reduce the number of adherent leukocytes [279].

It is important to note that the *in-vitro* and *in-vivo* studies are performed with acute exposure to hypertonic, glucose-containing peritoneal dialysis solutions. Whether or not these described acute processes have deleterious effects in conditions such as an inflammatory challenge is unknown. It is well recognized that in pathological states such as peritonitis the intraperitoneal leukocyte count may rapidly increase from a few cells to hundreds or thousands of cells per mm^3. The anti-adhesive effects of the solutions appear to be easily overcome in active inflammation. However, an intriguing question to consider is whether or not hyperosmolar, glucose-containing peritoneal dialysis solutions have a potential microvascular anti-inflammatory effect (as determined by leukocyte rolling and adhesion) during routine conditions.

It appears that glucose-containing peritoneal dialysis solutions have a negative impact on other aspects of leukocyte host defences. The activity of peripheral blood leukocytes as measured by chemiluminescence, phagocytosis and bacterial killing is suppressed by peritoneal dialysis solutions. This suppression is believed to be secondary to such factors as the solution's high osmolality and low pH [280]. It has also been shown that peritoneal dialysis solutions can decrease peritoneal macrophage function by decreasing the cell's phagocytic activity and respiratory burst [281]. The requirement for frequent exchanges may dilute the intraperitoneal immunoglobulin concentrations, thus rendering the patient more susceptible to infection [282]. Thus, glucose-containing peritoneal dialysis solutions appear to affect leukocytes both in terms of leukocyte–endothelial interactions and in terms of leukocyte function.

Summary

This section has attempted to define some of the immunological processes which occur in the microcirculation as related to leukocyte–endothelial interactions. Several inflammatory mediators promote leukocyte rolling and adhesion in the mesenteric microcirculation. In the presence of some inflammatory agents, leukocyte adherence may affect microvascular permeability, possibly through modulation of junctional adhesion proteins. Animal models have demonstrated that peritoneal dialysis solutions acutely affect leukocyte-endothelial interactions. Hyperosmolar, glucose-containing peritoneal dialysis solutions acutely decrease microvascular leukocyte adhesion, perhaps through the modulation of leukocyte adhesion molecules. The dynamic interplay between peritoneal dialysis solutions, leukocytes, inflammatory cytokines, and the endothelium all have important roles in determining a microvascular inflammatory response. This section has examined only events in the microcirculation. It should be emphasized that to form a complete picture of the immunological process occurring during peritoneal dialysis there must be integration of events occurring in the microcirculation with events occurring in the interstitium, mesothelium and peritoneal cavity.

Closing remarks

This chapter has presented an overview of the peritoneal microcirculation; it has detailed many concepts in microvascular physiology in relation to peritoneal dialysis. The challenge to future researchers will be to maximize the efficiency of peritoneal dialysis while protecting the peritoneal microvascular environment through which dialysis occurs. It is hoped that the long-term survival and the quality of life of our peritoneal dialysis patients will continue to improve as our knowledge of peritoneal physiology and clinical peritoneal dialysis advances.

References

1. Williams PL, Warwick R, eds. Gray's Textbook of Anatomy. Philadelphia, PA: WB Saunders, 1980, pp. 1319–89.
2. Nance FC. Diseases of the peritoneum, retroperitoneum, mesentery and omentum. In: Haubrichus, Schaffner F, Berk JE, eds. Gastroenterology. Philadelphia, PA: WB Saunders, 1995, pp. 3061–3.
3. Nolph KD, Twardowski Z. The peritoneal dialysis system. In: Nolph KD, ed. Peritoneal Dialysis. Boston, MA: Martinus Nijhoff, 1985, pp. 23–50.
4. Verger C. Peritoneal ultrastructure. In: Nolph KD, ed. Peritoneal Dialysis. Boston, MA: Martinus Nijhoff, 1985, pp. 95–113.
5. Henderson LW. The problem of peritoneal membrane area and permeability. Kidney Int 1973; 3: 409–10.
6. Mion CM, Boen ST. Analysis of factors responsible for the formation of adhesions during chronic peritoneal dialysis. Am J Med Sci 1965; 250: 675–9.
7. Knapowski J, Feder E, Simon M, Zabel M. Evaluation of the participation of parietal peritoneum in dialysis: physiological morphological and pharmacological data. Proc Eur Dial Trans Assoc 1979; 16: 155–64.
8. Rubin J, Clawson M, Planch A, Jones Q. Measurements of peritoneal surface area in man and rats. Am J Med Sci 1988; 295: 453–8.
9. Rubin J, Jones Q, Planch A, Stanek K. Systems of membranes involved in peritoneal dialysis. J Lab Clin Invest 1987; 110: 448–53.
10. Rubin J, Jones Q, Andrew M. An analysis of ultrafiltration during acute peritoneal dialysis in rats. Am J Med Sci 1989; 298: 383–9.
11. Rubin J, Jones Q, Planch A, Rushton F, Bower J. The importance of the abdominal viscera to peritoneal transport during peritoneal dialysis in the dog. Am J Med Sci 1986; 292: 203–8.
12. Rubin J, Jones Q, Planch A, Bower J. The minimal importance of the hollow viscera to peritoneal transport during peritoneal dialysis in the rat. Trans Am Soc Artif Intern Organs 1988; 34: 912–5.
13. Albert A, Takamatsu H, Fonkalsrud EW. Absorption of glucose solutions from the peritoneal cavity in rabbits. Arch Surg 1984; 119: 1247–51.
14. Zakaria ER, Carlsson O, Sjunnesson H, Rippe B. Liver is not essential for solute transport during peritoneal diaysis. Kidney Int 1996; 50: 298–303.
15. Zakaria ER, Carlsson O, Rippe B. Limitation of small solute exchange across the visceral peritoneum: effects of vibration. Perit Dial Int 1997; 17: 72–79.
16. Lukus G, Brindle SD, Greengard P. The route of absorption of intraperitoneally administered compounds. J Pharmacal Exp Ther 1971; 178: 562–6.
17. Nolph KD, Ghods AJ, Stone JV, Brown PA. The effects of intraperitoneally vasodilators on peritoneal clearances. Trans Am Soc Artif Intern Organs 1976; 22: 586–94.
18. Hirszel P, Lameire N, Bogaert M. Pharmacologic alterations of peritoneal transport rates and pharmacokinetics of the peritoneum. In: Gokal R, Nolph K, eds. The Textbook of Peritoneal Dialysis. Dordrecht: Kluwer, 1994, pp. 161–232.
19. Wideroe TE, Dahl KJ, Smeby LC et al. Pharmacokinetics of transperitoneal insulin transport. Nephron 1996; 74: 283–90.
20. Chambers R, Zwiefach BW. Functional activity of the blood capillary bed, with special reference to visceral tissue. Ann NY Acad Sci 1946; 46: 683–94.

21. Zweifach BW. The microcirculation of the blood. Sci Am 1959, January, pp. 54–60.

22. Richardson. Basic Circulatory Physiology. Boston, MA: Little, Brown, 1976, pp. 101–36.

23. Johnson PC, Wayland H. Regulation of blood flow in single capillaries. Am J Physiol 1967; 212: 1405–15.

24. Miller FN. The peritoneal microcirculation. In: Nolph K, ed. Peritoneal Dialysis. Boston, MA: Martinus Nijhoff, 1985, pp. 51–93.

25. Buez S. An open cremaster muscle preparation for the study of blood vessels by in vivo microscopy. Microvasc Res 1973; 5: 384–94.

26. Smuje L, Zweifach BW, Intaglietta M. Micropressure and capillary filtration coefficients in single vessels of the cremaster muscle in the rat. Microvasc Res 1970; 2: 96–110.

27. Gabella G (section ed.) Cardiovascular. In: Williams PL, Bannister L, Berry M, Collins P, Dyson M, Dussek J, Ferguson M, eds. Grays Anatomy. New York: Churchill Livingstone, 1995, p. 1465.

28. Renkin EM. Microcirculation and exchange. In: Patton HD, Fuchs AF, Hille B, Scher AM, Steiner R, eds. Testbook of Physiology. Philadelphia, PA: WB Saunders, 1989, pp. 860–78.

29. Chambers R, Zweifach BW. Topography and function of the mesenteric capillary circulation. Am J Anat 1944; 75: 173–2.

30. Taylor AE, Granger DN. Exchange of macromolecules across the circulation. In: Renkin EM, Michel CC, eds. Handbook of Physiology, Microcirculation; Section, Chapter 11. Baltimore, MD: American Physiological Society, 1984, pp. 467–500.

31. Harper SL, Bohlen HG, Granger DN. Vasoactive agents and the mesenteric microcirculation. Am J Physiol 1985; 249: G309–15.

32. Diana JN, Laughlin MH. Effect of ischemia on capillary pressure and equivalent pore radius in capillaries of the isolated dog hind limb. Circ Res 1974; 35: 77–101.

33. Korthuis RJ, Granger DN. Peritoneal dialysis: an analysis of factors which influence peritoneal mass transport. In: Stigmark B, ed. Peritoneum and Peritoneal Access. London: John Wiley, 1988, pp. 24–41.

34. Rippe B, Haraldson B. Capillary permeability in rat hindquarters as determined by estimations of capillary reflection coefficients. Acta Physiol Scand 1986; 127: 289–303.

35. Aune S. Transperitoneal exchange. IV. The effect of transperitoneal fluid transport on the transfer of solutes. Scand J Gastroenterol 1970; 5: 241–52.

36. Curry FE, Mason JC, Michel CC. Osmotic reflection coefficients of capillary walls to low molecular weight hydrophilic solutes measured in single perfused capillaries of the frog mesentary. J Physiol 1976; 261: 319–36.

37. Michel CC. Reflection coefficients in single capillaries compared with results from whole organs. Bibl Anat 1977; 15: 172–6.

38. Michel CC. Filtration coefficients and osmotic reflection coefficients of the walls of single frog mesenteric capillaries. J Physiol 1980; 309: 341–55.

39. Pyle WK, Moncrief JW, Popovich RP. Peritoneal transport evaluation in CAPD. In: Moncrief JW, Popovich RP, eds. Proc Second International Symposium on CAPD. New York: Masson, 1981, pp. 35–9.

40. Rippe B, Perry MA and Granger DN. Permselectivity of the peritoneal membrane. Microvasc Res 1985; 29: 89–102.

41. Rippe B, Stelin G, Ahlmen J. Basal permeability of the peritoneal membrane during continuous ambulatory peritoneal dialysis (CAPD). In: Advances in Peritoneal Dialysis. Proc. Second International Symposium on Peritoneal Dialysis. Amsterdam: Excerpta Medica, 1981, pp. 5–9.

42. Nakamura Y, Watalnd H. Macromolecular transport in the cat mesentery. Microvasc Res 1975; 9: 1–21.

43. Rippe B, Stelin G. Simulations of peritoneal solute transport during CAPD. Application of two pore formalism. Kidney Int 1989; 35: 1234–44.

44. Stelin G, Rippe B. A phenomenologic interpretation of the variations in dialysate volume with dwell time in CAPD. Kidney Int 1990; 38: 465–72.

45. Rippe B, Simonsen O, Stelin G. Clinical implications of a three-pore model of peritoneal transport. In: Khanna R, Nolph KD, Prowant BF, Twardowski ZJ, Oreopoulos D, eds. Advances in Peritoneal Dialysis, 1991, Vol. 7, Peritoneal Dialysis Bulletin, 1991, pp. 3–9.

46. Agree P, Preston GM, Smith BL et al. Aquaporin CHIP: the archetypal molecular water channel. Am J Physiol 1993; 265: F463–76.

47. Conolly DL, Shanahan CM, Weissberg PL. The aquaporins. A family of water channel proteins. Int J Biochem Cell Biol 1998, 30; 169–72.

48. Rippe B, Krediet R: Peritoneal physiology. Transport of solutes. In: Gokal R, Nolph K, eds. The Textbook of Peritoneal Dialysis. Dordrecht: Kluwer, 1994, pp. 68–132.

49. Akiba T, Ota T, Fushimi Ket al. Water channel AQP1, 3, and 4 in the human peritoneum and peritoneal dialysate. Adv Perit Dial 1977; 13: 3–6.

50. Carlsson O, Nielsen S, Zakaria E, Rippe B: In vivo inhibition of transcellular water channels (aquaporin-1) during acute peritoneal dialysis in rats. Am J Physiol 1996; 271 (Heart Circ Physiol 40): H2254–62.

51. Gabella G (section ed.) Cardiovascular. In: Williams PL, Bannister L, Berry M, Collins P, Dyson M, Dussek J, Ferguson M, eds. Grays Anatomy. New York: Churchill Livingstone, 1995, 1466.

52. Granger DN. Richardson PDI, Taylor AE. The effects of isoprenaline and bradykinin on capillary filtration in the cat small intestine. Br J Pharmacol 1979; 67: 361–6.

53. Granger DN, Kvietys PR, Wilborn WH, Mortillaro NA, Taylor AE. Mechanisms of glucagon-induced intestinal secretion. Am J Physiol 1980; 239: G30–38.

54. Mortillaro NA, Granger DN, Kvietys PR, Rutili G, Taylor AE. Effects of histamine and histamine antagonists on intestinal capillary permeability. Am J Pysiol 1981; 240: G381–6.

55. Bjork J, Lindbom L, Gerdin B, Smedegard G, Arfors KE, Benveniste J. PAF (platelet activating factor) increases microvascular permeability and affects endothelium–granulocyte interactions in microvascular beds. Acta Physiol Scand 1983; 119: 305–8.

56. Dahlen SE, Bjork J, Hedqvist P et al. Leukotrienes promote plasma leakage and leukocyte adhesion in postcapillary venules: in vivo effects with relevance to the acute inflammatory response. Proc Natl Acad Sci USA 1981; 78: 3887–91.

57. Bjork J, Hagli TE, Smedegard G. Microvascular effects of anaphylatoxin C3a and C5a. J Immunol 1985; 134: 1115–19.

58. Miller FN, Joshua IG, Anderson GL. Quantitation of vasodilator-induced macromolecular leakage by in vivo fluorescent microscopy. Microvasc Res 1982; 24: 56–7.

59. Roberts WG, Palade GE. Increased microvascular permeability and endothelial fenestration induced by vascular endothelial growth factor. J Cell Sci 1995; 108: 2369–79.

60. Atherton A, Born GVR. Relationship between the velocity of rolling granulocytes and that of blood flow in venules. J Physiol 1973; 233: 157–65.

61. Granger DN, Benoit JN, Suzuki M, Grisham MB. Leukocyte adherence to venular endothelium during ischemia-reperfusion. Am J Physiol 1989; 257: G683–8.

62. Perry MA, Granger DN. Role of CD11/CD18 in shear rate-dependent leukocyte–endothelial cell interactions in cat mesenteric venules. J Clin Invest 1991; 87: 1798–804.

63. Ley K, Gaehtyens P. Endothelial, not hemodynamic differences are responsible for preferential leukocyte rolling in rat mesenteric venules. Circ Res 1991; 69: 1034–41.

64. Granger DN, Kubes P. The microcirculation and inflammation: modulation of leukocyte–endothelial cell adhesion. J Leuk Biol 1994; 55: 662–75.

65. Bienvenu K, Hernandez L, Granger DN. Leukocyte adhesion and emigration in inflammation. Ann NY Acad Sci 1992; 664: 388–99.

66. Tonneson MG. Neutrophil–endothelial cell interactions: mechanisms of neutrophil adherence to vascular endothelium. J Invest Dermatol 1989; 93: 535–85.

67. Kishimoto TK, Jutila MA, Berry EL, Butcher EC. Neutrophil Mac-1 and MEL-14 adhesion proteins are inversely regulated by chemotactic factors. Science 1989; 45: 1238–41.

68. Bevilagua MP, Strengelin S, Gimbrone MA, Seed B. Endothelial leukocyte adhesion molecule 1: an inducible receptor for neutrophils related to complement regulatory proteins and lectins. Science 1989; 243: 1160–65.

69. McEver RP. Selectins: novel adhesion receptors that mediate leukocyte adhesion during inflammation. Thromb Haemostas 1991; 65: 223–8.

70. Smith GW. Molecular determinants of neutrophil–endothelial cell adherence reactions. Am J Respir Cell Molec Biol 1990; 2: 487–99.

71. Springer T, Anderson DC, Rosenthal, Rothelein R. Leukocyte Adhesion Molecules. New York: Springer-Verlag, 1989.

72. Luscher TF, Barton M. Biology of the endothelium. Clin Cardiol 1997; 20 (suppl. II): II-3–II–10.

73. Pepine CJ. Clinical implications of endothelial dysfunction. Clin Cardiol 1998; 21: 795–9.

74. Vallance P. Endothelial regulation of vascular tone. Prostgrad Med J 1992; 68: 697–701.

75. Furchgott RF, Zawadzki JV. The obligatory role of endothelial cells in the relaxation of arterial smooth muscle by acetylcholine. Nature 1980; 299: 373–6.

76. Palmer RM, Ashton DS, Moncada S. Vascular endothelial cells synthesize nitric oxide from L-arginine. Nature 1988; 333: 664–6.

77. Marietta MA. Nitric oxide synthase: aspects concerning structure and catalyst. Cell 1994; 78: 927–30.

78. Moncada S, Higgs A. The L-arginine–nitric oxide pathway. N Engl J Med 1993; 329: 2002–12.

79. Rees DD, Palmer RMJ, Schulz R, Hodson HF, Moncada S. Characterization of three inhibitors of endothelial nitric oxide synthase *in vitro* and *in vivo*. Br J Pharmacol 1990; 101: 746–52.

80. Vallance P, Leone A, Calver A, Collier J, Moncada S. Accumulation of an endogenous inhibitor of nitric oxide synthesis in chronic renal failure. Lancet 1992; 339: 572–5.

81. Vallance P, Leone A, Calver A, Collier J, Moncada S. Endogenous dimethylarginine as an inhibitor of nitric oxide synthesis. J Cardiovasc Pharmacol 1992; 20 (suppl. 12): S60–2.

82. Gardiner SM, Kemp PA, Bennett T, Palmer RMJ, Moncada S. Regional and cardiac hemodynamic effects of N^G,N^G-dimethyl-L-arginine and their reversibility by vasodilators in conscious rats. Br J Pharmacol 1993; 110: 1457–64.

83. White R, Barefield D, Ram S, Work J. Peritoneal dialysis solutions reverse the hemodynamic effects of nitric oxide synthesis inhibitors. Kidney Int 1995; 48: 1986–93.

84. Yanagisawa M. A novel potent vasoconstrictor peptide produced by vascular endothelial cells. Nature 1988; 332: 411–15.

85. Inoue A. The human endothelin family: three structurally and pharmacologically distinct isopeptides predicted by three separate genes. Proc Natl Acad Sci 1989; 86: 2863–7.

86. Battistini B, D'Orleans-Juste P, Sirois P. Biology of disease, endothelins: circulating plasma levels and presence in other biologic fluids. Lab Invest 1993; 68: 600–28.

87. Hosoda K. Organization, structure, chromosomal assignment, and expression of the gene encoding the human endothelin-A receptor. J Biol Chem 1992; 267: 18797–804.

88. Sakamoto A. Cloning and functional expression of human cDNA for the ETB endothelin receptor. Biochem Biophys Res Commun 1991; 178: 656–63.

89. Luscher TF, Oemar BS, Boulanger CM, Hahn AW. Molecular and cellular biology of endothelin and its receptors, part 1. J Hypertens 1993; 11: 7–11.

90. Luscher TF. Endothelin, endothelin receptors and endothelin antagonists. Curr Opin Nephrol Hypertens 1994; 3: 92–8.

91. Riezebos J, Watts IS, Vallance P. Endothelin receptors mediating functional responses in human small arteries and veins. Br J Pharmacol 1994; 111: 609–15.

92. Rohmeiss P, Photiadis J, Rohmeiss S, Unger T. Hemodynamic actions of intravenous endothelin in rats: comparison with sodium nitroprusside and methoxamine. Am J Physiol 1990; 258: H337–46.

93. Gellai M. Physiologic role of endothelin in cardiovascular and renal hemodynamics: studies in animals. Curr Opin Nephrol and Hypertens 1997; 6: 64–8.

94. Lebel M, Moreau V, Grose JH, Kingma I, Langlois S. Plasma and peritoneal endothelin levels and blood pressure in CAPD patients with or without erythropoietin relacement therapy. Clin Nephrol 1998; 49: 313–8.

95. Kubes P, Suzuki M, Granger DN. Nitric oxide: an endogenous modulator of leukocyte adhesion. Proc Natl Acad Sci USA 1991; 88: 4651–5.

96. Lopez-Farre A, Reisco A, Espinosa G et al. Effect of endothelin-1 on neutrophil adhesion to endothelial cells and perfused heart. Circulation 1993; 88: 1166–71.

97. McCarron RM, Wang L, Stanimirovic DB, Spatz M. Endothelin induction of adhesion molecule expression on human brain microvascular endothelial cells. Neurosci Lett 1993; 156: 31–4.

98. Markewitz B, Palazzo M, Li Y, White RG. Endothelin-1 increases leukocyte rolling in mesenteric venules. Abstract. Chest 1998; 114; 251S.

99. Tsukita S, Furuse M, Itoh M. Molecular dissection of tight junctions. Cell Struct Funct 1996; 21: 381–5.

100. Balda MS, Matter K. Tight junctions. J Cell Sci 1998; 111: 541–7.

101. Stevenson BR, Siliciano JD, Mooseker MS, Goodenough DA. Identification of ZO-1: a high molecular weight polypeptide associated with the tight junction (zona occludens) in a variety of epithelia. J Cell Biol 1986; 103: 755–66.

102. Furuse M, Hirase T, Itoh M et al. Occludin: a novel integral protein localizing at tight junctions. J Cell Sci 1993; 123: 1777–88.

103. Anderson JM, Van Itallie CM. Tight junctions and the molecular basis for regulation of paracellular permeability. Am J Physiol 1995; 269: G467–75.

104. Mitic LL, Anderson JM. Molecular architecture of tight junctions. Annu Rev Physiol 1998; 60: 121–42.

105. Denker BM, Nigam SK. Molecular structure and assembly of the tight junction. Am J Physiol 1998; 274: F1–9.

106. Hirase T, Staddon JM, Saitou M et al. Occludin as a possible determinant of tight junction permeability in endothelial cells. J Cell Sci 1997; 110: 1603–13.

107. Kevil CG, Okayma N, Trocha SD et al. Expression of zona occludens and adherens junctional proteins in human venous and arterial endothelial cells: role of occludin in endothelial solute barriers. Microcirculation 1998; 5: 197–210.

108. Martin-Padural, Lostaglio S, Schneemann M et al. Junctional adhesion molecule, a novel member of the immunoglobulin superfamily that distributes at intercellular junctions and modulates monocyte transmigration. J Cell Biol 1998; 142: 117–27.

109. Kemler R. From cadherins to catenins: cytoplasmic protein interactions and regulation of cell adhesion. Trends Genet 1993; 9: 317–21.

110. Klymkowsky MW, Parr B. The body language of the cells: the intimate connection between cell adhesion and behavior. Cell 1995; 83: 5–8.

111. Gumbiner BM. Cell adhesion: the molecular basis of tissue architecture and morphogenesis. Cell 1996; 84: 345–57.

112. Ali J, Liao F, Martiens E, Muller WA. Vascular endothelial cadherin (VE-cadherin): cloning and the role in endothelial cell–cell adhesion. Microcirculation 1997; 4: 267–77.

113. Kevil CG, Payne K, Mire E, Alexander JS. Vascular permeability factor/vascular endothelial cell growth factor-medi-

ated permeability occurs through disorganization of endothelial junctional proteins. J Biol Chem 1998; 273: 15099–103.

114. Alexander JS, Jackson SA, Chaney E, Kevil CG, Haselton FR. The role of cadherin endocytosis in endothelial barrier regulation: involvement of protein kinase C and actin–cadherin interactions. Inflammation 1998; 22: 419–33.

115. Bernfield M. Introduction. In: Porter R *et al.* eds. Basement Membranes and Cell Movement. London: Pitman. Ciba foundation Symposium 108, 1984, pp. 1–5.

116. Clementi F, Palade GE. Intestinal capillaries. I. Permeability to peroxidases and ferritin. J Cell Biol 1969; 41: 33–58.

117. Fox JR, Wayland H. Interstitial diffusion of macro-molecules in the rat mesentery. Microvas Tes 1979; 18: 255–74.

118. Johansson BR. Permeability of muscle capillaries to interstitially microinjected ferritin. Microvasc Res 1978; 16: 362–8.

119. Laurent TC. Interaction between proteins and glycosaminoglycans. Fed Proc 1977; 36: 24–7.

120. Watson PD, Grodins FS. An analysis of the effects of the interstitial matrix on plasma–lymph transport. Microvasc Res 1978; 16: 19–41.

121. Granger DN, Taylor AE. Permeability of intestinal capillaries to endogenous macromolecules. Am J Physiol 1980; 238: H457–64.

122. Majno G. Ultrastructure of the vascular membrane. In: Handbook of Physiology–Circulation, Section 2, Vol. 3. Baltimore: MD: Williams & Wilkins, 1965, pp. 2293–376.

123. Majno G, Palade GE. Studies on inflammation. I. The effect of histamine and serotinin on vascular permeability: an electron microscopic study. J Biophys Biochem Cytol 1961; 11: 571–606.

124. Nolph KD. Peritoneal anatomy and transport physiology. In: Maher JF, ed. Replacement of Renal Function by Dialysis, 3rd edn. Boston: MD: Kluwer, 1989, pp. 516–36.

125. Nolph KD, Miller F, Rubin J, Popovich R. New directions in peritoneal dialysis concepts and applications. Kidney Int 1980; 18: S111–16.

126. Flessner MF, Dedrick RL, Schultz JS. A distributed model of peritoneal–plasma transport: theoretical considerations. Am J Physiol 1984; 246: R597–607.

127. Flessner MD, Dedrick RL, Schultz JS. A distributed model of peritoneal–plasma transport: analysis of experimental data in the rat. Am J Physiol 1985; 248: F413–24.

128. Flessner MF, Fenstermacher JD, Dedrick RL, Blasberg RG. A distributed model of peritoneal–plasma transport: tissue concentration gradients. Am J Physiol 1985; 248: F425–35.

129. Douma CE, De Waart DR, Struijk DG, Krediet R. The nitric oxide donor nitroprusside intraperitoneally affects peritoneal permeability in CAPD. Kidney Int 1997; 51: 1885–92.

130. Flessner MF, Dedrick RL. Role of the liver in small-solute transport during peritoneal dialysis. J Am Soc Nephrol 1994; 5: 116–20.

131. Flessner MF. Small-solute transport across specific peritoneal tissue surfaces in the rat. J Am Soc Nephrol 1996; 7: 225–33.

132. Stephenson RB. Microcirculation and exchange. In: Patton HD, Fuchs AF, Hille B, Scher AM, Steiner R, eds. Textbook of Physiology. Philadelphia, PA: WB Saunders, 1989, pp. 911–923.

133. Wade OL, Combes B, Childes AW, Wheeler HO, Dournand D, Bradley SE. The effect of exercise on the splanchnic blood flow and splanchnic blood volume in normal man. Clin Sci 1956; 15: 457.

134. Korthuis RJ, Granger DN. Role of the peritoneal microcirculation in peritoneal dialysis: In: Nolph KD, ed. Peritoneal Dialysis, 3rd edn. Boston, MA: Kluwer, 1989.

135. Aune S. Transperitoneal exchange II. Peritoneal blood flow estimated by hydrogen gas clearance. Scand J Gastroenterol 1970; 5: 99–104.

136. Bulkey GB. Washout of intraperitoneal xenon: effective peritoneal perfusion as an estimateion of peritoneal blood glow.

In: Granger DN, Bulkey GB, eds. Measurement of Blood Flow: Application to the Splanchnic Circulation. Baltimore, MD: Williams & Wilkins, 1981, pp. 441–53.

137. Nolph KD, Popovich RP, Ghods AJ, Twardowski Z. Determinants of low clearances of small solutes during peritoneal dialysis. Kidney Int 1978; 13: 117–23.

138. Erb RW, Greene JA Jr, Weller JM. Peritoneal dialysis during hemorrhagic shock. J Appl Physiol 1967; 22: 131–5.

139. Texter E, Clinton JR. Small intestinal blood flow. Am J Dig Dis 1963; 8: 587–613.

140. Miller FN, Nolph KD, Harris PD, Rubin J, Wiegman DL, Joshua IG. Effects of peritoneal dialysis solutions on human clearances and rat arterioles. Trans Am Soc Intern Organs 1978; 24: 131–2.

141. Miller FN, Nolph KD, Harris PD *et al.* Microvascular and clinical effects of altered peritoneal dialysis solutions. Kidney Int 1979; 15: 630–9.

142. Nolph KD. Effects of intraperitoneal vasodilators on peritoneal clearances. Dial Transplant 1978; 7: 812.

143. Nolph KD, Ghods AJ, Brown PA, Twardowski ZJ. Effects of intraperitoneal nitroprusside on peritoneal clearances with variations in dose, frequency of administration, and dwell times. Nephron 1979; 24: 114–20.

144. Nolph KD, Ghods AJ, Van Stone J, Brown PA. The effects of intraperitoneal vasodilators on peritoneal clearances. Trans Am Soc Artif Intern Organs 1976; 22: 586.

145. Nolph KD, Ghods AJ, Brown PA *et al.* Effects of nitroprusside on peritoneal mass transfer coefficients and microvascular physiology. Trans Am Soc Artif Intern Organs 1977; 23: 210–18.

146. Ronco C, Feriani M, Chiaramonte S, Brendolan A, Milan M, La Greca G. Peritoneal blood flow: does it matter? Perit Dial Int 1996; 16 (suppl. 1): S70–5.

147. Kim M, Lofthouse J, Flessner MF. A method to test blood flow limitation of peritoneal–blood solute transport. J Am Soc Nephrol 1997; 8: 471–4.

148. Kim M, Lofthouse J, Flessner MF. Blood flow limitations of solute transport across the visceral peritoneum. J Am Soc Nephrol 1997; 8: 1946–50.

149. Rubin J, Nolph KD, Popovich RP, Moncrief JW, Prowant B. Drainage volume during continuous ambulatory peritoneal dialysis. Am Soc Artif Intern Org 1979; 22: 54–60.

150. Twardowski ZJ, Khanna R, Nolph KD. Osmotic agents and ultrafiltration in peritoneal dialysis. Nephron 1986; 42: 93–101.

151. Maher JF, Hirszel P, Lasrich M. An experimental model for study of pharmacologic and hormonal influences on peritoneal dialysis. Contrib Nephrol 1979; 17: 131–8.

152. Maher JF. Peritoneal transport rates: mechanisms, limitation and methods for augmentation. Kidney Int 1980; 18: S117–21.

153. Nolph KD, Mactier R, Khanna R, Twardowski ZJ, Moore H, McGary T. The kinetics of ultrafiltration during peritoneal dialysis. Kidney Int 1987; 32: 219–26.

154. Flessner MF, Schwab A. Pressure threshold for fluid loss from the peritoneal cavity. Am J Physiol 1996; 270: F377–90.

155. Flessner MF. Osmotic barrier of the parietal peritoneum. Am J Physiol 1994; 267: F861–70.

156. Grzegorzewska AE, Moore HL, Nolph KD, Chen TW. Ultrafiltration and effective peritoneal blood flow during peritoneal dialysis in the rat. Kidney Int 1991; 39: 608–17.

157. Granger DN. Richardson PDI, Taylor AE. The effects of isoprenaline and bradykinnin on capillary filtration in the cat small intestine. Br J Pharmocol 1979; 67: 361–6.

158. Granger DN, Kvietys PR, Wilborn WH, Mortillaro NA, Taylor AE. Mechanisms of glucagon-induced intestinal secretion. Am J Physiol 1980; 239: G30–8.

159. Mortillaro NA, Granger DN, Kvietys PR, Rutili G, Taylor AE. Effects of histamine and histamine antagonists on intestinal capillary permeability. Am J Pysiol 1981; 240: G381–6.

160. Granger DN, Perry MA, Kvietys PR, Taylor AE. Permeability of intestinal capillaries: effects of fat absorption and gastrointestinal hormones. Am J Physiol 1982; 242: G194–201.

161. Campion DS, North JDK. Effect of protein binding of barbiturates on their rate of removal during peritoneal dialysis. J Lab Clin Med 1965; 66: 549–63.

162. Cole DEC, Lirenman DS. Role of albumin enriched peritoneal dialysate in acute copper posioning. J Pediatr 1978; 92: 955–77.

163. Etteldorf JM, Dobbins WT, Summitt RL, Rainwater WT, Fischer RI. Intermittent peritoneal dialysis using 5% albumin in the treatment of salicylate intoxication in children. J Pediatr 1961; 58: 226–36.

164. Schultz JC, Crouder DG, Medart WS. Excretion of studies in ethylchlorovynol (placidil) intoxication. Arch Intern Med 1966; 117: 409–11.

165. El-Bassiouni EA, Mattocks AM. Acceleration of peritoneal dialysis with minimal N-myristyl-B-aminoproprionate. J Pharm Sci 1973; 62: 1314–16.

166. Kudla RM, ElBassiouni EA, Mattocks AM. Accelerated peritoneal dialysis of barbituarates, and salicylate. J Pharm Sci 1971; 60: 1065–7.

167. Mattocks AM. Accelerate removal of salicylate by additives in peritoneal dialysis fluid. J Pharm Sci 1969; 58: 595–9.

168. Hirszel P, Lasrich M, Maher JF. Arachidonic acid increases peritoneal clearances. Trans Am Soc Artif Intern Organs 1981; 27: 61–3.

169. Maher JF, Hirszel P, Lasrich M. Effects of gastrointestinal hormones on transport by peritoneal dialysis. Kidney Int 1979; 16: 130–6.

170. Lal SM, Nolph KD, Moore HS, Khanna R. Calcium channel blockers enhance urea transport without increasing protein loss. Clin Res 1986; 34: 40.

171. Vargemezis V, Pasadakis P, Thodis E. Effect of a calcium antagonist (verapamil) on the permeability of the peritoneal membrane in patients on continuous ambulatory peritoneal dialysis. Blood Purif 1989; 7: 309–13.

172. Penzotti SC, Mattocks MA. Acceleration of peritoneal dialysis by surface-acting agents. J Pharm Sci 1968; 57: 119–205.

173. Maher JF, Hirszel P, Lasrich M. Effects of gastrointestinal hormones on transport by peritoneal dialysis. Kidney Int 1979; 16: 130–6.

174. Hirszel P, Dodge K, Maher JF. Acceleration of peritoneal transport by cytochalasin D. Uremia Invest 1984; 8: 85.

175. Covey TJ. Ferous sulfate poisoning: a review, case summaries and therapeutic regimen. J Pediatr 1964; 64: 218–26.

176. Stanbaugh GH Jr, Homes AW, Gillit D. Iron chelation therapy in CAPD: A new effective treatment for iron overload disease in ESRD patients. Perit Dial Bull 1983; 3: 99–103.

177. Williams P, Khanna R, Crapper McLachlan DR. Enhancement of aluminum removal by desferrioxamine in a patient on continuous ambulatory peritoneal dialysis with dementia. Perit Dial Bull 1981: 73–7.

178. Knochel JP, Clayton E, Smith WL, Barry KG. Intraperitoneal THAM: an effective method to enhance phenobarbital removal during peritoneal dialysis. J Lab Clin Med 1964; 64: 257–68.

179. Knochel JP, Mason AD. Effect of alkalinization on peritoneal diffusion of uric acid. Am J Physiol 1966; 210: 1160–4.

180. Nolph KD, Ghods AJ, Van Stone J, Brown PA. The effects of intraperitoneal vasodilators on peritoneal clearances. Trans Am Soc Artif Intern Organs 1976; 22: 586–94.

181. Penzotti SC, Mattocks MA. Acceleration of peritoneal dialysis by surface-acting agents. J Pharm Sci 1968; 57: 1192–5.

182. Mattocks AM, Penzotti SC. Acceleration of peritoneal dialysis with minimum amounts of dioctyl sodium sulfosuccinate. J Pharm Sci 1972; 61: 475–6.

183. Maher JF, Hirszel P, Abraham JE. The effect of dipyridamole on peritoneal mass transport. Trans Am Soc Artif Intern Organs 1977; 23: 219–23.

184. Hare HG, Valtin J, Gosselin RE. Effects of drugs on peritoneal dialysis in the dog. J Pharmacol Exp Ther 1964; 145: 122–9.

185. Shear L, Harvey JD, Barry KG. Peritoneal sodium transport: enhancement by pharmological and physical agents. J Lab Clin Med 1966; 67: 181–8.

186. Mehbod H. Treatment of lead intoxication. Combined use of peritoneal dialysis and edentate calcium disodium. JAMA 1967; 201: 972–4.

187. Maher JF, Hohnadel DC, Shea C, Sisanzo F, Cassetts M. Effects of intraperitoneal diuretics on solute transport during hypertonic dialysis. Clin Nephrol 1977; 7: 96–100.

188. Grzegorzewska A, Baczyk K. Furosemide-induced increase in urinary and peritoneal excretion of uric acid during peritoneal dialysis in patients with chronic uremia. Artif Organs 1982; 6: 220–4.

189. Maher JF, Hirszel P, Lasrich M. Effects of gastrointestinal hormones on transport by peritoneal dialysis. Kidney Int 1979; 16: 130–6.

190. Nolph KD, Ghods AJ, Brown P, Van Stone JC. Factors affecting peritoneal dialysis efficiency. Dial Transplant 1977; 6: 52–6.

191. Felt J, Richard C, McCaffrey C, Lefy M. Peritoneal clearance of creatinine and insulin during dialysis in dogs. Effect of splanchnic vasodilators. Kidney Int 1979; 16: 459–69.

192. Hirszel P, Maher JF, Legrow W. Increased peritoneal mass transport with glucagon acting at the vascular surface. Trans Am Soc Artif Organs 1978; 24: 136–8.

193. Rasio EA. Metabolic control of permeability in isolated mesentery. Am J Physiol 1974; 226: 962–8.

194. Brown EA, Kliger AS, Goffinet J, Finkelstein FO. Effect of hypertonic dialysate and vasodilators on peritoneal dialysis clearances in rats. Kidney Int 1978; 12: 271–7.

195. Granger DN, Richardson PDI, Kvietys PR, Mortillaro NA. Intestinal blood flow. Gastroenterology 1980; 78: 837–63.

196. DeSanto NG, Capodicasa G, Capasso G. Development of means to augment peritoneal urea clearances: the synergic effects of combining high dialysate temperature and high dialysate flow rates with dextrose and nitroprusside. Artif Organs 1981; 5: 409–14.

197. Henderson LW, Nolph KD. Altered permeability of the peritoneal membrane after usng hypertonic peritoneal dialysis fluid. J Clin Invest 1969; 48: 992–1001.

198. Rasio EA. Metabolic control of permeability in isolated mesentery. Am J physiol 1974; 226: 962–8.

199. Brown ST, Aheran DJ, Nolph KD. Reduced peritoneal clearances in scleroderma increased by intraperitoneal isoproterenol. Ann Intern Med 1973; 78: 891–7.

200. Maher JF, Shea C, Cassetta M, Hohnadel DC. Isoproterenol enhancement of permeability. J Dial 1977; 1: 319–31.

201. Nolph KD, Miller L, Husted FC, Hirszel P. Peritoneal clearances in scleroderma and diabetes mellitus. Effects of intraperitoneal isoproterenol. Int Urol Nephrol 1976; 8: 154–61.

202. Shinaberger JH, Shear L, Clayton LE. Dialysis of intoxication with lipid soluble drugs: enhancement of glutethimide extraction with lipid dialysate. Trans Am Soc Artif Organs 1965; 11: 173–7.

203. Miller FN, Nolph KD, Harris PD. Effects of peritoneal dialysis solutions on human clearances and rat arterioles. Trans Am Soc Artif Intern Organs 1978; 24: 131–2.

204. Nolph KD. Effects of intrraperitoneal vasodilators on peritoneal clearances. Dial Transpl 1978; 7: 812.

205. Nolph KD, Ghods AJ, Brown PA, Twardowski ZJ. Effects of intraperitoneal nitroprusside on peritoneal clearances with variations in dose, frequency of administration, and dwell times. Nephron 1979; 24: 114–20.

207. Breborowicz A, Knapowski J. Augmentation of peritoneal dialysis clearances with procaine. Kidney Int 1984; 26: 392–6.

208. Maher JF, Hirszel P, Lasrich M. Modulation of peritoneal transport rates by prostaglandins. Adv Prostagland Thrombox Res 1980; 7: 695–700.

209. Hirszel P, Lasrich M, Maher JF. Peritoneal transport rates and inhibition of prostaglandin synthetase by mefenamic acid. Abstr Am Soc Artif Intern Organs 1980; 9: 48.

210. Parker HR, Schroeder JP, Henderson LW. Influence of dopamine and Regitine on peritoneal dialysis in unanesthetized dogs. Abstr Am Soc Artif Intern Organs 1978; 7: 43.

211. Alavi N, Lianos E, Andres G. Effect of protamine on the permeability and structure of rat peritoneum. Kidney Int 1982; 21: 44–53.

212. Avasthi PS. Effects of aminonucleoside on rat blood–peritoneal barrier permeability. J Lab Clin Med 1979; 94: 295–302.

213. Gutman RA, Nixon WP, McRae RL, Spencer HW. Effect of intraperitoneal and intravenous vasoactive amines on peritoneal dialysis: Study in anephric dogs. Trans Am Soc Artif Intern Organs 1976; 22: 570–3.

214. Hirszel P, Larisch M, Maher JF. Divergent effects of catecholamines on peritoneal mass transport. Trans Am Soc Artif Intern Organs 1979; 25: 110–13.

215. Raja RM, Kramer MS, Rosenbaum JL. Enhanced clearance with intraperitoneal nitroprusside in high flow recirculation peritoneal dialysis. Trans Am Soc Artif Intern Organs 1978; 24: 133–5.

216. Nolph KD, Rubin J, Wiegman DL, Harris PD, Miller FN. Peritoneal clearances with three types solutions. Nephron 1979; 24: 35–40.

217. Grzegorzewska A, Barcz M, Kriczi M, Antoniewicz K. Peritoneal blood flow and peritoneal transfer parameters during intermittent peritoneal dialyses performed with administration of sodium nitroprusside or chlorpromazine. Przegl Lek 1996; 53: 412–16.

218. Carlsson O, Rippe B. Enhanced peritoneal diffusion capacity of ^{51}Cr-EDTA during the initial phase of peritoneal dialysis: role of vasodilatation, dialysate 'stirring', and of interstitial factors. Blood Purif 1998; 16: 162–70.

218. Brown ST, Aheran DJ, Nolph KD. Reduced peritoneal clearances in scleroderma increased by intraperitoneal isoproterenol. Ann Intern Med 1973; 78: 891–7.

219. Miller FN, Nolph KD, Joshua IG, Rubin J. Effects of vasodilators and peritoneal dialysis solution on the microcirculation of the rat cecum. Proc Soc Exp Biol Med 1979; 161: 605–8.

220. Miller FN, Nolph KD, Joshua IG, Weigman DL, Harris PD, Anderson DB. Hyperosmolality, acetate and lactate: dilatory factors during peritoneal dialysis. Kidney Int 1981; 20: 397–402.

221. Miller FN, Joshua JG, Harris PD, Weigman DL, Jauchem JR. Peritoneal dialysis solutions and the microcirculation. Contrib Nephrol 1977; 17: 51–8.

222. Steenbergen JM, Bohlen HG. Sodium hyperosmolarity of intestinal lymph causes arteriolar vasodilation in part mediated by EDRF. Am J Physiol 1993; 265: H323–8.

223. MacAllister R, Vallance P. Nitric oxide in essential in renal hypertension. J Am Soc Nephrol 1994; 5: 1057–65.

224. Anderstam B, Katzarski K, Bergstrom J. Serum levels of N^G,N^G-dimethylarginine, a potential endogenous nitric oxide inhibitor in dialysis patients. J Am Soc Nephrol 1997; 8: 1437–9.

225. Breborowicz A, Wieczorowska-Tobis K, Korybalska K, Polubinska A, Radowski M, Oreopoulos D. The effect of a nitric oxide inhibitor (L-NAME) on peritoneal transport during peritoneal dialysis. Perit Dial Int 1998; 18: 188–92.

226. Douma CE, de Waart DR, Struijk DG, Krediet RT. Effect of amino acid based dialysate on peritoneal blood flow and permeability in stable CAPD patients: a potential role for nitric oxide? Clin Nephrol 1996; 45: 295–302.

227. Schmid-Schonbein GW, Usami S, Skalak R, Chien S. The interaction of leukocytes and erythrocytes in capillary and postcapillary vessels. Microvasc Res 1980; 19: 45–70.

228. Kishimoto TK. A dynamic model for neutrophil localization to inflammatory sites. J NIH Res 1991.

229. House SD, Lipowsky JJ. Leukocyte–endothelium adhesion: microhemodynamics in mesentery of the cat. Microvasc Res 1987; 34: 363–79.

230. Engler RL, Schmid-Schonbein, Pavelec RS. Leukocyte capillary plugging in myocardial ischemia and reperfusion in the dog. Am J Pathol 1983; 3: 98–111.

231. Worthen GS, Schwab B, Elson EL, Downey OP. Cellular mechanics of stimulated neutrophils: stiffening of cells induces retention in pores *in vitro* and long capillaries *in vivo*. Science 1989; 245: 183–6.

232. Carden DL, Smith JK, Korthuis RJ. Neutrophil mediated microvascular dysfunction in postischemic canine skeletal muscle: role of granulocyte adherence. Circ Res 1990; 66: 1436–44.

233. Harlan JM. Leukocyte–endothelial cell interactions. Blood 1985; 65: 513–25.

234. Gaboury J, Woodman RC, Granger DN, Reinhardt P, Kubes P. Nitric oxide prevents leukocyte adherence: role of superoxide. Am J Physiol 1993; 265: H862–7.

235. Gaboury J, Anderson D, Kubes P. Molecular mechanisms involved in superoxide-induced leukocyte–endothelial cell interactions *in vivo*. Am J Physiol 1994; 266: H637–42.

236. Del Maestro RF, Planker, Arfors KE. Evidence for the participation of superoxide anion radical in altering the adhesive interaction between granulocytes and endothelium *in vivo*. Int J Microcirc Clin Exp 1982; 1: 105–20.

237. Asako H, Kurose I, Wolf R *et al.* Role of H1-receptors and P-selectin in histamine-induced leukocyte rolling and adhesion in postcapillary venules. J Clin Invest 1994; 93: 1508–15.

238. Olofsson AM, Von Andrian UH, Ranezani L, Wolitzky B, Arfors KE. E-selectin mediates leukocyte rolling in interleukin-1 treated rabbit mesentery venules. FASEB J 1993; 7: A342 (abstract).

239. Mayadas TN, Johnson R, Rayburn H, Hynes RO, Wagner DD. Leukocyte rolling and extravasation are severely compromised in P-selectin-deficient mice. Cell 1993; 74: 541–54.

240. Wallace JL, McKnight W, Miyasaka M *et al.* Role of endothelial adhesion molecules in NSAID-induced gastric mucosal injury. Am J Physiol 1993; 265: G993–8.

241. Eppihimer MJ, Granger DN. Ischemia/reperfusion-induced leukocyte–endothelial interactions in postcapillary venules. Shock 1997; 8: 16–25.

242. Argenbright LW, Letts LG, Rothlein R. Monoclonal antibodies to the leukocyte membrane CD18 glycoprotein complex and to intercellular adhesion molecule-1 inhibit leukocyte–endothelial adhesion in rabbits J Leuk Biol 1991; 49: 253–7.

243. Kubes P, Suzuki M, Granger DN. Modulation of PAF-induced leukocyte adherence and increased microvascular permeability. Am J Physiol 1990: 259: G859–64.

244. Dillon PK, Fitzpatrick MF, Ritter AB, Duran WN. Effect of platelet-activating factor on leukocyte adhesion to microvascular endothelium. Time course and dose–response relationships. Inflammation 1988; 12: 563–73.

245. Bjork J, Hedqvist P, Arfors KE. Increase in vascular permeability induced by leukotriene B4; and the role of polymorphonuclear leukocytes. Inflammation 1982; 6: 189–200.

246. Kubes P, Grisham MB, Barrowman JA, Gaginella T, Granger DN. Leukocyte-induced vascular protein leakage in cat mesentery. Am J Physiol 1991; 261: H1872–9.

247. Asako H, Wolf R, Granger DN, Korthuis RJ. Phalloidin reduces leukocyte emigration and vascular permeability in postcapillary venules. Am J Physiol 1992; 263: H1637–42.

248. Suzuki M, Asako H, Kubes P, Jennings S, Grisham MB, Granger DN. Neutrophil-derived oxidants promote leukocyte adherence in postcapillary venules. Microvasc Res 1991; 42: 125–38.

249. Asako H, Kubes P, Wallace JL, Wolf RE, Granger DN. Indomethacin-induced leukocyte adhesion in mesenteric venules: role of lipoxygenase products. Am J Physiol 1992; 262: G903–8.

250. Arndt H, Smith CW, Granger DN. Leukocyte–endothelial cell adhesion in spontaneously hypertensive and normal rats. Hypertension 1993; 21: 667–73.

251. Granger DN, Kvietys PR, Perry MA. Leukocyte–endothelial cell adhesion induced by ischemia and reperfusion. Can J Physiol Pharmacol 1993; 71: 67–75.

252. Lehr HA, Hubner C, Nolte D, Kohlscutter A, Messmer K. Dietary fish oil blocks the microcirculatory manifestations of ischemia–reperfusion injury in striated muscle in hamsters. Proc Natl Acad Sci USA 1991; 88: 6726–30.

253. Miura S, Imaeda H, Shiozaki H, Suematsu M, Sekizuka E, Tsuchiya M. Attenuation of endotoxin-induced intestinal microcirculatory damage by eicosapentanoic acid. Am J Physiol 1993; 264: G828–34.

254. Grisham MB, Hernandez LA, Granger DN. Adenosine inhibits ischemia/reperfusion-induced leukocyte adherence and extravasation. Am J Physiol 1989; 257: H1334–9.

255. Asako H, Wolf R, Granger DN. Leukocyte adherence in rat mesenteric venules: effects of adenosine and methotrexate. Gastroenterology 1993; 104: 31–7.

256. Asako H, Kubes P, Wallace JL, Wolf RE, Granger DN. Modulation of leukocyte adhesion in rat mesenteric venules by aspirin and salicylate. Gastroenterology 1992; 103: 149–52.

257. Erlansson M, Bergqvist D, Persson NH, Svensjo E. Modification of postischemic increase of leukocyte adhesion and vascular permeability in the hamster by iloprost. Prostaglandins 1991; 41: 157–68.

258. Kubes P, Granger DN. Nitric oxide modulates microvascular permeability. Am J Physiol 1992; 262: H611–15.

259. Kurose I, Kubes P, Wolf RE et al. Inhibition of nitric oxide production: mechanisms of vascular albumin leakage. Circ Res 1993; 73: 164–71.

260. Lehr HA, Kress E, Menger MD et al. Cigarette smoke elicits leukocyte adhesion to endothelium in hamsters: inhibition by CuZn-SOD. Free Radic Biol Med 1993; 14: 573–81.

261. Suzuki M, Grisham MB, Granger DN. Leukocyte–endothelial cell interactions: role of xanthine oxidase-derived oxidants. J Leuk Biol 1991; 50: 488–94.

262. Arndt H, Russell JM, Kurose I, Kubes P, Granger DN. Mediators of leukocyte adhesion in rat mesenteric venules elicited by inhibition of nitric oxide sythesis. Gastroenterology 1993; 105: 675–80.

263. Lehr HA, Guhlmann A, Nolte D, Keppler D, Messmer K. Leukotrienes as mediators in ischemia–reperfusion injury in a microcirculation model in the hamster. J Clin Invest 1991; 87: 2036–41.

264. Asako H, Kubes P, Baethge BA, Wolf RE, Granger DN. Colchicine and methotrexate reduce leukocyte adherence and emigration in rat mesenteric venules. Inflammation 1992; 16: 45–56.

265. Kubes P, Kanwar S, Niu XF, Gaboury J. Nitric oxide synthesis inhibition induces leukocyte adhesion via superoxide and mast cells. FASEB J 1993; 7: 1293–9.

266. Kubes P, Suzuki M, Granger DN. Platelet activating factor-induced microvascular dysfunction: role of adherent leukocytes. Am J Physiol 1990; 258: G158–63.

267. Weiss S. Oxygen, ischemia and inflammation. Acta Physiol Scand 1986; 126 (suppl. 584): 9–38.

268. Weiss SJ. Tissue destruction by neutrophils. N Engl J Med 1989; 320: 365–76.

269. Reilly PM, Schiller HJ, Bulkley GB. Pharmacological approach to tissue injury by free radicals nd other reactive oxygen metabolites. Am J Surg 1991; 161: 488–503.

270. Kubes P, Suzuki M, Granger DN. Modulation of PAF-induced leukocyte adherence and increased microvascular permeability. Am J Physiol 1990; 259: G858–64.

271. Kubes P, Granger DN. Nitric oxide modulates microvascular permeability. Am J Physiol 1992; 262: H611–15.

272. Del Maschio A, Zanetti A, Corada M et al. Polymorphonuclear leukocyte adhesion triggers the disorganization of endothelial cell-to-cell adherens junctions. J Cell Biol 1996; 135: 497–510.

273. Gotsch U, Borges E, Bosse R et al. VE-cadherin antibody accelerates neutrophil recruitment in vivo. J Cell Sci 1997; 110: 583–8.

274. White R, Work J, Korthius R. The effect of a hypertonic peritoneal dialysis solution on leukocyte adhesion to post-capillary venules in the rat mesentery. FASEB J 1993; A343: 1985 (abstract).

275. Jonasson P, Bagge U, Wieslander A, Braide M. Heat sterilized PD fluid blocks leukocyte adhesion and increases flow velocity in rat peritoneal venules. Perit Dial Int 1996; 16 (suppl. 1): S137–40.

276. White R, Ram S. Peritoneal dialysis solution attenuates microvascular leukocyte adhesion induced by nitric oxide synthesis inhibition. Adv Perit Dial 1996; 53–6.

277. Kaupke CJ, Zhang J, Rajpoot D, Wang J, Zhou XJ, Vaziri ND. Effects of conventional peritoneal dialysates on leukocyte adhesion and CD11b, CD18 and CD14 expression. Kidney Int 1996; 50: 1676–83.

278. Nolte D, Bayer M, Lehr H et al. Attenuation of postischemic microvascular disturbances in striated muscle by hyperosmolar saline dextran. Am J Physiol 1992; 263: H1411–16.

279. White R, Work J, Korthuis R. The effect of a hyperosmolar non-glucose containing solution on leukocyte adhesion to postcapillary venules in the rat mesentery. FASEB J 1994; 1871 (abstract).

280. Duwe AK, Vas SI, Weatherhead JW. Effects of the composition of peritoneal dialysis fluid on chemiluminescence, phagocytosis, and bactericidal activity in vitro. Infect Immun 1981; 33: 130–5.

281. H van Bronswijk, Verbrugh HA, Heezius HCJM, J van der Meulen, Oe PL, Verhoef J. Dialysis fluids and local host resistance in patients on continuous ambulatory peritoneal dialysis. Eur Clin Microbiol Infect Dis 1988; 7: 368–73.

282. Verbrugh HA, Keane WF, Hoidal JR, Freiberg MR, Elliott GR, Peterson PK. Peritoneal macrophages and opsonins: antibacterial defense in patients undergoing chronic peritoneal dialysis. J Infect Dis 1983; 6: 1018–29.

283. Granger DN, Ulrich M, Perry MA, Kvietys PR. Peritoneal dialysis solutions and splanchnic blood flow. Clin Exp Pharmacol Physiol 1984; 11: 473–83.

5 | The physiology of peritoneal solute transport and ultrafiltration

R. T. KREDIET

The surface area of the peritoneum

Few studies have been published on the magnitude of the surface area of the peritoneum. Wegener mentioned a surface area of 1.72 m^2 in one adult woman [1] and Putiloff a value of 2.07 m^2 in one adult male [2]. More recent autopsy studies reported lower values [3–5]; the average peritoneal surface area in adults ranged from 1.0 m^2 [3] to 1.3 m^2 [5]. Using CT scanning in CAPD patients a value of 0.55 m^2 has been found [6], but this method needs further validation. Some studies reported relationships between peritoneal surface area and body weight and/or body surface area, while others did not. The ratio between peritoneal surface area and body weight in adults is about half of that found in newborn infants [3]. A difference between adults and infants is barely present when peritoneal surface area is related to body surface area [3].The peritoneal/body surface area averaged 0.6–0.8 in adults, and 0.5–0.6 in infants. About 60% of the peritoneum consists of visceral peritoneum, 10% of which covers the liver, 30% of mesenterium and omentum, and 10% is parietal peritoneum [3–5]. The latter includes the diaphragmatic peritoneum which comprises 3–8% of the total peritoneal surface area. Species differences are present, especially with regard to the contribution of diaphragmatic peritoneum, which is larger in humans than in rodents [5]. The contribution of the various parts of the peritoneum to solute transport during peritoneal dialysis may vary. Evisceration was found to cause a marked reduction in the transport of creatinine in rabbits [7], but not in rats [8, 9]. Effective peritoneal dialysis has been described in a neonate with extensive resection of the small intestine [10]. It has been hypothesized that the peritoneum covering the liver might be especially important in solute transport during peritoneal dialysis, because of the close proximity with the liver sinusoids, but this could not be confirmed in experimental studies in rats [11, 12]. The diaphragmatic part of the peritoneum is especially involved in the absorption of solutes and fluid from the peritoneal cavity into the lymphatic system [13]. Observations in rats have shown that the peritoneal surface area increases with the age of the animals, with a proportional increase in dialysate/plasma (D/P) ratios of urea and creatinine [14].

The proportion of the peritoneum that is involved in transport during peritoneal dialysis is not known. The above-mentioned evisceration experiments suggest that the relative contribution of the parietal peritoneum may be more important than that of the visceral peritoneum. Although similar diffusion rates were found during experiments in rats undergoing peritoneal dialysis using a diffusion chamber, placed at various parts of the peritoneum, it appeared that only 25–30% of the visceral peritoneum was in contact with the dialysis solution [11]. Furthermore, it has been shown in cats that commercial dialysis solutions increase blood flow to the mesentery, omentum, intestinal serosa and parietal peritoneum, without altering total splanchnic blood flow [15]. This study, using microspheres, points to hyperaemia of these tissues, thereby increasing the peritoneal capillary surface area.

It appears from the above data that the surface area of the peritoneal membrane involved in peritoneal dialysis is not a static property, but should be defined in a functional way. The functional surface area of the peritoneal membrane cannot be measured directly, but the functional cross-sectional exchange pore area divided by the effective diffusion path length can be estimated. This parameter takes not only the capillary surface area into account, but also the distance to the dialysate/mesothelial contact. Using kinetic modelling values of 117–250 m have been reported [16–19]. When the surface area of the peritoneum that is involved in transport is 0.6 m^2 and the unrestricted area over diffusion distance is set at 190 m, it can be calculated that the

R. Gokal, R. Khanna, R.Th. Krediet and K.D. Nolph (eds.), Textbook of Peritoneal Dialysis, 2nd Edition, 135–172.
© 2000 *Kluwer Academic Publishers. Printed in Great Britain.*

length from the capillary wall to the peritoneal cavity would be 3 mm in case of unrestricted diffusion in water. As the peritoneum is much thinner, this means that the resistance to diffusion of interstitial tissue must greatly exceed that of water. This will be discussed further in the following section.

Pathways and barriers

Solutes passing from the blood in the peritoneal capillaries to the dialysate-filled peritoneal cavity have to pass at least three structures that can offer resistance: the capillary wall, the interstitial tissue and the mesothelial cell layer (Fig. 1). Stagnant fluid layers at the mesothelial site have also been proposed as sites of resistance [20]. However, it has been calculated by Flessner that these are only a minor barrier to solute transport compared to the interstitial tissue [21]. The mesenterium is an important layer in the prevention of friction between abdominal organs, and is also involved in host defence. It is, however, not a main barrier to peritoneal transport of solutes and water. *In-vitro* studies on the diffusion properties of an isolated avascular part of mesentery, thus representing transport in a diffusion chamber across two layers of mesothelium divided by interstitial tissue, have shown that the diffusion of particles with a molecular weight up to 500 kDa was similar to the expected values on the basis of their molecular weights [22, 23]. A pore radius of 0.7 µm could be calculated [22]. *In-vivo* studies have

shown that, although permeability coefficients were lower than *in vitro* [24], intraperitoneally administered macromolecules could easily pass the mesothelial layer [25, 26]. The mesothelium of the parietal peritoneum was also no osmotic barrier [27].

The interstitial tissue in general consists of bundles of collagen within a mucopolysaccharide hydrogel. It has been described as a two-phase system, in which a colloid-rich, water-poor phase is in equilibrium with a water-rich, colloid-poor phase [28]. The mucopolysaccharides of the colloid-rich phase are mainly composed of glycosaminoglycans, either hyaluronan or proteoglycans fixed to their core proteins. The free fluid phase is interspaced between areas of the colloid-rich phase. It is assumed that water transports throughout the interstitial space, while small solutes are partly excluded from the colloid phase and protein transport is restricted to the tortuous, water-rich phase. The thickness of the peritoneum is variable depending on its localization. In the mesentery the average thickness from mesothelium to mesothelium is 30 µm, with exceptions up to 110 µm [29]. The parietal peritoneum is loosely attached to the abdominal wall and easily stripped. Its thickness is estimated to be 2 mm [30]. The visceral peritoneum is more dense and firmly attached to the underlying tissues [30]. Examining cross-sections of the gut reveals that the thickness of the serosa varies from 30 to 250 µm [31]. Assuming a contribution of the visceral peritoneum to solute transport of 30% [11], an average thickness of the peritoneal interstitium of 500 µm can be calculated. This corresponds to the findings of Flessner *et al.* in which the steepest concentration gradient of EDTA in various parts of the peritoneal interstitium was found 400–600 µm from the serosa [32]. This is a factor 6 less than the 3 mm calculated on the basis of the unrestricted area over diffusion distance. This difference is likely to represent the restriction of the interstitial tissue to diffusion, compared with diffusion in water. The question arises whether this interstitial restriction is size-selective, i.e. the proportional restriction of solutes with various molecular weights is more pronounced than can be expected on the basis of free diffusion of these solutes only. The *in-vitro* studies using an isolated mesentery suggested no size selectivity [22, 23], but the *in-vivo* study on an isolated rat mesentery provided evidence that the apparent diffusion coefficients of various neutral dextran fractions were progressively lower than those in water [33]. No size selectivity was found for low molecular weight solutes.

The capillary wall is probably the most important restriction barrier. Solute transport occurs size selec-

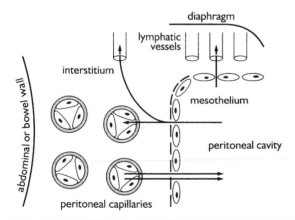

Figure 1. A schematic representation of the peritoneal membrane. Diffusion and transcapillary ultrafiltration occur in two directions. Transcapillary ultrafiltration from the peritoneal capillaries to the peritoneal cavity occurs through small interendothelial pores and transcellularly through water channels. Lymphatic absorption from the peritoneal cavity is partly directly into the subdiaphragmatic lymphatics and partly into the lymphatics that drain the mesothelium.

tively and is generally considered to take place through a system of pores [34, 35]. Although the vascular wall is likely to be heteroporous, the capillary wall can be considered to function mainly as an isoporous membrane in combination with a small amount of very large pores, as has been described for the glomerulus [36]. This combination is known as the two-pore theory of capillary transport [37–39]. This theory assumes the presence of small pores with radii of 40–50 Å that are involved in the transport of low molecular weight solutes. Interendothelial clefts with radii of 40 Å have been considered the anatomical equivalents of the small pores [40, 41], but this is still an assumption. Transport through plasmalemmal vesicles, that would form channels, has also been suggested in electronmicroscopy studies [42].

The two-pore model also consists of a small number of large pores with various radii, that are expressed as the average large-pore radius. The number of large pores is likely to be less than 0.1% of the total pore count and their average radius exceeds 150 Å. These pores are involved in the transport of macromolecules, such as serum proteins. The morphological equivalent of the large pores has not been established. Electronmicroscopic studies also suggested transport of macromolecules through plasmalemma vesicles [43]. Such a transport route would, however, require active metabolic processes and hence energy. Cooling experiments reduced the transcapillary passage of albumin only to the extent that cooling reduced passive transcapillary filtration, but not to the extent that would be expected due to decreased cell metabolism [44]. A light short-term fixation of vascular endothelial cells also did not reduce their permeability to albumin [45]. It follows from these experiments that the transcapillary transport of macromolecules is not an active process, but occurs by passive filtration and/or diffusion. Other possible morphological equivalents of the large-pore system are transcellular channels, vesicular–vacuolar organelles or interendothelial gaps. It has been shown that the interendothelial vesicles that can be seen with electronmicroscopy are actual invaginations from either side of the cell membrane [46] with the possibility of a connection, thereby forming a channel. This theory has more recently been extended by the description of vesicular–vacuolar organelles (VVO) that would account for the increased vascular permeability of tumour vessels [47, 48]. VVO are grape-like clusters of vesicles and vacuoles present in the cytoplasm of endothelial cells lining venules and small veins. The individual vesi-

cles and vacuoles are interconnected with each other and with the endothelial cell plasma membranes by means of fenestrae that may be open or closed by diaphragms. The function of these VVO is up-regulated by vascular endothelial growth factor [49].

Other candidates for the large pores are the postulated presence of very rare interendothelial clefts in which the adherence discontinuity is three to four times wider than in the ordinary clefts [38], or venular interendothelial gaps with radii of 500–5000 Å, that can be provoked by the administration of histamine [50]. Such gaps could also be induced by other locally produced vasodilating substances. All this evidence indicates that the large-pore radius is not a constant value, but that it can be subject to variations. In other words, the capillary wall is a heteroporous membrane that can be described by the combination of a large set of small pores with uniform radii and an additional small set of large pores with different radii. The radius calculated for the large pores is therefore an average value.

The two-pore model with a predominance of small pores of uniform size does not explain the discrepancy between sieving coefficients and osmotic reflection coefficients that is found in peritoneal dialysis. The sieving coefficient (S) describes the magnitude of convective solute transport (solute transport coupled to the transport of water; solvent drag), while the reflection coefficient (σ) of a solute to a membrane determines its osmotic effectiveness. Both can range between 0 and 1 for a semipermeable membrane. For a homoporous membrane the relationship between the two is: $S = (1 - \sigma)$. Various studies on convective transport of low molecular weight solutes have reported sieving coefficients (calculated as solute clearance/net volume flow) of 0.6–0.7 [51–55]. However, estimates of the reflection coefficient of glucose yield values ranging between 0.02 and 0.05 [56–60]. This apparent discrepancy has been explained by assuming the presence of water-conductive ultrasmall pores in the plasmalemma of endothelial cells with radii of 3–5 Å allowing the transport of water, but not of solutes [17, 61, 62]. This so-called three-pore model also explains why glucose is an effective osmotic agent during peritoneal dialysis despite its small size (radius 2–3 Å). According to this model about one-half of transcapillary ultrafiltration would occur through these ultrasmall pores, whereas the other half passes through the small interendothelial pores. Estimation in CAPD patients also showed that transcellular water transport contributed about 50%

to ultrafiltration, but with marked interindividual differences [63].

At the time of the above computer simulations a 28 kDa protein was discovered, present in the plasma membrane of red blood cells and *Xenopus* oocytes, that appeared to be involved in channel-mediated water transport [64]. This protein, originally called CHIP 28, and now aquaporin-1, was subsequently found to be the water channel in the proximal tubular cells of the kidney [65]; it is present both in the apical and basolateral membrane of these cells [66]. Water can be transported through it when an osmotic gradient is present. Aquaporin-1 is also present in various non-fenestrated epithelia [67]. As it could be detected in endothelial cells of peritoneal capillaries and venules, both at mRNA and at protein levels [68–71], aquaporin-1 may be the major water channel that constitutes the ultrasmall pore system [72]. Expression of the water channels aquaporin-3 and 4 has also been described in peritoneal tissue, but much less pronounced [69, 70]. The function of aquaporin-1 can be inhibited by mercury compounds [73]. The hypothesis that aquaporin-1 indeed represents the ultrasmall pores was supported by the finding that intraperitoneal administration of mercury chloride reduced transcellular water transport, both in rats [74] and in rabbits [75].

Mechanisms of solute transport

Diffusion and convection are the mechanisms involved in the transport of solutes during peritoneal dialysis. Diffusion through a membrane takes place when a concentration gradient is present. According to Fick's first law of diffusion, the rate of transfer of a solute is determined by the diffusive permeability of the peritoneum to that solute (the ratio between the free diffusion coefficient of that solute and the diffusion distance), the surface area available for its transport, and the concentration gradient:

$$J_s = \frac{D_f}{\Delta x} \cdot A \Delta C \qquad (1)$$

in which J_s is the rate of solute transfer, D_f is the free diffusion coefficient, Δx is the diffusion distance, A is the surface area and ΔC is the concentration gradient. $D_f A / \Delta x$ is called the permeability surface area product or the mass transfer area coefficient (MTAC). During peritoneal dialysis ΔC is the concentration difference between the plasma concentration of a solute (P) and its dialysate concentration

(D):

$$J_s = \text{MTAC}(P - D) \qquad (2)$$

Convective transport or solute drag occurs in conjunction with the transport of water, and thus during ultrafiltration. It is determined by the water flux (J_v), the mean solute concentration ($\bar{C}$) in the membrane and the solute reflection coefficient (σ):

$$J_s = J_v \bar{C}(1 - \sigma) \qquad (3)$$

For reasons of simplicity $\bar{C}$ is often approached as:

$$\bar{C} = (P + D)/2 \qquad (4)$$

Staverman's reflection coefficient σ is the fraction of the maximal osmotic pressure a solute can exert across a semipermeable membrane. It equals 1.0 for an ideal semipermeable membrane and 0 when the membrane offers no resistance to the transport of a solute. With an isoporous membrane $\sigma = 1 - S$ in which S is the sieving coefficient. S is the ratio between the concentration of a solute in the filtrate divided by its concentration in plasma when no diffusion occurs. The explanation for the discrepancy between S and σ values has been discussed in the section on pathways and barriers.

Size-selectivity

Diffusion of solutes across the peritoneal membrane is a size-selective process. It means that small molecules diffuse at a faster rate than large molecules due to differences in their free diffusion coefficients. The question whether the peritoneal membrane is a size-selective barrier in itself can be analysed by relating transport by diffusion of various solutes to their molecular weights. When a particle is an ideal sphere the relationship between its radius (r) and molecular weight (MW) is given by:

$$\text{MW} = \frac{4}{3} \pi r^3 \qquad (5)$$

The relationship between the free diffusion coefficient (D_f) of a solute and its radius is given in the Einstein–Stokes equation:

$$D_f = \frac{RT}{6\pi \eta r N} \qquad (6)$$

in which R is Bolzmann's gas constant, T is the absolute temperature, η is the viscosity of the solvent and N is Avagadro's number. This implies that, in the case of an ideal sphere, the free diffusion coefficient of a solute is related to the cubic root of its molecular weight:

$$D_f = aMW^{-0.33} \qquad (7)$$

in which a is a constant.

It is evident from the above that relationships between solute transport and molecular weight should be expressed as power functions:

$$y = ax^b \qquad (8)$$

or

$$\ln y = b \ln x + \ln a \qquad (9)$$

This implies that the power (b) is the slope of the correlation line that is obtained when x and y are plotted on a double-logarithmic scale. Most solutes are not ideal spheres. When the free diffusion coefficients in water of urea, glucose and inulin were plotted against their molecular weights on a double-logarithmic scale, the slope of the correlation line was -0.46 [76, 77]. This implies that values up to -0.46 are consistent with free diffusion across the peritoneal membrane. In that case only the surface area determines the maximal transport capacity. Values exceeding -0.46 imply size-selectively restricted diffusion. This means that the membrane itself (the pore size or the interstitium) offers an additional size-selective barrier to the transport of solutes. For the clearances of low molecular weight solutes up to β_2-microglobulin (MW 11.8 kDa) a value of -0.44 was found during intermittent peritoneal dialysis [78]. During CAPD we found a value of -0.50 (Fig. 2). These data give no indication for an important size-selective restriction barrier for low molecular weight solutes during peritoneal dialysis, but are more in favour of a transport process, similar to free diffusion in water, but in a colloid/water interstitial ground substance as vehicle for diffusion, instead of water. It follows from equation (6) that this will influence the magnitude of the diffusion rates, but the effects will be similar for all low molecular weight solutes. The functional or effective peritoneal surface area is mainly determined by the number of perfused peritoneal capillaries (the number of pores) in combination with interstitial resistances. No evidence is available that exogenous factors such as the hydration status of the interstitium would markedly influence MTAC of low molecular weight solutes. This contrasts with the observation that under basal circumstances only 25% of the peritoneal capillaries are perfused, and that this may be changed by exogenous stimuli (see section on regulation of peritoneal transport) [79]. In addition, it has been shown that splanchnic blood

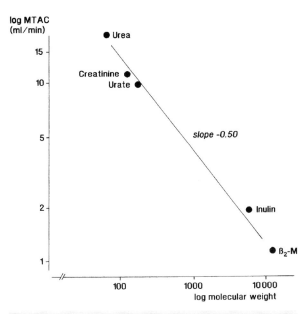

Figure 2. The power relationships of MTAC of low- and middle-molecular weight solutes with their molecular weights. Mean values are given. Based on data from references 87 and 93. See text for explanation.

volume, not the flow rate, is an important determinant of peritoneal solute transport capacity [80]. It can therefore be concluded that the peritoneal vascular surface area is the main determinant of the MTAC of low molecular weight solutes. Consequently, the MTAC of such a solute, for example creatinine, can be used as a functional measurement of the vascular peritoneal surface area. Changes in the MTAC of creatinine in individual patients are likely to reflect changes in their vascular peritoneal surface area.

Another approach to describe the size-selectivity of the peritoneal membrane is to relate MTAC of various solutes to their free diffusion coefficients in water, instead of to their molecular weights. This is based on the notion that the molecular weight of a solute is not the only determinant of its diffusion velocity. The density and the shape of a molecule can also have an effect. This is evident for non-protein macromolecules, such as dextrans. Based on the equation: radius $= 3.05 MW^{-0.47}$ [81], as derived from the data of Granath and Kvist [82], it can be calculated that the dextran fraction with a diffusion radius identical to that of β_2-microglobulin (MW 820 kDa) has a molecular weight of only 4.6 kDa. For α_2-macroglobulin (MW 820 kDa) the molecular weight of the corresponding dextran fraction is 176 kDa [83]. Since diffusion is the most important mechanism for the transport of low

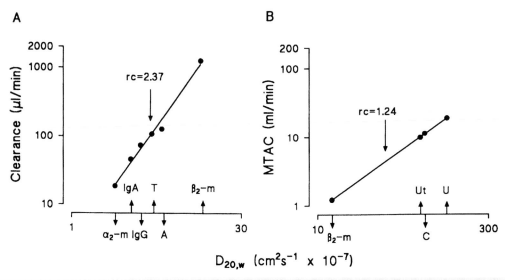

Figure 3. The power relationship between MTAC of urea (U), creatinine (C), urate (Ut) and β_2-microglobulin (β_2-m) and their free diffusion coefficient in water ($D_{20,w}$) is given in panel **A**, and the power relationship between the protein clearances of β_2-microglobulin, albumin (A), transferrin (T), IgG and α_2-macroglobulin (α_2-m) and their free diffusion coefficients in water is given in panel **B**. All values are plotted on a double logarithmic scale. The slope of the regression line represents the restriction coefficient. A restriction coefficient of 1.0 means that a linear relationship is present between clearances of solutes and their free diffusion coefficients in water. For the low molecular weight solutes a slope of 1.24 ± 0.03 and for the proteins a slope of 2.37 ± 0.04 were found. Published with permission from ref. 87 and from Blackwell Scientific Publications.

molecular weight solutes, and restricted diffusion may be the most important mechanism for the transport of macromolecules, the establishment of power relationships between the MTAC of solutes and their free diffusion coefficients in water, is a more rational approach than the use of the molecular weights. A power relationship was found for peritoneal clearances (C) of proteins and their free diffusion coefficients in water (D_w) [84], according to the equation:

$$C = aD_w^{rc} \tag{10}$$

in which the slope (rc) was called the peritoneal restriction coefficient. The restriction coefficient represents the size-selective permeability of the peritoneal membrane: high values mean a low permeability. The application of the restriction coefficient in individual patients was validated both for proteins [85] and for dextran fractions [86].

A restriction coefficient that equals 1.0 means a linear relationship between MTAC and free diffusion coefficients, and no hindrance by the size-selective restriction barrier. In this situation differences in free diffusion coefficients of solutes are the only determinants of the differences in their clearances, and so the functional (vascular) peritoneal surface area is the only membrane characteristic that determines the differences in solute transport. In a study in 10

Table 1. Relationship between parameters of solute transport and permeability characteristics of the peritoneal membrane

	Functional or vascular surface area	Size-selectivity or intrinsic permeability
MTAC or D/P ratio of low molecular weight solutes	+	−
Selectivity index or restriction coefficient to macromolecules	−	+

CAPD patients a mean value for the restriction coefficient of 1.24 was found for low molecular weight solutes and of 2.37 for serum proteins (Fig. 3) [87]. These figures have been confirmed in a larger group of patients [88]. This is consistent with a mainly size-unrestricted diffusion process for low molecular weight solutes and a size-selectively restricted transport for macromolecules. In Table 1 a summary is given of the relationship between the parameters of solute transport and the permeability characteristics of the peritoneal membrane. The functional surface area can be characterized by the

MTAC of creatinine. The size-selective permeability can be characterized by the calculation of the restriction coefficient. The functional surface area can be considered as a reflection of the number of pores, whereas the restriction coefficient mainly represents the size of the large pores and possible size-selective interstitial resistances.

Electric charge

Glycosaminoglycans exhibit a negative electric charge. This is especially important in the glomerular basement membrane where the strongly negative charged glycosaminoglycan side-chains of heparan sulphate proteoglycan are involved in the charge-selective glomerular permeability [89]. Using ruthenium red staining, fixed negative charges have also been demonstrated in peritoneal tissue of rats not exposed to peritoneal dialysis [90], but with a much lower density than in the glomerular basement membrane. They were especially found on the basal lamina of the capillary endothelial cells and also along interstitial collagen fibres. It is, however, not established whether, and how, they influence solute transport during peritoneal dialysis. Intraperitoneal administration of protamine sulphate to rabbits led to increased concentrations of total protein in the effluent, that could be prevented by simultaneous administration of heparin [91]. This was interpreted as an effect of neutralization of anionic sites by protamine. Such an effect would particularly favour the transport of the negatively charged albumin molecules. A direct toxic effect on mesothelial cells leading to release of tissue proteins, however, could not be excluded [92]. No evidence for charge selectivity was found in a study comparing the transport of the negatively charged serum albumin with a dextran fraction of a similar diffusion radius in CAPD patients [93]. An opposite finding was reported in a study in rabbits that compared the transport of intravenously administered neutral and charged dextrans [94]. The positively charged dextrans were especially hindered in their transperitoneal transport. This could be explained by the assumption that the colloid-rich phase of the peritoneal interstitium behaves as a cation exchange column, facilitating the transport of negatively charged solutes through the tissue and retarding that of cationic macromolecules. Such effects are likely to disappear during steady-state conditions, as present for serum proteins during CAPD. In that situation the concentrations of serum proteins in the interstitium are probably in equilibrium with their plasma concentrations. Therefore comparisons were made between the transport of proteins with (near)-identical sizes, but different charges. IgG subclasses range in isoelectric points between less than 6 and 8.7. Their clearances in CAPD patients, however, were not different [95]. Comparisons between the peritoneal clearances of albumin and transferrin, β_2-microglobulin and lysozyme also gave no indication for a charge-selective barrier [96]. Only the clearances of LDH subclasses suggested charge selectivity [97]. Observations during peritonitis showed that an alternative explanation is more likely. Fixed negative charges disappear during peritonitis [98]. However, during peritonitis in CAPD patients signs of increased charge selectivity for LDH were found [96]. This could be explained by release of LDH by the cells present in the peritoneal effluent.

Taken together, most evidence points to an absence of charge selectivity of the peritoneum in the transport of macromolecules. This may be explained by the lower density of fixed negative charges in the peritoneum compared to the glomerular basement membrane. Another possibility might be the occurrence of loss of negative charges caused by the continuous exposure of peritoneal tissues to high glucose concentrations during peritoneal dialysis. Such loss has been shown to occur in the glomerular basement membrane in patients with diabetic nephropathy [99, 100]. It is not known whether this phenomenon can also be observed in long-term peritoneal dialysis, or whether it has impact on peritoneal protein transport.

Peritoneal blood flow

The number of perfused peritoneal capillaries is dependent on peritoneal blood flow and blood volume [80]. Based on the anatomical situation, splanchnic blood flow is probably much more important than flow in the abdominal wall. Splanchnic blood flow averages 1200 ml/min in normal adults [101]. Its distribution over the various splanchnic organs is markedly influenced by the instillation of dialysate. Experiments in rats, using microspheres, showed marked increases in the blood flow to the mesentery, omentum, intestinal serosa and parietal peritoneum [15]. There was no effect on total splanchnic blood flow. Using the peritoneal clearance of hydrogen gas in rabbits [102] a value of 4.2 ml/min per kg body weight was found. Similar values could be calculated during peritoneal dialysis in rats with the microsphere technique [15]. Using the peritoneal clearance of carbon dioxide in rats an average value of 4.9 ml/min per kg was found after the instillation of an isotonic solution and of 8.1 ml/min per kg with a hypertonic dialysis fluid [103].

The relationship between peritoneal blood flow and solute transport in animals is only marginal. A reduction of blood flow in dogs by haemorrhagic hypotension caused only a 10–25% decrease in peritoneal urea clearance [104, 105]. Instillation of sodium chromate in rabbits induced hepatic venous stasis leading to a decreased blood flow, but increased solute transport [80], indicating that peritoneal blood volume is more important than peritoneal blood flow. Intravenous isoproterenol in dogs increased peritoneal blood flow, but had no effect on solute clearances [106]. Intraperitoneal isoproterenol resulted almost in a doubling of mesenteric blood flow, but this was accompanied by an increase in clearances of small solutes of only 20–30% [106]. More recent *in-vivo* studies using a diffusion chamber in rats combined with laser Doppler flowmetry showed that a 70% reduction of blood flow did not alter the transfer rate of urea and mannitol across the abdominal wall [107] or hollow viscera [108]. However, when blood flow was halted, the transport rates were reduced significantly. Only a reduction of the local blood flow to the liver induced significant decreases in solute transfer in this model [108], but the hepatic peritoneum makes up only a small portion of the effective exchange area. These studies imply that only a minimal blood flow is necessary for solute transport.

Estimation of peritoneal blood flow in peritoneal dialysis patients revealed lower values than in animals when expressed per kg body weight; it has been assumed to average 60–100 ml/min [109]. Studies in a limited number of intermittent peritoneal dialysis patients, using the peritoneal mass transfer area coefficient of carbon dioxide, yielded values ranging between 68 and 82 ml/min [110], or of about 150 ml/min [111]. Using the same technique in stable CAPD patients values ranging from 20 to 151 ml/min were found in three studies using 1.36% glucose [112–114]. The median value averaged 66 ml/min. A much lower value of 25 ml/min has been estimated in one study [115, 116]. This was based on the relationship between the hydrostatic pressure and the plasma protein concentration obtained with a hollow-fibre haemofilter, and extrapolated to the situation in peritoneal dialysis. These authors also reported a linear relationship between blood flow and small solute clearances or

ultrafiltration in an *in-vitro* perfusion model of small vascular loops of isolated human peritoneal tissue [117, 118]. The 'nearest capillary' hypothesis has been developed by the same group [119]. In this hypothesis it is assumed that the capillaries positioned closest to the mesothelium will be dilated and have low blood flow, while the most distal ones have the highest blood flow, but less effective diffusion due to interstitial resistances. The resulting 'effective' peritoneal blood flow would be a limiting factor for solute clearances. It is difficult to predict to what extent the above models and hypotheses are important in clinical peritoneal dialysis.

In agreement with the data obtained in animals, the effects of peritoneal blood flow on solute transport are probably limited. This is supported by the following studies. (1) Effective peritoneal dialysis is possible in patients with intractable heart failure following an acute myocardial infarction [120], a condition in which decreased splanchnic blood flow can be expected. (2) CAPD with a 1.1% amino acid solution increased peritoneal blood flow 55% compared to 1.36% glucose, but the increase in the MTAC of urea and creatinine averaged only 15% [112]. (3) Intraperitoneally administered nitroprusside had no effect on peritoneal blood flow [113, 121], but caused a marked increase in the MTAC of small solutes and macromolecules. These data make it likely that, similar to the situation in animals, peritoneal blood volume is more important than peritoneal blood flow in the transfer of solutes during peritoneal dialysis. Peritoneal blood volume can be increased by nitroprusside induced vasodilation and by an increased venous pressure. This increased venous pressure is probably the explanation for the fact that effective peritoneal dialysis has been described in patients with severe congestive heart failure [122–126] and in patients with liver cirrhosis [127].

The regulation of splanchnic blood flow is complex. Intrinsic and extrinsic control mechanisms are involved [128]. The intrinsic regulation consists of a pressure-flow autoregulation, while the venous pressure and the ingestion of meals also have effects [129]. The intrinsic regulation is mediated by myogenic factors, metabolic factors and locally produced substances such as vasoactive peptides and autocoids such as prostaglandins [128]. Extrinsic control mechanisms are predominantly mediated by the sympathic noradrenergic nerves and by circulating vasoactive substances, such as catecholamines, vasopressin and angiotensin II [128]. Alpha-adrenergic stimulation causes intestinal vasoconstriction, and stimulation of β_2-receptors leads to dilatation. Intra-arterial infusion of norepinephrine causes intestinal vasoconstriction and a decrease in capillary density [128]. A similar effect is present for epinephrine in high doses, but β_2-receptor-mediated vasodilation prevails after the administration of a low dose. Vasopressin and angiotensin II cause generalized vasoconstriction with a disproportionate reduction in mesenteric blood flow [130]. Vasopressin also causes a decrease in the density of perfused capillaries [128]. Angiotensin II is probably mainly involved in the control of mesenteric blood flow during volume depletion [131]. The administration of glucagon leads to splanchnic dilation [132], but its role in the regulation of splanchnic blood flow is not established [128]. The extrinsic control mechanisms of splanchnic blood flow regulation are mainly involved in the decrease that is present during shock and exercise [133].

The regulation of surface area and permeability

In the previous section it has been shown that peritoneal blood flow is unlikely to be the main factor in the regulation of the peritoneal vascular surface area and permeability. Therefore endogenous substances with vasoactive properties may be involved. Plasma levels of catecholamines, vasopressin, aldosterone and plasma renin activity are elevated in CAPD patients [134–136]. This does not necessarily imply increased sympathetic activity, but could also be the result of a decreased clearance [135]. Dialysate levels of catecholamines have been measured in one study [134]. The dialysate/plasma ratio was 0.69 for epinephrine and 1.17 for norepinephrine, suggesting local production in the peritoneal cavity. A correlation was found between the dialysate levels of norepinephrine and the effective peritoneal surface area, represented by the mass transfer area coefficient of creatinine. Because this finding is the opposite of the effects of intraperitoneally administered norepinephrine, as will be discussed below, it may be that the large effective surface area causes the release of norepinephrine.

Prostaglandins and cytokines are likely to be produced locally in the peritoneal cavity during peritoneal dialysis. This has been shown for the prostaglandins 6-keto-PGF1α, PGE2, PGF2α, TXB2 and 13,14-dihydro-15-keto-PGF2α [137–139]. The concentrations of the vasodilating prostaglandins exceeded that of the vasoconstricting ones. Drained peritoneal effluent also contains the cytokines TNFα [140, 141], interleukin-1 (IL-1) [142, 143], IL-6 [144–146] and IL-8 [146]. The presence of TNFα in the dialysate of uninfected CAPD patients is probably caused by diffusion from the circulation [140, 141], while the other cytokines mentioned above are produced locally within the peritoneal cavity. A relationship has been reported between very high dialysate IL-6 levels in stable CAPD patients and a low peritoneal restriction coefficient, representing a high intrinsic permeability to macromolecules [145]. In that study no relationship was found with the vascular peritoneal surface area. Marked elevations of prostaglandins and cytokines in dialysate are present during peritonitis [137–139, 144, 146, 147]. In addition, local production of TNFα also occurs during the acute phase of the inflammation [147]. It appeared that the increase in intrinsic permeability to macromolecules was especially correlated with dialysate PGE2 concentrations [147]. Intraperitoneal administration of indomethacin during peritonitis inhibited the increase of prostaglandins. This was accompanied by a reduction of the dialysate protein loss in one study [139], but this effect could not be confirmed in a longitudinal study during peritonitis [148]. Only a small effect on the peritoneal restriction coefficient for macromolecules was found [148]. Intraperitoneal indomethacin had no effect on peritoneal permeability characteristics in stable, uninfected peritoneal dialysis patients [149]. Relationships between cytokines in peritoneal effluent and permeability have been reviewed recently [150, 151].

Nitric oxide is the final common pathway for various vasodilating processes. It is very rapidly converted into nitrite and nitrate. Dialysate concentrations of these metabolites have therefore been used to study possible involvement of nitric oxide in the regulation of peritoneal permeability. In contrast to nitrite in plasma, which is converted to nitrate, nitrite in fresh and spent peritoneal dialysis fluids is stable [114], but its concentration is much lower than that of nitrate. Comparing MTAC of nitrate with those of other solutes made it likely that dialysate nitrate concentrations in stable uninfected CAPD patients were dependent only on diffusion from nitrate from the circulation to the dialysate-filled peritoneal cavity [152]. Increased dialysate nitrate concentrations have been found in some studies during the acute phase of peritonitis [132, 153], but not in all [114]. Relationships between nitrate levels and peritoneal permeability characteristics have not been found.

Possible effects of solutes, generally considered to be involved in the regulation of the permeability characteristics of the peritoneum, have been analysed by studying transport kinetics during peritoneal dialysis after their intraperitoneal or intravenous administration. These include: (1) the dialysate itself; (2) hormones, such as catecholamines, gastrointestinal hormones and vasopressin; and (3) histamine and prostaglandins.

The administration of hypertonic and acid dialysate in the rat causes arteriolar vasodilation in the cremaster muscle preceded by an initial vasoconstriction [154–156], and also vasodilation of caecum arterioles [157]. This effect was more pronounced for acetate-buffered than for lactate-buffered dialysate, and also more pronounced for glucose 1.5% than for glucose 0.5%-containing dialysate. The instillation of commercial dialysate in cats leads to a redistribution of splanchnic blood flow, especially to an increased flow in the mesentery, omentum, intestinal serosa and parietal peritoneum [15]. The application of an iso-osmotic bicarbonate-buffered solution, that was not vasoactive in the rat cremaster muscle model, to patients treated with intermittent peritoneal dialysis, had no effect on the functional peritoneal surface area when compared with commercial dialysate [158]; however, it led to an increase in the total protein concentration of the dialysate. In further studies it appeared that this effect could not be explained solely by the osmolarity or pH of the dialysis fluid [159]. A more recent study using a single 4 h exchange with a hypo-osmotic bicarbonate buffered solution confirmed the above findings for the clearances of individual plasma proteins [160]. However, clinical trials with bicarbonate-buffered glucose-containing solutions did not report alterations in the transport of low molecular weight solutes or dialysate protein loss [161–165].

Intravenously administered amino acids cause renal vasodilation [166, 167]. This effect is mediated by nitric oxide [168]. Therefore, effects on the permeability characteristics of the peritoneal membrane during CAPD could in theory be expected. However, the results of different studies on the use of amino acids are equivocal. In some studies, reviewed in ref. 169, no effect was found on peritoneal transport [170–172], while others reported increased peritoneal protein loss [173–175]. This was accompanied by increased dialysate concentrations of prostaglandin E_2. A study using a bicarbonate buffered amino acid solution reported no effect on MTAC of low molecular weight solutes, increased peritoneal D/P

ratios for serum proteins and increased dialysate concentrations of prostaglandins, IL-6, IL-8 and TNFα [164]. An effect on MTAC of low molecular weight solutes, reflecting the vascular surface area, was found in two studies [112, 176]. No increased protein clearances were present in these studies. Neither was an indication detectable for involvement of nitric oxide or prostagladins [112, 164]. It is noteworthy that with the exception of one study [173], all studies reporting increased protein loss and increased dialysate concentrations of prostaglandins used dialysis solutions prepared by one manufacturer. This suggests that differences in the composition of the dialysis solutions could explain the divergent effects on peritoneal permeability characteristics.

Increasing the glucose concentration of the dialysis solution from 1.36% to 3.86% has no effects on the indices of the vascular peritoneal surface area or the intrinsic size-selective permeability [87]. Only the clearance of β_2-microglobulin is greater, with 3.86% glucose due to higher convective transport across the small pores [87]. The use of the glucose polymer icodextrin also increased β_2-microglobulin clearance [63, 177–179], but its administration has no effects on other peritoneal permeability characteristics [63, 177].

Intravenous administration of norepinephrine in rabbits leads to a decrease in vascular surface area as judged from the clearances of urea and creatinine [180]. In contrast, intravenous glucagon increases the clearances of urea and creatinine [181, 182]. As glucagon, a peptide with a molecular weight of 3484 Da, was not effective after intraperitoneal administration, these findings support a direct effect on the peritoneal microvasculature. The effects of glucagon have also been confirmed in dogs [183]. Vasopressin, administered either intraperitoneally [184] or intravenously [185], leads to a fall in solute kinetics consistent with a decreased effective peritoneal surface area. Topical application of histamine causes arteriolar vasodilation with leakage of proteins both in skeletal muscles and in the mesenterial vasculature [186, 187]. This would suggest an action both on the vascular peritoneal surface area and on the permeability to macromolecules. Intraperitoneal administration of histamine in rats caused a 10–20% increase in the clearance of urea [188]. This effect was not confirmed in rabbits in another study, but a marked increase was reported for the protein loss in the dialysate [189]. The histamine-induced protein loss could be blocked by a combination of H_1 and H_2 receptor antagonists. These antagonists were not effective when given alone or during desoxycholate-induced chemical peritonitis.

The possible role of prostaglandins on the functional peritoneal surface area has been studied by intravenous and intraperitoneal administration of vasodilating and vasoconstricting prostaglandins in rabbits [190–192]. In general the effects were most pronounced after intraperitoneal administration. Arachidonic acid and the vasodilating prostaglandins led to an increase in the vascular peritoneal surface area, while the vasoconstricting PGF2α decreased the clearances of urea and creatinine. The oral administration of cyclo-oxygenase inhibitors had only a marginal effect. Combining these data with those obtained on effects of indomethacin in humans, suggests that prostaglandins are not important in the regulation of peritoneal surface area and permeability during uninfected CAPD with glucose-based solutions.

Intraperitoneal administration of the direct nitric oxide donor nitroprusside in intermittent peritoneal dialysis patients causes an increase in clearances and MTAC of low molecular weight solutes and also in peritoneal protein loss [193, 194]. This effect markedly exceeded that of other vasodilators such as isoproterenol and diazoxide [193]. Nitroprusside in combination with different buffer anions and varying pH, augmented peritoneal clearances in all solutions to a similar extent [195]. These effects of nitroprusside are also present during CAPD [113, 196]. In addition a decrease was found in the restriction coefficient to macromolecules [113]. Exposure of animal peritoneal tissues to nitroprusside caused opening of previously unperfused capillaries and increased the capillary pore area [194, 197]. These human and animal data all point to an effect of intraperitoneal nitroprusside on the peritoneal vascular surface area and the size-selective permeability to macromolecules. Involvement of nitric oxide in these processes was confirmed by an increase in the D/P ratio of the NO second messenger cGMP [113] and in the induction of an increased peritoneal albumin clearance after intraperitoneal administration of the nitric oxide substrate L-arginine in high dosages [198]. Administration of the NO inhibitor L-NMMA in this model had no effect on solute transport. These data suggest that nitric oxide is probably not involved in the regulation of peritoneal permeability during stable CAPD. The effects of nitroprusside should be regarded as a pharmacological phenomenon.

The peritoneal surface area and permeability are not only influenced by vasoactive substances, but physical phenomena might also affect them, such as position and intra-abdominal pressure. Most studies reported lower solute transport rates in the upright position than during recumbency [199–201], but another study did not report an effect of position [202]. Increasing the intraperitoneal pressure by the application of external pressure also decreased MTAC of low molecular weight solutes and clearances of serum proteins [203].

It can be concluded that many factors may be involved in the regulation of peritoneal surface area and permeability. Some of these factors have been identified but much uncertainty is present on the effects of many others.

Models and parameters of solute transport

Because of the very complex structure of the various barriers to the peritoneal transport of solutes and fluid, the so-called distributed models are probably the most complete ones to describe peritoneal exchange [32, 204, 205]. They are, however, very complicated and based on a large number of assumptions. A much simpler approach is to consider the peritoneal tissues involved in the exchange of solutes and fluids as a single membrane that separates two well-mixed pools: the blood compartment and the peritoneal cavity compartment. In this membrane concept the peritoneal dialysis system is compared with an artificial membrane having cylindrical, fluid-filled pores, similar to the situation for transcapillary transport.

With these so-called 'lumped' models the MTAC is determined. This parameter is the theoretical maximal clearance by diffusion at time zero, i.e. before solute transport has started. The MTAC can be calculated using very complicated models, but more simple equations can also be used. In general a distinction can be made between complicated numerical models and more simple analytical models (reviewed in ref. 206). The numerical models include those of Popovich and Pyle [207–209], Randerson and Farrell [210] and Smeby et al. [211]. The analytical models generally start with the same mass balance equation, in which the accumulation of solutes in the peritoneal fluid in time is given by: $d(VD)/dt$, in which V is the dialysis volume and t is time. As this is the result of diffusion and convection, the mass balance equation using equations (2)–(4) is:

$$\frac{d}{dt}(VD) = \text{MTAC}(P - D) + 0.5J_v(P + D)(1 - \sigma)$$

(11)

The most simple approach to solve this differential equation is to neglect the contribution of convective transport and to assume that the appearance rate of solutes in dialysate follows first-order kinetics. This is the basis of the Henderson and Nolph equation [212].

$$\text{MTAC} = \frac{V_t}{t} \ln \left[\frac{P - D_0}{P - D_t} \right]$$

(12)

In this equation V_t is usually the drained dialysate volume. This method can be used as a rough estimation. It is an especially good method during a period of isovolaemia, as described by Lindholm *et al.* [213]. Correction for convective transport leads to the following equation:

$$\text{MTAC} = \frac{V_t}{t} \ln \left[\frac{V_0^{1-f}(P - D_0)}{V_t^{1-f}(P - D_t)} \right]$$

(13)

in which f is a weighing factor between diffusion and convection, dependent on the transcapillary ultrafiltration, the sieving coefficient and the mass transfer area coefficient. When convection is relatively high compared to diffusion, f approaches zero. When diffusion is the principal transport mode, f rises to a limiting factor of 0.5. Garred *et al.* [214] developed a simple model based on multiple dialysate samplings, and assuming $f = 0$ and $S = 1$:

$$\text{MTAC} = \frac{V}{t} \ln \left[\frac{V_0(P - D_0)}{V_t(P - D_t)} \right]$$

(14)

This model could also be used taking samples only before instillation and after drainage, and taking the drained volume for V [215]. Waniewski *et al.* [216] pointed out that f values of 0.33 for a large degree of convective transport and of 0.5 for negligible convection are more justified. In addition plasma concentrations of small solutes should be corrected for aqueous solute concentrations, either by a correction factor of 1.05 or using the total protein concentration in plasma [217]. However, in a comparison between the effect of 1.36% dialysate glucose and 3.86% glucose on the calculation of MTAC values for urea,

creatinine and urate, the difference was marginal between $f = 0$, 0.33 or 0.5 [87]. In all three models no significant difference was found for the MTAC of creatinine between the 1.36% glucose study (little convection) and the 3.86% glucose study (more convection). This indicates that all simplified models that correct for convective transport give MTAC values that represent diffusion, and that they are not influenced by convection to a clinically relevant degree. It should be appreciated that all simplified models use the intraperitoneal volume, instead of the volume that would have been present in the absence of lymphatic absorption, and also do not correct for solute loss due to uptake in the lymphatic system. However, the two factors are likely to compensate each other more or less.

The MTAC is usually calculated on solute concentrations obtained during 4–6 h exchanges. However, a number of studies have shown that MTACs are somewhat higher during the initial phase of a dwell, compared to the subsequent hours [16, 59, 87, 218, 219]. The explanation for this phenomenon is not clear, but it may be an aspecific reaction to the instillation of fresh dialysis fluids. It is one of the reasons that assessment of the MTAC by using solute clearances obtained during short dwell times does not give accurate values. This technique was usually employed during intermittent peritoneal dialysis, and has also been used in CAPD patients [220]. Another problem with the use of short clearance periods is the relatively large contribution of time of inflow and drainage compared to the dialysis time, making it difficult to establish the precise dwell time. The contribution of convective transport will also be relatively large, leading to an inflated estimate of the MTAC.

Dialysate/plasma (D/P) ratios after a 4 h dwell and 24 h clearances are most often used in clinical practice. The time course of the D/P ratio of urea, creatinine and urate for a 1.36% glucose dialysis solution are shown in Fig. 4. It appears from this graph that D/P urea almost approaches 1.0. Consequently the peritoneal clearance of this solute will mainly be determined by the drained dialysate volume. Therefore, the 24 h peritoneal clearance of low molecular weight solutes does not reflect their MTAC, but provides an overall estimation of the removal of urea (expressed as Kt/V_{urea}) and of creatinine. They can therefore be used as estimates of the adequacy of peritoneal dialysis with regard to solute removal. This is further discussed in Chapter 13. Good relationships are present between D/P ratios and MTAC [221, 222], but deviations from linearity

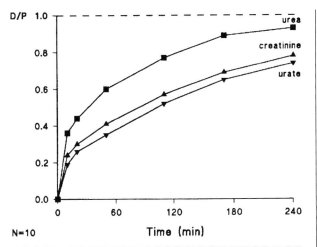

Figure 4. The time-course of dialysate/plasma (D/P) ratios of urea (MW 60 Da), creatinine (MW 113 Da) and urate (MW 168 Da). Mean values of 10 stable CAPD patients are given. Reprinted with permission from the Boerhaave Committee for postgraduate medical education of the faculty of medicine, Leiden University, The Netherlands.

are especially present in patients with very low and very high MTAC values [222]. D/P ratios overestimated the MTAC in the low ranges, whereas in the high ranges the MTAC values were underestimated. Both D/P ratios and MTAC have a high reproducibility in individual patients. This has been found for D/P ratios within a period of 3 months [223], but changes may occur in the long term [223, 224]. Using the simplified Garred model for the calculation of MTAC the intraindividual coefficient of variation averaged 7% [200].

Transport of low molecular weight solutes

Diffusion is quantitatively the most important transport mechanism for low molecular weight solutes, such as urea, creatinine, and uric acid. This is especially the case when the osmolality of the dialysate is low. Figure 5 shows the D/P ratios of urea and creatinine using 2.5% glucose-based dialysis solutions in the population of 86 patients studied by Twardowski et al. [225]. Normal values for the MTAC of urea, creatinine and uric acid as obtained in a cross-sectional study using 1.36% glucose dialysate in 86 adult patients [222] are given in Table 2. It appeared that some relationship was present between MTAC creatinine and body surface area, but the variation was rather large. This suggests some relationship between peritoneal surface area and body surface area, but also underlines the fact that many other factors may influence peritoneal solute transport, such as the vascular peritoneal surface area. Nevertheless, MTAC are preferably expressed per 1.73 m^2 body surface area.

Transport of electrolytes

The dialysate concentration of sodium decreases during the initial phase of a dialysis dwell using hypertonic solutions, followed by a gradual rise [54, 217, 219, 226–229]. The minimum value is usually reached after 1 h. It is likely that this apparent siev-

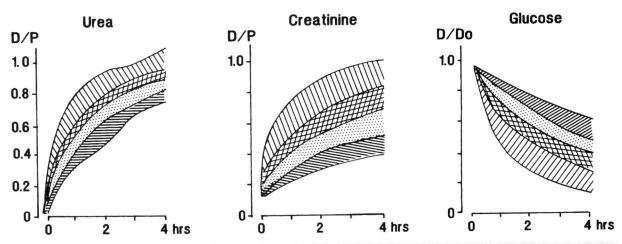

Figure 5. The results of 103 peritoneal equilibration test using glucose 2.5% dialysate. The upper zones of D/P ratios of urea and creatinine represent high transporters (> mean + SD), the adjacent zones high average transporters (between mean and mean + SD), the following zone (between mean and mean − SD) the low average transporters, and the lowest zone (< mean − SD) represents the low transporters. The same symbols, but in a mirrow view, indicate the same transport categories for D/Do glucose. Redrawn from ref. 225, with permission from the author and from Pergamon Press.

Table 2. Normal values for the MTACs of low molecular weight solutes and clearances (Cl) of serum proteins (data from ref. 222)

Parameter	Mean of normal distribution	95% confidence interval
Simplified Garred model		
MTAC$_{urea}$ (ml/min per 1.73 m^2)	16·0	10.7–21.2
MTAC$_{creatinine}$ (ml/min per 1.73 m^2)	9.4	5.5–13.4
MTAC$_{urate}$ (ml/min per 1.73 m^2)	7.9	3.9–11.8
Waniewski model		
MTAC$_{urea}$ (ml/min per 1.73 m^2)	17.5	11.5–23.5
MTAC$_{creatinine}$ (ml/min per 1.73 m^2)	10.2	5.7–14.7
MTAC$_{urate}$ (ml/min per 1.73 m^2)	8.6	4.1–13.0
Cl$_{\beta_2 m}$ (µl/min/1.73 m^2)	853	400–1310
Cl$_{alb}$ (µl/min/1.73 m^2)	89	34–144
Cl$_{IgG}$ (µl/min/1.73 m^2)	45	15–76
Cl$_{\alpha_2 m}$ (µl/min/1.73 m^2)	13	3–23

β_2m: beta-2-microglobulin, alb: albumin, α_2m: alpha-2-macroglobulin.

ing of sodium is caused by transcellular water transport through ultrasmall pores or, alternatively, temporal binding of Na$^+$ in the interstitial tissue. The time-course of the D/P ratio of Na$^+$ is shown in Fig. 6. Water transport rates are high during the initial phase of a hypertonic exchange; therefore, the decrease in dialysate Na$^+$ is a dilutional phenomenon [230]. This implies that during short dwells using hypertonic dialysate much more water than sodium is removed from the extracellular volume.

This can lead to hypernatraemia [231]. The gradual rise during the subsequent hours is probably caused by diffusion of sodium from the circulation. The effect of sodium diffusion on the D/P ratio of Na$^+$ is most marked in patients who also have high MTACs of other uncharged low molecular weight solutes [229].

The MTAC of sodium is difficult to calculate due to the small differences in dialysate and plasma concentrations. Using 3.86% dialysate glucose an average value of 4 ml/min has been reported during a period of isovolaemia [217, 227]. Using dialysate with a sodium concentration of 102–105 mmol/L average values of 7–8 ml/min have been found [59, 232]. Corrections for Gibbs–Donnan equilibrium were applied in these calculations. The MTAC of chloride was 9 ml/min [59]. Both for Na$^+$ (MW 23 Da) and Cl$^-$ (MW 35.5 Da) the MTAC values were considerably below those of urea (MW 60 Da), creatinine (MW 113 Da) and urate (MW 168 Da). As a consequence these electrolytes are transported at a lower rate than expected on the basis of their molecular weight. The molecular radii of anhydrated sodium (0.98 Å) and chloride (1.81 Å) are also smaller than those estimated during peritoneal dialysis, based on computer simulations (2.3 Å for sodium and chloride) [17]. It is conceivable that interactions of these ions with H$_2$O molecules, leading to a water shell, may cause transport characteristics that suggest a higher molecular weight. In the study by Imholz *et al.* the calculated radius of sodium during peritoneal dialy-

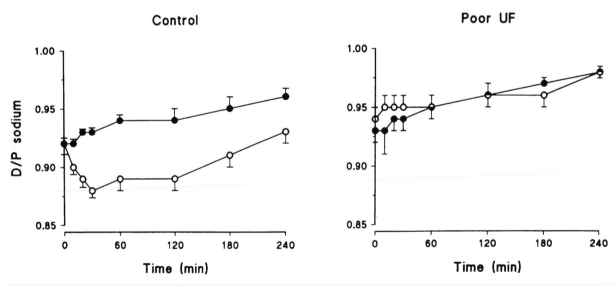

Figure 6. The D/P sodium ratios in a control group of 10 CAPD patients with normal net ultrafiltration (based on data from ref. 87), is given in the left panel. The D/P sodium ratios in a selected group of six CAPD patients with severe ultrafiltration failure without an obvious cause in the peritoneal equilibration test is given in the right panel. Mean and SEM values obtained with 1.36% glucose are presented as closed dots and those obtained with 3.86% glucose-based dialysate are presented as open dots. Published with permission from ref. 329 and from Multimed Inc.

sis was 2.68 Å and that of chloride 2.42 Å [59]. The lower MTAC of sodium than that of chloride is in accordance with the lower permeability coefficient of sodium compared to that of chloride, present for transport across synthetic lipid bilayer membranes *in vitro* [233].

The finding that sodium diffuses as a larger molecule during peritoneal dialysis has focused attention on the potential use of ultra-low sodium dialysis solutions to improve net ultrafiltration, especially as Nakayama *et al.* reported favourable results of such a solution in overhydrated CAPD patients [234]. In a study comparing dialysate with a normal sodium concentration with a dialysate containing sodium 102 mmol/L, that was made isosmotic by addition of more glucose, a slightly better net ultrafiltration was found with the low-sodium dialysate: about 100 ml during a 6 h dwell [59]. This difference could be explained by the calculated reflection coefficient of glucose (0.0326), that was slightly higher than the reflection coefficient of sodium (0.0297).

The clearance of potassium by diffusion during intermittent peritoneal dialyse averages about 17 ml/min [235]. Average MTAC values between 12 and 16 ml/min have been reported in CAPD patients [59, 217, 227], in between those of urea and creatinine. During the first hour of a dwell the value is 24 ml/min [59]. The most probable explanation for these high values is release of potassium from the cells that line the peritoneal cavity. This may be promoted by the initial low pH and/or by the hyperosmolality of the instilled dialysate. It is also supported by the finding of sieving coefficients of potassium exceeding 1.0 [176, 216]. It can be concluded that charged electrolytes are transported at lower rates than expected on the basis of their molecular weights, irrespective of the charge being positive or negative. For potassium release from intracellular sources during the initial phase of a dialysis dwell is likely to occur.

The standard peritoneal dialysis solutions contain 1.75 mmol/L Ca^{2+} and 0.75 mmol/L Mg^{2+}. The normal ionized concentrations of these electrolytes in plasma are 1.25 mmol/L for Ca^{2+} and 0.55 mmol/L for Mg^{2+}. Consequently peritoneal dialysis will lead to mass transfer from the dialysate to the circulation by diffusion, especially when dialysis solutions inducing little convective transport are used. A positive mass transfer for Ca^{2+} of 0.96 mmol/4 h exchange and for Mg^{2+} of 0.21 mmol/4 h exchange has been found in stable CAPD patients using 1.36% glucose-based dialysate [236]. The balance will approach zero when 3.86% glucose is used because of convective transport from blood to dialysate, counterbalancing the diffusion [236, 237].

The MTAC of bicarbonate (MW 61 Da) has been reported to average 18 ml/min in intermittent peritoneal dialysis [238]. This may be an overestimation because of the short dwell time employed. From a more recent study using 24 h collections an average value of 9.5 ml/min can be calculated [239]. The bicarbonate loss with the dialysate is slightly greater than the lactate gain using 35 mmol/L lactate [236], but a dialysis alkali yield of 31 mmol/day has been found in CAPD patients using 40 mmol/L lactate [239]. The total mass transfer of bicarbonate from the circulation to the dialysate is determined by the plasma bicarbonate concentration and the ultrafiltration rate [240, 241]. Bicarbonate loss is especially increased during high ultrafiltration rates due to additional convective transport.

Transport of macromolecules

Macromolecules, such as serum proteins, are transported from the circulation to the peritoneal cavity at a much lower rate than low molecular weight solutes. Therefore, their dialysate concentrations are low and do not reach equilibrium with serum. Consequently their clearances can be used as an approximation of MTAC. Normal values for the clearances of β_2-microglobulin (MW 11.8 kDa), albumin (MW 69 kDa), IgG (MW 150 kDa) and α_2-macroglobulin (MW 820 kDa) are given in Table 2. The transport of macromolecules is size-selective, both for proteins and uncharged dextran molecules [93, 242]. Similar to low molecular weight solutes, the relationship between clearances and molecular weights can be described as a power relationship [242, 243]. The slope of the regression line between molecular weights and clearances is however much steeper (−0.69) than that between molecular weights and free diffusion coefficients (−0.36) [242]. This indicates that the transperitoneal transport of macromolecules is hindered by a size-selective restriction barrier within the peritoneal membrane. Unlike the transport of low molecular weight solutes, that is mainly dependent on the functional surface area of the peritoneum, the transport of macromolecules is determined both by surface area and intrinsic size-selective permeability.

It is still controversial whether the main transport mechanism of macromolecules during peritoneal dialysis is by convection [244, 245] or by restricted diffusion [50, 93, 246, 248]. *In-vitro* studies using endothelial monolayers on polycarbonate filters suggest that macromolecular transport in this system is caused by both diffusion and convection [248]. Restricted diffusion was especially present with highly confluent monolayers on filters with pores of about 400 Å, a situation probably similar to that in peritoneal dialysis. Convection requires fluid transport. This can occur by hydrostatic forces and by osmotic forces. An effect of osmotically induced convection has been demonstrated only for the low molecular weight protein β_2-microglobulin, but not for larger proteins such as albumin, transferrin, IgG and α_2-macroglobulin, which are transported through the large pores [87]. A mathematical approach has been used in an attempt to demonstrate that proteins larger than 50 Å reach the peritoneal cavity exclusively by hydrostatic convection through the large pore system [61]. However, this can occur only when the pressure in the peritoneal blood vessels exceeds that in the interstitial tissue. The intraperitoneal pressure during CAPD averages 8 mmHg during recumbency [203]. This value is lower than that in the arterioles, but similar to that in the venules. This implies that the localization of the large pores determines whether hydrostatic convection across them is likely to occur. Increasing the intraperitoneal pressure by 10 mmHg with the application of external compression decreased the clearances of proteins [203]. This effect was most pronounced for proteins with the highest molecular weights, suggesting an effect on the size of the pores. The measured data could be explained by convection through large pores with a radius of about 180 Å, but also by diffusion through large pores with an average radius of 1000 Å. The large venular interendothelial gaps with radii from 500 Å to 5000 Å, which can be found after the application of vasoactive substances, such as histamine [50], suggest that the latter value is not unrealistic.

It can be concluded that the peritoneal transport of albumin and larger proteins presumably occurs through the large pore system, and is size-selectively restricted. The mechanism involved may be restricted diffusion, or hydrostatic-induced convection, or a combination of the two, as has already been suggested by Renkin [249]. The localization and size of the large pore system determine which mechanism prevails.

Transport from the peritoneal cavity

Low molecular weight solutes

The disappearance rate of intraperitoneally administered low molecular weight solutes from the dialysate is dependent on their molecular weights [77, 250]. This suggests a mainly diffusive process. As a consequence the absorption of lactate during a 4 h dialysis dwell was found to average 82% of the instilled quantity (data from ref. 77). For glucose a mean value of 66% has been reported, irrespective of the glucose concentration used in the dialysate [251]. This could range between 51% and 80% in individual patients. When the disappearance of glucose is expressed as the ratio between the dialysate concentration after a 4 h dwell and the initial dialysate concentration (D/D_0), as is usually done during PET tests, values ranging from 0.12 to 0.60 can be found [225]. Other low molecular weight solutes that can be used as osmotic agents during peritoneal dialysis, such as glycerol and amino acids, are also absorbed according to their molecular weights. The absorption of glycerol (MW 92 Da) averages 84% after a 6 h dwell [252], and that of amino acids (mean MW 145 Da) 73–90% [171, 253]. The absorption of these solutes by diffusion occurs mainly in the portal circulation [254].

Babb *et al.* were the first to study bidirectional solute transport [255]. This was done by comparing mass transfer area coefficients of radiolabelled sucrose and vitamin B_{12} in the same patients after intravenous and intraperitoneal administration. Higher MTAC values were found after intraperitoneal administration. Similar results have been reported for the clearances of the non-protein-bound antibiotics fosfomycin [256] and cefamandole [257], as well as for inulin [258, 259]. A difference between MTAC values after intravenous and intraperitoneal administration of the same order of magnitude is present when transport rates of endogenous creatinine and albumin are compared to those of intraperitoneally administered solutes with an almost identical molecular weight [250, 260]. These data are summarized in Table 3. When we assume that the peritoneal restriction barrier is symmetric in its hindrance to diffusion, i.e. there is bidirectional equivalency to diffusive mass transfer, then a molecular-weight-independent, convective transport out of the peritoneal cavity of 1–2 ml/min should be present for solutes that are administered intraperitoneally. Although such a bidirectional equivalency to diffusion has not been proven definitely, it is supported by the fact that the absolute difference between intravenous and intraperitoneal administration is always of the same order of magnitude, irrespective of the size of the solutes. However, the relative difference (compared to the MTAC after intravenous administration) ranges from 16% for low molecular weight solutes such as creatinine, to more than 1000% for albumin. When diffusion would

Table 3. Comparison of bidirectional transport of solutes with similar molecular weights. Transport rates are expressed as mass transfer area coefficients (MTAC). Only paired data are used

Solute (IV/IP)	Molecular weight (dalton)	IV administration (ml/min)	IP administration (ml/min)	Absolute difference (ml/min)	Relative difference (%)
MTAC creatinine/5-flucytosine[a]	113/129	16.10	19.20	3.10	19
MTAC sucrose[b]	360	5.48	7.56	2.08	38
MTAC vitamin B_{12}[b]	1355	3.30	4.85	1.55	47
MTAC inulin[c]	5500	1.83	3.17	1.35	74
Cl albumin/haemoglobin[d]	69 000/68 000	0.12	1.53	1.43	1192

Data taken from refs [a]250, [b]255, [c]258, [d]260.

not occur equally in both directions, but would always be systematically higher for intraperitoneally administrated solutes, a constant relative difference would have been expected. Furthermore, Leypoldt et al. compared the bidirectional transport of creatinine in rabbits using a kinetic model that included convective solute transport by lymphatic absorption out of the peritoneal cavity, and found identical MTAC values [261]. This confirms the presence of a size-independent transport out of the peritoneal cavity from 1 to 2 ml/min.

The higher solute transport rates after intraperitoneal administration due to convection, imply that MTAC calculations do not represent diffusion only, when they are calculated with simplified models that do not take into account convective transport out of the peritoneal cavity. This convective leak is probably caused by the lymphatic drainage from the peritoneal cavity, and by transmesothelial transport to the peritoneal interstitial tissue induced by abdominal pressure. The contribution of convection to diffusive transport is relatively small for low molecular weight solutes, but becomes increasingly more important the higher the molecular weight of a solute. The convection/diffusion ratio is about 0.1 for glucose, 1.0 for inulin [258], but 10 for intraperitoneally administered autologous haemoglobin [260], making the disappearance rate of macromolecules relatively independent of molecular size (see below).

It can be concluded that the absorption of intraperitoneally administered molecules is partly size-selective (diffusion) and partly non-size-selective (convection). The relative contribution of convection increases the higher the molecular weight of the solute. Size-selectivity is therefore most pronounced for solutes with a molecular weight of less than 500.

Effects of bidirectional anion transport on acid–base status

Lactate used in peritoneal dialysis fluids usually consists of a racemic mixture of L- and D-lactate. One study reported a greater absorption of L-lactate than

of D-lactate in chronic peritoneal dialysis patients [262], similar to the stereospecificity of the blood–brain barrier [263]. However, in more recent studies similar peritoneal absorption rates were found for L- and D-lactate [264]. Absorbed L-lactate is converted by L-lactate dehydrogenase to pyruvate and then metabolized to bicarbonate. Lactate dehydrogenase is stereospecific and does not convert D-lactate. Accumulation of D-lactate could in theory cause metabolic acidosis. Such a D-lactate acidosis has been described in patients after extensive bowel surgery with bacterial overgrowth [265, 266]. In this situation the abnormal gut flora produced very large amounts of D-lactate. D-lactate can be metabolized in mammals, although slowly, probably by the enzyme D-2-hydroxy acid dehydrogenase [265]. Yet the capacity of the liver to metabolize D-lactate is probably sufficient for intravenous or intraperitoneally administered lactate solutions. Infusion of L- and D-lactate in the portal circulation of dogs showed hepatic extraction rates that were not different for both isomers [267]. Also, metabolic acidosis due to accumulation of D-lactate has not been found in peritoneal dialysis patients [238, 264, 267]. Impairment of lactate metabolism probably occurs only in patients with poor hepatic function [268].

Net base balance in patients treated with peritoneal dialysis is mainly dependent on the difference between the dialysate base gain (the difference between the mass transfer of bicarbonate and lactate) and the production of metabolic acids. As the latter is related to the breakdown of proteins, a relationship with the protein equivalent of nitrogen appearance (PNA) can be expected. Gotch et al. showed that the PNA multiplied by 0.77 corresponds well to the production of metabolic acids in stable patients [269]. Indeed, a negative relationship has been found between blood bicarbonate concentration and the estimated metabolic acid production [240]. The lactate mass transfer from the peritoneal cavity will be greatest during the beginning of a dwell, when the dialysate lactate concentration is highest. As a consequence, increasing the dialysis dose by performing more exchanges will increase the alkali gain. This explains the metabolic alkalosis that has been described in patients treated with high-dose CAPD [270]. The potential of bicarbonate-containing dialysis solutions in correcting acid–base disorders of CAPD patients is not essentially different from that of lactate-based fluids [241]. The net bicarbonate gain appeared to correlate with the ultrafiltration rate, the plasma bicarbonate level and the dialysate bicarbonate concentration [271]. Similar to lactate-based solutions, the ultrafiltration rate was the predominant parameter. A dialysis solution with a combination of bicarbonate and lactate as buffer also showed good control of acid–base status [163, 165].

The use of acetate as a buffer has now been abandoned because of its association with the development of peritoneal sclerosis [272–274]. Comparison of acetate- with lactate-based dialysis solutions showed that the rise in pH after instillation was more rapid with lactate [275]. Using acetate 18 min were required to reach a dialysate pH of 7, while this was only 7 min for lactate. The most probable explanation is the higher buffer capacity of acetate ($pK_A = 4.76$) compared to lactate ($pK_A = 3.86$) at pH = 5.6. This difference in pK_A is the reason for the much higher content of titrable acid in acetate than in lactate-buffered dialysis fluid [275].

Macromolecules

Particles, such as blood cells and bacteria, that are introduced into the peritoneal cavity, are absorbed in the diaphragmatic lymphatics (reviewed in ref. 277). It is therefore not surprising that a proportion of intraperitoneally administered macromolecules, during peritoneal dialysis, also disappears from the peritoneal cavity. Gjessing used dextran 70, 60 g/L as a dialysis solution in peritoneal dialysis patients treated with 30 min dwells. The recovery of dextran 70 in the dialysate averaged 92% after the dwell, while the plasma concentration increased to 1 g/L after 8 h dialysis and even to 4 g/L after 24 h [277]. Recoveries of intraperitoneally administered macromolecules of 70–90% after 4–7 h dwells in patients have been reported for radioiodine-tagged serum albumin [219, 278–282], for unlabelled human albumin [283], for dextran 70, 10 g/L [284] and 1 g/L [285], and for autologous haemoglobin [259, 281]. In only one study has a recovery of

autologous haemoglobin in excess of 95% been reported [286]. A high recovery of one batch of unlabelled human albumin was found in another study [287]. This was shown to be caused by a high transport of endogenous albumin, because this particular batch contained a high concentration of pre-kallikrein activator that caused an inflammatory reaction.

The disappearance rate of intraperitoneally administered macromolecules is independent of molecular size, both in animals [25, 288, 289] and in CAPD patients [290]. Furthermore, it is linear in time [285, 291]. In one study it was influenced by the osmolarity of the dialysis solution [281], but other studies could not confirm this [87, 291]. The disappearance rate is increased after the instillation of large dialysate volumes [77], and after the application of external pressure [203, 292]. It is likely that a proportion of the intraperitoneally administered macromolecules is taken up directly into the subdiaphragmatic lymphatic vessels, as has been shown in experiments using india ink [293]. Transmesothelial uptake, especially in the anterior abdominal wall, has been shown in rats using radiolabelled fibrinogen [294] and radiolabelled albumin [26]. Uptake of radiolabelled albumin in peritoneal tissues is also likely to be present in peritoneal dialysis patients [278]. The macromolecules transported to the interstitial tissue are probably taken up slowly in the lymphatic system, as continuous intraperitoneal administration of dextran 70 in CAPD patients had no effect on the magnitude of its disappearance rate from the peritoneal cavity [285].

In summary, the above data from the literature point to the presence of a non-size-selective mechanism for the disappearance of macromolecules from the peritoneal cavity. They are partly taken up directly by the subdiaphragmatic lymphatic vessels and partly in the peritoneal interstitium. Subsequent uptake into the lymphatics that drain the interstitial tissues is likely to occur.

Fluid transport

Transcapillary ultrafiltration

Fluid transport during peritoneal dialysis consists of water transport from the peritoneal capillaries into the peritoneal cavity by transcapillary ultrafiltration and by fluid loss out of the peritoneal cavity. The latter consists of transcapillary back-filtration and by fluid uptake into the lymphatic system. As a consequence, the changes in the *in-situ* intraperitoneal volume are determined by the magnitude of the transcapillary ultrafiltration and lymphatic absorption. The water removal from the body at the end of a dwell period, defined as net ultrafiltration, is therefore the difference between the cumulative transcapillary ultrafiltration and fluid uptake into the lymphatic system.

The transport of water across the capillary wall occurs through the small pore system and probably through ultra-small transcellular water channels (see section on pathways and barriers). The small pores are mainly involved in transport by hydrostatic and colloid osmotic forces, transport through the ultra-small pores is dependent on the osmotic gradient across the endothelial cells. It has been assumed that, during CAPD, 40% of the filtered fluid volume passes through transcellular water channels [61]. According to Starling's law, the transcapillary ultrafiltration rate in peritoneal dialysis is determined by the ultrafiltration coefficient of the peritoneal membrane and the driving forces between the peritoneal capillaries and the abdominal cavity. These forces are exerted by hydrostatic, crystalloid osmotic and colloid osmotic pressure gradients. The dependency of the transcapillary ultrafiltration rate (TCUFR) can be described by the following equation:

$$TCUFR = UFC(\Delta P - \Delta \Pi + \sigma \Delta O) \qquad (15)$$

in which UFC is the peritoneal ultrafiltration coefficient, ΔP is the hydrostatic pressure gradient, $\Delta \Pi$ is the colloid osmotic pressure gradient, σ the reflection coefficient and ΔO the crystalloid osmolality gradient. The ultrafiltration coefficient of the peritoneum is the product of the hydraulic permeability and surface area. Little is known about determinants of the hydraulic permeability, which is most likely dependent on the combination of intracapillary pressure, and the number and size of the pores. The state of the interstitial tissue, possibly containing sites of fibrosis, may also be one of the determinants. In computer simulations of peritoneal transport values of 0.04 and 0.08 ml/min per mmHg have been calculated for the ultrafiltration coefficient [62].

The hydrostatic pressure in the peritoneal capillaries is assumed to be 17 mmHg [295]. The intraperitoneal pressure during CAPD has been reported to average 2 mmHg [296] and 8 mmHg [200, 203] in the supine position, depending on the choice of reference point. It exceeds 20 mmHg while walking [296], and is dependent on the instilled dialysate volume [297]. This implies that the hydrostatic pressure gradient is determined mainly by the intra-

peritoneal pressure. The colloid osmotic pressure in the peritoneal capillaries probably averages 26 mmHg [295]. In CAPD patients who have a mean serum albumin concentration of 34 g/L [298] a value of 21 mmHg can be calculated [63]. The contribution of the dialysate to the colloid osmotic pressure gradient can be neglected because of its low protein content. The crystalloid pressure gradient is mainly determined by glucose. The effectiveness of this osmotic agent depends on the resistance the membrane exerts on its transport. This is expressed as the osmotic reflection coefficient (see section on pathways and barriers); it can range from 1 (no passage, ideal semipermeable membrane) to 0 (passage not hindered, no osmotic effect). In case of a reflection coefficient of 1, every mosmol exerts an osmotic pressure of 19.3 mmHg according to van't Hoff's law. The reflection coefficient for glucose during CAPD is probably between 0.02 and 0.05 [56–60], so very low. It must be appreciated, however, that these are mean values. The reflection coefficient for glucose across the ultra-small pores will be 1.0, and will approach zero across the large pores. This might explain why glucose is an effective osmotic agent despite its small size.

The hyperosmolality of commercial dialysis fluid when compared to uraemic plasma is about 45 mosmol/kg H_2O for the lowest glucose concentration (1.36%) and 180 mosmol/kg H_2O for the highest glucose concentration (3.86%). The osmotic pressure exerted by these solutions across the peritoneal membrane can therefore be estimated as 45×0.03 (reflection coefficient) $\times 19.3 = 23$ mmHg (lowest glucose concentration), and similarly 104 mmHg (highest glucose concentration). The various pressure gradients are summarized in Table 4. The values for the crystalloid osmotic pressure gradients are the maximum values, as present during the initial phase of a dialysis dwell. They will decrease in time due to absorption of glucose from the dialysate. This glucose absorption averages 61% of the instilled quantity during a 4 h dwell [222] and 75% after 6 h [227]. The absolute, but not the relative, absorption is influenced by the glucose concentration used [299]. As a consequence the transcapillary ultrafiltration rate has its maximum value at the start of dialysis and decreases during the dwell. The figures given in Table 4 imply that dialysate with a low glucose concentration will induce only a small amount of osmosis-induced transcapillary ultrafiltration. The maximal transcapillary ultrafiltration rate with 1.36% glucose during the initial phase of a dwell averages 2.7 [112] to 4.3 ml/min

Table 4. Pressure gradients across the peritoneal membrane during the initial phase of a peritoneal dialysis exchange

	Pressure in peritoneal capillaries	Pressure in dialysate-filled peritoneal cavity	Pressure gradient
Hydrostatic pressure (mmHg)	17	8 recumbent	9
Colloid osmotic pressure (mmHg)	21	0.1	−21
Osmolality (mosmol/kg H₂O)	305	347 (glucose 1.36%) 486 (glucose 3.86%)	
Maximal crystalloid osmotic pressure gradient (mmHg)		(glucose 1.36%) (glucose 3.86%)	24 105

The reflection coefficient of low molecular weight solutes is set at 0.03.

[62]. With 3.86% glucose-based dialysate the initial transcapillary ultrafiltration during 4 h dwells averages 12–16 ml/min [62, 87, 228, 300]. Mean values for transcapillary ultrafiltration during 4 h dwells average 1.0–1.2 ml/min for 1.36% glucose [87, 112, 222], and 3.4 ml/min for 3.86% glucose [87]. Substituting the maximal transcapillary ultrafiltration rate obtained with 3.86% glucose in the left term of equation (15) and the pressure gradients given in Table 4 in the right term, provides the following:

$$15(\text{ml/min}) = \text{UFC}[(17 - 8) - (21)$$
$$+ 0.03(486 - 305) \times 19.3] \text{ mmHg}$$

It follows from this that the peritoneal ultrafiltration coefficient during 3.86% glucose-based dialysate averages 0.16 ml/min per mmHg. This value, representing water transport through the small and ultra-small pore system, is about twice as high as the figure of 0.08 ml/min per mmHg used in computer simulations [62]. The most likely explanation for this difference is the apparent paradox that water channels contribute only to a limited extent to the total surface area, but allow the transport of large quantities of water by crystalloid osmosis. Multiplication of the UFC with σ glucose yields the osmotic conductance to glucose, which is 4.8 μl/min per mmHg, a value very similar to those used in computer simulations [17].

Dextrins are glucose polymers that can also be applied as osmotic agents during peritoneal dialysis. Icodextrin is a disperse mixture of dextrins with an average molecular weight of 16.8 kDa that is currently used in clinical practice [301]. Due to its high molecular weight, icodextrin is likely to induce colloid osmosis [302]. This implies that macromolecules are able to induce transcapillary ultrafiltration even in an isotonic or hypotonic solution.

The process of colloid osmosis is based upon the principle that fluid flow across a membrane which is permeable to small solutes, occurs in the direction of relative excess of impermeable large solutes, rather than along a concentration gradient. Consequently dialysis solutions containing macromolecules to remove fluid from the body will induce water transport through the small pore system. When such a solution is not hypertonic, no water transport will be induced through the ultra-small water channels. The pressure gradients across the peritoneal membrane that can be expected using a 7.5% icodextrin-based dialysis solution are shown in Table 5. It follows from this table that the maximum pressure gradient across the peritoneal membrane is 42 mmHg, which is higher than the 12 mmHg exerted by 1.36%/1.5% glucose, but markedly less than the 93 mmHg exerted by 3.86%/4.25% glucose. However, because of its lower absorption than glucose, the gradient will remain present for a much longer time. Using 7.5% icodextrin a UFC of 0.05 ml/min per mmHg can be calculated. This value can be employed to estimate the back-filtration of dialysis fluid into the capillaries by the colloid osmotic pressure gradient: back-filtration rate = 0.05 (9 − 21) = 0.6 ml/min. In a previous study using a dialysis solution without an osmotic agent, the overall back-filtration rate was 0.9 ml/min during a 4 h dwell [160]. It was highest during the start of the dwell (2.6 ml/min), because the solution was hypotonic to uraemic plasma, and averaged 0.4 ml/min during the last 2 h. A value of about 1 ml/min can be calculated on data from a study using intraperitoneal 0.9% NaCl [278].

The absorption of icodextrin averaged 19% during an 8 h exchange [303]. Therefore, the transcapillary ultrafiltration rate induced by it is almost stable during an exchange [63, 304] and averages 1.4–2.3 ml/min [63, 304]. This could explain why

Table 5. Pressure gradients across the peritoneal membrane during the initial phase of a peritoneal dialysis exchange using 7.5% icodextrin

	Pressure in peritoneal capillaries	Pressure in dialysate-filled peritoneal cavity	Pressure gradient
Hydrostatic pressure (mmHg)	17	8 recumbent	9
Colloid osmotic pressure (mmHg)	21	66	45
Osmolality (mosmol/kg H$_2$O)	305	285	
Maximal crystalloid osmotic pressure gradient (mmHg)			$(285 - 305) \times 0.03 \times 19.3 = -12$

It is assumed that the molecular weight of icodextrin is 16 800 and the reflection coefficient is 0.767. The reflection coefficient of low molecular weight solutes is set at 0.03.

icodextrin-based dialysis solutions are especially effective during dwells of 8–12 h [305].

Lymphatic absorption

Direct measurement of the lymphatic flow from the peritoneal cavity is impossible in humans; therefore, indirect methods have been used. They include the disappearance rate (clearance) of intraperitoneally administered macromolecules from the peritoneal cavity, and their appearance rate in the circulation. Using the disappearance rate it is assumed that the administered macromolecule is removed from the peritoneal cavity by absorption into the lymphatic system. Human albumin [283], radioiodinated serum albumin (RISA) [219, 227, 306], autologous haemoglobin [228, 260, 281, 286] and dextran 70 [284] have all been used. This approach is justified because the disappearance rate of these solutes is constant in time [285, 291] and independent of molecular size [290] (see also the section on transport from the peritoneal cavity). Using these tracers average values of 1.0–1.5 ml/min have been found in CAPD patients [219, 222, 227, 260, 283, 284, 306]. The validity of this method has been questioned, because the appearance rate of intraperitoneally administered RISA in the circulation is only about 20% of the disappearance rate [278, 279]. However, half this difference can be explained by the fact that only 40–50% of the total albumin mass is intravascular [307]. Local accumulation of intraperitoneal RISA has been found in the anterior abdominal wall of rats [26], most likely caused by transmesothelial transport. It is probable that macromolecules in the peritoneal interstitial tissue will eventually be taken up into the lymphatic system, as has been made plausible in mice [308]. This is supported by the observation that saturation of the peritoneal interstitium in CAPD patients by

continuous administration of dextran 70 did not alter the appearance rate of this macromolecule [285].

Direct measurement of lymphatic flow from the peritoneal cavity has been studied by the group of Johnston, both in anaesthetized and conscious sheep [309–312]. In these animals the right lymphatic duct could not be cannulated. Anaesthesia appeared to have a pronounced effect on the flow in the cannulated lymphatics, probably because of reduced movements of the diaphragm. The mean lymph flow in conscious sheep ranged from 1 to 1.5 ml/h per kg body weight, depending on estimations for flow in the right lymphatic duct. Comparisons of these measured flow rates with disappearance and appearance rates of RISA in sheep are difficult, because the disappearance rate of RISA was very high and the RISA appearance rate was 60% of the disappearance rate, i.e. a much smaller difference than in human CAPD patients. The amount of RISA administered intraperitoneally, recovered in the blood and in the drained lymphatic vessels was always equal to the amount lost from the peritoneal cavity during a 6 h dwell. This is not supportive of marked accumulation of RISA in the anterior abdominal wall. The flow from the caudal mediastinal lymph node can be raised 200% in the awake sheep model by intraperitoneal administration of fluid [313]. In analogy, the disappearance rate of intraperitoneally administered autologous haemoglobin is higher in CAPD patients after the administration of a 3 L dialysate volume than with a volume of 2 L [77]. Increasing the intraperitoneal pressure in rats that underwent peritoneal dialysis also increased the RISA disappearance rate [292]. However, it had no effect on its appearance rate in the systemic circulation. Combining this observation with those in awake sheep and CAPD patients suggests that the disappearance rate of macromolecules is a clinically more relevant way of assessing lymphatic absorption in CAPD patients than the appearance rate.

It has been suggested that fluid transport associated with the disappearance of macromolecules should not be called lymphatic flow or lymphatic absorption, but simply fluid loss [314]. This is a simplification, because reabsorption of fluid into the capillaries by the colloid osmotic pressure gradient is not associated with the transport of macromolecules, as has been shown in studies using normal saline [278], or hypotonic dialysate without an osmotic agent [160]. The amount of saline absorbed during a 7 h dwell was 24% in the former study, but the amount of RISA that had disappeared was only 17%. In the latter study the dialysate concentration of intraperitoneally administered dextran 70 increased 10% during a 4 h dwell, most likely because of transcapillary back-filtration of water, caused by the colloid osmotic pressure gradient. This underlines that fluid loss from the peritoneal cavity is coupled mainly to the disappearance of macromolecules (lymphatic absorption), but is also partly uncoupled (back-filtration by colloid osmosis). Based on these data it can be concluded that the disappearance rate of intraperitoneally administered macromolecules cannot be used alone as a measurement of lymph flow through the subdiaphragmatic lymphatics, but also cannot be used as an overall indicator of fluid loss from the peritoneal cavity, irrespective of the mechanism involved. It is plausible that the disappearance rate can be used as a functional approach for the calculation of the effective lymphatic absorption from the peritoneal cavity during CAPD. Consequently all pathways of lymphatic drainage from the peritoneal cavity, both subdiaphragmatic and interstitial, are included in the definition of the effective lymphatic absorption rate. The term 'effective' is analogous to the effective renal plasma flow, where a clearance is used to estimate flow.

Intraperitoneal pressure is likely to be one of the determinants of the effective lymphatic absorption. Intraperitoneal administration of saline in rats causes an increase in the number of patent subdiaphragmatic stomata, not present when the intraperitoneal pressure was kept constant [315]. A relationship has also been found between intraperitoneal pressure in CAPD patients and the disappearance rate of intraperitoneally administered dextran 70 [316]. Increasing the intraperitoneal pressure 10 mmHg, by external compression, leads to a marked increase in the effective lymphatic absorption rate [203], and consequently a lower net ultrafiltration. Net ultrafiltration is also somewhat (16%) lower in the upright position compared to recumbency [200], caused by the combination of a small increase in the dextran disappearance rate and a slight decrease in the transcapillary ultrafiltration rate. The effects of higher intraperitoneal pressure in the upright position are probably counterbalanced by the effect of gravity leading to a decreased contact between the dialysate and the subdiaphragmatic lymphatics. The coefficients of intra-individual variation of the parameters of fluid transport average 17% [200]. The time-course of transcapillary ultrafiltration, effective lymphatic absorption and net ultrafiltration (the difference between the two) is shown in Fig. 7 for 1.36%/1.5% glucose, 3.86%/4.25% glucose and 7.5% icodextrin. The transcapillary ultrafiltration rate on glucose-based solutions is negatively related to the MTAC creatinine (representing a large vascular surface area), but the relationship is positive when an icodextrin-based solution is used, as shown in Fig. 8. These relationships can be explained by the different properties of the two osmotic agents. The presence of a large vascular surface area allows high water transport rates, as many pores are available for transport. This explains the effects of icodextrin. For glucose-based solutions, however, the positive effects on water transport are counteracted by high glucose absorption rates, leading to a rapid disappearance of the osmotic gradient.

Assessment of fluid transport in individual patients

Fluid transport is preferably investigated using a standardized 4 h dwell with a 3.86%/4.25% glucose-based dialysis solution [317]. This is justified, because: (1) net ultrafiltration with the most hypertonic solution is less subject to error than that obtained with less hypertonic fluids; and (2) a better estimation of the sieving of Na^+ is possible. The use of 3.86%/4.25% glucose does not influence D/P ratios [318] or MTAC [87], compared to a 1.36%/1.5% glucose dialysis solution. Analysis of data from literature on 3.86%/4.25% glucose dialysate suggests that net ultrafiltration of less than 400 ml/4 h with this solution can be considered clinically important ultrafiltration failure, although the various studies applied different methodologies [87, 219, 318, 319]. For 2.27%/2.5% glucose, net ultrafiltration less than 100 ml/4 h [223] and for 1.36%/1.5% solutions a value of less than minus 400–500 ml/4 h [222, 318] can be considered as impaired ultrafiltration, but especially the latter are very much subject to interference with other factors. Analysis of sodium dip

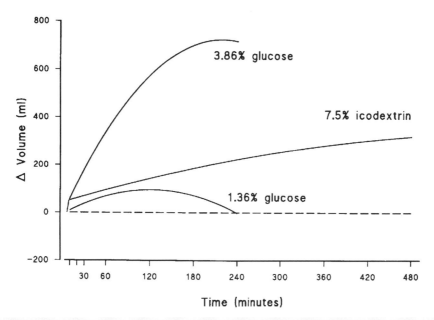

Figure 7. The time-course of the intraperitoneal volume during a 4 h exchange with 1.36% glucose, a 4 h exchange with 3.86% glucose and an 8 h exchange with 7.5% icodextrin-based dialysis solution. Median values are given. Based on refs 63, 112, and 304.

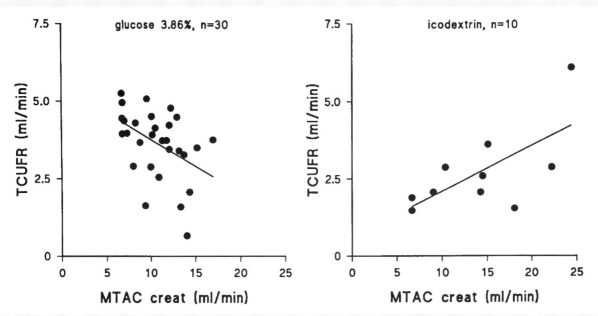

Figure 8. The different relationships between the MTAC creatinine, representing the vascular peritoneal surface area and the transcapillary ultrafiltration rate obtained during 4 h exchanges with 3.86% glucose (left panel) and 7.5% icodextrin (right panel). The icodextrin data are from ref. 63, the glucose data are from a randomly selected group of stable CAPD patients who underwent a standard peritoneal permeability analysis. Note that a high MTAC creatinine is associated with a low transcapillary ultrafiltration rate on glucose and with a high transcapillary ultrafiltration rate on icodextrin.

during a 3.86%/4.25% exchanges provides information on channel-mediated water transport.

The addition of a macromolecular tracer to a peritoneal dialysis solution allows the calculation of the transcapillary ultrafiltration, the lymphatic absorption and the net ultrafiltration rate. It also allows the calculation of the residual volume after drainage of the peritoneal cavity. The latter can easily be determined by adding a specific volume (V_x) of fresh solution intraperitoneally, followed by immediate draining. By comparing the concentration of solutes in this rinsing bag and comparing them to those in the drained (test) bag, the residual volume (V_r) can be calculated by: $V_r = V_x \times [C_2/C_1 - C_2)]$, in which C_1 represents the concentration in the (test) bag and C_2 that in the rinsing bag. In a comparison between various endogenous solutes present in drained dialysate and intraperitoneally administered inulin and dextran 70, a good correlation was found between the residual volume determined with the two exogenous solutes [320]. All endogenous low molecular weight solutes and proteins overestimated the residual volume, probably due to mass transport during the procedure. After correction for mass transport, albumin appeared the most useful endogenous marker for the estimation of the residual volume.

Causes of ultrafiltration failure

Verger *et al.* [321] proposed two categories of ultrafiltration failure: type 1 was associated with intact and even high mass transfer area coefficients or D/P ratios of low molecular weight solutes, while type 2 was associated with impaired solute transport. It has now become evident that type 2 is extremely rare and possibly only present in a minority of patients with peritoneal sclerosis [322]. Low ultrafiltration is overrepresented in patients with high D/P ratios [323].

In principle four main causes of ultrafiltration failure can be distinguished: (1) the presence of a large vascular surface area, (2) a decreased osmotic conductance to glucose, (3) the presence of a high disappearance rate of intraperitoneally administered macromolecules ('lymphatic absorption'), and (4) an extremely small peritoneal surface area, e.g. due to multiple adhesions. Combinations of causes are also possible, such as (1) and (2) [324, 325] and (1) and (3) [324]. All studies have shown that the presence of a large vascular surface area is by far the most frequent cause of ultrafiltration failure, especially in long-term patients [219, 222, 319, 326]. It is likely to be present in more than half of the patients with this condition [219, 222]. Although a large number of perfused peritoneal capillaries would allow high water transport rates, because a large number of small pores and water channels is available, this effect is counteracted by fast absorption of the osmotic agent leading to a rapid disappearance of the osmotic gradient.

A decreased osmotic conductance of the peritoneal membrane to glucose ($LpS + \sigma$) can be another cause of low ultrafiltration. It can either be the result of a decrease in the peritoneal ultrafiltration coefficient (LpS) or of a reduction of σ-glucose, which is mainly

determined by the number and function of aquaporins. It is unknown whether a decrease in hydraulic permeability (Lp) of the interstitial peritoneal tissue is an abnormality that can occur during peritoneal dialysis. Its existence is not supported by data on solute transport, because the size-selectivity of the peritoneum for low molecular weight solutes is not affected by the duration of peritoneal dialysis [88]. Only for macromolecules was an increased size-selectivity found with the duration of peritoneal dialysis [88, 327]. It is also unclear whether a reduced expression of aquaporin-1 exists as a cause of impaired ultrafiltration. One patient has been described with ultrafiltration failure due to an abolition of transcellular water transfer, but with a normal expression of aquaporin-1 in a peritoneal biopsy [71]. This would suggest that structural alterations in aquaporin-1 leading to impairment of its function would be the most important cause of decreased hydraulic permeability of the peritoneal membrane. It is evident that more data on this subject are required.

The prevalence of impaired channel-mediated water transport in patients with ultrafiltration failure is unknown. It was present in six patients with severe ultrafiltration failure with no obvious cause in the peritoneal equilibration test [328]. These patients had almost no sieving of sodium and a reduced difference in net ultrafiltration obtained with 3.86%/4.25% glucose and 1.36%/1.5% glucose. In another study in which a diffusion correction was applied for the Na^+ gradient, impaired channel-mediated water transport contributed to other causes of ultrafiltration failure in three out of eight patients with this condition [324]. In an ongoing study D/P $Na^+_{60\,min}$ without correction for diffusion was 0.903 in nine patients with net ultrafiltration < 400 ml/4 h with 3.86%/4.25% glucose, which was significantly greater than the value of 0.873 in 15 patients with normal ultrafiltration. However, the difference disappeared after a diffusion correction was made, using either the MTAC urate or the MTAC creatinine [329]. The duration of peritoneal dialysis is likely to affect aquaporin-mediated water transport. Comparing the ultrafiltration coefficients obtained with 3.86%/4.25% glucose and 7.5% icodextrin, it appeared that a linear relationship was present between the ultra-small pore ultrafiltration coefficient and the time on CAPD [63]. In patients who developed peritoneal sclerosis we also found evidence for decreasing transcellular water transport, as judged from the difference in net ultrafiltration between 3.86%/4.25% glucose and 1.36%/1.5% glucose dialysate [322, 330]. It can be concluded that impaired aquaporin-mediated water transport can contribute to ultrafiltration failure, especially in long-term peritoneal dialysis, but more data are necessary to estimate its prevalence.

Impaired net ultrafiltration due to high water transport rates associated with the disappearance of intraperitoneally administered macromolecules was found in two out of the nine patients with ultrafiltration failure described by Heimbürger et al. [219]. Combining previously published results [324] with those of an ongoing multicentre study in the Netherlands a dextran disappearance rate exceeding 2 ml/min was found in seven out of 19 patients with ultrafiltration failure (net UF <400 ml/4 hs on 3.86%/4.25% glucose), often in combination with the presence of a large peritoneal surface area. Up to now no evidence is present suggesting that the prevalence of this cause of impaired peritoneal fluid removal would increase with the duration of peritoneal dialysis. The presence of a small surface area as a cause of low ultrafiltration rates is very rare, and present only in patients with multiple adhesions and in some patients with peritoneal sclerosis [322, 331]. No quantitative data are available on the prevalence of ultrafiltration loss due to an extremely small surface area.

Peritoneal permeability in systemic diseases

Uraemia

The uraemic state is probably associated with more permeable serosal membranes than is the non-uraemic situation. This is illustrated by the easy development of pleural and pericardial effusions. Increased capillary permeability has also been reported in the lungs during chronic uraemia [332]. A similar increase has been found for the permeability characteristics of the peritoneal membrane during 3 h dialysis exchanges, when three patients with chronic renal failure were compared to four patients with normal renal function who were dialysed because of psoriasis [333]. The uraemic patients had higher transport rates for uric acid, phosphate and protein than those with psoriasis, indicating a larger effective peritoneal surface area in the uraemic patients. The intrinsic permeability to macromolecules was not investigated in this study. On the other hand decreased clearances of urea and creatinine have been reported during intermittent peritoneal dialysis in patients with severe hyperparathyroidism [334]. In acute renal failure due to rhabdomyolysis caused by heat stress and exercise, decreased peritoneal clearances have also been reported for creatinine and uric acid, but not for urea [335].

Diabetes mellitus

Patients with diabetes mellitus have an abnormal microcirculation. Capillary basement membrane alterations with thickening and loose areas of the fibrillar meshwork are especially common [336]. Increased microvascular permeability to proteins is also present [337]. Peritoneal clearances of exogenously administered radiolabelled albumin in rats undergoing peritoneal dialysis have been found higher in animals with alloxan-induced diabetes mellitus than in those with gentamicin-induced renal failure [338]. This was especially the case in the rats with the most severe diabetes. The findings in animal models cannot simply be applied for the situation in chronic peritoneal dialysis patients. The continuous exposure to extremely high dialysate glucose concentrations leads to diabetiform membrane alterations, such as reduplicated basement membranes [339], and neoangiogenesis [340] with deposition of collagen IV [341]. This may obscure differences between diabetic and non-diabetic patients that might have been present in the initial phase of peritoneal dialysis. Therefore, the various studies should be interpreted with caution.

Low peritoneal clearances of creatinine and urate have been reported in one patient with severe diabetes mellitus treated with intermittent peritoneal dialysis [342]. In contrast, the MTAC values of urea, creatinine and glucose in a larger group of diabetic CAPD patients were similar to those of patients with renal failure due to a primary renal disease [343–345] (Table 6). In one study a dependency of D/P creatinine on peritonitis incidence has been described [346]: patients with a high incidence have higher D/P ratios than non-diabetic patients and patients with a low incidence had lower ratios. Reduced ultrafiltration was present during periods of hyperglycaemia [346]. Patients studied during the initial period of CAPD had higher D/P ratios for creatinine than non-diabetic controls in one study [346], and lower transcapillary ultrafiltration rates in another one [347]. Peritoneal protein losses in diabetic CAPD patients are not different from those of other patients [348–350]. As serum albumin concentrations are often low in some of them [307], this can mask increased permeability to macromolecules. In accordance with the findings in alloxan-induced diabetes in rats [338], clearances of albumin, transferrin and IgG have been reported

Table 6. Comparison of peritoneal permeability characteristics between 46 patients with a primary renal disease and 38 patients with systemic diseases. Permeabiltiy to low molecular weight solutes is expressed as mass transfer area coefficient (MTAC), that of proteins as clearance (Cl). Mean values $\pm$ SEM are given

	Primary renal disease ($n = 46$)	Systemic lupus erythematosus ($n = 7$)	Systemic sclerosis ($n = 2$)	Diabetes mellitus ($n = 23$)	Amyloidosis ($n = 6$)
MTAC creatinine (ml/min)	9 ± 0.4	10 ± 1	12 ± 1	10 ± 1	$14 \pm 2^*$
MTAC glucose (ml/min)	9 ± 0.4	11 ± 1	10 ± 1	11 ± 1	13 ± 2
Cl albumin (μl/min)	92 ± 6	92 ± 19	118 ± 11	97 ± 7	110 ± 21
Cl IgG (μl/min)	50 ± 3	47 ± 12	61 ± 2	53 ± 5	59 ± 13

$^* p < 0.05$ versus primary renal disease.

30% higher in diabetic than in non-diabetic CAPD patients [242]. However, when larger numbers of patients were studied, the difference was no longer significant (Table 6). The explanation for this is probably the large variability in the effective peritoneal surface area and intrinsic permeability in the patients with a primary renal disease.

Systemic lupus erythematosus

Low clearances for urea, creatinine and urate have been reported in one patient with fulminant systemic lupus erythematosus (SLE) and severe hypertension, treated with intermittent peritoneal dialysis [342]. More recent data show that the prognosis of SLE patients on renal replacement therapy is similar to those with a primary renal disease [351]. In the literature more detailed data on CAPD in SLE have only been reported in 16 patients [352–354]. Solute transport rates were published in four CAPD patients, indicating a normal vascular surface area and a decreased intrinsic permeability to macromolecules [344, 345]. This could not be confirmed when larger number of patients were studied (Table 6).

Systemic sclerosis

Patients with systemic sclerosis can be treated with peritoneal dialysis, despite their low life expectancy [351]. Low peritoneal clearances of low molecular weight solutes have been reported in one patient on intermittent peritoneal dialysis [356], but essentially normal values were found in another one [357]. CAPD treatment has also been described to give good metabolic control [358] and acceptable clearances of low molecular weight solutes [359]. Data on solute transport in two patients are given in Table 6.

Amyloidosis and paraproteinemia

Peritoneal dialysis as renal replacement therapy in patients with amyloidosis and/or paraproteinaemia has given satisfactory clinical results [354, 359]. Evidence for a large peritoneal surface area has been reported in four patients with amyloidosis [343, 355]. This may be of importance because peritoneal dialysis can be used to remove immunoglobulins and light chains from the body, thereby preventing further amyloid formation, hyperviscosity syndromes and, perhaps in some cases, reverse renal insufficiency in patients with nephrotoxic light chain-induced renal failure [361, 362]. Solute transport data in six patients with amyloidosis are given in Table 6.

It can be concluded that the presence of a systemic disease has no uniform effect on the permeability characteristics of the peritoneal membrane during CAPD, although some patients may present with abnormal high or low MTAC values. However, such abnormal values can also be found in patients with a primary renal disease. This implies that peritoneal dialysis should not be abandoned in patients with systemic diseases, because of the expectation of an abnormal peritoneal permeability.

Peritoneal permeability during infections peritonitis

Inflammation causes hyperaemia, and therefore changes in the permeability characteristics of the peritoneal membrane are likely to occur. 'Membrane failure', as judged from deteriorating biochemical control has been reported in four of 35 IPD patients with peritonitis [363]. In contrast, increased clearances of creatinine and urea during peritonitis have been found in four IPD patients who were studied both in the absence of, and in the presence of, peritonitis [364]. As the effluent volume was similar, increased permeability caused by inflammation was the most likely explanation.

The most striking clinical finding in CAPD patients with peritonitis is impaired net ultrafiltration, leading to weight gain and other signs of fluid overload [365]. This phenomenon is associated with increased transport of low molecular weight solutes and increased absorption of glucose [76, 114, 366–370]. These phenomena point to an increased vascular peritoneal surface area caused by hyperaemia. This leads to rapid disappearance of the osmotic gradient, and thus to reduced net ultrafiltration. In this situation a high molecular weight osmotic agent should be able to induce more transcapillary ultrafiltration. This was recently confirmed by the use of icodextrin, which led to increased, instead of decreased, net ultrafiltration during peritonitis [371]. Using autologous haemoglobin as a volume marker, it was shown that the maximal intraperitoneal volume during peritonitis is reached at about 1 h after instillation of the dialysis fluid, compared to 2.5 h after recovery [76]. This may explain why a decrease in net ultrafiltration has not been observed during peritonitis in IPD patients. The steep rise in the intraperitoneal volume during the initial phase of a dwell is caused by high transcapillary ultrafiltration rates during this period, as shown with dextrin 70 [114]. A contribution of an increased fluid absorption from the peritoneal cavity is equivocal. It was suggested in a study using autologous haemoglobin as a volume marker [76, 372] and also, but to a minor degree, in a study using kinetic modelling of fluid transport [18]. However, in a more recent study using dextran 70 no effect of the inflammatory reaction on peritoneal fluid absorption could be established [114]. The alterations in peritoneal transport during peritonitis return to normal values within 1–2 weeks after recovery from the infection [370, 373].

Protein loss in the dialysis effluent is also markedly increased during peritonitis [76, 242, 364, 368, 373, 374]. In contrast to CAPD the losses in IPD can be as high as 48 g per dialysis and often remain elevated for several weeks [373]. These proteins could be produced locally, or originate from the circulation [374]. Serum proteins are quantitatively the most important in peritoneal effluent. The increment in their clearances of more than 100%, during peritonitis, favours increased transport [76, 242], due both to the increased effective surface area and increased peritoneal permeability to macromolecules [242]. In a longitudinal study in CAPD patients with peritonitis, Zemel et al. showed an increase in the vascular peritoneal surface area and a decrease in the restriction coefficient to macromolecules during the acute phase of the inflammation [147]. The decreased restriction coefficient, pointing to an increased permeability of the peritoneum, returns to normal values within 1–2 days [114, 147], but the vascular surface area remains increased for a longer time.

Possible causes for the changes in surface area and permeability include endotoxin and complement activation [375], as well as prostaglandins [114, 138, 139, 147], IL-6 [144, 147], TNFα [141, 147] and local production of nitric oxide [114, 152, 153]. Inhibition of the inflammatory reaction with indomethacin reduced dialysate prostaglandin concentration, and had some effect on the restriction coefficient to macromolecules [148]. The importance of the relative contributions of all these mediators in the functional alterations of the peritoneal membrane during infectious peritonitis is not known.

Peritoneal transport during long-duration peritoneal dialysis

Many studies on peritoneal membrane transport characteristics are difficult to interpret since patients may be taken off peritoneal dialysis, e.g. for peritonitis, while impaired peritoneal transport function may have been present, but was not regarded as the main cause for discontinuation. In addition not all studies used standardized dwells. Impaired transport of water and solutes has been reported as a reason for drop-out in 16% of patients from three dialysis populations in which the mean follow-up was 14 months [376], 15 months [377] and 24 months [378]. Ultrafiltration failure was reported in half of these patients and inadequate clearances in the other half. However, peritoneal clearances of low molecular weight solutes during a situation of near-equilibrium between dialysate and plasma concentrations such as in CAPD, are mainly determined by the drained volume [379]. Consequently patients with the highest D/P ratios of creatinine may have the lowest peritoneal mass transfer of urea and creatinine due to small drained volumes [324]. It is therefore likely that ultrafiltration failure as a reason for drop-out has been underestimated in the above-mentioned epidemiological studies. Higher figures for drop-out because of ultrafiltration failure are also found when the period of follow-up is longer. In the analysis of Kawaguchi et al. ultrafiltration failure was the reason for withdrawal from CAPD in 24% of the total CAPD population, but in 51% of the patients who had been treated with CAPD for more than 6 years [380].

It follows from the above data that impaired ultrafiltration is the most frequent transport abnormality in CAPD. Its prevalence is dependent on the duration of treatment. Using a clinical definition Heimbürger *et al.* estimated it to be present in 3% of the patients after 1 year, but in 31% after 6 years [219]. Clinical definitions are subject to bias, as overhydration can also occur due to excessive fluid intake or a reduced urine production. Using a standardized 4 h exchange with 3.86%/4.25% glucose, and defining ultrafiltration failure as net ultrafiltration <400 ml/4 h, a prevalence of 23% was found in a cross-sectional study in patients with a median duration of CAPD of 19 months (range 0.3–178) [324]. A prevalence of 35% was detected in unselected patients treated for more than 4 years in an ongoing multicentre study using the same definition (unpublished). It can be concluded that ultrafiltration failure is an especially important problem in long-term peritoneal dialysis patients. The various causes have been discussed in the section on causes of ultrafiltration failure.

A large number of rather small studies on the time-course of peritoneal permeability characteristics has been published, often with a short duration of follow-up. Eight longitudinal studies with at least 10 patients and a follow-up of more than 3 years are summarized in Table 7 [381–392]. It appears from these studies that the ones employing standardized 4 h dwells in unselected patients followed from the start of CAPD found increases in D/P ratios

and MTAC of creatinine and reduced net ultrafiltration. The other studies that did not report this merely used peritoneal clearances. It is likely that in these studies the reduced ultrafiltration and the increased D/P ratios may have counteracted each other, thereby obscuring the effect of dialysis duration on the peritoneal membrane. No study has shown an increase or decrease in peritoneal total protein loss in relation with the duration of peritoneal dialysis [386, 387, 393–395]. When peritoneal clearances of individual serum proteins were examined, no effect of the time on peritoneal dialysis was found [319, 327, 396]. However, when the clearances of these proteins were used to calculate the peritoneal restriction coefficient for macromolecules (see section on size-selectivity), an increase of this parameter was found in long-term CAPD patients [88, 327]. Such an increase was not found in the restriction coefficient calculated on MTAC of low molecular weight solutes [88]. The increase in the restriction coefficient to macromolecules was not present after 2 years of CAPD [396], but was evident after 4 years [88, 327]. It points to an increased size-selectivity of the peritoneal membrane. Whether this is caused by a reduction in the average radius of the large pore system, or by interstitial changes, is unknown.

The alterations in peritoneal transport that can be found in long-term peritoneal dialysis patients are also present in a large proportion of those with peritoneal sclerosis [322, 397, 398]. This suggests that the peritoneal membrane changes that can be detected in long-term peritoneal dialysis may progress to peritoneal sclerosis. As far as the transport function is concerned, ultrafiltration failure, high

Table 7. Summary of published longitudinal studies on the effects of the duration of CAPD on peritoneal transport characteristics. Only studies with >10 patients and a follow-up >3 years were used

Year	Number of patients	Duration of follow-up (years)	Standardized 4 h dwell	Effect on low molecular weight solute transport	Effect on net ultrafiltration	Ref.
1986–98	90	17	yes	MTAC creat ↑ MTAC urea =	↓	381–385
1989	134	8	no	Cl creat ↑	=[a]	386
1990	35	5	no	MTAC creat =	=	387
1990	31	4	no	Cl creat =	=[a]	388
1990[b]	32	>3	no	Cl urea ↑	?	389
1992[b]	10	>5	no	Cl urea =	=	390
1994[b]	23	>7	no	D/P creat =	↓ or =[c]	391
1996	67	4	yes	D/P creat ↑	↓	392

[a]Some of the patients dropped out, because of ultrafiltration failure.
[b]Only patients were included who had survived 3, 5 or 7 years, and these were analysed retrospectively.
[c]A decreased ultrafiltration was found only in patients who had been treated with acetate-based dialysate in the past.

MTAC or D/P ratios of low molecular weight solutes and an increased restriction coefficient to macromolecules are the most prominent findings. These suggest the development of an increased vascular peritoneal surface area in combination with a reduced permeability or size-selectivity. The finding of an increased number of peritoneal microvessels in long-term peritoneal dialysis is in accordance with the peritoneal transport findings [340].

References

1. Wegener G. Chirurgische Bemerkungen über die peritoneale Hole, mit besondere Berucksichtigung der Ovariotomie. Arch Klin Chir 1877; 20: 51–9.
2. Putiloff PV. Materials for the study of the laws of growth of the human body in relation to the surface area: the trial on Russian subjects of planigraphic anatomy as a mean of exact anthropometry. Presented at the Siberian branch of the Russian Geographic Society, Omsk, 1886.
3. Esperanca MJ, Collins DL. Peritoneal dialysis efficiency in relation to body weight. J Paediatr Surg 1966; 1: 162–9.
4. Rubin JL, Clawson M, Planch A, Jones Q. Measurements of peritoneal surface area in man and rat. Am J Med Sci 1988; 245: 453–8.
5. Pawlaczyk K, Kuzlan M, Wieczorowska-Tobis K *et al.* Species-dependent topography of the peritoneum. Adv Perit Dial 1996; 12: 3–6.
6. Chagnac A, Herskovitz P, Hamel I, Weinstein T, Hirsch J, Gafter U. Measurement of the peritoneal membrane surface area (PMSA) in PD patients: further validation of the method. J Am Soc Nephrol 1998; 9: 190A (abstract).
7. Bell JL, Leypoldt JK, Frigon RP, Henderson LW. Hydraulically-induced convective solute transport across the rabbit peritoneum. Kidney Int 1990; 38: 19–27.
8. Rubin J, Jones Q, Planch A, Stanck K. Systems of membranes involved in peritoneal dialysis. J Lab Clin Med 1987; 110: 448–53.
9. Fox SD, Leypoldt JK, Henderson LW. Visceral peritoneum is not essential for solute transport during peritoneal dialysis. Kidney Int 1991; 40: 612–20.
10. Alon U, Bar-Maor JA, Bar-Joseph G. Effective peritoneal dialysis in an infant with extensive resection of the small intestine. Am J Nephrol 1988; 8: 65–7.
11. Flessner MF. Small solute transport across specific peritoneal tissue surfaces in the rat. J Am Soc Nephrol 1996; 7: 225–32.
12. Zakaria ER, Carlsson O, Sjunnesson H, Rippe B. Liver is not essential for solute transport during peritoneal dialysis. Kidney Int 1996; 50: 298–303.
13. Khanna R, Mactier R, Twardowski ZJ, Nolph KD. Peritoneal cavity lymphatics. Perit Dial Bull 1986; 6: 113–21.
14. Kuzlan M, Pawlaczyk K, Wieczorowska-Tobis K, Korybalska K, Breborowicz A, Oreopoulos DG. Peritoneal sarface area and its permeability in rats. Perit Dial Int 1997; 17: 295–300.
15. Granger DN, Ulrich M, Perry MA, Kvietys PR. Peritoneal dialysis solutions and feline splanchnic blood flow. Clin Exp Pharmacol Physiol 1984; 11: 473–82.
16. Rippe B, Stelin G, Haraldsson B. Understanding the kinetics of peritoneal transport. In: Hatano M, ed. Nephrology. Tokyo, Springer, 1991, pp. 1563–72.
17. Rippe B, Stelin G, Haraldsson B. Computer simulations of peritoneal fluid transport in CAPD. Kidney Int 1991; 40: 315–25.
18. Haraldsson B. Assessing the peritoneal dialysis capacities of individual patients. Kidney Int 1995; 47: 1187–98.
19. Douma CE, Imholz ALT, Struijk DG, Krediet RT. Similarities and differences between the effects of amino acids and nitroprusside on peritoneal permeability during CAPD. Blood Purif 1998; 16: 57–65.
20. Nolph KD, Miller F, Rubin J, Popovich R. New directions in peritoneal dialysis concepts and applications. Kidney Int 1980; 18 (suppl. 10): S111-16.
21. Flessner MF. Peritoneal transport physiology: insights from basic research. J Am Soc Nephrol 1991; 2: 122–35.
22. Nagel W, Kuschinsky W. Study of the permeability of the isolated dog mesentery. Eur J Clin Invest 1970; 1: 149–54.
23. Rasio EA. Metabolic control of permeability in isolated mesentery. Am J Physiol 1974; 226: 962–8.
24. Frokjaer-Jensen J, Christensen O. Potasium permeability of the mesothelium of frog mesentery. Acta Physiol Scand 1979; 105: 228–38.
25. Flessner MF, Dedrick RL, Schulz JS. Exchange of macromolecules between peritoneal cavity and plasma. Am J Physiol 1985; 248: H15–25.
26. Flessner MF, Fenstermacher JD, Blasberg RG, Dedrick RL. Peritoneal absorption of macromolecules stadied by quantitative autoradiography. Am J Physiol 1985; 248: H26–32.
27. Flessner MF. Osmotic barrier of the parental peritoneum. Am J Physiol 1994; 267 (Renal Fluid Electrolyte Physiol 36): F861–70.
28. Wiederhielm CA. The interstitial space. In: Fung YC, Perrone N, Andeker M, eds. Biomechanics: its foundations and objectives. Englewood Cliffs, NJ: Prentice-Hall, 1972, pp. 273–286.
29. Baron MA. Structure of the interstitial peritoneum in man. Am J Anat 1941; 69: 439–96.
30. Williams PL, Warwick R, Dyson M, Bannister CH. Gray's anatomy, 37th edn. Edinburgh: Churchill Livingstone, 1989, p. 1336.
31. Di Fiore MSH. Atlas of human histology. Philadelphia, PA: Lea and Febiger, 1981.
32. Flessner MF, Fenstermacher JD, Dedrick RL, Blasberg RG. A distributed model of peritoneal–plasma transport. Tissue concentration gradients. Am J Physiol 1985; 248: F425–35.
33. Fox JR, Wayland H. Interstitial diffusion of macromolecules in the rat mesentery. Microvasc Res 1979; 18: 255–76.
34. Grotte G. Passage of dextran molecules across the blood–lymph barrier. Acta Chir Scand 1956; 211 (suppl.): 1–84.
35. Mayerson HS, Wolfram CG, Shirley Jr HH, Wasserman K. Regional differences in capilairy permeability. Am J Physiol 1960; 198: 155–60.
36. Deen WM, Bridges CR, Brenner BM, Myers BD. Heteroporous model of glomerular size selectivity: application to normal and nephrotic humans. Am J Physiol 1985; 249: F374–89.
37. Renkin EM. Relation of capillary morphology to transport of fluid and large molecules: a review. Acta Physiol Scand 1979; 463 (suppl.): 81–91.
38. Bundgaard M. Transport pathways in capillaries; in search of pores. Annu Rev Physiol 1980; 42: 325–36.
39. Rippe B, Haraldsson B. Transport of macromolecules across microvascular walls: the two-pore theory. Physiol Rev 1994; 74: 163–219.
40. Karnovsky MJ. The ultrastructural basis of capillary permeability studied with peroxidase as a tracer. J Cell Biol 1967; 35: 213–36.
41. Rippe B, Haraldsson B. How are macromolecules transported across the capillary wall? News Physiol Sci 1987; 2: 135–8.
42. Simionescu N, Simionescu M, Palade GE. Permeability of muscle capillaries to exogenous myoglobin. J Cell Biol 1973; 57: 424–52.
43. Simionescu N, Simionescu M, Palade GE. Permeability of muscle capillaries to small heme-peptides. J Cell Biol 1975; 64: 586–607.
44. Haraldsson B, Johansson BR. Changes in transcapillary exchange induced by perfusion fixation with glutaraldehyde, followed by simultaneous measurements of capillary filtration

coefficient, diffusion capacity and albumin clearance. Acta Physiol Scand 1985; 124: 99–106.

45. Rippe B, Kamiya A, Folkow B. Transcapillary passage of albumin; effects of tissue cooling and of increases in filtration and plasma colloid osmotic pressure. Acta Physiol Scand 1979; 105: 171–87.

46. Frokjaer-Jensen J. Three-dimensional organization of plasmalemmal vesicles in endothelial cells. An analysis by serial sectioning of frog mesenteric capillaries. J Ultrastruct Res 1980; 73: 9–20.

47. Kohn S, Nagy JA, Dvorak HF, Dvorak AM. Pathways of macromolecular tracer transport across venules and small veins. Structural basis for the hyperpermeability of tumor blood vessels. Lab Invest 1992; 67: 596–607.

48. QuHong, Nagy JA, Senger Dr, Dvorak HF, Dvorak AM. Ultrastructural localization of vascular permeability factor/vascular endothelial growth factor (VPF/VEGF) to the abluminal plasma membrane and vesico-vacuolar organelles of tumor microvascular endothelium. J Histochem Cytochem 1995; 43: 381–9.

49. Dvorak HF, Brown LF, Detmar M, Dvorak AM. Vascular permeability factor/vascular endothelial growth factor, microvascular hypepermeability, and angiogenesis. Am J Pathol 1995; 146: 1029–39.

50. Fox J, Galey F, Wayland H. Action of histamine on the mesenteric microvasculature. Microvasc Res 1980; 19: 108–26.

51. Henderson LW. Peritoneal ultrafiltration dialysis: enhanced urea transfer using hypertonic peritoneal dialysis fluid. J Clin Invest 1966; 45: 950–5.

52. Nolph KD, Hano JE, Teschan PE. Peritoneal sodium transport during hypertonic peritoneal dialysis. Ann Intern Med 1969; 70: 931–41.

53. Rubin J, Klein E, Bower JD. Investigation of the net sieving coefficient of the peritoneal membrane during peritoneal dialysis. ASAIO J 1982; 5: 9–15.

54. Chen TW, Khanna R, Moore H, Twardowski ZJ, Nolph KD. Sieving and reflection coefficients for sodium salts and glucose during peritoneal dialysis. J Am Soc Nephrol 1991; 2: 1092–100.

55. Leypoldt JK, Blindauer KM. Peritoneal solvent drag reflection coefficients are within the physiological range. Blood Purif 1994; 12: 327–36.

56. Rippe B, Perry MA, Granger DN. Permselectivity of the peritoneal membrane. Microvasc Res 1985; 29: 89–102.

57. Krediet RT, Imholz ALT, Struijk DG, Koomen GCM, Arisz L. Ultrafiltration in continuous ambulatory peritoneal dialysis. Perit Dial Int; 1993; 13 (suppl. 2): S59–66.

58. Zakaria ER, Rippe B. Osmotic barrier properties of the rat peritoneal membrane. Acta Physiol Scand 1993; 149: 355–64.

59. Imholz ALT, Koomen GCM, Struijk DG, Arisz L, Krediet RT. Fluid and solute transport in CAPD patients using ultralow sodium dialysate. Kidney Int 1994; 46: 333–40.

60. Leypoldt JK. Interpreting peritoneal osmotic reflection coefficients using a distributed model of peritoneal transport. Adv Perit Dial 1993; 9: 3–7.

61. Rippe B, Stelin G. Simulations of peritoneal solute transport during CAPD. Application of two-pore formalism. Kidney Int 1989; 35: 1234–44.

62. Stelin G, Rippe B. A phenomenological interpretation of the variation in dialysate volume with dwell time in CAPD. Kidney Int 1990; 38: 465–72.

63. Ho-dac-Pannekeet MM, Schouten N, Langedijk MJ et al. Peritoneal transport characteristics with glucose polymer based dialysate. Kidney Int 1996; 50: 979–86.

64. Preston GM, Carroll TP, Guggino WB, Agre P. Appearance of water channels in *Xenopus* oocytes expressing red cell CHIP 28 protein. Science, Washington DC 1992; 256: 385–7.

65. Dempster JA, van Hoek AN, van Os CH. The quest for water channels. News Physiol Sci 1992; 7: 172–6.

66. Nielsen S, Agre P. The aquaporin family of water channels in the kidney. Kidney Int 1995; 48: 1057–68.

67. Agre P, Preston GM, Smith BL et al. Aquaporin CHIP: the archetypal molecular water channel. Am J Physiol 1993; 265: F463–76.

68. Pannekeet MM, Mulder JB, Weening JJ, Struijk DG, Zweers MM, Krediet RT. Demonstration of aquaporin-chip in peritoneal tissue of uremic and CAPD patients. Perit Dial Int 1996; 16 (suppl. 1): S54–7.

69. Hayakawa H, Hasegawa H, Takahashi H, Suzuki M. Kawaguchi Y, Sakai O. Participation of water channels in peritoneal water transport. J Am Soc Nephrol 1995; 6: 511A (abstract).

70. Akiba P, Ota T, Fushimi K et al. Water channel APQP1, 3 and 4 in the human peritoneum and peritoneal dialysate. Adv Perit Dial 1997; 13: 3–5.

71. Goffin E, Combet S, Jamar F, Cosyns J-P, Devuyst O. Expression of aquaporin-1 (AQP1) in a long-term peritoneal dialysis patient with impaired transcellular water transport. Am J Kidney Dis 1999; 33: 383–8.

72. Ho-dac-Pannekeet MM, Krediet RT. Water channels in the peritoneum. Perit Dial Int 1996; 16: 255–9.

73. Krepper MA. The aquaporin family of molecular water channels. Proc Natl Acad Sci USA 1994; 91: 6255–8.

74. Carlsson O, Nielsen S, Zakaria ER, Rippe B. *In vivo* inhibition of transcellular water channels (aquaporin-1) during acute peritoneal dialysis in rats. Am J Physiol 1996; 271 (Heart Circ Physiol 40): H2254–62.

75. Zweers MM, Douma CE, van der Wardt AB, Krediet RT, Struijk DG. Amphotericin B, HgCl₂ and peritoneal transport in rabbits. Perit Dial Int 1998: 18: 141 (abstract).

76. Krediet RT, Zuyderhoudt FMJ, Boeschoten EW, Arisz L. Alterations in the peritoneal transport of water and solutes during peritonitis in continuous ambulatory peritoneal dialysis patients. Eur J Clin Invest 1987; 17: 43–52.

77. Krediet RT, Boeschoten EW, Struijk DG, Arisz L. Differences in the peritoneal transport of water, solutes and proteins between dialysis with two- and with three-litre exchanges. Nephrol Dial Transplant 1988; 2: 198–204.

78. Lasrich M, Maher JM, Hirszel P, Maher JF. Correlation of peritoneal transport rates with molecular weight: a method for predicting clearances. ASAIO J 1979; 2: 107–13.

79. Nolph KD, Ghods A, Brown P et al.Effects of nitroprusside on peritoneal mass transfer coefficients and microvascular physiology. Trans Am Soc Artif Intern Organs 1977; 23: 210–18.

80. Pietrzak I, Hirszel P, Shostak A, Welch PG, Lee RE, Maher JF. Splanchnic volume, not flow rate, determines peritoneal permeability. Trans Am Soc Artif Intern Organs 1989; 35: 583–7.

81. Leypoldt JK, Frigon RP, De Vore KW, Henderson LW. A rapid renal clearance methodology for dextran. Kidney Int 1987; 31: 855–60.

82. Granath KA, Kvist BE. Molecular weight distribution analysis by gel chromatography on sephadex. J Chromatogr 1967; 28: 69–81.

83. Krediet RT, Struijk DG, Zemel D, Koomen GCM, Arisz L. The transport of macromolecules across the human peritoneum during CAPD. In: La Greca G, Ronco C, Feriani M, Chiaramonte S, Conz P, eds. Peritoneal Dialysis. Milan: Wichtig Ed., 1991, pp. 61–9.

84. Zemel D, Krediet RT, Koomen GCM, Struijk DG, Arisz L. Day-to-day variability of protein transport used as a method for analyzing peritoneal permeability in CAPD. Perit Dial Int 1991; 11: 217–23.

85. Krediet RT, Zemel D, Struijk DG, Koomen GCM, Arisz L. Individual characterization of the peritoneal restriction barrier to the transport of serum proteins. In: Ota K. Maher JF, Winchester JF, et al., eds. Current Concepts in Peritoneal Dialysis. Amsterdam: Excerpta Medica, 1992, pp. 49–55.

86. Krediet RT, Zemel D, Struijk DG, Koomen GCM, Arisz L. Individual characterization of the peritoneal restriction barrier to macromolecules. Adv Perit Dial 1991; 7: 15–20.

87. Imholz ALT, Koomen GCM, Struijk DG, Arisz L, Krediet RT. The effect of dialysate osmolarity on the transport of low molecular weight solutes and proteins during CAPD. Kidney Int 1993; 43: 1339–46.

88. Ho-dac-Pannekeet MM, Koopmans JG, Struijk DG, Krediet RT. Restriction coefficients of low molecular weight solutes and macromolecules during peritoneal dialysis. Adv Perit Dial 1997; 13: 17–22.

89. Van den Born J, Van den Heuvel LPWJ, Bakker MAH, Veerkamp JH, Assmann KJ, Berden JHM. A monoclonal antibody against GBM heparan sulfate induces an acute selective proteinuria in rats. Kidney Int 1992; 41: 115–23.

90. Gotloib L, Bar-Sella P, Jaichenko J, Shustack A. Ruthenium-red-stained polyanionic fixed charges in peritoneal microvessels. Nephron 1987; 47: 22–8.

91. Galdi P, Shostak A, Jaichenko J, Fudin R, Gotloib L. Protamine sulfate induces enhanced peritoneal permeability to proteins. Nephron 1991; 57: 45–51.

92. Alavi N, Lianos E, Andres G, Bentzel CJ. Effect of protamine on the permeability and structure of rat peritoneum. Kidney Int 1982; 21: 44–53.

93. Krediet RT, Koomen GCM, Koopman MG et al. The peritoneal transport of serum proteins and neutral dextran in CAPD patients. Kidney Int 1989; 35: 1064–72.

94. Leypoldt JK, Henderson LW. Molecular charge influences transperitoneal macromolecule transport. Kidney Int 1993; 43: 837–44.

95. Krediet RT, Struijk DG, Koomen GCM et al. Peritoneal transport of macromolecules in patients on CAPD. Contrib Nephrol 1991; 89: 161–74.

96. Buis B, Koomen GCM, Imholz ALT et al. Effect of electric charge on the transperitoneal transport of plasma proteins during CAPD. Nephrol Dial Transplant 1996; 11: 1113–20.

97. Haraldsson B. The peritoneal membrane acts as a negatively charged barrier restricting anionic proteins. J Am Soc Nephrol 1993; 4: 407 (abstract).

98. Gotloib L, Shustuk A, Jaichenko J. Loss of mesothelial electronegative fixed charges during murine septic peritonitis. Nephron 1989; 51: 77–83.

99. Vernier RL, Steffels MW, Sisson-Ros S, Mauen SM. Heparan sulfate proteoglycan in the glomerular basement membrane in type 1 diabetes mellitus. Kidney Int 1992; 41: 1070–80.

100. Tamsma JT, Van den Born J, Bruijn JA et al. Expression of glomerular extracellular matrix components in human diabetic nephropathy: decrease of heparan sulphate in the glomerular basement membrane. Diabetologia 1994; 37: 313–20.

101. Bradley SE. Variations in hepatic flow in man during health and disease. N Engl J Med 1949; 240: 456–61

102. Aune S. Transperitoneal exchange. Peritoneal blood flow estimated by hydrogen gas clearance. Scand J Gastroenterol 1970; 5: 99–104.

103. Grzegorzewska AE, Moore HL, Nolph KD, Chen TW. Ultrafiltration and effective peritoneal blood flow during peritoneal dialysis in the rat. Kidney Int 1991; 39: 608–17.

104. Erbe RW, Greene Jr JA, Weller JM. Peritoneal dialysis during hemorrhagic shock. J Appl Physiol 1967; 22: 131–5.

105. Greene Jr JA, Lapco L, Weller JM. Effect of drug therapy of hemorrhagic hypotension on kinetics of peritoneal dialysis in the dog. Nephron 1970; 7: 178–83.

106. Felt J, Richard C, McCaffrey C, Levy M. Peritoneal clearance of creatinine and inulin during dialysis in dogs: effect of splanchnic vasodilators. Kidney Int 1979; 16: 459–69.

107. Kim M, Lofthouse J, Flessner MF. A method to test blood flow limitation of peritoneal blood solute transport. J Am Soc Nephrol 1997; 8: 471–4.

108. Kim M, Lofthouse J, Flessner MF. Blood flow limitations of solute transport across the visceral peritoneum. J Am Soc Nephrol 1997; 8: 1946–50.

109. Maher JF. Transport kinetics in peritoneal dialysis. Perit Dial Bull 1983 (suppl.): S4–6.

110. Nolph KD, Popovich RP, Ghods AJ, Twardowski ZJ. Determinants of low clearances of small solutes during peritoneal dialysis. Kidney Int 1978; 13: 117–23.

111. Grzegorzewska AE, Antoniewicz K. An indirect estimation of effective peritoneal capillary blood flow in peritoneally dialyzed uremic patients. Perit Dial Int 1993; 13 (suppl. 2): S39–40.

112. Douma CE, De Waart DR, Struijk DG, Krediet RT. Effect of aminoacid based dialysate on peritoneal blood flow and permeability in stable CAPD patients: a potential role for nitric oxide? Clin Nephrol 1996; 5: 295–302.

113. Douma CE, De Waart DR, Struijk DG, Krediet RT. The nitric oxide donor nitroprusside intraperitoneally affects peritoneal permeability in CAPD. Kidney Int 1997; 51: 1885–92.

114. Douma CE, De Waart DR, Struijk DG, Krediet RT. Are phospholipase A_2 and nitric oxide involved in the alterations in peritoneal transport during CAPD peritonitis? J Lab Clin Med 1998; 132: 329–40.

115. Ronco C, Brendolan A, Braglantini L et al. Studies on ultrafiltration in peritoneal dialysis: influence of plasma proteins and capillary blood flow. Perit Dial Bull 1986; 6: 93–7.

116. Ronco G, Feriani M, Chiaramonte S et al. Pathophysiology of ultrafiltration in peritoneal dialysis. Perit Dial Int 1990; 10: 119–26.

117. Ronco C, Brendolan A, Crepaldi C et al. Ultrafiltration and clearance studies in human isolated peritoneal vascular loops. Blood Purif 1994; 12: 233–42.

118. Ronco C, Feriani M, Chiaramonte S, Brendolan A, Milan M, La Graeca G. Peritoneal blood flow: does it matter? Perit Dial Int 1996; 16 (suppl. 1): S70–5.

119. Ronco C. The 'nearest capillary' hypothesis: a novel approach to peritoneal transport physiology. Perit Dial Int 1996; 16: 121–5.

120. Malach M. Peritoneal dialysis for intractable heart failure in acute myocardial infarction. Am J Cardiol 1972; 29: 61–3.

121. Grzegorzewska AE, Antoniewicz K. Peritoneal blood flow and peritoneal transfer parameters during dialysis with administration of drugs. Adv Perit Dial 1995; 11: 28–32.

122. Raja RM, Krasnoff O, Moros JG et al. Repeated peritoneal dialysis in the treatment of heart failure. J Am Med Assoc 1970; 213: 1533–5.

123. Kim D, Khanna R, Wu G, Fountas P, Druck M, Oreopoulos DG. Successful use of continuous ambulatory peritoneal dialysis in refractory heart failure. Perit Dial Bull 1985; 5: 127–30.

124. Rubin J, Ball R. CAPD as treatment of severe congestive heart failure in the face of chronic renal failure. Arch Intern Med 1986; 146: 1533–5.

125. Stegmayr BG, Banga R, Lundberg L, Wikdahl A-M, Plum-Wirell M. PD treatment for severe congestive heart failure. Perit Dial Int 1996; 16 (suppl. 1): S231–5.

126. Ryckelynck J-P, Lobbedez T, Valette B et al. Peritoneal ultrafiltration and refractory congestive heart failure. Adv Perit Dial 1997; 13: 93–7.

127. Durant P-Y, Bénévent D, Issad B, Chanliau J, Kessler M. Peritoneal dialysis in 15 cirrhotic patients with chronic renal failure: long term study. Perit Dial Int 1997; 17 (suppl. 1): S59 (abstract).

128. Crissinger KD, Granger DN. Gastrointestinal blood flow. In: Yamada T, ed. Textbook of Gastroenterology. Philadelphia, PA: Lippincott, 1991, pp. 447–74.

129. Brandt JL, Castleman L, Ruskin HD, Greenwald J, Kelly JJ Jr, Jones A. The effect of oral protein and glucose feeding on splanchnic blood flow and oxygen utilization in normal and cirrhotic subjects. J Clin Invest 1955; 34: 1017–25.

130. Rocha E, Silva M, Rosenberg M. The release of vasopressin in response to haemorrhage and its role in the mechanism of blood pressure regulation. J Physiol (Lond) 1969; 202: 535–57.

131. Suvannapara A, Levens NR. Local control of mesenteric blood flow by the renin–angiotensin system. Am J Physiol 1988; 225: G267–74.

132. Rayford PL, Miller TA, Thompson J. Secretin, cholecysto-kinin and newer gastrointestinal hormones. N Engl J Med 1976; 244: 1093–100.

133. Wade OL, Combes B, Childs AW, Wheeles HO, Cournand A, Bradley SE. The effect of exercise on the splanchnic blood flow and splanchnic blood volume in normal man. Clin Sci 1956; 15: 457–63.

134. Selgas R, Munoz IM, Conesa J et al. Endogenous sympathetic activity in CAPD patients: its relationship to peritoneal diffusion capacity. Perit Dial Bull 1986; 6: 205–8.

135. Ratge D, Augustin R, Wisser H. Plasma catecholamines and α- and β-adrenoceptors in circulating blood cells in patients on continuous ambulatory peritoneal dialysis. Clin Nephrol 1987; 28: 15–21.

136. Zabetakis PM, Kumar DN, Gleim GW et al. Increased levels of plasma renin, aldosterone, catecholamines and vasopressin in chronic ambulatory peritoneal dialysis (CAPD) patients. Clin Nephrol 1987; 28: 147–51.

137. Steinhauer HB, Grünter B, Schollmeyer P. Stimulation of peritoneal synthesis of vasoactive prostaglandins during peritonitis in patients on continuous ambulatory peritoneal dialysis. Eur J Clin Invest 1985; 15: 1–15.

138. Steinhauer HB, Günter B, Schollmeyer P. Enhanced peritoneal generation of vasoactive prostaglandins during peritonitis in patients undergoing CAPD. In: Maher JF, Winchester JF, eds. Frontiers in Peritoneal Dialysis. New York: Field, Rich, 1986, pp. 604–9.

139. Steinhauer HB, Schollmeyer P. Prostaglandin-mediated loss of proteins during peritonitis in continuous ambulatory peritoneal dialysis. Kidney Int 1986; 29: 584–90.

140. Hain H, Jorres A, Gahl M, Pustelnik A, Müller C, Köttgen E. Peritoneal permeability for proteins in uninfected CAPD patients: a kinetic study. In: Ota K et al., eds. Current Concepts in Peritoneal Dialysis. Amsterdam: Excerpta Medica, 1992, pp. 59–66.

141. Zemel D, Imholz ALT, De Waart DR, Dinkla C, Struijk DG, Krediet RT. Appearance of tumor necrosis factor α and soluble TNF-receptors I and II in peritoneal effluent of CAPD. Kidney Int 1994; 46: 1422–30.

142. Shaldon S, Koch KM, Quellhorst E, Dinarello CA. Hazards of CAPD: interleukin-1 production. In: Maher JF, Winchester JF, eds. Frontiers in Peritoneal Dialysis. New York: Field, Rich, 1986, pp. 630–3.

143. Shaldon S, Dinarello CA, Wyler DJ. Induction of interleukin-1 during CAPD. Contr Nephrol 1987; 57: 207–12.

144. Goldman M, Vandenabeele P, Moulart J et al. Intraperitoneal secretion of interleukin-6 during continuous ambulatory peritoneal dialysis. Nephron 1990; 56: 277–80.

145. Zemel D, ten Berge RJM, Struijk DG, Bloemena E, Koomen GCM, Krediet RT. Interleukin-6 in CAPD patients without peritonitis: relationship to the intrinsic permeability of the peritoneal membrane. Clin Nephrol 1992; 37: 97–103.

146. Lin CY, Lin CC, Huang TP. Several changes of interleukin-6 and interleukin-8 levels in drain dialysate of uremic patients with continuous ambulatory peritoneal dialysis during peritonitis. Nephron 1993; 63: 404–8.

147. Zemel D, Koomen GCM, Hart AAM, ten Berge RJM, Struijk DG, Krediet RT. Relationships of THFα, interleukin-6 and prostoglandins to peritoneal permeability for macromolecules during longitudinal follow-up of peritonitis in continuous ambulatory peritoneal dialysis. J Lab Clin Med 1993; 122: 686–96.

148. Zemel D, Struijk DG, Dinkla C, Stolk LM, ten Berge RJM, Krediet RT. Effects of intraperitoneal cyclooxygenase inhibition in inflammatory mediators in dialysate and peritoneal membrane characteristics during peritonitis in continuous ambulatory peritoneal dialysis. J Lab Clin Med 1995; 126: 204–15.

149. Douma CE. Nitric oxide and peritoneal permeability in peritoneal dialysis. Thesis. University of Amsterdam, 1997: 105–14.

150. Zemel D, Krediet RT. Cytokine patterns in the effluent of continuous ambulatory peritoneal dialysis: relationship to peritoneal permeability. Blood Purif 1996; 14: 198–216.

151. Ho-dac-Pannekeet MM, Krediet RT. Inflammatory changes *in vivo* during CAPD: what can the effluent tell us? Kidney Int 1996; 50 (suppl. 56): S12–16.

152. Douma CE, De Waart DR, Zemel D et al. Nitrate in stable CAPD patients and during peritonitis. Adv Perit Dial 1995; 11: 36–40.

153. Yang CW, Hwang TL, Wu CH et al. Peritoneal nitric oxide is a marker of peritonitis in patients on continuous ambulatory peritoneal dialysis. Nephrol Dial Transplant 1996; 11: 2466–71.

154. Miller FN. Effects of peritoneal dialysis on rat microcirculation and peritoneal clearances in man. Dial Transplant 1978; 7: 818–38.

155. Miller FN. The peritoneal microcirculation. In: Nolph KD, ed. Peritoneal Dialysis, 2nd edn. Boston, MA: Nijhoff, 1985, pp. 51–93.

156. Miller FN, Nolph KD, Joshua IG, Wiegman DL, Harris PD, Andersen DB. Hyperosmolality, acetate, and lactate: dilatory factors during peritoneal dialysis. Kidney Int 1981; 20: 397–402.

157. Miller FN, Nolph KD, Joshua IG. The osmolality component of peritoneal dialysis solutions. In: Legrain M, ed. Continuous Ambulatory Peritoneal Dialysis. Amsterdam: Excerpta Medica, 1980, pp. 12–17.

158. Rubin J, Nolph KD, Arfania D et al. Clinical studies with a nonvasoactive peritoneal dialysis solution. J Lab Clin Med 1979; 93: 910–15.

159. Miller FN, Nolph KD, Sorkin ML, Gloor HJ. The influence of solute composition on protein loss during peritoneal dialysis. Kidney Int 1983; 23: 35–9.

160. Struijk DG, Krediet RT, Imholz ALT, Koomen GCM, Arisz L. Fluid kinetics in CAPD patients during dialysis with a bicarbonate based hypoosmolar solution. Blood Purif 1996; 14: 217–26.

161. Feriani M, Dissegna D, La Graeca G, Passlick-Deetjen J. Short-term clinical study with bicarbonate-containing peritoneal dialysis solution. Perit Dial Int 1993; 13: 296–301.

162. Passlick-Deetjen J, Kirchgessner J. Bicarbonate: the alternative buffer for peritoneal dialysis. Perit Dial Int 1996; 16 (suppl. 1): S109–13.

163. Coles GA, Gokal R, Ogg C et al. A randomized controlled trial of a bicarbonate- and a bicarbonate/lactate-containing dialysis solution in CAPD. Perit Dial Int 1997; 17: 48–51.

164. Plum J, Fuszhöller A, Schoenicke G et al. *In vivo* and *in vitro* effects of amino-acid-based and bicarbonate-buffered peritoneal dialysis solutions with regard to peritoneal transport and cytokines/prostanoids dialysate concentrations. Nephrol Dial Transplant 1997; 12: 1652–60.

165. Coles GA, O'Donoghue DJ, Prichard N et al. A controlled trial of two bicarbonate-containing dialysis fluids for CAPD – Final report. Nephrol Dial Transplant 1998; 13: 3165–71.

166. Graf H, Stumvoll HK, Luger A, Prager R. Effects of amino acid infusion on glomerular filtration rate. N Engl J Med 1983; 308: 159–60.

167. Ter Wee PM, Geerlings W, Rosman JB, Sluiter WJ, Van der Geest E, Donker AJM. Testing renal reserve filtration capacity with an amino acid solution. Nephron 1985; 41: 193–9.

168. Tolins JP, Raij L. Effects of amino acid infusion on renal hemodynamics. Role of endothelium-derived relaxing factor. Hypertension 1991; 17: 1045–51.

169. Krediet RT, Douma CE, Ho-dac-Pannekeet MM et al. Impact of different dialysis solutions on solute and water transport. Perit Dial Int 1997; 17 (suppl. 2): S17–26.

170. Lindholm B, Werynski A, Bergström J. Peritoneal dialysis with aminoacid solutions: fluid and solute transport kinetics. Artif Org 1988; 12: 2–10.

171. Goodship THJ, Lloyd S, McKenzie PW *et al*. Short-term studies on the use of amino acids as an osmotic agent in continuous ambulatory peritoneal dialysis. Clin Sci 1987; 73: 471–8.

172. Bruno M, Bagnis C, Marangella M, Rovera L, Cantaluppi A, Linari F. CAPD with an amino acid dialysis solution: a long-term cross-over study. Kidney Int 1989; 35: 1189–94.

173. Young GA, Dibble JB, Taylor AE, Kendall S, Brownjohn AM. A longitudinal study of the effects of amino acid-based CAPD fluid on amino acid solution and protein losses. Nephrol Dial Transplant 1989; 4: 900–5.

174. Steinhauwer HB, Lubrick-Birkner I, Kluthe R, Baumann G, Schollmeyer P. Effect of amino-acid based dialysis solution on peritoneal permeability and prostanoid generation in patients undergoing continuous ambulatory peritoneal dialysis. Am J Nephrol 1991; 12: 61–7.

175. Steinhauer HB, Lubrich-Birkner I, Kluthe R, Hörl WH, Schollmeyer P. Amino acid dialysate stimulator prostaglandin E$_2$ generation in humans. Adv Perit Dial 1988; 4: 21–6.

176. Waniewski J, Werynski A, Heimbürger O, Park MS, Lindholm B. Effects of alternative osmotic agents on peritoneal transport. Blood Purif 1993; 11: 248–64.

177. Mistry CD, O'Donoghue DJ, Nelson S, Gokal R, Ballardi FW. Kinetic and clinical studies of β$_2$-microglobulin in continuous ambulatory peritoneal dialysis: influence of renal and enhanced peritoneal clearances using glucose polymer. Nephrol Dial Transplant 1990; 5: 513–19.

178. Imholz ALT, Brown CB, Koomen GCM, Arisz L, Krediet RT. The effects of glucose polymers on water removal and protein clearances during CAPD. Adv Perit Dial 1993; 9: 25–30.

179. Krediet RT, Douma CB, Imholz ALT, Koomen GCM. Protein clearance and icodextrin. Perit Dial Int 194; 14 (suppl. 2): S39–44.

180. Hirzsel P, Lasrich M, Maher JF. Augmentation of peritoneal mass transport by dopamine. J Lab Clin Invest 1979; 94: 747–54.

181. Hirzsel P, Maher JF, Le Grow W. Increased peritoneal mass transport with glucagon acting at the vascular surface. Trans Am Soc Artif Intern Organs 1978; 24: 136–8.

182. Maher JF, Hirzsel P, Lasrich M. Effects of gastrointestinal hormones on transport by peritoneal dialysis. Kidney Int 1979; 16: 130–6.

183. Felt J, Richard C, McCaffrey C, Levy M. Peritoneal clearance of creatinine and inulin during dialysis in dogs: effect of splanchnic vasodilators. Kidney Int 1979; 16: 459–69.

184. Hare HG, Valtin H, Gosselin RE. Effect of drugs on peritoneal dialysis in the dog. J Pharmacol Exp Ther 1964; 145: 122–9.

185. Henderson LW, Kintzel JE. Influence of antidiuretic hormone on peritoneal membrane area and permeability. J Clin Invest 1971; 40: 2437–43.

186. Fox J, Galey F, Wayland H. Action of histamine on the mesenteric microvasculature. Microvasc Res 1980; 19: 108–26.

187. Miller FN, Joshua IG, Anderson GL. Quantitation of vasodilator-induced macromolecular leakage by *in vivo* fluorescent microscopy. Microvasc Res 1982; 24: 56–67.

188. Brown EA, Kliger AS, Goffinet J, Finkelstein FO. Effect of hypertonic dialysate and vasodilators on peritoneal dialysis clearances in the rat. Kidney Int 1978; 13: 271–7.

189. Shostak A, Chakrabarti E, Hirzsel P, Maher JF. Effects of histamine and its receptor antagonists on peritoneal permeability. Kidney Int 1988; 34: 786–90.

190. Maher JF, Hirzsel P, Lasrich M. Modulation of peritoneal transport rates by prostaglandins. Adv Prostagland Thrombox Res 1980; 7: 695–700.

191. Hirzsel P, Lasrich M, Maher JF. Arachidonic acid increases peritoneal clearances. Trans Am Soc Artif Intern Organs 1981; 27: 61–3.

192. Maher JF, Hirzsel P, Lasrich M. Prostaglandin effects on peritoneal transport. In: Gahl GM, Kessel M, Nolph KD, eds. Advances in Peritoneal Dialysis. Amsterdam: Excerpta Medica, 1981, pp. 64–9.

193. Nolph KD, Ghods AJ, Van Stone J, Brown PA. The effects of intraperitoneal vasodilators on peritoneal clearances. ASAIO Trans 1976; 22: 586–94.

194. Nolph KD, Ghods AJ, Brown PA *et al*. Effects of nitroprusside on peritoneal mass transfer coefficients and microvascular physiology. ASAIO Trans 1977; 23: 210–18.

195. Nolph KD, Ghods AJ, Brown PA, Twardowski ZJ. Effects of intraperitoneal nitropusside on peritoneal clearances in man with variation in dose, frequency of administration and dwell times. Nephron 1979; 24: 114–20.

196. Lee HB, Park MS, Chung SH *et al*. Peritoneal solute clearances in diabetics. Perit Dial Int 1990; 10: 85–8.

197. Miller FN, Joshua IG, Harris PD, Wiegman DL, Jauchem JR. Peritoneal dialysis solutions and the microcirculation. Contrib Nephrol 1979; 17: 51–58.

198. Douma CE, Zweers MM, De Waart DR, Van der Wardt AB, Krediet RT, Struijk DG. Substrate and inhibitor for nitric oxide synthase during peritoneal dialysis in rabbits. Perit Dial Int 1999; 19 (suppl 2): S358–64.

199. Curatola G, Zoccali C, Crucitti S *et al*. Effect of posture on peritoneal clearance in CAPD patients. Perit Dial Int 1988; 8: 58–9.

200. Imholz ALT, Koomen GCM, Voorn WJ, Struijk DG, Arisz L, Krediet RT. Day-to-day variability of fluid and solute transport in upright and recumbent positions during CAPD. Nephrol Dial Transplant 1998; 13: 146–53.

201. Zanozi S, Winchester JF, Kloberdanz N *et al*. Upright position and exercise lower peritoneal transport rates. Kidney Int 1983; 23: 165.

202. Otero A, Esteban J, Canovas L. Does posture modify solute transport in CAPD? Perit Dial Int 1992; 12: 399–400.

203. Imholz ALT, Koomen GCM, Struijk DG, Arisz L, Krediet RT. Effect of increased intraperitoneal pressure on fluid and solute transport during CAPD. Kidney Int 1993; 44: 1078–85.

204. Flessner MF, Dedrick RL, Schultz JS. A distributed model of peritoneal plasma transport: theoretical considerations. Am J Physiol 1984; 246: R597–607.

205. Seasmes EL, Moncrief JW, Popovich RP. A distributed model of fluid and mass transfer in peritoneal dialysis. Am J Physiol 1990; 258: 958–72.

206. Lysaght MJ, Farrell PC. Membrane phenomena and mass transfer kinetics in peritoneal dialysis. J Membr Sci 1984; 44: 5–53.

207. Popovich RP, Moncrief JW. Kinetic modeling of peritoneal transport. Contr Nephrol 1974; 17: 59–72.

208. Pyle WK, Popovich RP, Moncrief JW. Mass transfer in peritoneal dialysis. In: Gahl GM, Kessel M, Nolph KD, eds. Advances in Peritoneal Dialysis. Amsterdam: Excerpta Medica, 1981, pp. 41–6.

209. Pyle WK. Mass transfer in peritoneal dialysis. Thesis, University of Texas at Austin, University Microfilms International, Ann Arbor, Michigan, 1982.

210. Randersson DH, Farrell P. Mass transfer properties of the human peritoneum. ASAIO J 1980; 3: 140–6.

211. Smeby LC, Wideroe T-E, Jorstad S. Individual differences in water transport during continuous peritoneal dialysis. ASAIO J 1981; 4: 17–27.

212. Henderson LW, Nolph KD. Altered permeability of the peritoneal membrane after using hypertonic peritoneal dialysis fluid. J Clin Invest 1969; 48: 992–1001.

213. Lindholm B, Werynski A, Bergström J. Kinetics of peritoneal dialysis with glycerol and glucose as osmotic agents. ASAIO Trans 1987; 33: 19–27.

214. Garred LJ, Canaud B, Farrell PC. A simple kinetic model for assessing peritoneal mass transfer in chronic ambulatory peritoneal dialysis. ASAIO J 1983; 6: 131–7.

215. Krediet RT, Boeschoten EW, Zuyderhoudt FMJ, Strackee J, Arisz L. Simple assessment of the efficacy of peritoneal trans-

port in continuous ambulatory peritoneal dialysis patients. Blood Purif 1986; 4: 194–203.

216. Waniewski J, Werynski A, Heimbürger O, Lindholm B. Simple models for description of small solute transport in peritoneal dialysis. Blood Purif 1991; 9: 129–41.

217. Waniewski J, Heimbürger O, Werynski A, Lindholm B. Aqueous solute concentrations and evaluation of mass transport coefficients in peritoneal dialysis. Nephrol Dial Transplant 1992; 7: 50–6.

218. Lindholm B, Werynski A, Bergström J. Kinetics of peritoneal dialysis with glycerol and glucose as osmotic agents. ASAIO Trans 1987; 10: 19–27.

219. Heimbürger O, Waniewski J, Werynski A, Traneaus A, Lindholm B. Peritoneal transport in CAPD patients with permanent loss of ultrafiltration capacity. Kidney Int 1990; 38: 495–506.

220. Rubin J, Nolph KD, Arfania D, Brown P, Prowant B. Follow-up of peritoneal clearances in patients undergoing continuous ambulatory peritoneal dialysis. Kidney Int 1979; 16: 619–23.

221. Heimbürger O, Waniewski J, Werynski A, Park MS, Lindholm B. Dialysate to plasma solute concentration (D/P) versus peritoneal transport parameters in CAPD. Nephrol Dial Transplant 1994; 9: 47–59.

222. Pannekeet MM, Imholz ALT, Struijk DG et al. The standard peritoneal permeability analysis: a tool for the assessment of peritoneal permeability characteristics in CAPD patients. Kidney Int 1995; 48: 866–75.

223. Davies SJ, Brown B, Bryan J, Russel GI. Clinical evaluation of the peritoneal equilibration test: a population-based study. Nephrol Dial Transplant 1993; 8: 64–70.

224. Nolph KD. Clinical implications of membrane transport characteristics on the adequacy of fluid and solute removal. Perit Dial Int 1994; 14 (suppl. 3): S78–81.

225. Twardowski ZJ, Nolph KD, Khanna R et al. Peritoneal equilibration test. Perit Dial Bull 1987; 7: 138–47.

226. Nolph KD, Twardowski ZJ, Popovich RP, Rubin J. Equilibration of peritoneal dialysis solutions during long-dwell exchanges. J Lab Clin Med 1979; 93: 246–56.

227. Heimbürger O, Waniewski J, Werynski A, Lindholm B. A quantitative description of solute and fluid transport during peritoneal dialysis. Kidney Int 1992; 41: 1320–32.

228. Canaud B, Liendo-Liendo C, Claret G, Mion H, Mion C. Etude 'in situ' de la cinétique de l'ultrafiltration en cours de dialyse péritoneale avec périodes de diffusion prolongé. Néphrologie 1980; 1: 126–32.

229. Wang T, Waniewski J, Heimbürger O, Werynski A, Lindholm B. A quantitative analysis of sodium transport and removal during peritoneal dialysis. Kidney Int 1997; 52: 1609–16.

230. Raja RM, Cantor RE, Boreyko C, Bushehri H, Kramer MS, Rosenbaum JL. Sodium transport during ultrafiltration peritoneal dialysis. Trans Amer Soc Artif Intern Organs 1972; 18: 429–33.

231. Nolph KD, Hano JE, Teschan PE. Peritoneal sodium transport during hypertonic peritoneal dialysis. Ann Intern Med 1989; 70: 931–41.

232. Leypoldt JK, Charney DI, Cheung AK, Naprestek CL, Akin BH, Shockley TR. Ultrafiltration and solute kinetics using low sodium peritoneal dialysate. Kidney Int 1995; 48: 1959–66.

233. Stryer L. Biochemistry, 2nd edn. Freeman, San Francisco, CA: Freeman, 1981, p. 205.

234. Nakayama M, Yokoyama K, Kubo H et al. The effect of ultra-low sodium dialysate in CAPD. A kinetic and clinical analysis. Clin Nephrol 1996; 45: 188–93.

235. Brown ST, Ahearn J, Nolph KD. Potassium removal with peritoneal dialysis. Kidney Int 1973; 4: 67–9.

236. Merchant MR, Hutchinson AJ, Butler SJ, Boulton H, Hincliffe R, Gokal R. Calcium, magnesium mass transfer and lactate balance study in CAPD patients with reduced calcium/magnesium and high lactate dialysis fluid. Adv Perit Dial 1992; 8: 365–8.

237. Martis L, Serkes KD, Nolph KD. Calcium carbonate as a phosphate binder: is there a need to adjust peritoneal dialysate calcium concentrations for patients using $CaCO_3$? Perit Dial Int 1989; 9: 325–8.

238. Richardson RMA, Roscoe JM. Bicarbonate, L-lactate and D-lactate balance in intermittent peritoneal dialysis. Perit Dial Bull 1986; 6: 178–85.

239. Uribarri J, Buquing J, Oh MS. Acid–base balance in chronic peritoneal dialysis patients. Kidney Int 1995; 47: 269–73.

240. Feriani M. Adequacy of acid–base correction in continuous ambulatory peritoneal dialysis patients. Perit Dial Int 1994; 14 (suppl. 3): S133–8.

241. Feriani M, Ronco C. La Graeca G. Acid–base balance with different CAPD solutions. Perit Dial Int 1996; 16 (suppl. 1): S126–9.

242. Krediet RT, Zuyderhoudt FMJ, Boeschoten EW, Arisz L. Peritoneal permeability to proteins in diabetic and non-diabetic continuous ambulatory peritoneal dialysis patients. Nephron 1986; 42: 133–40.

243. Bonomini V, Zucchelli P, Mioli V. Selective and unselective protein loss in peritoneal dialysis. Proc Eur Dial Transplant Assoc 1967; 4: 146–9.

244. Taylor AE, Granger DN. Exchange of macromolecules across the microcirculation. In: Renkin EM, Michell CC, eds. Handbook of Physiology. Section 2: The Cardiovascular System. Bethesda, Maryland: American Physiological Society, 1984, pp. 467–520.

245. Rippe B, Haraldsson B. Fluid and protein fluxes across small and large pores in the microvasculature. Applications of two-pore equations. Acta Physiol Scand 1987; 131: 411–28.

246. Nolph KD, Miller FN, Pyle WK, Popovich RP, Sorkin MI. An hypothesis to explain the ultrafiltration characteristics of peritoneal dialysis. Kidney Int 1981; 20: 543–48.

247. Leypoldt JK, Blindauer KM. Convection does not govern plasma to dialysate transport of protein. Kidney Int 1992; 42: 1412–18.

248. Schaeffer RC Jr, Bitrick MS, Holberg III WC, Katz MA. Macromolecular transport across endothelial monolayers. Int J Microcirc: Clin Exp 1992; 11: 181–201.

249. Renkin EM. Relation of capillary morphology to transport of fluid and large molecules: a review. Acta Physiol Scand 1979; (suppl. 463): 81–91.

250. Krediet RT, Boeschoten EW, Struijk DG, Arisz L. Pharmacokinetics of intraperitoneally administered 5-fluorocytosine in continuous ambulatory peritoneal dialysis. Nephrol Dial Transplant 1987; 2: 453.

251. Krediet RT, Boeschoten EW, Zuyderhoudt FMJ, Arisz L. The relationship between peritoneal glucose absorption and body fluid loss by ultrafiltration during continuous ambulatory peritoneal dialysis. Clin Nephrol 1987; 27: 51–5.

252. Heaton A, Ward MK, Johnston DG, Nicholson DV, Alberti KGMM, Kerr DNS. Short-term studies on the use of glycerol as an osmotic agent in continuous ambulatory peritoneal dialysis (CAPD). Clin Sci 1984; 67: 121–30.

253. Williams PF, Marliss EB, Andersson GH et al. Amino acid absorption following intraperitoneal administration in CAPD patients. Perit Dial Bull 1982; 2: 124–30.

254. Lukas G, Brindle SD, Greengard P. The route of absorption of intraperitoneally administered compounds. J Pharmacol Exp Ther 1971; 178: 562–6.

255. Babb AL, Johansen PJ, Strand MJ, Tenckhoff H, Scribner BH. Bi-directional permeability of the human peritoneum to middle molecules. Proc Eur Dial Transplant Assoc 1973; 10: 247–61.

256. Bouchet JL, Albin H, Quentin C et al. Pharmacokinetics of intravenous and intraperitoneal fosfomycin in continuous ambulatory peritoneal dialysis. Clin Nephrol 1988; 29: 35–40.

257. Janicke DM, Morse GD, Apicella MA, Jusko WJ, Walshe JJ. Pharmacokinetic modelling of bidirectional transfer

during peritoneal dialysis. Clin Pharmacol Ther 1986; 40: 209–18.

258. Struijk DG, Krediet RT, Koomen GCM, Boeschoten EW, Reijden HJ van der, Arisz L. Indirect measurement of lymphatic absorption with inulin in continuous ambulatory peritoneal dialysis (CAPD) patients. Perit Dial Int 1990; 10: 141–5.

259. Struijk DG, Imholz ALT, Krediet RT, Koomen GCM, Arisz L. The use of the disappearance rate for the measurement of lymphatic absorption during CAPD. Blood Purif 1992; 10: 182–8.

260. Krediet RT, Struijk DG, Boeschoten EW, Hoek FJ, Arisz L. Measurement of intraperitoneal fluid kinetics in CAPD patients by means of autologous hemoglobin. Neth J Med 1988; 33: 281–90.

261. Leypoldt JK, Pust AH, Frigon RP, Henderson LW. Dialysate volume measurements required for determining peritoneal solute transport. Kidney Int 1988; 34: 254–61.

262. Rubin J, Adair C, Johnson B, Bower J. Stereospecific lactate absorption during peritoneal dialysis. Nephron 1982; 31: 224–8.

263. Nemoto EM, Severinghaus JW. Stereospecific permeability of rat blood–brain barrier to lactic acid. Stroke 1974; 5: 81–4.

264. Nolph KD, Twardowski ZJ, Khanna R et al. Tidal peritoneal dialysis with racemic or L-lactate solutions. Perit Dial Int 1990; 10: 161–4.

265. Oh MS, Pheleps KR, Traube M, Barbosa-Saldivar JL, Boxhill C, Carrol HJ. D-lactic acidosis in a man with the short-bowel syndrome. N Engl J Med 1979; 301: 249–52.

266. Stolberg L, Rolfe R, Gitlin N et al. D-lactate acidosis due to abnormal gut flora. N Engl J Med 1982; 306: 1344–48.

267. Fine A. Metabolism of D-lactate in the dog and in man. Perit Dial Int 1989; 9: 99–101.

268. Dixon SR, McKean WI, Pryor JE, Irvine ROH. Changes in acid–base balance during peritoneal dialysis with fluid containing lactate ions. Clin Sci 1970; 39: 51–60.

269. Gotch FA, Sargent JA, Keen ML. Hydrogen ion balance in dialysis therapy. Artif Organs 1982; 6: 388–395.

270. Tattersall TE, Dick S, Doyle S, Greenwood RN, Farrington K. Alkalosis and hypomagnesaemia: unwanted effects of a low calcium CAPD solution. Nephrol Dial Transplant 1995; 10: 258–62.

271. Feriani M, Passlick-Deetjen J, La Graeca G. Factors affecting bicarbonate transfer with bicarbonate-containing CAPD solution. Perit Dial Int 1995; 15: 336–41.

272. Rottembourg J, Gahl GM, Pognet JL et al. Severe abdominal complications in patients undergoing continuous ambulatory peritoneal dialysis. Proc Eur Dial Transplant Assoc 1983; 20: 236–42.

273. Slingeneyer A, Mion, Mourad G, Canaud B, Faller B, Béraud JJ. Progressive sclerosing peritonitis: a late and severe complication of maintenance peritoneal dialysis. Trans Am Soc Artif Intern Organs 1983; 29: 633–40.

274. Rottembourg J, Issad B, Langlois P, de Groc F, Legrain M. Sclerosing encapsulating peritonitis during CAPD. Evaluation of potential risk factors. In: Maher JF, Winchester JF, eds. Frontiers in peritoneal dialysis. New York: Field, Rich, 1986, pp. 643–9.

275. Pedersen FB, Ryttov N, Deleuran P, Dragsholt C, Kildeberg P. Acetate versus lactate in peritoneal dialysis solutions. Nephron 1985; 39: 55–8.

276. Khanna R, Mactier R, Twardowski ZJ, Nolph KD. Peritoneal cavity lymphatics. Perit Dial Bull 1986; 6: 113–21.

277. Gjessing J. The use of dextran as a dialyzing fluid in peritoneal dialysis. Acta Med Scand 1969; 185: 237–9.

278. Daugirdas JT, Ing TS, Gandhi VC, Hano JE, Chen WT, Yuan L. Kinetics of peritoneal fluid absorption in patients with chronic renal failure. J Lab Clin Med 1980; 95: 351–61.

279. Rippe B, Stelin G, Ahlmen J. Lymph flow from the peritoneal cavity in CAPD patients. In: Maher JF, Winchester JF, eds. Frontiers in Peritoneal Dialysis. New York: Field, Rich, 1986, pp. 24–30.

280. Spencer PC, Farrell PC. Solute and water transfer kinetics in CAPD. In: Gokal R, ed. Continuous Ambulatory Peritoneal Dialysis. Edinburgh: Churchill Livingstone, 1986, pp. 38–55.

281. De Paepe M, Belpaire F, Schelstraete K, Lameire N. Comparison of different volume markers in peritoneal dialysis. J Lab Clin Med 1988; 111: 421–9.

282. Lindholm B, Heimbürger O, Waniewski J, Werynski A, Bergström J. Peritoneal ultrafiltration and fluid reabsorption during peritoneal dialysis. Nephrol Dial Transplant 1989; 4: 805–13.

283. Mactier RA, Khanna R, Twardowski ZJ, Moore H, Nolph KD. Contribution of lymphatic absorption to loss of ultrafiltration and solute clearances in continuous ambulatory peritoneal dialysis. J Clin Invest 1987; 80: 1311–16.

284. Krediet RT, Struijk DG, Koomen GCM, Arisz L. Peritoneal fluid kinetics during CAPD measured with intraperitoneal dextran 70. ASAIO Trans 1991; 37: 662–7.

285. Struijk DG, Koomen GCM, Krediet RT, Arisz L. Indirect measurement of lymphatic absorption in CAPD patients is not influenced by trapping. Kidney Int 1992; 41: 1668–75.

286. Brouard R, Tozer TN, Baumelou A, Gambertoglio JG. Transfer of autologous haemoglobin from the peritoneal cavity during peritoneal dialysis. Nephrol Dial Transplant 1992; 7: 57–62.

287. Struijk DG, Bakker JC, Krediet RT, Koomen GCM, Stekkinger P, Arisz L. Effect of intraperitoneal administration of two different batches of albumin solutions on peritoneal solute transport in CAPD patients. Nephrol Dial Transplant 1991; 6: 198–202.

288. Hirszel P, Shea-Donohue T, Chakrabarti E, Montcalm E, Maher JF. The role of the capillary wall in restricting diffusion of macromolecules. Nephron 1988; 44: 58–61.

289. Cheek TR, Twardowski ZJ, Moore HL, Nolph KD. Absorption of inulin and high-molecular weight gelatin isocyanate solutions from peritoneal cavity of rats. In: Avram MM, Giordano C, eds. Ambulatory Peritoneal Dialysis. New York: Plenum, 1990, pp. 149–52.

290. Krediet RT, Struijk DG, Koomen GCM, Hoek FJ, Arisz L. The disappearance of macromolecules from the peritoneal cavity during continuous ambulatory peritoneal dialysis (CAPD) is not dependent on molecular size. Perit Dial Int 1990; 10: 147–52.

291. Nolph KD, Mactier R, Khanna R, Twardowski ZJ, Moore H, McGary T. The kinetics of ultrafiltration during peritoneal dialysis: the role of lymphatics. Kidney Int 1987; 32: 219–26.

292. Rippe B, El Rashied Z. Peritoneal fluid and albumin kinetics in the rat; effects of increases in intraperitoneal hydrostatic pressure. Perit Dial Int 1993; 13 (suppl. 1): S74.

293. Mactier RA, Khanna R, Twardowski ZJ, Moore H, Nolph KD. Influence of phosphatidylcholine on lymphatic absorption during peritoneal dialysis in the rat. Perit Dial Int 1988; 8: 179–86.

294. Flessner MF, Parker RJ, Sieber SM. Peritoneal lymphatic uptake of fibrinogen and erythrocytes in the rat. Am J Physiol 1983; 244: H89–96.

295. Rose BD. Clinical Physiology of Acid–Base and Electrolyte Disorders, 2nd edn. New York:, McGraw-Hill, 1984, p. 33.

296. Twardowski ZJ, Khanna R, Nolph KD et al. Intra-abdominal pressures during natural activities in patients treated with continuous ambulatory peritoneal dialysis. Nephron 1986; 44: 129–35.

297. Twardowski ZJ, Prowant BF, Nolph KD, Martinez AJ, Lampton LM. High volume, low frequency continuous ambulatory peritoneal dialysis. Kidney Int 1983; 23: 64–70.

298. Krediet RT, Koomen GCM, Struijk DG, Van Olden RW, Imholz ALT, Boeschoten EW. Practical methods for assessing dialysis efficiency during peritoneal dialysis. Kidney Int 1994; 46 (suppl. 48): S7–13.

299. Krediet RT, Boeschoten EW, Zuyderhoudt FMJ, Arisz L. The relationship between peritoneal glucose absorption and

body fluid loss by ultrafiltration during continuous ambulatory peritoneal dialysis. Clin Nephrol 1987; 27: 51–5.

300. Rubin J, Nolph KD, Popovich RP, Moncrieff JW, Prowant B. Drainage volumes during continuous ambulatory peritoneal dialysis. ASAIO J 1979; 2: 54–60.

301. Alsop RM. History, chemical and pharmaceutical development of icodextrin. Perit Dial Int 1994; 14 (suppl. 2): S5–12.

302. Mistry CD, Gokal R. Can ultrafiltration occur with a hypoosmolar solution in peritoneal dialysis?: the role for 'colloid' osmosis. Clin Sci 1993; 85: 495–500.

303. Gokal R, Mistry CD, Peers E, MIDAS Study Group. A United Kingdom multicenter study of icodextrin in continuous ambulatory peritoneal dialysis. Perit Dial Int 1994; 14 (suppl. 2): S22–7.

304. Douma CE, Hirallall JK, De Waart DR, Struijk DG, Krediet RT. Icodextrin with nitroprusside increases ultrafiltration and peritoneal transport during long CAPD dwells. Kidney Int 1998; 53: 1014–21.

305. Mistry CD, Gokal R, Peers E, MIDAS Study Group. A randomized multicenter clinical trial comparing isosmolar icodextrin with hyperosmolar glucose solutions in CAPD. Kidney Int 1994; 46: 496–503.

306. Lindholm B, Heimbürger O, Waniewski J, Werynski A, Bergström J. Peritoneal ultrafiltration and fluid reabsorption during peritoneal dialysis. Nephrol Dial Transplant 1989; 4: 805–13.

307. Kaysen GA, Schoenfeld PY. Albumin homeostasis in patients undergoing continuous ambulatory peritoneal dialysis. Kidney Int 1984; 25: 107–14.

308. Nagy JA. Lymphatic and nonlymphatic pathways of peritoneal absorption in mice: physiology versus pathology. Blood Purif 1992; 10: 148–62.

309. Abernathy HJ, Clin W, Hay JB, Rodela H, Oreopoulos D, Johnston MG. Lymphatic removal of dialysate from the peritoneal cavity of anesthetized sheep. Kidney Int 1991; 40: 174–81.

310. Johnston MG. Studies on lymphatic drainage of the peritoneal cavity in sheep. Blood Purif 1992; 10: 122–31.

311. Tran LP, Rodella H, Abernathy NJ et al. Lymphatic drainage of hypertonic solution from the peritoneal cavity of anesthetized and conscious sheep. J Appl Physiol 1993; 74: 859–67.

312. Tran LP, Rodella H, Hay JB, Oreopoulos DG, Johnston MG. Quantitation of lymphatic drainage of the peritoneal cavity in sheep: comparison of direct cannulation techniques with indirect methods to estimate lymph flow. Perit Dial Int 1993; 13: 270–9.

313. Drake RE, Gabel JC. Diaphragmatic lymph vessel drainage of the peritoneal cavity. Blood Purif 1992; 10: 132–5.

314. Shockley TR, Ofsthun NJ. Pathways for fluid loss from the peritoneal cavity. Blood Purif 1992; 10: 115–21.

315. Tsilibary EC, Wissig SL. Lymphatic absorption from the peritoneal cavity: regulation of patency of mesothelial stomata. Microvasc Res 1983; 25: 22–9.

316. Abensur H, Romao JE Jr, Brando de Almeida Prado E, Kakahaski E, Sabbaga E, Marcoudes M. Influence of the hydrostatic intraperitoneal pressure and the cardiac function on the lymphatic absorption rate of the peritoneal cavity in CAPD. Adv Perit Dial 1993; 9: 41–5.

317. Rippe B. How to measure ultrafiltration failure: 2.27% or 3.86% glucose? Perit Dial Int 1997; 17: 125–128.

318. Virga G, Amici G, DaRin G, Vianello A, Calconi G, Da Porto A, Bocci C. Comparison of fast peritoneal equilibration test with 1.36 and 3.86% dialysis solutions. Blood Purif 1994; 12: 113–20.

319. Krediet RT, Boeschoten EW, Zuyderhoudt FMJ, Arisz L. Peritoneal transport characteristics of water, low molecular weight solutes and proteins during long-term continuous ambulatory peritoneal dialysis. Perit Dial Bull 1986; 6: 61–5.

320. Imholz ALT, Koomen GCM, Struijk DG, Arisz L, Krediet RT. Residual volume measurements in CAPD patients with

exogenous and endogenous solutes. Adv Perit Dial 1992; 8: 33–8.

321. Verger C, Larpent L, Celicout B. Clinical significance of ultrafiltration failure on CAPD. In La Graeca G, Chiaramonte S, Fabris A, Feriani M, Ronco C, eds. Peritoneal Dialysis. Milan: Wichtig Ed., 1986, pp. 91–4.

322. Krediet RT, Struijk DG, Boeschoten EW et al. The time course of peritoneal transport kinetics in continuous ambulatory peritoneal dialysis patients who develop sclerosing peritonitis. Am J Kidney Dis 1989; 13: 299–307.

323. Wang T, Heimbürger O, Waniewski J, Bergström J, Lindholm B. Increased peritoneal permeability is associated with decreased fluid and small-solute removal and higher mortality in CAPD patients. Nephrol Dial Transplant 1998; 13: 1242–49.

324. Ho-dac-Pannekeet MM, Atasever B, Struijk DG, Krediet RT. Analysis of ultrafiltration failure in peritoneal dialysis patients by means of standard peritoneal permeability analysis. Perit Dial Int 1997; 17: 144–50.

325. Waniewski J, Heimbürger O, Werynski A, Lindholm B. Osmotic conductance of the peritoneum in CAPD patients with permanent loss of ultrafiltration capacity. Perit Dial Int 1996; 16: 488–96.

326. Widerøe TE, Smeby LC, Mjåland S, Dahl K, Berg LJ, Aas TW. Long-term changes in transperitoneal water transport during continuous ambulatory peritoneal dialysis. Nephron 1984; 38: 238–47.

327. Struijk DG, Krediet RT, Koomen GCM et al. Functional characteristics of the peritoneal membrane in long-term continuous ambulatory peritoneal dialysis. Nephron 1991; 59: 213–20.

328. Monquil MCJ, Imholz ALT, Struijk DG, Krediet RT. Does impaired transcellular water transport contribute to net ultrafiltration failure during CAPD? Perit Dial Int 1995; 15: 42–8.

329. Zweers MM, Struijk DG, Krediet RT. Correcting sodium sieving for diffusion from circulation. Perit Dial Int 1999; 15: 65–72.

330. Krediet RT. Loss of membrane permeability: a threat for CAPD. In: Andreucci VE, Fine LG, eds. International Yearbook of Nephrology, 1997. New York: Oxford University Press, 1997, pp. 153–62.

331. Verger C, Celicout B. Peritoneal permeability and encapsulating peritonitis. Lancet 1985; 1: 986–7.

332. Crosbie WA, Snowden S, Parsons V. Changes in lung capillary permeability in chronic uremia. Br Med J 1972; 4: 388–90.

333. Rubin J, Rust P, Brown P, Popovich RP, Nolph KD. A comparison of peritoneal transport in patients with psoriasis and uremia. Nephron 1981; 29: 185–9.

334. Diaz-Buxo JA, Farmer CD, Walker PJ, Chandler JT, Holt KL. Effect of hyperparathyroidism on peritoneal clearances. Trans Am Soc Artif Intern Organs 1982; 28: 276–9.

335. Nolph KD, Whitcomb ME, Schrier RW. Mechanisms for inefficient peritoneal dialysis in acute renal failure associated with heat stress and exercise. Ann Intern Med 1969; 71: 317–26.

336. Osterby R. Basement membrane morphology in diabetes mellitus. In: Ellenberg M, Rifkin H, eds. Diabetes Mellitus, Theory and Practice, 3rd edn. New York: Medical Examination Publishing Co., 1983, pp. 323–42.

337. Parving H. Increased microvascular permeability to plasma proteins in short- and long-term juvenile diabetes. Diabetes 1976; 25 (suppl. 2): 884–9.

338. Zimmerman AL, Sablay LB, Aynedjian HS, Bank N. Increased peritoneal permeability in rats with alloxan-induced diabetes mellitus. J Lab Clin Med 1984; 103: 720–30.

339. Di Paolo N, Sacchi G. Peritoneal vascular changes in continuous ambulatory peritoneal dialysis (CAPD): an *in vivo* model for the study of diabetic microangiopathy. Perit Dial Int 1989; 9: 41–5.

340. Mateijsen MAM, van der Wal AC, Hendriks PMEM, Zweers MM, Mulder J, Krediet RT. Vascular and interstitial changes in the peritoneum of CAPD patients with peritoneal sclerosis. J Am Soc Nephrol 1997; 8: 268A–9A.

341. Honda K, Nitta K, Horita S, Yumura W, Nikei W. Morphological changes in the peritoneal vasculature of patients on CAPD with ultrafiltration failure. Nephron 1996; 72: 171–6.

342. Nolph KD, Stolz ML, Maher JF. Altered peritoneal permeability in patients with systemic vasculitis. Ann Intern Med 1971; 75: 753–5.

343. Krediet RT. Peritoneal permeability in continuous ambulatory peritoneal dialysis. Dissertation, Amsterdam: University of Amsterdam, 1986.

344. Selgas R, Madero R, Munoz J, Huarte E, Rinon C, Miquel JL, Sanchez-Sécilia L. Functional peculiarities of the peritoneum in diabetes mellitus. Dial Transplant 1988; 17: 419–36.

345. Rubin J, Nolph KD, Arfania D, Brown P, Moore H, Rust P. Influence of patient characteristics on peritoneal clearances. Nephron 1981; 27: 118–21.

346. Lamb EJ, Worrall J, Buhler R, Harwood S, Catell WR, Dawnay AB. Effect of diabetes and peritonitis on the peritoneal equilibration test. Kidney Int 1995; 47: 1760–7.

347. Serlie MJM, Struijk DG, de Blok K, Krediet RT. Differences in fluid and solute transport between diabetic and non diabetic patients at the onset of CAPD. Adv Perit Dial 1997; 13: 29–32.

348. Rubin J, Nolph KD, Arfania D, Brown P, Moore H, Rust P. Influence of patients characteristics on peritoneal clearances. Nephron 1981; 27: 118–21.

349. Rottembourg J, El Shahat Y, Agrafiotis A *et al.* Continuous ambulatory peritoneal dialysis in insulin-dependent diabetic patients: a 40-month experience. Kidney Int 1983; 23: 40–5.

350. Rubin J, Walsh D, Bower JD, Diabetes, dialysate losses, and serum lipids during continuous ambulatory peritoneal dialysis. Am J Kidney Dis 1987; 10: 104–8.

351. Fassbinder W, Brunner FP, Brynger H *et al.* Combined report on regular dialysis and transplantation in Europe 20, 1989. Nephrol Dial Transplant 1991; 6: 5–35.

352. Correia P, Cameron JS, Ogg CS, Williams DG, Bewick M, Hicks JA. End-stage renal failure in SLE with nephritis. Clin Nephrol 1984; 22: 293–302.

353. Wu GG, Gelbast DR, Hasbargen JA, Inman R, McNamee P, Oreopoulos DG. Reactivation of systemic lupus in three patients undergoing CAPD. Perit Dial Bull 1986; 6: 6–9.

354. Cantaluppi A. CAPD and systemic diseases. Clin Nephrol 1988; 30 (suppl. 1): S8–12.

355. Krediet RT, Boeschoten EW, Zuyderhoudt FMJ, Arisz L. Permeability of the peritoneum to proteins in CAPD patients with systemic disease. Proc Eur Dial Transplant Assoc 1985; 22: 405–9.

356. Brown ST, Ahearn DJ, Nolph KD. Reduced peritoneal clearances in scleroderma increased by intraperitoneal isoproterenol. Ann Intern Med 1973; 78: 891–4.

357. Robson M, Oreopoulos DG. Dialysis in scleroderma. Ann Intern Med 1978; 88: 843.

358. Winfield J, Khanna R, Reynolds WJ, Gordon DA, Finkelstein S, Oreopoulos DG. Management of end-stage scleroderma renal disease with continuous ambulatory peritoneal dialysis. Report of two cases. Perit Dial Bull 1982; 2: 174–7.

359. Copley JB, Smith BJ. Continuous ambulatory peritoneal dialysis and scleroderma. Nephron 1985; 40: 353–6.

360. Browning MJ, Banks RA, Harrison P *et al.* Continuous ambulatory peritoneal dialysis in systemic amyloidosis and end-stage renal disease. J R Soc Med 1984; 77: 189–92.

361. Rosansky SJ, Waddell PH. CAPD in the treatment of primary amyloidosis. Perit Dial Bull 1983; 3: 217–18.

362. Rosansky SJ, Richards FW. Use of peritoneal dialysis in the treatment of patients with renal failure and paraproteinemia. Am J Nephrol 1985; 5: 361–5.

363. Heale WF, Letch KA, Dawborn JK, Evans SM. Long term complications of peritonitis. In: Atkins RC, Thomson NM, Farrell PC, eds. Peritoneal Dialysis. Edinburgh: Churchill Livingstone, 1981, pp. 284–90.

364. Rubin J, McFarland S, Hellems EW, Bower JD. Peritoneal dialysis during peritonitis. Kidney Int 1981; 19: 460–4.

365. Prowant BF, Nolph KD. Clinical criteria for diagnosis of peritonitis. In: Atkins RC, Thomson NM, Farrell PC, eds. Peritoneal Dialysis. Edinburgh: Churchill Livingstone, 1981, pp. 257–63.

366. Smeby LC, Wideröe TE, Jörstad S. Individual differences in water transport during peritonitis. ASAIO J 1981; 4: 17–27.

367. Raja RM, Kramer MS, Rosenbaum JL, Bolisay C, Krug M. Contrasting changes in solute transport and ultrafiltration with peritonitis in CAPD patients. Trans Am Soc Artif Intern Organs 1981; 27: 68–70.

368. Rubin J, Ray R, Barnes T, Bower J. Peritoneal abnormalities during infectious episodes of continuous ambulatory peritoneal dialysis. Nephron 1981; 29: 124–7.

369. Smeby LC, Wideröe TE, Svartås TM, Jörstad S. Changes in water removal due to peritonitis during continuous ambulatory peritoneal dialysis. In: Gahl GM, Kessel M, Nolph KD, eds. Advances in Peritoneal Dialysis. Amsterdam: Excerpta Medica, 1981, pp. 287–92.

370. Raja RM, Kramer MS, Barber K. Solute transport and ultrafiltration during peritonitis in CAPD patients ASAIO J 1984; 7: 8–11.

371. Gokal R, Mistry CD, Peers EM, MIDAS Study Group. Peritonitis occurrence in a multicenter study of icodextrin and glucose in CAPD. Perit Dial Int 1995; 15: 226–30.

372. Krediet RT, Arisz L. Fluid and solute transport across the peritoneum during continuous ambulatory peritoneal dialysis (CAPD). Perit Dial Int 1989; 9: 15–25.

373. Blumenkrantz MJ, Gahl GM, Kopple JD *et al.* Protein losses during peritoneal dialysis. Kidney Int 1981; 19: 593–602.

374. Dulaney JT, Hatch Jr FE. Peritoneal dialysis and loss of proteins: a review. Kidney Int 1984; 26: 253–62.

375. Miller FN, Hammerschmidt DE, Anderson GL, Moore JN. Protein loss induced by complement activation during peritoneal dialysis. Kidney Int 1984; 25: 480–85.

376. Gokal R, Jakubowski C, King J *et al.* Outcome in patients on continuous ambulatory peritoneal dialysis: 4 year analysis of a prospective multicenter study. Lancet 1987; 2: 1105–8.

377. Canusa Peritoneal Dialysis Study Group. Adequacy of dialysis and nutrition in continuous ambulatory peritoneal dialysis: association with clinical outcomes. J Am Soc Nephrol 1996; 7: 198–207.

378. Genestier J, Hedelin G, Schaffer P, Faller B. Prognostic factors in CAPD patients: a retrospective study of a 10-year period. Nephrol Dial Transplant 1995; 10: 1905–11.

379. Krediet RT, Douma CE, van Olden RW, Ho-dac-Pannekeet MM, Struijk DG. Augmenting solute clearance in peritoneal dialysis. Kidney Int 1998; 54: 2218–35.

380. Kawaguchi Y, Hasegawa T, Nakayama M, Kubo H, Shigematu T. Issues affecting the longevity of the continuous peritoneal dialysis therapy. Kidney Int 1997; 52 (suppl. 62): S105–7.

381. Selgas R, Rodrigues-Carmona A, Martinez ME *et al.* Peritoneal mass transfer in patients on long-term CAPD. Perit Dial Bull 1984; 4: 153–6.

382. Selgas R, Rodrigues-Carmona A, Martinez ME *et al.* Follow-up of peritoneal mass transfer properties in long-term CAPD patients. In: Maher JF, Winchester JF, eds. Frontiers in Peritoneal Dialysis. New York: Field, Rich, 1986, pp. 53–5.

383. Selgas R, Muños J, Cigarran S *et al.* Peritoneal functional parameters after five years on continuous ambulatory peritoneal dialysis (CAPD): the effect of late peritonitis. Perit Dial Int 1989; 9: 329–32.

384. Selgas R, Fernandez-Ryes M-J, Bosque E *et al.* Functional longevity of the human peritoneum: how long is continuous

peritoneal dialysis possible? Results of a prospective medium long-term study. Am J Kidney Dis 1994; 23: 64–73.

385. Selgas R, Bajo M-A, Paiva A *et al.* Stability of the peritoneal dialysis patients. Adv Renal Replacement Ther 1998; 5: 168–78.

386. Pollock CA, Ibels LS, Caterson RJ, Mahoney JF, Waugh DA, Cocksedge B. Continuous ambulatory peritoneal dialysis. Eight years of experience at a single center. Medicine 1989; 68: 293–308.

387. Kush RD, Hallett MD, Ota K *et al.* Long-term continuous ambulatory peritoneal dialysis; mass transfer and nutritional and metabolic stability. Blood Purif 1990; 8: 1–13.

388. Bordoni E, Lombardo V, Bibiano L *et al.* Peritoneal clearances, ultrafiltration and diuresis in long-term continuous ambulatory peritoneal dialysis. In: Avram MM, Giordano C, eds. Ambulatory Peritoneal Dialysis. New York: Plenum, 1990, pp. 87–90.

389. Chan PCK, Chan CY, Wu PG, Cheng IKP, Chan MK. Long-term peritoneal clearances in patients on continuous ambulatory peritoneal dialysis. Int J Artif Organs 1990; 13: 707–8.

390. Lameire NH, Vanholder R, Veyt D, Lambert M-C, Ringoir S. A longitudinal, five year survey of urea kinetic parameters in CAPD patients. Kidney Int 1992; 42: 426–32.

391. Faller B, Lameire N. Evaluation of clinical parameters and peritoneal function in a cohort of CAPD patients followed over 7 years. Nephrol Dial Transplant 1994; 9: 280–6.

392. Davies SJ, Bryan J, Philips L, Russel GI. Longitudinal changes in peritoneal kinetics: the effects of peritoneal dialysis and peritonitis. Nephrol Dial Transplant 1996; 11: 498–506.

393. Rubin J, Nolph KD, Arfania D, Brown P, Prowant B. Follow-up of peritoneal clearances in patients undergoing continuous ambulatory peritoneal dialysis. Kidney Int 1979; 16: 619–23.

394. Park MS, Lee J, Lee MS, Baick SH, Hwang SD, Lee HB. Peritoneal solute clearances after four years of continuous ambulatory peritoneal dialysis (CAPD). Perit Dial Int 1989; 9: 75–8.

395. Coronel F, Tornero F, Mucia M *et al.* Peritoneal clearances, protein losses and ultrafiltration in diabetic patients after four years on CAPD. Adv Perit Dial 1991; 7: 35–8.

396. Struijk DG, Krediet RT, Koomen GCM, Boeschoten EW, Hoek FJ, Arisz L. A prospective study of peritoneal transport in CAPD patients. Kidney Int 1994; 45: 1739–44.

397. Hendriks PMEM, Ho-dac-Pannekeet MM, van Gulik TM *et al.* Peritoneal sclerosis in chronic peritoneal dialysis patients: analysis of clinical presentation, risk factors and peritoneal transport kinetics. Perit Dial Int 1997; 17: 136–43.

398. Krediet RT. The peritoneal membrane in chronic peritoneal dialysis. Kidney Int 1999; 55: 341–56.

6 | Peritoneal lymphatics

R. A. Mactier and R. Khanna

Introduction

The peritoneal lymphatics serve as a route for continuous absorption of fluids and solutes from the peritoneal cavity by convective flow [1, 2]. The important role of lymphatic drainage from the peritoneal cavity in the pathogenesis of ascites due to liver disease or malignancy is well established [3–16] and the considerable absorptive capacity of the peritoneal lymphatics has been utilized to perform intraperitoneal blood transfusions in the fetus and in children [17–21]. However, the initial kinetic studies on peritoneal dialysis iatrogenic 'ascites' tended to focus only on fluid and solute exchange between the peritoneal microcirculation and the instilled dialysis solution, and neglected the role of the peritoneal lymphatics [22–39]. The efficiency of peritoneal dialysis is assessed clinically by measuring solute clearances and *net* ultrafiltration volumes. These indices of dialysis efficacy represent the cumulative balance of transperitoneal transport into and out of the peritoneal cavity and therefore incorporate the role of back-filtration from the peritoneal cavity. Absorption from the peritoneal cavity can occur by two mechanisms: uptake via the peritoneal cavity lymphatics (translymphatic absorption) or uptake by the peritoneal capillaries (transcapillary absorption).

Translymphatic absorption

Many of the studies of translymphatic absorption were performed in the era before CAPD.

Lymphatic pathways of the peritoneal lymphatics

Lymphatic drainage from the peritoneal cavity is primarily via specialized end lymphatic openings (stomata) located in the subdiaphragmatic perito-

neum [40–43]. Moreover, absorption of intraperitoneal fluid is greatest from the right hemidiaphragm overlying the liver [42]. In contrast, absorption by the lymphatic capillaries within the interstitium of the mesentery, omentum and parietal peritoneum makes a relatively minor contribution to total peritoneal lymphatic drainage [2, 43, 44].

The lymphatic capillaries leading from the subdiaphragmatic stomata coalesce to form a plexus of collecting lymphatics within the muscular portion of the diaphragm. This subperitoneal plexus also communicates with the lymphatics from the pleural surface. From the diaphragm and the diaphragmatic lymph nodes, most of the lymphatic trunks accompany the internal mammary vessels to the anterior mediastinal lymph nodes around the thymus (Fig. 1) and thereafter return almost 80% of the peritoneal lymphatic drainage to the venous circulation via the right lymph duct [2, 45]. Some of the efferent lymphatics from the anterior mediastinal nodes may, however, occasionally drain to the central veins on the left side either in association with or separate from the thoracic duct. The lymphatic drainage from the remainder of the peritoneum, including part of the subdiaphragmatic peritoneum, returns to the systemic circulation through the thoracic duct [2]. Consequently cannulation of the thoracic duct during peritoneal dialysis in the rat collected less than 30% of total estimated lymphatic absorption [46]. The major substernal and other minor lymphatic pathways from the peritoneal cavity are summarized schematically in Fig. 2.

Subdiaphragmatic stomata

Von Recklinghausen in 1863 was the first to suggest that carbon particles, red blood cells, proteins and fluid were transported directly from the peritoneal cavity into the lymphatics of the diaphragm via openings in the subdiaphragmatic peritoneum, which he called stomata [47]. Other investigators

R. Gokal, R. Khanna, R.Th. Krediet and K.D. Nolph (eds.), Textbook of Peritoneal Dialysis, 2nd Edition, 173–192.
© 2000 *Kluwer Academic Publishers. Printed in Great Britain.*

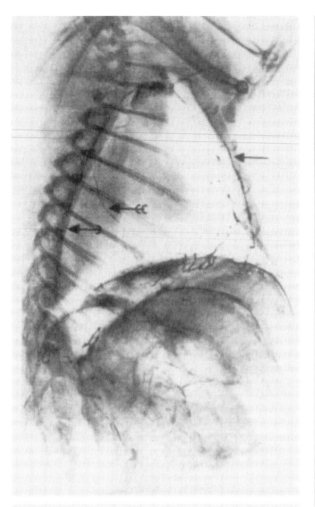

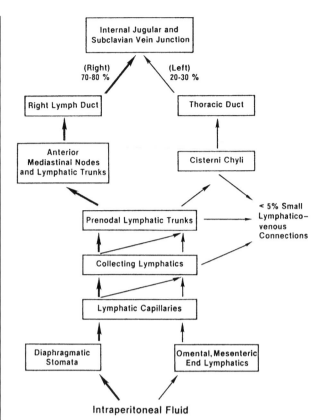

Figure 2. Anatomical pathways of lymphatic absorption of intraperitoneal fluid. (Reproduced with permission from ref. 108.)

Figure 1. Lateral x-ray following intraperitoneal Thorotrast. The diaphragmatic lymphatics drain predominantly into the parasternal lymphatics (←). The paravertebral lymphatics (←⟶) and a small tortuous mediastinal lymphatic (←◄) are also opacified. (Reproduced with permission from ref. 40.)

subsequently claimed that the stomata were artefacts [48–50] but the presence of these specialized terminal lymphatics in experimental animals and humans has since been confirmed by light and electron microscopy [51–56].

The lacunae of the terminal lymphatics of the subdiaphragmatic peritoneum are separated from the peritoneal cavity only by a thin triple-layer, consisting of small, rounded and interdigitating mesothelium, a loose network of connective tissue and lymphatic endothelium [52, 54]. Scanning and transmission electron microscopy have shown that the stomata permit absorption of intraperitoneal particles, cells, colloids and fluid into the underlying lymphatic lacunae via extracellular pathways [52, 57] (Fig. 3). The mesothelial cells which overlie

the lymphatic lacunae are smaller and separate from each other more readily than the cells in the surrounding mesothelium [52, 58]. Internally the lacunar mesothelial cells have bands of actin filaments arranged along their base [54]. The stomata are formed by the separation of adjacent mesothelial cells and, in the rat, can accommodate spherical particles up to 22.5 μm in diameter [59]. At the stomata the submesothelial basement membrane and the underlying lattice of connective tissue become fenestrated [60] and allow the mesothelial cells to adjoin the lymphatic endothelial cells to form a channel from the peritoneal cavity to the lumen of the underlying lacuna [61, 62].

Mechanism of lymphatic absorption

The rate at which intraperitoneal fluid is absorbed by the peritoneal cavity lymphatics is dependent upon the excursions of the diaphragm during respiration [63–65]. As the diaphragm relaxes during

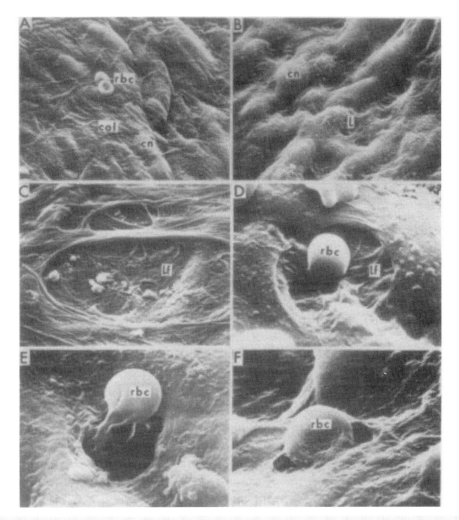

Figure 3. Scanning electron microscopy of red blood cells passing through the subdiaphragmatic stomata.
A Non-absorbing surface in the rat diaphragm; rbc, red blood cell; col, collagen fibres; cn, mesothelial cell nucleus. ×780.
B Absorbing surface overlying lymphatic lacunae (L) in the rat diaphragm. ×1200.
C Rabbit diaphragm showing the roof of a lacuna (Lf).
D Red blood cell passing through a slit in the roof of lacuna in the rabbit diaphragm. ×3120.
E Red blood cell passing between mesothelial cells in the rat diaphragm. ×4200.
F As for **E**. ×3780.
(Reproduced with permission from ref. 57.)

expiration, the adjacent mesothelial and endothelial cells in the roofs of the lymphatic lacunae separate from each other and intraperitoneal fluid is absorbed as suction is created by the distension of the lacunae. In inspiration the contraction of the diaphragm closes the gaps between the overlying mesothelial and endothelial cells and the contents of the lacunae are emptied into the efferent lymphatics. The presence of the abundant actin filaments in the cytoplasm of both the mesothelial and endothelial cells, however, suggests that there may be an active as well as a passive mechanism for maintaining the patency of the stomata [63, 64]. Backflow of the absorbed fluid into the peritoneal cavity is prevented during inspiration by the overlapping of the endothelial cells in the roofs of the lacunae [53, 54] (Fig. 4). Forward flow, induced by lymphatic contractility and changes in intrathoracic pressure, is maintained by the presence of valves in the efferent lymphatics [53, 54, 65]. The higher lymphatic absorption rate from the right hemidiaphragm is probably due to compression of the liver against the subdiaphragmatic stomata during respiration [58]. The ultrastructure and the mechanism of absorption of the peritoneal cavity lymphatics are reviewed in greater detail elsewhere [66].

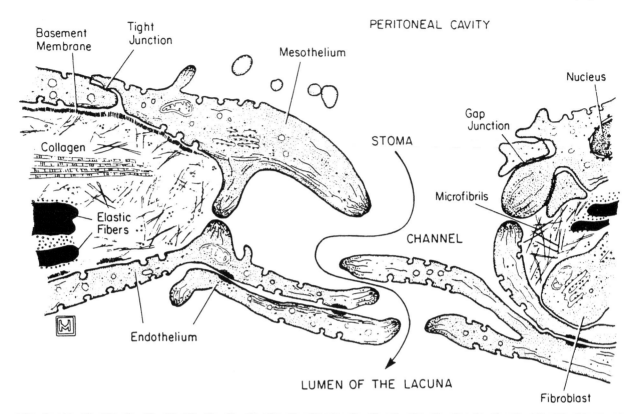

Figure 4. Diagram of a typical stoma and underlying channel linking the peritoneal cavity with the lumen of a lymphatic lacuna. (Reproduced with permission from ref. 54.)

Function of peritoneal cavity lymphatics

The lymphatics draining the peritoneal cavity act as a one-way system returning excess intraperitoneal fluid and protein to the systemic circulation. The sum of the hydrostatic and osmotic pressure gradients across the peritoneum normally favours a minor net inflow of fluid into the peritoneal cavity [31]. Bidirectional transperitoneal transfer of small solutes occurs by diffusion and by solvent drag. However, macromolecules (molecular weight greater than 20 000) exhibit minimal direct reabsorption into the peritoneal capillaries [67] and consequently, after unidirectional transport from the peritoneal microcirculation in the peritoneal cavity, are returned to the venous circulation by convective flow into the lymphatics. Normally peritoneal lymphatic drainage of serous fluids equals its rate of formation and only a small volume of isosmotic fluid is maintained within the peritoneal cavity.

The second major function of the lymphatics is their contribution to the host defences of the peritoneal cavity. Absorption by the peritoneal cavity lymphatics and phagocytosis by the resident intraperitoneal and omental macrophages are the first lines of defence after an inoculum of bacteria gains entry to the peritoneal cavity [68, 69]. The macrophages in the omentum provide an effective defence against bacteria but the omental lymphatics play only a minor role in the absorption of the fluid from the peritoneal cavity [44]. Likewise, it is important to emphasize that although the lymphatics carrying fluid and solutes from the intestinal mucosa traverse the mesentery before draining into the cisterna chyli and the thoracic duct, they are not significantly involved in absorption of isosmotic fluid from the peritoneal cavity *per se* [2, 43].

Absorptive capacity of the peritoneal lymphatics

The lymphatics draining the peritoneal cavity, therefore, are virtually the only pathway for absorption of intraperitoneal isosmotic fluid, biologically inert particles, colloids and cells [2, 58, 65, 70]. Consequently the absorptive capacity of the peritoneal cavity lymphatics has been evaluated in normal animals from the constant rate of uptake of isosmotic fluid (plasma or whole blood) infused into the perito-

Table 1. Rates of isosmotic fluid absorption from the peritoneal cavity in different species

Species	Infusion volumes	Infused solution	Absorption rate	Ref.
Rat	20 ml (per kg)	Homologous plasma	6 ml/kg per hour	74
Rabbit	20 ml (per kg)	Homologous plasma	3.5 ml/kg per hour	74
Cat	50 ml (2.4–2.7 kg)	Homologous serum	4.2–6.0 ml/h	43

Table 2. Factors influencing lymphatic absorption from the peritoneal cavity

1   Intraperitoneal fluid volume
2   Intraperitoneal hydrostatic pressure
3   Rate and depth of respiration
4   Posture
5   Intestinal peristalsis
6   Patency of the diaphragmatic and mediastinal lymphatics
7   Lymphatic vessel outflow pressure

neal cavity [41–43, 71–78]. Representative values from these studies indicate that lymphatic absorption rates from the peritoneal cavity in animals are considerable (Table 1). However, the rate of absorption of intraperitoneal crystalloid solutions decreases exponentially after infusion due to transcapillary absorption until osmotic equilibrium is reached, and thereafter remains almost constant [79, 80]. The importance of the peritoneal cavity lymphatics has been emphasized by studies showing that obliteration of the subdiaphragmatic peritoneum [43, 73] or ligation of the parasternal lymphatic trunks [74] greatly reduces the rate of intraperitoneal fluid absorption.

Factors controlling peritoneal lymphatic absorption

Several physiological factors have been shown in studies in animals before the introduction of CAPD to alter the rate of lymphatic absorption from the peritoneal cavity. Hyperventilation, which was induced by breathing carbon dioxide, increased, whereas anaesthesia and acute phrenic neurectomy reduced lymphatic absorption [77, 78, 81, 82]. Lymphatic and peritoneal transcapillary absorption were both enhanced by increasing intraperitoneal hydrostatic pressure [76] and decreased after paracentesis [83]. Upright posture with small intraperitoneal volumes reduced the rate of lymphatic flow, although absorption still occurred due to propulsion of the intraperitoneal fluid towards the diaphragm by intestinal peristalsis [74]. Indeed, the circulation of intraperitoneal fluid towards the diaphragm is the most likely explanation for the relative frequency of abscess formation in the right subphrenic space following entry of bacteria into the peritoneal cavity [84]. Fowler successfully localized infection in the pelvis of patients with diffuse peritonitis by elevating the head of their beds by 12–15 inches [85]. Even though obstruction of the peritoneal cavity lymphatics by fibrin or fibrosis may

decrease lymphatic absorption after infectious peritonitis, chemical peritonitis induced by sodium hypochlorite was observed to increase the rate of lymphatic absorption in the recovery period [86]. This rise in lymphatic flow may be related to rapid regeneration of end lymphatics after injury. Lymphatic flow is reduced if outflow pressure is increased by catheter insertion or raised central venous pressure [87]. The factors known to influence peritoneal lymphatic drainage are summarized in Table 2.

Transcapillary absorption

Prior to absorption into the peritoneal capillaries located mainly within the deeper layers of the interstitium intraperitoneal fluid and solutes must traverse at least six identified anatomical resistance sites: fluid films within the peritoneal cavity, mesothelium and its basal lamina, interstitial matrix, endothelial basement membrane, endothelial layer and fluid films within the capillary lumen [22]. Fluid movement between the peritoneal cavity and peritoneal capillaries is determined by the balance of hydrostatic and osmotic pressure gradients across these resistance sites. Transperitoneal absorption is only strictly analogous to transcapillary uptake within other tissues if solutes and water permeate equally in either direction across the peritoneal barrier.

The peritoneum acts as a composite membrane (capillary endothelium, interstitium and mesothelium) which exhibits functional as well as anatomical asymmetry. Phylogenetic evidence indicates that the peritoneum evolved as an excretory organ and therefore may not permit ready absorption of intraperitoneal fluid or solutes [88, 89]. The presence of phospholipids (surfactant) within peritoneal fluid which is synthesized and secreted by the mesothelium suggests that the mesothelial surface has fluid-repellent properties [90–92]. Small solutes are absorbed by diffusive transport which is dependent on solute size, charge and configuration, whereas large solutes of molecular weight greater than 20 000 demonstrate minimal absorption into the peritoneal capillaries [67]. Macromolecules would accumulate within the peritoneal cavity if there was no alternative absorptive pathway.

Role of lymphatic absorption in ascites

Ascites develops when the net transperitoneal inflow of fluid into the peritoneal cavity exceeds the rate of fluid efflux via the peritoneal cavity lymphatics [3–8]. The fluid flux rate across the peritoneum (J_w) is determined by the product of peritoneal hydraulic permeability (L_P), the effective membrane area (A) and the sum of osmotic ($\Delta\pi$) and hydrostatic (ΔP) transmembrane pressure gradients. That is:

$$J_w = L_P A (\Delta\pi + \Delta P) \tag{1}$$

Accordingly, net inflow of fluid into the peritoneal cavity is observed in conditions where there is a rise in hepatic sinusoidal and portal venous hydrostatic pressure, a reduction in serum albumin concentration and/or an increase in peritoneal permeability. The net transcapillary accumulation of intraperitoneal fluid is countered by its continuous reabsorption by the peritoneal cavity lymphatics at a rate influenced by the volume of ascites, the intraperitoneal hydrostatic pressure, the patency of the lymphatic pathways and central venous pressure (Table 2). The continuous bidirectional transport of fluid in ascites, however, precludes direct estimation of lymphatic drainage from the rate of absorption of isosmotic fluid as in normal animals (Table 1).

The peritoneal lymphatic absorption rate in ascites has been estimated indirectly from the rate of mass transfer of labelled colloids from the peritoneal cavity to the systemic circulation. This formulation is dependent on prior observations that intraperitoneal macromolecules (molecular weight greater than 20 000) are returned to the venous circulation almost exclusively by the peritoneal lymphatics [2, 67, 93, 94] and that isosmotic intraperitoneal fluid is drained by the peritoneal lymphatics without change in the concentration of index macromolecules [75, 76, 95–97]. Nevertheless, peritoneal to plasma mass transfer rates of radioiodinated serum albumin [9, 10, 97] and other radiocolloids [10–13] have provided a valid comparison of the relative peritoneal lymphatic flow rates in patients with hepatic [9, 10, 97], malignant [10–13] and dialysis-associated ascites [9]. Estimations of peritoneal lymphatic

Table 3. Transcapillary fluid influx and effective lymphatic absorption rates in ascites

Form of ascites	Net transcapillary fluid influx rate	Lymphatic absorption rate
Hepatic	+ + + +	+ +
Malignant	+	−
Nephrogenic	+	−
Peritoneal dialysis	+ + +	+

+, increase; −, decrease.

absorption by this method in 10 patients with hepatic ascites ranged from 24 to 223 ml/h and averaged 80 ml/h [9, 10, 97]. Presumably the large intraperitoneal fluid volume ensures constant contact of fluid with the undersurface of the diaphragm and the concurrent rise in intraperitoneal pressure enhances convective movement of fluid into the diaphragmatic lymphatics. In contrast, metastatic invasion of the subdiaphragmatic peritoneum is not uncommon in patients with intra-abdominal malignancy [98, 99] and may at least partially obstruct lymphatic drainage from the peritoneal cavity [14, 15]. Peritoneal lymphatic absorption in 22 patients with malignant ascites ranged from 1 to 63 ml/h and averaged only 11 ml/h [10]. Mediastinal lymphoscintigraphy in patients with malignant ascites often failed to demonstrate patent diaphragmatic lymphatics or identify mediastinal lymph nodes [10–13]. Moreover, the calculated lymphatic absorption rate correlated with the concurrently performed lymphoscintigram [10]. Likewise, patients with schistosomal hepatic fibrosis and ascites have significant fibrous thickening of the subdiaphragmatic peritoneum, which most likely limits flow into the diaphragmatic lymphatics [16]. In support of this mechanism, obliteration of the diaphragm with fibrous tissue significantly increased the incidence of and severity of ascites in animals with infrahepatic portal hypertension [100]. Ascites due to a transient reduction in lymphatic drainage has been reported in a patient transferring from CAPD to haemodialysis because of refractory peritonitis [101]. The role of lymphatic absorption in the pathophysiology of these different forms of ascites is summarized in Table 3.

Role of lymphatic absorption in peritoneal dialysis kinetics

The terminology used to describe the kinetics of peritoneal dialysis has been modified to incorporate

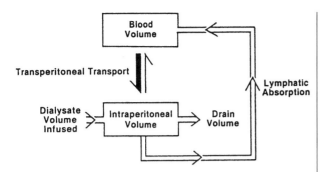

Figure 5. Schematic representation of the role of lymphatic absorption in the kinetics of peritoneal dialysis. (Reproduced with permission from ref. 108.)

the role of the peritoneal cavity lymphatics [102–105]. The measurable net ultrafiltration volume represents the net change in the intraperitoneal fluid volume at the end of the dwell time and, assuming that the residual volume remains constant, equals the dialysate drain volume minus the infusion volume. However, the net ultrafiltration volume is in effect the difference between cumulative net transcapillary ultrafiltration into the peritoneal cavity and total effective lymphatic absorption out of the peritoneal cavity during the dwell time (Fig. 5). These two formulations of net ultrafiltration may be designated directly measured and calculated net ultrafiltration (UF), respectively. That is:

Measured net UF

= drain volume − infusion volume

Calculated net UF

= cumulative net transcapillary UF

− effective lymphatic absorption

Cumulative net transcapillary ultrafiltration defines the total net influx of fluid from the peritoneal microcirculation into the peritoneal cavity during the dwell time in response to the osmotic pressure of the dialysis solution. This definition allows for bidirectional transcapillary water movement during the dwell time but acknowledges that inflow into the peritoneal cavity dominates and that only the net fluid flux can be measured. The resultant net inflow of fluid would equal measured net ultrafiltration if it was not for cumulative drainage into the lymphatics and interstitial tissue during the dwell time (Fig. 5).

In patients with ascites lymphatic drainage exceeds 50 ml/h unless the diaphragmatic or mediastinal lymphatics are obstructed by tumour or fibrosis

[10]. Intraperitoneal fluid volumes during peritoneal dialysis are routinely greater than 2 L and should also ensure continuous contact of fluid with the undersurface of the diaphragm. Furthermore, the patency of the peritoneal cavity lymphatics should be preserved in peritoneal dialysis provided that the subdiaphragmatic parietal peritoneum only undergoes the same minor histological changes as are observed in the parietal peritoneum lining the anterior abdominal wall [106–108]. In peritoneal dialysis as well as chronic hepatic ascites the thoracic duct and other mediastinal lymph vessels may gradually dilate and so promote lymph flow from the peritoneal cavity [6].

In hypertonic peritoneal dialysis the intraperitoneal fluid volume begins to decrease before isosmolarity of the dialysis solution and plasma is observed [29, 32], indicating that net fluid absorption occurs before net transcapillary ultrafiltration is complete (Fig. 6). The dialysis solution becomes isosmolar with plasma before glucose equilibrium because of solute sieving with transcapillary ultrafiltration [24, 25, 109].

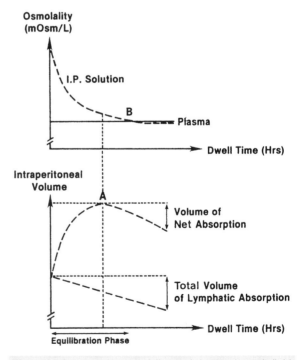

Figure 6. Changes in osmolality and intraperitoneal fluid volume following infusion of a hypertonic dextrose dialysis solution. The peak intraperitoneal volume (point A) precedes osmolar equilibrium (point B). Thereafter net fluid absorption represents effective lymphatic absorption in excess of net transcapillary ultrafiltration. (Reproduced with permission from ref. 108.)

The total transperitoneal osmotic pressure gradient is the sum of products of the concentration gradient and the peritoneal reflection coefficient of each solute. Accordingly, a higher peritoneal reflection coefficient of glucose, compared with other small molecular weight solutes [110] tends to maintain an osmotic pressure gradient into the dialysis solution after isosmolarity is reached and thereby allows net transcapillary ultrafiltration to continue at a slow rate until osmotic pressure equilibrium is approached later in the dwell time. This mechanism has also been invoked to explain the net ultrafiltration observed following intraperitoneal infusion of electrolyte-free 5% dextrose solution (252 mOsm/L) [110]. Since the dialysis solution becomes hypo-osmolar to the plasma towards the end of the dwell time [105], this further suggests that net transcapillary ultrafiltration continues after osmolar equilibrium is first observed. Consequently the reduction in intraperitoneal volume (ΔV) after peak ultrafiltration really represents the effective lymphatic absorption rate (L) in excess of the concurrent net transcapillary ultrafiltration rate (J_w in equation (1)). Thus,

$$\Delta V = L_P A (\Delta \pi + \Delta P) - L \qquad (2)$$

Direct measurements of drain volumes after sequential dwell times in 29 CAPD patients showed that the rate of decrease in the intraperitoneal volume ranged from 8 to 89 ml/h and averaged 39 ml/h [28, 29]. The net absorption rate was not significantly different, irrespective of whether 2 L volumes of 1.5%, 2.5% or 4.25% dextrose dialysis solution were instilled [28, 29]. Moreover, net absorption rates during dialysis with 2.5 L infusion volumes also averaged 37 ml/h in 16 CAPD patients [26].

In conclusion, by analogy with ascites and by extrapolation from previous studies of drain volumes after infusion of isotonic and hypertonic solutions, the average daily effective lymphatic absorption rate during CAPD may be predicted to approach 1 L/day.

Methods of estimating lymphatic absorption in peritoneal dialysis

Two indirect methods have been described for measuring lymphatic drainage during dialysis [46, 67, 102–105, 111–132]. Both apply the same physiological functions of the peritoneal cavity lymphatics. By assuming that intraperitoneal marker colloids are returned to the systemic circulation exclusively by the lymphatics without increase or decrease in concentration of index colloids [2, 67, 75, 93–97], the lymphatic absorption rate may be estimated either from the mass transfer rate of marker colloids from the peritoneal cavity to the blood [46, 67, 102] or from their rate of disappearance from the peritoneal cavity [103–105, 111–132].

Mass transfer rates of intraperitoneal colloids to the blood

The first method essentially represents the peritoneal to blood clearance of a radio-labelled colloid. That is:

$$L = \frac{V_D \times \Delta C_D}{C_P} \qquad (3)$$

where:

L = total lymphatic flow during the time of the study

V_D = volume of distribution of the tracer colloid (plasma volume)

ΔC_D = rise in plasma concentration of the tracer colloid

C_P = time averaged mean intraperitoneal concentration of the tracer colloid

Using this approach the average lymphatic absorption rate in 10 CAPD patients was only 0.21 ml/min per 1.73 m^2 body surface area [102]. The absolute lymphatic absorption rates during CAPD most likely were underestimated in this study since the plasma volume of the CAPD patients was extrapolated from their body weight and, most importantly, the plasma appearance rate of radioiodinated serum albumin, as in similar studies in patients with ascites [97, 133, 134] was only 20% of the peritoneal disappearance rate. As well as confirming that there is an initial lag phase before the plasma concentration of the radiocolloid begins to increase linearly [9, 10, 46, 97], Spencer and Farrell have shown that the mass transfer of intraperitoneal radioiodinated albumin to the blood in CAPD patients was significantly greater after 24 h than after the end of a 4 hour study exchange [33]. Thus, transfer of radio-colloids continues after the washout exchange at the end of the study time and cannot be accurately timed to the duration of the exchange. These factors may explain why lymphatic flow rates calculated by this method are much lower than direct observations of absorption of intraperitoneal plasma or whole blood in the same animal model [41, 46].

Estimates by this method represent the *lower* limit of lymphatic absorption rates in peritoneal dialysis.

Mass transfer rates of colloids from the peritoneal cavity

Alternatively the effective lymphatic absorption rate (L) may be estimated from the mass transfer rate of intraperitoneal macromolecules from the peritoneal cavity. That is:

$$L = \frac{(V_0 \times C_0) - (V_t \times C_t)}{C_P} \qquad (4)$$

where:

V_0 and V_t = intraperitoneal fluid volumes at times 0 and t

C_0 and C_t = intraperitoneal concentration of marker colloid at times 0 and t

C_P = time-averaged mean intraperitoneal concentration of marker colloid

This mass balance equation avoids the error in calculating lymphatic flow in the previous method due to delayed transfer of radiolabelled colloids from the diaphragm and interstitial lymphatics to the blood. This method, however, not only depends on the assumption that intraperitoneal macromolecules are absorbed exclusively from the peritoneal cavity by the convective flow via the lymphatics, but further assumes that all of the intraperitoneal marker colloid lost from the peritoneal cavity is absorbed by the non-restrictive pathways of the lymphatics. In connective tissue spaces, back-diffusion of colloids into capillaries is negligible, the osmolality and the concentration of protein in the tissue fluid and end lymphatic lymph are equal and absorption of tissue protein is fully accounted for by lymphatic flow [135–138]. Several observations indicate that these findings also pertain to intraperitoneal fluid and colloid kinetics and that intraperitoneal fluid absorption may be estimated from the rate of loss of an intraperitoneal marker colloid.

1. Cannulation or ligation of both the right lymph duct and thoracic ducts prevents T-1824 labelled protein from reaching the blood [2, 74].
2. Obliteration of the subdiaphragmatic peritoneum markedly reduces the absorption of intraperitoneal colloid [73, 74].
3. The concentration of marker colloids remains unchanged during absorption of intraperitoneal isosmotic fluid [41, 46], suggesting that colloids

are absorbed with fluid by convective transport presumably through lymphatic pathways.

4. Fractional peritoneal absorption of albumin and IgG [97] and gelatins and dextrans of different molecular weights [139, 140] are similar, further suggesting that absorption of macromolecules is a size-independent convective process. In contrast transport of macromolecules from the circulation to the peritoneal cavity in peritoneal dialysis is a size-selective restricted process [140].
5. The intraperitoneal content of radioiodinated serum albumin during hypertonic peritoneal dialysis decreases at a linear rate averaging 3% per hour [102] and, late in the dwell time, correlates with net fluid absorption [32, 102, 129].

However, with microquantities of radiocolloid, a significant proportion of the administered dosage may be adsorbed to the peritoneal mesothelium, dialysis bag and administration set or be absorbed by the adjacent subperitoneal tissues [46, 141]. The addition of a large quantity of unlabelled colloid, such as albumin, instead of microamounts of radiolabelled colloid, may obviate this potential error [104, 105, 111, 115].

Cumulative net transcapillary ultrafiltration can be estimated concurrently from the dilution of the initial dialysate marker colloid concentration [103] since the intraperitoneal colloid concentration is unchanged by lymphatic absorption of intraperitoneal fluid [93, 94] and thus any decrease in the dialysate colloid concentration during the dwell time results from net influx of marker colloid free ultrafiltrate from the peritoneal microcirculation. However, allowance must be made for the effect of tracer disappearance on its dilution by the ultrafiltrate [142].

The peritoneal disappearance rate may overestimate actual lymph flow if, under non-steady state conditions, tracer enters and accumulates in the adjacent tissues [46, 67, 103]. However, measurements of lymphatic absorption were not reduced after prior repeated intraperitoneal administration of the tracer colloid, dextran, which suggests that there is no significant effect of tracer trapping in the submesothelial tissues [132] in spite of the elevated intraperitoneal pressure in CAPD [143]. The dextran disappearance rates before and after saturation of the peritoneal interstitium with dextran were similar at 1.1 ± 0.6 and 1.0 ± 0.4 ml/min [132]. Alternatively lymphatic absorption in CAPD has been evaluated by comparing transperitoneal transport of a lower molecular weight solute following both intravenous (mainly diffusive transport) and intraperitoneal administration (diffusive and lymphatic transport). It was assumed that inulin would be less likely to be trapped in the interstitum and the difference between the mass transfer area coefficients of intraperitoneal and intravenous inulin averaged 1.5 ml/min [123], which corresponds to estimates of lymphatic absorption using the disappearance rate of macromolecules (see Table 5).

Estimates of lymphatic absorption derived from the mass transfer rates of colloids from the peritoneal cavity represent the *upper* limit of lymphatic flow in peritoneal dialysis patients.

Computer simulations of transperitoneal fluid transport

Theoretic lymphatic absorption rates have been derived by a computer model based upon a three-pore model of the peritoneal barrier [144, 145]. Using this model, if fluid reabsorption from the peritoneal cavity to blood is constant at 1.25 ml/min and peritoneal membrane sieving coefficients for small solutes are at least 0.3, theoretic values for lymphatic absorption during peritoneal dialysis in humans varied between 0.3 and 0.75 ml/min. The computer predictions of intraperitoneal volume versus time data make a good fit with clinical measurements in adult patients [145].

Cannulation of the major lymphatic vessels

Direct measurement of *total* lymph flow from the peritoneal cavity during peritoneal dialysis cannot be performed. Cannulation of the major lymphatics draining the peritoneal cavity has been studied recently during peritoneal dialysis in experimental animals but not in humans [146–149]. This approach has provided comparisons of the different methods used for estimating lymphatic absorption and has been used to evaluate the relationship between fluid loss rates and lymphatic absorption rates from the peritoneal cavity. This methodology permits a more direct measurement of lymph flow but has several limitations:

1. It is not possible to cannulate all of the major lymphatic pathways draining the peritoneal cavity. In the sheep model only the thoracic and caudal lymphatic ducts are cannulated and drainage via the right lymph duct and small lymphaticovenous communications remains unmeasured [146, 147]. Despite cannulation of two of the major lymphatic vessels, over half of

recovered tracer colloid lost from the peritoneal cavity reached the blood compartment via the right lymph duct, other minor lymphatic pathways or direct entry into the blood stream [146, 147]. Absorption directly into the systemic circulation was unlikely to be significant since the recovery rate in the blood compartment of labelled intraperitoneal red blood cells in the lymphatic cannulation studies was similar to radiolabelled albumin.

2. Tracer colloids or cells may be entrapped in the lymph nodes draining the peritoneal cavity [46].
3. Cannulation of lymphatics may alter outflow pressure and reduce lymph flow [150].
4. Anaesthesia reduces lymphatic absorption substantially [81, 82, 146, 147] and therefore results of studies in conscious animals are much more likely to reflect dialysis conditions.

In conscious sheep (n = 6) lymph flow rates measured by cannulation of the thoracic and caudal ducts averaged 1.02 ± 0.19 ml/h per kg during exchanges using 50 ml/kg 4.25% dextrose dialysis solution [148]. After including an estimate for drainage via the right lymph duct, lymph flow rates increased to 1.52 ± 0.21 ml/h per kg [148]. Much lower estimates of total lymph drainage were observed in anaesthetized sheep (n = 6) using 50 ml/kg 1.5% dextrose dialysis solution [147]. Lymph flow values were significantly higher in conscious than in anaesthetized animals [148, 149].

Comparison of methods of estimating lymphatic absorption

None of the above methods directly measures total lymphatic flow from the peritoneal cavity during peritoneal dialysis. Comparative data for each method of measuring peritoneal lymph flow in a sheep model of peritoneal dialysis are summarized in Table 4 [149]. The estimates of lymph flow during peritoneal dialysis in conscious sheep using the same

Table 4. Peritoneal lymph flow rates during peritoneal dialysis in conscious sheep (adapted from ref. 148)

Method of estimating lymph flow	Lymph flow (ml/kg per hour)
Plasma appearance rate of tracer	1.42 ± 0.11
Peritoneal disappearance rate of tracer	2.40 ± 0.62
Cannulation of thoracic and caudal ducts (right lymph duct = zero)	1.02 ± 0.19
Cannulation of thoracic and caudal ducts (right lymph duct = caudal)	1.52 ± 0.21

dialysis parameters varied widely, but only the estimates from the peritoneal disappearance of tracer and the unadjusted cannulation studies differed significantly (Table 4).

The peritoneal disappearance rate of tracer equates with fluid loss via bulk flow (convection) from the peritoneal cavity [151]. Accordingly if the peritoneal disappearance rate of tracer is an accurate estimate of lymph flow, all of the calculated fluid loss from the peritoneal cavity is ascribed to translymphatic uptake [103, 116, 118–121, 124–128]. If the alternative methods of estimating lymphatic drainage are more precise only a proportion of the fluid losses are considered to leave the peritoneal cavity by true lymphatic flow [46, 102, 145–149].

A unifying interpretation of fluid losses and lymphatic drainage rates from the peritoneal cavity has been proposed [152]. Fluid and macromolecules are transported from the peritoneal cavity by bulk flow (convection) into the peritoneal lymphatics and interstitium due to intraperitoneal hydrostatic pressure, but sieving within the interstitium then leads to absorption of much of the fluid into the peritoneal capillaries and the macromolecules are removed by the interstitial lymphatics [152].

Fluid losses from the peritoneal cavity during peritoneal dialysis in adult humans are acknowledged to approximate 1.0–1.5 ml/min and to be clinically relevant [105–120, 122–129]. Similar fluid loss rates from the peritoneal cavity have been incorporated into modelled predictions of peritoneal dialysis ultrafiltration kinetics and small solute clearances [153]. The proportion of fluid absorption attributed to peritoneal lymphatic drainage is dependent upon the method used to measure lymph flow rates. To circumvent this unresolved debate convective fluid losses from the peritoneal cavity have been termed effective lymphatic absorption by Krediet and co-workers [125, 132, 140, 154–156] or total fluid absorption by Lindholm and co-workers [122, 129, 157]. Hitherto in this chapter fluid absorption from the peritoneal cavity has been defined as backfiltration to acknowledge that fluid loss occurs by bulk flow into the lymphatics and surrounding interstitial tissues and may be considered analogous to back-filtration in haemodialysers. Emphasis on attempting to subdivide fluid losses from the peritoneal cavity into lymphatic and non-lymphatic bulk flow has tended to confound the negative impact of back-filtration on the kinetics of peritoneal dialysis.

Effective lymphatic absorption rates (back-filtration) in peritoneal dialysis

Effective lymphatic absorption rates estimated from the disappearance rate of intraperitoneal colloids exceed 1 ml/min in most adult CAPD patients (Table 5) [32, 110, 112, 125, 126, 129, 140, 158, 167]. These effective lymphatic absorption rates are higher than net fluid absorption rates in CAPD patients estimated from sequential drain volumes after exchanges of increasing duration [26, 28]. A transperitoneal glucose and osmolar concentration gradient persists after the peak intraperitoneal volume is attained, which may allow transcapillary ultrafiltra-

Table 5. Back-filtration rates derived from the peritoneal disappearance rates of intraperitoneal macromolecules in adults during exchanges using 2 L of 1.36% dextrose dialysis solution

Marker solute	Molecular weight	Effective lymph flow (ml/min $\pm$ SEM)	Ref.
Dextran	30 500	1.56 $\pm$ 0.42	140
Autologous haemoglobin	34 000	1.59 $\pm$ 0.15	112
Dextran	50 500–57 000	1.71 $\pm$ 0.30	140
RISA	69 000	1.20 $\pm$ 0.30	129
Polydisperse dextran 70	–	1.30 $\pm$ 0.30	125
RISA	69 000	1.47 $\pm$ 0.15	32
Dextran 70	70 000	1.32 $\pm$ 0.10	158

Table 6. Effective lymphatic flow (back-filtration) rates derived from the disappearance rate of intraperitoneal macromolecules in adult CAPD patients during exchanges using 2 L of 2.27% dextrose dialysis solution or 2 L of 3.86% dextrose dialysis solution*

Marker solute	Effective lymph flow (ml/min $\pm$ SEM)	No. of patients	Ref.
Unlabelled human albumin	1.47 $\pm$ 0.15	10	110
[125]I-polyvinylpyrrollidone (PVP)	1.27 $\pm$ 0.25	5	126
Dextran 70*	1.42 $\pm$ 0.15	10	158
RISA*	1.77 $\pm$ 0.60	23	167
RISA*	2.19 $\pm$ 0.38	8[†]	167
RISA*	4.65 $\pm$ 0.93	4[‡]	167

*Studies using 3.86% dextrose dialysis solution.
[†]Eight patients with poor peritoneal ultrafiltration capacity due to high diffusive mass transfer coefficients.
[‡]Four patients with poor peritoneal ultrafiltration capacity due to high effective lymphatic absorption (back-filtration).

tion to continue at a slow rate provided that the peritoneal reflection coefficient for glucose is sufficient to generate an adequate osmotic pressure gradient.

Lymphatic absorption in many of the above studies may be higher than in active CAPD patients since fluid contact with the subdiaphragmatic peritoneum is more extensive with the patient supine than when the patient is ambulatory [74]. Alternatively upright posture may enhance back-filtration by increasing intraperitoneal pressure [143]. In 15 patients who remained in the upright position or sitting throughout the study dwell time, the lymphatic absorption rate calculated from the peritoneal disappearance of dextran 70 averaged 1.03 ± 0.45 ml/min [131]. Extrapolated to continuous peritoneal dialysis modalities back-filtration on average reduces daily peritoneal urea and creatinine clearances by approximately 10–15% and net ultrafiltration volumes by 40–50% [116, 126]. Consequently computer models have incorporated similar back-filtration rates to predict small solute clearances and net ultrafiltration volumes in peritoneal dialysis [153].

Factors controlling back-filtration in peritoneal dialysis

The rate of disappearance of tracer macromolecules has been utilized to assess which variables influence fluid absorption rates from the peritoneal cavity in peritoneal dialysis. The elimination rates of radiocolloid during 2 L exchanges with 1.36%, 2.27% and 3.86% anhydrous dextrose dialysis solutions were not significantly different, with values of 1.47 ± 0.15, 1.28 ± 0.16 and 1.30 ± 0.25 ml/min respectively [32]. Back-filtration rates using 1.36% glucose and 3.86% glucose in the same CAPD patients were similar at 1.32 ± 0.10 and 1.42 ± 0.15 ml/min respectively [154]. Studies with 2 L volumes of different osmotic agents (dextrose, ultra-low sodium dialysate, amino acids, glycerol and glucose polymer) demonstrated similar back-filtration rates [118, 155, 156]. Hence neither the osmolarity nor osmotic agent of the dialysis solution significantly influences back-filtration rates in peritoneal dialysis.

Back-filtration rates were elevated from 1.87 ± 0.23 to 3.39 ± 0.31 ml/min ($p < 0.01$) when the infusion volume of 1.36% dextrose dialysis solution was increased from 2 to 3 L [113]. Increased back-filtration with higher intraperitoneal volumes has been confirmed in other studies [128, 157].

During peritonitis calculated fluid reabsorption rates were 2.11 ± 0.25 ml/min compared with 1.05 ± 0.25 ml/min in the recovery period 20–40 days later ($p < 0.01$) [114]. During exchanges in adults and children using exchanges with comparable dialysate volumes back-filtration rates in children were 1.13 ± 0.20 ml/min per m² body surface area and in adults 0.75 ± 0.15 ml/min per m² body surface area [115]. Back-filtration rates in children using dextran as the marker colloid were similar to those of adults [127, 158], whereas back-filtration rates using autologous haemoglobin were higher than reported values for adults corrected for body surface area [159]. Back-filtration rates in 34 adult CAPD patients were found to be unrelated to patient age, sex, body surface area, duration of peritoneal dialysis or past history of peritonitis [128]. These studies indicate that back-filtration is increased in peritoneal dialysis using higher dialysate volumes [113, 128, 157] and during episodes of peritonitis [114].

Net ultrafiltration volumes are inversely related to intraperitoneal pressure in CAPD patients [160, 161]. Intraperitoneal pressure has been shown to be inversely related to transcapillary ultrafiltration and to correlate with back-filtration rates [161, 162]. From animal studies raised central venous pressure may be expected to reduce lymphatic flow rates but this has not yet been evaluated in CAPD patients [87].

Posture had only a minor effect on fluid kinetics in eight CAPD patients [163]. Upright posture results in a minor decrease in net ultrafiltration volumes when compared to recumbency due to a combination of slightly higher effective lymphatic absorption rates and slightly lower transcapillary ultrafiltration with upright posture [163]. Continuous vibration of the abdominal wall with a small electric vibrator enhanced small solute mass transfer area coefficients but had no effect on net ultrafiltration volumes or lymphatic absorption in a rat model of peritoneal dialysis [164]. Attenuation of spontaneous contractions of the lymphatic vessels using intraperitoneal isoprenaline had no effect on effective lymphatic drainage [165].

Consequences of back-filtration during peritoneal dialysis

The physiological roles of the peritoneal cavity lymphatics in the absorption of intraperitoneal isosmotic fluid, macromolecules, particles and bacteria are normally beneficial. However, back-filtration has mainly adverse effects on the clinical application of long-dwell peritoneal dialysis as an effective form of renal replacement therapy.

Loss of Ultrafiltration

Back-filtration of intraperitoneal fluid throughout the dwell time reduces the potential drain volume, and thus net ultrafiltration, in all CAPD patients. Since net transcapillary ultrafiltration occurs mainly during the first hours of each exchange when using small molecular weight solutes as an osmotic agent, while back-filtration is continuous throughout the dwell time, effective lymphatic absorption has a greater influence on ultrafiltration kinetics in CAPD than in intermittent peritoneal dialysis with rapid exchanges. In short-dwell exchanges cumulative net transcapillary ultrafiltration greatly exceeds lymphatic drainage and consequently the reduction in the dialysate drain volume resulting from back-filtration is relatively minor. Wide interindividual [35, 36] and intraindividual [37] variation in net ultrafiltration has been observed in CAPD patients even if the dwell time, osmolality and volume of exchanges are standardized. Poor peritoneal ultrafiltration capacity has usually been ascribed to high peritoneal permeability area, rapid absorption of glucose from the dialysate, early dissipation of the transperitoneal osmolar gradient and thus reduced cumulative net transcapillary ultrafiltration [35–37, 39]. In addition, since transperitoneal osmotic pressure is equivalent to the sum of the products of the osmolar gradient and the peritoneal reflection coefficient of each solute, the lower peritoneal reflection coefficient for glucose in patients with high peritoneal permeability area will further reduce transcapillary ultrafiltration by generating reduced osmotic pressure at any given glucose concentration gradient. Such patients with high effective peritoneal surface area or MTAC for small solutes will have an earlier and reduced peak ultrafiltration volume and may develop Type 1 ultrafiltration failure.

Interpatient differences in peritoneal ultrafiltration capacity after long-dwell exchanges may, however, depend on back-filtration as well as peritoneal permeability area.

Studies of ultrafiltration kinetics in two groups of CAPD patients with high and average peritoneal transport rates showed that the disappearance rates of intraperitoneal marker macromolecules (back-filtration) were similar (83 ± 16 ml/h in patients with average peritoneal solute transport rates and 89 ± 9 ml/h in patients with high peritoneal perme-

ability area [116]). The former group, as expected, had higher net transcapillary ultrafiltration and net ultrafiltration volumes. Therefore, despite equal absolute fluid absorption rates, back-filtration causes a proportionately greater reduction in ultrafiltration capacity in patients with higher than average peritoneal permeability area (Fig. 7).

Studies in a total of 73 CAPD patients with true loss of peritoneal ultrafiltration capacity have identified four patterns of ultrafiltration failure [34, 105, 111, 166–174]. It was not possible to delineate the pattern of ultrafiltration failure in six other patients reported in these studies [171, 174]. The most common cause of loss of ultrafiltration is a decrease in transcapillary ultrafiltration as a result of rapid absorption of dialysate glucose and early loss of the transperitoneal osmotic gradient (Type 1 membrane failure), whereas failure of ultrafiltration due to a reduction in transcapillary ultrafiltration in a patient with low peritoneal permeability-area is rare (Table 7). Sclerosing peritonitis may be associated with either Type 1 or Type 2 membrane failure.

However, a significant proportion of patients with loss of ultrafiltration capacity have average transcapillary ultrafiltration but high back-filtration rates from the peritoneal cavity (Table 7). A further group of patients with ultrafiltration failure has been characterized [166], in which net ultrafiltration is low in spite of average effective membrane area, back-filtration and residual volumes. The absence of solute sieving in this group of patients, as manifest by the minimal reduction in dialysate sodium concentration during the first hour of an exchange, is most likely due to impaired transcellular water transport in response to an adequate transperitoneal osmotic gradient [166]. This most recently described cause of poor ultrafiltration capacity has been termed 'Type 4' failure in Table 7. Nevertheless the underlying pathophysiological mechanisms of these patterns of ultrafiltration failure remain unknown in most patients. The prevalence of ultrafiltration failure in patients using only lactate-based dialysis fluids increases with the duration of dialysis; 3% of patients after 1 year of CAPD, 10% after 3 years and 31% after 6 years, excluding patients with temporary loss of ultrafiltration capacity due to peritoneal catheter malposition or dialysate leaks [168]. It remains uncertain whether factors such as temporal changes in the mesothelium, the glycation of peritoneal structural proteins or dialysate effluent phospholipid concentrations determine peritoneal ultrafiltration capacity.

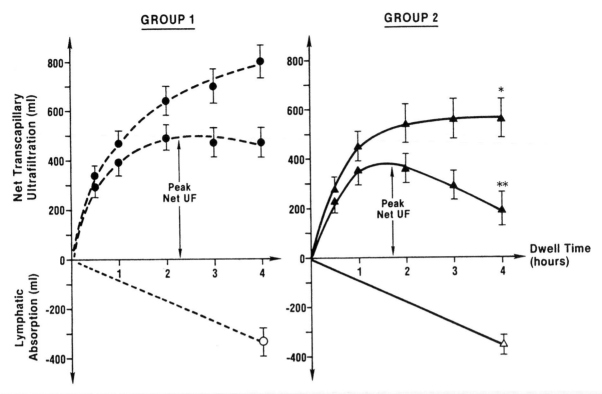

Figure 7. Comparison of cumulative effective lymphatic absorption, net ultrafiltration and cumulative net transcapillary ultrafiltration (mean ± SEM) during 4 h exchanges using 2 L of 2.5% dextrose dialysis solution in CAPD patients with average (group 1] and high (group 2] peritoneal permeability × area. (Reproduced with permission from ref. 116.) (** < 0.01; *p < 0.05).

Table 7. Mechanisms of poor peritoneal ultrafiltration capacity reported in 73 CAPD patients with ultrafiltration failure (number of CAPD patients with each type of UF failure)

High MTAC (Type 1)	Low MTAC (Type 2)	High back-filtration (Type 3)	Low transcellular water transport (Type 4)	Ref.
3	–	2	–	34
4	–	–	–	110
–	–	1	–	111
–	–	–	6	166
8	–	4	–	167
7	–	2	–	168
3	–	2	–	169
4	1	–	–	170
6	–	5	–	171
5	–	2	–	172
–	–	1	–	173
3	–	4	–	174
Totals				
43	1	23	6	

Reduction in solute mass transfer

The continuous absorption of dialysate solutes by back-filtration decreases solute mass transfer significantly during CAPD [105, 116, 175–177]. Peritoneal solute clearances are calculated as the product of daily drain volume and drain dialysate solute concentration divided by the mean serum solute concentration, while reverse solute clearances may be estimated from the product of daily back-filtration and mean dialysate solute concentration divided by the mean serum solute concentration. Extrapolated to four exchanges using 2 L of 2.5% dextrose dialysis solution per day, back-filtration in 18 CAPD patients reduced the potential daily drain volume by 18 ± 2%, potential daily urea clearance by 14 ± 1.4% and potential daily creatinine clearance by 13.3 ± 1.5% (Fig. 8) [116]. Similar observations have been reported by other groups [126]. These findings indicate that estimates of transperitoneal solute transport, which are based on the dialysate drain volume and solute concentration, are erroneously low, since no allowance has been made for back-filtration throughout the dwell time. Accord-

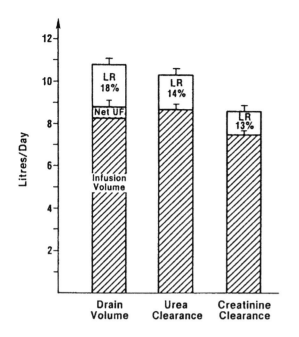

Figure 8. Contribution of back-filtration to loss of potential drain volume, urea clearance and creatinine clearance (mean ± SEM) in adult CAPD patients (n = 18] using four exchanges of 2.5% dextrose dialysis solution per day. (Reproduced with permission from ref. 116.)

ingly the efficiency of the peritoneum as a dialysing membrane is greater than previously recognized [27, 33, 34, 178–181] and the inclusion of the effect of dialysate back-filtration in models of transperitoneal urea transport was shown to increase the mass transfer area coefficient significantly [175]. Practical approaches for decreasing back-filtration from the peritoneal cavity are limited. The clinical results of attempting to use phospholipids or neostigmine to reduce back-filtration and to augment ultrafiltration and solute clearances have been conflicting [120, 124, 130, 182–192]. Bethanechol orally in nine CAPD patients [193] and bicarbonate glycylglycine peritoneal dialysis solution in normal rabbits [194] enhanced ultrafiltration volumes; this was attributed to reduced back-filtration rates. Hyaluronic acid added to the dialysate has been shown to reduce fluid absorption and improve ultrafiltration volumes in a rat model of peritoneal dialysis [195].

Absorption of intraperitoneal bacteria

The uptake of intraperitoneal bacteria by the peritoneal cavity lymphatics is well established [196, 197].

Nevertheless, blood cultures are infrequently positive during CAPD-associated peritonitis [198] and secondary pulmonary infections or right-sided endocarditis are very rare complications of peritonitis [69, 198]. The bacteria are presumably filtered and effectively trapped by the mediastinal lymph nodes. In a sterile peritonitis model of peritoneal dialysis in conscious sheep cannulation of the caudal mediastinal and thoracic ducts showed that the major route of removal of inflammatory cells from the peritoneal cavity is through the diaphragmatic lymphatics [199].

Absorption of intraperitoneal polymers and particles

The uptake of large solutes and particles by convective flow into the peritoneal cavity lymphatics has several implications for peritoneal dialysis. Alternative less absorbable osmotic agents than glucose have been sought to reduce the undesired metabolic sequelae of dialysate glucose absorption and, most importantly, to induce sustained net transcapillary ultrafiltration [31, 200]. However, lymphatic drainage results in systemic absorption of all polymer osmotic agents [200–204], regardless of their molecular weight, which may hinder the development of safe and effective alternative osmotic agents to glucose. Icodextrin is currently recommended for use only in one exchange per day, to limit systemic absorption and accumulation. Human albumin would be an ideal osmotic agent since its systemic absorption would be beneficial rather than potentially harmful.

Particulate material entering the peritoneal cavity in the dialysis solution will also be absorbed by the peritoneal cavity lymphatics. Thus contaminants in commercial dialysis solutions should be avoided, to prevent their systemic accumulation and toxicity as well as their potentially adverse effects on the peritoneal membrane [114, 205].

The continuous uptake of tracer macromolecules from the peritoneal cavity requires that estimates of the dialysate volume using the single-injection indicator-dilution method must be corrected for the peritoneal disappearance rate of the index colloid [206, 207].

Conclusion

Back-filtration rates during peritoneal dialysis are greater than 1.0 ml/min in most patients and have a major influence on the kinetics of ultrafiltration in long-dwell exchanges. On average back-filtration reduces net ultrafiltration volumes each day by 40–50%, and urea and creatinine clearances per day by approximately 15%. Nevertheless the currently available range of glucose-containing dialysis solutions has been developed to induce sufficient net transcapillary ultrafiltration to offset back-filtration and so achieve adequate daily peritoneal ultrafiltration and small solute clearances in the majority of CAPD patients.

Acknowledgement

The secretarial assistance of Linda Grier is greatly appreciated.

References

1. Allen L. Lymphatics and lymphoid tissues. Annu Rev Physiol 1967; 29: 197–224.
2. Courtice FC, Steinbeck AW. The lymphatic drainage of plasma from the peritoneal cavity of the cat. Austral J Exp Biol Med Sci 1950; 28: 161–9.
3. Hyatt RE, Smith JR. The mechanisms of ascites: physiological appraisal. Am J Med 1954; 16: 434–48.
4. Courtice FC. Ascites: the role of the lymphatics in the accumulation of ascitic fluid. Med J Aust 1959; 26: 945–51.
5. Witte MH, Witte CL, Dumont AE. Progress in liver disease: physiological factors involved in the causation of cirrhotic ascites. Gastroenterology 1971; 61: 742–50.
6. Dumont AE, Mulholland JH. Flow rate and composition of thoracic duct lymph in patients with cirrhosis. N Engl J Med 1960; 263: 471–4.
7. Barrowman JA. Liver lymph. In: Barrowman JA, ed. Physiology of the Gastrointestinal Lymphatic System. Cambridge: Cambridge University Press, 1978, pp. 229–55.
8. Witte CL, Witte MH, Dumont AE. Lymph imbalance in the genesis and perpetuation of the ascites syndrome in hepatic cirrhosis. Gastroenterology 1980; 78: 1059–68.
9. Morgan AG, Terry SI. Impaired peritoneal fluid drainage in nephrogenic ascites. Clin Nephrol 1981; 15: 61–5.
10. Bronskill MJ, Bush RS, Ege GN. A quantitative measurement of peritoneal drainage in malignant ascites. Cancer 1977; 40: 2375–80.
11. Coates G, Bush RS, Aspin N. A study of ascites using lymphoscintigraphy with 99m Tc sulfur colloid. Radiology 1973; 107: 577–83.
12. Atkins HL, Hauser W, Richards P. Visualization of mediastinal lymph nodes after intraperitoneal administrations of 99m Tc sulfur colloid. Nuclear-medizin 1970; 9: 275–8.
13. Kroon BBR. Overhet ontstaan en de chirurgische behandeling van maligne ascites. MD thesis, University of Amsterdam, 1986.
14. Feldman GB, Knapp RC. Lymphatic drainage of the peritoneal cavity and its significance in ovarian cancer. Am J Obstet Gynecol 1974; 119: 991–4.
15. Feldman GB. Lymphatic obstruction in carcinomatous ascites. Cancer Res 1975; 35: 325–32.
16. Ismail AH, Mohamed FS. Structural changes of the diaphragmatic peritoneum in patients with schistosomal hepatic fibrosis in relation to ascites. Lymphology 1986; 19: 82–7.
17. Clausen J. Studies on the effect of intraperitoneal blood transfusion. Acta Paediatr 1940; 27: 24–33.
18. Cole WC, Montgomery JC. Intraperitoneal blood transfusion. Report of 237 transfusions in 117 patients in private practice. Am J Dis Child 1929; 37: 497–510.
19. Siperstein DM, Sansby JM. Intraperitoneal transfusion with citrated blood. Am J Dis Child 1923; 25: 107–29.
20. Scopes JW. Intraperitoneal transfusion in blood in newborn babies. Lancet 1963; 1: 1027–8.
21. Liley AW. Intrauterine transfusion of the foetus in haemolytic disease. Br Med J 1963; 2: 1107–9.
22. Nolph KD, Popovich RP, Ghods AJ, Twardowski Z. Determinants of low clearances of small solutes during peritoneal dialysis. Kidney Int 1978; 13: 117–23.
23. Nolph KD, Miller F, Rubin J, Popovich R. New directions in peritoneal dialysis concepts and applications. Kidney Int 1980; 18: S111–16.
24. Nolph KD. Solute and water transport during peritoneal dialysis. Perspect Perit Dial 1983; 1: 4–8.
25. Nolph KD, Miller FN, Pyle WK, Popovich RP, Sorkin M I. An hypothesis to explain the ultrafiltration characteristics of peritoneal dialysis. Kidney Int 1981; 20: 543–48.
26. Twardowski Z, Janicka L. Three exchanges with a 2.5 liter volume for continuous ambulatory peritoneal dialysis. Kidney Int 1981; 20: 281–4.
27. Pyle WK, Popovich RP, Moncrief JW. Mass transfer evaluation in peritoneal dialysis. In: Moncrief JW, Popovich RP, eds. CAPD Update. New York: Masson, 1981, pp. 35–52.
28. Twardowski Z, Ksiazek A, Majadan M et al. Kinetics of continuous ambulatory peritoneal dialysis (CAPD) with four exchanges per day. Clin Nephrol 1981; 15: 119–30.
29. Rubin J, Nolph KD, Popovich RP, Moncrief JW, Prowant B. Drainage volumes during continuous ambulatory peritoneal dialysis. ASAIO J 1979; 2: 54–60.
30. Krediet RT, Boeschoten EW, Zuyderhoudt RMJ, Arisz L. The relationship between peritoneal glucose absorption and body fluid loss by ultrafiltration during continuous ambulatory peritoneal dialysis. Clin Nephrol 1987; 27: 51–5.
31. Twardowski AJ, Khanna R, Nolph KD. Osmotic agents and ultrafiltration in peritoneal dialysis. Nephron 1986; 42: 93–101.
32. Lindholm B, Werynski A, Bergstrom J. Kinetics of peritoneal dialysis with glycerol and glucose osmotic agents. ASAIO Trans 1987; 33: 19–27.
33. Spencer PC, Farrell PC. Solute and water kinetics in CAPD. In: Gokal R, ed. Continuous Ambulatory Peritoneal Dialysis. Edinburgh: Churchill Livingstone, 1986, pp. 38–55.
34. Krediet RT, Boeschoten EW, Zuyderhoudt FMJ, Arisz L. Peritoneal transport characteristics of water, low-molecular weight solutes and proteins during long-term continuous ambulatory peritoneal dialysis. Perit Dial Bull 1986; 6: 61–5.
35. Nikolakakis N, Rodger RSC, Goodship THJ et al. The assessment of peritoneal function using a single hypertonic exchange. Perit Dial Bull 1985; 5: 186–8.
36. Smeby LC, Wideroe TE, Jorstad S. Individual differences in water transport during continuous peritoneal dialysis. ASAIO J 1981; 4: 17–27.
37. Wideroe TE, Smeby LC, Mjaaland S, Dahl K, Berg KJ, Aas TW. Long-term changes in transperitoneal water transport during continuous ambulatory peritoneal dialysis. Nephron 1984; 38, 238–47.
38. Raja RM, Khanna MS, Barber K. Solute transport and ultrafiltration during peritonitis in CAPD patients. ASAIO J 1984; 7: 8–11.
39. International Co-operative Study. A survey of ultrafiltration in continuous ambulatory peritoneal dialysis. Perit Dial Bull 1984; 4: 137–42.
40. Olin T, Saldeen T. The lymphatic pathways from the peritoneal cavity: a lymphangiographic study in the rat. Cancer Res 1964; 24: 1700–11.

41. Courtice FC, Simmonds WJ. Physiological significance of lymph drainage of the serous cavities and lungs. Physiol Rev 1954; 34: 419–48.
42. Higgins GM, Graham AS. Lymphatic drainage from the peritoneal cavity in the dog. Arch Surg 1929; 19: 453–65.
43. Raybuck HE, Allen L, Harms WS. Absorption of serum from the peritoneal cavity. Am J Physiol 1960; 199: 1021–24.
44. Simer PH. The drainage of particulate matter from the peritoneal cavity by lymphatics. Anat Rec 1944; 88: 175–92.
45. Courtice FC, Harding J, Steinbeck AW. The removal of free red blood cells from the peritoneal cavity of animals. Aust J Exp Biol Med Sci 1953; 31: 215–25.
46. Flessner MF, Parker RJ, Sieber SM. Peritoneal lymphatic uptake of fibrinogen and erythrocytes in the rat. Am J Physiol 1983; 244: H89–96.
47. Von Recklinghausen F. Zur Fettresorption. Arch Pathol Anat Physiol Klin Med 1863; 26: 172–208.
48. MacCallum WG. On the mechanism of absorption of granular material from the peritoneum. Bull John Hopkins Hosp 1903; 14: 105–15.
49. Cunningham RS. Studies in absorption from serous cavities IV. On the passage of blood cells and particles of different size through the walls of the lymphatics in the diaphragm. Am J Physiol 1922; 62: 248–52.
50. Hertzler AE. The morphogenesis of the stigmata and stomata occurring in peritoneal and vascular endothelium. Trans Am Microsc Soc 1901; 22: 63–82.
51. Allen L. The peritoneal stomata. Anat Rec 1937; 67: 89–103.
52. French JE, Florey HW, Morris B. The absorption of particles by the lymphatics of the diaphragm. Q J Exp Physiol 1960; 45: 88–103.
53. Casley-Smith JR. Endothelial permeability – the passage of particles into and out of diaphragmatic lymphatics. Q J Exp Physiol 1964; 49: 365–83.
54. Tsilibary EC, Wissig SL. Light and electron microscope observations of the lymphatic drainage units of the peritoneal cavity of rodents. Am J Anat 1987; 180: 195–207.
55. Tsilibary EC, Wissig SL. Absorption from the peritoneal cavity: SEM study of mesothelium covering the peritoneal surface of the muscular portion of the diaphragm. Am J Anat 1977; 149: 127–33.
56. Hedenstedt S. Elliptocyte transfusions as a method in studies on blood destruction, blood volume and peritoneal resorption. Acta Chir Scand 1947; 95 (suppl. 128): 105–34.
57. Morris B, Murphy MJ, Bessis M. The passage of red blood cells from the peritoneal cavity. In: Yoffey JM, Courtice FC, eds. Lymphatics, Lymph and Lymphoid Tissue. London: Academic Press, 1970, p. 303.
58. Florey HW. Reactions of, and absorption by, lymphatics with special reference to those of the diaphragm. Br J Exp Pathol 1927; 8: 479–90.
59. Allen L. On the penetrability of the lymphatics of the diaphragm. Anat Rec 1956; 124: 639–57.
60. Allen L, Weatherwood T. Role of fenestrated basement membrane in lymphatic absorption from the peritoneal cavity. Am J Physiol 1959; 197: 551–4.
61. Leak LV, Rahil K. Permeability to the diaphragmatic mesothelium: the ultrastructural basis for stomata. Am J Anat 1978; 151: 557–94.
62. Tsilibary EC, Wissig SL. Structural plasticity in the pathway for lymphatic drainage from the peritoneal cavity. Microvasc Res 1979; 17: S144.
63. Bettendorf U. Lymph flow mechanism of the subperitoneal diaphragmatic lymphatics. Lymphology 1978; 11: 111–16.
64. Tsilibary EC, Wissig SL. Lymphatic absorption from the peritoneal cavity: regulation of patency of mesothelial stomata. Microvasc Res 1983; 25: 25–39.
65. Allen L, Vogt E. A mechanism of lymphatic absorption from serous cavities. Am J Physiol 1937; 119: 776–82.
66. Khanna R, Mactier R, Twardowksi ZJ, Nolph KD. Anatomy of peritoneal cavity lymphatics. Perit Dial Bull 1986; 6: 113–21.
67. Flessner MF, Dedrick RL, Schultz JS. Exchange of macromolecules between peritoneal cavity and plasma. Am J Physiol 1985; 248: H15–25.
68. Dunn DL, Barke RA, Knight NB, Humphrey EW, Simmons RL. Role of resident macrophages, peripheral neutrophils and translymphatic absorption in bacterial clearance from the peritoneal cavity. Infect Immun 1985; 49: 257–64.
69. Keane WF, Peterson PK. Host defence mechanisms of the peritoneal cavity and continuous ambulatory peritoneal dialysis. Perit Dial Bull 1984; 4: 122–7.
70. Simer PH. The passage of particulate matter from peritoneal cavity into the lymph vessels of the diaphragm. Anat Rec 1948; 101: 333–51.
71. Clark AJ. Absorption from the peritoneal cavity. J Pharmacol Exp Ther 1920; 16: 415–28.
72. Courtice FC, Steinbeck AW. The rate of absorption of heparinized plasma and of 0.9% NaCl from the peritoneal cavity of the rabbit and guinea-pig. Aust J Exp Biol Med Sci 950; 28: 171–82.
73. Allen L, Raybuck HE. The effects of obliteration of the diaphragmatic lymphatic pleuxus on serous fluid. Anat Rec 960; 137: 25–32.
74. Courtice FC, Steinbeck AW. The effects of lymphatic obstruction and of posture on the absorption of protein form the peritoneal cavity. Aust J Exp Biol Med Sci 1951; 29: 451–8.
75. Bolton C. Absorption from the peritoneal cavity. J Pathol Bacterial 1921 24: 429–45.
76. Zink J, Greenway CV. Control of ascites absorption in anesthetized cats: effects of intraperitoneal pressure, protein and furosemide diuresis. Gastroenterology 1977; 73: 1119–24.
77. Morris B. The effect of diaphragmatic movement on the absorption of red cells and protein from the peritoneal cavity. Aust J Exp Biol Med Sci 1953; 31: 239–46.
78. Higgins GM, Beaver MG, Lemon WS. Phrenic neurectomy and peritoneal absorption. Am J Anat 1930; 45: 137–57.
79. Shear L, Castellot J, Barry KG. Peritoneal fluid absorption: effect of dehydration on kinetics. J Lab Clin Med 1965; 66: 232–43.
80. Shear L, Swartz C, Shinaberger JA, Barry KG. Kinetics of peritoneal fluid absorption in adult man. N Engl J Med 1965; 272: 123–27.
81. Schad H, Brechtelsbaver H. Thoracic duct lymph flow and composition in conscious dogs and the influence of anesthesia and passive limb movement. Plugers Arch 1977; 371: 25–31.
82. Elk JR, Adair T, Drake RE, Gabel JC. The effect of anesthesia and surgery on diaphragmatic lymph vessel flow after endotoxin in sheep. Lymphology 1990; 23: 145–8.
83. Shear L, Ching S, Gabuzda GJ. Compartmentalisation of ascites and oedema in patients with hepatic cirrhosis. N Engl J Med 1970; 282: 1391–6.
84. Hau T, Ahrenholz DH, Simmons RL. Secondary bacterial peritonitis: the biologic basis of treatment. Curr Probl Surg 1979; 16: 1–65.
85. Fowler GR. Diffuse septic peritonitis, with special reference to a new method of treatment, namely, the elevated head and trunk posture, to facilitate drainage into the pelvis. With a report of nine consecutive cases of recovery. Med Rec 1900; 57: 617–23.
86. Levine S. Post-inflammatory increase of absorption from peritoneal cavity into lymph nodes: particulate and oily inocula. Exp Mol Pathol 1985; 43: 124–34.
87. Drake RE, Gabel JC. Abdominal lymph flow response to intra-peritoneal fluid in awake sheep. Lymphology 1991; 24: 77–81.
88. Dobbie JW. From philosopher to fish: the comparative anatomy of the peritoneal cavity as an excretory organ and its significance for peritoneal dialysis in man. Perit Dial Int 1988; 8: 3–6.
89. Di Paolo N. The peritoneal mesothelium: an excretory organ. Perit Dial Int 1989; 9: 151–3.

90. Dobbie JW, Pavlina T, Lloyd J *et al*. Phosphatidylcholine synthesis by peritoneal mesothelium: its implications for peritoneal dialysis. Am J Kidney Dis 1988; 12: 31–8.

91. Grahame GR, Torchia MC, Dankevich KA *et al*. Surface active material in peritoneal effluent of CAPD patients. Perit Dial Bull 1985; 5: 109–11.

92. Breborowicz A, Sombolos K, Bodela H *et al*. Mechanism of phosphalidylcholine action during peritoneal dialysis. Perit Dial Bull 1987; 7: 6–9.

93. Lill SR, Parsons RH, Bohac I. Permeability of the diaphragm and fluid resorption from the peritoneal cavity in the rat. Gastroenterology 1979; 76: 997–1001.

94. Aune S. Transperitoneal exchange IV. The effect of transperitoneal fluid transport on the transfer of solutes. Scand J Gastroenterol 1970; 5: 241–52.

95. Courtice FC, Steinbeck AW. Absorption of protein from the peritoneal cavity. J Physiol 1951; 114: 336–55.

96. Nicoll PA, Taylor AE. Lymph formation and flow. Annu Rev Physiol 1977; 39: 73–95.

97. Henriksen JH, Lassen NA, Parving H, Winkler K. Filtration as the main transport mechanism of protein exchange between plasma and the peritoneal cavity in hepatic cirrhosis. Scan J Clin Invest 1980; 40: 503–13.

98. Goranson LR, Johnson K, Olin T. Parasternal scintigraphy with technetium-99m sulfide colloid in human subjects: a comparison between two techniques. Acta Radiol Diag 1974; 15: 639–49.

99. Bergman F. Carcinoma of the ovary; a clinicopathological study of 86 autopsied cases with special reference to mode of spread. Acta Obstet Gynecol Scand 1966; 45: 211–31.

100. Raybuck HE, Weatherwood T, Allen L. Lymphatics in the genesis of ascites in the rat. Am J Physiol 1960; 198: 1207–10.

101. Harber M, Page C, Streather C, O'Doherty M, Barton I. Restoration of peritoneal lymphatic drainage leading to spontaneous resolution of haemodialysis ascites. Nephrol Dial Transplant 1994; 9: 716–17.

102. Rippe B, Stelin G, Ahlmen J. Lymph flow from the peritoneal cavity in CAPD patients. In: Maher JF, Winchester JF, eds. Frontiers in Peritoneal Dialysis. New York: Field, Rich, 1986, pp. 24–30.

103. Mactier RA, Khanna R, Twardowski Z, Nolph KD. Role of peritoneal cavity lymphatic absorption in peritoneal dialysis. Kidney Int 1987; 32: 165–72.

104. Nolph KD, Mactier RA, Khanna R, Twardowski ZJ, Moore H, McGary T. Kinetics of peritoneal ultrafiltration: the role of lymphatics. Kidney Int 1987; 32: 219–26.

105. Mactier RA, Khanna R, Twardowski ZJ, Nolph KD. Contribution of lymphatic absorption to loss of ultrafiltration and solute clearances in CAPD. J Clin Invest 1987; 80: 1311–16.

106. Dobbie JW, Zaki M, Wilson L. Ultrastructural studies on the peritoneum with special reference to chronic ambulatory peritoneal dialysis. Scott Med J 1981; 26: 213–23.

107. Di Paolo N, Sacchi G, De Mia M *et al*. Morphology of the peritoneal membrane during peritoneal dialysis. Nephron 1986; 44: 204–11.

108. Verger C, Brunschvigg O, Le Carpentier Y, Laverone A. Structural and ultrastructural peritoneal membrane changes and permeability alterations during CAPD. Proc EDTA 1981; 18: 199–203.

109. Nolph KD, Hano JE, Teschan PE. Peritoneal sodium transport during hypertonic peritoneal dialysis: physiologic mechanisms and clinical implications. Ann Intern Med 1969; 70: 931–41.

110. Knochel JP. Formation of peritoneal fluid hypertonicity during dialysis with isotonic glucose solutions. J Appl Physiol 1969; 27: 233–6.

111. Mactier RA, Khanna R, Twardowski ZJ, Nolph KD. Failure of ultrafiltration in CAPD due to excessive lymphatic absorption. Am J Kidney Dis 1987; 10: 461–6.

112. Krediet RT, Struijk DG, Boeschoten EW *et al*. Autologous haemoglobin for the measurement of intraperitoneal volume and lymphatic absorption in CAPD. Perit Dial Int 1988; VIII Annual CAPD Abstracts, 83A.

113. Krediet RT, Boeschoten EW, Struijk DG, Arisz L. Differences in the peritoneal transport of water, solutes and proteins between dialysis with two or with three litre exchanges. Nephrol Dial Transplant 1988; 2: 198–204.

114. Krediet RT, Struijk DG, Boeschoten EW, Arisz L. The effect of peritonitis on lymphatic fluid absorption from the peritoneal cavity. Nephrol Dial Transplant 1988; 3: 556A.

115. Mactier RA, Khanna R, Moore H, Russ J, Nolph KD, Groshong T. Kinetics of peritoneal dialysis in children: role of lymphatics. Kidney Int 1988; 34: 82–8.

116. Mactier RA. The role of lymphatic absorption in peritoneal dialysis. MD thesis, University of Glasgow, 1988.

117. Lindholm B, Werynski A, Bergstrom J. Peritoneal dialysis with amino acid solutions: fluid and solute transport kinetics. Artif Organs 1988; 12: 2–10.

118. De Paepe M, Matthys D, Lameire N. Measurement of peritoneal lymph flow in CAPD using different osmotic agents. Perit Dial Int, 1989; IX Annual CAPD Abstracts, 44A.

119. Mactier RA, Khanna R. Absorption of fluid and solutes from the peritoneal cavity. Theoretic and therapeutic implications and applications. Trans ASAIO 1989; 35: 122–31.

120. Struijk DG, Van der Reijden HJ, Krediet RT, Koomen GCM, Arisz L. Effect of phosphatidylcholine on peritoneal transport and lymphatic absorption in a CAPD patient with sclerosing peritonitis. Nephron 1989; 51: 577–8.

121. Breborowicz A, Rodela H, Oreopoulos DG. Effect of various factors on peritoneal lymphatic flow in rabbits. Perit Dial Int 1989; 9: 85–90.

122. Lindholm B, Heimburger O, Waniewski J, Werynski A, Bergstrom J. Peritoneal ultrafiltration and fluid reabsorption during peritoneal dialysis. Nephrol Dial Transplant 1989; 4: 805–13.

123. Stuijk DG, Krediet RT, Koomen GCM, Boeschoten EW, Reijden HJ, Arisz L. Indirect measurement of lymphatic absorption with inulin in CAPD patients. Perit Dial Int 1990; 10: 141–5.

124. Chan PCK, Tam SCF, Cheng IKP. Oral neostigmine and lymphatic absorption in a myasthenia gravis patient on CAPD. Perit Dial Int 1990; 10: 93–6.

125. Krediet RT, Struijk DG, Koomen GCM, Arisz L. Peritoneal fluid kinetics during CAPD measured with intraperitoneal dextran 70. ASAIO Trans 1991; 37: 662–7.

126. Lysaght MJ, Moran J, Lysaght CB, Schindhelm K, Farrell PC. Plasma water filtration and lymphatic uptake during peritoneal dialysis. ASAIO Trans 1991; 37: M402–4.

127. Schroder CH, Reddingius RE, Van Dreumel JAM, Theeuwes AGM, Monnens LAH. Transcapillary ultrafiltration and lymphatic absorption during childhood continuous ambulatory peritoneal dialysis. Nephrol Dial Transplant 1991; 6: 571–3.

128. Chan PCK, Wu PG, Tam SCF, Ip MSM, Fang GX, Cheng IKP. Factors affecting lymphatic absorption in Chinese patients on CAPD. Perit Dial Int 1992; 11: 147–51.

129. Heimburger O, Waniewski J, Werynski A, Lindholm B. A quantitative description of solute and fluid transport during peritoneal dialysis. Kidney Int 1992; 41: 1320–32.

130. Hasbargen JA, Hasbargen BJ, Fortenbery EJ. Effect of intraperitoneal neostigmine on peritoneal transport characteristics in CAPD. Kidney Int 1992; 42: 1398–1400.

131. Abensur H, Romad JE, Prado EBA, Kakehashi ET, Sabbaga E, Marcondes M. Use of dextran 70 to estimate peritoneal lymphatic absorption rate in CAPD. Adv Perit Dial 1992; 8: 3–6.

132. Struijk DG, Koomen GCM, Krediet RT, Arisz L. Indirect measurement of lymphatic absorption in CAPD patients is not influenced by trapping. Kidney Int 1992; 41: 1668–75.

133. Dykes PW, Jones JH. Albumin exchange between plasma and ascitic fluid. Clin Sci 1968; 34: 185–97.

134. Daugirdas JT, Ing TS, Gandhi VC, Hano JE, Chen WT, Yuan L. Kinetics of peritoneal fluid absorption (from the

peritoneal cavity) in patients with chronic renal failure. J Lab Clin Med 1980; 95: 351–61.

135. Arfors KE, Rutili G, Svensjo E. Microvascular transport of macromolecules in normal and inflammatory conditions. Acta Physiol Scand 1979; 463: S93–103.

136. Taylor AE, Gibson WH, Granger HJ, Guyton AC. The interaction between intercapillary and tissue forces in the overall regulation of interstitial fluid volume. Lymphology 1973; 6: 192–208.

137. Rutili G, Arfors KE. Interstitial fluid and lymph protein concentration in the subcutaneous tissue. Bibl Anat 1975; 13: 70–1.

138. Noer I, Lassen NA. Evidence of active transport (filtration?) of plasma proteins across the capillary walls in muscle and subcutis. Acta Physiol Scand 1979; 463: 105–10.

139. Cheek TR, Twardowski ZJ, Moore HL, Nolph KD. Absorption of inulin and high molecular weight gelatin isocyanate solution from peritoneal cavity of rats. In: Avram MM, Giordano C, eds. Ambulatory Peritoneal Dialysis (Proceedings of the Fourth International Congress of Peritoneal Dialysis). New York: Plenum, 1990, p. 149.

140. Krediet RT, Struijk DG, Koomen GCM, Hoek FJ, Arisz L. The disappearance of macromolecules from the peritoneal cavity during CAPD is not dependent on molecular size. Perit Dial Int 1990; 10: 147–52.

141. Flessner MF, Fentschermacher JD, Blasberg RG, Dedrick RL. Peritoneal absorption of macromolecules studied by quantitative autoradiography. Am J Physiol 1985; 248: H26–32.

142. Waniewski J, Heimburger O, Park MS, Werynski A, Lindholm B. Impact of tracer disappearance on transcapillary ultrafiltration and net dialysate volume change. Perit Dial Int 1992 (suppl. 12): S14.

143. Twardowski ZJ, Khanna R, Nolph KD et al. Intra-abdominal pressures during natural activities in patients treated with continuous ambulatory peritoneal dialysis. Nephron 1986; 44: 129–35.

144. Stelin G, Rippe B. A phenomenological interpretation of the variation in dialysate volume with dwell time in CAPD. Kidney Int 1990; 38: 465–72.

145. Rippe B, Stelin G, Haraldsson B. Computer simulations of peritoneal fluid transport in CAPD. Kidney Int 1991; 40: 315–25.

146. Abernethy NJ, Chin W, Hay JB, Rodela H, Oreopoulos D, Johnston MG. Lymphatic drainage of the peritoneal cavity in sheep. Am J Physiol (Renal, Fluid Electrolyte Physiol 29) 1991; 260: 353–8.

147. Abernethy NJ, Chin W, Hay JB, Rodela H, Oreopoulos D, Johnston MG. Lymphatic removal of dialysate from the peritoneal cavity of anesthetized sheep. Kidney Int 1991; 40: 174–81.

148. Tran LP, Rodela H, Abernethy NJ, Yuan ZY, Hay JB, Oreopoulos D, Johnston MG. Lymphatic drainage of hypertonic dialysis solution from the peritoneal cavity: comparison between anesthetized and conscious sheep. J Appl Physiol 1993; 74: 859–67.

149. Tran L, Rodela H, Hay JB, Oreopoulos D, Johnston MG. Quantitation of lymphatic drainage of the peritoneal cavity in sheep: comparison of direct cannulation techniques with indirect methods to estimate lymph flow. Perit Dial Int 1993; 13: 270–9.

150. Laine GA, Allen SJ, Katz J, Gabel JC, Drake RE. Outflow pressure reduces lymph flow rate from various tissues. Microvasc Res 1987; 33: 135–42.

151. Shockley TR, Ofsthun NJ. Pathways for fluid loss from the peritoneal cavity. Perit Dial Int 1992; (S2): S6.

152. Fressner MF. Peritoneal transport physiology: insights from basic research. J Am Soc Nephrol 1991; 2: 122–35.

153. Flessner MF. Computerized kinetic modeling: a new tool in the quest for adequacy in peritoneal dialysis. Perit Dial Int 1997; 17: 581–5.

154. Imholz AL, Koomen GC, Struijk DG, Arisz L, Krediet RT. Effect of dialysate osmolarity on the transport of low-molecular weight solutes and proteins during CAPD. Kidney Int 1993; 43: 1339–46.

155. Ho-dac-Pannekeet MM, Schouten N, Langendijk MJ et al. Peritoneal transport characteristics with glucose polymer based dialysate. Kidney Int 1996; 50: 979–86.

156. Imholz AL, Koomen GC, Struijk DG, Arisz L, Krediet RT. Fluid and solute transport in CAPD patients using ultralow sodium dialysate. Kidney Int 1994; 46: 333–40.

157. Wang T, Heimburger O, Cheng H, Waniewski J, Bergstrom J, Lindholm B. Effect of increased dialysate fill volume on peritoneal fluid and solute transport. Kidney Int 1997; 52: 1068–76.

158. Reddingius RE, Schroder CH, Willems JL, Lelivelt M, Kohler BE, Krediet RT, Monnens LA. Measurement of peritoneal fluid handling in children on continuous ambulatory peritoneal dialysis using dextran 70. Nephrol Dial Transplant 1995; 10: 866–70.

159. Reddingius RE, Schroder CH, Willems HL et al. Measurement of peritoneal fluid handling in children on continuous ambulatory peritoneal dialysis using autologous hemoglobin. Perit Dial Int 1994; 14: 42–7.

160. Durand PY, Chanliau J, Gamberoni J, Hestin D, Kessler M. Intraperitoneal pressure, peritoneal permeability and volume of ultrafiltration in CAPD. Adv Perit Dial 1992; 8: 22–5.

161. Imholz AL, Koomen GC, Struijk DG, Arisz L, Krediet RT. Effect of an increased intraperitoneal pressure on fluid and solute transport during CAPD. Kidney Int 1998; 44: 1078–85.

162. Abensur H, Romao Jr JE, Prado EBA, Kakehashi E, Sabbaga E, Marcondes M. Influence of hydrostatic intraperitoneal pressure and cardiac function on the lymphatic absorption rate of the peritoneal cavity in CAPD. Adv Perit Dial 1993; 9: 41–5.

163. Imholz AL, Koomen GC, Voorn WJ, Struijk DG, Arisz L, Krediet RT. Day-to-day variability of fluid and solute transport in upright and recumbent positions during CAPD. Nephrol Dial Transplant 1998; 13: 146–53.

164. Utsunomiya T, Kumano K, Sakai T, Yamashita A. Effect of direct pulsatile peritoneal dialysis on peritoneal permeability and lymphatic absorption in the rat. Jpn J Nephrol 1995; 37: 24–8.

165. Abensur H, Romao Jr JE, Prado EB, Kakehashi E, Sabbaga E, Marcondes M. Influence of spontaneous contractions of the lymphatic vessels on the lymphatic absorption rate of the peritoneal cavity in CAPD. Adv Perit Dial 1993; 9: 16–20.

166. Monquil MC, Imholz AL, Struijk DG, Krediet RT. Does impaired transcellular water transport contribute to net ultrafiltration failure during CAPD? Perit Dial Int 1995; 15: 42–8.

167. Heimburger O, Waniewski J, Werynski A, Park MS, Lindholm B. Lymphatic absorption in CAPD patients with loss of ultrafiltration capacity. Blood Purif 1995; 13: 327–39.

168. Heimburger O, Waniewski J, Werynski A, Tranaeus A, Lindholm B. Peritoneal transport in CAPD patients with permanent loss of ultrafiltration capacity. Kidney Int 1990; 38: 495–506.

169. Kumano K, Suyama K, Sakai T. Increased lymphatic absorption as a cause of ultrafiltration failure in long-term CAPD patients. Perit Dial Int 1992; 12(S2): S14.

170. Kim D, Maduluko GC, Thome F, Cattran DC, Fenton SSA. The spectrum of ultrafiltration failure and its pathogenesis among CAPD patients. Kidney Int 1985; 27: 181A.

171. Davies SJ, Brown B, Bryan J, Russell GI. Clinical evaluation of the peritoneal equilibration test: a population-based study. Nephrol Dial Transplant 1993; 8: 64–70.

172. Pollock CA, Ibels LS, Hallett MD et al. Loss of ultrafiltration in continuous ambulatory peritoneal dialysis. Perit Dial Int 1989; 9: 107–10.

173. Suyama K, Kumano K, Go M, Sakai T. Ultrafiltration failure in a peritoneal dialysis patient due to a marked increase in lymphatic absorption a case report. Jpn J Urol 1994; 85: 664–7.

174. Ho-dac-Pannekeet MM, Atasever B, Struijk DG, Krediet RT. Analysis of ultrafiltration failure in peritoneal dialysis patients by means of standard peritoneal permeability analysis. Perit Dial Int 1997; 17: 144–50.

175. Graff J, Fugleberg S, Joffe P, Brahm J, Fogh-Andersen N. An evaluation of twelve nested models of transperitoneal transport of urea: the one-compartment assumption is valid. Scand J Clin Lab Invest 1995; 55: 331–9.

176. Fugleberg S, Graff J, Joffe P et al. Transperitoneal transport of creatinine. A comparison of kinetic models. Clin Physiol 1994; 14: 443–57.

177. Hallet M, Lysaght M, Farrell P. The role of lymphatic drainage in peritoneal mass transfer. Artif Organs 1989; 13: 23–34.

178. Randerson DH, Farrell PC. Mass transfer properties of the human peritoneum. ASAIO J 1980; 3: 140–6.

179. Popovich RP, Moncrief JW. Transport kinetics. In: Nolph KD, ed. Peritoneal Dialysis, 2nd edn. Boston, MA: Martinus Nijhoff, 1985, pp. 115–58.

180. Garred LJ, Canaud B, Farrell PC. A simple kinetic model for assessing peritoneal mass transfer in chronic ambulatory peritoneal dialysis. ASAIO J 1983; 6: 131–7.

181. Selgas R, Rodriguez-Carmona A, Martinez ME et al. Peritoneal mass transfer in patients on long-term CAPD. Perit Dial Bull 1984; 4: 153–6.

182. Mactier RA, Khanna R, Moore H, Twardowski Z, Nolph KD. Pharmacological reduction of lymphatic absorption from the peritoneal cavity increases net ultrafiltration and solute clearances in peritoneal dialysis in the rat. Nephron 1988; 50: 229–32.

183. Mactier RA, Khanna R, Twardowski Z, Moore H, Nolph K. Influence of phosphatidylcholine on lymphatic absorption during peritoneal dialysis in the rat. Perit Dial Int 1988; 8: 179–86.

184. Di Paolo N, Buoncristiani U, Capotondo L et al. Phosphatidylcholine and peritoneal transport during peritoneal dialysis. Nephron 1986; 44: 365–70.

185. Dombros N, Balaskas E, Savidis N, Tourkantonis A, Sombolos K. Phosphatidylcholine increases ultrafiltration in CAPD patients. Perit Dial Bull 1987; 7: S24.

186. Sturijk D, Van Der Reijden H, Krediet R, Koomen G, Arisz L. Effect of phosphatidylcholine on peritoneal transport on lymphatic absorption in a patient with sclerosing peritonitis. Nephron 1989; 51: 577–8.

187. Di Paolo B, Chakrabarti E, Maher JF. Phosphatidylcholine does not affect peritoneal transport of intact rabbits. Perit Dial Int 1989; 9: 211–3.

188. De Vecchi A, Castelnovo C, Guerra L, Scalamogna A. Phosphatidylcholine administration in CAPD patients with reduced ultrafiltration. Perit Dial Int 1989; 9: 207–10.

189. Chan H, Abraham G, Oreopoulos DG. Oral lecithin improves ultrafiltration in patients on peritoneal dialysis. Perit Dial Int 1989; 9: 203–5.

190. Querques M, Procaccini DA, Pappani A, Strippoli P, Passion EA. Influence of phosphatidylcholine on ultrafiltration and solute transfer in CAPD patients. ASAIO Trans 1990; 36: M581–3.

191. Chan PC. Effect of phosphatidylcholine on ultrafiltration in patients on CAPD. Nephron 1993; 59: 100–3.

192. Krack G, Viglino G, Cavalli PL et al. Intraperitoneal administration of phosphatidylcholine improves ultrafiltration in CAPD patients. Perit Dial Int 1992; 12: 359–64.

193. Baranowska-Daca E, Torneli J, Popovich RP, Moncrief JW. Use of bethanechol chloride to increase available ultrafiltration in CAPD. Adv Perit Dial 1995; 11: 69–72.

194. Yatzidis H. Enhanced ultrafiltration in rabbits with bicarbonate glycylglycine peritoneal dialysis solution. Perit Dial Int 1993; 13: 302–6.

195. Wang T, Cheng H, Heimburger O, Chen C, Bergstrom J, Lindholm B. Effect of different concentrations of intraperitoneal hyaluron on peritoneal fluid kinetics. Perit Dial Int 1998; 18 (S1): S8.

196. Steinberg B. Infections of the Peritoneum. New York: Paul Hoeber, 1944.

197. Durham HE. The mechanism of reaction to peritoneal infection. J Pathol Bact 1897; 4: 338–82.

198. Vas SI. Peritonitis. In: Nolph KD, ed. Peritoneal Dialysis, 2nd edn. Boston, MA: Martinus Nijhoff, 1985, pp. 403–39.

199. Yuan Z, Rodela H, Hay JB, Oreopoulos D, Johnston MG. Lymph flow and lymphatic drainage of inflammatory cells from the peritoneal cavity in a casein–peritonitis model in sheep. Lymphology 1994; 27: 114–28.

200. Wu G. Osmotic agents for peritoneal dialysis solutions. Perit Dial Bull 1982; 2: 151–4.

201. Higgins JT, Gross ML, Somani P. Patient tolerance and dialysis effectiveness of a glucose polymer containing peritoneal dialysis solution. Perit Dial Bull 1984; 4: S131–3.

202. Mistry CD, Mallick NP, Gokal R. Ultrafiltration with an isosmotic solution during long peritoneal dialysis exchanges. Lancet 1987; 2: 178–82.

203. Twardowski ZJ, Nolph KD, Khanna R, Hain H, Moore H, McGarry TJ. Charged polymers as osmotic agents for peritoneal dialysis. Materials Research Society Symposium Proceedings 1986; 55: 319.

204. Winchester JF, Stegink LD, Ahmad S et al. A comparison of glucose polymer and dextrose as osmotic agents in CAPD. In: Maher JF, Winchester JF, eds. Frontiers in Peritoneal Dialysis. New York: Field, Rich, 1986, pp. 231–40.

205. Junor BJR, Briggs JD, Forwell MA, Dobbie JW, Henderson IS. Sclerosing peritonitis: role of chlorhexidine in alcohol. Perit Dial Bull 1985; 5: 101–4.

206. Mactier RA. Measurement of dialysate volumes in peritoneal dialysis. Perit Dial Int 1989; 9: 155–7.

207. Pust AH, Leypoldt JK, Frigon RP, Henderson LW. Peritoneal dialysate volume determined by indicator dilution measurements. Kidney Int 1988; 33: 64–70.

7 | Pharmacological alterations of peritoneal transport rates and pharmacokinetics in peritoneal dialysis

N. LAMEIRE, W. VAN BIESEN, P. HIRSZEL AND M. BOGAERT

Introduction

In the first part of the chapter the effects of pharmacological manipulations on peritoneal transport will be discussed. Increased understanding of peritoneal transport mechanisms may lead to the development of clinically useful methods to augment peritoneal transport efficiency. In this chapter only pharmacological tools for influencing peritoneal transport will be discussed. A detailed discussion of the physiology of peritoneal transport is provided in another chapter of this book.

In the second part of this chapter the pharmacokinetic concepts underlying transperitoneal drug transport and their implications for rational and safe use of drugs in patients treated with peritoneal dialysis will be discussed. Basic concepts of pharmacokinetics will be shortly reviewed, as a starting point to elaborate further on general pharmacokinetic principles in patients with decreased renal function and in patients on peritoneal dialysis. Tables with data and guidelines for prescription of specific drugs will also be provided.

Peritoneal membrane transport

Diffusive transport

According to the three-pore model proposed by Rippe [1], the principal peritoneal exchange route for water and water-soluble substances is a protein-restrictive pore pathway of radius 40–55 Å, accounting for approximately 99% of the total exchange (pore) area and approximately 90% of the total peritoneal ultrafiltration coefficient (LpS). For their passage through the peritoneal membrane, proteins are confined to so-called 'large pores' of radius approximately 250 Å, which are extremely few in number (0.01% of the total pore population) and more or less non-restrictive with respect to protein

transport. The third pathway of the three-pore model accounts for only about 2% of the total LpS and is permeable to water but impermeable to solutes, a so-called 'water-only' (transcellular?) pathway. These ultra-small transcellular pores (< 5 Å) are probably specialized water channels, consisting of intermembrane proteins, the so-called aquaporins. The presence of these aquaporins has been demonstrated in the peritoneal capillaries and venules in human [2] and rat [3] peritoneal membranes.

As detailed in other chapters in this book, solute transport in peritoneal dialysis occurs by the mechanisms of diffusion and convection.

Transport of low molecular weight solutes during peritoneal dialysis is primarily diffusive, whereas convective transport becomes more important with their increasing molecular weight. The absorption of intraperitoneally administered macromolecules is linear in time, irrespective of molecular size or concentration. Total removal of a solute is dependent not only on the peritoneal transport rate but also on the total drained dialysate volume. The latter is determined by the instilled volume and the net ultrafiltration. Transport across any membrane is determined by the surface area available for transport and by the intrinsic permeability of the membrane. The effective peritoneal surface area used for transport of solutes is determined both by the number of perfused capillaries (and thus by splanchnic blood flow) [4], and by the contact of the dialysate with the peritoneal surface [5].

The intrinsic permeability of the peritoneum reflects its size-selectivity. This is probably mainly determined by the large pore size and can be characterized by the so-called restriction coëfficient to macromolecules [6, 7].

In terms of the three-pore theory, the effective peritoneal surface area, measured by the MTAC of small molecules, can be used to represent the number of pores available for transport, whereas the restriction coëfficient represents the average large pore

R. Gokal, R. Khanna, R.Th. Krediet and K.D. Nolph (eds.), Textbook of Peritoneal Dialysis, 2nd Edition, 193–251.
© 2000 Kluwer Academic Publishers. Printed in Great Britain.

diameter. For the ultra-small pores the sieving of sodium can be used as a functional parameter. Thus, these three parameters should be included in the evaluation of the impact of a given drug on peritoneal transport

Convective transport

Solute is also convected into the peritoneum by ultrafiltration. The pores through capillary walls restrict the passage of protein, but solutes as large as inulin are sieved appreciably during peritoneal ultrafiltration. In contrast with diffusive transport, convective transport rate is independent of molecular size if, of course, below the cut-off limit of the membrane. The hydrostatic pressure of the blood is normally opposed by the plasma oncotic pressure and by the interstitial hydrostatic pressure minus the interstitial osmotic pressure. Although little is known about the hydraulic permeability of the peritoneum, it is thought to be dependent on interstitial tissue structures and the number of pores. Convective transport can also be pharmacologically altered by manipulation of these physicochemical factors.

Lymphatic absorption

Lymphatics are the primary route for absorption from the peritoneum of isotonic dialysate including macromolecules, particles and formed blood elements [8]. Most absorption occurs via the subdiaphragmatic lymphatics with smaller amounts via the mesenteric lymphatic vessels [9]. Yet, before reaching lymphatic channels, macromolecules are probably distributed in the large peritoneal tissue compartment [10]. Absorption from the peritoneum of macromolecules such as albumin, haemoglobin, fibrinogen and polydisperse dextran 70 has been reported [11–16] and used as a measure of peritoneal lymphatic flow rates [17–19]. The lymphatic flow rate in CAPD patients is about 11 ml/h based on radioiodinated serum albumin studies [13], or about 1–2.5 ml/min based on the disappearance rate of intraperitoneal macromolecules [18, 19]. Peritoneal lymph flow is significantly increased during peritonitis [14]. The peritoneal absorption of polydispersed neutral dextrans does not show size discrimination, adding evidence that the major route is by lymphatic transport [16, 20]. To obtain net peritoneal ultrafiltration the lymphatic absorption must be subtracted from the gross peritoneal ultrafiltration volume and abnormally high peritoneal

absorption may be an important cause of clinically significant loss of net ultrafiltration.

Role of electric charges on the peritoneal membrane

Anionic sites predominantly composed of heparan sulphate and chondroitin sulphate are a constant feature of basement membranes of the microvasculature [21]. They are particularly abundant in fenestrated capillaries, some of which have been identified in human parietal and diaphragmatic peritoneum [22]. These anionic charges could, at least theoretically, restrict the diffusive and convective passage of charged solutes through the membrane. There is a paucity of data concerning the influence of the peritoneal membrane anionic sites on transport of charged macromolecules across the peritoneum.

Leypoldt and Henderson [23] studied the effect of molecular charge on transperitoneal macromolecule transport using dextrans, and have demonstrated that transport rates for cationic dextrans were less than for either neutral or anionic dextrans. These results differ from what one should expect. On the other hand, negatively charged amino acids such as glutamic acids show a slower transperitoneal mobility compared to neutral or positively charged amino acids [24]. In contrast, based on the determination of peritoneal clearances of 10 different proteins and their isoforms, Buis *et al.* [25] concluded that the peritoneal membrane was not a charge-selective barrier for the transport of macromolecules between blood and dialysate. The effect of electrically charged drugs on peritoneal transport will be discussed later.

Pharmacological alterations of peritoneal transport

Better knowledge of the pharmacological alterations that occur in peritoneal dialysis patients may be useful for several of the reasons that are summarized in Table 1.

1. Comorbidity is high in renal failure and these patients are exposed to a multitude of drugs that may affect the peritoneal transport of solutes and water. Knowledge of the effects of such agents on transport parameters can influence the appropriate selection of a drug.
2. There may be need for augmenting the peritoneal diffusive capacity. A redefinition of adequacy

Table 1. Factors affecting peritoneal drug clearance after systemic administration

Dialysate properties
  Flow rate
  Temperature
  pH
  Osmotic content

Drug properties
  Molecular weight
  Ionic charge
  Volume of distribution
  Protein binding
  Extrarenal clearance
  Lipid or water solubility

Characteristics of the peritoneal membrane
  Surface and charge
  Permeability
    Peritonitis
    Sclerosis
  Peritoneal blood flow
  Stagnant layers
  Ultrafiltration

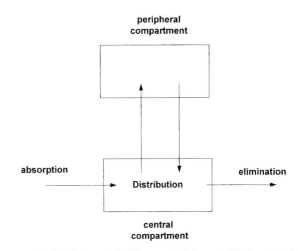

Figure 1. Schematic representation of a two-compartment model.

targets of peritoneal dialysis has emerged over recent years. Many studies have focused attention on optimizing the quantity of solute clearance in an attempt to improve clinical outcome. Dialysis dose is currently quantified in terms of small solute clearance (fractional urea (Kt/V)) and creatinine clearance rate. Although considerable controversy remains as to the exact clearance targets, theoretical and clinical evidence suggests that failure to attain clearance targets is associated with increased morbidity and mortality [26]. Moreover, under certain circumstances when peritoneal dialysis could be useful, increased catabolism may increase the nitrogen load and augmented transport may be required.

3. A major cause of cardiovascular morbidity and mortality, and also of technique failure, in peritoneal dialysis is the inadequate removal of fluid across the peritoneal membrane. A better knowledge of fluid transport (filtration and transcapillary and lymphatic absorption) may open possibilities for pharmacological manipulation of the peritoneal ultrafiltration capacity, or chemical modification of the dialysate, in order to prevent excessive fluid reabsorption from the peritoneal cavity.

4. To date, much research is devoted to improvement of the biocompatibility of the peritoneal dialysis fluid. Adverse interactions of these fluids with the peritoneal membrane provoke chemical modifications of the membrane which may even end in peritoneal fibrosis. Treatment with vasoactive and/or anti-inflammatory agents could be attempted in order to decrease these adverse effects.

5. When peritoneal dialysis is used to remove exogenous toxins it is usually mandatory that removal rates be maximal. Conversely, when protein loss is excessive it may be judicious to decrease the transport rates, at least of larger solutes.

6. Finally, pharmacological manipulation of peritoneal transport has increased our understanding of peritoneal physiology.

This part of the chapter will describe the several pharmacological manipulations on peritoneal transport, seeking enhanced understanding of transport mechanisms and clinically useful methods to either augment transport or to preserve the structural and functional integrity of the membrane. Figure 1 is a schematic representation of the several different interventions to alter peritoneal solute and water removal.

Drugs acting on the peritoneal blood flow and their impact on solute transport

Greatly improved mass transport must depend on augmentation of blood flow or peritoneal permeability or area, just as haemodialyser efficiency increases with larger surface area dialysers, more permeable membranes and higher blood flow rates.

Mesenteric blood flow

Blood flow to the visceral peritoneum derives predominantly from the mesenteric circulation. About

60% of peritoneal surface can be ascribed to the mesentery of the oesophago-rectal viscera, with nearly 15% covering the liver and approximately 15% being parietal [27].

The parietal peritoneum is perfused by vasculature of the abdominal wall. Mesenteric blood flow rates average about 10% of the cardiac output [28]. The 'effective' blood flow rate to the human peritoneum has been estimated to average between 60 and 100 ml/min [29].

It should be recalled that estimations of peritoneal blood flow in peritoneal dialysis patients reveal lower values than in animals when expressed per kg body weight. Based on studies of peritoneal mass transfer area coefficient of carbon dioxide, values ranging from 68 to 82 ml/min [30] or about 150 ml/min have been obtained [31].

In stable CAPD patients, values ranging from 20 to 151 ml/min with a median value of 66 ml/min were found [32–34]. All these values assume that gas clearances represent the 'effective' peritoneal blood flow.

When mesenteric blood flow is doubled, the clearances of small solutes such as urea increase by 30–50% [35], consistent with a resting blood flow that exceeds the maximal rate at which the capillary diffusion capacity can completely clear the perfusing blood [36]. This is compatible with the results obtained by Douma *et al.* [34], finding an increase in MTAC of small molecules without a change in peritoneal 'effective' blood flow as measured by the MTAC of CO_2.

The splanchnic vascular bed can sequester blood, excluding it from, or releasing it into, the circulation as systemic volume changes. Thus, haemodynamic effects of drugs can influence splanchnic blood volume and flow rate considerably. Because drugs usually affect the splanchnic blood flow and volume *pari passu*, changes in peritoneal transport that result from the altered volume can be misinterpreted as flow-rate-mediated. There is also evidence to suggest that splanchnic blood volume, rather than flow rate, determines the degree of peritoneal mass transfer [4]. For example, the volume contraction induced by the systemic administration of dihydroergotamine results in lower peritoneal clearances of potassium, urea and phosphate [37], and this effect is due to a reduction in blood volume. On the other hand, both volume expansion by dextrose infusion [38] and sodium chromate-induced hepatic venous stasis increase these parameters. Current opinion prevails that, under physiological conditions, peritoneal blood flow does not limit the transfer of solutes.

However, the effective blood flow available for transport will only be a fraction of the total blood flow through the tissues surrounding the peritoneal cavity, because most of the exchange capillaries are too far from the cavity to be active in the exchange process [39], or they are contained in tissues not in contact with the solution in the cavity [40]. In contrast, in the 'nearest capillary' theory of Ronco *et al.* [41], it is hypothesized that the capillaries positioned closest to the mesothelium are dilated and have a low blood flow, while the most distal capillaries have a higher blood flow, but with a less effective diffusion due to interstitial resistances. The resulting 'effective' peritoneal blood flow in this hypothesis would be a limiting factor for solute clearance.

Recent experiments by Flessner and his associates [42] have further tested this hypothesis with a technique to assess the effect of blood flow on the mass transfer of small solutes across the parietal and visceral peritoneum [43]. As was found for the parietal wall, a 60–70% blood flow reduction from control values does not limit solute transfer in the hollow viscera such as stomach and caecum, but causes significant changes in the mass transfer across the liver surface. Because the liver makes up only a small portion of the effective exchange area, overall transperitoneal solute transfer should not be greatly affected by significant decreases in blood flow.

As outlined in Chapter 5, most data obtained in experimental animals, as well as in humans, suggest that the effects of small peritoneal blood flow changes on solute transport are probably limited.

It is important to remember that, as in any other microvascular beds, the peritoneal microcirculation consists of arterioles, capillaries and venules. The arterioles give rise directly to the capillaries (5–10 μm in diameter), or to *metarterioles* (10–20 μm in diameter), which then give rise to capillaries. The metarterioles can either bypass the capillary bed, and thus serve as thoroughfare channels to the venules, or serve as direct conduits to supply the capillary bed. Cross-connections are often made between arterioles and between venules, as well as in the capillary network.

The regulation of the mesenteric circulation is very complex.

The *extrinsic* control of the mesenteric circulation is predominantly mediated by the sympathetic noradrenergic nerves, and by circulating vasoactive substances, such as catecholamines, vasopressin, and angiotensin. The mesenteric vasculature is accompanied by autonomic neuroelements from the coeliac plexus with primary neurocontrol by sympathetic innervation. Increased sympathetic activity constricts the mesenteric arterioles and capacitance vessels. These responses are mediated by α-adrenergic receptors, which are predominant in the mesenteric circulation; however, β-adrenergic receptors are also present [44]. Vasoactive responses of the mesenteric vascular bed to pharmacological manipulations are well established. The vasocontrictor response that normally occurs with appropriate stimuli can be prevented by blocking α-receptors of the mesenteric vascular bed with phenoxybenzamine. These vessels also contain dopaminergic receptors.

The *intrinsic* regulation consists of autoregulation, while the venous pressure and the ingestion of meals also have an effect. Food ingestion increases intestinal blood flow and this functional hyperaemia is mediated by certain gastrointestinal hormones such as gastrin and cholecystokinin. Autoregulation of blood flow, i.e. the maintenance of a constant blood flow over a range of perfusion pressures, is not as well developed in the intestinal circulation as in other vascular beds, such as those in the brain and kidney. The principal mechanism responsible for mesenteric autoregulation is metabolic, i.e. any intervention that results in an oxygen supply that is inadequate for the requirements of the tissue prompts the formation of vasodilator metabolites. However, a myogenic mechanism probably also participates.

Adenosine is a potent vasodilator in the mesenteric vascular bed and may be the principal metabolic mediator of autoregulation.

Influence of drugs reducing peritoneal blood flow

Catecholamines. To explore vasoactive effects on peritoneal transport, catecholamines have been studied in animals undergoing peritoneal dialysis. Gutman *et al.* [45] noted lower increments in dialysate urea with large intraperitoneal doses of dopamine in dogs, but did not measure dialysate volume. Because blood pressure increased, the lower urea accumulation in the dialysate was attributed to splanchnic vasoconstriction. To offset vasoconstriction, Parker *et al.* [46] added an α-adrenergic blocker to the dialysis fluid. With intraperitoneal phentolamine and intravenous dopamine, peritoneal clearances increased in dogs. In human patients, however, Chan *et al.* [47] observed no effect of low (4 mg/L) or high doses (20–160 mg/L) of intraperitoneal dopamine on dialysate urea, creatinine or phosphate.

In rabbits, intraperitoneal dopamine caused dose-related (0.6–1.8 mg/kg) increases in peritoneal urea clearance [48]. The increments occurred with lower doses than those used by Gutman *et al.* [45] and drug concentrations (10–30 mg/L) within the range studied by Chan *et al.* [47].

Intravenous 1-norepinephrine significantly decreased peritoneal clearances of urea and creatinine in unanesthetized rabbits [47, 48]. Dose-dependent decrements correlated with the pressor response [49]. Comparable pressor doses of intravenous dopamine increased clearances of urea and creatinine to 145% of control values, whereas low doses had minimal and inconsistent effects [49]. Osmotic water flux increased only slightly (from 0.18 to 0.24 ml/kg per minute) but significantly. Because dopamine vasoconstricts venules relatively more than arterioles as compared to norepinephrine [50], augmented water flux could be mediated by increased hydrostatic pressure rather than a change in hydraulic permeability. The augmented transport is attributed to dopamine receptor-mediated mesenteric vasodilation and, in part, by general α-adrenergic vasoconstriction increasing blood pressure, while mesenteric blood flow is maintained. Although dopamine may not be suitable for augmenting efficiency of routine peritoneal dialysis, these data strongly suggest that dopamine should be preferable to 1-norephinephrine when vasopressor therapy is required during peritoneal dialysis. Only minimal increments in fluid and solute flux occurred with ibopamine, an oral dopamine analogue, whether given by mouth, intravenously or intraperitoneally to normal rabbits [51]. Interestingly, the dialysate to plasma ratio for norepinephrine was 1.17 in CAPD patients, suggesting local production in the peritoneal cavity [52].

An unexpected correlation was found between the dialysate levels of norepinephrine and the effective peritoneal surface area, represented by the mass transfer area coefficient for creatinine.

Vasopressin and angiotensin. Vasopressin and angiotensin cause a generalized vasoconstriction with a disproportionate reduction in mesenteric blood flow [53].

Parenteral administration of vasopressin to anaesthetized dogs decreased peritoneal clearances of small solutes, consistent with a hormonally mediated reduction in mesenteric blood flow [54, 55]. Since inulin clearance increased slightly under these circumstances, a concurrent increase in membrane permeability has been postulated [56], in accord with the accelerated transport that occurs in isolated membrane preparations [57].

Angiotensin II is probably mainly involved in the control of mesenteric blood flow during volume depletion [58]. The effect of angiotensin II (AII) on peritoneal permeability and lymphatic absorption in the rat was studied by Go *et al.* [59]; AII was added to the dialysate and it decreased the transcapillary ultrafiltration rate from 15.7 ± 2.8 ml/4 h dwell in control to 5.7 ± 1.5 ml/4 h dwell. Lymphatic absorption was increased in a dosedependent fashion with no change in clearances of urea nitrogen or inorganic phosphate.

Drugs increasing peritoneal blood flow

When peritoneal blood flow and clearances have been reduced by disease, transport rates may be restored towards normal by treating the specific abnormality. For example, the mesenteric blood flow rate varies directly with cardiac output, and treatment of heart failure should improve peritoneal clearances.

Loss of blood volume by haemorrhage reduces peritoneal transport of urea and potassium in the dog [60]. When blood pressure and volume are restored towards normal by infusing blood or saline, clearances return to normal. After haemorrhagic hypotension, clearances are not increased by raising blood pressure with norepinephrine, nor is transport affected adversely by lowering the blood pressure further with phenoxybenzamine [61]. These studies suggest that blood pressure *per se* does not greatly influence the efficiency of peritoneal dialysis, and that the latter depends more on adequate splanchnic volume and perfusion.

Although the mechanisms of a decrease in solute transport by a reduction in peritoneal blood flow are important, much more attention has been paid to the study of the possibilities for augmenting peritoneal transport by systemic or intraperitoneal administration of vasodilating drugs. Many studies suggest that peritoneal clearances will increase only if a vasodilator selectively affects the splanchnic vasculature or is applied locally, e.g. by intraperitoneal instillation. When administered intravenously such drugs may cause widespread vasodilation, decreasing blood pressure, splanchnic perfusion and splanchnic volume, thereby lowering peritoneal transport rates. To date, membrane-active agents have augmented transport only when applied locally, i.e. instilled intraperitoneally.

Increased splanchnic perfusion augments peritoneal clearances of larger solutes at least as much as the transport of smaller solutes. This suggests an increase in peritoneal surface area or permeability resulting from vasodilation, attributed to dilation of the functional peritoneal capillaries combined with perfusion of more capillaries. Spreading the same wall mass over a larger circumference decreases the wall thickness and stretches pores. Intercellular junctions widen, accelerating mass transport [62]. Raising blood flow by local application of vasodilators also opens previously closed capillaries, increasing the surface area available for transport [63, 64]. In the resting state blood may circulate predominantly through metarterioles. Enhanced perfusion opens more capillaries, exposing blood to a more permeable surface. Furthermore, vasodilators with a predominant venular site of action may cause greater increases in diffusion rates, but arteriolar dilators may increase the ultrafiltration rate. By increasing blood flow, diffusion and ultrafiltration may occur throughout a greater length of the capillaries than occurs under resting conditions.

Depending on the nature of the vasodilating agent there may be an increase (arteriolar relaxation), decrease (lowered venular tone), or no change (balanced effects) in capillary hydrostatic pressure. This hydrostatic pressure may affect capillary diameter, volume and permeability and is a major determinant of the filtration rate through the capillary. The solute transfer of small molecules, measured by their mass transfer area coefficients, is usually markedly increased during the first 15 min of peritoneal dialysis dwells. Besides being caused by initial arteriolar vasodilation and, hence, recruitment of capillary surface area, other explanations for this rapid increase are possible. These include an initial discharge (or saturation) of solutes from (in) the interstitium or an increased mixing, i.e. 'macrostirring' caused by the exchange procedure *per se* [65].

These possibilities have recently been investigated during acute PD in rats, by assessing the mass transfer coefficient for ^{51}Cr-EDTA as a function of time [65]. The discharge effect was studied by saturating the peritoneal interstitium with ^{51}Cr-EDTA by intravenous tracer infusion prior to each dwell. The potential effect of initial vasodilation was studied by adding isoproterenol to the dialysis fluid. Finally, the potential influence of an increased interstitial 'macrostirring', induced by high glucose concentrations, was investigated by comparing 1.36% glucose with 3.86% glucose dialysate. The conclusion of these experiments was that vasodilation, but not interstitial discharge (or loading), may explain the sharp rise in mass transfer occurring during the initial part of PD dwells. In addition, 'macrostirring', induced by the exchange procedure *per se*, may also be important.

Specific drugs may directly affect the permeability of the capillary or the mesothelium [66]. Drugs that influence membrane charge, cell volume, cell metabolism or intercellular junction may directly influence peritoneal permeability without affecting flow rates.

Isoproterenol. Isoproterenol, a β-adrenergic agonist, relaxes the mesenteric vascular bed. In patients with reduced peritoneal clearance, Nolph *et al.* improved transport rates by adding isoproterenol (0.06 mg/L) to the dialysis solution [67, 68]. Mean clearances increased to the lower range of normal but only transiently, and not all patients improved significantly [69]. No systemic effects of intraperitoneal isoproterenol were detected even with cardiac monitoring. Such use of isoproterenol has been explored in greater detail in animals. In acute studies in anaesthetized dogs, intraperitoneal isoproterenol increased urea and creatinine clearance by 45% and 30%, respectively, but subpressor intravenous doses did not augment transport [45]. In unanaesthetized rabbits, 0.04 mol/kg of intraperitoneal isoproterenol raised urea and creatinine clearance by 50% , but osmotically induced water flux was unaffected [70]. No systemic effects were observed.

Despite raising mesenteric blood flow to 188% of control by intravenous isoproterenol, Felt *et al.* [35] found no increase in clearances. With intraperitoneal isoproterenol a comparable flow increase raised peritoneal inulin and creatinine clearances by 27% and 18%, respectively. The disparity in blood flow and clearance changes suggests that capillary blood volume may be as important as blood flow in mediating changes in permeability.

Vasodilator gastrointestinal hormones. *Secretin* is a polypeptide gastrointestinal hormone that increases mesenteric blood flow by as much as 100% above baseline when given in pharmacological doses [71]. Secretin, like cholecystokinin, increases predominantly hepatic blood flow. Slight increments in urea and creatinine clearances occurred with intravenous secretin and cholecystokinin [72]. Intravenous, but not intraperitoneal, secretin (10 U/kg) increased osmotic water flux in rabbits from 0.19 to 0.29 ml/kg/min [72]. The endogenous release of cholecystokinin or secretin or their intra-arterial infusion relaxes precapillary sphincters and increases the capillary filtration coefficient from 0.05 to 0.10 ml/min/mmHg/100 g [73].

Gastrin, structurally similar to cholecystokinin, also increases mesenteric blood flow [71]. The effects of secretin and cholecystokinin on mesenteric blood flow are additive and potentiated by theophylline [74]. This hormonal mesenteric vasodilation is attributed to direct relaxation of vascular tone, presumably mediated by cyclic AMP.

Glucagon is structurally similar to secretin, but has a more potent effect on the mesenteric circulation. When administered intravenously, immediately before dialysis, glucagon significantly increased peritoneal clearances of urea and creatinine in non-anaesthetized rabbits [72, 75]. The same dose given intraperitoneally did not affect clearances. Since this large molecule should traverse the peritoneum slowly, hormonal activity presumably occurs at the endothelial rather than at the mesothelial surface. Nevertheless, much higher doses given intraperitoneally do increase clearance somewhat.

In dogs, intravenous infusion of about 30 μg/kg/h glucagon increased mesenteric arterial blood flow and peritoneal inulin but not creatinine clearance, unlike intraperitoneal instillation [35]. Glucagon did not affect peritoneal water flux during dialysis in rabbits [72]. The separation of the effects of all these gastrointestinal hormones on diffusive and on convective transport suggests the possible use of different pharmacological agents acting additively.

Prostaglandins. The prostaglandins are unsaturated 20-carbon lipids biosynthesized from arachidonic acid and other precursors by the cyclooxygenase (COX) enzymes. COX exists in two distinct isoforms: COX1, a constitutive form, and COX-2, which can be up-regulated by inflammatory mediators [76].

There is recent evidence that the mesothelial cells, when exposed to cytokines, show a time-dependent increase in the levels of both COX-1 and COX-2 mRNA, with the greatest increase being seen for COX-2. These data demonstrate specific stimulation of eicosanoid metabolism in human peritoneal mesothelial cells (HPMC) by peritoneal macrophage-derived cytokines, indicating the possible importance of these mediators in the activation of intraperitoneal prostaglandin synthesis [77].

Depending on the local concentration of the specific terminal enzymes, e.g. endoperoxide reductase leading to PGF2α or endoperoxide isomerase leading to PGE2, a given product predominates in a given tissue. Regional blood flow is one determinant of enzyme activity. In the circulation the prostaglandins are degraded during a single passage through the lung, thereby acting only locally with the exception of prostacyclin and thromboxanes which have half-lives of a few minutes. Prostaglandins of the PGA, PGE or PGI series are vasodilators, whereas $PGF2\alpha$ and thromboxanes are potent vasoconstrictors [78, 79]. These prostaglandins act locally in arterial walls to influence vascular tone and modulate the response of vascular smooth muscle to other vasoactive agents [80], for example by modifying vasoconstrictor responses [79].

Intraperitoneal instillation of PGA1 or PGE1 increased peritoneal clearances of urea and creatinine moderately in non-anaesthetized rabbits, whereas 125 µg/kg of PGE2 significantly raised creatinine clearance to 132% and urea clearance to 180% of control values [81]. In contrast, intraperitoneal administration of the vasoconstrictor $PGF2\alpha$ (125 µg/kg) decreased peritoneal clearances to 80% (urea) and 82% (creatinine) of control [81]. These prostaglandins did not affect fluid flux and were ineffective when given intravenously. Neither intravenous nor intraperitoneal administration of prostacyclin affected peritoneal solute or water transport significantly over a dose range from 25 to 125 µg/kg, nor did prostacyclin show pronounced effects on peritoneal transport under baseline conditions. Oral pretreatment with 10–21 mg/kg of sulphinpyrazone, a potent stimulator of prostaglandin synthetase, did not alter peritoneal clearances significantly [82]. When mefenamic acid, a prostaglandin synthetase inhibitor, was administered intravenously or intraperitoneally to unanaesthetized rabbits in doses sufficient to inhibit platelet function, neither the peritoneal clearances of creatinine or urea nor water flux changed [82]. Oral pretreatment of rabbits with indomethacin blocked platelet aggregation but did not change clearance or ultrafiltration rates significantly [82]. Intraperitoneal indomethacin increases the size of pinocytotic vesicles and narrows intercellular spaces in the rabbit, however [83]. Alteration of prostaglandin synthetase affects both vasoconstrictor and vasodilator prostaglandins. Hence, regional blood flow may remain unchanged. Yet when vasodilator prostaglandin activity predominates to compensate for increased renin-angiotensin activity or ischaemic vascular disease, aspirin and indomethacin decrease regional blood flow. However, the reduction of clearances induced by intravenous 1-norepinephrine, which should be accompanied by vasodilator prostaglandin stimulation, is exaggerated by pretreatment with indomethacin in only half of the animals so studied. These results suggest that endogenous prostaglandins do not play a major role in regulating peritoneal blood flow under ordinary circumstances. However, in patients who depend on vasodilator prostaglandins to maintain organ perfusion, blockade of prostaglandin synthetase could impair transport, and a history of exposure to such drugs should be sought if clearances are low. Intraperitoneally, the prostaglandin precursor arachidonic acid (1.5–5.6 mg/kg) increased creatinine clearance by 36% and urea clearance by 24%, suggesting an effect of endogenous prostaglandins, but systemic use of indomethacin did not block this increase [82, 84].

In patients with peritonitis the increased solute transport rates are accompanied by augmented prostaglandin release, abnormalities that can be blocked by indomethacin [85]. This effect was not confirmed in a longitudinal study in peritonitis [86].

Nitroprusside. The observation by Nolph *et al.* [69], that intraperitoneal nitroprusside increases peritoneal mass transport, has been confirmed in multiple laboratories in several species [5, 87–89]. Urea and creatinine clearances increase as much as 50% above control with greater increments in inulin clearances and protein loss, consistent with enhanced peritoneal permeability or area or both, rather than simply increased solute delivery. Osmotic ultrafiltration increases only slightly [5] or not at all as rapid glucose absorption dissipates the osmotic gradient. Nitroprusside-induced increases in mass transport are dose-dependent and can be seen with as little as 1.0 mg/L [90]. It has also been suggested that increments in peritoneal mass transfer coefficients with topical nitroprusside can indicate peritoneal vascular reserve [91]. In most studies systemic effects of nitroprusside have not been detected and intravenously the drug does not accelerate peritoneal mass transport. The transport increment is sustained for several exchanges, and on discontinuation may persist somewhat for up to 2 h. Augmented transport represents an increase in permeance of the peritoneum (mass transfer coefficient × area) due to capillary, especially venular, dilation and from opening of previously non-perfused capillaries [64, 90]. Although nitroprusside is metabolized to thiocyanate, this toxic metabolite is rapidly dialysed and no evidence of accumulation has been observed with repeated nitroprusside instillation.

Other vasodilators. No consistent change in peritoneal clearance of urea or creatinine was observed in patients given 20–40 mg of *hydralazine* intraperitoneally, which decreased blood pressure slightly [69]. Hydralazine (168 Da) should be rapidly absorbed from the peritoneal fluid, but its pharmacological action may depend on biotransformation to an active compound. Hence, widespread vasodilation may occur despite local application with no preferential effect on splanchnic blood flow or volume.

Theophylline acts as a non-selective antagonist of two types of adenosine receptors which mediate opposite effects on vascular tone [92]. In rabbits, changes in solute and water fluxes were inconsistent after intraperitoneal or intravenous aminophylline in doses exceeding the therapeutic range [93]. Presumably widespread vasodilation blunted any potential gain in peritoneal blood flow.

Diazoxide caused a modest increase in peritoneal clearances of urea and creatinine and a significant decrement in blood pressure when administered intraperitoneally to patients at a dose of 100–300 mg [69]. An increase in ultrafiltration rate approaching 50% of control values was inconsistently found.

The intraperitoneal administration of 5 mg of *phentolamine* did not influence peritoneal solute transport rates in five patients so investigated, nor did it affect osmotic water flux [69].

In anaesthetized rats, *histamine* (4–8 µg) raised only modestly (9% to 16%) the clearances of urea and inulin, whereas 3 µg of bradykinin augmented these clearances by 13% and 25%, respectively [87]. Histamine causes overt capillary dilation and increases permeability with protein exudation, which can be blocked in rabbits by both H1 and H2 receptor antagonists [94]. Minimal effects of histamine on small solute transport may reflect decreased plasma volume due to protein loss. In isolated rat mesentery, viewed by television microscopy after fluorescein labelling, protein exudation is also demonstrable with histamine [62]. Dilation is most prominent in the venous end of the capillary and similar changes are noted with nitroprusside.

The effects of *calcium channel blockers* on peritoneal mass transport have been studied by several investigators. In the anaesthetized rat model, verapamil and diltiazem, given locally, modestly but significantly increased peritoneal clearances of urea without enhancing protein losses [95]. A more recent animal study [96] explored the effects of the intraperitoneal administration of three calcium channel blockers (nicardipine, diltiazem, and verapamil). All three vasodilators caused a decrease in blood pressure, which was associated with a decrease in net ultrafiltration rate. The three calcium antagonists increased peritoneal net fluid absorption rate

in a dose-dependent way. Nicardipine and verapamil increased the permeability to urea and glucose but not to protein. Diltiazem caused no change in permeability.

Significant augmentation of small solute clearances and ultrafiltration associated with diminished glucose reabsorption were reported with intraperitoneal verapamil and nifedipine in CAPD patients [97, 98]. In hypertensive CAPD patients, oral nifedipine administered in blood pressure-controlling doses brought about significant augmentation of peritoneal clearance of creatinine and β_2-microglobulin, associated with higher glucose reabsorption, while the rate of ultrafiltration remained unaffected [99]. These studies suggest that calcium channel blockers act on the arteriolar end of peritoneal capillaries without a consistent effect on venular permeability.

In rats, modest increases in urea clearance and glucose absorption and a marked exaggeration of protein loss was seen following intraperitoneal instillation of very large doses of captopril, an *angiotensin-converting enzyme inhibitor* [100]. These increments, despite drug-induced systemic hypotension, may reflect increased blood flow, surface area, or permeability. In the above-mentioned study by Kumano *et al.* [96], captopril was also investigated after intraperitoneal administration to animals. Captopril increased membrane permeability to small and large molecular solutes, with a consequent decrease in ultrafiltration rate.

In a clinical study [101], six CAPD patients with hypertension received intraperitoneal enalaprilat and five of them also received oral enalapril. After intraperitoneal enalaprilat, blood pressure declined significantly, and plasma angiotensin-converting enzyme (ACE) activity was suppressed below detectable limits. There were no changes in peritoneal transport characteristics.

In contrast, in another study in CAPD patients, glucose, creatinine and β_2-microglobulin transport rates were increased after oral administration of hypotensive doses of enalapril [99]. Smaller doses of oral captopril significantly reduced peritoneal protein loss in diabetic CAPD patients, with only a small decrease in their mean blood pressure [102].

No consistent change in small solutes transport were seen after modest doses of intraperitoneal *papaverine* [103].

The influences of a variety of other agents on peritoneal mass transport have been explored.

Atrial natriuretic peptide (ANP) is a hormone with well-known diuretic and vasodilating properties. It has recently been reported that ANP could increase peritoneal fluid formation and increase peritoneal solute clearance. The effect of ANP on peritoneal fluid and solute transport kinetics has recently been investigated in the rat [104]. Addition of ANP to peritoneal dialysis solution significantly increases peritoneal fluid removal by decreasing peritoneal fluid absorption rate by 51%.

The peritoneal transport rates of potassium and iodide-131 increased when *streptokinase* or *serotonin* was administered systemically to anaesthetized dogs [54]. Whether these agents affect peritoneal permeability directly, or augment blood flow, remains to be determined.

In sedated rabbits dialysed with a hypertonic dialysis solution, 0.25% *procaine hydrochloride* increased peritoneal urea and inulin clearances by more than 60% [105]. The effect persisted for at least 1 h after procaine was discontinued. Procaine may augment transport by vasodilation. However, the addition of procaine to either side of the isolated mesothelium increased transport, after a transient decrease. This effect may be due to disruption of the microfilaments of tight junctions between cells.

The nitric oxide system and the peritoneal circulation and transport. Nitric oxide (NO) is the final common pathway for many of the vasodilating processes, including nitroprusside. NO is synthesized in the endothelial cells from L-arginine via NO synthase, and it activates guanalylyl cyclase in the vascular smooth muscle to increase the cyclic guanosine cyclase (cGMP) concentration, which produces relaxation by decreasing cytosolic free calcium. Besides the expression of aquaporins (see later), Devuyst *et al.* [106] also investigated the expression of endothelial nitric oxide synthase (eNOS) in 19 peritoneal samples from normal subjects ($n = 5$), from uraemic patients treated by haemodialysis ($n = 7$) or peritoneal dialysis ($n = 4$), and from non-uraemic patients ($n = 3$), using Western blotting and immunostaining. eNOS was located in all types of endothelium and was up-regulated in the three patients with ascites and/or peritonitis.

NO is very rapidly converted into nitrite and nitrate and the dialysate concentrations of both products have been used to estimate peritoneal NO production. In contrast to nitrite in plasma, which is rapidly converted to nitrate, nitrite in fresh and spent dialysis fluid is stable [107]. However, interpretation of such results should be made with caution. It is likely that the L-arginine–NO pathway is not the only route for generating nitrate, and that

nitrate and nitrite are not accepatable measures of biologically active NO [108].

It is well known that different isoforms of NO synthase exist; the two most relevant ones in peritoneal dialysis being eNOS and iNOS. The latter is induced whenever immunological stimulation is present. Peritoneal macrophages are an important source of iNOS [109, 110]. For example, treatment with LPS caused at least a 20-fold increase in the amount of iNOS mRNA in the liver or in macrophages isolated from the peritoneum in rats [111].

Recently Combet *et al.* [112] were able to demonstrate a strong increase in total NOS activity in an experimental model of peritonitis in the rat. This increase was inversely correlated with peritoneal free-water permeability. It is thus conceivable that the elevated levels of nitrate in peritonitis are derived from iNOS activity and not from the 'haemodynamically active' pool of eNOS.

With these reservations in mind, nitrate in plasma and dialysate was measured [113] in six stable CAPD patients and in eight CAPD patients with 11 peritonitis episodes in the acute phase and after recovery. The correlation between the MTAC of nitrate and the MTAC of creatinine indicated diffusion from the circulation and not local production of NO in the stable patients. The median dialysate/ plasma (D/P) ratio of nitrate in the acute phase of peritonitis was 1.47 (range 0.96–2.55), which was higher than after recovery: 1.07 (0.99–1.75), $p < 0.05$. No relationship was found between the D/P ratio of nitrate and the D/P ratio of TNFα (tumour necrosis factor). It was suggested that D/P ratios of nitrate exceeding 1.0 during the acute phase of peritonitis are probably the result of local NO production, which may contribute to the marked vasodilation during peritonitis.

To investigate the effects of intraperitoneal nitroprusside, a NO donor, on peritoneal permeability and perfusion, 10 stable CAPD patients were studied twice within 1 week with glucose-based dialysate (1.36% Dianeal), with and without addition of nitroprusside 4.5 mg/L [34].

The MTAC values of low molecular weight solutes were greater with nitroprusside compared to the control dwell, pointing to an increase in effective peritoneal surface area. There was a dramatic increase in the clearances of serum proteins with a decrease in the restriction coefficient for macromolecules. This implies an increase in the intrinsic permeability of the peritoneal membrane. Kinetic modelling, using computer simulations, revealed that nitroprusside led to an increase of both the large-pore radius and the small-pore radius, and of the unrestricted area over diffusion distance. Peritoneal blood flow estimated by mass transfer of CO_2 was not different with and without nitroprusside. The D/P ratio of cGMP was greater after addition of nitroprusside, pointing to local generation of cGMP, induced by NO.

The theoretical positive effect of nitroprusside on ultrafiltration and the small solute clearances is, however, counteracted by an increase in glucose absorption. The absorption of the glucose polymer icodextrin is much lower in comparison with glucose-based dialysis solutions and the effect of a 7.5% icodextrin dialysis solution with and without the addition of 4.5 mg/L nitroprusside was studied during 8 h CAPD dwells [33].

With nitroprusside the resulting net ultrafiltration increased, while the mass transfer area coefficient of urea increased by 15% and that of creatinine by 26%, consistent with the expected enlargement of the vascular peritoneal surface area. The increase in protein clearances was more pronounced for larger proteins. The nitroprusside-induced increase in MTAC of creatinine and in ultrafiltration caused an increase in creatinine clearance from 4.2 ml/min to 5.0 ml/min during the 8 h dwell. This means that nitroprusside, when used for the long dwells together with icodextrin, adds 3 L/week to the peritoneal clearance of creatinine.

In *in-vivo* experiments on isolated rat mesentery, PD solutions reverse the haemodynamic effects of inhibitors of NO synthesis [114]. It was found that such inhibition with arginine analogues produced strong vasoconstriction of the mesenteric arterioles, suggesting that basal levels of NO control blood flow through the mesenteric arterioles.

Breborowicz et al. [115] studied peritoneal transport of small and large solutes, and net ultrafiltration in rats during PD with glucose 3.86% solution, where 0.5–5 mg/ml L-NAME was used as an additive to dialysis fluid. In addition, the effect of L-NAME (5 mg/ml) given intraperitoneally during acute peritonitis induced by lipopolysaccharides (5 μg/ml) was evaluated. L-NAME increased the peritoneal selectivity and net ultrafiltration.

Lipopolysaccharides alone induced a significant decline in net ultrafiltration while, together with L-NAME, no changes in transperitoneal transport of small and large molecules was observed, nor a significant decline in net ultrafiltration. L-NAME given intraperitoneally reduced both local and systemic production of NO, which might explain its effects on peritoneal transport.

Dipyridamole. Dipyridamole rapidly but transiently vasodilates [116] and has a sustained antiplatelet effect, which may explain the restoration of clearances towards normal in patients with intravascular platelet aggregations [117]. Peritoneal transport of urea and creatinine increase by 43% and 70%, respectively, in patients with normal vasculature given 300 mg/day of dipyridamole orally [118]. Modest increments in the clearances of uric acid and inulin also occur, but are delayed for a few days [119]. In rabbits, dipyridamole given intravenously (0.5 mg/kg) or intraperitoneally (2.5 mg/kg) increased urea and creatinine clearances by 39% and 16%, respectively [117]. The limited effectiveness and the transient vasodilator response of dipyridamole are reflected by two randomized control studies which did not demonstrate significant increases in peritoneal transport [56, 120]. Several vascular diseases (vasculitis, diabetes mellitus, lupus, etc.) can impair the mesenteric arterial circulation and reduce peritoneal transport rates [121]. Reduced peritoneal transport rates complicating these diseases are improved by dipyridamole [122]. The augmentation of peritoneal transport rates persists after dipyridamole vasodilation abates, and is attributed to its antiplatelet effect. Peritoneal clearances of patients with normal vasculature improve only minimally and transiently with dipyridamole administered orally or intraperitoneally [117]. Nevertheless, dipyridamole may be useful for selected patients when systemic disease with platelet thrombi affects mesenteric vessels, and an oral agent is preferred.

The impaired peritoneal transport that complicates irreversible systemic vascular lesions can also improve with the local application of vasodilators such as isoproterenol [67, 68]. There is no evidence that increased clearances result from improvement in the vascular disease, but rather may be attributed to vasodilation of diseased vessels.

Alterations of the electric charges

Charged macromolecules may interact with peritoneal anionic sites, altering membrane ultrastructure and permeability. In rats, local administration of protamine, a polycation, markedly increases peritoneal permeability to inulin and, to a lesser extent, urea, associated with a partial disruption of the mesothelial junctions [123]. In rabbits, protamine-induced rise in peritoneal permeability to proteins can be reversed by heparin, which provides additional evidence for the physiological importance of negative electric charges on the membrane [124].

Also in rats, cationic poly-*l*-lysine augments peritoneal permeability for urea, inulin and albumin, while with the anionic poly-*l*-glutamic acid there was an opposite trend [125]. These results were confirmed in a rabbit model by Pietrzak *et al.* [126], who showed that intraperitoneal administration of poly-*l*-lysine is associated with a significant increase in ultrafiltration rate and higher peritoneal permeability to protein and dextran. The ultrafiltrate sodium concentration was also increased, implying that elimination of the hindrance of anionic charges on the peritoneal transport barrier allowed sodium to follow water flux more proportionately.

Agents such as poly-*l*-lysine, polybrene and procaine hydrochloride block the negative charges on the capillary walls and higher mass transports ensue, especially for charged solutes [127]. A poly-*l*-lysine-induced modest increase in the transfer rate of large uncharged molecules such as dextrans may be attributed to an effect on pore dimensions.

These findings contrast with those of Breborowicz *et al.* [128], who found decreased hydraulic permeability of the mesothelium *in vitro* when exposed to cationic ferritin or alcian blue. *In-vitro* studies of isolated mesothelium, however, may not relate closely to *in-vivo* conditions, in which the capillary wall and interstitium are the more important transfer barriers. Further evaluation of polycations as transport accelerators, particularly for patients with impaired peritoneal transfer capacity, is undoubtedly warranted.

Influence of pharmacological substances on peritoneal convective transport

Solute is also convected into the peritoneum by ultrafiltration. The pores through capillary walls restrict the passage of protein but little compositional change occurs with smaller solutes such as urea. Solutes as large as inulin are sieved appreciably during peritoneal ultrafiltration. As outlined above, according to the three-pore model [1], the existence of a third, ultra-small pore could explain the dissociation between water and sodium transport observed during peritoneal dialysis, mainly when using hypertonic dialysis solutions. Aquaporin-1 has recently been recognized as the molecular correlate to such channels and positive staining for aquaporin-1 has recently been reported in the endothelial cells of the peritoneum of normal and uraemic subjects [2, 106]. The transcellular water channel AQP-1 exists as a tetramer, probably composed of three non-glycosylated subunits and one bearing a large polyoctosaminoglycan [129]. Chronic exposure to high glu-

cose concentrations may lead to glycosylation of the other units. Glycosylated AQP-1 can be demonstrated by Western blotting and immunostaining [106].

Aquaporins can be inhibited by mercurials, and in a study by Carlsson *et al.* [3], $HgCl_2$ was applied locally to the peritoneal cavity in rats, dialysed with a hypertonic 3.86% glucose solution. $HgCl_2$ treatment reduced water flow and inhibited the sieving of Na^+ without causing any untoward changes in microvascular permeability, compared with that of control rats. The peritoneal ultrafiltration was greatly inhibited in the $HgCl_2$-treated animals, further supporting the theory that water channels had been blocked.

At least eight isoforms of aquaporins are now described, and besides aquaporin 1, aquaporins 3 and 4 are also present in the peritoneum [130].

Some drugs can also specifically affect the capillary filtration coefficient, i.e. the volume filtered per unit of pressure per unit of time (ml/mmHg/min). The rate of ultrafiltration is largely determined, however, by the osmotic gradient across the peritoneum induced by dextrose. The gross ultrafiltration rate and solute mass transfer are offset by dialysate absorption; hence, lowering lymphatic flow rates raises net ultrafiltration and peritoneal clearance of solutes.

Diuretics

The addition of 1 mg/kg of furosemide to hypertonic peritoneal dialysis solution augmented sodium movement, accompanying osmotically induced water flux in rabbits [131]. Normally, electrolytes do not accompany water in the same concentration as exists in plasma water, suggesting that membrane charge impedes transport, a phenomenon that is interrupted by furosemide. Intraperitoneal furosemide also caused a 27% increase in peritoneal urea clearance, but no demonstrable changes in transport rates occur in patients undergoing intermittent peritoneal dialysis when treated systemically with this diuretic. Moreover, oral administration of furosemide did not affect sodium, potassium or water transport in patients undergoing continuous ambulatory peritoneal dialysis [132]. Furosemide, however, does increase the peritoneal transport of uric acid and of barbiturates [133]. Intraperitoneally, 1.25 mg/kg of ethacrynic acid did not affect sodium flux accompanying the bulk flow of water across the peritoneum, but augmented urea clearance to about 165% of baseline [131]. Patients treated by CAPD may experience a restoration of lost ultrafiltration capacity after treatment by furosemide or by haemo-filtration [134]. A specific effect of furosemide has been postulated, but correction of an over-expanded splanchnic volume by decreasing glucose absorption was able to restore the ultrafiltration capacity.

Amphotericin B

Amphotericin B increases the rate of ultrafiltration per osmotic gradient, i.e. the ultrafiltration coefficient [135]. Above 0.5 mg/kg there is no dose effect, and it is effective only from the serosal side [135, 136]. Amphotericin B creates channels in biological membranes for solute and water penetration. Increments in peritoneal solute clearances with amphotericin B are only modest and can be accounted for by enhanced convection [135]. Peritoneal mass transport of sodium also increases. Because osmotic ultrafiltrate during peritoneal dialysis is hyponatric, the sodium gradient so established is an impediment to water transport that is cancelled by amphotericin B [136].

Intraperitoneal use of use of amphotericin B has been reported to increase ultrafiltration during *short peritoneal dwell* in rabbits. However, in the rat model amphotericin B did not increase peritoneal fluid removal after 4 h of dwell. Higher D/P ratios and K_{BD} values, as well as higher clearances for potassium, were observed in the treated groups, suggesting a possible local release of potassium due to the cytoxic effect of amphotericin B. It was therefore concluded that amphotericin B is not useful for the improvement of peritoneal dialysis efficiency [137].

Beta-blockers

Recently, use of β-blockers has been associated with peritoneal ultrafiltration failure [138]. Of 13 patients with ultrafiltration failure, 12 had used β-blockers, compared to 18 patients without these problems, where only two patients used these drugs. In a comment by Krediet [139], possible mechanisms explaining this observation are reviewed. From a theoretical point of view, either a decrease in portal venous pressure or an increase in lymphatic absorption is a possible mechanism.

Increasing ultrafiltration rates by miscellaneous drugs

Secretin increases the hydraulic permeability of the peritoneal membrane [140]. This selective action on the splanchnic bed occurs from the vascular side only. The aminonucleoside, puromycin, which causes glomerular lesions with increased macromolecular permeability, also induces this effect on peritoneal capillaries [141]. After a few days puromycin causes a proteinaceous ascites in rats, with faster permeation of labelled test solutes than in control rats. The prolonged effect of such a permeability-augmenting drug could be commendable, but other non-glomerular capillary beds are probably also affected, which would make it hazardous even in anephric patients.

Chlorpromazine (2 mg/L) intraperitoneally increases the ultrafiltration rate and solute clearance, largely by increased convection and presumably by its surfactant effect [142]. This drug decreased surface tension of the dialysate.

Neostigmine decreases the rate of lymphatic flow and thereby increases net ultrafiltration in rats [143]. Anticholinesterase agents have complex haemodynamic effects which could influence peritoneal transport and increase gastrointestinal motility, which would enhance dialysate mixing.

The osmotic gradient across the peritoneum is the major determinant of the rate of ultrafiltration per surface area. This gradient depends mainly on the dialysate dextrose concentration but is also influenced by sodium and urea gradients, plasma oncotic pressure and the rate of dextrose absorption. Higher ultrafiltration rates due to diminished glucose reabsorption were reported with intraperitoneal calcium channel blockers in CAPD patients [97, 98]. Ronco et al. [41] suggested that maximal rates of ultrafiltration are inhibited by the steep curvilinear rise in plasma protein oncotic pressure in the peritoneal capillaries, reflecting the limited blood flow rate. Maher et al. [144] demonstrated that the ultrafiltration coefficient decrease in rabbits as intraperitoneal dwell is prolonged, suggesting some concentration polarization, which could be corrected by increasing turbulence at the membrane interfaces [144]. Increased absorption of dextrose will accompany most manipulations that enhance solute permeability and hence dissipate the glucose osmotic gradient faster, reducing ultrafiltration. Insulin is required to maintain low plasma glucose levels and achieve the maximal gradient. Exogenous insulin added intraperitoneally does not increase the glucose mass transfer coefficient [145]. Because excessive glucose absorption can be hazardous, alternative osmotic agents have been evaluated. Amino acids added to the dialysate offer a nutritional advantage but may be expensive. Dextrans, glucose polymers and cross-linked gelatins are large enough to permeate the peritoneum poorly, thereby maintaining the osmotic gradient throughout long dwell exchange [146], but are eliminated slowly after absorption.

Lymphatic absorption

Lymphatics are the primary route for absorption from the peritoneum of isotonic dialysate including macromolecules, particles and formed blood elements [8]. Most absorption occurs via the subdiaphragmatic lymphatics, with lesser amounts via the mesenteric lymphatic vessels [9]. Yet before reaching lymphatic channels macromolecules are probably distributed in the large peritoneal tissue compartment [10]. Absorption from the peritoneum of macromolecules such as albumin, haemoglobin, fibrinogen and polydisperse dextran 70 has been reported [11–16] and has been used as a measure of peritoneal lymphatic flow rates [13, 14, 17–19]. The lymphatic flow rate in CAPD patients is about 11 ml/h based on radioiodinated serum albumin studies [13], or about 1–2.5 ml/min, based on the disappearance rate of intraperitoneal macromolecules [18, 19]. During peritonitis, peritoneal lymph flow is significantly increased [14].

The peritoneal absorption of polydispersed neutral dextrans does not show size discrimination, adding evidence that the major route is by lymphatic transport [16, 20]. The rate of lymphatic flow from the peritoneum correlates positively with ventilation (diaphragmatic movement) and negatively with end-expiratory pressure; it decreases with erect posture and with dehydration [147]. Lymphatic absorption subtracts from the gross peritoneal ultrafiltration volume. In the rat peritoneal dialysis model, neostigmine increased net ultrafiltration and solute transport by reducing the cumulative lymphatic absorption, without an increase in total transcapillary ultrafiltration [143]. Lower doses of intraperitoneal neostigmine failed to influence lymphatic absorption in CAPD patients [148], but the animal data were confirmed by a case report of a CAPD patient suffering from myasthenia gravis who required high oral dosage of this drug [149]. In another animal study phosphatidylcholine augmented net ultrafiltration and solute clearances without increasing flux of water and solutes into the peritoneal cavity, thus acting by reducing lymphatic reabsorption [150]. Similar results were reported in a recent clinical study [151] and it has been suggested that phosphatidylcholine affects peritoneal fluid kinetics through its cholinergic action [152]. These studies indicate that limiting lymphatic

absorption is a potential mechanism for augmenting peritoneal clearances that should be explored further.

The study of different additives to the dialysate

It is known that peritoneal fluid absorption substantially decreases the efficiency of peritoneal dialysis. Consequently, improving the dialysis efficiency of the peritoneum has been one of the major research activities in recent decades.

In CAPD patients peritoneal fluid absorption reduced potential net ultrafiltration by $83.2 \pm 10.2\%$, urea clearance by $16.9 \pm 1.9\%$ and creatinine clearance by $16.5 \pm 1.9\%$ in one 6 h exchange. The contribution of peritoneal fluid absorption to low dialysis efficiency is more significant in high transporters and when 1.36% glucose solution is used [153]. Therefore, reducing the peritoneal fluid absorption should be an effective way to improve the adequacy (as regards removal of both small solutes and fluid) of PD, especially when high dialysate fill volumes are used. Peritoneal fluid absorption is mainly driven by the intraperitoneal hydrostatic pressure [154, 155].

Hyaluronan

Using the rat model it has been found that peritoneal absorption was significantly reduced and peritoneal small solute clearance substantially increased by adding to the peritoneal dialysate 0.01% *hyaluronan*, a long polysaccharide chain that consists of repeating disaccharide units of N-acetylglucosamine and glucuronic acid [156, 157]. It is speculated that the effect of hyaluronan is due to the accumulation of a restrictive filter 'cake' of hyaluronan chains at the tissue–cavity interface [158].

Hyaluronan plays an important role in tissue hydraulic conductivity and has been shown to exhibit a high resistance against water flow. It can thus act in tissue as a barrier against rapid changes in tissue water content [159], impeding the efflux from the peritoneal cavity. This effect of hyaluronan is both size- and concentration-dependent [160].

It is also possible that exogenous high molecular weight hyaluronan stabilizes the endogenous hyaluronan, which forms a stagnant layer at the mesothelial cell surface [161]. Effluent dialysate from CAPD patients stimulates production of hyaluronic acid by human mesothelial cells and acts synergistically with cytokines, such as IL-1 [162]. It has been shown that normal human mesothelial cells *in vitro* surround themselves with a particular matrix, 'coat', containing mainly hyaluronan [163]. These promising results now need to be confirmed in clinical studies.

N-acetylglucosamine

Related to the effects of hyaluronan, it is relevant to draw attention to the studies with *N*-acetylglucosamine (NAG) either as osmotic agent for peritoneal dialysis [164, 165] or as an additive to classical dialysate. Chronic peritoneal dialysis with dialysis solution supplemented with NAG (50 mmol/L) causes accumulation of glycosaminoglycans in the peritoneal interstitium, which results in a change of peritoneal permeability [166].

Supplementation of the dialysate with NAG could enhance the synthesis of hyaluronan by the mesothelial cells, since hyaluronan contains both glucuronic acid and NAG. In rats, equivalent concentrations of NAG and glucose were associated not only with a greater ultrafiltration with NAG [165], but also with a greater *in-vitro* synthesis of hyaluronan [164].

Chronic peritoneal dialysis in rats with a solution supplemented with NAG showed an accumulation of polyanionic glucosaminoglycans in the submesothelial interstitium which must be associated with a decreased hydraulic permeability of that tissue [167]. Enhanced intraperitoneal synthesis of glycosaminoglycans increases the permselectivity of the peritoneum and preserves its function during chronic PD [168–170].

Chondroitin sulphate (CS)

Chondroitin sulphate, another naturally occurring polyanionic polymer glycosaminoglycan, has been tested as an alternative osmotic agent or has been added to saline [171] or conventional dialysis solution to enhance peritoneal ultrafiltration [169]. In the presence of CS, net peritoneal ultrafiltration increased, while absorption of glucose and horseradish peroxidase from the peritoneal cavity decreased [172, 173].

Recently it was found that intraperitoneal CS increased the MTAC of small molecules while preserving the peritoneal ultrafiltration capacity [174].

It is postulated that the polyanionic CS molecules are trapped in the peritoneal interstitium, thus decreasing its hydraulic conductivity and permeability, which in turn increases net fluid removal during peritoneal dialysis because of its slower absorption from the peritoneal cavity.

Phosphatidylcholine

In 1985 Grahame *et al.* detected the presence of surface-active material (phospholipids) in the peritoneal effluent of CAPD patients [175].The surface-active material, lining the peritoneal membrane, is mostly composed of phosphatidylcholine (lecithin). Peritoneal efficiency may be altered by the constant removal of phosphatidylcholine and other phospholipids in the dialysate effluent [175].

A decrease in dialysate phospholipids was reported in patients with a low ultrafiltration capacity and in those with peritonitis [176]. Intraperitoneal phosphatidylcholine promptly raised the ultrafiltration rate, while after oral administration about 30 days were required to achieve this effect. The authors suggest that lecithin administration restored the normal peritoneal surfactant lining [176]. To explain augmentation of ultrafiltration after phosphatidylcholine, another group proposed that these phospholipid molecules bind to the anionic sites on the luminal side of the mesothelium, creating a water-repellent surface which diminishes the thickness of the unstirred dialysate. This would augment diffusion of solutes from blood to the peritoneum while the hydrophobic lecithin molecules would impede water absorption, favouring ultrafiltration [177].

In rabbits, phosphatidylcholine increases net ultrafiltrate volume [177], an effect that becomes significant only after hours of peritoneal dialysis, and does not show up during hourly exchanges.

Clinical studies have shown that a phosphatidylcholine premixed dialysis solution significantly enhances ultrafiltration also in patients without ultrafiltration loss [151], but other results were controversial [178, 179].

Besides its surfactant effect, phosphatidylcholine may impede lymphatic absorption [150]. In rat experiments, administration of 50 mg/L phosphatidylcholine to a glucose dialysate of 4.25% glucose leads to a reduction in lymphatic absorption without increased transperitoneal transport of water [150].

However, in *in-vitro* experiments phosphatidylcholine was cytotoxic to human mesothelial cells, as indicated by the release of lactate dehydrogenase from their cytosol. Cells exposed to phosphatidylcholine had a diminished capacity for taking up ^{86}Rb from medium and had decreased fibrinolytic properties and increased procoagulant activity. These results suggest that the positive short-term effect of the addition of phosphatidylcholine to the dialysis solution (i.e. an increase in ultrafiltration) may be masked by its deleterious action on human mesothelial cell membrane [180].

Dioctyl sodium sulphosuccinate (DSS)

Dioctyl sodium sulphosuccinate (DSS) is a surfactant and has been shown to increase peritoneal small solute clearance. Penzotti and Mattocks [181, 182] accelerated peritoneal transport of labelled urea and creatinine in sedated rabbits by adding a variety of surface-acting agents including DSS and setyl trimethyl ammonium chloride. Dunham *et al.* [183] found a dose-dependent rise in creatinine and urea clearances when docusate sodium was given intraperitoneally to tranquillized rabbits. The effect persisted for 5 h. DSS was found to increase peritoneal fluid and small solute removal whereas the peritoneal solute transport rate did not change [184].

Cytochalasins

These molecules disrupt microfilaments of cellular junctions. Cytochalasin D given intraperitoneally raises the clearances of creatinine and urea in the rabbit, consistent with augmented diffusion through intercellular gaps [185]. Similarly, cytochalasin B, D and E increase permeability of the peritoneum to urea, inulin and albumin in rats [186]. Only cytochalasin B effects were clearly reversible, which may relate to its unique ability to affect carrier proteins of the cell membrane.

Antioxidants and free radical scavengers

Breborowicz *et al.* [187] tested the effect of L-2-oxothiazolidine-4-carboxylate (procysteine), a precursor of intracellular cysteine, on the function of human mesothelial cells in culture. Procysteine stimulated the proliferation of these cells and decreased their spontaneous death rate. The cells, when pretreated with procysteine, were resistant to injury by free radicals. Procysteine also reversed the cytotoxic effects of a mixture of essential and non-essential amino acids on the cells. The same drug was also studied in an *in-vivo* model of lipopolysaccharide (LPS)-induced peritonitis in rats [188]. The addition of LPS to dialysis fluid increased the white blood cell count and the nitrite level (index of NO synthesis) in the dialysate. Simultaneous addition of procysteine to the dialysis fluid prevented an increase of white blood cells, but not of nitrites in the dialysate. The intraperitoneal inflammation was accompanied by a decrease in net transperitoneal ultrafil-

tration, an increase in the absorption of glucose, and a loss of protein into the dialysate. Procysteine partially reversed the effect of peritonitis on net ultrafiltration. Peritoneal leukocytes from rats exposed to LPS showed a reduced concentration of glutathione, an effect that was reversed in the presence of the drug. These results show that the addition of procysteine to dialysis fluid modified the peritoneal reaction to acute inflammation. The same group [189] showed that supplementation of intraperitoneally infused saline with vitamin E decreased the peroxidation of peritoneum estimated as the malondialdehyde (MDA) level in rats' omentum. However, the permeability of the peritoneum to glucose and protein in vitamin E-treated rats was increased. Vitamin E appeared to be cytotoxic to human mesothelial cells, as measured by inhibition of their proliferation, and this effect was irreversible.

Influence of drugs on peritoneal mesothelial cells

The short-term effects of antineoplastic agents such as methotrexate, doxorubicin and mitoxantrone on the integrity of human peritoneal mesothelial cells (HPMC) membrane and mechanisms of intracellular potassium transport were assessed [190]. There was no evidence of significant cytotoxicity to either methotrexate, doxorubicin or mitoxantrone. However, methotrexate diminished Na,K,ATPase activity and simultaneously enhanced ^{86}Rb transport via a furosemide-sensitive pathway. Mitoxantrone reduced the furosemide-sensitive ^{86}Rb influx in a dose-dependent manner. These data demonstrate that antineoplastic agents interfere with HPMC function which might contribute to the oncostatic-induced peritoneal toxicity.

The same group investigated the effects of insulin on the $Na^+/K(+)$-ATPase expression and activity in human peritoneal mesothelial cells [191]. A time- and dose-dependent increase in the $Na^+/K(+)$-ATPase activity was found. This effect appears to be mediated by an increase in $[Na^+]_i$ and is not related to alterations in $Na^+/K(+)$-ATPase subunit mRNA expression.

Transport acceleration of specific solutes

Removal of barbiturates may be accelerated by increasing dialysate pH with Tris buffer, thereby influencing the rate of non-inonic diffusion [146]. Alkalinization of peritoneal dialysate by THAM also raised uric acid transport [192]. Drugs that counteract the membrane anionic charge should enhance removal of charged solutes. Adding albumin to peritoneal dialysis solution enhances removal of barbiturates [193], etchchlorvynol [194] and salicylate [195], and is expected to augment the clearance of numerous other drugs that circulate bound to plasma proteins, such as quinine and phenytoin. For lipophilic drugs such as glutethimide and short-acting barbiturates, transport can be enhanced by adding lipid to the dialysate [196]. In general, for treating severe overdosage, the removal of drugs by peritoneal dialysis is too slow. Specific effects such as chelation, however, may influence concentrations of drugs and certain uraemic metabolites.

Peritoneal protein loss attenuation

In a preliminary study, captopril significantly reduced protein loss into the peritoneum in diabetic CAPD patients, presumably by modulating vasoconstrictive responses of peritoneal capillaries [102]. In rabbits a marked increase in protein elimination into the peritoneum occurred after addition of histamine, an effect blocked by its antagonist [94]. Because histamine may be involved in the pathogenesis of hypersensitivity reactions to drugs, leachables or contaminants of the dialysis solution, antihistamine agents could be of value in such circumstances.

Several lines of evidence support the role of intact anionic sites on the peritoneal transport barrier in the restriction of the passage of charged macromolecules to the peritoneal cavity. Partial neutralization of anionic sites may account for the findings from an animal study in which dialysate pH adjustment from 5.6 up to 7.4 significantly increased peritoneal protein loss in the presence of nitroprusside [64]. Another group demonstrated that, in rabbits, transperitoneal protein loss was substantially enhanced by protamine. Neutralization of protamine with heparin prevented this effect [124]. In a recent animal study [197], blood to peritoneum transport rates of cationic DEAE dextran were less that those of both neutral dextran and dextran sulphate. The effects of chondroitin sulphate have been described above.

Conclusions

It is easy for clinicians as well as basic scientists to forget that the peritoneum, unlike synthetic haemodialysis membranes, is alive. The mesenteric circulation is remarkable for its size and complexity, and until recently not much was known about its physiology. The numerous drugs and hormones that affect mesenteric blood flow and membrane physiology have predictable effects on peritoneal transport parameters [198, 199]. Patients undergoing chronic dialysis often take several drugs, many of which have haemodynamic and membrane transport effects. The influences of these agents on the peritoneum must be ascertained. Patients treated for acute problems, for example in an intensive-care unit, are exposed to an even greater abundance of drugs potentially altering transport. Rational use of drugs and other physiological manipulations in patients maintained by peritoneal dialysis requires an understanding of their effects on peritoneal blood flow and permeability. It is naive to consider the peritoneum as an inert membrane with constant blood flow and transport characteristics. Further investigation of the interactions of drugs and the peritoneum may identify optimal methods for augmenting transport efficiency safely.

Pharmacokinetic aspects of peritoneal transport of drugs

This part of the chapter has been divided in two major sections: the first section covers some basic pharmacokinetic concepts in the presence of normal and abnormal renal function. More detailed information on this subject is available in standard textbooks and reviews on pharmacokinetics [200–202]. Also in this first section a general discussion on the major factors determining the transperitoneal transport of drugs after systemic and intraperitoneal administration will be provided.

In the second section the pharmacokinetic data obtained with drugs, commonly used in continuous ambulatory or automated peritoneal dialysis (CAPD or APD) patients, have been listed in tables. Following each table, recommendations for possible dose adaptations in peritoneal dialysis patients are provided.

Basic pharmacokinetics

Drugs produce their therapeutic or toxic effects in biological systems by reacting with receptor sites or other sites of action located in target tissues. The intensity of these effects is, in most cases, determined by the concentration of the drug in the direct environment of the site of action (the 'biophase'). It is not possible to determine drug concentrations in the biophase. However, all tissues are supplied by blood (or plasma). Although often a complex relationship exists between the drug concentration in the biophase and that in plasma water, the latter is an alternative and more accessible site to measure the drug concentration. Responses to a particular drug are therefore commonly related to the concentration of the drug (or in some cases of its metabolites), in plasma water. After administration of a drug, absorption from the site of administration to the plasma (in case of extravascular administration), distribution from the plasma to organs and tissues, elimination by biotransformation (predominantly in the liver) or by excretion of the chemically unaltered parent drug (predominantly via the kidneys), take place. However, after biotransformation, the metabolites are often excreted by the kidneys, even when the parent drug is not. In the situation in which the metabolite(s) is pharmacologically active, dose adaptation in renal failure of drugs which are not primarily eliminated by the kidney may be necessary. As a consequence of these events, drug concentrations in plasma water, and in the biophase, change with time, as does the pharmacological effect.

In addition, drugs can be bound to proteins, and their effect may depend on the free/protein-bound ratio. With the usual methods, however, total plasma drug concentrations are measured, i.e. free drug and drug bound to plasma proteins together. If the protein binding of the drug is constant, total drug concentration in plasma water can be used as an index of free drug concentration. If, however, the protein binding of the drug has changed, e.g. because of renal failure or by interaction with other drugs, this relationship will change and the intensity of effect will be smaller or larger than expected for a particular total plasma drug concentration.

Compartmental models

Pharmacokinetics involve the mathematical description of the time-course of the concentration of the drug (and, in some cases, its metabolites), in biological fluids after its administration. In most models, compartments are used; it is important to realize that a pharmacokinetic compartment does not necessarily correspond to a given anatomical body fluid compartment. The time-course of the plasma drug concentrations can usually be adequately described by a one-compartment model, in which the body is viewed as one space, in which the drug is distributed rapidly and homogeneously. Although this is an

oversimplification, such a one-compartment model is often satisfactory for the study of the pharmacokinetics of a drug, e.g., in order to determine its optimal dosage.

A two-compartment model (Fig. 1) consists of a central and a peripheral compartment. The central compartment includes the plasma, but also the extracellular fluid of highly perfused organs such as heart, lung, liver and kidney. The peripheral compartment involves the compartment in which the drug is distributed at a slower rate. Transfer between the two compartments is slow, and changes in concentration in one compartment will only be accompanied by changes in the other compartment with a certain delay. What parts of the organism belong to the central or to the peripheral compartment will depend upon the physicochemical characteristics of the drug, and of the general condition of the tissues involved. In a patient with sepsis, for example, the separation between central ('vascular') and peripheral ('interstitial tissue') compartments has greatly disappeared by the generalized hyperpermeability of the capillaries. Although three- and even more-compartmental models describe the situation more correctly, they are difficult to handle and their use is usually not needed.

Plasma concentration–time-course

In Fig. 2 the time-course of the plasma concentrations of a drug after intravenous injection of a single dose is shown for both a one-compartmental and a two-compartmental model. Factors such as

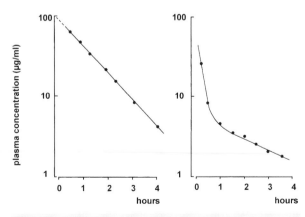

Figure 2. Plasma concentrations as a function of time; in the *left panel* the logarithm of the plasma concentration is plotted for a drug for which a one-compartmental analysis is appropriate. In the *right panel*, log plasma concentrations are shown for a two-compartmental analysis. After the distribution phase there is a linear decay of the concentration, corresponding to the elimination phase.

absorption, distribution, elimination and excretion usually follow first-order kinetics. When first-order kinetics apply, the changes in concentration occurring are proportional to the drug concentration at that particular moment. After absorption and distribution are completed, the fall of the plasma concentration is only determined by elimination. As illustrated in Fig. 2, if elimination follows first-order kinetics, the log concentration-versus-time curve in a two-compartment model is a straight line. From the plasma concentration–time curve a number of pharmacokinetic parameters can be calculated. These are useful in the procedures for dose adaptation in different situations.

The elimination half-life of the drug ($t_{1/2}$), is the time taken for the plasma concentration as well as the amount of drug in the body to decrease by 50%. A closely related parameter is the elimination constant (K_e), where:

$$K_e = 0.693/t_{1/2} \tag{1}$$

The apparent volume of distribution (V_d) of a drug relates the total amount of drug in the body to the concentration of drug in plasma at the same moment.

The volume of distribution (V_d) can be calculated from:

$$V_d = D/C_0 \tag{2}$$

where D equals the dose given and C_0 equals the plasma concentration at the time 0, the time of administration. The volume of distribution can be calculated only when the dose of the drug entering the body is known; that means when the drug is either given intravenously or if the exact amount absorbed is known.

The distribution volume provides an estimate of the extent of distribution of the drug throughout the body. If there is important uptake of the drug by the tissues, a distribution volume several times larger than the total body fluid volume (approximately 42 L for a body weight of 70 kg) can be found.

One of the important factors determining the size of the apparent distribution volume is the degree of plasma protein binding. The relationship between the apparent volume of distribution of a drug and its protein binding is as follows:

$$V_D = V_B + V_T(F_B/F_T) \tag{3}$$

V_B and V_T are the volumes of water in blood and in tissues, respectively, and F_B and F_T are the fractions of free drug in blood and tissues, respectively. An increase in F_B without a proportional increase in F_T would produce an increase in the apparent volume of distribution.

The apparent distribution volume can also be calculated from the area under the plasma concentration versus time-curve (AUC), and K_e:

$$V_d = D/\text{AUC} \times K_e$$

or $\tag{4}$

$$V_d = (D \times t_{1/2})/(\text{AUC} \times 0.693)$$

Total body clearance or total plasma clearance is the volume of plasma that is cleared completely of the drug per unit time: it gives an estimate of the efficiency of the elimination of the drug by organs such as liver or kidney. Total body or plasma clearance is the sum of the clearances by the individual elimination routes, mainly biotransformation in the liver and excretion by the kidneys. For some substances elimination takes place only via the kidney, and then total body clearance equals renal clearance.

Total body clearance (Cl_{tot}) can be calculated by means of the equations:

$$Cl_{tot} = 0.693V_d/t_{1/2} \tag{5}$$

$$Cl_{tot} = D/\text{AUC} \tag{6}$$

Although clearance can be calculated from V_d and $t_{1/2}$, it does not depend on these parameters. On the other hand, half-life of elimination is dependent not only upon the clearance, but also upon the volume of distribution. Although gentamicin and digoxin are both cleared by the kidneys to approximately the same extent as creatinine (this means at a rate of approximately 120 ml/min in a normal situation), the elimination half-life of digoxin is 36 h, while that of gentamicin is only 2 h. This is due to the fact that the distribution volume of digoxin is more than 500 L, while that of gentamicin is only about 15 L. When elimination in different situations is compared (for example in patients with renal failure compared to healthy individuals, or in pre-dialysis patients compared to those on dialysis), clearances and not only half-lives should be calculated whenever possible.

Elimination half-life should not be confused with duration of action. The latter is determined by the time during which drug concentrations are above a minimal effective concentration (MEC). The duration of drug action is dependent not only on the elimination half-life of the drug but also on the dose given, bioavailability and of the drug distribution.

Total body clearance can be measured exactly only after intravenous drug administration or when the bioavailability, *F*, is known. Drugs are, however, often administered orally without knowing their exact bioavailability.

While the pharmacokinetics of a drug are usually studied after single-dose administration, it is of utmost importance to know what happens after chronic administration of a drug. For some drugs at the moment of the second administration the amount still present in the body is negligible, so that after the second administration concentrations in the plasma will be similar to those after the first administration. This is for example the case when, in patients with normal renal function, gentamicin (with an elimination half-life of 2 h) is administered three times a day. When, however, drugs are administered at dosing intervals shorter than 4 half-lives, an important fraction of what was introduced with the first administration is still present at the time of the second dosage. Consequently, the concentration after the second dose will be higher than that after the first dose, i.e. accumulation of the drug occurs. In that case, steady-state concentrations are obtained only after a number of administrations. The time to reach steady-state plasma concentrations depends only on the half-life, and is approximately four to five times the half-life of the drug. For example for digoxin, with its half-life of 1.5 days, this works out at approximately 1 week. If the steady-state levels are to be achieved earlier, a loading dose of the drug must be given. The extent of accumulation (i.e. how much higher the steady-state levels will be than those after the first administration) depends on the half-life and the dosing interval.

Pharmacokinetic alterations in patients with decreased renal function

In patients with renal failure the fate of a drug can be altered profoundly. Gastrointestinal absorption after oral administration of a drug may be impaired in uraemic patients because gastrointestinal pH or motility are altered. Biotransformation of drugs can be decreased or increased in uraemic patients. There is also much interest in alterations in plasma protein binding of drugs in these patients. For a number of acidic drugs, which are mainly bound to plasma albumin, binding is often markedly decreased, due either to a decrease in albumin concentration in the plasma or to a decrease in the affinity at the binding sites; the decrease in affinity can be due to structural changes of the albumin molecules or to the presence of endogenous inhibitors. Some basic drugs bind mainly to α_1-acid glycoprotein (α_1-AGP). In renal failure the binding of these drugs may be increased due to the elevated α_1-AGP concentrations in the plasma. These changes in protein binding can markedly affect the calculated pharmacokinetic parameters, and they can in some circumstances lead to changes in free drug concentration in plasma, to changes in efficacy and to side-effects.

Most important of course is the decrease in renal excretion of the drug. The renal clearance of a drug is usually decreased proportionally to the decrease in glomerular filtration rate. If renal excretion is the only elimination route of the drug, total body or plasma clearance will be reduced to the same extent. For substances that are only partly eliminated by the kidneys, the alteration in total body clearance will depend upon the relative importance of the renal versus the non-renal elimination. It should, however, be re-emphasized that it is not because a drug is not eliminated via the kidney, that total body clearance is not altered in patients with renal failure. For example, hepatic clearance can also be affected by a change in protein binding or because of accumulation of other molecules.

However, the volume of distribution of drugs in these patients is often also different due to the changes in binding in plasma or in tissues. The plasma half-life, which depends on both V_d and Cl, is therefore not always a good parameter of the drug clearance in these patients. For example, digoxin is not bound to a significant extent to plasma proteins, but it is bound extensively to tissues of the kidneys, liver and myocardium. This binding is decreased in patients with renal failure. As apparent from equation (3), a decrease in drug tissue binding without a corresponding decrease in drug plasma binding results in a decrease in the apparent volume of distribution. In several studies it has been observed that the volume of distribution of digoxin is significantly smaller in patients with chronic renal failure (230–280 L vs 500 L in normals).

The pharmacokinetic changes in chronic renal failure can, mainly after chronic administration of a drug, lead to important changes in total and free plasma concentrations, if the dose is not adjusted. Drug concentrations in the body can be much higher and the time to reach steady state (at a higher level) can be increased, if the half-life is prolonged. This explains why in patients with renal failure a loading dose is often needed. Thus, for many drugs, dose adjustments will be necessary in chronic renal failure. The mean steady-state levels (C_{ss}) which will be achieved in a given situation can be calculated with the following equation:

$$C_{ss} = (F \times D)/(Cl_{tot} \times T) \tag{7}$$

where F = fraction absorbed, T = the dosing interval and D the maintenance dose. This can also be expressed as:

$$Css = (1.44F \times D \times t_{1/2})/(V_d \times T) \tag{8}$$

From these equations the maintenance dose needed for a given C_{ss} can be calculated. The many nomograms available for calculation of maintenance doses are based on these principles.

The loading dose (D^*), i.e. the dose needed to obtain a given C_{ss} at once, can be calculated by the equation

$$D^* = V_d \times C_{ss} \tag{9}$$

Pharmacokinetic alterations in patients on peritoneal dialysis

Peritoneal dialysis can alter the pharmacokinetics of a drug, depending upon the route of administration of the drug and rate of removal via the dialysate. This can necessitate dose adaptations.

Pharmacokinetics of drugs after systemic administration: assessment

Plasma and dialysate concentrations can be measured as a function of time. To evaluate whether systemic kinetics are affected by dialysis, serum half-life, volume of distribution and total body clearance (and in some cases residual renal clearance) can be calculated and compared to the values obtained in terminal chronic renal failure patients without dialysis. The amount recovered from the peritoneal dialysate over the period of time (A_{per}), can be used to assess the need for dose adaptation. This amount should be viewed in relation to that lost in the body over the same period of time by other routes, such as hepatic biotransformation or residual renal excretion.

The peritoneal dialysis clearance (Cl_{per}) can be calculated from the equation:

$$Cl_{per} = (A_{per}\,t_1 - t_2)/\mathrm{AUC}\,t_1 - t_2 \tag{10}$$

where $A_{per}\,t_1 - t_2$ is the amount recovered in the dialysate over a given time period and AUC $t_1 - t_2$ is the area under the plasma concentration curve over the same time period. The peritoneal clearance should be compared to the total body clearance (Cl_{tot}). Indeed, the increased plasma clearance that can be found with dialysis is dependent of the perito-

neal clearance of the drug, the residual renal clearance and the non-renal clearance.

Factors influencing peritoneal drug clearance. The dialysis clearance of a systemically administered drug in the peritoneal dialysis setting will depend upon factors that are summarized in Table 1. The peritoneal membrane characteristics have been described in the first part of this chapter. Only some of the other factors will be discussed below.

The most important factor in determining the magnitude of the peritoneal clearance of a drug, is the *dialysate flow rate*, which is around 6–7 ml/min in CAPD. Small solute peritoneal clearances are largely dialysate flow-dependent. This explains why, during the rapid exchanges in APD programmes, clearances of solutes with low molecular weight are increased. During the long dwells of CAPD the transport rate of small solutes per unit of time is high at the beginning of the dwell and decreases with time because diffusion equilibrium is either obtained or approached. With increasing molecular weight of the solute the transport rate during the dwell becomes more homogeneous. During the rapid exchanges of continuous cyclic peritoneal dialysis (CCPD) (for example four exchanges of 2.5 L over 8 h overnight, followed by a long diurnal dwell time of 10–12 h), the dialysate flow rate can be around 15–20 ml/min, values much greater than those for CAPD. However, the concentration of most systemically administered drugs achieved in the drained dialysate after 2 h will be much lower than after long dwells so that the total amount of drug removed over 24 h in CCPD will be not much different from CAPD.

Another important factor determining the rate of diffusion across the peritoneal membrane is the *molecular weight* of the drug. The molecular weights of most drugs range between 100 and 700 Da, with some notable exceptions such as vancomycin (MW 1450), insulin (MW 6000) and erythropoietin (MW 30 400). The diffusion of a solute from blood to dialysate is inversely proportional to the square root of the solute mass, both in α-haemodialysis and peritoneal dialysis [203, 204].

Another factor is the extent of drug–protein binding, since only unbound, free drug is available for diffusion. A drug with a high plasma protein binding usually shows a low peritoneal clearance. The effect of plasma protein binding on the peritoneal transport of intravenously administered β-lactam antibiotics has been investigated in rats [205]. The antibiotic concentration–time profiles obtained in the dialysate were compatible with the concept that only unbound antibiotic is available for peritoneal transport. Although Flessner *et al.* [206] reported that bovine serum albumin is transferred through the peritoneal tissues from plasma to the peritoneal cavity in rats, the capillary membrane permeability of cephalosporins was 5–17-fold higher than that of albumin. Therefore, even if molecules bound to albumin can be transported through the peritoneal membrane, the contribution of this fraction is probably minor. For practical purposes this implies that the peritoneal membrane plays no important role in the transport of endogenous substances highly bound to proteins [207]. Dialysate concentrations of proteins are lower than serum concentrations and the protein binding of drug molecules in the peritoneal compartment is believed to be of minor clinical significance [208]. Based upon these considerations a reasonably accurate formula for the prediction of the peritoneal clearance in CAPD after systemic administration of drugs has been proposed [209], where:

$$Cl_{per} \; (ml/min) = 75 \sqrt{(f_U)}/\sqrt{(MW)} \qquad (11)$$

In this formula, f_U represents the free fraction in the serum and MW the molecular weight of the drug. This formula is valid for a 2 L dialysate and a 6 h dwell, in the absence of peritonitis. Erythromycin, for example, has a molecular weight of 730 and a free fraction of 0.30; therefore, the peritoneal clearance is estimated to be 1.52 ml/min. The validity of the formula was tested by comparing the predicted values with the observed clearances in 19 clinical studies. A linear regression analysis yielded a correlation coefficient of 0.958.

A drug with a low molecular weight (< 500 kDa) and with a low plasma protein binding can have a clinically relevant peritoneal dialysis clearance.

Need for dose adaptation after systemic drug administration in peritoneal dialysis. The dialysability of a drug in any dialysis strategy is clinically relevant only when at least two conditions are fulfilled. First, the dialysis clearance should be at least 30% higher than the endogenous total plasma clearance; otherwise the additive effect of dialysis clearance on overall drug elimination is negligible [210]. Second, the distribution volume of the drug should be less than 1 L/kg bodyweight. If V_d is larger, only a small fraction of the drug is available in the plasma for elimination via dialysis, and the amount of drug removed is small, even for a high clearance. Since in terminal chronic renal failure for most drugs, the total endo-

genous drug plasma clearance is higher than 20–30 ml/min, and the distribution volume is more than 1 L/kg body weight, the peritoneal drug clearance rarely contributes significantly to drug removal in the CAPD setting. Therefore, additional dose adaptations for CAPD beyond the recommendations for terminal chronic renal failure are very rarely necessary. Notable exceptions are drugs with a small distribution volume, low protein binding and a small total plasma clearance in uraemia.

As outlined above, the dialysate flow rate is greater during the rapid exchanges in some automated peritoneal dialysis regimens. Dialysis clearances during the short dwell times could be higher, because sink conditions tend to be maintained. It could be that during the rapid exhanges a significant fraction of a systemically given drug is removed through the peritoneum. Pharmacokinetic investigations in modern CCPD settings have not been conducted, and currently there are no formal drug-dosing guidelines for patients receiving these dialysis modalities. However, based on the theoretical calculations explained above, we suspect that the daily peritoneal removal of most drugs also in APD is as a rule clinically unimportant.

The presence of peritonitis does not significantly influence the magnitude or rapidity of drug transport into the peritoneal cavity after systemic administration. For example, the peritoneal clearances of netilmicin and of ciprofloxacin in patients with or without peritonitis were not different [211, 212].

Studies after systemic administration of a drug are of interest not only to evaluate the need for dose adaptations to maintain adequate systemic concentrations, but also for knowing the dialysate drug concentrations. The low peritoneal drug clearance does not exclude that, for example, for an antibiotic, therapeutically effective concentrations can be achieved in the dialysate after systemic administration, due to the low volume (2–3 L) in which the drug diffuses.

The rapidity with which therapeutic concentrations are achieved in the dialysate may be influenced by the presence of peritonitis. For example, after intravenous administration, therapeutic vancomycin concentrations in the dialysate are reached after 30 min of dwell in peritonitis patients, versus 2–4 h in a non-inflamed peritoneum [213].

The concentrations of antibiotic drugs that are achieved in the dialysate after systemic as well as after intraperitoneal administration must be viewed against their activities against the strains that are isolated from patients with peritonitis. As recently pointed out by several workers, used peritoneal dialysis fluid is a better medium to test these activities than the classically used broth [214–216]. Furthermore, recent work has shown that culturing conditions, dialysate manipulations, and adherence capacity of germs are critical factors affecting antibiotic activity [217].

For drugs that are metabolized by equilibrium-rated reactions to metabolites which are removed by peritoneal dialysis, a higher total clearance of the parent drug may also be present during peritoneal dialysis, even if the drug itself is not found in the dialysate. Thus the absence of the drug in drained dialysate does not mean that total clearance of that drug is not altered by CAPD. An example of this phenomenon was recently described for mycophenolate acid and its metabolite mycophenolate glucuronide, where a significant amount of mycophenolate acid was removed in the dialysate, almost completely in its glucuronidated form [218].

Pharmacokinetics of drugs after intraperitoneal administration

Peritoneal transport is also of interest with regard to intraperitoneal administration of drugs. For example, the intraperitoneal doses of insulin or erythropoietin required to achieve adequate systemic concentrations, or of antibiotics for local treatment of peritonitis, need to be carefully calculated. There are two sources of blood supply to the organs of the peritoneal cavity, one to the parietal and the other to the visceral peritoneum; both layers are rich in lymphatic circulation. The venous blood of visceral peritoneum returns to the portal circulation, while the venous return from the parietal peritoneum drains into the systemic rather than into the portal circulation. Earlier pharmacokinetic studies have indicated that, after intraperitoneal injection, drugs such as atropine, caffeine, glucose, glycine and progesterone are absorbed predominantly via the visceral peritoneum [219]. Therefore these drugs, when introduced intraperitoneally, are subject to immediate handling by the liver and some of them might undergo a first-pass metabolism.

After intraperitoneal administration of drugs, concentrations can be measured as a function of time in both dialysate and plasma. In view of the low peritoneal clearance of drugs after systemic administration, the rapid drug disappearance out of the peritoneum when the drug is given via the intraperitoneal route is at first sight surprising. It is, however, merely the consequence of pharmaco-kinetic factors, i.e. volume of distribution and protein binding. The contrast between the small dialysate volume and the very large distribution volume of the drug in the body, leads to a high concentration gradient. This is illustrated for vancomycin in Fig. 3 (adapted from Bailie et al. [220]).

Studies after intraperitoneal administration of glycopeptides have shown that bioavailability increases with dwell time. The data in Fig. 4 (from ref. 221) show that bioavailability is highly variable at early dwell times so that, to ensure consistent absorption of an intraperitoneally administered drug, short dwell times are not recommended. This may be relevant for APD patients who receive antibiotics intraperitoneally during the rapid exchanges. It is likely

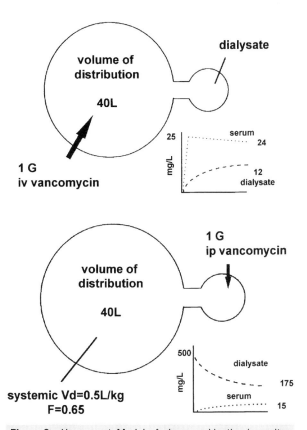

Figure 3. *Upper part:* Model of pharmacokinetics in peritoneal dialysis after intravenous administration of 1 g of vancomycin into a theoretical volume of distribution of 40 L (0.5 L/kg in an 80 kg patient). The inset shows the relationship of serum and dialysate concentrations over the duration of the 4-h dwell, which started at the same time as the intravenous administration. *Lower part:* Model of pharmacokinetics of vancomycin in peritoneal dialysis after intraperitoneal administration of 1 g of vancomycin into a 2 L exchange in a patient with a theoretical volume of 40 L. The inset shows the relationship of serum and dialysate concentrations over the 4-h duration of the vancomycin-containing exchange.

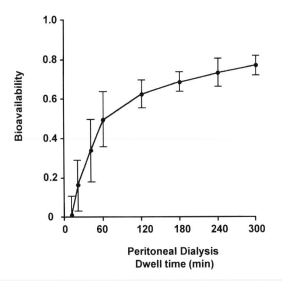

Figure 4. Relationship between systemic bioavailability and dwell time when teicoplanin is administered intraperitoneally. Bioavailability was calculated by comparison of AUC values following single intraperitoneal and intravenous doses, as well as from the amount of drug remaining within the peritoneal cavity with time. (From Brouard *et al.* [221], with permission.)

Table 2. Factors affecting transperitoneal drug absorption after intraperitoneal administration

Dialysate properties
  Flow rate
  Temperature
  Volume
  Chemical composition
  pH

Drug properties
  Molecular weight
  Ionic charge
  Volume of distribution
  Binding to membrane
  Lipid or water solubility

Characteristics of the peritoneal membrane
  Surface and charge
  Permeability
    Peritonitis
    Sclerosis
  Peritoneal blood flow
  Lymphatic absorbtion
  Stagnant layers

that these patients may not be receiving their full dosages due to decreased dwell time in the peritoneal cavity.

The high protein binding of some drugs in the plasma, versus a negligible protein binding in the dialysate, further promotes this apparent one-way diffusion from dialysate to blood.

Factors affecting transperitoneal drug absorption after intraperitoneal administration. These factors are summarized in Table 2; only a few of them will be discussed here; some of them have been described in the first part of this chapter. An important factor influencing drug transport after intraperitoneal administration is the *electric charge* of a drug. As outlined in the first part of this chapter, there exist anionic charges on the peritoneal basement membrane and capillaries subjacent to it [22, 222]. These charges, residing on the heparan or chondroitin sulphate components of cellular membranes, are greatly reduced under conditions of local or generalized inflammation (i.e. during peritonitis and sepsis) [223]. Intraperitoneal protamine, a highly cationic molecule, neutralizes these anionic fixed charges and enhances the peritoneal permeability to anionic plasma proteins [124]. The presence or absence of these peritoneal anionic charges can influence transperitoneal absorption of cationic drug molecules such as aminoglycosides. We and others have,

however, shown a much-enhanced transperitoneal absorption of gentamicin, netilmicin and tobramycin during peritonitis [211, 224, 225] (see below). These observations are difficult to explain if electric charges are important in their transport. Similarly, conflicting effects on the transport of gentamicin with intraperitoneal heparin, a negatively charged drug, have been reported. One earlier study reported lower blood gentamicin concentrations with intraperitoneal heparin [226], while a more recent study revealed that heparin caused an increase in transport of uncharged molecules such as urea and creatinine and of the positively charged gentamicin [227].

As was explained earlier, the importance of electric charges on transperitoneal transport is conflicting. Kuzuya *et al.* [228] used different xanthines, with comparable molecular weight (180–208 Da), but with different charges. They found that hydrophobicity plays an important role in peritoneal permeability.

It is possible that incorporation of proteoglycans such as heparin, hyaluronic acid or chondroitin sulphate in the peritoneal membrane alters peritoneal transport by mechanisms other than by electrical charge, as was shown by Hadler [229]. The effects of these molecules on peritoneal transport will be discussed separately in another section of this chapter.

As the electrical charge of a molecule in solution depends upon the pH of the fluid, theoretically at least, drug transport characteristics could change when bicarbonate-containing dialysate solutions are used. It is, however, accepted that the conventional (acidic) glucose-containing dialysate solutions rapidly correct their pH to physiological values after instillation. Studies in rats have shown that a significant proportion of the transport of macromolecules from the peritoneal cavity to the plasma is via convective transport via *peritoneal lymphatic absorption* [230, 231].

Recombinant human growth hormone (GH) (MW 21 000) was intraperitoneally instilled and showed an immediate absorption with peak serum GH levels obtained between 4 and 8 h following administration [232]. It is highly probable that this drug is, at least partly, transported via the lymphatics. The pharmacokinetics of erythropoietin and heparin will be described later.

As reviewed by a number of authors [140, 207, 233, 234] the systemic absorption of intraperitoneal antibiotics varies from 50% to 80% within a dwell period of 6 h in CAPD. The amount absorbed can easily be measured by subtracting, from the amount of drug initially instilled, the amount of drug that is present in the first peritoneal outflow. This, however, assumes that there is no *degradation of the drug* over the time interval in the dialysate. Most commonly used antibiotics are stable in peritoneal dialysate, either alone or in combination, or in the presence of additives such as insulin or heparin [235–239]. However, for some cephalosporins a degradation of 12–16%, and for rifampicin a degradation of 6%, was found in CAPD solutions or in effluent over 6 h [237]. This may lead to an overestimation of the amount of drug absorbed after intraperitoneal administration. Vancomycin is not stable at basic pH, and complex formation may occur after addition to bicarbonate-containing dialysate.

Studies by us and others have demonstrated a faster and more important absorption of antibiotics such as aminoglycosides, vancomycin, piperacillin and various β-lactam antibiotics in *peritonitis* patients. [211, 224, 225, 240–242].

Figue 5, taken from the paper by De Paepe and Lameire [224], illustrates the difference between peritonitis and non-peritonitis. It is also apparent, that after intraperitoneal administration of gentamicin, the decrease in dialysate concentration is much more pronounced than the increase in plasma concentrations. This is not surprising as the volume of distribution of the body is much larger than the volume of the peritoneal dialysis fluid. Equal concentrations of gentamicin in serum and dialysate were achieved at approximately 24 h. The clinical rele-

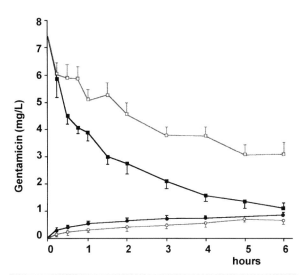

Figure 5. Concentrations (mean ± SEM) of gentamicin in serum (○) and dialysate (□) in five patients without peritonitis and in serum (●) and dialysate (■) in five patients with peritonitis. Gentamicin was added in a concentration of 7.5 mg/L to the dialysate at time 0.

vance of the higher systemic availability during peritonitis is questionable for drugs with a wide therapeutic toxic margin. However, if a drug with a narrow therapeutic index is only negligibly cleared after transport to the systemic circulation, systemic accumulation after repetitive intraperitoneal administration of the drug could occur. After chronic administration of gentamicin into the peritoneal dialysis fluid for 2–3 weeks, plasma concentrations approach end of dwell-time dialysate concentrations [224]. This can lead to potentially toxic concentrations and necessitates dose reduction.

After intraperitoneal administration of a single dose of 0.6 mg/kg of gentamicin, both total body clearance and the mean serum concentrations at 24 h were significantly lower in patients with, compared to patients without, *residual renal function* [243].

Adverse effects. Rapid transperitoneal drug absorption may cause adverse systemic effects. The 'red man syndrome' has been described after rapid intraperitoneal administration of 1 g of vancomycin diluted in 2 L of dialysate [244]. Drugs, when given intraperitoneally in therapeutic doses, may also cause peritoneal irritation. This has been described with a fixed combination of cilastatin/imipenem [207], amphotericin B [245–248], certain brands of vancomycin [249], methylene blue [250] and angiotensin I [251].

Effect of peritoneal dialysis on drug plasma protein binding

There are only a few studies in which the influence of peritoneal dialysis, notably CAPD, on drug binding has been assessed. Drug protein binding of acid drugs in peritoneal dialysis patients is expected to be lower than in undialysed or haemodialysis patients. This may be secondary to the often poor nutritional status of these patients, as reflected by serum albumin concentrations in the lower normal range, the continuous peritoneal losses of proteins during the dialysis process, and accumulating endogenous compounds competing for occupation of binding sites. Changes in protein binding and total and free concentrations of digitoxin have been reported for CAPD and haemodialysis patients. The binding of digitoxin was $94.7 \pm 1.5\%$ in CAPD, significantly less than that observed in haemodialysis patients $(96.2 \pm 1.3\%)$. Following a 0.1 mg oral dose of digitoxin, the mean free serum concentrations in CAPD and haemodialysis were 0.8 and 0.9 ng/ml respectively, which is not significantly different [252].

Relevant to this problem is the case of severe toxic myopathy and associated hyperkalaemia that we observed in a CAPD patient treated with a dose of clofibrate that was not adapted to the decrease in protein binding of that drug [253]. We can expect that in some malnourished peritoneal dialysis patients the binding to serum albumin of several acid drugs may be lowered, possibly leading to elevated free drug concentrations. Protein binding of the antifungal drug ketoconazole was also lower in CAPD patients (98.5%) than in control subjects (99%) [254].

The influence of CAPD on the concentrations of α_1-AGP in serum and dialysate and on the serum binding of two basic drugs (oxprenolol and propranolol) and of one acidic drug (phenytoin) has been reported [255]. Before starting CAPD treatment the protein binding of oxprenolol and propranolol was higher, related to the elevated serum levels of α_1-AGP concentrations in uraemia [256], while the binding of phenytoin was lower than in healthy volunteers. During the first week after starting CAPD, the serum α_1-AGP concentrations rose with a concomitant increase in the binding of oxprenolol and propranolol. Subsequently, however, the α_1-AGP levels and the binding of oxprenolol and propranolol decreased to the values found before starting CAPD. The binding of phenytoin, which was lower than in normal healthy volunteers, did not show any change during CAPD.

It must, however, be emphasized that, in general, changes in plasma protein binding of a drug only exceptionnally lead to relevant changes in plasma drug concentrations. Changes in free drug concentration are immediately associated with changes in the distribution volume of the drug which 'buffer' against major fluctuations in free drug plasma concentrations.

Peritoneal pharmacokinetics of common drugs and dose recommendations

Description of the tables

In the following tables the pharmacokinetics are described per class of drug studied during CAPD or continuous cycling peritoneal dialysis (CCPD). The tables also provide data on protein binding, elimination half-life, distribution volume and total plasma clearance for each drug in the presence of normal renal function, and on elimination half-life and total plasma clearance in end-stage chronic renal disease (ESRD). For this information we have used data published in standard textbooks [201, 202, 257, 258].

The pharmacokinetic data have been collected from reports published up to the beginning of 1999. Many papers contain results obtained in cross-over studies after either intravenous, oral or intraperitoneal administration. Therefore, the data published per individual paper have been included in the tables. The dose/route column indicates the dose and the route of drug administration in each respective study. When available, the loading dose or maintenance dose is given. Data on serum half-life $(t_{1/2})$, maximal – or, occasionally, steady state (SS) – serum concentrations achieved, total plasma clearance and peritoneal clearance are given. A comparison of these values with data obtained in normal renal function and in terminal renal failure shows the effect of peritoneal dialysis on these parameters. Finally, the percentage of dose either removed from the body by PD (in case of systemic administration) or absorbed across the peritoneal membrane (after intraperitoneal administration) is provided, whenever it has been calculated.

Each table is accompanied by a brief discussion of the need for dose adjustment in peritoneal dialysis, for drugs that are frequently used in these patients. Table 3 provides a glossary of the abbreviations used in the tables.

Table 3. Abbreviations used in Tables 4–10. All data are given as mean ± standard error or standard error of mean

Cl	Clearance
ESRD	End-stage renal disease
IP	Intraperitoneal administration
IV	Intravenous administration
LD	Loading dose
MD	Maintenance dose
MTC	Mass transfer coefficient
O	Oral administration
PB	Protein binding
perit+	In presence of peritonitis
SD	Single dose

Pharmacokinetic data in CAPD

Tables 4 to 10 summarize the pharmacokinetic data on systemic and intraperitoneal drug administration in CAPD.

Cardiovascular drugs (Table 4)

Based on the pharmacokinetic data, dose adaptation for *digoxin* is not necessary in CAPD patients beyond that for end-stage renal disease.

Data on pharmacokinetics of *ACE inhibitors* are scarce. In a study of five patients on CAPD, captopril was detectable in the dialysate after a single dose of 50 mg. However, the impact on total elimination varied widely between individuals [288]. After 24 h, only 0.5% of a dose of 2.5 mg quinaprilat was removed by peritoneal dialysis. The elimination half-life of quinaprilat is prolonged in patients with renal failure, and an inhibition of >90% of ACE was observed after administration of 2.5 mg of quinaprilat in CAPD patients. This dose can thus be recommended as starting dose in CAPD patients [199, 275].

Fosinoprilat was found to be cleared only to a limited extent by peritoneal dialysis. Fosinoprilat, however, is also cleared by biliary secretion, that might compensate for the reduced renal clearance. In six CAPD patients serum ACE activity remained significantly suppressed at 24 and 48 h after administration of 10 mg fosinoprilat [276]. The moderate pharmacokinetic alterations observed in these patients compared to those with normal renal function suggest that in most CAPD patients initial dose modifications are not necessary.

β-lactam antibiotics and glycopeptides (Table 5)

In general the amount of *penicillin* lost in the peritoneal cavity after systemic administration is negligi-

ble; on the other hand the transperitoneal absorption can be as high as 90% in the presence of peritonitis.

First-, second- and third-generation cephalosporins have been extensively studied. Based on the adequate dialysate levels that are achieved after oral administration (cephadrine or cephalexin), some authors have used this group of antibiotics as first choice for initial treatment of peritonitis either as single drug or in combination with other drugs [359–365]). Inspection of the concentration versus time curve, after intraperitoneal administration of 1 g *ceftazidime*, demonstrates that serum concentrations reach therapeutic levels within 30 min and are maintained for more than 24 h. A distribution volume of 16 L was found. Overall, use of 1–1.5 g once daily or 15 mg/kg body weight has been recommended [326, 327].

Cefotaxime is metabolized in the liver to an active metabolite, which is primarily excreted by glomerular filtration and tubular secretion. However, dose reduction is necessary only when the creatinine clearance falls below 5 ml/min. Several studies explored the pharmacokinetics of cefotaxime in CAPD [366]: a high proportion of the intraperitoneally administered cefotaxime is absorbed into the circulation and therapeutic serum levels can be obtained after intraperitoneal administration; no further dose adaptation is needed for patients on CAPD.

The clearance of *cefepime*, a third-generation cephalosporin, is 15 ml/min in CAPD patients, with a peritoneal dialysis-related clearance of 4 ml/min [303]. For intravenous administration 1–2 g every 48 h is recommended [302]. It has a low protein binding value, and a relatively low volume of distribution; therefore, a once-daily intraperitoneal administration is probably not recommended, and the intravenous route should be preferred.

Cefpirome can be administered both intraperitoneally and intravenously. Dialysis clearance by peritoneal dialysis is negligible.

Moxolactam is a semisynthetic β-lactam antibiotic with activity against a broad range of Gram-positive and Gram-negative aerobic and anaerobic bacteria. This antibiotic exists as two stereoisomers with different antimicrobial activities. Several pharmacokinetic studies in CAPD patients have shown that, after intravenous administration, dosage adjustment to account for loss of moxalactam via the peritoneal cavity is not necessary. It appears further that there are no significant differences between R-Mox and S-Mox kinetics in CAPD patients [367].

For *piperacilline*, whether or not in combination with tazobactam, dose adaptations should be made

Table 4. Pharmacokinetic studies with cardiovascular drugs in CAPD

	Normal renal function				ESRD			PD					
	PB (%)	$t_{1/2}$ (h)	V_{dis} (L/kg)	Cl_{tot} (ml/min)	$t_{1/2}$ (h)	Cl_{tot} (ml/min)	Dosage/route	$t_{1/2}$ (h)	C_{max} (mg/ml)	Cl_{tot} (ml/min)	Cl_{per} (ml/min)	Percentage dose removed or absorbed	Refs
Digoxin	20–30	36	7.1 ESRD 4.2!	160	100	35	0 0.125 mg daily 5 days SS (n=1)	97.9 at 2 h	3.2 ng/ml	12.6	2.0	<4/24 h	259
							0 0.50 mg	–	3.8 ± 2.3 ng/ml at 0.56 h	–	3.0 ± 1	1/24 h	260
							0 0.1 mg/day SS	–	–	–	3.9 ± 1.3	<2/24 h	261
							0 0.125 mg every 2–3 days	54–141	–	11–52	2.3–3.1	<10/4 days	262
							0 0.125 mg per day	–	–	–	3.6 ± 0.4	7.6 ± 0.9/24 h	263
Digitoxin	90 86–89 ESRD	145	0.5	3	200	2	0 0.1 mg/day SS	7.5 days	–	3.5	0.7 ± 0.3	<2/24 h	261
Quinidine	80–85	6	2	270	6	270	0 350 mg 4 ×/day	5.4	–	154.2	0.79	0.6/24 h	264
Denopamine							0 10 mg SD	4.6 ± 2.5	0.0123 ± 0.0067	–	0.10 ± 0.05	<0.1/6 h	265
Labetalol	50	7	5.6	1700	13	1198	IV 0.7–1 mg/kg	13.05 ± 6.32	–	1397.2 ± 272.3	1.94 ± 0.65	0.14/72 h	266
Propranolol	93	3.5	3	695	3.5	695	0 320 mg/day	–	–	–	–	3.3/24 h	267
							0 20 mg/day	–	–	–	–	5.2/24 h	
Atenolol	<5	5.5	0.7	176	73	13	IV 20 mg	27.6 ± 2.18	–	21 ± 1.4	2.53 ± 0.3	6/24 h	268
Esmolol	–	0.2	3.2	19950	–	–	IV 150 mg/kg/min for 4 h	0.1 ± 0.06	0.8 (0.5) Css (80 kg)	20504 ± 11448	0	0	269
Betaxolol	55	14–22	6	327	30	200	–	27	–	–	–	–	270
Nifedipine	90–95	2	1.4	1100	2.6	1100	0 2 × 20 mg/day	4.2 ± 1.1	448 ± 118	–	4.3 ± 2.7	<1/24 h	271
Isosorbide-5-nitrate	16–28	0.2–0.5	1.8	–	0.2–0.5	–	0 3 × 20 mg/day	–	–	–	–	1–6/24 h	272
Diltiazem	80–85	4.0	5.3	1400	3.4	1400	0 60 mg	3.09 ± 1.15	95.8 ± 63.8 (3 h)	2653 1316 (70 kg)	1.5 ± 1.0	<0.1/24 h	273

Drug							Dose						Ref
Captopril	25–30	1.9	3	1277	35	69	0 50 mg SD		0.387 ± 0.0075			<1%/6 h	274
Free captopril								1 ± 0.3	2.77 ± 0.43				
Total								1.0 ± 0.3	0.107 ± 0.067				
Quinapril*	—	1*	—	—	0.9*	—	0 20 mg SD			2207 ± 1621	—	0 / 2.6 ± 1.2/24 h	199
Quinaprilat	97*	—		—	12.5*	—	0 2.5 mg	20.1 ± 10.1	0.689 ± 0.124	19 ± 8.3	—	—	275
Quinaprilat	90							34.1	64.3	11.9		—	
Fosinoprilate	95	15	0.15	—	19–28	—	0 10 mg	19.5 ± 7.5	0.202 ± 0.071	70.6 ± 38.5	0.09 ± 0.07; 1.5; <5 ml/min	2 ± 1.4/48 h	276
Guanfacine	30	17	4	—	14	—		—	—	—	2.2	—	277
Tocainide	10–15	11–14	3.2	182	17–43	100	0 400 mg SD	15 ± 5	3.2 ± 1	83 ± 36		2.2 ± 2/24 h	278
Flecainide	40	14–26	8.7	567	19–26	357	0 100 mg/day	40	—	30		1/24 h	279
Procainamide	14 / 15	3 / 2	2	810	14 / 8	200	0 625 mg SD	34.1 / 26	64.3 / 1.9–4.8	11.9 / 143	0.28–5.55	— / <5/days	280 / 281
N-acetylprocainamide	10	6	1.5	200	4.2	29	0 500 mg	42.8	—	29.8	1.74–7.20	<5	
Furosemide	95	0.5	0.12	162	1.4	105	SD – perit	10.5 ± 1.2	12.8 ± 2.1		0.5 ± 0.1	0.9 ± 0.2/24 h	282
							+ perit	11.6 ± 3.3	6.6 ± 0.4		0.5 ± 0.1	0.6 ± 0.1/24 h	
							SD – perit, 0 80 mg	12.5 ± 3.4	7.7 ± 06		0.4 ± 0.1	0.6 ± 0.1/24 h	283
							SD – perit, IV 80 mg	3.87 ± 1.26	3.2 ± 1.4		—	—	284
							SD – perit	2.7 ± 0.83	—		—		
Theophylline	60	8.7	0.45	46	7.3	67		4.7	—	60 ± 18	1.5	<1/24 h	285
Mexiletine	64	5–9	5–6	846	22	200	IV 250 mg	10.5	—	25.6/kg	9.22/kg	<1%	286

* Data from ref. 287.

Table 5. Pharmacokinetic studies with β-lactams and glycopeptide antibiotics in CAPD

	Normal renal function				ESRD		Dosage/route	PD					Refs
	PB (%)	$t_{1/2}$ (h)	V_{dis} (L/kg)	Cl_{tot} (ml/min)	$t_{1/2}$ (h)	Cl_{tot} (ml/min)		$t_{1/2}$ (h)	C_{max} (mg/ml)	Cl_{tot} (ml/min)	Cl_{per} (ml/min)	Percentage dose removed or absorbed	
I. Beta-lactams													
Ampicillin	16–20	1.2	0.48	325	14	30	IV 2 g IP 1 g/L	9.5 ± 2.2 9.6 ± 2.6	170.3 ± 56.6 48 ± 7.6	25 ± 7.7 25 ± 7.7	2.7 ± 0.5	11.3 ± 2.2/48 h 60 ± 13/48 h	289
Sulbactam	–	0.25	0.2	250	21	–	IV 1 g IV 1 g	9.7 ± 2.2 9.4 ± 3.2	87.5 ± 29.9/5–6 h 27.8 ± 4.1/5–6 h	22.6 ± 3.2 22.6 ± 3.2	3.4 ± 0.4	152 ± 1.9/48 h 68 ± 13/48 h	290
Imipenem	13–21	1	–	205	1	205	IV 500 mg SD IP 500 mg/L	3.28 ± 0.59	29.3 ± 10.5	66.8 ± 18.1	–	3.2 ± 0.5 79 ± 8	
Cilastatin Imipenem	13–21	1	0.31	238	3.7–4.8	54	IV 500 mg SD IV 500 mg SD IV 1000 mg SD IV 500 mg IV 1000 mg	8.84 ± 3.8 6.2 ± 1.4 6.9 ± 1.1 22.6 ± 6.4 15.4 ± 5.0	34.8 ± 6.5 29.5 ± 12.2 69.5 ± 9.5 51.9 ± 13.4 110.8 ± 20.3	24 ± 14.9 76.3 ± 23.5 50.6 ± 15.6 8.1 ± 1.8 10.7 ± 1.4	4.8 ± 0.6 5.4 ± 0 5.4 ± 0.6 5.4 ± 1.2	5.2 ± 0.5 – –	291
Piperacillin	21	1	0.21	188	3.3	57	IV 2 g SD IP 500 mg/L – petit + perit IV 1 g SD IP 1 g/L + perit	2.43 ± 0.84 2.41 ± 0.49	104.4 ± 26.1 6.8 ± 2.9/2.6 h 8.9 ± 2	104 ± 37.7 – 100.2 ± 13.8 –	3.17 ± 0.67 – 2.7 ± 0.8 –	2.5 ± 0.7/6 h 67.8 ± 8.5/6 h 83.4 ± 4.6/6 h – 96.3/6 h	242
Tazobactam Temocillin	– 63–88	0.89 ± 4.5 5–6	15.91 ± 1.9 0.29	219 ± 25 44	3.58 ± 46.5 16–28	49.5 ± 8 9	IV 3 g SD IV 0.375 g IV 15 mg/kg SD	2.12 ± 26.3 6.36 ± 876.1 13.4 ± 3.9	270 ± 31 28.6 ± 5.7 –	65 ± 12.9 36.9 ± 11.8 9.3 ± 1.8	3.6 3.8 –	5.5/28 h 10.7/28 h 8 ± 2.6/24 h	293 294 295
Cefamandole	67–80	0.7	0.16	109	15	9	IP 500 mg/L SD IV 1 g SD IP 500 mg IV 1 g	10.4 ± 7.3 9.02 ± 1.0/1 h 8.1 ± 1.2 6.1 ± 1.7	31.3 ± 4.7/6 h 65 ± 10 33 ± 3/6 h	20 ± 6.2 24.4 ± 6.4 25.4 ± 6.6 21.9 ± 9.7	3.2 ± 1.6 1.48 ± 0.41 2.5 ± 0.7 0.92 ± 0.25	71.7 ± 12.8/6 h 5 ± 2/24 h 71 ± 10/6 h 5 ± 2.4/54 h	296 297 298 299
Cefazolin	70–85	1.8	0.14	60	27	5	IV 10 mg/kg SD IP 10 mg/kg IP 500 mg/L LD 250 mg/L MD perit + 125 mg/L perit +	33.1 ± 1.0 29.2 ± 16.2	– 30 54.8 ± 6.7 110.9 ± 6.7 141.3 ± 51.9	5.7 ± 0.6 5.85 ± 0.7 7.8 2.8 ± 1.5	1.0 ± 0.4 0.81 ± 0.14 –	73.7/4 h 88/6 h 65/24 h –	300 301
Cefepime							IV 1 g SD IV 2 g SD	17.6 ± 2.9 18.8 ± 1.6	62.9 ± 15.8 124 ± 14	15.4 ± 4.9 14 ± 1.3	3.86 ± 0.59 4.35 ± 0.69	25/72 h	302
Cefepime Cefodizime	88	1.3–2.3	20.5 ± 4.8	89–178	13.5 ± 2.6	18.7 ± 5.18	IV 1 g SD IV 1 g SD IP 500 mg/L SD	17.6 ± 2.9 4.1–6.8 4–9.8	62.9 ± 15.8	15.4 ± 4.9 1.6–31.7 19.7–39.2	– 0.3–0.9 –	– 1.2–6.4/24 h 41–100/24 h	303 304
Cefoperazone	65–90	1.8	0.22	100	2.9	78	IV 1 g IP 1 g/L IV 1 g day 1–3 IP 2 × 1 g/2 L 2 days	2.65 ± 0.39	104.2 ± 29.1 33.2 ± 5.3/6 h	80 ± 20 70.1 ± 19.2	6.9 ± 1.0	95 ± 12/10 h 63.8 ± 4.8 –	305 306
Cefoperazone Sulbactam Cefoperazone							IV 2 g ± 0.82 IV 1 g/L	2.08 ± 21.2 2.33 ± 0.96	280.9 ± 33.4 38.9 ± 12.4/2–4 h	71.9 71.9 ± 33.4	0.55 ± 0.08	1.0/48 h 64 ± 14/6 h	307

Drug	Study data	Sample	Dosage						Ref
Sulbactam Cefoperazone	36		IV 1 g	6.86 ± 1.67	82.2 ± 16.2	33.4 ± 5.3	3.6 ± 0.2	11.1 ± 1.4/48 h	308
	1		IP 0.5 g/L	6.26 ± 1.45	82.2 ± 2.0	33.4 ± 5.3	–	70 ± 10/6 h	309 310
		135	IP 62.5 mg/L for 10 days + perit	–	10 at 24 h	–	–	–	
Cefotaxime	322		IV 30 mg/kg	1.8 ± 1.2	–	65 ± 25	3.2	–	311
			IV 2 g	2.6 ± 0.3	–	88 ± 39	2.4 ± 0.8	–	312
	0.28		IP 1 g/L	3.1 ± 1.3	10–12/2–3 h	87.2 ± 34.3	1.93 ± 1.0	2.18/6 h 90/9 h	
	2.5		1 g	–	–	–	–		
Cefotaxime (CFT)		CFT	IP 0.5 g/L	2.31 ± 0.20	15 ± 1.5/2 h	118.7 ± 12.3	6.7 ± 1.3	4.9 ± 0.7/24 h	312
		DAC*		11.4 ± 1.9	9.7 ± 1.4/6 h	–	3.6 ± 0.9	2.6 ± 0.6/24 h	
		CFT	IV 1 g	2.3 ± 0.3	322.9 ± 105.2	–	–	58.7 ± 6.4/4 h	313
		DAC		13.2 ± 4.3	37.8 ± 19.4	81 ± 31	1.82 ± 0.43	–	
		CFT	IV 2 g	2.24 ± 1.04	29.7 ± 9.2/4–8 h	–	2.84 ± 0.7	–	314
		DAC		18.9 ± 21.7	19.5 ± 12.6/7.1 h	71.2 ± 29.3	11.5 ± 6.9	74.6 ± 21.3/6 h	
		CFT	IP 1 g/L	2.57 ± 1.03	156/5 min	–	3.46 ± 1.03	3.5/6 h	314
		DAC		25.3 ± 33.8	17.4/2 h	–	–	65/6 h	315
		CFT	IV 1 g	1.59 ± 0.47	9.1/2 h	–	–	90/24 h 67/24 h	316
		CFT	IP 0.5 g/L	–	–	250.8 ± 59.5	–	1.4–4.2/6 h	
		CFT	IP 250 mg/L + perit	–	–	94.8 ± 23.4	–		
		CFT	− perit	–	–	11–103	–		
		CFT DAC	IV 1 g	2.3 ± 8.2	10–60	–	–		
*Desacetyl Cefotaxime Cefotaxime		CFT	IP 500 mg/L (2 children)	1.83–2.49	11.9–13.1/4.08 and 2.22 h	79–62	1.14–2.81	56.6 and 64.8/5 h	317
		DAC		11–8.1	5.16–9.29 /5.73–5.33	–	1.88–4.15		
		CFT	IP 500 mg/L + perit (children)						
Cefotetan Cefotiam	78–91 3.7 0.15 39 35	4	IV 1 g	15.5 ± 1.9	26.9 ± 7.8	6.5–20	1.1–3.2	5–9/24 h	318
			IV 1 g	8.1 ± 2.4	–	20.9 ± 3.8	3.3 ± 0.2	6 ± 1.1/5 h	319 320 241
			IV 1 g	5.1	103	–		–	
Cefoxitin	50–60 0.9 0.3 290 22	12	IV 2 g	7.8 ± 1.1	197	20.4 ± 1.45	1.44 ± 0.25	71.2/24 h	321
			IP 4 × 50 mg/L/24 h	20.2 ± 3.7	15	13 ± 3.3	4.1 ± 2.3		322
			4 × 100 mg/L/24 h		7				
Cefpirome Cefsulodin			IV 1 g SD	15.4 ± 1.9	–	15.4 ± 2.4	1.62 ± 1.5	12.4–96 h	323
			IV 1 g	11.6 ± 4.7	–	14.7 ± 5.4	4.3 ± 1.7	8.7 ± 13/5 h	320
			IP 1 g − perit	11.2 ± 1.9	–	26.5 ± 9	–	81 ± 3.6/5 h	
			+ perit	9.4 ± 1.3	–	23.9 ± 11.1	–	84 ± 6/5 h	
Ceftazidime	10–17 2 0.24 130 25	7	IP 4 × 125 mg/L − perit	–	9.27–22.24 (6–24 h)	–	1.47–4.13	–	324
			+ perit	–	13.1–25.3 (6–24 h)	–	2.43–3.89	65–75/24 h	
Ceftazidime			IV 1 g	–	–	8.7	3–4	4.3–7/4–6 h	325
			IV 1 g	1.9		–	–	–	326
			IP 15 mg/kg single dwell	22 ± 5		14.1 ± 4.25	5.74 ± 1.6		327
Ceftazidime Ceftazidime	10–17 2 0.24 130 25	7	IV 1 g	1.9		8.7	–	–	326
			IP 15 mg/kg single dwell	22 ± 5		14.1 ± 4.25	5.74 ± 1.6	–	327

* Desacetyl Cefotaxime

Table 5. (Continued.)

	Normal renal function				ESRD		PD						
	PB (%)	$t_{1/2}$ (h)	V_{dis} (L/kg)	Cl_{tot} (ml/min)	$t_{1/2}$ (h)	Cl_{tot} (ml/min)	Dosage/route	$t_{1/2}$ (h)	C_{max} (mg/ml)	Cl_{tot} (ml/min)	Cl_{per} (ml/min)	Percentage dose removed or absorbed	Refs
Ceftizoxime	31	1.4	0.4	190	35	6	IV 500 mg	10.2 ± 5.8	—	27.7	2.9	4.8 ± 2.1/6 h	328
							IV 1 g	12 ± 4.8	—	22.8	3.4	4.4/6 h	
							IP 250 mg/L		12.5/5 h			78 ± 4	
Ceftriaxone	85–95	6–9	0.09	15	12–57	8	IV 3 g	9.7 ± 5.1	411 ± 137/0.25 h	—	—	—	329
							IV 1 g	12.3 ± 4.4	412 ± 354	17.1 ± 7.4	2.8 ± 0.7	4.5 ± 2.9/72 h	330
							IP 1 g	13.7 ± 10.1/42 h	38.8 ± 11.6	14 ± 5.6	0.6 ± 0.4	44 ± 13/4 h	
Cefdinir							O 100 mg	10.8–21.9	1.64–4.43	—	—	—	331
Quinupristin-Dalfopristin	23–32	0.93 ± 0.15	1.07 ± 0.27	780 ± 120	—	—	IV 7.5 mg/kg	0.83 ± 0.13	2.89 ± 0.85	710 ± 200	—	—	332
Dalfopristin	50–56	0.71 ± 0.18	0.77 ± 0.34	770 ± 180	—	—		0.76 ± 0.29	8.52 ± 3.25	670 ± 360	—	—	
Ceftriaxone							IV 2 × 2 g at 24 h interval −perit	9.8 ± 1.9	285 ± 69	13.3 ± 5	0.67 ± 0.5	—	333
							+perit	14.8 ± 12.7	272 ± 54	15 ± 10	2.05 ± 1	—	
							IP 500 mg/L	10.5 ± 2.3	58.9	14.8	—	70.6 ± 7.9/4–6 h	334
							IP 1 g/L	12.7 ± 2.9	71.1	10.1 ± 3.0 ml/kg/h	0.69 ± 0.2 ml/kg/h	71.4/5 h	335
							IP 1 g/L						
							IV 1 g	12.2	—	7.4 (4–12.9)	—	—	336
Cefuroxime	33	1.3	0.2	140	20	15	IV 15 mg/kg	14.7 ± 1.1	24.2 ± 6.4	21.5 ± 1.2	3.59 ± 0.8	—	337
							IV 500 mg −perit	15.1 ± 1.9	—	—	4.2–2.9 ± 1.2–1.3	—	338
							IP 250 mg/L −perit	14.4 ± 2.1	12.1 ± 2.2	20.3 ± 1.4	2.3–6.5	70	
							IP 1 × 250 mg/L LD +125 mg/L MD		43.2 ± 7.5 SS	—	9.9–12.4		
Cephalexin	18.5 37	0.8	0.26	263	20	10	O 500 mg SD	8.6 ± 0.9	97.8 ± 24.2/4 h	18.4 ± 2.71	2.29 ± 0.63	16.5/day 1	299
							O 1–2 g/days for 3 days				55 ± 19.4 in dialysate day 1	−25.5/day 2	339
Cephalothin	60–65	0.6	0.26	350	10	21	IP 100 mg/L 4 exch/24 h	—	5.6 ± 2.2/24 h	—	—	—	340
							IV 1 g + IP 250 mg/L	17.1 ± 6.0 ±6.0	100.3 ± 39.2	11.1 ± 12.7	—	—	301
							IV 1 g		111.0	—	—	—	241
							IP 0.5 g/L	3.0	18.4/2 h	—	—	—	
Cephradine	7.5 19	1.0	0.31	323	12	20	O 500 mg SD	16.7 ± 2.9	—	—	2.8–3.5	6.9/48 h	341
Moxolactam	50	2.5	0.3	97	20	12	IV 1 g		123 ± 9	10.6 ± 2.0	2.7 ± 0.5	17.4 ± 3.1/24 h ±60/4 h	342
							IP 0.5 g/L	13.2 ± 2.9	38.6 ± 12.7/4 h	11.5 ± 2.4	2.3 ± 0.5		343
							IV 1–2 g SD						
							R MOX	17.3 ± 3.4		12.9 ± 6.9 (ml/kg/h)	1.1 ± 0.6		344
							S MOX	18 ± 3.3		13 ± 5.5 (ml/h/kg)	1.27 ± 0.62		

Drug							Dose/Route					$t_{1/2}$	Ref
Moxolactam	10	7	0.47	55	240	2	IP 0.5–1g/L SD	–	–	–	–	71 ± 18	330
							R MOX	–	–	–	–	79 ± 18	
							S MOX	17.9 ± 4.2	171 ± 62/0.08 h	12.8 ± 7.7	2.1 ± 0.5	20.2 ± 8.3/48 h	
							IV 1 g SD	15.4 ± 4.1	34.1 ± 8.5/4.3 h	–	–	57 ± 16/4 h	63
							IP 0.5 g/L SD						
II. Glycopeptides													
Vancomycin							IP 500 mg/L	81	23.7 ± 6.5	9.4 ± 1.9	2.4 ± 0.08	53/6 h	345
							IV 10 mg/kg				1.48 ± 3.6	–	346
							IP 10 mg/kg 2 L	65.8 ± 10.7	6.3	15.1 ± 2.0	2.50 ± 0.33	65/4 h	347
							IV 10 mg/kg	90.2 ± 24.2		6.45 ± 1.1	1.35 ± 0.35		
							IP 500 mg/L LD	–	9.1/5 h			71.3/6 h	348
							IP 500 mg/L + perit	62.3	35.3 ± 19.1/6 h			–	349
							300 mg/kg per 2 L IP —perit	–	–			50.8/6 h	240
							300 mg/kg per 2 L IP —perit	–	–			73.9/6 h	
							IV 25 mg/kg + perit	115 ± 6	56.8 ± 4.7	7.2 ± 0.3	1.4 ± 1.05	–	350
							IV 15 mg/kg	111 ± 22	S57.1 ± 9.3	5.0 ± 1.4	1.2 ± 0.5	46/6 h	351
							IP 30 mg/kg	91.7 ± 28	S30.4 ± 7.2	5.0 ± 1.3	1.7 ± 0.9	–	352
							IP 1 g/2 L LD		15.5 ± 12.3/4 h	8.52	–	–	353
							IP 15 mg/kg LD		16.2 ± 1.75			70 ± 15/3 h	
							IP 37.5 mg/L CAPD + perit	–	13.3 ± 4.5				
Vancomycin	95	41–62	0.84–1.13	36.438	124	<2	IP 37.5 mg/L CAPD – perit	–	8.8 ± 2.5	–	–	39 ± 13/3 h	220
							IP 15 mg/kg/2 L LD +MD 25 mg/L		17.8 ± 2.2/1–6 h			63 ± 10.1/4 h	
							IP 25 mg/L no LD		0.27 ± 0.42/6 h			71.9 ± 17.5/4 h	
							IV 1 g perit +	103.9 ± 57.2	–	4.09 ± 0.45	3.84* ± 0.75 *max perit	–	213
Teicoplanin							IV 3 mg/kg	162 ± 52	–	5.15 ± 1.34 ml/h/kg	0.34 ± 0.02 ml/h/kg	6.8 ± 1.2/6 days	354
							IV 6 mg/kg	242 (202–273)	–	5.7 ± 2.00.2	−0.4	–	355
							IV 3 mg/kg	135	4.84 ± 1.43/6 h	–	–	7.1 ± 1.2/6 h	356
							IP 6 mg/kg		8.0 ± 0.6			81.5 ± 10.7	357
							IV 3 mg/kg	377 ± 109	31.6 ± 5.2	2.76 ± 1.08	0.25 ± 0.21	3/5 h 9/2 weeks	221
							IV 6 mg/kg	266.4 ± 51.9	56.5 ± 7.0	0.04/kg	0.007/kg	6.1 ± 0.7/46 h	357
							IP 3 mg/kg	338 ± 60	6.6 ± 1.8/4 h		0.13 ± 0.07	77 ± 21	221
Teicoplanin	95	41–62	0.84–1.13	5–10	124	<2	IP 20 mg/L	508	9	2.5	–	–	358

according to residual creatinine clearance. During CAPD, 5.5% of piperacilline and 10.7% of the tazobactam are removed by the dialysate over 28 h [294].

The two major drugs in the class of *glycopeptide antibiotics* are *vancomycin* and *teicoplanin*.

Staphylococcus aureus and *Staphylococcus epidermidis* are almost always susceptible to vancomycin. Concentrations of 5 µg/ml or less are inhibitory although some strains require 10–20 µg/ml. Vancomycin is a large molecule (around 1500 Da) and has a low serum binding. In end-stage renal disease its half-life is very prolonged [200–250 h]. Pharmacokinetic studies after intravenous administration in CAPD patients show a low peritoneal clearance, which, however, increases during peritonitis. Although it has been claimed that CAPD does not require dose adjustment, serum drug levels should be followed in patients with substantial residual renal function [368]. As the volume of distribution of vancomycin (0.5 L/kg) is large in comparison with the intraperitoneal volume, there remains a high concentration gradient between dialysate and plasma after intraperitoneal administration (figure 12 from ref. 368). Therefore, vancomycin is rapidly absorbed into the circulation. When the dialysate is drained, and new dialysate is instilled, it rapidly becomes saturated with vancomycin from the blood, and adequate intraperitoneal levels of vancomycin are obtained. Because of this phenomenon, a single high dose (15 mg/kg) of vancomycin is sufficient to obtain adequate dialysate levels. Whether, from a microbiological point of view, vancomycin is still the antibiotic of first choice in the treatment of peritoneal dialysis-related peritonitis, is a matter of debate. The growing concern on the emergence of vancomycin-resistant enterococci in the United States has forced the Ad Hoc Advisory Committee to classify vancomycin from agent of choice to agent to be avoided (see Chapter 17, on peritonitis). Other centres, however, having a high incidence of methicillin-resistant staphylococci (MRSA), have recommended a centre-tailored therapeutic approach of peritonitis where vancomycin is still regarded as the first choice [369].

As mentioned above, chemical peritonitis after intraperitoneal administration has been observed; it rarely occurs with vancomycin commercialized by the Lilly company.

Teicoplanin is a glycopeptide that is mainly excreted via the renal route and has a prolonged terminal half-life in renal failure. In peritoneal dialysis patients with peritonitis the serum half-life was 508 ± 193 h, and the volume of distribution was 0.48 L/kg [358]. The pharmacokinetic data of teicoplanin in normal and severely impaired renal function in Table 6 are derived from a review by Rowland [370].

Fluoroquinolones, aminoglycosides, trimethoprim-sulphamethoxazole and miscellaneous antibiotics (Table 6)

Pharmacokinetic data of some of these antibiotics have been recently reviewed [211]. *Fluoroquinolones* have a large antibacterial spectrum, including Gram-negative bacteria and staphylococci. Most fluoroquinolones are well absorbed after oral administration and have a favourable pharmacokinetic profile. Janknegt [406] has summarized the pharmacokinetic and clinical studies with ciprofloxacin, ofloxacin, pefloxacin and fleroxacin in CAPD patients.

In a CAPD patient, therapy with quinolones requires dose adjustment as for patients with end-stage renal failure. However, high drug intraperitoneal concentrations can be achieved after intravenous or oral administration, making these substances, at least theoretically, attractive alternatives to conventional treatment of CAPD peritonitis (for review and dose recommendations see refs 406 and 407).

The pharmacokinetics after intraperitoneal administration in CAPD have been studied for ofloxacin, pefloxacin and ciprofloxacin; the latter has also been studied in CCPD [408]. During CAPD the half-lives of ciprofloxacin, pefloxacin and ofloxacin are 10 h, 17–21 h and 25 h, respectively. Adequate peritoneal ofloxacin levels were reported in the second and third exchanges after a single intraperitoneal dose of 200 mg in the first exchange [381]. For fleroxacine a mean dialysate to plasma concentration ratio of 0.5–0.6 can be expected after a short dwell of 4 h [375]. Therapeutic concentrations in the peritoneal fluid can be achieved in CAPD patients using an oral loading dose of 800 mg fleroxacin and a daily maintenance dose of 400 mg. Fractions of dose of quinolones removed by CAPD range between 1% and 2% at 24 h after dosing [373, 375, 376], probably due to the large volume of distribution of these agents. As the intraperitoneal levels of quinolones are reportedly low during the first 24 h of oral therapy, an intraperitoneal loading dose is recommended [407]. It is of note that the concomitant administration of antacids significantly reduces the gastrointestinal absorption of the quinolones.

After systemic administration of *aminoglycosides* a substantial fraction of the administered dose is removed over 24–48 h. The peritoneal clearance adds approximately 20–30% to the total removal from the body and clinically relevant concentrations in the dialysate are achieved after intravenous administration. This significant peritoneal clearance is due to the low protein binding and the small volume of distribution of these drugs. It is recommended that plasma levels should be measured regularly, especially in repeated usage [243].

For all aminoglycosides tested, an important absorption has been observed after intraperitoneal administration; there is a significantly higher systemic bioavailability in peritonitis compared to non-peritonitis patients. Continuous intraperitoneal administration of aminoglycosides in patients with peritonitis leads to more or less constant plasma levels and carries the risk for otovestibular toxicity and further decrease in residual renal function [409]. In order to decrease this potential ototoxicity and nephrotoxicity, once-daily administration seems to be preferable. Once-daily dosing with aminoglycosides is possible due to their important post-anti-biotic effect. After intraperitoneal administration of 0.6 mg/kg gentamicin, serum elimination half-life was 35.8 h, and distribution volume was 0.23 ± 0.08 L/kg [243]. A higher dose, 1 mg/kg, was recommended to obtain sufficient plasma and dialysate levels during 24 h. Studies on stability of aminoglycoside antibiotics in peritoneal dialysate have also been performed [410]. Netilmicin, sisomicin and gentamicin were moderately stable (51–76% activity at 24 h), amikacin was less stable (38–50% activity at 24 h) and tobramycin was the least stable (15–30% activity at 24 h).

Aztreonam, a monobactam antibiotic, is effective against Gram-negative bacteria, with, compared to aminoglycosides, greater safety and a more predictable action in dialysate. The pharmacokinetics of aztreonam have been studied after both intravenous and intraperitoneal administration in CAPD patients. Based on these data several authors have recently described favourable results in Gram-negative peritonitis, including some *Pseudomonas* infections, with the intraperitoneal administration of aztreonam alone [402, 411], or in combination with cefuroxime [412] or vancomycin [411, 413].

The pharmacokinetics of *roxithromycin* were determined following a single oral dose to patients on peritoneal dialysis. Serum elimination half-life was doubled compared to healthy individuals. Less than 5% of the dose was recovered in dialysate over 48 h, and dialysate concentrations were low. Administration every 48 h is recommended [399].

Pharmacokinetic data on other *macrolides* are not available in peritoneal dialysis patients. It is of note that macrolides can inhibit metabolization, and thus affect the plasma levels of many other drugs. Serious adverse interactions are therefore possible, and dose adaptations for these medications (e.g. cyclosporin, oral contraceptives), are necessary when macrolides are administered.

The two agents used in anaerobic infections, *metronidazole* and *ornidazole* have a low peritoneal clearance and only 10% and 6% of the dose respectively, are removed by the peritoneum [403, 405]. The dosage in CAPD patients is therefore the same as in undialysed, uraemic patients [404].

Antiviral and antifungal drugs (Table 7)

Acyclovir has significant activity against HSV-1, HSV-2 and *Varicella zoster* virus (VZV). Acyclovir seems to have a three-compartment pharmacokinetic profile in CAPD patients [433]. Mean total plasma clearance was 46 ml/h per kg, 12% of which was due to peritoneal dialysis. Acyclovir has an apparent distribution volume of 62.5 L, with a protein binding of less than 20%. Stathoulopoulou et al. [434] found that the doses recommended for end-stage renal failure patients (1600 mg) led to supratherapeutic levels of acyclovir in CAPD patients, increasing the risk of neurotoxicity, which was reported in two patients [435]. Based on computer modelling, a daily oral dose of 600–800 mg is recommended [434].

Ganciclovir is extensively used as an antiviral agent for cytomegalovirus (CMV) infections in immunocompromised patients. Studies of the pharmacokinetics of ganciclovir in patients with renal impairment are, however, scarce. Sommadossi et al. [436] reported higher, although highly variable, values for distribution volume in patients with renal failure (V_d 0.41 ± 1.5 L/kg) compared to normal volunteers. Ganciclovir has a low molecular weight (255 Da) and a low protein binding (1–2%) and is thus effectively cleared by haemodialysis. However, due to the large volume of distribution compared to the dialysate volume, removal of ganciclovir by peritoneal dialysis is negligible, and the doses should be adapted as for patients with renal failure. It is of note that, due to an important tubular secretion, CAPD patients with residual renal function have a ganciclovir clearance higher than the creatinine clearance [417].

Table 6. Pharmacokinetic studies with quinolones, aminoglycosides, trimethoprim-sulphamethoxazole, and miscellaneous antibiotics

Drug	Normal renal function				ESRD		Dosage/route	PD					Refs
	PB (%)	$t_{1/2}$ (h)	V_{dis} (L/kg)	Cl_{tot} (ml/min)	$t_{1/2}$ (h)	Cl_{tot} (ml/min)		$t_{1/2}$ (h)	C_{max} (mg/ml)	Cl_{tot} (ml/min)	Cl_{per} (ml/min)	Percentage dose removed or absorbed	
Ciprofloxacin	40	3–4	2.8	652	16.8	300	0 750 mg (n = 6)	16.8 ± 5.1	3.61 ± 1.56	373.5 ± 213.4	—	0.4–1.6/48 h	371
							0 4 × 250 mg	8.44 ± 3.23	—		—	1/48 h	212
							– perit	7.19 ± 1.75				1.5/48 h	
							+ perit 0 4 × 250 mg every 12 h	11 ± 1	2.3 ± 0.2	256 ± 47	4.16 ± 0.33	2/48 h	372
Ciprofloxacin Fleroxacin	18	4.6 ± 0.9 8.6	7.33 ± 5.67 1.5	86.3 ± 43.8 168	11.1 ± 2.8 24.7	19.6 ± 7.6 63	0 750 mg IV 100 mg SD	8.9 ± 3.1	3.36 ± 1.12	33.0 ± 28.6	8.8 ± 6.5	7.8 ± 3.6/96 h	373
							0 400 mg SD	28.6 ± 6.7	4.9 ± 0.06	0.58 ± 0.13/kg	0.05 ± 0.01/kg		374
Fleroxacin Ofloxacin	25–30	8.9–13.5 6* ± 1.2	1.23* ± 0.11	122–168 180.5* ± 12.1	13–21 18.4* ± 12.1	68.4* ± 35.1	0 300 mg	25.1 ± 2.54		3.55 ± 0.43		<10	375
							0 200 mg	26.8 ± 2.5		35.2 ± 8.2	4.0 ± 0.5	4.2/24 h ± 0.5	376
							0 250 mg					5.8/24 h	377
							0 200 mg SD	35 ± 4.19		29.3 ± 11.2	4.5 ± 0.8	5/24 h	378
							IP 10 mg/L SD					15/96 h	379
							– perit 4 × 20 mg/2 L MD IP 10 mg/L SD		0.57 ± 0.07/24 h			81.9 ± 1.5/4 h	380
Ofloxacin Pefloxacin	25–30 25*	6 ± 1.2 8*	1.23 1.9*	180.5 137*	18.4 ± 12.1 12.1* ± 1.7	68.4* ± 35.1 117*	– perit 4 × 20 mg/2 L MD 0 200 mg	22.1	17.8 ± 0.17	35.9	2.15	84.7 ± 1.5/3 h	381
							0 400 mg SD	19.2 ± 3.3	3.55	1.0 ± 0.2 (ml/min/kg)	0.06 ± 0.01	<10	383
Pefloxacin							IV 400 mg SD	17.4 ± 2.3	6.4 ± 0.4			—	384
							IP 200 mg/L		3.5 ± 0.8/65 kg	1.3 ± 0.3 (ml/min/kg)	0.09 ± 0.02	—	
Gentamicin	<10	2	0.24	95	60	2	0 400 mg SD	19 ± 5.8	5.6 ± 1.3	39.1 ± 11.1	2.7	2.3–3.7/24 h	385
							IV 1 mg/kg	27.4 ± 11.7	4.5 ± 1.0			0 in 3/5 patients	
							IP 1 mg/kg	27.9	3.64 (6 h)			84/6 h	
							IP 50 mg/L	36 ± 9	3.9 ± 1.5 (6 h)		2.94 ± 0.4	20.2 ± 9/24 h	386
							IP 7.5 mg/L		0.6 (6 h)		5.7 ± 0.4 mass transfer	64/6 h	224
							– perit						
							+ perit		0.8 (6 h)		16.4 ± 1.9 mass transfer	79.3/6 h	
Tobramycin	<10	2.5	0.23	80	60	3	0.6 mg/kg	35.8		7.36 ± 1.49	5.74 ± 1.5		243
							IV 1.1–1.5 mg/kg	34.6 ± 7.4		8.0 ± 1.0	3.8 ± 0.4	13–26/24 h	387
							IV 1.5 mg/kg	39.5 ± 18		7.6 ± 3.1	1.11 ± 0.8	52/6 h	346
							IP 1.5 mg/kg/2 L	35.1 ± 12	1.8	9.8 ± 4.0	1.96 ± 1.6	30/48 h	388
							IV 2 mg/kg	25.7 ± 46.5	9.8 ± 3/0.3 h	7.3 ± 2 70 kg	3.4 ± 1 70 kg	73 ± 10.6 h	
							IP 2 mg/kg/2 L CCPD 2 L cycles per hour IP 160 mg/2 L		5.6 ± 2/6 h				
							– perit		5.9 ± 1.4/40 h		12.8 ± 1.2	44 ± 4.4/48 h	225
							+ perit		6.5 ± 1.3/40 h		17.4 ± 1.1	55 ± 3.6/48 h	
							IP 5 mg/L		1.3–2.1 ± 0.12/24 h	6.8		48/48 h	300

Drug						Dose					Ref
Tobramycin	35	2.5				IP 50 mg/L LD IP 7.5 mg/L MD IP 1.93 mg/kg/2 L LD IP 0.96 mg/kg/2 L IP 20 mg/2 L	4.3/6 h 3.7 6.6 ± 1.1	5.6 — 6.9 ± 1.2		85/6 h 50 ss —	389 390
Streptomycin	80	2.5	0.26	80	3	IP 100 mg/L LD IP 30 mg/L MD IV 7.5 mg/kg	5.5/5 h 4.8 18.6–26.8/24 h		—	75/6 h	391
Amikacin	<10	2.5	0.25	85	3	IP 7.5 mg/kg	42.2 ± 14.2	3.9 ± 1.0 /1.73 m² 4.6 ± 1.2	2.0 ± 1.0 /1.73 m² 2.7 ± 0.4	—	392
Netilmicin	<10	2.0	0.25	90	5	IP 7.5 mg/kg/2 L IV 100 mg	19.6 ± 6.1/5.6 h	37.2 ± 13.2	3.38 ± 0.37 4.9 ± 1.1	53 ± 14/5 h	211
Netilmicin		2.0	0.23	88	2	– perit + perit	— 1.9 ± 9.9	18.1 ± 3.7 19.6 ± 2.0 1.4 ± 9.0		23 ± 2.7/48 h 27.9 ± 5.2/48 h	393
Kanamycin	<10	2	0.23	95	2	IP 1.5 mg/kg followed by IP 40 mg/day IP 50 mg/L – perit + perit	— 3.1 ± 0.3 4.3 ± 0.4		11.4 ± 0.9 mass transfer 17.2 ± 2.1 mass transfer	67 ± 4/4 h 83 ± 2/4 h	394
Trimethoprim	40–70	13	2	125	25	O 80 mg	24		2.32 ± 0.39 (night) 4.65 ± 1.25 (day)		395
Sulphamethoxazole	40–90	10	0.2	30	35	O 400 mg 4 × day	15		1.64 ± 0.58 (night) 4.29 ± 0.95 (day)		
Trimethoprim						O 320 mg IV 320 mg O 320 mg	27.7 28.6 ± 10.6 27 ± 8.8	31.1 29.3 ± 11 39.1 ± 20	0.88 0.77 ± 0.36 0.77 ± 0.35	2.75/24 h 2.7/24 h 73	396
Sulphamethoxazole						O 1600 mg IV 1600 mg IP	12.8 ± 1.9 13.0 11.8 ± 2.2	11.9 ± 3.2 11.8 ± 3.1 15.3 ± 5.0	0.62 ± 0.25 0.62 ± 0.25 0.53 ± 0.08 14 ± 2.5	5.24/24 h 5.17/24 h 65	
Fosfomycin	<10%	1.5–2		—		IV 1 g IP 0.5 g	38.4 ± 8.7 — /5 h	7.0 ± 1.4 —	3.2 ± 0.2 —	60/3 h 37.2 ± 3.6 68.4 ± 6.0	397 398
Roxithromycine	50–60	10–14		—	2.3–6.8	O 300 mg IV 1 g	20.6 ± 8.7 —	37–118 23.8 ± 2.5	0.9–1.8 2.1 ± 0.29	1.0–3.1 9/48 h	399 400
Aztreonam		1.8	0.2	80	22	IP 500 mg/L IP 500 mg/L IP 1.5 g/L single LD + pert	30 ± 3.3/3 h 42.5 ± 12.4/6 h 83 (61–96)/2 h	— 30.4	10.05 ± 3.7 —	72.9 ± 2.4/6 h 90.8 ± 3/8 h 86–95	401 402
Metronidazole	20	7	0.7	82	82	IV 750 mg	10.93 ± 2.01	50.17 ± 18.6 (ml/kg/h)	4.49 ± 0.88	10/48 h	403
Metronidazole	6.0–8.8	10–14	0.53–1.1	68–87	55–183	IV 500–800 mg single dose O 250–2000	5.6			10	404
Ornidazole	6.1–14.7	1.8	0.52–0.96	68–81	—	IV 500 mg	11.8 ± 0.9	47.9 ± 6.3	3.0 ± 0.4	6.2 ± 1.1/48 h	405

Table 7. Pharmacokinetic data with antiviral and antifungal drugs in CAPD

Drug	Normal renal function PB (%)	t₁/₂ (h)	V_{dis} (L/kg)	Cl_{tot} (ml/min)	ESRD t₁/₂ (h)	Cl_{tot} (ml/min)	Dosage/route	PD t₁/₂ (h)	C_{max} (mg/ml)	Cl_{tot} (ml/min)	Cl_{per} (ml/min)	Percentage dose removed or absorbed	Refs
Acyclovir	15	2–3	0.6	300	19.5	25	IV 200 mg/kg (n=1)	14.7	–	48.6	3.6	7.3/24 h	414
							IV 5 mg/kg (n=1) SD	17.1	7.7	48.3	4.4	5.7/24 h	415
							IV 1 g (n=2); IV 0.5 g (n=2)	13.2 ± 4.7	–	39.7 ± 10	3.4 ± 0.2	–	416
Ganciclovir					6.3	35.5	IP 1 g/2L; 5 mg/kg IV	10.8 ± 2.9	–	64.6 ± 7.5	–	61 ± 10 probably not relevant	417
Foscarnet		4.5					O 200 mg SD	41.4–45.8	–	8.8–9.8	4.5–5.8	5–30	418
Zidovudine							O 200 mg	1.8 ± 0.5	5.3 ± 2.4	1059 ± 511	0	0	419
Zidovudine							O 200 mg (n=5) SD				5	<1/24 h	419
GZVD* Zidovudine	30	1.1	1.4	1500	1.4	737	SD 200 mg	–	–	–	15	20/24 h	420
							SD 200 mg O (n=1)	7.9	1.36	856	4.2	0.5/14 h	420
							SD 100 mg O	26	0.2	2079	5.8	0.14/14 h	
							SD 200 mg ZVD	19.9	9.06	–	3.6	8.5/14 h	
							100 mg ZVD	7.1	6.78	–	3.7	4/14 h	
Didanosine		1.56 ± 0.43 / 1.54 ± 0.38		13.0 ± 1.6	3.6 ± 0.8	3.4 ± 1.2	300 mg IV; 300 mg per os	3.11 ± 0.88 / 3.88 ± 1.26	9.17 ± 4.54 / 2.16 ± 1.32	3.2 ± 1.2	?		421
Amphotericin B	90–95	24	0.46	15	40	9	50 mg IV/4 h	S: 10* D: 0.1–0.2* S: 0.2 (1–12 h)					422
							10 mg IV	D: 0.2					423
Fluconazole	11	33	0.71	–	98	–	O 100 mg	85	S: 1439 ± 246 D: 1050 (6–24) 790 (24–48 h)	–	5.53 ± 1.03	18/48	424
							IP 150 mg/2 L; IP 50 mg/2 L	80 / 72	S: 2123 ± 360 S: 885 ± 136 S ?	8.75 ± 2 / 7.63 ± 1.2	4.3 ± 0.4 / 4.41 ± 0.49		425
Fluorocytosine	4	5	0.7	113	85	7	LD 30–40 mg/kg 4 days; MD 15 mg/kg O 4 days		D ? SSs: 24–86				426
							LD 3.5 g 2 days; 2.5 g 2 days; MD 1 g day		SSs: 25–33				427
							IP 100 mg/L – perit		1.78		16.1 ± 2 mass transfer	81 ± 2/4 h	428
							+ perit		–		19.0 mass transfer	93/4 h	
							LD 0 2 g +IP 100 mg/2 L		S: 25–33 D: 29–43				

Drug				Dose		Serum/dialysate conc.			Ref.
Itraconazole	99.8	21–38	—	25	0 200 mg SD	—	S: 0.08	— 0	0	429
Ketoconazole	99	3	—	—	0 400 mg/day (n=1) 0 200 mg/day for 4 days 0 400 mg/D for 4 days 0 200 mg SD − perit + perit	3.51	SC_{max} 2.0 ± 11.3 DC_{max} < 0.1 SC_{max} 1.6 ± 0.5 DC_{max} < 0.1 DC_{max} 0.021 (ND–0.073) DC_{max} 0.015 (0.010–0.019)	—	—	430 431 432
Ketoconazole	99	3	—	—	400 mg SD − perit + perit 0 400 mg SD	2.4 ± 0.8	C_{max} D: 0.029 (0.014–0.056) D: 0.074 (0.032–0.115) C_{max} 2.3 ± 1.7	—	< 1	256

No pharmacokinetic data for peritoneal dialysis patients are available for *foscarnet*, and dose adaptations are recommended as in end-stage renal failure. One case report described a serum half-life of 45.8 h for a patient on CAPD (normal patients 4.5 h). CAPD clearance of foscarnet was calculated to be 4.5 ml/min with a total clearance of 8.8 ml/min [418].

Studies in a limited number of CAPD patients treated with *Zidovudine* (ZDV) suggest that no further modification from the renal failure dosage regimen is necessary [420, 437]; however, great interpatient variability in its pharmacokinetics was noted [437].

Didanosine is an antiretroviral agent used for treatment of HIV infections. In patients with renal failure, elimination half-life was reported to be prolonged to 3.6 ± 0.8 h as compared to 1.5 ± 0.5 h in patients with normal renal function. CAPD has little effect on the removal of didanosine; dose reduction to one-fourth of the daily dose is thus recommended (a single administration), in patients on CAPD as well as in non-dialysed end-stage renal failure patients [421].

Information on the pharmacokinetics of *antifungal drugs* in peritoneal dialysis patients is disappointingly scarce. Most studies are limited to occasional measurements of serum and/or dialysate levels during treatment for fungal peritonitis.

Amphotericin B is highly protein-bound and circulates in the blood in a complex of high molecular weight (200 000–300 000). It penetrates very poorly in the peritoneal fluid after systemic administration. The data are, however, conflicting [438–440]. Chemical peritonitis causing abdominal pain after intraperitoneal administration of amphotericin B has been observed [245–248]. It has been proposed that for intraperitoneal use the dialysate should be adjusted to a neutral pH to prevent aggregation [441]. Amphotericin B has been used in an intravenous dose of 0.5 to 1 mg/kg body weight, combined with an intraperitoneal dose of 2–3 mg/L dialysate [442]. Amphotericin B induces the formation of pores and channels in the cell membrane, causing leakage of potassium and magnesium. This is probably the reason why the drug increases transcapillary ultrafiltration [135, 443]; however, the chemical drug-induced peritonitis may also play a role in this observation [444]. Studies of the absorption of amphotericin B after intraperitoneal instillation are lacking, although the large distribution volume and the high protein binding are expected to favour its transfer to the blood stream.

Systemically administered *fluorocytosine* penetrates well into the peritoneal fluid [438]. The usual loading dose of 20–30 mg/kg in uraemic patients is followed by a maintenance doses of 15 mg/kg. Serum levels of fluorocytosine should be monitored since toxicity is expected when serum levels exceed 100–125 µg/ml. This has mainly been tried with intraperitoneal administration of 100–200 mg/2 L, together with amphotericin B intravenously [247, 445] or in a dose of 150 mg/L in combination with oral ketoconazole 400 mg daily [446].

Fluconazole is effective for both superficial and systemic fungal infections. The pharmacokinetic profile of orally administered fluconazole shows a low plasma protein binding, and a long plasma half-life, allowing once-daily dosing. The bioavailability is excellent. A good penetration of fluconazole into the peritoneal dialysate after a single oral dose of 100 mg in CAPD patients has been found [424]. When given systemically the dose should be the same as in undialysed patients [447]. When administered intraperitoneally the recommended dose is 150 mg in a single 2 L dwell, every 48 h.

A single-dose pharmacokinetic study of *itraconazole* has been performed in patients with ESRD, including five CAPD patients [429]. The systemic pharmacokinetics of itraconazole were not affected by CAPD and the drug could not be detected in the peritoneal dialysate. Oral administration of *ketoconazole* in CAPD patients revealed extremely low peritoneal clearances. After oral administration of 400 mg ketoconazole, Johnson *et al.* [254] reported mean serum concentrations of 2.3 µg/ml, while the D/P ratio was only 0.03 after 5 h. Other studies confirmed this low penetration in the dialysate after oral administration [448].

In conclusion, from a pharmacokinetic point of view, fluconazole, preferably in combination with another agent, should be the drug of choice to treat fungal peritonitis in peritoneal dialysis patients [448].

Drugs used in gastroenterology (Table 8)

H$_2$ antagonists are frequently described in patients with ESRD and treated with dialysis, including chronic peritoneal dialysis. Studies have been performed with *cimetidine*, *rantidine* and *famotidine* [449–452]. Dosage reduction necessary for undialysed patients should be applied for patients on peritoneal dialysis. No pharmacokinetic data on *nizatidine* or *roxatidine* in CAPD are available. These drugs have, however, been studied in chronic

renal failure [459]. It can be presumed that these drugs have a negligible peritoneal clearance.

To our knowledge *omeprazole*, a proton-pump inhibitor, has not been studied in CAPD patients. In patients with severe chronic renal failure its pharmacokinetics are not significantly different from those in healthy subjects [456, 460] and the drug is not detected in dialysis fluid during haemodialysis [461]. One can therefore expect that omeprazole could be administered in uraemic and CAPD patients at the usual dose of 20 mg/day. *Lansoprazole* and *pantoprazole* are also completely metabolized. The elimination half-life of lansoprazole seemed to be prolonged in patients with moderate, but not in those with severe, renal dysfunction. Haemodialysis did not seem to influence the plasma concentrations of lansoprazole, probably due to a very high protein binding (97–99%) [457]. Lansoprazole also has some renally cleared active metabolites. The data with pantoprazole in patients with renal impairment are difficult to interpret, and further studies are required to clarify the controversial observations made until now [456]. Haemodialysis does not appear to significantly influence the pharmacokinetics of pantoprazole or its main metabolite M2 in patients with end-stage renal disease [458].

With *cisapride*, a gastrokinetic drug, in a dose of 5 mg/L dialysate four times per day, excellent results were obtained in two diabetic CAPD patients suffering from gastroparesis. The intraperitoneal dose produced the same plasma levels as the oral or intravenous doses of 30 mg and 10 mg, respectively [453]. In haemodialysis patients the terminal half-life of cisapride was 9.6 ± 3.3 h and the volume of distribution 4.8 ± 3.3 L/kg. Cisapride was not found in the dialysate, in contrast with its metabolite norcisapride. The authors conclude that dose adaptation is not necessary [454]. It is of note that intoxication with cisapride, leading to cardiac arrhythmias, has been described in patients using ketoconazole, fluconazole, itraconazole, miconazole, and antibiotics from the macrolide family. These drugs should not be coadministered with cisapride [462].

Erythropoietin (Tables 9a–c)

A number of interesting pharmacokinetic studies have been performed with erythropoietin (Epo) in peritoneal dialysis. When administered subcutaneously, Epo is slowly absorbed with a T_{max} around 20–24 h. The subcutaneous bioavailability compared to intravenous dosing ranges between 10% and 36%. Peritoneal dialysis itself has no significant effect on the removal of erythropoietin.

Table 8. Pharmacokinetic data with H_2-antagonists, metoclopramide and cispramide

	Normal renal function				ESRD			PD					
	PB (%)	$t_{1/2}$ (h)	V_{dis} (L/kg)	Cl_{tot} (ml/min)	$t_{1/2}$ (h)	Cl_{tot} (ml/min)	Dosage/route	$t_{1/2}$ (h)	C_{max} (mg/ml)	Cl_{tot} (ml/min)	Cl_{per} (ml/min)	Percentage dose removed or absorbed	Refs
Cimetidine	13–25	1.5–2	0.8–1.2	313–808	3–5	193	IV 300 mg	6.9 ± 0.18	–	167.1 ± 8.06	3.01 ± 0.57	1.6 ± 0.23/24 h	449
							IV 300 mg	4.3	–	191 ± 55	4.2 ± 3.1	2.2 ± 1.4/24 h	450
Ranitidine	15	1.5–3	1.1–1.9	568–709	6–9	103–230	IV 50 mg	7.06 ± 0.96	–	126 ± 67.5	3.2 ± 0.7	1.3/24 h	451
							O 150 mg	10.02 ± 1.71	904 ± 529/4.2 h		2.6 ± 0.6	0.9/24 h	
Famotidine	15–20	2.5–3.5	1.1–1.4	412	9–18	40–60	IV 20 mg	15.5 ± 4.0	–	–	–	4.5 ± 1.1/24 h	452
Cisapride	98*	7–10*	2.4*	–	15*	385*	O 30 mg every 6 h	–	–	–	–	–	453
							IV 10 mg every 6 h	–	0.031–0.04 (serum)	–	–	–	
								–	0.007–0.008 (dialysate)	–	–	–	
							IP 5 mg/L every 6 h	–	0.028–0.053 (serum)	–	–	–	
Cisapride	98	36 440	2.4		9.6 ± 3.3	380 ± 161	O 20 mg		probably not altered	–			454
Metoclopramide	–	3	3.4	916	14	196	O 15 mg ($n=1$)	34.65	66.4	–	3.54	–	455
							IV 15 mg ($n=1$)	30.13	329	61.6	1.47	3/6 h	
							IP 15 mg/2 L ($n=1$)	30.13	146.2	–	–	97/6 h	
Lansaprazole	96	1.2–2.9					O 15–30 mg	1.6	probably not altered				456, 457
Pantoprazole	98	0.9–1.9	0.15–0.17	60–130	not altered				probably not altered				458
Omeprazole	95	0.7–2.1			0.7–2.1				probably not altered				456

* From refs 495 and 496.

Table 9A. Pharmocokinetics of intravenously administered erythropoietin in peritoneal dialysis

PD regimen	Dose	C_{max} (U/L)	T_{max} (h)	$t_{1/2}$ (h)	AUC (U/1 h)	V_d (L)	Cl_{tot}	Percentage dose lost	References
6 CAPD	300	7688 ± 1103	0.5	11.2 ± 0.4	81 004 ± 9523	5.0 ± 1.0/24 h	0.52 ± 0.008 ml/min/kg	2.63 ± 0.45/24 h	463
9 CAPD	100	1595 ± 104 (11–145)	0.4 ± 0.1	8.7 ± 1.0	16 909 ± 1217	4.9 ± 0.6	6.7 ± 0.5 ml/min	–	464
10 CAPD	100	2000	–	5.1 ± 0.6	–	–	–	–	465
7 CAPD	100	1440 (1088–1994)	–	8.3 (6.6–13)	14 623 (10 286–19 562)	4.5	6.0 (4.7–9.7) ml/min/1.73 m²	–	466
12 IPD	100	1923 ± 197	0.3	5.6 ± 0.3	–	3.7 ± 0.6	8.1 ± 1.4 ml/min	–	467
8 CAPD	120	3959 ± 758	0.25	8 ± 2 (6.2–10.2)	45 102 ± 11 405 (0–24 h)	0.033 ± 0.013 1/kg	0.047 ± 0.017 ml/min/kg	2.3/24 h (1.7–3)	468
6 CAPD	100	1602	–	6.1	13 592	–	–	–	469

In animal studies an enhanced absorption after intraperitoneal administration of Epo was found [472, 473]. However in human pharmacokinetic studies on intraperitoneal administration of erythropoietin a very low bioavailability (ranging from 2.5% to 8.5%) was found when diluted in 2 L of dialysate, but this increased to 41.4 ± 7.2%, when administered into a dry abdomen [467, 471]. The problem of low bioavailability of intraperitoneal erythropoietin when diluted in dialysate can be overcome by using high dosages of Epo or low volumes of dialysate. Frenken *et al.* [474] utilized 100 U/kg intraperitoneally, diluted in 1 L of dialysate over a 9 h dwell thrice weekly and observed a slow but significant increase in haematocrit; Nasu *et al.* [475] reported an excellent haematocrit response when Epo in a high dose of 300 U/kg, diluted in 2 L dialysate, was given.

Intraperitoneal administration of *iron dextran* leads to an efficient absorption of iron. However, severe toxicity to the peritoneal membrane was found, precluding the use of concentrations higher than 2 mg/L [476]. Whether lower dosing schemes (0.125 mg/L), with no proven toxicity, are able to restore iron stores remains to be proven [477]. Until now, intraperitonael administration of iron dextran seems not to be recommendable.

Miscellaneous drugs (Table 10)

An interesting observation was made on the removal of *ethosuximide* and *phenobarbital* in an epileptic child by peritoneal dialysis [478]. During a peritonitis episode the daily dialysis time of 8 h (CCPD) was increased to 24 h and the patient developed convulsions. Apparently a substantial amount of both anticonvulsant medications was removed via the peritoneal dialysate and supplementary doses of both drugs were needed to stabilize the patient.

Leaky *et al.* [487] described a 3-year-old asthmatic boy who developed acute renal failure, necessitating acute peritoneal dialysis. His plasma *theophylline* concentrations remained therapeutic; yet the child developed the symptoms of theophylline toxicity while undergoing peritoneal dialysis. Excessively high plasma concentrations of the principal theophylline metabolite, 1,3-dimethyluric acid, were found. The high concentrations decreased only when renal function recovered. Apparently peritoneal dialysis is not able to remove this theophylline metabolite.

In a pharmacokinetic study of *flurbiprofen*, CAPD patients were used as representative patients with

Table 9B. Pharmocokinetics of subcutaneously administered erythropoietin in peritoneal dialysis

PD regimen	Dose	C_{max} (U/L)	T_{max} (h)	AUC (U/1 h)	Bioavailability (%)	References
6 CAPD	300	484 ± 75	24	8230 ± 1312 (0–24 h)	10.2 ± 1.0/24 h	463
9 CAPD	100	81 (11–145)	12	–	14/24 h; 31/72 h	465
12 IPD	100	32 ± 4	28 ± 5	–	14.9 ± 4.8	467
8 CAPD	120	176 ± 75	18	9610 ± 4862 (0–24 h)	21.5 (11.3–36)	468
6 CAPD	100	114	–	3316	24.0	469
10 CAPD	50	81 ± 13 mU/L	24	1492 ± 165 mU/1 h	–	470

Table 9C. Pharmocokinetics of intraperitoneally administered erythropoietin in peritoneal dialysis

	Dose (U/kg)	Vol dialysate	Dwell (h)	C_{max} (U/L)	T_{max} (h)	AUC (U/1 h)	Bioavailability (%)	References
6 CAPD	300	2	4	108 ± 18	8–12	1981 ± 271 (0–24 h)	2.5 ± 0.2	463
3 CAPD	300	2	12	170 ± 13	12	2933 ± 413 (0–24 h)	3.6 ± 0.5	
9 CAPD	100		12	52 ± 14	12 ± 0.2	1426 ± 366	8.5 ± 1.9	464
3 CAPD	100	2	10	80	12	56% of AUC after SC inj.	–	465
7 CAPD	100	2	12	23 (18–55)	14 (6.3–18)	808 (426–1652)	6.8 (2.2–12)	466
12 IPD	100	dry cavity	–	213 ± 27	17 ± 2.3	–	41.4 ± 7.2	467
8 CAPD	50 000 U	1.5–2	8	375 ± 123	12	6432 ± 2150 (0–24 h)	2.9 (1.2–6.8)	468
10 CAPD	50	2	8	36 ± 4	12–24	803 ± 67 mU/1 h	–	470
6 CAPD	400	50 ml of (saline undiluted)	8	1500 (estimated)	12	$52\,399 \pm 6865$ mU/ml/h	> 9-fold increase vs diluted	471
6 CAPD	400	2 diluted	8	300 (estimated)	12	5739 ± 1292 mU/m/h	–	

end-stage renal disease. Neither flurbiprofen nor its metabolites was detected in the dialysate [488].

Peritoneal dialysis patients have a decreased clearance of *ethinyl oestradiol*, leading to slightly higher serum concentrations compared to women with normal renal function [486]. Serum half-life was 8.4 ± 4.1 vs 3.4 ± 1.6 h in peritoneal dialysis patients and normal individuals respectively after single oral dose, and 15.7 ± 3.3 vs 14.3 ± 2.3 after a multiple dose.

Data on the pharmacokinetics of *benzodiazepines* in peritoneal dialysis are scarce. The triazolobenzodiazepine *alprazolam* has been studied in normal subjects and dialysis patients [489]. CAPD patients had longer serum half-lives than controls and haemodialysis patients. There were also higher free fractions of the drug. CAPD patients should thus be monitored for side-effects and the dose should be adjusted accordingly. For *midazolam*, only data in renal failure patients were found. Protein binding was decreased compared to normal subjects, resulting in a doubling of the free fraction of the drug [418]. Since clearance is mostly hepatic, this increased fraction may explain why total midazolam

clearance was higher in renal failure patients. Dose modification may thus not be necessary in renal failure for midazolam [483]. However, some reports of sustained activity of midazolam due to accumulation of metabolites in renal failure were reported in ICU patients with renal failure [490].

Zolpidem is an imidazopyridine which differs in structure from benzodiazepines. Zolpidem is approximately 92% bound to plasma proteins. The free fraction increases to 14.9% in uraemic patients, while the volume of distrubution increases, and elimination half-life doubles [485]. Although exact data are not available, dose reduction in CAPD patients thus seems to be prudent.

Mycophenolate mofetil is a prodrug of the new immunosuppressive agent mycophenolic acid. After initiation of peritoneal dialysis in patients with GFR < 10 ml/min, the area under the concentration curve decreased substantially. The calculated clearance increased from 8.1 ml/min per kg in non-dialysed patients to 14.6 ml/min per kg in CAPD patients. Mycophenolate acid itself was found in only trace amounts in the dialysate. However, mycophenolate glucuronide, a metabolite of mycopheno-

Table 10. Pharmocokinetics of miscellaneous drugs in CAPD

	Normal renal function				ESRD		Dosage/route	PD				Percentage dose removed or absorbed	Refs
	PB (%)	$t_{1/2}$ (h)	V_{dis} (L/kg)	Cl_{tot} (ml/min)	$t_{1/2}$ (h)	Cl_{tot} (ml/min)		$t_{1/2}$ (h)	C_{max} (mg/ml)	Cl_{tot} (ml/min)	Cl_{per} (ml/min)		
Ethosuximide	0	60	–	10	–	–	0.3 × 400 mg CCPD (child)	–	–	–	–	50/24 h	478
Phenobarbital	66	70	0.75	9	100	6	0.2 × 250 mg day 6 CCPD (child)	–	21	–	–	40/24 h	478
Phenytoin	87–93	18	0.57	25	9	125	0.3 × 100 mg	–	16.6 mm/L SS	–	1.77	–	479
							0.3 × 200 mg	–	22.6 mm/L SS	–	1.70	–	
							0.4 × 100 mg	–	26.1	–	1.60	–	
1.25 di-OH vit D								0.27.4 IP 19.2	0.116 IP 121	0.15.3 IP 18.4	–	–	480
1-alpha-OH-vit D							80 mg/kg	IV 109.4 ± 129.5	NM ?				481
Clodronate							300 mg IV	182 ± 138		26.0 ± 19.3	2.4 ± 0.6	7	482
Mycophenolate–Mofetil							0.2 × 1 g			14.6 ± 3.4	6.5 ± 1.6		218
Alprazolam	68.4	10–14.5	0.72–1.05	44–67	11.5	70	0.1 mg				–		483
Triazolam		2.56 ± 4.06	1.31 ± 0.1	330 ± 110	2.29	–	0.5 mg						483
Midazolam		1.36 ± 2.29	0.38–1.14	323–645		680	0.5–20 mg		680				483
	95–97.5					–	–	–					484
Loprazolam		6.3–14.8		230			0.0.5–2 mg						483
Zolpidem	92	1.5–2.4	0.54–0.68	15.7	3–4.8		0.5–20 mg		probably as in ESRD				485
Ethinyl oestradiol		3.4 ± 1.6		1007 ± 754				8.4 ± 4.1	9.3 ± 0.7	518 ± 307			486

late, was found to be removed by peritoneal dialysis for up to 2 g/12 h, representing removal of 1.2 g of mycophenolic acid [218].

CAPD treatment is associated with peritoneal losses of *vitamin D metabolites*, contributing to the low serum levels of 25-OH-D3 and 25-OH-D binding capacity [481, 482]; losses of 1,25(OH)2D3 and 24,25(OH)2D3 in the dialysate average 6–8% of the plasma pool per day [491].

Intraperitoneal calcitriol raises serum calcium and depresses serum PTH more effectively than increasing dialysis fluid calcium [492]. The calcitriol and alfacalcidol should, however, be injected directly through the catheter port and not into the dialysate, as a substantial amount is otherwise adsorbed to the PVC bags [493, 494].

Salusky *et al.* [493] have studied the pharmacokinetics of calcitriol after intravenous, oral and intraperitoneal administration of 60 ng/kg in CAPD and CCPD patients. The serum calcitriol levels were similar after 24 h for the different routes of administration. The bioavailability of calcitriol (AUC 0–24 h) was 50–60% greater after intravenous than after oral or intraperitoneal administration. Comparable results were obtained by Jones *et al.* and Joffe *et al.* [480, 481], who determined appearance of 1,25-OH vitamin D3 after oral, intravenous and intraperitoneal administration of alfacalcidol [481]. Radioisotope tracer studies indicated that 35–40% of the hormone adheres to plastic components of the peritoneal dialysate delivery system. The authors modified the technique of intraperitoneal calcitriol administration by direct instillation of the drug in the Tenckhoff catheter and by increasing the intraperitoneal dose to 120 ng/kg. With this method an AUC equal to the AUC obtained after intravenous injection was observed [493].

Biphosphonates are becoming increasingly popular for treatment of osteoporosis, morbus Paget and hypercalcaemia. The major route of elimination of *clodronate* is renal excretion. Hence, the dose of clodronate should be reduced in renal failure. In a study by Saha *et al.* [482], CAPD removed clodronate poorly from the circulation (7% of administered dose over 24 h), and most of the clearance was attributed to skeletal deposition of the drug. This uptake was related to parathormone levels. Clearance of clodronate after a single intravenous injection was 2.4 ± 0.6 ml/min. The volume of distribution was 0.49 ± 0.34 L/kg, and elimination half-life was 16.9 ± 4.7 h. D/P for clodronate was approximately 0.4 after a 6 h dwell. Data on *pamidronate* in peritoneal dialysis are not available, but most probably the same recommendations as for clodronate can be made, and dose adaptations as in patients with severe renal failure should be made.

Insulin

Earlier studies demonstrated that intraperitoneal insulin is absorbed into the portal venous circulation [495] and that intraperitoneal insulin leads to a persistent positive portal–systemic difference [496]. A substantial portion (50%) of the portal venous insulin is degraded during first passage through the liver. Such intraperitoneal treatment appears to improve glucose control and glucose stability without increasing the risk of hypoglycaemia [497–501]. Recent studies have shown that the intrapatient variation of the plasma-free insulin was markedly lower with continuous intraperitoneal than with continuous subcutaneous or intramuscular insulin administration [502, 503]. This could be attributed to the considerably smaller insulin depot after intraperitoneal than after subcutaneous administration.

Insulin is one of the most commonly administered intraperitoneal drugs in peritoneal dialysis patients. As already pointed out in the introductory section of this chapter, intraperitoneal insulin administration is most effective in patients on peritoneal dialysis if it is given into an empty peritoneal cavity, at least 30 min before the dialysate is instilled [504]; this creates a high peritoneum to plasma concentration gradient and avoids the adsorption of insulin to the peritoneal fluid bags. When radiolabelled insulin was added to the 2 L dialysate bags only 35% of the dose entered the peritoneal cavity [505]. In contrast, about 84% of 16 U of unlabelled insulin added per bag reached the peritoneal cavity when administered directly through a port on the Tenckhoff catheter [506]. Intraperitoneal insulin is rapidly absorbed and is detected in the peripheral blood within 15 min of administration, and peak serum insulin levels are observed 30–45 min after administration into an empty peritoneal cavity [112, 231]. These peak values are delayed until 90–120 min when insulin is added to the dialysate [507]. However, due to the partial hepatic inactivation of intraperitoneal insulin, absorption kinetics and efficacy of intraperitoneal and systemic insulin are difficult to compare by measurement of peripheral blood insulin levels. At least in the experimental animal, the magnitude of the serum level is dependent on the intraperitoneal dose [508]. Studies by Rubin *et al.* [145] have shown that the addition of intraperitoneal insulin has no effect on solute clearances, ultrafiltration volume or glucose absorption from the dialysis solution in CAPD patients. Wideröe *et al.* [231] found that fluid volume and osmolality of the solution in the peritoneal cavity decrease the transport rate of insulin, but not its bioavailability. A better blood glucose regulation after 120 min was found with intraperitoneal administration in dialysate as compared to administration into an empty abdomen [231]. Several protocols for administration of intraperitoneal insulin during CAPD have been reviewed [509].

Heparin

Heparin has an average MW of 15 kDa and consists of a heterogeneous group of anionic mucopolysaccharides, called glycosaminoglycans. Heparin is the most frequently used drug in peritoneal dialysis, for the purpose of preventing fibrin formation and catheter obstruction.

In the period when mainly intermittent peritoneal dialysis was used, doses from 100 U to 2500 U heparin or more per litre dialysate over varying lengths of time from a few days to many months have been recommended [510–514]. Furman *et al.* [515] performed a pharmacokinetic study of intraperitoneal heparin. Intraperitoneal heparin was assayed as the activated-partial-thromboplastin time (APTT) of dialysate added to control plasma. The half-life of disappearance from the peritoneal cavity ranged between 8.26 and 12.77 h in four patients. This study was one of the first to show that systemic blood coagulation was unaffected by a single intraperitoneal dose of 10 000 U of heparin. The authors doubted the usefulness of intraperitoneal heparin as an anticoagulant because of the low dialysate concentrations of the heparin cofactor antithrombin III (ATIII). Other investigators [516, 517] showed that heparin did transfer across the rabbit peritoneal membrane and to a slight extent in CAPD patients [518]. In a CAPD patient with deep-vein thrombosis, long-term intraperitoneal application of low molecular weight heparin in a dose of 8000 antifactor Xa units/2 L, resulted in adequate and therapeutic plasma levels as measured by antifactor Xa units [519]. Recently it was demonstrated that the intraperitoneal administration of heparin (1000–2500 U/ L) without addition of ATIII was sufficient for prevention of intraperitoneal fibrin formation in CAPD patients [518, 520].

Desferrioxamine

A pharmacokinetic study of desferrioxamine and its iron and aluminium chelates has been performed in CAPD patients [521]. Desferrioxamine (10 mg/kg) was administered either intramuscularly or intraperitoneally. The AUC calculated from 0 to 12 h was about 20% lower after the intraperitoneal than after the intramuscular administration. An advantage of the peritoneal administration was, however, the progressive increase in plasma concentrations, without an unduly high peak. The fact that 8–12 h after administration the concentrations of desferrioxamine in plasma and peritoneal fluid were approximately the same, is consistent with the low binding of desferrioxamine to plasma proteins.

Desferrioxamine was given intravenously and intraperitoneally in a CAPD patient in order to remove iron. Forty-five per cent of the total amount instilled was recovered in the outflow dialysate [522]. An intraperitoneal dose of 750 mg/day or 1250 mg on alternate days led to removal of 73 mg and 39.6 mg iron, respectively, as compared with 75 mg removal per week after an intravenous dose of 1500 mg thrice weekly.

Several authors have used intraperitoneal desferrioxamine successfully to remove aluminium in peritoneal dialysis patients [523–525]. Intraperitoneal doses of 40 mg/kg were used over a 10 h dwell in one study [525] and 0.5 g into each 2 L dialysate to a total dose of 6 g was applied in another study [526]. In the latter study the aluminium clearance with desferrioxamine was 3.1 ml/min vs 2.5 ml/min without desferrioxamine. The enhanced removal of aluminium by peritoneal dialysis persists for several days after single administration of the chelator.

Vitamins

Boeschoten *et al.* [527] have summarized earlier studies on vitamin status and vitamin losses in the dialysate in IPD and CAPD patients. They have performed a more complete analysis of plasma and 24 h dialysate losses of vitamin A, B1, B2, B6, B12, C, folic acid, E and β-carotene in 44 CAPD patients. Vitamins B12, A and E and carotenoids were not detectable in dialysate. In contrast, vitamins B2, B3, B6, C and folic acid were excreted in the 24 h dialysate in amounts higher than in 24 h urine of individuals with normal renal function. The loss of vitamin B1 in dialysate was low. These authors recommend vitamin supplementations in CAPD patients for vitamins B1, B6, C and folic acid.

References

1. Rippe B. A three-pore model of peritoneal transport. Perit Dial Int 1993; 13 (suppl. 2): S35–8.

2. Pannekeet MM, Mulder JB, Weening JJ, Struijk DG, Zweers MM, Krediet RT. Demonstration of aquaporin-CHIP in peritoneal tissue of uremic and CAPD patients. Perit Dial Int 1996; 16 (suppl. 1): S54–7.

3. Carlsson O, Nielsen S, Zakaria ER, Rippe B. *In vivo* inhibition of transcellular water channels (aquaporin-1) during acute peritoneal dialysis in rats. Am J Physiol 1996; 271: H2254–62.

4. Pietrzak I, Hirszel P, Shostack A, Welch PG, Lee RE, Maher JF. Splanchnic volume, not flow rate, determines peritoneal permeability. Trans Am Soc Artif Intern Organs 1989; 35: 583–7.

5. Nolph KD, Ghods A, Brown P *et al.* Effects of nitroprusside on peritoneal mass transfer coefficients and microvascular physiology. Trans Am Soc Artif Intern Organs 1977; 23: 210–217.

6. Zemel D, Krediet RT, Koomen GCM, Struijk D, Arisz L. Day to day variability of peritoneal transport used as a method for analyzing peritoneal permeability in CAPD. Perit Dial Int 1991; 11: 217–23.

7. Struijk D, Krediet RT, Koomen GCM *et al.* Functional characteristics of the peritoneal membrane in long-term continuous ambulatory peritoneal dialysis. Nephron 1991; 59: 213–20.

8. Dumont AE, Robbins E, Martelli A, Iliescu H. Platelet blockade of particle absorption from the peritoneal surface of the diaphragm. Proc Soc Exp Biol Med 1981; 167: 137–42.

9. Dedrick RL, Fenstermacher JD, Blasberg RG, Sieber SM. Peritoneal absorption of macromolecules. In: Maher JF, Winchester JF, eds. Frontiers in Peritoneal Dialysis. New York: Field, Rich, 1986, pp. 41–6.

10. Lindholm B, Werynski A, Bergström J. Fluid transport in peritoneal dialysis. Int J Artif Organs 1990; 13: 352–8.

11. Daugirdas JT, Ing TS, Gandhi VC, Hano JE, Chen WT, Yuan L. Kinetics of peritoneal fluid absorption in patients with chronic renal failure. J Lab Clin Med 1980; 95: 351–61.

12. Flessner MF, Parker RJ, Sieber SM. Peritoneal lymphatic uptake of fibrinogen and erythrocytes in the rat. Am J Physiol 1983; 224: H89–96.

13. Rippe B, Stelin G, Ahlmen J. Lymph flow from the peritoneal cavity in CAPD patients. In: Maher JF, Winchester JF, eds. Frontiers in Peritoneal Dialysis. New York: Field, Rich, 1999, pp. 24–30.

14. Brouard R, Tozer TN, Baumelou A, Gambertoglio JF. Transfer of autologous hemoglobin from peritoneal cavity during peritoneal dialysis. Nephrol Dial Transplant 1992; 7: 57–62.

15. Carlsson O, Nielsen S, Zakaria el R, Rippe B. *In vivo* inhibition of transcellular water channels (aquaporin-1) during acute peritoneal dialysis in rats. Am J Physiol 1996; 271: H2254–62.

16. Krediet RT, Struijk DG, Koomen GC, Hoek FJ, Arisz L. The disappearance of macromolecules from the peritoneal cavity during continuous ambulatory peritoneal dialysis is not dependent on molecular size. Perit Dial Int 1990; 10: 147–52.

17. Mactier RA, Nolph KD, Khanna R, Twardowski ZJ, Moore H, McGary T. Lymphatic absorption in peritoneal dialysis in the rat. Lymphology 1987; 20: 47.

18. De Paepe M, Matthys D, Lameire N. Measurement of peritoneal lymph flow in CAPD using different osmotic agents. In: Khanna R, Nolph KD, Prowant BF, Twardowski ZJ, Oreopoulos DG, eds. Advances in Peritoneal Dialysis, 1989, pp. 2–15.

19. Koomen GC, Krediet RT, Leegwater ACI, Arisz L, Hoek FJ. A fast reliable method for the measurement of intraperitoneal dextran used to calculate lymphatic absorption. In: Khanna R, Nolph KD, Prowant BF, Twardowski ZJ, Oreopoulos DG, eds. Advances in Peritoneal Dialysis, 1991, pp. 10–14.

20. Hirszel P, Shea-Donohue T, Chakrabarti EK, Montcalm E, Maher JF. The role of the capillary wall in restricting diffusion of macromolecules. A study of peritoneal clearance of dextran. Nephron 1988; 49: 58–61.

21. Charonis AS, Wissig SL. Anionic sites in basement membranes. Differences in their electrostatic properties in continuous and fenestrated capillaries. Microvasc Res 1983; 25: 265–85.

22. Gotloib L, Shustack A, Jaichenko J. Ruthenium-red-stained anionic charges of rat and mice mesothelial cells and basal lamina: the peritoneum is a negatively charged dialyzing membrane. Nephron 1988; 48: 65–70.

23. Leypoldt JK, Henderson LE. Molecular charge influences transperitoneal macromolecule transport. Kidney Int 1993; 43: 837–44.

24. Nakao T, Ogura M, Takahashi H, Okada T. Charge-affected transperitoneal movement of amino acids in CAPD. Perit Dial Int 1996; 16 (suppl. 1): S90.

25. Buis B, Koomen GC, Imholz AL *et al.* Effect of electric charge on the transperitoneal transport of plasma proteins during CAPD (see comments). Nephrol Dial Transplant 1996; 11: 1113–20.

26. Keshaviah P. Adequacy of CAPD: a quantitative approach. Kidney Int 2000; 42 (suppl. 38): S160–4.

27. Rubin J, Clawson M, Planch A, Jones Q. Measurements of peritoneal surface in man and rat. Am J Med Sci 1988; 295: 453–58.

28. Grayson J, Mendel D. Physiology of the Splanchnic Circulation. Baltimore, MD: Williams & Wilkins, 1965.

29. Aune S. Transperitoneal exchange. II: Peritoneal blood flow estimated by hydrogen gas clearances. Scand J Gastroenterol 1970; 5: 99–104.

30. Nolph KD, Popovich R, Ghods J, Twardowski ZJ. Determinants of low clearances of small solutes during peritoneal dialysis. Kidney Int 1978; 13: 117–23.

31. Grzegorzewska AE, Antoniewicz K. An indirect estimation of effective peritoneal capillary blood flow in peritoneally dialyzed uremic patients. Perit Dial Int 1993; 13 (suppl. 2): S39–40.

32. Douma CE, de Waart DR, Struijk DG, Krediet RT. Effect of amino acid based dialysate on peritoneal blood flow and permeability in stable CAPD patients: a potential role for nitric oxide? Clin Nephrol 1996; 45: 295–302.

33. Douma CE, Hiralall JK, de Waart DR, Struijk DG, Krediet RT. Icodextrin with nitroprusside increases ultrafiltration and peritoneal transport during long CAPD dwells (see comments). Kidney Int 1998; 53: 1014–21.

34. Douma CE, de Waart DR, Struijk DG, Krediet RT. The nitric oxide donor nitroprusside intraperitoneally affects peritoneal permeability in CAPD. Kidney Int 1997; 51: 1885–92.

35. Felt J, Richard C, McCaffrey C, Levy M. Peritoneal clearance of creatinine and inulin during dialysis in dogs: effect of splanchnic vasodilators. Kidney Int 1979; 16: 459–69.

36. Renkin EM. Exchange of substances through capillary walls. In: Wolstenholme GEW, ed. Ciba Foundation Symposium. Boston: Little, Brown, 1969, pp. 50–66.

37. Shostak A, Hirszel P, Chakrabarti EK, Maher JF. Dihydroergotamine lowers peritoneal transfer rates; a hypovolemic transport decrease. In: Avram MM, Giordano C, eds. Ambulatory Peritoneal Dialysis. New York: Plenum, 1990, pp. 79–82.

38. Maher JF, Bennett RR, Hirszel P, Chakrabarti EK. The mechanism of dextrose-enhanced peritoneal transport. Kidney Int 1985; 28: 16–20.

39. White R, Korthuis R, Granger DN. The peritoneal microcirculation in peritoneal dialysis. In: Gokal R, Nolph KD, eds. The Textbook of Peritoneal Dialysis. Dordrecht: Kluwer, 1994, pp. 45–68.

40. Flessner MF. Small-solute transport across specific peritoneal tissue surfaces in the rat. J Am Soc Nephrol 1996; 7: 225–33.

41. Ronco C, Chiaramonte S, Brendolan A, Milan M, La Greca G. Peritoneal blood flow: does it matter? Perit Dial Int 1996; 16 (suppl. 1): S70–5.

42. Kim M, Lofthouse J, Flessner MF. A method to test blood flow limitation of peritoneal–blood solute transport. J Am Soc Nephrol 1997; 8: 471–4.

43. Kim M, Lofthouse J, Flessner MF. Blood flow limitations of solute transport across the visceral peritoneum. J Am Soc Nephrol 1997; 8: 1946–50.
44. Swan KG, Reynolds DG. Adrenergic mechanisms in the canine mesenteric circulation. Am J Physiol 1971; 220: 1779–85.
45. Gutman RA, Nixon WP, McRae R, Spencer HW. Effect of intraperitoneal and intravenous vasoactive amines on peritoneal dialysis: study in anephric dogs. Trans Am Soc Artif Intern Organs 1976; 22: 570–3.
46. Parker HR, Schroeder JP, Henderson LW. Influence of dopamine and regitine on peritoneal dialysis in unanesthetized dogs. Am Soc Artif Intern Organs 1978; 7: 43 (abstract).
47. Chan MK, Varghese Z, Baillod RA, Moorhead JF. Peritoneal dialysis: effect of intraperitoneal dopamine. Dial Transplant 1980; 9: 380–4.
48. Hirszel P, Lasrich M, Maher JF. Divergent effects of catecholamines on peritoneal mass transport. Trans Am Soc Artif Intern Organs 1979; 25: 110–12.
49. Hirszel P, Lasrich M, Maher JF. Augmentation of peritoneal mass transport by dopamine. Comparison with norepinephrine and evaluation of pharmacologic mechanisms. J Lab Clin Med 1979; 94: 747–54.
50. Goldberg LI. Cardiovascular and renal actions of dopamine: potential clinical applications. Pharmacol Rev 1972; 24: 1–29.
51. Maher JF, DiPaolo N, Shostack A, Hirszel P. Pharmacology of peritoneal transport. In: Khanna R, Nolph KD, Prowant BF, Twardowski ZJ, Oreopoulos DG, eds. Advances in CAPD. Toronto: University of Toronto Press, 1987, pp. 3–6.
52. Selgas R, Munos IM, Conesa J et al. Endogenous sympathetic activity in CAPD patients: its relationship to peritoneal diffusion capacity. Perit Dial Bull 1986; 6: 205–8.
53. Rocha E, Silva M, Rosenberg M. The release of vasopressin in response to hemorrhage and its role in the mechanism of blood pressure regulation. J Physiol (Lond) 1969; 202: 553–7.
54. Hare HG, Valtin H, Gosselin RE. Effect of drugs on peritoneal dialysis in the dog. J Pharmacol Exp Ther 1964; 145: 122–9.
55. Henderson LW, Kintzel JE. Influence of antidiuretic hormone on peritoneal area and permeability. J Clin Invest 1971; 50: 2437–43.
56. Rubin J, Adair C, Bower J. A double-blind trial dipyridamole in CAPD. Am J Kidney Dis 1985; 5: 262–6.
57. Shear L, Harvey JD, Barry KG. Peritoneal sodium transport: enhancement by pharmacologic and physical agents. J Lab Clin Med 1966; 67: 181–8.
58. Suvannapara A, Levens AR. Local control of mesenteric blood flow by the renin–angiotensin system. Am J Physiol 1988; 225: G267–74.
59. Go M, Kumano K, Sakai T. Effect of angiotensin II (AII) on peritoneal transport during peritoneal dialysis in rat. Nippon-Jinzo-Gakkai-Shi 1992; 34: 921–9.
60. Erbe RW, Greene JA Jr, Weller JM. Peritoneal dialysis during hemorrhagic shock. J Appl Physiol 1967; 22: 131–5.
61. Greene JA Jr, Lapco R, Weller JM. Effect of drug therapy of hemorrhagic hypotension on kinetics of peritoneal dialysis in the dog. Nephron 1970; 7: 178–83.
62. Wayland H. Transmural and interstitial molecular transport. Proc Int Symp Continuous Ambulatory Peritoneal Dialysis 1980; 18–27.
63. Nolph KD. Peritoneal anatomy and transport physiology. In: Drukker W, Parsons FM, Maher JF, eds. Replacement of Renal Function by Dialysis. The Hague: Martinus Nijhoff, 1983, pp. 440–56.
64. Miller FN, Nolph KD, Harris PD et al. Microvascular and clinical effects of altered peritoneal dialysis solutions. Kidney Int 1979; 15: 630–9.
65. Carlsson O, Rippe B. Enhanced peritoneal diffusion capacity of ^{51}Cr-EDTA during the initial phase of peritoneal dialysis dwells: role of vasodilatation, dialysate 'stirring', and of interstitial factors. Blood Purif 1998; 16: 162–70.
66. Breborowicz A, Knapowski J. Local anesthetic bupivicaine increases the transperitoneal transport of solutes. Part II: *In vitro* studies. Perit Dial Bull 1984; 4: 224–8.
67. Brown ST, Ahearn DJ, Nolph KD. Reduced peritoneal clearance in scleroderma increased by intraperitoneal isoproterenol. Ann Int Med 1973; 78: 891–4.
68. Nolph KD, Miller L, Husted FC, Hirszel P. Peritoneal clearance in scleroderma and diabetes mellitus: effects of intraperitoneal isoproterenol. Int Urol Nephrol 1976; 8: 161–9.
69. Nolph KD, Ghods AJ, Van Stone J, Brown PA. The effects of intraperitoneal vasodilators on peritoneal clearances. Trans Am Soc Artif Intern Organs 1976; 22: 586–93.
70. Maher JF, Shea C, Cassetta M, Hohnadel DC. Isoproterenol enhancement of peritoneal permeability. J Dial 1977; 1: 319–31.
71. Thulin L, Samnegard H. Circulatory effects of gastrointestinal hormones and related peptides. Acta Chir Scand 1978; 482 (suppl.): 73–4.
72. Maher JF, Hirszel P, Lasrich M. The effects of gastrointestinal hormones on transport by peritoneal dialysis. Kidney Int 1979; 16: 131–6.
73. Biber B, Fara J, Lundgren O. Vascular reactions in the small intestine during vasodilation. Acta Physiol Scand 1973; 89: 449–56.
74. Fara JW. Effects of gastrointestinal hormones on vascular smooth muscle. Am J Digest Dis 1975; 20: 346–53.
75. Hirszel P, Maher JF, LeGrow W. Increased peritoneal mass transport with glucagon acting at the vascular surface. Trans Am Soc Artif Intern Organs 1978; 24: 136–8.
76. Vane J, Bakhle Y, Botting R. Cyclooxygenases 1 and 2. Annu Rev Pharmacol Toxicol 1998; 38: 97–120.
77. Topley N, Petersen MM, Mackenzie R et al. Human peritoneal mesothelial cell prostaglandin synthesis: induction of cyclooxygenase mRNA by peritoneal macrophage-derived cytokines. Kidney Int 1994; 46. 900–9.
78. Nakano J, McCurdy JR. Hemodynamic effects of prostaglandins E1, A1, and F2 in dogs. Proc Soc Exp Biol Med 1968; 128: 39–42.
79. Messina EJ, Kaley G. Microcirculatory responses to prostacyclin and PGE2 in the rat cremaster muscle. Adv Prostaglandin Thromb Res 1980; 7: 719–22.
80. Vane JR, McGiff JC. Possible contributions of endogenous prostaglandins to the control of blood pressure. Circ Res 1975; 36/37 (suppl. 1): 68–75.
81. Maher JF, Hirszel P, Lasrich M. Modulation of peritoneal transport rates by prostaglandins. Adv Prostaglandin Thromb Res 1980; 7: 695–700.
82. Maher JF, Hirszel B, Lasrich M. Prostaglandin effects on peritoneal transport. Proc 2nd Symp Perit Dial 1981; 2: 65–9.
83. Mileti M, Bufano G, Scaravonati P, Pecchini F, Carnevale G, Lanzarini P. Effect of indomethacin on the peritoneum of rabbits on peritoneal dialysis. Perit Dial Bull 1983; 3: 194–5.
84. Hirszel P, Lasrich M, Maher JF. Arachidonic acid increases peritoneal clearances. Trans Am Soc Artif Intern Organs 1981; 27: 61–3.
85. Steinhauer HB, Schollmeyer P. Prostaglandin-mediated loss of proteins during peritonitis in continuous ambulatory peritoneal dialysis. Kidney Int 1986; 29: 584–90.
86. Zemel D, Struijk DG, Dinkla C, Stolk LM, ten Berge IJ, Krediet RT. Effects of intraperitoneal cyclooxygenase inhibition on inflammatory mediators in dialysate and peritoneal membrane characteristics during peritonitis in continuous ambulatory peritoneal dialysis. J Lab Clin Med 1995; 126: 204–15.
87. Brown EA, Kliger AS, Goffinet J, Finkelstein FO. Effect of hypertonic dialysate and vasodilators on peritoneal dialysis clearances in the rat. Kidney Int 1978; 13: 271–7.
88. Hirszel P, Maher JF, Chamberlin M. Augmented peritoneal mass transport with intraperitoneal nitroprusside. J Dial 1978; 2: 131–142.
89. Raja RM, Kramer MS, Rosenbaum J. Enhanced clearance with intraperitoneal nitroprusside in high flow recirculation

peritoneal dialysis. Trans Am Soc Artif Intern Organs 1978; 24: 133–5.

90. Nolph KD, Ghods AJ, Brown PA, Twardowski ZJ. Effects of intraperitoneal nitroprusside on peritoneal clearances in man with variations of dose frequency of administration and dwell times. Nephron 1979; 24: 114–20.

91. Selgas R, Carmona AR, Martinez ME *et al.* Peritoneal vascular reserve characterization through nitroprusside-induced modification of peritoneal mass transfer coefficients. Int J Artif Organs 1985; 8: 181–6.

92. Londos C, Cooper DMF, Wolff J. Subclasses of external adenosine receptors. Proc Natl Acad Sci USA 1980; 77: 2551–4.

93. Maher JF, Cassetta M, Shea C, Hohnadel DC. Peritoneal dialysis in rabbits. A study of transperitoneal theophylline flux and peritoneal permeability. Nephron 1978; 20: 18–23.

94. Shostak A, Chakrabarti EK, Hirszel B, Maher JF. Effects of histamine and its receptor antagonists on peritoneal permeability. Kidney Int 1988; 34: 786–90.

95. Lal SM, Nolph KD, Moore FL, Khanna R: Effects of calcium channel blockers (verapamil, diltiazem) on the permeability of the peritoneal membrane in patients on continuous ambulatory peritoneal dialysis. Trans Am Soc Artif Intern Organs 1986; 32: 564–6.

96. Kumano K, Go M, Sakai T. Effects of vasodilators on peritoneal solute and fluid transport in rat peritoneal dialysis. Adv Perit Dial 1996; 12: 27–32.

97. Vargemezis V, Pasadakis P, Thodis E. Effect of a calcium antagonist (verapamil) on the permeability of the peritoneal membrane in patients on continuous ambulatory peritoneal dialysis. Blood Purif 1989; 7: 309–13.

98. Balaskas EV, Dombros N, Savidis N, Pidonia I, Lazaridis A, Tourkantonis A. Nifedipine intraperitoneally increases ultrafiltration in CAPD patients. In. Ota K, Maher JF, Winchester J, Hirszel B, eds. Current Concepts in Peritoneal Dialysis. Amsterdam: Excerpta Medica, 1992, pp. 427–32.

99. Favazza A, Montanaro D, Messa P, Antonucci F, Gropuzzo M, Mioni G. Peritoneal clearances in hypertensive patients after oral administration of clonidine, enalapril and nifedipine. Perit Dial Int 1992; 12: 287–91.

100. Lal SM, Moore HL, Nolph KD. Effects of intraperitoneal captopril on peritoneal transport in rats. Perit Dial Bull 1987; 7: 80–5.

101. Ripley EB, Gehr TW, Kish CW, Sica DA. Hormonal, blood pressure, and peritoneal transport response to short-term ACE inhibition. Perit Dial Bull 1994; 14. 378–83.

102. Coronel F, Hortal L, Naranjo P, Cruceyra A, Barrientos A. Captopril, proteinuria and peritoneal protein leakage in diabetic patients. Nephron 1989; 51: 443.

103. Ilker NY, Ozgur S, Cetin S. Effects of papaverine on solute transport in peritoneal dialysis. Int Urol Nephrol 1989; 21: 119–20.

104. Wang T, Cheng H, Heimbürger O *et al.* Atrial natriuretic factor increases peritoneal fluid removal. J Am Soc Nephrol 1997; 8: 183A (abstract).

105. Breborowicz A, Knapowski J. Augmentation of peritoneal dialysis clearance with procaine. Kidney Int 1984; 26: 392–6.

106. Devuyst O, Nielsen S, Cosyns JP *et al.* Aquaporin-1 and endothelial nitric oxide synthase expression in capillary endothelia of human peritoneum. Am J Physiol 1998; 275: H234–42.

107. Douma CE, de Waart DR, Struijk DG, Krediet RT. Are phospholipase A2 and nitric oxide involved in the alterations in peritoneal transport during CAPD peritonitis? J Lab Clin Med 1998; 132: 329–40.

108. Baylis C, Vallance P. Measurement of nitrite and nitrate levels in plasma and urine-what does this measure tell us about the activity of the endogenous nitric oxide system? Curr Opin Nephrol Hypertens 1998; 7: 59–62.

109. Akubeu J, Stochs SJ. Endrin-induced production of nitric oxide by rat peritoneal macrophages. Toxicol Lett 1992; 62: 311–16.

110. Moncada S. Induction of nitric oxide synthase in rat peritoneal neutrophils and its inhibition by dexamethasone. Eur J Immunol 1991; 21: 2523–7.

111. Morrissey JJ, McCracken R, Kaneto H, Vehaskari M, Montani D, Kahr S. Location of an inducible nitric oxide synthase mRNA in the normal kidney. Kidney Int 1994; 45: 998–1005.

112. Combet S, Van Landschoot M, Moulin P *et al.* Regulation of aquaporin-1 and nitric oxide synthase isoforms in a rat model of acute peritonitis. J Am Soc Nephrol 1999; 10: 2185–96.

113. Douma CE, de Waart DR, Zemel D *et al.* Nitrate in stable CAPD patients and during peritonitis. Adv Perit Dial 1995; 11: 36–40.

114. White R, Barefield D, Ram S, Work J. Peritoneal dialysis solutions reverse the hemodynamic effects of nitric oxide synthesis inhibitors. Kidney Int 1995; 48: 1986–93.

115. Breborowicz A, Wieczorowska-Tobis K, Korybalska K, Polubinska A, Radkowski M, Oreopoulos DG. The effect of a nitric oxide inhibitor (L-NAME) on peritoneal transport during dialysis in rats. Perit Dial Bull 1998; 18: 188–92.

116. Sano N, Satoh S, Hashimoto K. Differences among dipyridamole, carbochromen and lidoflazine in responses of the coronary and the renal arteries. Jpn J Pharmacol 1972; 22: 857–65.

117. Maher JF, Hirszel P, Abraham J, Galen MA, Chamberlin M, Hohnadel DC. The effect of dipyridamole on peritoneal mass transport. Am Soc Artif Intern Organs 1977; 23: 219–23.

118. Ryckelynck JP, Pierre D, DeMartin A, Rottembourg J. Amélioration des clairances péritonéales par le dipyridamole. Nouv Presse Méd 1978; 7: 472.

119. Rubin J, Adair C, Barnes T, Bower JD. Augmentation of peritoneal clearance by dipyridamole. Kidney Int 1982; 22: 658–61.

120. Reams GP, Young M, Sorkin M, Twardowski ZJ, Gloor H, Nolph KD. Effects of dipyridamole on peritoneal clearances. Uremia Invest 1986; 9: 27–33.

121. Nolph KD, Stoltz ML, Maher JF. Altered peritoneal permeability in patients with systemic vasculitis. Ann Intern Med 1973; 75: 753–5.

122. Maher JF, Hirszel P. Augmentation of peritoneal clearances by drugs. In: Legrain M, ed. Proc Int Symp Contin Ambul Perit Dial. Amsterdam: Excerpta Medica, 1980, pp. 42–6.

123. Alvai H, Lianos E, Andres G. Effect of protamine on the permeability and structure of rat peritoneum. Kidney Int 1982; 21: 44–53.

124. Galdi P, Shustack A, Jaichenko J, Fudin R, Gotloib L. Protamine sulfate induces enhanced peritoneal permeability to proteins. Nephron 1991; 57: 45–51.

125. Capodicasa G, Capasso G, Anastasio P, Lanzetti N, Giordano C. Changes on peritoneal permeability by charged poly-amino acids. Perit Dial Bull 1987; 7: S13.

126. Pietrzak I, Hirszel B, Maher JF. Poly-*l*-lysine, a cationic macromolecule, increases peritoneal hydraulic and solute permeability. In: Ota K, Maher JF, Winchester J, Hirszel B, eds. Current Concepts in Peritoneal Dialysis. Amsterdam: Excerpta Medica, 1992, pp. 433–8.

127. Maher JF, Pietrzak I, Hirszel P. Role of anions in restricting peritoneal transfer rates. Arq Med 1989; 2: 347–9.

128. Breborowicz A, Rodela H, Bargman J, Oreopoulos DG. Effect of cationic molecules on the permeability of the mesothelium *in vitro*. Perit Dial Bull 1987; 7: S9.

129. Agre P, Bonhivers M, Borgnia MJ. The aquaporins: blueprints for cellular plumbing systems. J Biol Chem 1998; 273: 14659–62.

130. Akiba T, Ota T, Fushimi K *et al.* Water channel AQP1, 3, and 4 in the human peritoneum and peritoneal dialysate. Adv Perit Dial 1997; 13: 3–6.

131. Maher JF, Hohnadel DC, Shea C, DiSanzo F, Cassetta M. Effects of intraperitoneal diuretics on solute transport during hypertonic dialysis. Clin Nephrol 1977; 7: 96–100.

132. Scarpioni L, Ballocchi S, Bergonzi G, Fontana F, Poisetti P, Zanazzi MA. High-dose diuretics in CAPD. Perit Dial Bull 1982; 2: 177–8.

133. Grzegorzewska A, Baczyk K. Furosemide-induced increase in urinary and peritoneal excretion of uric acid during peritoneal dialysis in patients with chronic uremia. Artif Organs 1982; 6: 220–4.

134. Bazzato G, Coli U, Landini S *et al.* Restoration of ultrafiltration capacity of peritoneal membrane in patients on CAPD. Int J Artif Organs 1984; 7: 93–6.

135. Maher JF, Hirszel B, Bennett RR, Chakrabarti EK. Amphotericin B selectively increases peritoneal ultrafiltration. Am J Kidney Dis 1984; 4: 285–8.

136. Maher JF, Hirszel B, Bennett RR, Chakrabarti EK. Augmentation of peritoneal hydraulic permeability by amphotericin B: locus of action. Perit Dial Bull 1984; 4: 229–31.

137. Wang T, Heimbürger O, Bergström J, Lindholm B. Amphotericin B does not increase peritoneal fluid removal. Perit Dial Int 1998; 18 (suppl. 1) (abstract).

138. Stegmayr BG. Beta-blockers may cause ultrafiltration failure in peritoneal dialysis patients. Perit Dial Int 1997; 17: 541–5.

139. Krediet RT. Beta-blockers and ultrafiltration failure – Perit Dial Int 1997; 17: 528–31.

140. Paton TW, Cornish WR, Manuel MA, Hardy BG. Drug therapy in patients undergoing peritoneal dialysis. Clinical pharmacokinetic considerations. Clin Pharmacokin 1985; 10: 404–26.

141. Avasthi PS: Effects of aminonucleoside on rat blood peritoneal barrier permeability. J Lab Clin Med 1979; 94: 295–302.

142. Indrapasit S, Sooksriwongse C. Effects of chlorpromazine on peritoneal clearances. Nephron 1985; 40: 341–3.

143. Mactier RA, Khanna R, Moore H, Twardowski ZJ, Nolph KD. Pharmacological reduction of lymphatic absorption from the peritoneal cavity increases net ultrafiltration and solute clearances in peritoneal dialysis. Nephron 1988; 50: 229–32.

144. Maher J, Hirszel P, Shostack A, DiPaolo N, Chakrabarti EK. Prolonged intraperitoneal dwell decreases ultrafiltration coefficient in rabbits. Am J Kidney Dis 1988; 12: 62–5.

145. Rubin J, Reed V, Adair C, Bower J, Klein E. Effect of intraperitoneal insulin on solute kinetics in CAPD: insulin kinetics in CAPD. Am J Med Sci 1986; 291: 81–7.

146. Twardowski Z.J, Khanna R, Nolph KD: Osmotic agents and ultrafiltration in peritoneal dialysis. Nephron 1986; 42: 93–101.

147. Khanna R, Mactier RA, Twardowski ZJ, Nolph KD. Peritoneal cavity lymphatics. Perit Dial Bull 1986; 6: 113–21.

148. Hasbargen JA, Hasbargen BJ, Fortenberg EJ, James JK. Effects of intraperitoneal neostigmine on peritoneal transport characteristics in CAPD. Kidney Int 1992; 42: 1398–400.

149. Chan PCK, Tam SCF, Cheng IKP. Oral neostigmine and lymphatic absorption in a myasthenia gravis patient on continuous ambulatory peritoneal dialysis. Perit Dial Int 1990; 10: 93–6.

150. Mactier RA, Khanna R, Twardowski ZJ, Moore H, Nolph KD. Influence of phosphatidylcholine on lymphatic absorption during peritoneal dialysis in the rat. Perit Dial Int 1988; 8: 179–86.

151. Krack G, Viglino G, Gandolfo C, Cantaluppi A, Peluso F. Intraperitoneal administration of phosphatidylcholine improves ultrafiltration in continuous ambulatory peritoneal dialysis patients. Perit Dial Int 1992; 12: 359–64.

152. Ersoy FF, Khanna R, Moore H. Effect of phosphatidylcholine on peritoneal fluid kinetics. Perit Dial Int 1992; 12 (suppl. 2): S3.

153. Mactier RA, Khanna R. Absorption of fluid and solutes from the peritoneal cavity: Theoretic and therapeutic implications. ASAIO Trans 1989; 35: 122–31.

154. Flessner MF. Peritoneal transport physiology: insights from basic research. J Am Soc Nephrol 1991; 2: 122–35.

155. Rippe B, Krediet RT. Peritoneal physiology – transport of solutes. In: Gokal R, Nolph KD, ed. Textbook of Peritoneal Dialysis. Dordrecht: Kluwer, 1994, pp. 69–113.

156. Wang T, Heimbürger O, Waniewski J, Bergström J, Lindholm B. Time dependence of solute removal during a single exchange. Adv Perit Dial 1997; 13: 23–8.

157. Wang T, Cheng H, Heimbürger O, Waniewski J, Bergström J, Lindholm B. Hyaluronan prevents the decrease in net fluid removal caused by increased dialysate fill volume. Kidney Int 1998; 53. 496–502.

158. Wang T, Chen C, Heimbürger O, Waniewski J, Bergström J, Lindholm B. Hyaluronan decreases peritoneal fluid absorption in peritoneal dialysis. J Am Soc Nephrol 1997; 8: 1915–20.

159. Fraser JRE, Laurent TC, Laurent UBG. Hyaluronan: its nature, distribution, function and turnover. J Intern Med 1997; 242: 27–33.

160. Wang T, Cheng H, Heimbürger O *et al.* Hyaluronan decreases peritoneal fluid absorption: effect of molecular weight and concentration of hyaluronan. Kidney Int 1999; 55: 667–73.

161. Dobbie JW, Anderson JD. Ultrastructure, distribution, and density of lamellar bodies in human peritoneum. Perit Dial Int 1996; 16: 488–96.

162. Breborowicz A, Korybalska K, Grzybowski A *et al.* Synthesis of hyaluronic acid by human peritoneal mesothelial cells: effect of cytokines and dialysate. Perit Dial Int 1996; 16: 374–8.

163. Heldin P, Pertoft H. Synthesis and assembly of the hyaluronan-containing coats around normal human mesothelial cells. Exp Cell Res 1993; 208: 422–9.

164. Breborowicz A, Wieczorowska-Tobis K, Kuzlan M *et al.* N-acetylglucosamine: a new osmotic solute in peritoneal dialysis solutions. Perit Dial Int 1997; 17 (suppl. 2): S80–3.

165. Wu G, Breborowicz A, Korybalska K, Tam P, French I. Use of N-acetyl-glucosamine as osmotic agent for peritoneal dialysis. Perit Dial Int 1996; 16: (suppl. 2): S16.

166. Wu G, Wieczorowska-Tobis K, Polubinska A *et al.* N-acetylglucosamine changes permeability of peritoneum during chronic peritoneal dialysis in rats. Perit Dial Bull 1998; 18: 217–24.

167. Comper WD, Laurent TC. Physiological function of connective tissue polysaccharides. Physiol Rev 1978; 58: 255–325.

168. Wieczorowska-Tobis K, Breborowicz A, Martis L, Oreopoulos DG. Protective effect of hyaluronic acid against peritoneal injury. Perit Dial Bull 1995; 15: 81–3.

169. Breborowicz A, Wieczorowska K, Martis L, Oreopoulos DG. Glycosaminoglycan chondroitin sulphate prevents loss of ultrafiltration during peritoneal dialysis in rats. Nephron 1994; 67: 346–50.

170. Bazzato G, Fracasso A, Baggio B. Use of glycosaminoglycans to increase efficiency of long-term continuous peritoneal dialysis. Lancet 1995; 346: 740–1.

171. Breborowicz A, Wieczorowska K, Knapowski J, Martis L, Serkes KD, Oreopoulos DG. Chondroitin sulphate and peritoneal permeability. Adv Perit Dial 1992; 8: 11–14.

172. Breborowicz A, Radkowski M, Knapowski J, Oreopoulos DG. Effects of chondroitin sulphate on fluid and solute transport during peritoneal dialysis in rats. Perit Dial Int 1991; 11: 351–4.

173. Breborowicz A, Wieczorowska K, Knapowski J, Martis L, Serkes KD, Oreopoulos DG. Chondroitin sulphate and peritoneal permeability. Adv Perit Dial 1992; 8: 11–14.

174. Van Biesen W, Waterloos M, Vogeleere P, Naggi A, Lameire N. Use of chondroitin sulphate as additive to glucose containing dialysate. Perit Dial Int 1999; 19: S11 (abstract).

175. Grahame G, Torchia M, Dankewich K, Ferguson I. Surface active material in peritoneal effluent of CAPD patients. Perit Dial Bull 1985; 5: 109–11.

176. DiPaolo N, Buoncristiani U, Capotundo L, Saggiotti E, Sansoni E, Bernini M. Phosphatidylcholine and peritoneal

transcript during peritoneal dialysis. Nephron 1986; 44: 365–70.

177. Breborowicz A, Sombolos K, Rodela H, Ogilvie R, Bargman J, Oreopoulos DG. Mechanism of phosphatidylcholine action during peritoneal dialysis. Perit Dial Bull 1987; 7: 9.

178. De Vecchi A, Castelnovo J, Guerra L, Scalamonga A. Phosphatidylcholine administration in continuous ambulatory peritoneal dialysis patients with reduced ultrafiltration. Perit Dial Int 1989; 9: 207–10.

179. De Alvaro F, Selgas R. Oral phosphatidylcholine effects on peritoneal MTCs in CAPD patients. Abstracts of the 15th EDTA Congress, 1988; 93 (abstract).

180. Breborowicz A, Witowski J, Knapowski J, Serkes KD, Martis L, Oreopoulos DG. Effect of phosphatidylcholine on the function of human mesothelial cells *in vitro*. Nephron 1993; 63: 15–20.

181. Penzotti SC, Mattocks AM. Effects of dwell time, volume of dialysis fluid and added accelerators on peritoneal dialysis of urea. J Pharm Sci 1975; 60: 1520–2.

182. Penzotti SC, Mattocks AM. Acceleration of peritoneal dialysis by surface-active agents. J Pharm Sci 1968; 57: 1192–5.

183. Dunham CB, Hak LJ, Hull JH, Mattocks AM. Enhancement of peritoneal permeability of the rat by intraperitoneal use of docusate sodium. Kidney Int 1981; 20: 563–8.

184. Wang T, Qureshi A, Heimbürger O *et al.* Dioctyl sodium sulphosuccinate increases net ultrafiltration in peritoneal dialysis. Nephrol Dial Transplant 1997; 12: 1218–22.

185. Hirzsel B, Dodge K, Maher JF. Acceleration of peritoneal solute transport by cytochalasin D. Uremia Invest 1985; 8: 85–9.

186. Alavi N, Lianos E, van Liew JB, Mookerjee BK, Bentzel CJ. Peritoneal permeability in the rat: modulation by microfilament-active agents. Kidney Int 1985; 27: 411–19.

187. Breborowicz A, Witowski J, Martis L, Oreopoulos DG. Enhancement of viability of human peritoneal mesothelial cells with glutathione precursor: L-2-oxothiazolidine-4-carboxylate. Adv Perit Dial 1993; 9: 21–4.

188. Korybalska K, Breborowicz A, Wieczorowska-Tobis K *et al.* Alterations of intraperitoneal inflammation by the addition of L-2-oxothiazolidine-carboxylate. Adv Perit Dial 1997; 13: 197–200.

189. Wieczorowska-Tobis K, Breborowicz A, Witowski J, Martis L, Oreopoulos DG. Effect of vitamin E on peroxidation and permeability of the peritoneum. J Physiol Pharmacol 1996; 47: 535–43.

190. Witowski J, Breborowicz A, Knapowski J. Effect of methotrexate, doxorubicin and mitoxantrone on human peritoneal mesothelial cell function *in vitro*. Oncology 1995; 52: 60–5.

191. Witowski J, Breborowicz A, Topley N, Martis L, Knapowski J, Oreopoulos DG. Insulin stimulates the activity of $Na^+/K(+)$-ATPase in human peritoneal mesothelial cells. Perit Dial Int 1997; 17: 186–93.

192. Knochel JP, Clayton LE, Smith WL, Barry KG. Intraperitoneal THAM: an effective method to enhance phenobarbital removal during peritoneal dialysis. J Lab Clin Med 1964; 64: 257–68.

193. Campion DAS, North JDK. Effect of protein binding of barbiturates on their rate of removal during peritoneal dialysis. J Lab Clin Med 1965; 66: 549–63.

194. Schultz JC, Crouder DG, Medart WS. Excretion studies in ethchlorvynol (Placidyl) intoxication. Arch Intern Med 1966; 117: 409–11.

195. Etteldorf JN, Dobbins WT, Summit RL, Rainwater WT, Fisher RL. Intermittent peritoneal dialysis using 5% albumin in the treatment of salicylate intoxication in children. J Pediatr 1961; 58: 226–36.

196. Shinaberger JH, Shear L, Clayton LE, Barry KG, Knowlton M, Goldbaun LR. Dialysis for intoxication with lipid-soluble drugs: enhancement of glutethimide extraction with lipid dialysate. Trans Am Soc Artif Intern Organs 1965; 11: 173–7.

197. Leypoldt JK, Henderson LW. Molecular charge influences macromolecular transport. Kidney Int 1993; 43: 837–44.

198. Ho-dac Pannekeet MM, Krediet RT. Water channels in the peritoneum (editorial). Perit Dial Int 1996; 16: 255–9.

199. Swartz RD, Starmann B, Horvath A, Olson S, Posvar EL. Pharmacokinetics of quinapril and its active metabolite quinaprilate during continuous ambulatory peritoneal dialysis. J Clin Pharmacol 1990; 30: 1136–40.

200. Rowland M, Tozer TN. Clinical Pharmacokinetics – Concepts and Applications. Baltimore, MD: Williams & Wilkins, 1995.

201. Benet LZ, Kroetz DL, Sheiner LB. Pharmacokinetics – The dynamics of drug absorption, distribution, and elimination. In: Hardman JG, Limbird LE, Molinoff PB, Ruddon RW, Goodman Gilman A, eds. Goodman & Gilman's The Pharmacological Basis of Therapeutics. New York: McGraw-Hill, 1996, pp. 3–27.

202. Benet LZ, Obie S, Schwartz JB. Design and optimization of dosage regimens; pharmacokinetic data. In: Hardman JG, Limbird LE, Molinoff PB, Ruddon RW, Goodman Gilman A, eds. Goodman & Gilman's The Pharmacological Basis of Therapeutics. New York: McGraw-Hill, 1996, pp. 1707–92.

203. Lasrich M, Maher JM, Hirzsel P, Maher JF. Correlation of peritoneal transport rates with molecular weight: a method for predicting clearances. ASAIO J 1979; 2: 107–13.

204. Maher JF. Peritoneal transport rates: mechanisms, limitations and methods for augmentation. Kidney Int 1980; 18: S117–20.

205. Deguchi Y, Nakashima E, Ishikawa F *et al.* Peritoneal transport of betalactam antibiotics: effects of plasma protein binding and the inter species relationship. J Pharm Sciences 1988; 77: 559–64.

206. Flessner MF, Dedrick RL, Schultz JS. Exchange of macromolecules between peritoneal cavity and plasma. Am J Physiol 1985; 248: H21–5.

207. Keller E, Reetze P, Schollmeyer P. Drug therapy in patients undergoing continuous ambulatory peritoneal dialysis. Clinical pharmacokinetic considerations. Clin Pharmacokin 1990; 18: 104–17.

208. Morse GD, Rowinski CA, Lieveld PE, Walshe JJ. Drug protein binding during continuous ambulatory peritoneal dialysis. Perit Dial Int 1988; 6: 144–7.

209. Janknegt R, Nube MJ. A simple method for predicting drug clearances during CAPD. Perit Dial Bull 1985; 5: 254–5.

210. Lee CC, Marbury TC. Drug therapy in patients undergoing hemodialysis. Clinical pharmacokinetic considerations. Clin Pharmacokin 1984; 9: 42–66.

211. Lameire N, Belpaire FM. Pharmacokinetics of antibiotics against gram-negative infections in continuous ambulatory peritoneal dialysis. Perit Dial Int 1993; 13 (suppl. 2): S371–6.

212. Fleming LW, Moreland TA, Scott AC, Stewart WK, White LD. Ciprofloxacin in plasma and peritoneal dialysate after oral therapy in patients in CAPD. J Antimicrob Chemother 1987; 19: 494–503.

213. Harford AM, Sica DA, Tartaglione T, Polk RE, Dalton HP, Poynor W. Vancomycin pharmacokinetics in continuous ambulatory peritoneal dialysis patients with peritonitis. Nephron 1986; 43: 217–22.

214. Verbrugh HA, Keane WF, Conroy WE, Peterson PK. Bacterial growth and killing in chronic ambulatory peritoneal dialysis fluids. J Clin Microbiol 1984; 20: 199–203.

215. Weissauer-Condon C, Engels I, Daschner FD. *In vitro* activity of four new quinolones in Mueller–Hinton broth and peritoneal dialysis fluid. Eur J Clin Microbiol 1987; 6: 324–6.

216. Halstead DC, Guzzo J, Giardina JA, Geshan AE. *In vitro* bactericidal activities of gentamicin, cefazolin, and imipenem in peritoneal dialysis fluids. Antimicrob Agents Chemother 1989; 33: 1553–6.

217. Wilcox MH, Smith DGE, Evans JA, Denyer SP, Finck RG, Williams P. Influence of carbon dioxide on growth and antibiotic susceptibility of coagulase-negative staphylococci cultures in human peritoneal dialysate. J Clin Microbiol 1990; 28: 2183–6.

218. Morgera S, Neumayer HH, Fritsche L *et al*. Pharmacokinetics of mycophenolate mofetil in renal transplant recipients on peritoneal dialysis. Int J Clin Pharmacol Ther Toxicol 1998; 36: 159–63.

219. Lukas G, Brindle SD, Greengard P. The route of absorption of intraperitoneally administered compounds. J Pharmacol Exp Ther 1971; 178: 562–6.

220. Bailie GR, Eisele G, Venezia RA, Yoeum D, Hollister A. Prediction of serum vancomycin concentrations following intraperitoneal loading doses in continuous ambulatory peritoneal dialysis patients with peritonitis. Clin Pharmacokin 1992; 22: 298–307.

221. Brouard R, Kapusnik JE, Gambertoglio JF *et al*. Teicoplanin pharmacokinetics and bioavailability during peritoneal dialysis. Clin Pharmacol Ther 1989; 45: 674–81.

222. Gotloib L, Bar-Sella P, Jaichenko J, Shostack A. Ruthenium-red stained polyanionic fixed charges in peritoneal microvessels. Nephron 1987; 47: 22–8.

223. Gotloib L, Shustack A, Jaichenko J. Loss of mesothelial and microvascular fixed anionic charges during murine experimentally induced septic peritonitis. Nephron 1989; 51: 77–83.

224. De Paepe M, Lameire N. Peritoneal pharmacokinetics of gentamicin in man. Clin Nephrol 1983; 19: 107–9.

225. Rubin J, Deraps GD, Walsh D, Adair C, Bower J. Protein losses and tobramycin absorption in peritonitis treated by hourly peritoneal dialysis. Am J Kidney Dis 1986; 8: 124–7.

226. Regany C, Schaberg D, Kiroy W. Inhibitory effect of heparin on gentamicin concentrations of blood. Antimicrob Agents Chemother 1972; 4: 329–32.

227. Ponce SP, Barata JD, Santos R. Interference of heparin with peritoneal solute transport. Nephron 1985; 39: 47–9.

228. Kuzuya T, Hasegawa T, Shiraki R, Nabeshima T. Structure-related pharmacokinetics of xanthines after direct administration into the peritoneal cavity of rats. Biol Pharmacol Bull 1997; 20: 1051–5.

229. Hadler N. Enhanced diffusivity of glucose in a matrix of hyaluronic acid. J Biol Chem 1980; 255: 3532–5.

230. Mactier RA, Moore H, Khanna R, Shah J. Effect of peritonitis on insulin and glucose absorption during peritoneal dialysis in diabetic rats. Nephron 1990; 54: 240–4.

231. Wideröe TE, Dahl KJ, Smeby LC *et al*. Pharmacokinetics of transperitoneal insulin transport. Nephron 1996; 74: 283–90.

232. Fine RN, Fine SE, Sherman BM. Absorption of recombinant human growth hormone (rhGH) following intraperitoneal instillation. Perit Dial Int 1989; 9: 91–3.

233. Lameire N, Bogaert M. Peritoneal pharmacokinetics and pharmacological manipulation of peritoneal transport. In: Gokal R, ed. Contiuous Ambulatory Peritoneal Dialysis. Edinburgh: Churchill Livingstone, 1986, pp. 56–93.

234. Maher JF. Influence of continuous ambulatory peritoneal dialysis on elimination of drugs. Perit Dial Bull 1987; 7: 159–67.

235. Sewell DL, Golper TA. Stability of antimicrobial agents in peritoneal dialysate. Antimicrob Agents Chemother 1982; 21: 528–9.

236. Sewell DL, Golper TA, Brown SD, Nelson E, Knower M, Kimbrough RD. Stability of single and combination antimicrobial agents in various peritoneal dialysates in the presence of insulin and heparin. Am J Kidney Dis 1983; 3: 209–12.

237. Janknegt R, Koks CHW, Nube MJ. Stability of antibiotics in CAPD fluid. Perit Dial Bull 1985; 5: 78.

238. Kehoe WA, Weber JN, Fries DS. The stability and comparability of clindamycin phosphate and gentamicin sulfate alone and in combination with peritoneal dialysis solution. Perit Dial Bull 1988; 8: 153–4.

239. Mason NA, Johnson CE, O'Brien MA. Stability of ceftazidime and tobramycin sulfate in peritoneal dialysis solution. Am J Hosp Pharm 1993; 49: 1139–42.

240. Bastani B, Spijker DA, Westervelt FB. Peritoneal absorption of vancomycin during and after resolution of peritonitis in continuous ambulatory peritoneal dialysis patients. Perit Dial Bull 1988; 8: 135–6.

241. Imada A, Itagaki N, Hasegawa H, Horiuchi A. Comparative study of the pharmacokinetics of various beta-lactams after intravenous and intraperitoneal administration in patients undergoing continuous ambulatory peritoneal dialysis. Drugs 1988; 35: 82–7.

242. Ryckelynck JP, Debruyne D, Hurault de Ligny B, Moulin M. Pharamacocinétique de la pipéracilline en dialyse péritonéale continue ambulatoire. Pathol Biol 1988; 36: 507–10.

243. Low CL, Bailie GR, Evans A, Eisele G, Venezia RA. Pharmacokinetics of once-daily IP gentamicin in CAPD patients. Perit Dial Int 1996; 16: 379–84.

244. Husserl F, Back S. Intraperitoneal vancomycin and the 'red man' syndrome. Perit Dial Bull 1987; 7: 262 (letter).

245. Fabris A, Biasioli S, Borin D, Brendolan A, Chiaramonte S. Fungal peritonitis in peritoneal dialysis: our experience and review of treatment. Perit Dial Bull 1984; 4: 75–7.

246. Mandell IN, Ahern MJ, Klier AS, Andriole VI. *Candida* peritonitis complicating peritoneal dialysis: successful treatment with low dose amphotericin B therapy. Clin Nephrol 1976; 6: 192–6.

247. Struijk DG, Krediet RT, Boeschoten EW, Rietra O, Arisz L. Antifungal treatment of Candida peritonitis in continuous ambulatory peritoneal dialysis. Am J Kidney Dis 1987; 9: 66–70.

248. Benevent D, El Akoum N, Lagarde C. Danger de l'administration intrapéritonéale de l'amphotéricine B au cours de la dialyse péritonéale continue ambulatoire. La Presse Méd 1984; 13: 1844.

249. Piraino B, Bernardini J, Johnston J, Sorkin M. Chemical peritonitis due to intraperitoneal vancomycin (Vancoled). Perit Dial Bull 1987; 7: 156–9.

250. Steiner RW. Adverse effects of intraperitoneal methylene blue. Perit Dial Bull 1983; 3: 43 (letter).

251. Bonner G, Lukowski K. Angiotensin I in peritoneal dialysis fluid improved hypotension. Clin Nephrol 1987; 27: 99–101.

252. Peters U, Risler T, Grabensee B. Pharmacokinetics of digoxin with end-stage renal failure treated with continuous ambulatory peritoneal dialysis. Kidney Int 1981; 20: 159 (abstract).

253. Demedts W, Desaer JP, Belpaire F, Ringoir S, Lameire N. Life-threatening hyperkalemia associated with clofibrate-induced myopathy in a CAPD patient. Perit Dial Bull 1983; 3: 15–16.

254. Johnson RJ, Blair AD, Ahmad S. Ketoconazole kinetics in chronic peritoneal dialysis. Clin Pharmacol Ther 1985; 37: 325–7.

255. Belpaire FM, Van de Velde EJ, Fraeyman NH, Bogaert MG, Lameire N. Influence of continuous ambulatory peritoneal dialysis on serum alpha-1-acid glycoprotein concentrations and drug binding. Eur J Clin Pharmacol 1988; 35: 339–43.

256. Haughy DB, Krafat CJ, Matzke GR, Keane WF, Halstenson CE. Protein binding of disopyramide and elevated alpha-1-glycoprotein concentrations in serum obtained from dialysis patients and renal transplant patients. Am J Nephrol 1985; 5: 35–9.

257. Shuler C, Golper TA, Bennett WM. Prescribing drugs in renal disease. In: Brenner BM, ed. The Kidney. Philadelphia, PA: WB Saunders, 1996, pp. 2653–702.

258. Hirszel B, Lameire N, Bogaert M. Pharmacology and pharmacokinetics in peritoneal dialysis. In: Nolph KD, Gokal R, eds. Textbook of Peritoneal Dialysis. Dordrecht: Kluwer, 1994, pp. 161–232.

259. Pancorbo S, Comty C. Digoxin pharmacokinetics in continuous ambulatory peritoneal dialysis. Ann Intern Med 1980; 93: 639.

260. De Paoli Vitali E, Casol D, Tessarin C, Tisone GF, Cavogna R. Pharmacokinetics of digoxin in CAPD. In: Gahl GM, Kessel M, Nolph KD, eds. Advances in Peritoneal Dialysis. Amsterdam: Excerpta Med, 1981, pp. 85–7.

261. Risler T, Peters U, Passlick J, Grabensee B, Krokou J. Pharmacokinetics of digoxin and digitoxin in patients on chronic ambulatory peritoneal dialysis. In: Gahl GM, Kessel M, Nolph KD, eds. Advances in Peritoneal Dialysis. Amsterdam: Excerpta Med, 1981, pp. 88–9.

262. De Paepe M, Belpaire F, Bogaerts Y. Pharmacokinetics of digoxin in CAPD. Clin Exp Dial Apheresis 1982; 6: 65–73.

263. Gloor HJ, Moore H, Nolph KD: The peritoneal handling of digoxin during CAPD. Perit Dial Bull 1982; 2: 13–16.

264. Chin TWF, Pancorbo S, Compty C. Quinidine pharmacokinetics in contiuous ambulatory peritoneal dialysis. Clin Exp Dial Apheresis 1981; 5: 391–7.

265. Yamakado M, Umezu M, Nagano M, Tagawa H. Pharmacokinetics of denopamine in patients on continuous ambulatory peritoneal dialysis. In: Ota K, Maher JF, Winchester J, eds. Current Concepts in Peritoneal Dialysis. Amsterdam' Excerpta Med, 1992, pp. 441–4.

266. Halstenson CE, Opsahl JA, Pence TV *et al.* The disposition and dynamics of labetolol in patients on dialysis. Clin Pharmacol Ther 1986; 40: 462–8.

267. Parrott KA, Alexander SE, Stennett DJ. Loss of propranolol via CAPD in two patients. Perit Dial Bull 1984; 2: 110 (abstract).

268. Salahudeen AK, Wilkinson R, McAinsh J, Batemax DN. Atenolol pharmacokinetics in patients on continuous ambulatory peritoneal dialysis. Br J Clin Pharmacol 1984; 18: 457–60.

269. Flaherty JF, Wong B, La Follette G, Warnock DG, Hulse JD, Gambertoglio JG. Pharmacokinetics of esmolol and ASL-8123 in renal failure. Clin Pharmacol Ther 1989; 45: 321–7.

270. Bianchetti G, Padovani P, Thenot JP, Thiercelin JF, Martin-Dupont C, Morselli L. Betaxolol disposition in chronic renal insufficiency, hemodialysis and ambulatory peritoneal dialysis. Eur J Clin Invest 1982; 12S: 3A (abstract).

271. Spital A, Scandling JD. Nifedipine in continuous ambulatory peritoneal dialysis. Arch Intern Med 1983; 143: 2025 (letter).

272. Evers J, Bonn R, Boertz A *et al.* Pharmacokinetics of isosorbide-5-nitrate during hemodialysis and peritoneal dialysis. Eur J Clin Pharmacol 1987; 32: 503–5.

273. Grech-Belanger O, Langlois S, Leboeuf E. Pharmacokinetics of diltiazem in patients undergoing contiuous ambulatory peritoneal dialysis. J Clin Pharmacol 1988; 28: 477–80.

274. Fujimora A, Kajiyama H, Ebihara A, Iwashita K, Nomura Y, Kawahara Y. Pharmacokinetics and pharmacodynamics of captopril in patients undergoing continuous ambulatory peritoneal dialysis. Nephron 1986; 44: 324–8.

275. Wolter K, Fritschka E. Pharmacokinetics and pharmacodynamics of quinaprilat after low dose of quinapril in patients with terminal renal failure. Eur J Clin Pharmacol 1993; 44 (suppl. 1): S53–6.

276. Gehr TWB, Sica DA, Grasela DM, Fakhry I, Davis J, Duchin KL. Fosinopril pharmacokinetics and pharmacodynamics in chronic ambulatory peritoneal dialysis. Eur J Clin Pharmacol 1991; 41: 165–9.

277. Rottembourg J, Issad B, Guerret M, Lavene D, Baumelou A, Kiechel JR. Particularités d'utilisation de la guanfacine chez l'insuffisant rénal traité par dialyse péritonéale continue ambulatoire. In: Structures cérébrales et contrôle tensionnel. Paris: Sandoz, 1983, pp. 165–72.

278. Raehl CL, Beirne GJ, Moorthy AV, Patel AK. Tocainide pharmacokinetics during continuous ambulatory peritoneal dialysis. Am J Cardiol 1987; 60: 747–50.

279. Bailie GR, Waldek S. Pharmacokinetics of flecainide in a patient undergoing continuous ambulatory peritoneal dialysis. J Clin Pharmacol Ther 1988; 13: 121–4.

280. Low CL, Phelps KR, Bailie GR. Relative efficacy of haemoperfusion, haemodialysis and CAPD in the removal of procainamide and NAPA in a patient with severe procanamide toxicity. Nephrol Dial Transplant 1996; 11: 881–4.

281. Sica DA, Yonce C, Small R, Cefali E, Harford A, Poynor W. Pharmacokinetics of procainamide in continuous ambula-

282. tory peritoneal dialysis. Int J Clin Pharmacol Ther Toxicol 1988; 26: 59–64.

282. Bourtron H, Singlas E, Brocard JF, Charpentier B, Fries D. Pharmacocinétique clinique du furosémide au cours de la dialyse péritonéale continue ambulatoire. Thérapie 1985; 40: 155–9.

283. Baumelou A, Singlas E, Merdjan H *et al.* Pharmacocinétique des médicaments administrés par voie générale chez les malades traités par dialyse péritonéale continue ambulatoire. Sém Urol Néphrol 1985; 11: 124–36.

284. Martin V, Winne R, Prescott LF. Frusemide disposition in patients on continuous ambulatory peritoneal dialysis. Br J Clin Pharmacol 1991; 31: 227–8.

285. Lee CSG, Peterson JC, Marbury TC. Comparative pharmacokinetics of theophylline in peritoneal dialysis and hemodialysis. J Clin Pharmacol 1983; 23: 274–80.

286. Jones TE, Reece PA, Fisher GC. Mexiletine removal by peritoneal dialysis. Eur J Clin Pharmacol 1983; 25: 839–40.

287. Olson S, Horvath A, Michniewicz B. The clinical pharmacokinetics of quinapril. Angiology 1989; 40: 351–9.

288. Hoyer J, Schulte KL, Lenz T. Clinical pharmacokinetics of angiotensin converting enzyme inhibitors in renal failure. Clin Pharmacokin 1993; 24: 230–54.

289. Blackwell BG, Leggett JE, Johnston CA, Zimmerman SW, Craig WA. Ampicillin and Sulbactam pharmacokinetics and pharmacodynamics in continuous ambulatory peritoneal dialysis. Perit Dial Int 1990; 10: 221–6.

290. Somani P, Freimer EH, Gross ML, Higgins JT. Pharmacokinetics of Imipenem–Cilastatin in patients with renal insufficiency undergoing continuous ambulatory peritoneal dialysis. Antimicrob Agents Chemother 1988; 36: 530–4.

291. Chan CY, Lai KN, Lam AW, Li PKT, Chung WWM, French GL. Pharmacokinetics of parenteral imipenem/cilastatin in patients on continuous ambulatory peritoneal dialysis. J Antimicrob Chemother 1991; 27: 225–32.

292. Debruyne D, Ryckelynck JP, Hurault de Ligny B, Moulin M. Pharmacokinetics of piperacillin in patients on peritoneal dialysis with and without peritonitis. J Pharmacokine Sci 1990; 79: 99–102.

293. Johnston CA, Halstenson CE, Kelloway JS *et al.* Single dose pharmacokinetics of piperacillin and tazobactam in patients with renal disease. Clin Pharmacol Ther 1992; 51: 32–41.

294. Johnson CA, Halstenson CE, Kelloway JS *et al.* Single-dose pharmacokinetics of piperacillin and tazobactam in patients with renal disease. Clin Pharmacol Ther 1992; 51: 32–41.

295. Boelaert J, Daneels R, Schurgers M *et al.* Effect of renal function and dialysis on temocillin pharmacokinetics. Drugs 1985; 29 (suppl. 5): 109–13.

296. Pancorbo S, Compty C. Pharmacokinetics of cefamandole in patients undergoing continuous ambulatory peritoneal dialysis. Perit Dial Bull 1983; 3: 135–7.

297. Janicke DM, Morse GD, Apicella MA, Jusko WJ, Walshe JJ. Pharmacokinetic modeling of bidirectional transfer during peritoneal dialysis. Clin Pharmacol Ther 1986; 40: 209–18.

298. Bliss M, Mayersohn M, Arnold T, Logan J, Michael UF, Jones W. Disposition kinetics of cefamandole during continuous ambulatory peritoneal dialysis. Antimicrob Agents Chemother 1986; 29: 649–53.

299. Bunke CM, Aronoff GR, Brier ME, Sloan R, Luft FC. Cefalozin and cephalexin kinetics in continuous ambulatory peritoneal dialysis. Clin Pharmacol Ther 1983; 33: 66–72.

300. Paton TW, Manuel A, Cohen LB, Walker SE. The disposition of cefazolin and tobramycin following intraperitoneal administration in patients on CAPD. Perit Dial Bull 1983; 3: 73–6.

301. Morrison G, Audet P, Peingold R, Murray T. Cefazolin: the cephalosporin antibiotic of choice in CAPD patients. Kidney Int 1999; 21: 174 (abstract).

302. Barbhaiya RH, Knupp CA, Pfeffer M *et al.* Pharmacokinetics of cefepime in patients undergoing continuous

ambulatory peritoneal dialysis. Antimicrob Agents Chemother 1992; 36: 1387–91.

303. Okamoto MP, Nakahiro RK, Chin A, Bedikian A. Cefepime clinical pharmacokinetics. Clin Pharmacokin 1993; 25: 88–102.

304. Mendes P, Lameire N, Rozenkranz B, Malerczyk V, Damm D. Pharmacokinetics of cefodizime during continuous ambulatory peritoneal dialysis. J Antimicrob Chemother 1990; 26 (suppl. C): 89–93.

305. Keller E, Jansen A, Pels K, Hoppe-Seyler G, Schurgers M. Intraperitoneal and intravenous cefoperazone kinetics during continuous ambulatory peritoneal dialysis. Clin Pharmacol Ther 1984; 35: 208–13.

306. Hodler JE, Geleazzi RL, Frey B, Rudhardt M, Seiler AJ. Pharmacokinetics of cefoperazone in patients undergoing chronic ambulatory peritoneal dialysis: clinical and pathophysiological implications. Eur J Clin Pharmacol 1984; 26: 609–12.

307. Johnston CA, Zimmerman SW, Reitberg DP, Whall TJ, Leggett JE, Craig WA. Pharmacokinetics and pharmacodynamics of Cefoperazone-Sulbactam in patients on continuous ambulatory peritoneal dialysis. Antimicrob Agents Chemother 1988; 32: 51–6.

308. Leehey DJ, Leid R, Chan AY, Ing TS. Cefoperazone in the treatment of peritonitis in continuous ambulatory peritoneal dialysis. Artif Organs 1988; 12: 482–3.

309. Schuring R, Kampf D, Spieber W, Weihermuller K, Becker H. Cefotaxime pharmacokinetics in peritoneal dialysis. In: Gokal GM, Kessel M, Nolph KD, eds. Advances in Peritoneal Dialysis. Amsterdam: Excerpta Medica, 1981, pp. 96–8.

310. Alexander D, Bamertoglio J, Barriere S, Warnock D, Schoenfeld P. Cefotaxime pharmacokinetics during continuous ambulatory peritoneal dialysis. Clin Pharmacol Ther 1984; 35: 225 (abstract).

311. Matouscovic K, Moravek J, Vitko S, Prat V, Horcickova M. Pharmacokinetics of intravenous and intraperitoneal cefotaxime in patients undergoing CAPD. Perit Dial Bull 1985; 5: 33–5.

312. Albin HC, Demotes-Mainrad FM, Bouchet JL, Vincon GA, Martin-Dupont C. Pharmacokinetics of intravenous and intraperitoneal cefotaxime in chronic ambulatory peritoneal dialysis. Clin Pharmacol Ther 1985; 38: 285–9.

313. Heim KL, Halstenson CE, Comty C, Affrime MB, Matzke GR. Disposition of cefotaxime and desacetyl cefotaxime during continuous ambulatory peritoneal dialysis. Antimicrob Agents Chemother 1986; 30: 15–19.

314. Hasegawa H, Imada A, Horiuchi A, Nishii Y, Fukushima M, Kurokawa E. Pharmacokinetics of cefotaxime in patients undergoing hemodialysis and continuous ambulatory peritoneal dialysis. J Antimicrob Chemother 1984; 14 (suppl. B): 135–42.

315. Petersen J, Stewart RDM, Catto GRD, Edward N. Pharmacokinetics of intraperitoneal cefotaxime treatment of peritonitis in patients on continuous ambulatory peritoneal dialysis. Nephron 1985; 40: 78–82.

316. Overgaard S, Lokkegaard N, Scroder S, Fugleberg S, Nielsen-Kudsk F. Cefotaxime disposition pharmacokinetics during peritoneal dialysis. Pharmacol Toxicol 1987; 60: 321–4.

317. Raap CM, Nahata MC, Mentser MA, Mahan JD, Puri SK, Hubbard JA. Cefotaxime and metabolite disposition in two pediatric continuous ambulatory peritoneal dialysis patients. Ann Pharmacother 1992; 26: 341–3.

318. Bald M, Rascher W, Bonzel KA, Muller-Wiefel DE. Pharmacokinetics of intraperitoneal cefotaxime in children with peritonitis undergoing continuous ambulatory peritoneal dialysis. Perit Dial Int 1990; 10: 311–13.

319. Browning MJ, Holt HA, White LO et al. Pharmacokinetics of cefotetam in patients with end-stage renal failure on maintenance dialysis. J Antimicrob Chemother 1986; 18: 103–6.

320. Brouard R, Tozer TN, Merdjan H, Guillemin A, Beaumelou A. Transperitoneal movement and pharmacokinetics of cefo-

tiam and cefsulodin in patients on continuous ambulatory peritoneal dialysis. Clin Nephrol 1988; 30: 197–206.

321. Greaves WL, Kreeft JH, Ogilvie RI, Richards GK. Cefoxitin disposition during peritoneal dialysis. Antimicrob Agents Chemother 1981; 22: 253–5.

322. Arvidsson A, Alvan G, Tranaeus A, Malmborg AS. Pharmacokinetic studies of cefoxitin in continuous ambulatory peritoneal dialysis. Eur J Clin Pharmacol 1985; 28: 333–7.

323. Veys N, Lameire N, Malerczyk V, Lehr K, Rozenkranz B. Single dose pharmacokinetics of Cefpirome in hemodialysed patients and patients treated by CAPD. Clin Pharmacol Ther 1993; 54: 395–401.

324. Ryckelynck JP, Vergnaud M, Hurault de Ligny B, Allogche G, Malbruny B, Morel C. Pharmacocinétique de la ceftazidime par voie intrapéritonéale en dialyse péritonéale continue ambulatoire. Pathol Biolog 1986; 34: 328–31.

325. Comstock TJ, Straughn B, Kraus AP, Meyer MC, Finn AL, Chubb JM. Ceftazidime pharmacokinetics during continuous peritoneal dialysis (CAPD) and intermittent peritoneal dialysis (IPD). Drug Intell Clin Pharm 1983; 17: 453 (abstract).

326. Stea S, Bachelor T, Cooper M, de Souza P, Koenig K, Bolton WK. Disposition and bioavailability of ceftazidime after intraperitoneal administration in patients receiving continuous ambulatory peritoneal dialysis. J Am Soc Nephrol 1996; 7: 2399–402.

327. Grabe DW, Bailie GR, Eisele G, Frye RF. Pharmacokinetics of intermittent intraperitoneal ceftazidime. Am J Kidney Dis 1999; 33: 111–17.

328. Gross ML, Somani P, Ribner BS, Raeader R, Freimer EH, Higgins JT. Ceftizoxime elimination kinetics in continuous ambulatory peritoneal dialysis. Clin Pharmacol Ther 1983; 34: 673–80.

329. Burgess ED, Blair AD. Pharmacokinetics of ceftizoxime in patients undergoing continuous ambulatory peritoneal dialysis. Antimicrob Agents Chemother 1983; 24: 237–9.

330. Albin HC, Ragnaud JM, Demotes-Mainrad FM, Vincon GA, Couzineau M, Wone C. Pharmacokinetics of intravenous and intraperitoneal ceftriaxone in chronic ambulatory peritoneal dialysis. Eur J Clin Pharmacol 1986; 31: 479–83.

331. Tomino Y, Fukui M, Hamada C, Inoue S, Osada S. Pharmacokinetics of cefdinir and its transfer to dialysate in patients with chronic renal failure undergoing continuous ambulatory peritoneal dialysis. Arzneim Forsch/Drug Res 1998; 48: 862–7.

332. Johnson CA, Taylor III CA, Zimmerman SW et al. Pharmacokinetics of quinupristin-dalfopristin in continuous ambulatory peritoneal dialysis patients. Antimicrob Agents Chemother 1999; 43: 152–6.

333. Favre H, Probst P. Pharmacokinetics of ceftriaxone after intravenous and intraperitoneal ceftriaxone after intravenous administration to CAPD patients with and without peritonitis. Chemoterapia 1987; 6 (suppl. 2): 273–4.

334. Zaruba K, Rastorfer M, Probst P. Pharmacokinetics of ceftriaxone in continuous ambulatory peritoneal dialysis patients after intraperitoneal administration. Chemoterapia 1987; 6 (suppl. 6): 267–70.

335. Koup JR, Keller E, Neumann H, Stoeckel K. Ceftriaxone pharmacokinetics during peritoneal dialysis. Eur J Clin Pharmacol 1986; 30: 303–7.

336. Ti TY, Fortin L, Kreeft JH, East DS, Ogilvie RI, Somerville PJ. Kinetic disposition of intravenous ceftriaxone in normal subjects and patients with renal failure on hemodialysis or peritoneal dialysis. Antimicrob Agents Chemother 1984; 25: 83–7.

337. Chan MK, Browning AK, Poole CMJ et al. Cefuroxime pharmacokinetics in continuous and intermittent peritoneal dialysis. Nephron 1985; 41: 161–5.

338. Dahl K, Walstad RA, Wideröe TE. The effect of peritonitis on the transperitoneal transport of cefuroxime in patients on CAPD treatment. Nephrol Dial Transplant 1990; 5: 272–81.

339. Davis GM, Forland SC, Cutler RE. Serum and dialysate concentrations of cephalexin following repeated dosing in CAPD patients. Am J Kidney Dis 1985; 6: 177–80.

340. Munch R, Steurer J, Luthy R, Siegenthaler W, Kuhlmann U. Serum and dialysate concentrations of intraperitoneal cephalothin in patients undergoing chronic ambulatory peritoneal dialysis. Clin Nephrol 1983; 20: 40–3.

341. Johnston CA, Welling PG, Zimmerman SW. Pharmacokinetics of oral cephradine in continuous ambulatory peritoneal dialysis patients. Clin Nephrol 1984; 35: 57–61.

342. Singlas E, Boutron HF, Merdjan J, Brocard JF, Pocheville M, Fries D. Moxolactam kinetics during chronic ambulatory peritoneal dialysis patients. Clin Pharmacol Ther 1983; 34: 403–7.

343. Jones TE, Milne RW, Mudaliar Y, Sansom LN. Moxolactam kinetics during continuous ambulatory peritoneal dialysis after intraperitoneal administration. Antimicrob Agents Chemother 1985; 28: 293–8.

344. Morse G, Janicke D, Cafarell R et al. Moxolactam epimer disposition in patients undergoing continuous ambulatory peritoneal dialysis. Clin Pharmacol Ther 1985; 38: 150–6.

345. Pancorbo S, Compty C. Peritoneal transport of vancomycin in 4 patients undergoing continuous ambulatory peritoneal dialysis. Nephron 1982; 31: 37–9.

346. Bunke CM, Aronoff GR, Brier ME, Sloan RS, Luft FC. Tobramycin kinetics during continuous ambulatory peritoneal dialysis. Clin Pharmacol Ther 1983; 34: 110–16.

347. Blevins RD, Halstenson CE, Salem NG, Matzke GR. Pharmacokinetics of vancomycin in patients undergoing continuous ambulatory peritoneal dialysis. Antimicrob Agents Chemother 1984; 25: 603–6.

348. Rogge MC, Johnston CA, Zimmerman SW, Welling PG. Vancomycin disposition during continuous ambulatory peritoneal dialysis: a pharmacokinetic analysis of peritoneal drug transport. Antimicrob Agents Chemother 1985; 27: 578–82.

349. Mounier M, Benevent D, Denis F. Pharmacocinétique de la vancomycine chez les patients insuffisants rénaux chroniques en dialyse péritonéale continue ambulatoire. Pathol Biolog 1985; 33: 542–4.

350. Whitby M, Edwards R, Astan E, Finck RG. Pharmacokinetics of single dose intravenous vancomycin in CAPD peritonitis. J Antimicrob Chemother 1987; 19: 351–7.

351. Suzuki K, Twardowski ZJ, Nolph KD, Khanna R. Absorption of iron dextran from the peritoneal cavity of rats. Adv Perit Dial 1995; 11: 57–9.

352. Neal D, Bailie GR. Clearance from dialysate and equilibration of intraperitoneal vancomycin in continuous ambulatory peritoneal dialysis. Clin Pharmacokin 1990; 18: 485–90.

353. Rubin J. Vancomycin absorption from the peritoneal cavity during dialysis-related peritonitis. Perit Dial Int 1990; 10: 283–5.

354. Traina GL, Gentile MG, Fellin G et al. Pharmacokinetics of teicoplanin in patients on continuous ambulatory peritoneal dialysis. Eur J Clin Pharmacol 1986; 31: 501–4.

355. Jankneght R, Koelman HH, Nube MJ. Pharmacokinetics of rifampicin and teicoplanin during CAPD. Med Sci Res 1987; 15: 171–2.

356. Bonati M, Traina GL, Rosina R. Pharmacokinetics of intraperitoneal teicoplanin in patients with chronic renal failure on continuous ambulatory peritoneal dialysis. Br J Clin Pharmacol 1988; 25: 761–6.

357. Guay DRP, Awni WM, Halstenson CE, Kenny MT, Keane WF, Matzke GR. Teicoplanin pharmacokinetics in patients undergoing continuous ambulatory peritoneal dialysis. Antimicrob Agents Chemother 1989; 33: 2012–15.

358. Finch RG, Holliday AP, Innes A et al. Pharmacokinetic behavior of intraperitoneal teicoplanin during treatment of peritonitis complicating continuous ambulatory peritoneal dialysis. Antimicrob Agents Chemother 1996; 40 (letter): 1971–2.

359. Boeschoten EW, Rietra PJGM, Krediet RW, Visser MJ, Arisz L. CAPD peritonitis: a prospective randomized trial of oral versus intraperitoneal treatment with cephradine. J Antimicrob Chemother 1985; 16: 789–97.

360. Drew PJT, Casewell MW, Desai N, Houang ET, Simpson CN, Marsh F. Cephalexin for the oral treatment of CAPD peritonitis. J Antimicrob Chemother 1984; 13: 153–9.

361. Knight KR, Polak A, Crump J, Mashell R. Laboratory diagnosis and treatment of CAPD peritonitis. Lancet 1982; 2: 1301–4.

362. Ragnaud JM, Roche-Béziam MC, Marceau C et al. Traitement des péritonites en dialyse péritonéale continue ambulatoire par une dose unique quotidienne de 1 g de céfotiam par voie intrapéritonéale. Pathol Biol 1986; 34: 512–16.

363. Gray MK, Goulding S, Eykyn SJ. Intraperitoneal vancomycin and ceftazidime in the treatment of CAPD peritonitis. Clin Nephrol 1985; 23: 81–4.

364. Beaman M, Solaro L, McGonigle RJS, Michael J, Adu D. Vancomycin and ceftazidime in the treatment of CAPD peritonitis. Nephron 1989; 51: 51–5.

365. Ragnaud JM, Roche-Béziam MC, Dupon M, Marceau C, Wone C. Traitement des péritonites en dialyse périonéale continue ambulatoire par la ceftriaxone intrapéritonéale. Pathol Biol 1986; 36: 552–6.

366. Andrassy K. Pharmacokinetics of cefotaxime in dialysis patients. Diagn Microbiol Infect Dis 1995; 22: 85–7.

367. Morse GD, Janicke DM, Cafarell R et al. Moxolactam epimer disposition in patients undergoing continuous ambulatory peritoneal dialysis. Clin Pharmacol Ther 1985; 38: 150–6.

368. Bailie GR, Eisele G. Vancomycin in peritoneal dialysis-associated peritonitis. Sem Dial 1996; 9: 417–23.

369. Van Biesen W, Vanholder R, Vogelaers D et al. The need for a center-tailored treatment protocol for peritonitis. Perit Dial Int 1998; 18: 274–81.

370. Rowland M. Clinical pharmacokinetics of teicoplanin. Clin Pharmacokin 1990; 18: 184–209.

371. Shalit I, Greenwood RB, Marks MI, Pederson JA, Frederick DL. Pharmacokinetics of single dose oral ciprofloxacin in patients undergoing CAPD. Antimicrob Agents Chemother 1986; 30: 152–6.

372. Golper TA, Hartstein AI, Morthland VH, Christensen JM. Effects of antacids and dialysate dwell times on multiple-dose pharmacokinetics of oral ciprofloxacin in patients on CAPD. Antimicrob Agents Chemother 1987; 31: 1787–90.

373. Kowalsky SF, Echols M. Pharmacokinetics of ciprofloxacin in subjects with varying degrees of renal function and undergoing hemodialysis or CAPD. Clin Nephrol 1993; 39: 53–8.

374. Stuck AE, Frey FJ, Heizmann P, Brandt R, Weiderkamm E. Pharmacokinetics and metabolism of intravenous and oral fleroxacin in subjects with normal and impaired renal function and in patients on CAPD. Antimicrob Agents Chemother 1989; 33: 373–81.

375. Stuck AE, Donbosco K, Frey FJ. Fleroxacin clinical pharamokinetics. Clin Pharmacokin 1992; 22: 116–31.

376. Lameire N, Rosenkranz B, Malerczyk V, Lehr KH, Veys N, Ringoir S. Ofloxacin pharmacokinetics in chronic renal failure and dialysis. Clin Pharmacokin 1991; 21: 357–71.

377. Passlick J, Wonner R, Keller E, Essers L, Grabensee B. Single and multiple dose kinetics of ofloxacin in patients on CAPD. Perit Dial Int 1989; 9: 267–72.

378. Flor S. Pharmacokinetics of ofloxacin. Am J Med 1989; 87 (suppl. 6C): 24–30.

379. Rosenkranz B, Malerczyk V, Zamba K, Jungbluth H, Lameire N. Pharmacokinetics of ofloxacin in CAPD. Kidney Int 1991; 39: 1239 (abstract).

380. Kampf D, Borner K, Hain H, Conrad W. Multiple-dose kinetics of ofloxacin after intraperitoneal application in CAPD patients. Perit Dial Int 1991; 11: 317–21.

381. Cheng IK, Chau PY, Kumana CR, Chan CY, Kou M, Siu LK. Single-dose paharmacokinetics of intraperitoneal

Ofloxacin in patients on continuous ambualtory peritoneal dialysis. Perit Dial Int 1993; 13 (suppl. 2): S383–5.

382. Lode H, Hoffkin G, Prinineg C *et al.* Comparative pharmacokinetics of new quinolones. Drugs 1987; 34 (suppl. I): 21–5.

383. Schmit JL, Hary L, Bou P *et al.* Pharmacokinetics of single-dose intravenous, oral and intraperitoneal pefloxacin in patients on chronic ambulatory peritoneal dialysis. Antimicrob Agents Chemother 1991; 35: 1492–4.

384. Nikolaidis P, Walker SE, Dombros N, Tourkantonis A, Paton TW, Oreopoulos DG. Single dose pefloxacin pharmacokinetics and metabolism in patients undergoing continuous ambulatory peritoneal dialysis. Perit Dial Int 1991; 11: 59–63.

385. Somani P, Shapiro RS, Stockard H, Higgins JT. Unidirectional absorption of gentamicin from the peritoneum during continuous ambulatory peritoneal dialysis. Clin Pharmacol Ther 1982; 32: 113–21.

386. Pancorbo S, Comty C. Pharmacokinetics of gentamicin in patients undergoing continuous ambulatory peritoneal dialysis. Antimicrob Agents Chemother 1981; 19: 605–7.

387. Paton TW, Manuel M, Walker SE. Tobramycin disposition in patients on continuous ambulatory peritoneal dialysis. Perit Dial Bull 1982; 2: 179–81.

388. Walshe JJ, Morse GD, Janicke DM, Apicella MA. Crossover pharmacokinetic analysis comparing intravenous and intraperitoneal administration of tobramycin. J Infect Dis 1986; 153: 796–9.

389. Halstenson CE, Matze GR, Comty CM. Intraperitoneal administration of tobramycin during CAPD. Kidney Int 1984; 25: 256 (abstract).

390. Rubin J. Tobramycin absorption from the peritoneal cavity. Perit Dial Int 1990; 10: 295–7.

391. Sennesael JJ, Maes VA, Pierard D, Debeukelaer SH, Verbeelen DL. Streptomycin pharmacokinetics in relapsing mycobacterium xenopi peritonitis. Am J Nephrol 1990; 10: 422–5.

392. Smeltzer BD, Schwartzman MS, Bertino JS. Amikacin pharmacokinetics during continuous ambulatory peritoneal dialysis. Antimicrob Agents Chemother 1988; 32: 236–40.

393. Anding K, Krumme B, Pelz K, Bohler J, Hollmeyer P. Pharmacokinetics and bactericidal activity of a single daily dose of netilmicin in the treatment of CAPD-associated peritonitis. Int J Clin Pharmacol Ther Toxicol 1996; 34: 465–9.

394. Krediet RT, Boeschoten EW, Arisz L. Kanamycin as marker for middle-molecular solute transport in CAPD patients with and without peritonitis. Blood Purif 1987; 5: 291 (abstract).

395. Martea M, Hekster YA, Vree TB, Voets AJ, Berden JHM. Pharmacokinetics of cephradine, sulfamethoxazole and trimethoprim and their metabolites in a patient with peritonitis undergoing continuous ambulatory peritoneal dialysis. Pharm Wkbl 1987; 9: 110–16.

396. Walker SE, Paton TW, Churchill DN, Ojo B, Manuel M, Wright N. Trimethoprim–sulfamethoxazole pharmacokinetics during continuous ambulatory peritoneal dialysis. Perit Dial Int 1989; 9: 51–5.

397. Rubin J, Planch A. Absorption of sulfamethoxazole and albumin from the peritoneal cavity. Trans Am Soc Artif Intern Organs 1990; 36: 834–7.

398. Bouchet JL, Albin HC, Quentin CL *et al.* Pharmacokinetics of intravenous and intraperitoneal fosfomycin in continuous ambulatory peritoneal dialysis. Clin Nephrol 1988; 29: 35–40.

399. Lam YWF, Flaherty JF, Yumena L, Schoenfeld PY, Gambertoglio JF. Roxithromycin disposition in patients on continuous ambulatory peritoneal dialysis. J Antimicrob Chemother 1995; 36: 157–63.

400. Gerig JS, Bolton ND, Swabb EA, Scheld WM, Bolton WK. Effect of hemodialysis and peritoneal dialysis on aztreonam pharmacokinetics. Kidney Int 1984; 26: 308–18.

401. Nikolaidis P, Dombros N, Alexion P, Balaskas EV, Tourkantonis A. Pharmacokinetics of aztreonam administered IP in continuous ambulatory peritoneal dialysis patients. Perit Dial Int 1989; 9: 57–9.

402. Brown J, Altmann P, Cunningham J, Shaw E, Marsh F. Pharmacokinetics of once daily intraperitoneal aztreonam and vancomycin in the treatment of CAPD peritonitis. J Antimicrob Chemother 1990; 25: 141–7.

403. Guay DR, Meatherall RC, Baxter H, Jacyk WR, Penner B. Pharmacokinetics of metronidazole in patients undergoing continuous ambulatory peritoneal dialysis. Antimicrob Agents Chemother 1984; 25: 306–10.

404. Lau AH, Lam NP, Piscitelli SC, Wilkes L, Danziger LH. Clinical pharmacokinetics of metronidazole and other nitroimidazole anti-infectives. Clin Pharmacokin 1992; 23: 328–64.

405. Merdjan H, Beaumelou A, Diquet B, Singlas E. Pharmacokinetics of ornidazole in patients with renal insufficiency: influence of hemodialysis and peritoneal dialysis. Br J Clin Pharmacol 1985; 19: 211–17.

406. Janknegt R. CAPD peritonitis and fluoroquinolones: a review. Perit Dial Int 1991; 11: 53–8.

407. Nikolaidis P. Quinolones: pharmacokinetics and pharmacodynamics. Perit Dial Int 1993; 13 (suppl. 2): S377–9.

408. De Fijter CWH, Biemond A, Oe LP *et al.* Pharmacokinetics of ciprofloxacin after intraperitoneal administration of uninfected patients undergoing CCPD. Adv Perit Dial 1992; 8: 18–21.

409. Chong TK, Oiraino B. Vestibular toxicity due to gentamicin in peritoneal dialysis patients. Perit Dial Int 1991; 11: 152–5.

410. Glew RH, Pavuk RA. Stability of vancomycin and aminoglycoside antibiotics in peritoneal dialysis concentrate. Nephron 1981; 28: 241–3.

411. Dratwa M, Glupczynski Y, Lameire N *et al.* Treatment of Gram-negative peritonitis with aztreonam in patients undergoing continuous ambulatory peritoneal dialysis. Rev Infect Dis 1991; 13: S645–7.

412. Fuiano G, Sepe V, Viscione M, Nani E, Conte G. Effectiveness of single daily intraperitoneal administration of aztreonam and cefuroxime in the treatment of peritonitis in continuous ambulatory peritoneal dialysis. Perit Dial Int 1989; 9: 273–5.

413. Cheng IKP, Chan CY, Wong WT. A randomized prospective comparison of oral ofloxacin and intraperitoneal vancomycin plus aztreonam in the treatment of bacterial peritonitis complicating continuous ambulatory peritoneal dialysis. Perit Dial Int 1991; 11: 27–30.

414. Seth SK, Visconti JA, Herbert LA, Krasny HC. Acyclovir pharmacokinetics in a patient on continuous ambulatory peritoneal dialysis. Clin Pharmacol 1985; 4: 320–2.

415. Shah GM, Winer RL, Krasny HC. Acyclovir pharmacokinetics in a patient on continuous ambulatory peritoneal dialysis. Am J Kidney Dis 1986; 7: 507–10.

416. Burgess ED, Gill MJ. Intraperitoneal administration of acyclovir in patients receiving continuous ambulatory peritoneal dialysis. J Clin Pharmacol 1990; 30: 997–1000.

417. Swan SK, Munat MY, Wigger MA, Bennett WM. Pharmacokinetics of ganciclovir in a patient undergoing hemodialysis. Am J Kidney Dis 1991; 17: 69–72.

418. Alexander AC, Akers A, Matzke GR, Aweeka FT, Fraley DS. Disposition of foscarnet during peritoneal dialysis. Ann Pharmacother 1996; 30: 1106–9.

419. Schwenk MH, Halstenson CE, Simpson ML, Pence TV, Reynolds DJ. Pharmacokinetics of zidovudine in an AIDS patient during continuous ambulatory peritoneal dialysis. Am Coll Clin Pharm 1990; Kansas City: (abstract).

420. Gallicano KD, Tobe S, Sahai J *et al.* Pharmacokinetics of single and chronic dose zidovudine in two HIV positive patients undergoing continuous ambulatory peritoneal dialysis. J Acquir Immune Defic Syndr Hum Retrovirol 1992; 5: 242–50 (abstract).

421. Knupp CA, Hak LJ, Coakley DF *et al.* Disposition of dida-nosine in HIV-seropositive patients with normal renal function or chronic renal failure: influence of hemodialysis and continuous ambulatory peritoneal dialysis. Clin Pharmacol Ther 1996; 60: 535–42.

422. Kerr CM, Perfect JR, Cran PC *et al.* Fungal peritonitis in patients on continuous ambulatory peritoneal dialysis. Ann Int Med 1983; 99: 334–7 (abstract).

423. Fraser AK, O'Connor JP. Peritoneal penetration of ampho-tericin B. Perit Dial Bull 1984; 4: 265 (abstract).

424. Debruyne D, Ryckelynck JP, Morelin M *et al.* Pharmaco-kinetics of fluconazole in patients undergoing continuous ambulatory peritoneal dialysis. Clin Pharmacokin 1990; 18: 491–8 (abstract).

425. Debruyne D, Ryckelynck JP. Fluconazole serum, urine and dialysate levels in CAPD patients. Perit Dial Int 1999; 12: 328–9 (letter).

426. Cecchin E, Panarello G, de March IS. Fungal peritonitis in ambulatory peritoneal dialysis. Ann Intern Med 1984; 100: 321 (letter).

427. Jones JM, Greenfeld RA. Administration of flucytosine to a patient on CAPD. Perit Dial Bull 1982; 2: 46–7.

428. Krediet RT, Boeschoten EW, Struijk DG, Arisz L. Pharm-acokinetics of intraperitoneally administered 5-fluoro-cytosine in continuous ambulatory peritoneal dialysis. Nephrol Dial Transplant 1987; 2: 453 (abstract).

429. Boelaert J, Schurgers M, Matthys E, Daneels R, van Peer A. Intraconazole pharmacokinetics in patients with renal dys-function. Antimicrob Agents Chemother 1988; 32: 1595–7.

430. Doherty D, Seth S, Bay W. Fungal peritonitis and ketocona-zole levels in a CAPD patient. Perit Dial Bull 1984; 4: S20 (abstract).

431. McGuire N, Port FK, Kauffman CA. Ketoconazole pharm-acokinetics in continuous ambulatory peritoneal dialysis. Perit Dial Int 1984; 4: 199–201.

432. Valainis GT, Morford DW. Ketoconazole levels in perito-neal fluid. Perit Dial Bull 1985; 5: 136 (letter).

433. Boelaert J, Schurgers M, Daneels R, Van Landuyt HW, Weatherley BC. Multiple dose pharmacokinetics of intra-venous acyclovir in patients on continuous ambulatory peri-toneal dialysis. J Antimicrob Chemother 1987; 20: 69–76.

434. Stathoulopoulou F, Almond MK, Dhillon S, Raftery MJ. Clinical pharmacokinetics of oral acyclovir in patients on continuous ambulatory peritoneal dialysis. Nephron 1996; 74: 337–41.

435. Davenport A, Goel S, Mackenzie JC. Neurotoxicity of acyclovir in patients with end-stage renal failure treated with continuous ambulatory peritoneal dialysis. Am J Kidney Dis 1992; 20: 647–9.

436. Sommadossi JP, Bevan R, Ling T *et al.* Clinical pharmaco-kinetics of ganciclovir in patients with normal and impaired renal function. Rev Infect Dis 1988; 3 (suppl. 10): 507–14.

437. Kremer D, Munar MY, Kohlhepp SJ *et al.* Zidovudine pharmacokinetics in five HIV seronegative patients under-going continuous ambulatory peritoneal dialysis. Pharmaco-therapy. 1992; 12: 56–60 (abstract).

438. Muther RS, Bennett WM. Clearance of amphotericin B and 5-fluorocytosine by peritoneal dialysis. Western J Med 1980; 133: 157–60.

439. Peterson LR, Hall WH, Kelty RH, Votava HJ. Therapy of candida peritonitis: penetration of amphotericin B into peri-toneal fluid. Postgrad Med J 1978; 54: 340–2.

440. Kravitz SP, Berry PL. Successful treatment of aspergillus peritonitis in a child undergoing continuous ambulatory peritoneal dialysis. Arch Intern Med 1986; 146: 2061–2.

441. Khanna R, Oreopoulos DG, Vas S, McCready W, Dombros N. Fungal peritonitis in patients undergoing chronic intermittent or continuous peritoneal dialysis. Proc EDTA 1980; 17: 291–6.

442. Rault R. Candida peritonitis complicating chronic peritoneal dialysis. A report of five cases and review of the literature. Am J Kidney Dis 1983; 2: 544–7.

443. Maher JF, Hirszel B, Chakrabarti EK, Bennett RR. Con-trasting effects of amphotericin B and the solvent sodium desoxycholate on peritoneal transport. Nephron 1986; 43: 38–42.

444. Imholz AL, Koomen GC, Struijk DG, Arisz L, Krediet RT. The effect of amphotericin B on fluid kinetics and solute transport in CAPD patients. Adv Perit Dial 1993; 9: 12–15.

445. Eisenberg ES. Intraperitoneal flucytosine in the management of fungal peritonitis in patients on continuous ambulatory peritoneal dialysis. Am J Kidney Dis 1988; 11: 465–7.

446. Slingeneyer A, Laroche B, Steel F, Canaud B, Beraud JJ, Mion C. Oral ketoconazole plus IP 5-fluorocytosine as a sole treatment of fungal peritonitis in CAPD. Perit Dial Bull 1984; 4: S60 (abstract).

447. Levine JD, Bernard DB, Idelson BA, Farnham H, Saunders C, Sugar AM. Fungal peritonitis complicating continuous ambulatory peritoneal dialysis: successful treatment with fluconazole, a new orally active antifungal agent. Am J Med 1989; 86: 825–7.

448. Fabris A, Pellanda MV, Gardin C, Contestabile A, Bolzo-nella R. Pharmacokinetics of antifungal agents. Perit Dial Int 1993; 13, (suppl. 2): S380–2.

449. Paton TW, Manuel M, Walker SE. Cimetidine disposition in patients on continuous ambulatory peritoneal dialysis. Perit Dial Bull 1982; 2: 73–6.

450. Kogan FJ, Sampliner RE, Myersohn M, Kazama RM, Hones W, Michael UF. Cimetidine disposition in patients undergoing continuos ambulatory peritoneal dialysis. J Clin Pharmacol 1983; 20: 252–6.

451. Sica DA, Comstock T, Harford A, Eshelman F. Ranitidine pharmacokinetics in continuous ambulatory peritoneal dialysis. Eur J Clin Pharmacol 1987; 32: 587–91.

452. Gladziwa U, Klotz U, Krishna DR, Schmitt H, Glockner WM, Mann H. Pharmacokinetics and dynamics of famoti-dine in patients with renal failure. Br J Clin Pharmacol 1988; 26: 315–21.

453. Lazarovitz AI, Page D. Intraperitoneal cisapride for the treatment diabetes with gastroparesis and end-stage renal disease. Nephron 1990; 56: 107–9.

454. Gladziwa U, Bares R, Klotz U *et al.* Pharmacokinetics and pharmacodynamics of cisapride in patients undergoing hemodialysis. Clin Pharmacol Ther 1991; 50: 673–81.

455. Gora ML, Visconti JA, Seth S, Shields B, Bay W. Pharma-cokinetics of intraperitoneal metoclopramide in a patient with renal failure. Clin Pharmacol 1992; 11: 174–6.

456. Andersson T. Pharmacokinetics, metabolism and inter-actions of acid pump inhibitors. Clin Pharmacokin 1996; 31: 9–28.

457. Barradell LB, Faulds D, McTavish D. Lansoprazole – a review of its pharmacodynamic and pharmacokinetic prop-erties and its therapeutic efficacy in acid-related disorders. Drugs 1992; 44: 225–50.

458. Fitton A, Wiseman L. Pantoprazole – a review of its pharma-cological properties and therapeutic use in acid-related dis-orders. Drugs 1996; 51: 460–82.

459. Lameire N, Rosenkranz B, Brockmeier D. Pharmacokinetics of histamine (H2)-receptor antagonists, including roxatidine, in chronic renal failure. Scand J Gastroenterol 1988; 23 (suppl. 146): 100–10.

460. Naesdal J, Anderson T, Bodemar G, Larrson R, Regardt CG. Pharmacokinetics of C14-omeprazole in patients with impaired renal function. Clin Pharmacol Ther 1986; 40: 344–51.

461. Howden CW, Payton CD, Meredith A *et al.* Antisecretory effect and oral pharmacokinetics of omeprazole in patients with chronic renal failure. Eur J Clin Pharmacol 1985; 28: 637–40.

462. Bedford TA, Rowbotham DJ. Cisapride–drug interactions of clinical significance. Drug Saf 1996; 15: 167–75.

463. Boelaert JR, Schurgers ML, Matthys EG, Belpaire FM, Daneels RF. Comparative pharmacokinetics of recombinant

erythropoietin administration by the intravenous, subcutaneous and intraperitoneal routes in continuous ambulatory peritoneal dialysis patients. Perit Dial Int 1989; 9: 95–8.

464. Gahl GM, Passlick J, Pustelnik A, Kampf D, Grabensee B. Intraperitoneal versus intravenous recombinant erythropoietin in stable CAPD patients. Proc 6th Congr EDTA-ERA Gothenburg 1990, 199 (abstract).

465. Hughes RT, Cotes PM, Oliver DO *et al.* Correction of anemia of chronic renal failure with erythropoietin : pharmacokinetic studies on hemodialysis and CAPD. Contrib Nephrol 1989; 76: 123–30.

466. Kampf D, KahlA, Passlick J, Pustelnik A, Eckardt KU. Single-dose kinetics of recombinant human erythropoietin after intravenous , subcutaneous and intraperitoneal administration. Contrib Nephrol 1989; 76: 106–11.

467. Kromer G, Solf A, Ehmer B, Kaufmann B, Quellhorst E. Single dose pharmacokinetics of recombinant human erythropoietin comparing intravenous, subcutaneous and intraperitoneal administration in IPD patients. Kidney Int 1990; 37: 311.

468. Macdougall IC, Roberts DE, Neubert P, Dharmasena AD, Coles GA, Williams JD. Pharmacokinetics of recombinant human erythropoietin in patients on continuous ambulatory peritoneal dialysis. Lancet 1989; 1: 425–7.

469. Stockenhuber F, Loibl U, Gottsauner-Wolf M *et al.* Pharmacokinetics and dose response after intravenous and subcutaneous administration of recombinant erythropoietin in patients on regular hemodialysis treatment or continuous ambulatory peritoneal dialysis. Nephron 1991; 59: 399–402.

470. Lui SF, Chung WWM, Leung CB, Chan K, Lai KN. Pharmacokinetics and pharmacodynamics of subcutaneous and intraperitoneal administration of recombinant human erythropoietin in patients on continuous ambulatory peritoneal dialysis. Clin Nephrol 1990; 33: 47–51.

471. Bargman J, Jones JE, Petro JM. The pharmacokinetics of intraperitoneal erythropoietin administered undiluted or diluted in dialysate. Perit Dial Int 1992; 12: 269–72.

472. Nissenson AR. Erythropoietin and peritoneal dialysis: the efficacy of intraperitoneal dosing. Perit Dial Int 1992; 12: 350–2.

473. Bargman J, Breborowicz A, Rodela H, Sombolos K, Oreopoulos DG. Intraperitoneal administration of recombinant human erythropoietin in uremic animals. Perit Dial Int 1988; 8: 249–52.

474. Frenken LAM, Struijk DG, Coppens PJ, Tiggeler RG, Krediet RT, Koene RA. Intraperitoneal administration of recombinant human erythropoietin. Perit Dial Int 1992; 12: 378–3.

475. Nasu T, Mitui H, Shinohara Y, Hayashida S, Ohtuka H. Effect of erythropoietin in CAPD patients: comparison between intravenous and intraperitoneal administration. Perit Dial Int 1992; 12: 373–7.

476. Park SE, Twardowski ZJ, Moore HL, Khanna R, Nolph KD. Chronic administration of iron dextran into the peritoneal cavity of rats. Perit Dial Int 1997; 17: 179–85.

477. Pecoits-Filho RFS, Twardowski ZJ, Kim YL, Khanna R, Moore H, Nolph KD. The absence of toxicity in intraperitoneal iron dextran administration: a functional and histological analysis. Perit Dial Int 1998; 18: 64–70.

478. Marquardt ED, Ishisaka DY, Batra KK, Chin B. Removal of ethosuximide and phenobarbital by peritoneal dialysis in a child. Clin Pharm 1992; 11: 1030–1.

479. Hess B, Keusch G, Fluckinger J, Binswanger U. Zur Pharmakokinetik von Phenytoin bei kontinuerlicher ambulanter Peritonealdialyse. Schweiz Med Wochenschr 1984; 114: 16–19.

480. Jones CL, Vieth R, Spino M *et al.* Comparisons between oral and intraperitoneal 1,25-dihydroxyvitamin D3 therapy in children treated with peritoneal dialysis. Clin Nephrol 1994; 42: 44–9.

481. Joffe P, Cintin C, Ladefoged SD, Rasmussen SN. Pharmacokinetics of 1-alpha-hydroxycholecalciferol after intraperitoneal, intravenous and oral administration in patients undergoing peritoneal dialysis. Clin Nephrol 1994; 41: 364–9.

482. Saha HHT, Ala-Houhala IO, Liukko-Sipi SH, Ylitalo P, Pasternack AI. Pharmacokinetics of clodronate in peritoneal dialysis patients. Perit Dial Int 1998; 204 (abstract 209).

483. Garzone PD, Kroboth PD. Pharmacokinetics of the newer benzodiazepines. Clin Pharmacokin 1989; 16: 337–64.

484. Calvo R, Suarez JM, Rodriguez-Sasiain JM, Martinez I. The influence of renal failure on the kinetics of intravenous midazolam: an 'in vitro' and 'in vivo' study. Res Comm Chem Pathol Pharmacol 1992; 78: 311–20.

485. Salvà P, Costa J. Clinical pharmacokinetics and pharmacodynamics of zolpidem – therapeutic implications. Clin Pharmacokin 1995; 29: 142–53.

486. Price TM, Dupuis RE, Carr BR, Stanczyk FZ, Lobo RA, Droegemueller W. Single- and multiple-dose pharmacokinetics of a low-dose oral contraceptive in women with chronic renal failure undergoing peritoneal dialysis. Am J Obstet Gynecol 1993; 168: 1400–6.

487. Leaky TEB, Elias-Jones AC, Coates PE, Smith KL. Pharmacokinetics of theophylline and its metabolites during acute renal failure. Clin Pharmacokin 1991; 21: 400–8.

488. Cefali EA, Poynor WJ, Sica D, Cox S. Pharmacokinetic comparison of flurbiprofen in end-stage renal disease subjects and subjects with normal renal function. J Clin Pharmacol 1991; 31: 814.

489. Schmith V, Piraino B, Smith RB, Kroboth PD. Alprazolam in end-stage renal disease. J Clin Pharmacol 1991; 31: 571–9.

490. Bauer TM, Ritz R, Haberthür C *et al.* Prolonged sedation due to accumulation of conjugated metabolites of midazolam. Lancet 1995; 346: 145–7.

491. Shany S, Rapoport J, Goligorsky M, Yankowitz N, Zuili I, Chaimovitz C. Losses of 1,25- and 24,25-dihydroxy-cholecalciferol in the peritoneal fluid of patients treated with continuous ambulatory peritoneal dialysis. Nephron 1984; 36: 111–13.

492. Delmez JA, Dougan CS, Gearing BK *et al.* The effects of intraperitoneal calcitriol on calcium and parathyroid hormone. Kidney Int 1987; 31: 795–9.

493. Salusky IB, Goodman WG, Horst R *et al.* Pharmacokinetics of calcitriol in continuous ambulatory peritoneal and cycling peritoneal dialysis patients. Am J Kidney Dis 1990; 16: 126–32.

494. Joffe P, Ladefoged SD, Cintin C, Lehmann H. 1-alpha-hydroxycholecalciferol adsorption to peritoneal dialysis bags: influence of time, glucose concentration, temperature, and albumin. Nephrol Dial Transplant 1992; 7: 1249–51.

495. Schade DS, Eaton RP, Davis T *et al.* The kinetics of peritoneal insulin absorption. Metabolism 1981; 30: 149–55.

496. Nelson JA, Stephen R, Landau ST, Wilson DE, Tyler FH. Intraperitoneal insulin administration produces a positive portal systemic blood insulin gradient in unanesthetized, unrestrained swine. Metabolism 1982; 31: 969–72.

497. Schade DS, Eaton RP, Friedman N, Spencer W. The intravenous, intraperitoneal and subcutaneous routes of insulin delivery in diabetic man. Diabetes 1979; 28: 1069–72.

498. Selam JJ, Slingeneyer A, Hedon B, Mares P, Berand JJ, Mirouze J. Long-term ambulatory peritoneal insulin infusion of brittle diabetes with portable pumps: comparison with intravenous and subcutaneous routes. Diabetes Care 1983; 6: 105–11.

499. Kritz J, Hagmuller H, Lovett R, Irsigler K. Implanted constant basal rate insulin infusion devices for type 1 (insulin-dependent) diabetic patients. Diabetologica 1983; 25: 78–81.

500. Micossi P, Bosi E, Cristallo M *et al.* Chronic continuous intraperitoneal insulin infusion (CIPII) in type I diabetic patients non-satisfactorily responsive to continuous subcutaneous insulin infusion (CSII). Acta Diabetol Lat 1986; 23: 155–64.

501. Saudek CD, Selam JL, Pitt HA *et al.* A preliminary trial of the programmable implantable medication system for insulin delivery. N Engl J Med 1986; 31: 574–9.

502. Vaag A, Handberg A, Lauritzen M *et al.* Variation in absorption of NPH-insulin due to intramuscular injection. Diabetes Care 1990; 13: 74–6.

503. Wredling R, Liu D, Lins PE, Adamson U. Variation of insulin absorption during subcutaneous and intraperitoneal infusion of insulin-dependent diabetic patients with unsatisfactory long-term glycemic response to continuous subcutaneous insulin infusion. Diabète Métab 1991; 17: 456–9.

504. Balducci A, Slama G, Rottembourg J, Baumelou A, Delage A. Intraperitoneal insulin in uremic diabetics undergoing continuous ambulatory peritoneal dialysis. Br Med J 1981; 283: 1021–3.

505. Wideröe TE, Smeby LC, Berg KJ, Jorstad S, Svartas TM. Intraperitoneal (^{125}I) insulin absorption during intermittent and continuous peritoneal dialysis. Kidney Int 1983; 23: 22–8.

506. Peetoom JJ, Willekens FLA, Meinders AE. Absorption and biological effect of intraperitoneal insulin administration in patients with terminal renal failure treated by continuous ambulatory peritoneal dialysis. Neth J Med 1985; 28: 435–1.

507. Shapiro DJ, Blumenkranz MJ, Levin SR, Coburn JW. Absorption and action of insulin added to peritoneal dialysate in dogs. Nephron 1979; 23: 174–80.

508. Rubin J, Bell AH, Andrews M, Jones Q, Planck A. Intraperitoneal insulin – a dose responsive curve. Am Soc Artif Intern Organs 1989; 35: 17–21.

509. Beardsworth SF, Ahmad R, Terry E, Karim K. Intraperitoneal insulin: a protocol for administration during CAPD and review of published protocol. Perit Dial Bull 1988; 8: 145–51.

510. Brewer TE, Caldwell FT, Patterson RM, Flanigan WJ. Indwelling peritoneal (Tenckhoff) dialysis catheters – experience with 24 patients. Am J Med 1972; 219: 1011–15.

511. Heal MR, England AG. Four years experience with indwelling silastic cannulae for long-term peritoneal dialysis. Br Med J 1973; 4: 596–600.

512. Lankisch PG, Tonnis JH, Fernandez-Redo E *et al.* Use of Tenckhoff catheter for peritoneal dialysis in terminal renal failure. Br Med J 1973; 4: 712–13.

513. Tenckhoff H. Catheter implantation. Dial Transplant 1972; 1: 18–21.

514. Tenckhoff H. Chronic peritoneal dialysis manual. University of Washington School of Medicine, Seattle, 1974.

515. Furman KJ, Gomperts ED, Hockley J. Activity of intraperitoneal activity of heparin during peritoneal dialysis. Clin Nephrol 1978; 9: 15–18.

516. Canavese C, Salomone M, Mangiorotti G *et al.* Heparin transfer across the rabbit peritoneal membrane. Clin Nephrol 1986; 26: 116–20.

517. Gotloib L, Grassweller P, Rodella H *et al.* Experimental models for studies of continuous peritoneal dialysis in uremic rabbits. Nephron 1982; 31: 254–9.

518. Takahashi S, Shimada A, Okada K *et al.* Effect of intraperitoneal administration of heparin to patients on continuous ambulatory peritoneal dialysis. Perit Dial Int 1991; 11: 81–3.

519. Schrader J, Tonnis HJ, Scheler F. Long-term intraperitoneal application of low molecular weight heparin in a continuous ambulatory peritoneal dialysis patient with deep vein thrombosis. Nephron 1986; 42: 83–4.

520. Tabata T, Shimada H, Emoto M *et al.* Inhibitor effects of heparin and/or antithrombin III on intraperitoneal fibrin formation in continuous ambulatory peritoneal dialysis. Nephron 1990; 56: 391–5.

521. Allain P, Chalcil D, Mauras Y *et al.* Pharmacokinetics of desferrioxamine and of its iron and aluminum chelates in patients on peritoneal dialysis. Clin Chim Acta 1988; 173: 313–16.

522. Falk RJ, Mattern WD, Lamanna RW *et al.* Iron removal during continuous ambulatory peritoneal dialysis. Kidney Int 1983; 24: 110–12.

523. Payton D, Junor BJR, Fell GS. Successful treatment of aluminium encephalopathy by intraperitoneal desferrioxamine. Lancet 1984; 1: 1132–3.

524. Andreoli SP, Dunn D, Demyer W, Sherrard DJ, Bergstein JM. Intraperitoneal deferoxamine therapy for aluminum intoxication in a child undergoing continuous ambulatory peritoneal dialysis. J Pediatr 1985; 107: 760–3.

525. Hercz G, Salusky IB, Norris KC, Coburn JW. Aluminum removal by peritoneal dialysis: intravenous vs intraperitoneal deferoxamine. Kidney Int 1986; 30: 944–8.

526. O'Brien AAJ, McParland C, Keogh JAB. The use of intravenous and intraperitoneal desferrioxamine in aluminum osteomalacia. Nephrol Dial Transplant 1987; 2: 117–19.

527. Boeschoten EW, Schrijver J, Krediet RT, Schreuers WHP, Arisz L. Deficiencies of vitamins in CAPD patients: the effect of supplementation. Nephrol Dial Transplant 1988; 2: 187–93.

8 | Peritoneal dialysis solutions and systems

M. FERIANI, L. CATIZONE AND A. FRACASSO

Introduction

This chapter is divided in three sections in order to review all components of the CAPD system: (a) the container or bag and its related problems (A.F.), (b) the solution in the bag and its modern developments (M.F.), (c) the connection between the bag and the peritoneal catheter that permits the fluid to come in contact with the peritoneal membrane (L.C.).

The container

The major developments in the CAPD programme in the past 20 years are due mainly to the introduction of plastic materials in the manufacture of CAPD containers [1]. The material first proposed in 1978 was polyvinyl chloride (PVC) added to esters of phthalic acid plasticizers (Pl) to make it more soft, flexible and transparent. PVC remains the most used plastic material in medical devices, other than CAPD bags, to date. Several studies carried out in the past 30 years, however, have emphasized many problems related to the human or environmental toxicity of this product. Therefore new materials to substitute Pl–PVC have been searched for.

The ideal plastic material for medical use should have the characteristics summarized in Table 1.

Table 1. Ideal plastic material for medical devices

Soft, flexible and transparent
Wall totally collapsible
Do not contain plasticizers
High resistance to heat (steam sterilization at 121°C)
Low permeability to water vapour
Very low permeability to gases
Totally inert
High mechanical resistance
Disposal easy and harmless to the environment
Low cost
No interaction with solutes or drugs

Polyvinyl chloride

PVC was first patented in 1913 [2] and first produced industrially in 1931. It has gained widespread application not only for medical devices but for many other uses in various fields. The raw materials employed in the manufacture of PVC are derived from sodium chloride (57%) and natural gas (43%). The PVC production process [3] (Fig. 1) starts from liquid natural gas that is heated in furnaces called crackers. The cracking process produces ethylene and propylene. The application of an electric cracking to aqueous salt solution determines the production of chlorine and caustic soda. While the caustic soda is destined for other uses, chlorine and ethylene react together to produce an intermediate product, ethylene dichloride, that is catalytically cracked to form vinyl chloride (VC). Afterwards, polymerization takes place in suspension to produce S-PVC or, as emulsion, to provide a paste – making PVC polymers. The S-PVC is an odourless white powder and is employed in medical devices. The lower molecular weight (MW) S-PVC is used for

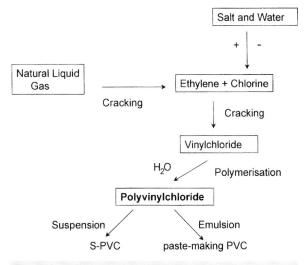

Figure 1. PVC polymer production.

R. Gokal, R. Khanna, R.Th. Krediet and K.D. Nolph (eds.), Textbook of Peritoneal Dialysis, 2nd Edition, 253–305.
© 2000 *Kluwer Academic Publishers. Printed in Great Britain.*

rigid PVC compounds, while the higher MW types, that provide a greater mechanical strength with a wide range of MW and porous polymer morphologies, are used for plasticized PVC composition. This material, although it shows a small degree of crystallinity, is very stiff (rigid) and strong as a result of polar interaction between chlorine and hydrogen atoms. For making PVC soft and flexible small Pl molecules are added to the PVC polymer. The plasticizer does not neutralize the polarity but provides an alternative to the chlorine–hydrogen interaction with lubricating effects. The result is a polymer that is soft and flexible.

The annual demand for PVC in Europe is approximately 5 million tons with an annual increase of 2–5%; the PVC demand for manufacture of biomedical devices is about 45 000 tons, less than 1% of the total amount. The plasticizer bound to PVC for increasing its usefulness in perhaps 95% of all applications is diethylhexyl phthalate (DEHP) (Fig. 2), the percentage of this plasticizer present in the final product depends on the degree of flexibility required and often equals or exceeds that of the base polymers (20–70%) [4].

The characteristics of PVC foils for use in peritoneal dialysis (PD) are listed in Table 2. Depending on the percentage of Pl content, PVC has a good resistance to breakage with good flexibility and transparency and, moreover, production costs are very low.

One of the disadvantages of PVC is its permeability to water vapour. This influences the stability of the solution contained in the bag. The evaporation leads to an increased concentration of the infusion solutions upon storage. This phenomenon can be reduced by storing bags in a carton, or by overwrapping the PD set with laminate foils [5]. When overwrapping is used, it has been demonstrated that

Table 2. Mechanical and chemical properties of PVC

Mechanical properties

Strength (resistance to breakage)	Good
Flexibility	Good
Transparence	Good
Cost	Low

Chemical properties

Permeability to water vapour	High
Stability of solutions (after 2 years of storage)	Poor
Interaction between drugs and containers, i.e.:	High
Insulin (after 20 min of storage)	49%
Heparin (after 20 min of storage)	2%
Extraction of plasticizers	High
Permeability to gasses	
O_2	High
CO_2	High
Sterilization	121°C
Waste dangerous	

water evaporation can be reduced to approximately 1% per year. This leads to an acceptable stability for 3 years. Several studies have demonstrated that, when drugs are added to solutions contained in plastic bags, their concentrations tend to decline with time due to their adsorption to the wall; they may even 'disappear' from the solution [6, 7]. The mechanism responsible for drug adsorption to the PVC is not yet completely understood. It seems that the degree of ionization or liposolubility of drugs, as well as the temperature of the solution, plays an important role in determining this phenomenon [8]. For instance, when insulin is added to a solution contained in PVC bags its concentration falls to 49% after 20 min of storage at 21°C, while under the same conditions, heparin concentration falls to only 2% of the infused dosage.

The permeability of PVC–Pl to gases is high. This aspect, on the other hand, is considered helpful in some circumstances; like blood storage. Since 1970, it has been known that diethylhexylphthalate (DEHP) is present in blood stored in PVC–Pl bags in concentration of about 0.25 mg/100 ml blood/day [4]. It seems that oxygen exchange associated to Pl dismission and their incorporation into the red cell membrane [9], is able to improve the survival of erythrocytes and their osmotic fragility and flexibility [10]. In PD, on the other hand, the passage of CO_2 and O_2 through the plastic wall has been described to induce oxidative processes in highly unstable solutions such as amino acid and bicarbonate. For this reason special attention in manufacturing the containers, e.g. overwrapping or a separate bag for bicarbonate are needed.

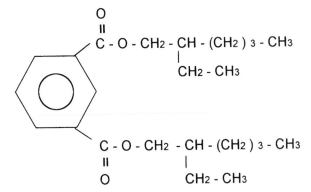

Figure 2. Diethyl-hexyl-phthalate.

The PVC–Pl bags in PD are sterilized by steaming at a temperature of about 121°C. This procedure, however, leads to a pH decrease of the solution and the appearance in suspension of acidic impurities and decomposition products from PVC oxidation, such as formic acid or acetic acid [11]. Sterilization with ethylene oxide is not an alternative because of problems related to allergic reactions in patients, and production of ethylene chlorhydin, a toxic substance which is very difficult to remove [12].

The wide use of disposable Pl–PVC materials, especially in medicine, has led to much interest in their toxicity for both humans and the environment. Since DEHP is not chemically bound to PVC a leakage of this compound from the plastic matrix into solutions rich in lipid or protein was demonstrated as early as 1967 [13, 14]. This opened a large field of investigation as to the toxicity of the degradation products of PVC and plasticizers.

Environmental hazard

The large amount of disposable plastic material products in hospitals has led the involved personnel to question the potential environmental hazard of plastics when they ultimately become waste. This process can be by landfill disposal, incineration or recycling.

Landfill disposal. The landfill disposal of municipal waste is generally not considered dangerous. The gas emission and the leaking of degradation products into air, soil and water, however, must be considered. A relationship between PVC and its principal product of degradation, vinylchloride monomer (VCM) is not definitely established, since the main sources of VCM are the chlorine-containing solvents [15]. As far as Pl are concerned, several studies have demonstrated that air levels of DEHP are generally considered quite low. Giam *et al.* [16] reported levels of phthalates in air in the Gulf of Mexico and North Atlantic areas of $0.4 \, g/m^3$ and $2 \, ng/m^3$ respectively. Since phthalates are aromatic and oxygenated, they are highly reactive to hydroxyl radical attack in the atmosphere. Pl show a relatively low solubility in water (0.01 mg%). The US EPA has estimated a steady-state ambient water concentration of about 0.02 mg/L; 10 µg/L DEHP in drinking water may, however, be a more realistic upper limit value [17]. It is estimated that phthalate esters are adsorbed onto the organic matter in soil. The US EPA suggests a water/soil ratio between 1:150 and 1:3000 [17] but *in-vitro* studies have shown that microorganisms are able to aerobically degrade

up to 41% of the DEHP in 30 days, but no degradation occurred under anaerobic conditions [18]. A limitation of this waste disposal procedure is the increasing shortage of landfill sites, and principally, landfill is not the method of choice for the disposal of hospital waste.

Waste incineration. Two major problems are caused by PVC incineration: emission of hydrochloric acid and dioxyne formation. During the incineration process PVC releases hydrochloric, acid which is a component of the acid rains that are, in turn, one of the major causes of forest death. The HCl formation, however, is only a minor part of the acid emission responsible for the acid rains, which consist of nitric acid, sulphuric acid, and hydrochloric acid of which 50–70% is due to PVC [19]. The HCl emission in offgases from the incinerator has been calculated as about $900 \, mg/m^3$ and almost half of this amount is due to PVC incineration. Since, for example, in the Netherlands the law provides a maximum HCl emission of $50 \, mg/m^3$ [19], wet scrubbing of offgases to remove HCl is necessary with or without PVC.

The word dioxin suddenly became famous in 1976 after the Seveso disaster. The term dioxin includes more than 210 different substances, the structure of which is based on dibenzodioxine and dibenzofluorane. The toxicity of these substances is very high and is species-specific. In humans acute skin and eye irritations have been described. These products are accumulated in adipose tissues and can be extracted by breast milk. Dioxin is known to be a side-product of incomplete combustion with production of phenolic non-chlorinated precursors; after chlorination a *de-novo* synthesis of dioxin occurs. PVC incineration has been indicated as a source of chlorine necessary for *de-novo* synthesis of dioxin [19]. The available literature data, however, are contradictory; the chlorine production from municipal waste is greatly in excess of the amounts needed for dioxin formation, even without any PVC [20].

Recycling. Recycling of plastics is considered one of the more promising solutions for the disposal of waste. All thermoplastics, including PVC, can be recycled, although the quality of the regenerated product is not that of the original material. Up to now, regenerated plastic products are not allowed for pharmaceutical purposes. At the moment, although pharmaceutical industries or specialized recycling companies already recycle up to 95% of plastic scrap (not for medical use) this process is not economically convenient. The environmental aspects of waste, however, will give greater impulse to research towards solving this inconvenience in the near future [21]. Another problem in recycling plastic infusion bags or sets is the difficulty in separating different materials, e.g. metal or natural rubber components, from PVC. Research in this area has been carried out for optimizing the procedure to obtain better quality and lower costs.

Human toxicity

The toxicity of Pl–PVC for humans has been studied extensively over the past 30 years, after Pl traces in biological fluids stored in Pl–PVC bags were found [4]. The two principal compounds of this plastic membrane considered toxic are VCM and DEHP, the more used Pl.

VCM. The first study on VCM toxicity was conducted in the early 1970s by Villa and his group [22], who demonstrated VCM cancerogenicity in an experimental model. Afterwards, VCM was suspected to be cancerogenic in men after the observation of a higher incidence of liver cancer in operators exposed to high air VCM levels in PVC production plants. It is now generally accepted that VCM is able to cause a rare but lethal form of liver angiosarcoma [23]. Tumours of the brain and the central nervous system, and neoplasms of the lymphatic and haematopoietic system [24], as well as pulmonary disfunction [25] have also been described after VCM inhalation. These reports, however are, based on observations in men working in PVC plants and exposed to a large quantity of VCM. Recently, other studies have demonstrated that the monomer can migrate from food containers, with a possible human exposure to up to 100 μg/day [26]. In humans VCM is metabolized into chloroethylene oxide that is considered the most mutagenic metabolite [27]; the mechanism involved seems to be the alkylation of DNA. A VCM dose not exceeding 5 ppm is not considered to increase cancer incidence; the European pharmacopoeias, however, consider concentrations of 1 ppm more safe.

Plasticizers. Diethylhexyl phthalate (DEHP) is, up to now, the most used plasticizer. Other Pl, however have been proposed, e.g. dinonyl and didecil-phthalate, adipic acid esters, e.g. diethylhexyl adipate and citric acid esters, e.g. acetyltributyl acetate (ATBC). The newer Pl used in manufacturing PVC bags are esters of trimellinate such as tri-(2-ethylhexyl)-trimellinate (TOTM). These Pl migrate from PVC to

a lesser extent than DEHP [28]. They have the same inhibitory effect on erythrocyte deterioration [12], but unlike DEHP they are able to increase platelet survival from 3 to 5 days [29].

The possible routes of Pl exposure are: oral, intravenous and peritoneal. As emphasized above for VCM, DEHP can also migrate from PVC overwrapping packages for food or drinking water. It has been shown that 1.5 μg of DEHP can be found in 1 L of drinking water. Children are also exposed to Pl leaking from toys, so they could adsorb 200–2000 μg of Pl per day [30]. After oral administration DEHP is rapidly and extensively adsorbed in the upper digestive tract by lipase hydrolysis [31]. The major derivatives of DEHP are mono-(2-ethylhexyl)phthalate (MEHP), 2-ethylhexanol (2-EH) and phthalic acid (PA). Almost 50% of the administered dose of Pl is eliminated after 8–12 h of application, either as metabolite or in unmetabolized form by the kidney and faeces in healthy subjects [32]. Intravenous administration has been largely studied in polytransfused and haemodialysed patients. Lanina *et al.* [33] showed in 1991 that migration of DEHP into blood stored in PVC bags is time-dependent with different percentages of migration according to the blood component. After 21 days of storage, plasma contains about 50 mg/L of DEHP, total blood 37 mg/L and erythrocytes about 20 mg/L. In frozen condition, however, plasma contains only 3.85 mg/L of DEHP. Since the kidney is the major route of Pl excretion, these compounds tend to accumulate in patients with impairment of renal function. Obviously, the most exposed subjects are those receiving haemodialysis (HD). In several studies the Pl exposure of HD patients was investigated [34, 35]. Exposure on DEHP and its major metabolite MEHP has been quantified as ranging from 250 mg to 50 g per year [34]. Mettang *et al.* showed serum levels in 21 patients on HD of DEHP, MEHP and 2-EH leaching from sets and tubing into the blood stream. The highest values were found at the end of HD treatment. After the 3-day dialysis-free interval, serum levels of these substances decreased continuously, thus suggesting a route of excretion different from the kidney [36]. DEHP excretion has also been demonstrated in biliary secretion and by metabolic degradation to numerous MEHP derivatives [37] and PA. The metabolism and consequent toxicity of DEHP is dose-dependent and species-specific. In rodents further Pl metabolization takes place through oxidation to produce ketones and carboxylic acid [31], while in men glucuronates of MEHP are formed

[38]. This difference in the degree and type of conjugation seems to be the reason why toxicity in humans is less extensive than in rodents. A distinction has to be made between acute and chronic toxicity and also between the various routes of administration.

Acute oral toxicity in animal models is very low; the only sign in rodents is diarrhoea which is partly due to the oil composition of Pl. No reports are available in humans. Chronic exposure of animals to DEHP (Table 3), however, have pointed out a toxicity involving major organs such as liver, kidneys and reproductive system. Testicular atrophy has been reported in rats fed with a high dose of DEHP [39]. MEHP and other monoester metabolites of Pl can probably selectively remove testicular zinc and thereby lead to tubular atrophy. Zinc is essential for maintaining the structure and function of gonads, and its deficiency is known to produce testicular atrophy in both humans and experimental animals [40]. The effect of Pl on female fertility is controversial and considered dose-dependent, while embryo and fetal toxicity, as well as teratogenic, effects, have been reported [41]. The US National Toxicology Program Study on DEHP toxicity reported that ingestion of high doses of this compound (300–1200 mg/kg BW) increases the incidence of hepatocarcinoma in rodents while the same aspect is not evident in other species. In rodents, peroxisomal proliferation was noted after DEHP exposure [42]. These organelles have recently received much interest regarding their involvement in the carcinogenic process [43]. DEHP is responsible for peroxisomal β-oxidation by inducing an increment of lipid

deposition in the liver and also DNA stimulation leading to pronounced proliferation of peroxisomes [44]. Several studies have demonstrated that DEHP does not interact directly with DNA, so it is considered a nongenotoxic tumour promoter but not a tumor initiator [45]. Data on peroxisomal proliferation in humans are not extant, although preliminary results suggest a DEHP-mediated peroxisome proliferation in human cells transplanted into experimental animals. Obviously a threshold-risk assessment in humans is necessary. Mutagenicity of DEHP was found *in vitro* with chromosomal aberration in cultured cells [46]. *In-vivo* tests reported negative results with DEHP or MEHP. Finally, Crocker and co-workers found polycystic degeneration of the kidneys after oral administration of low doses of DEHP for 1 year in rats [47].

Acute DEHP toxicity has been described in rats after intravenous infusion of a high dose of Pl. The symptoms were characterized by respiratory distress due to pulmonary oedema, haemorrhage and polymorphonuclear infiltration, characteristic of a syndrome called 'shock lung' [48]. The importance of the physical form of the DEHP was emphasized in this study. When high doses of Pl were infused dissolved in ethanol they were readily tolerated, while when DEHP was injected dissolved in donor blood, lung abnormalities were seen with much lower DEHP doses. In humans a similar but less virulent form of pulmonary distress has been described in polytransfused patients who evidenced pulmonary oedema and respiratory distress of unknown origin [49]. Chronic exposure to intravenous DEHP has been investigated in an experimental model by Jacobson *et al.* [30]. Two groups of monkeys were treated for 3 years with blood transfusion (PVC bags) or only exposed to polypropylene. Liver necrosis and lymphocytic portal infiltration were found only in PVC-exposed animals. In humans high concentrations of DEHP were found in post-mortem biopsies of polytransfused patients in lung, spleen, liver and kidney [4]. In HD patients, where Pl exposure can be present for more than 20 years, DEHP toxicity has been associated with an increase in liver size and elevation of hepatic enzymes, as well as acute hepatitis without any sign of infectious hepatitis [50]. The symptoms improved when PVC was substituted with PVC-free material, and started again when the patients were re-exposed to the previous tubing system. Necrosing dermatitis and uraemic pruritus in HD patients were also associated to Pl exposure [51, 52], although other studies were not able to demonstrate any relationship between pruritus and DEHP concentration [53]. In another

Table 3. Acute and chronic DEHP toxicity

	Acute	Chronic
Per os	Diarrhoea	Testicular atrophy Embryo-fetal toxicity Genotoxicity Mutagenicity Teratogenic effect Hepatocarcinogenicity
Intravenous	Shock lung Pulmunary oedema Respiratory distress	Liver necrosis Liver dysfunction Hepatitis Necrotic dermatitis, pruritus Acquired polycystic kidney
Intraperitoneal	Peritoneal sclerosis Cytokine production Phagocytosis inhibition	Organ deposition Eosinophilic peritonitis

observation Crocker *et al.* hypothesized a correlation between DEHP and acquired polycystic kidney disease in long term HD patients. A high concentration of DEHP was also found in kidney biopsies from these patients.

Intraperitoneal toxicity of plasticizers

The situation in peritoneal dialysis (PD) is completely different. DEHP and its metabolites show a low solubility in aqueous solutions and their concentration is approximately 1000 times lower than in blood. The highest level of contamination (Table 4) is seen for the cyclohexaonone compound used as adhesive. Formic and acetic acid have been identified as impurities from PVC bags [55]. Nässberger *et al.* [50] showed in 1987 that DEHP dismission in CAPD bags was time-dependent and that the MEHP concentration was much higher than that of DEHP in PD solutions. It was postulated that a greater hydrolysation of DEHP than of MEHP occurred due to the autoclaving sterilization process.

The DEHP exposure of CAPD patients has been calculated by the same authors as about 10–40 mg per year. In a study in 1996 Mettang *et al.* [53] evaluated (Fig. 3) the DEHP and its most important metabolites concentration in PD fluid before, during and after an intraperitoneal dwell. While the DEHP concentration did not show any variation during the period studied, the MEHP steadily decreased during the dwell and seemed to be rapidly adsorbed by the peritoneal membrane. In this study the authors found a MEHP concentration in PD fluid higher than DEHP. The high concentrations of PA found in dialysate support the hypothesis of a peritoneal route of PA excretion. When serum Pl concentrations in HD and PD patients are compared, lower

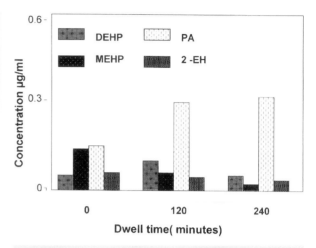

Figure 3. Concentrations of DEHP, MEHP, PA and 2-EH in CAPD solution at 0, 120 and 240 min of dwell [36].

MEHP and PA concentrations are found in PD patients (Fig. 4). Whether this was due to increased excretion or minor exposure to Pl has to be elucidated. Another important question is whether Pl can be stored in chronic renal failure (CRF) patients. Chen *et al.* showed in DEHP storage in lung, fat and spleen of nephrectomized dogs; the same authors found a low DEHP concentration in kidney, lung, liver and spleen of two patients who had been on dialysis before dying [56]. Fracasso *et al.* in 1986 studied the toxicological effects of three different plasticizers: DEHP, didodecyl-phthalate (DDIP) and benzylbutyl-phthalate (BBP) on membrane transport in an *in-vitro* [57] and *in-vivo* [58] study. In the *in-vitro* model of water transport, Pl were able to inhibit the vasopressin-stimulated or cyclic AMP-stimulated water transport in toad bladder. This effect was time- and dose-dependent and occurred after the generation of cyclic AMP. In the *in-vivo* study the authors investigated the toxicity of intraperitoneally injected Pl in four groups of rats in which one had normal renal function, one had

Table 4. Identified impurities in two brands of NaCl intravenous solutions contained in PVC bags (from Nässberger *et al.* [50])

	ACO (F3M019)	Travenol (830617J31)
Phthalic acid (µg/ml)	0.026	0.027
Cyclohexanone (µg/ml)	ND	35.0
Phenol (µg/ml)	0.024	0.029
Phthalide (µg/ml)	0.016	0.580
Benzoic acid (µg/ml)	0.029	ND
Benzaldehyde (µg/ml)	0.005	0.013
Bisphenol-A (µg/ml)	ND	0.32
Butyl hydroxyanisol (µg/ml)	0.058	ND
MEHP (µg/ml)	0.454	ND
DEHP (µg/ml)	0.007	0.005

ND: not detected.

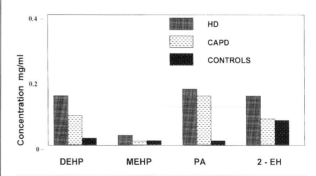

Figure 4. Concentration of DEHP, MEHP, PA and 2-EH in serum of patients on HD, CAPD and controls [36].

chronic renal failure (CRF) and one had CRF and received intraperitoneal Pl. The fourth group consisted of sham-operated animals which received Pl. In an extra group of CRF animals, very low doses of Pl were given. The results showed marked peritoneal sclerosis in low and high dosage Pl CRF animals with, at light microscopy, multiple layers of swollen cell and polymorphonucleate infiltration. The electron microscopy demonstrated a thickening of the interstitial tissue, collagen deposition and fibroblast infiltration with disappearance of microvilli. The evaluation of peritoneal transport efficacy showed reduction of ultrafiltration capacity. The same evaluation showed no difference in Pl-treated groups with normal renal function compared to normal animals. In a further analysis of body accumulation of DEHP high Pl concentrations were found in the peritoneal membrane, kidney and peritoneal fluid of Pl–CRF rats. In an *in-vitro* study of monocytes incubated with DEHP the same authors demonstrated increased cytokine production. They found an increase of interleukin 1α and interleukin 1β which could be responsible for the induction of peritoneal fibrosis [59]. The phthalate involvement in leukocyte function was also evaluated by Mettang *et al.* [36], who demonstrated a MEHP- and PA-induced inhibition of leukocyte phagocytic function at low pH. The mechanism responsible for this alteration is not known. It seems, however, that Pl are able to inhibit the respiratory chain at the level of the cytocrome C reductase, so determining an impairment of leukocyte functions for an inhibitory effect of the Pl on the oxidative metabolism of leukocytes. Eosinophilic peritonitis, as expression of an immune reaction to Pl–PVC PD containers, has also been hypothesized [55].

The conclusions that can be drawn on Pl–PVC toxicity are that the direct toxicity of this substance in humans is contradictory and still not well known, while its environmental hazard is a well-studied problem that has to be solved.

Alternative materials

The alternatives studied for making PVC material less toxic, while maintaining the same characteristics of flexibility and transparency, were first of all to substitute the DEHP with a different, less toxic plasticizer. As described above, a newer and more used Pl is tri-(2-ethylhexyl)-trimellinate. More recently, two new plastic materials have been proposed for medical use: Clear-Flex® and coextruded polyolefins.

Clear-Flex®

The first plastic material employed in the substitution of PVC was the Clear-Flex®, produced in Italy in 1983. This is a trilaminate structure composed by a three-layer film with the following composition: *polyethylene* (inner layer), *nylon* (middle layer) and *polypropylene* (outer layer) spliced to each other with a substance containing polyurethane. The three layers of the Clear-Flex® foil present some specific characteristics that determine the effectiveness of this material in PD: (1) the polyethylene comes into direct contact with the solution and is a totally non-toxic inert polymer, (2) nylon is a strong gas barrier and possesses high mechanical strength, (3) polypropylene drastically reduces the permeability to water vapour.

The mechanical and physicochemical characteristics are listed in Table 5. This material does not contain Pl, is perfectly transparent, collapsible and inert. It can be steam sterilized at 121°C, is highly resistant to mechanical injuries and totally harmless to the environment. In particular, during incineration the products of combustion (H_2O, CO_2, etc.) are similar to those obtained by burning natural organic materials such as wood.

Moreover, it has a water and vapour permeability 5–6 times lower than PVC. In Fig. 5 a comparative study is reported on the permeability of PVC and Clear-Flex® saline solutions with and without overwrapping. The plastic vapour permeability, measured as a percentage of weight loss over a period of 3 years with stable temperature and humidity, showed that leakage was higher in PVC bags, which was most evident when the containers were not overwrapped. The weight of trilaminate bags remained stable with only small differences between those overwrapped and those not overwrapped (unpublished data).

With regard to gas permeability, Clear-Flex® has been demonstrated to be highly impermeable to gases. O_2 permeability, in fact, is 17–19 times lower

Table 5. Clear-Flex physicochemical characteristics

Do not contain plasticizers
Perfectly transparent
High mechanical resistance
High resistance to heat (sterilized at 121°C)
Low permeability to water vapour
Low permeability to gases
Walls totally collapsible
Totally inert material
Safe disposal

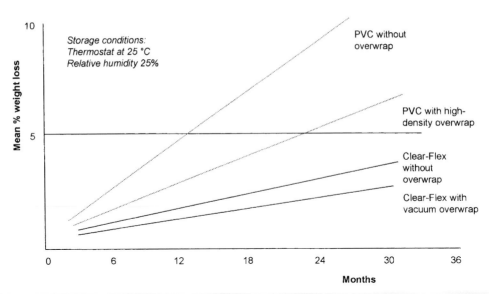

Figure 5. Permeability to water vapour. Comparison of Clear-Flex and PVC.

than that of PVC: 8–9 cc/m²/24 h and 155 cc/m²/ 24 h respectively, while CO_2 permeability is similar. This means that oxidizable and highly unstable solutions such as amino acids, as well as solutions that must be stored in the presence of CO_2, e.g. sodium bicarbonate, can better be supplied in Clear-Flex®.

The interaction between drugs and Clear-Flex® has been widely studied. It has been demonstrated that absorption by this material is negligible, and in many cases similar to that of glass. For example, ampicillin as well as gentamicin, showed no difference in concentration after 30–120 min of storage [60]. Insulin showed the same behaviour with concentrations of about 96% after 20 min of storage [61].

Particulate materials have been found in various concentrations in PD fluid stored in PVC bags. This is an important problem, since their incorporation in the peritoneal membrane has been proposed as one of the causes of peritoneal fibrosis. Verger *et al.* described the presence of small foreign bodies in up to 38% of peritoneal biopsies performed [62], and Di Paolo *et al.* hypothesized that this foreign material could be derived from plastic particles present in the solution [63]. In 1987 Cantù *et al.* evaluated the effect of heat on PVC and Clear-Flex® peritoneal dialysis bags [64]. The authors found (Fig. 6) a progressive increase of small particles in the PD fluid, much more evident in PVC bags.

It is well known that PD fluid is not fully biocompatible. One of the factors affecting the PD fluid biocompatibility is the chemical contamination of dialysis fluid by its container [65]. In a recent retrospective clinical study, Fracasso *et al.* [66] evaluated the PD efficiency in two groups of patients treated with PVC and Clear-Flex® PD solutions over a period of 2 and 4 years (Fig. 7). Urea and creatinine dialysate-to-plasma (D/P) ratios were lower in the PVC group after 4 years of treatment. The ultrafiltration was lower in the PVC group, especially after 4 years. The D/D_0 of glucose in the Clear-Flex® group remained stable during the period of observation, while it increased in the PVC group, especially after 4 years of dialysis. These findings suggest that Clear-Flex® contributes to the maintenance of a better permselectivity of the peritoneal membrane for a longer period.

In another study carried out by Carozzi *et al.* in 1992 [67], *in-vitro* effects of peritoneal solutions, stored in conventional PVC and Clear-Flex® bags, on peritoneal T-lymphocyte, fibroblast and mesothelial cell function were evaluated. The fibroblast proliferation activity (Table 6), evaluated by measuring their ability to incorporate [³H], demonstrated that Clear-Flex® PD samples only marginally stimulated fibroblast activity. The collagen stimulating synthesis expressed by increased secretion of interferon-γ and interleukin 1 by T-lymphocytes and macrophages, was considerably increased after contact with dialysate contained in PVC bags. Prostaglandin E_2 is considered an indicator of peritoneal tissue stability because of its ability to inhibit cell proliferation. Its production was considerably reduced in PVC solution. The conclusion of this study was that there are some substances in peritoneal fluid contained in PVC bags able to stimulate collagen,

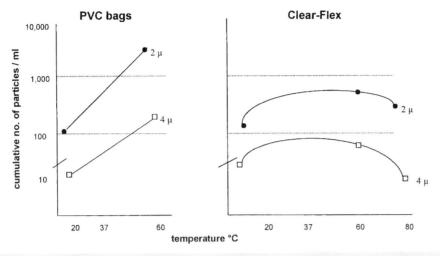

Figure 6. Particles found in PVC and Clear-Flex bags after heating at various temperature [62].

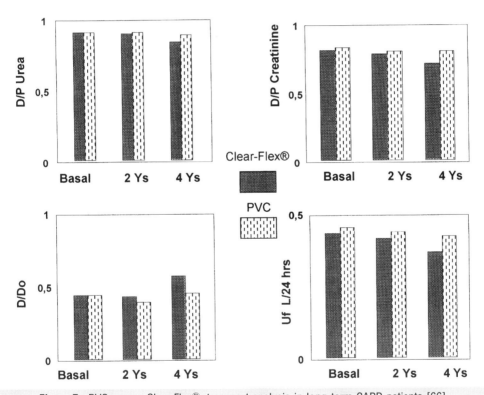

Figure 7. PVC versus Clear-Flex®, transport analysis in long-term CAPD patients [66].

Table 6. PVC versus clear-flex® biocompatibility (from Carozzi *et al.* [67])

| | Fibroblast proliferation [³H] thymidine | Collagen synthesis | | Cell proliferation inhibition PGE₂ |
		Interfon-γ	Interleukin-1	
Basal	+	+	+	+ + + +
PVC	+ + + +	+ + + +	+ + + +	+
Clear-flex®	+/±	+/±	+/±	+ + +

fibroblast and cellular proliferation, so inducing peritoneal fibrosis. Those phenomena were present to a lesser extent when peritoneal fluid contained in Clear-Flex® bags was tested.

The toxicological hazard of Clear-Flex® is mostly tied to the material used as adhesive. It has been demonstrated that polyurethane can produce methylenedianiline (MDA) during steam sterilization, that could be found in small quantities into the solution [68]. This compound is considered toxic for humans and it has been associated with colon and bladder carcinomas and lynphosarcomas in workers exposed to aromatic polyurethane. Its metabolite MDA, moreover, has also been suspected of causing hepatitis and allergic dermatitis [69]; however, until now neoplasms attributed to MDA in patients treated with peritoneal dialysis have not been reported.

Polyolefins. Polyolefins are polymers constructed exclusively from hydrogen and carbon atoms. The polyolefins employed for medical uses are polyethylene (PEL), polypropylene (PPL) and their copolymers. The low-density PEL is the polyolefin mostly used for medical devices. However, its characteristics of low flexibility and transparency have limited its employment to rigid and opaque containers and tubings. Three other polyolefins have to be taken into consideration: high-density polyethylene (HDPE) that presents a highly crystalline structure and a high haze level, PPL that can be produced in very clear sheets but its stiffness and brittleness are unacceptable and finally, ethylene vinyl acetate. Although the latter has good collapsibility and resistance properties, it cannot be considered because of its poor heat resistance. HDPE and PPL, even though they have some interesting properties such as resistance to high temperature and an adequate barrier to water vapour, are opaque and poorly flexible. The latter aspect can be improved by alloying them with elastomer derivatives of ethylene and polypropylene such as butyl rubber, polysobutylene, ethylene-polypropylene rubber and ethylene-propylene diene rubber. All of these alloys can be processed in foils with properties of flexibility and transparency that are determined by their blend morphology.

More recently an important development in polyolefin technology has allowed production of plastic foils with properties and performances similar or superior to plasticized PVC [70].

A special catalyst in a pool of liquid propylene joins propylene monomers into polymer chains. The chains can be assembled in several different structures, depending on the orientation of the different molecules, that form a microstructure able to influence the physicochemical properties of the final product. The chains can have a regular (isotactic) structure, when the monomers connect themselves head to tail and with other similar chains. In this case at the melting point of approximately 160°C they fit together to form crystals. The crystals are small and the polymer chains can be part of two adjacent crystals by giving to the isotactic conventional PPL the observed strength and stiffness. Other PPL molecules consist of monomers joined together entirely randomly. In this atactic structure, PPL monomers have the same chances of attaching in either head-to-head or head-to-tail orientation, to form a so-called amorphous PPL. These polymer chains, by combining with other polymers in orderly fashion, resist forming crystals; thus they lack the rigid structure of crystals with very low tensile strength, but compared with isotactic PPL, greater softness and flexibility. This flexibility derives from the non-polar and different tridimensional configuration of the PPL chains and also, because of the absence of crystals, there is no melting point. This new technique, called REXflex flexible polyolefin (FPO), has allowed variations in the amount of crystallinity during the polymerization process of PPL. The control of crystallinity allows control of flexibility without the necessity to add plasticizers as in PVC. Another advantage of this technique is that the more amorphous the polymer is, the easier it is for other polymers to be added, to modify its properties. Since so many modifications of polyolefin structure are possible, by varying their composition, different layers of polyolefins with different physical characteristics can be produced.

By employing this technique a multi-layer co-extruded plastic foil has been developed, called Biofine®. This has been employed in the manufacture of peritoneal dialysis bags. It consists of seven layers of polyolefins with different characteristics co-extruded and not laminated, that, for the natural adhesion existing between the different PPL layers, does not need the presence of adhesives. All these layers have a thickness of 100 μm compared with the 355 μm of the normal mono-PVC. Thus the containers will have a lower weight with a saving in terms of costs for plastic material and waste production. This membrane is flexible, transparent, has good drop resistance and is completely atoxic and inert. It presents a good barrier for water and gases similar to that of trilaminates so they do not need overwrap. Because of the absence of polarity, which is characteristic of the polyolefins, this material does not react with medicaments that can be kept. Another advantage is its temperature stability. In contrast to the other polyolefins Biofine® can withstand steam sterilization temperatures of 121°C while maintaining its physical integrity [71]. Particularly interesting are the ecological aspects of Biofine®. It offers significant advantages for disposal by incineration and, to a lesser extent, disposal in landfill. Biofine® is chemically inert and, being composed of polymers free of small molecules such as Pl, is stable in landfill. Very important is the recycling: especially when a complete PD system is manufactured with Biofine®, it is not necessary to separate all the components of the set, making recycling easier and less expensive. All the Biofine® components are hydrocarbon products (>99%). Therefore when incinerated they produce a heat of combustion comparable to fuel oil, with combustion products similar to any other saturated hydrocarbon fuel such as CO, CO_2 and H_2O.

In conclusion, the ecological hazards of Pl–PVC stimulated research into new plastic materials with characteristics similar to those of PVC but less harmful to the environment. In this category both Clear-Flex® and Biofine® have physicochemical properties similar and sometimes superior to PVC. In peritoneal dialysis the employment of these alternative materials is considered eligible for either better biocompatibility or better respect for the environment.

Container shape

The traditional CAPD bag consists of a single plastic chamber in which a solution of glucose and ionized molecules (electrolytes and buffer) is contained. When new substances have been proposed in order to improve clinical results or biocompatibility of the solution, some problems arose from chemical stability of such a solution in which several different molecules are sterilized and stored together.

Historically, the first proposal of a different shape for the CAPD bag was forwarded by Feriani et al. [72] (Fig. 8). These authors suggested the use of a double-chamber bag to sterilize and store bicarbonate and divalent cations such as calcium and magnesium.

During the autoclaving, these molecules precipitate as carbonate salts and glucose caramelizes due to the high pH of the solution.

A solution containing bicarbonate may reach a pH of 8.4. Under this condition bicarbonate and carbonate may exist according to the following

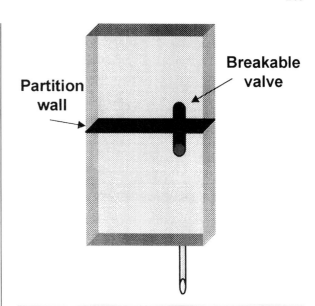

Figure 8. Schematic representation of a double-chamber bag.

equilibrium:

$$Na^+ + HCO_3^- \leftrightarrow Na^+ + CO_3^= + H^+$$

Since divalent anions such as Ca and Mg are also present in the dialysate, the following equilibrium will be achieved:

$$NaHCO_3 + CaCl_2 \leftrightarrow CaCO_3 + NaCl + HCl$$

When the pH of the solution is higher than 7, $CaCO_3$ will begin to precipitate, thus reducing the bicarbonate concentration. A high CO_2 content may avoid this precipitation, shifting the following reaction to the left:

$$Ca(HCO_3)_2 \leftrightarrow CaCO_3 + H_2O + CO_2$$

Thereby a soluble salt of calcium is formed.

Since CO_2 is volatile, the CO_2 content of the solution tends to be reduced over a prolonged period of time, facilitating $CaCO_3$ formation. This problem can be solved by the separation of Ca and bicarbonate into two containers and mixing them just before use.

Small amounts of an acid in the solution containing calcium, permit one to achieve a high CO_2 content in the final mixed dialysate. This is shown in the equation.

$$NaHCO_3 + AH \leftrightarrow ANa + H_2O + CO_2$$

In single-pass haemodialysis this problem has been solved by the so-called 'three-stream method', in which an acid and a basic (bicarbonate) solution are continuously mixed with treated water. The acid solution, which contains an organic acid, calcium, magnesium and glucose, lowers the pH of the final solution. As a consequence the carbonate ion concentration becomes so low that the solubility product of calcium and magnesium carbonate is not exceeded.

This concept was adapted to intermittent peritoneal dialysis by Ing *et al.* [73] and subsequently modified to a 'two-stream method' in which equal volumes of an acid and basic (bicarbonate) solution are simultaneously delivered by a roller pump to produce the final solution [74]. Later, these authors described [75] a new method of producing a bicarbonate solution, and used it during an intermittent peritoneal dialysis (IPD) session [76]. The bicarbonate content of a glass syringe was added to an acid solution placed in a second container to yield 2 L of the final dialysate. No problems were encountered during the clinical IPD session. Independently, a single container, which is divided into two compartments (one containing the acid and one containing the basic solutions) by a partition wall, has been developed for CAPD solutions [72]. A breakable valve in the partition wall is broken by an external pressure just before use, thus allowing the mixing of the two solutions. The final dialysate pH value was around 7.4. Clinical results are reported in another section of this chapter. This approach has been applied to other problems connected to the chemical instability of glucose in PD solutions.

It has been well known since 1912 that heat sterilization and long storage induces degradation of glucose in several products, some of them giving a yellow-brown colour to the solution [77]. This reaction is called the Maillard reaction (Fig. 9). In solution 99% of glucose is in its cyclic form while 1% is in an aldehydic form. If an amino group is present in the solution the aldehydic form of glucose reacts with it, forming a Schiff base that in turn becomes an Amadori glycosylation product. These reactions are responsible for the typical discoloration of the fluid and occur also *in vivo*, since tissue proteins have many exposed amino groups [78]. *In vivo*, advanced glycosilated end products (AGE) are formed from Amadori products after a complex series of chemical rearrangements. The clinical consequences are presented in other chapters of this book. For these reasons glucose/amino acid or polyglucose/amino acid solutions can be prepared only in a double-chamber bag.

If there are no amino groups in the solution, the aldehyde form of glucose is dehydrated to enediol and then to furan compounds, of which 5-hydroxy-

methylfurfural (5-HMF) is the most important [79]. These compounds can be further degraded to unsatured dicarbonyl products. Again these compounds yield discoloration of the solution. In order to reduce glucose degradation products as much as possible, 5-HMF is continuously monitored during the production of commercial fluids. Nevertheless levels increase with time of storage. 5-HMF is probably not the most toxic product of glucose degradation but only a precursor of more cytotoxic substances. However, 5-HMF is the easiest substance to be detected and measured. Elevated levels of 5-HMF in CAPD bags have been associated with infusion pain and reduction of ultrafiltration [80]; thus it is likely that glucose degradation products are among the pathogenetic agents in long-term degeneration of the peritoneal membrane.

Lower pH, higher glucose concentration and the absence of catalysing substances such as calcium and magnesium are chemical strategies that could be applied in order to reduce the formation of glucose degradation products during the heat sterilization [81]. In a two-chamber bag all these requirements could be met. Glucose is sterilized alone in one of the two chambers in a very acidic medium and without electrolytes. After mixing the two chambers, a standard CAPD fluid is obtained and the concentration of the most cytotoxic aldehydes is reduced to below the detection limit. The clinical use of this solution in four stable CAPD patients has been reported to reduce inflow pain, and to increase the concentration of cancer antigen 125 in the effluent, suggesting an increase in total mesothelial cell mass [82].

Solutions

Solute removal in PD is achieved both by diffusion and convection. The first mechanism takes place because of the concentration gradient between the blood of the peritoneal capillary and the PD solution infused in the abdomen. The solution infused in the peritoneal cavity tends to equilibrate with plasma water over time, and is removed at the end of one exchange after partial or complete equilibration. The composition of the dialysis solution allows one to remove, balance or even infuse solutes from and into the patient. The electrochemical concentration gradient is the driving force that allows such a passive diffusion [83]. In addition, fluid movement across the peritoneal membrane may occur when a transmembrane pressure gradient is generated between the blood and the dialysate compartments.

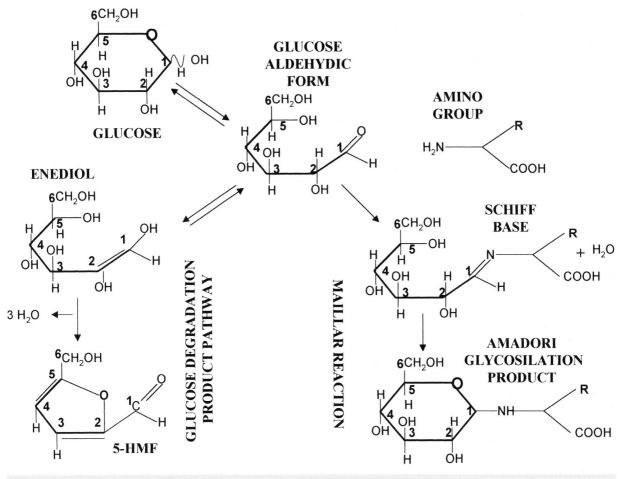

Figure 9. Glucose pathways towards degradation product and Maillard reaction.

Since a negative fluid balance is required in uraemic patients, an osmotic agent is added to the dialysis solution to increase its osmolality. In such a condition an osmotic pressure gradient is created and ultrafiltration occurs. As a consequence, solutes are moving across the membrane transported in the bulk flow and convective transport takes place [84, 85].

The composition of PD solution is therefore the key factor that governs both diffusion and convection, as well as the removal of the fluid excess from the body. In this way, utilizing different solutions, blood purification, acid–base control, electrolyte correction and body fluid balance can be adequately achieved [86].

Several types of PD solution are produced for clinical use today. The fluids are sterilized in varying volumes and glucose is added at various concentrations as an agent to vary dialysate osmolality. Solutions were originally provided in glass containers and subsequently in large plastic tanks. PD fluids

are today supplied in collapsible plastic bags of different sizes and shapes. Surprisingly enough, the composition of dialysis solutions available for clinical use today is very similar to that of the solution used in the late 1950s in Seattle by Boen *et al.* [87] (Table 7).

Clinical studies have recently suggested that PD solutions may not be completely adequate to achieve metabolic correction of the patient, and may create

Table 7. Composition of the peritoneal dialysis fluid

	Boen [87]	Commercial PD fluid
Sodium (mmol/L)	135	132–134
Potassium (mmol/L)		0–2
Calcium (mmol/L)	1.5	1.0–1.75
Magnesium (mmol/L)	0.75	0.25–0.75
Chlorine (mmol/L)	107.5	95–106
Acetate (mmol/L)	35	
Lactate (mmol/L)		35–40
Glucose (g/dl)	2.0 and higher	1.36–4.25

various negative effects on peritoneal membrane function and morphology. These aspects will be detailed in Chapter 18. They have spurred new interest in possible improvements of PD fluids, with regard to new constituents with lower degrees of cellular toxicity, and to the clinical application of new buffers and osmotic agents with a lower degree of side-effects. Therefore clinical trials on new PD solutions have begun in different countries, and new developments are under technical and clinical evaluation. In detail, more physiological concentrations of calcium and magnesium have been demonstrated to be of clinical benefit in several patients.

Substances such as glycerol, icodextrin amino acids and various mixtures of osmotic agents have been studied as alternatives to glucose. They have been chemically evaluated and clinically tested to elucidate possible advantages compared to glucose. Acetate has been replaced by lactate as buffer and the physiological buffer, bicarbonate, has recently been proposed. Different types of sterilization have been evaluated and the noxious effects of glucose degradation products in heat-sterilized solutions have been pointed out.

As the morphological and functional evaluation of the peritoneal mesothelium became possible by *in-vitro* cultured mesothelial cells and molecular biology studies of the various cells involved in the peritoneal membrane, subclinical damage to various structures has become evident. These lesions may be responsible for the short and long-term damage to the peritoneal membrane and the need for a more physiological and less irritating PD solution appears absolutely clear. The impact of PD fluid on the living membrane of peritoneum is therefore the critical point of today's art of PD.

Electrolytes

Electrolyte balance cannot fully be handled in end-stage renal failure [88]. Unphysiological values of serum electrolytes can result in life-threatening complications in uraemic patients [89]. Hyperkalaemia may occur frequently in uraemic patients and the parallel disturbance of acid–base homeostasis may further contribute to a severe disequilibrium between intracellular and extracellular concentrations [90]. Sodium, potassium and magnesium must be removed, or in some cases added, to the patient, via the dialytic fluid in order to normalize the pools in the body and to achieve adequate homeostasis. Calcium uptake from the gastrointestinal tract is reduced, and hypocalcaemia is a common pattern

in uraemia if oral calcium and/or vitamin D supplementation is not provided during conservative therapy. PD fluid is tailored to achieve adequate correction of these derangements and to obtain a restoration of the normal electrolyte composition of the body.

Sodium

Sodium concentration in PD fluids ranges between 130 and 137 mmol/L. In addition, during industrial preparation procedures, 5% variation from the reported sodium concentration can be present. Clinical studies have demonstrated that in CAPD different dialysate sodium concentrations (from 132 to 141 mmol/L) have no significant effect on serum sodium concentration [91]. This could be explained by the peculiar characteristics of the electrolyte transport in CAPD.

Dialytic sodium balance is both a function of diffusion and a result of combined convective transport [92]. Sodium movement by diffusion across the peritoneal membrane may result in net uptake or removal, depending on the concentration gradient between dialysis solution and plasma water [93]. PD may also remove sodium by convection during ultrafiltration. However, the net sodium removal per litre of ultrafiltrate (about 70 mmol/L) is much less than one could expect from the extracellular fluid concentration. This effect seems to be due to the low sieving coefficient for sodium of the peritoneal membrane [94–97], even though the Donnan equilibrium may play an important additional role [98]. Recently [99, 100] the sieving of sodium has been attributed to the presence of ultrasmall or transcellular pores which have been morphologically identified as aquaporins (see Chapter 5).

In the clinical routine the importance of convective transport of sodium may be such that the concentration in the serum is a negligible factor. Studies have demonstrated that when a wide range of drainage volumes, i.e. of ultrafiltration rates, is observed, sodium removal does not correlate with serum concentration [93]. However, since in a stable patient the daily drainage volume is fairly constant, Nolph *et al.* have constructed nomograms to predict dialytic sodium balance at various serum and dialysate sodium concentrations (Fig. 10). In such conditions, daily variations in net sodium balance are mostly a function of serum concentration: an increase in dietary sodium intake will result in a parallel increase in serum sodium, that will consequently lead to an increase in dialytic sodium removal. These

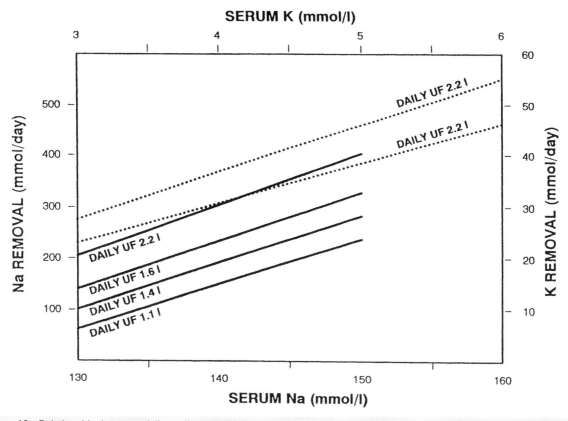

Figure 10. Relationship between daily sodium (solid lines) and potassium (dotted lines) removal and their respective serum concentrations at different daily ultrafiltration rates (modified from Nolph *et al.* [93]).

changes in net daily removal secondary to changes in serum concentration represent an intrinsic autoregulatory mechanism for adjustment of removal rates [93].

On the other hand, when body fluid expansion is isonatric, due to a positive balance of both sodium and water, the correction will be made in two steps. First, the increase of ultrafiltration by the increased number of hypertonic exchanges will result in a hyponatric dialysate with a net removal of water. Second, in this condition an increase of serum sodium concentration will progressively occur and this will lead to increased dialytic sodium removal.

When dialysate sodium concentration is maintained at 132 mmol/L, a normal daily sodium intake of 150 mmol can be easily managed with four CAPD exchanges/day with about 1200 ml/day of ultrafiltration [93]. When present, residual renal function can substantially contribute to sodium removal. It has been reported that, in the absence of major hormonal derangements, urinary sodium content is relatively constant at 70 mmol/L [101].

Since clinical studies have not reported specific side-effects when using the currently available

CAPD solutions with 132–134 mmol/L of sodium, only a few studies have been designed to explore the possible effects of variation of sodium content in CAPD solutions.

Colombi [101] calculated the sodium removal at different urinary volumes and at different daily ultrafiltration rates using a 134 mmol/L sodium CAPD solution in the presence of a serum concentration of 138 mmol/L. In these conditions a daily ultrafiltration of 1100 ml and a urinary volume of 500 ml should maintain the serum sodium concentration constant if sodium intake is about 150 mmol/day. The author suggests that a reduction of dialysate sodium concentration to 130 mmol/L should be considered for patients without residual renal function. De Vecchi *et al.* [102] used a dialysate sodium concentration of 137 mmol/L in 38 unselected patients, to correct orthostatic hypotension. The average orthostatic systolic pressure increased from 129 to 139 mmHg without statistical significance. Three patients required an increase of previous antihypertensive therapy, while no significant changes in the sense of thirst or peripheral oedemas were recorded. In three hypotensive patients dialysate sodium concentration was increased to 142 mmol/L. One patient became hypertensive and one patient normotensive, while no changes were registered in the last patient. The authors concluded that a 137 mmol/L sodium solution could enable better control of mild symptomatic hypotension, while a 142 mmol/L sodium concentration is not always effective in the treatment of severe hypotension in CAPD patients.

Recently a solution with a very low sodium concentration (98 mmol/L) has been proposed [103] to correct fluid overload in patients with insufficient ultrafiltration. The use of this solution once or twice daily led to a reasonable body weight reduction without hypotension or fatigue. A three times higher sodium removal and a significant increase in transcapillary ultrafiltration by using an ultralow sodium solution (102 mmol/L) as compared with a conventional 2.5% glucose solution has been investigated by Imholz *et al.* [104]. Besides other important implications on the mechanisms of solute and water transport, this study demonstrated that this approach could be beneficial for CAPD patients with fluid and sodium overload. A subsequent clinical study in six overhydrated patients with sodium excess, treated once a day for seven consecutive days with a solution containing 98 mmol/L of sodium, confirmed the effectiveness of the ultralow sodium solution [105]. The major results were a 2.5% reduction in body weight, a 12.3% decrease in mean arterial pressure, a 86.5% increase in daily ultrafiltration and a marked (131%) increase in sodium removal.

Different sodium concentrations can also be required when the dialytic regimen is different, as in the case of automated peritoneal dialysis (APD). During short dwell-time exchanges, convection plays a prime role and, as mentioned before, a hyponatric ultrafiltrate is produced in the early phases of one exchange. Consequently, in rapid cycling techniques, water is removed faster than sodium and hypernatraemia may occasionally occur [94–97]. During rapid hypertonic exchanges the use of solutions with 140 mmol/L of sodium resulted in severe thirst, hypertension [106] and hypernatraemia over 160 mmol/L [107]. Raja *et al.* [95] suggested that hypernatraemia can be avoided by utilizing a sodium concentration of 115–120 mmol/L in a 7% dextrose dialysis solution or a concentration of 125–130 mmol/L in a 4.25% dextrose solution. In such conditions an isonatric ultrafiltrate can be obtained. Similar results have been reported by Ahearn *et al.* [97]. More recently Shen *et al.* [108]

proposed a sodium concentration of 118 mmol/L for 2.5% glucose solutions and 109 mmol/L for 4.25% glucose solutions. However, such solutions with lower sodium concentrations have never been commercially available. Furthermore, an increased sense of thirst and difficult blood pressure control have been observed in patients on nightly automated peritoneal dialysis by using dialysis solutions with 132 mmol/L of sodium [109].

Potassium

Hyperkalaemia is one of the most harmful complications in end-stage renal failure. Dialysis treatment must therefore contribute to achieve and maintain an adequate potassium balance. Potassium balance in PD is a function of several factors: among them, serum potassium concentration, insulin bioavailability, cell membrane Na/K pump activity, dialysate potassium concentration and acid–base correction.

The potassium concentration in the commercially available CAPD fluids ranges between 0 and 2 mmol/L. However, solutions without potassium are commonly used in the clinical routine.

Net potassium balance across the peritoneal membrane follows the same chemical–physical principles described for sodium. However, since potassium is absent in the dialysis solution the gradient for diffusion is maximized. Since potassium concentration in extracellular fluid is low, the removal by convection is generally negligible and diffusion is the most important mechanism for net potassium removal [110].

Dialysate potassium should theoretically equilibrate with plasma faster than sodium because of the lower molecular weight and the smaller hydrated radius. However, even after long dwell-times, dialysate potassium does not completely equilibrate with serum [102]. This is because several factors (such as Donnan's equilibrium, membrane sieving and others) may interfere with complete equilibration. On the other hand, serum potassium measurements may be artifactually high because of leaching of potassium from red cells during serum separation [103].

Nomograms to predict daily potassium removal based on serum potassium concentration have been published (Fig. 10). It can be seen that convection minimally increases net potassium removal as previously observed in IPD sessions with hypertonic dialysate [111].

In regular CAPD treatment about 30 mmol/day are lost in the dialysate [112]. About 20 mmol/L of urine are generally added to dialytic removal in case of preserved residual renal function [101]. This overall amount is considerably lower than the usual daily intake of 70–80 mmol. Nevertheless, most patients have a normal serum potassium, which can be explained by increased excretion in the stools [113]. Increased intestinal excretion may become particularly important in patients with high potassium intake, since excretion in the stools is highly correlated with the serum concentration [114]. Insulin levels are also important since the activity of the hormone promotes cellular uptake and tends to restore intracellular–extracellular gradients for the electrolyte.

In previous studies a CAPD solution containing 4 mmol/L of potassium induced hyperkalaemia in about 50% of treated patients who required ionic exchange resin administration [115]. With the commonly used potassium-free CAPD solutions, hypokaliaemia is found in 10–36% of patients [116, 117] even though the intracellular muscle potassium [118] and total body potassium [119, 120] contents have been reported to be normal or slightly increased. It is not clear whether, in such conditions, the hypokalaemic state may be a consequence of an anabolic state, or may reflect a poor nutritional intake [121]. A possible condition of hyperpolarization of the cells with increased transcellular potassium gradient might also contribute to explain this observation.

Magnesium

Magnesium is an important cation involved in several enzymatic reactions. The serum concentration of magnesium in dialysis patients depends on dietary intake and on the concentration of the cation in the dialysis solution. Hypermagnesaemia is a common finding in dialysis patients [122]. While it is almost impossible to show abnormalities related to modestly elevated magnesium concentrations, hypomagnesaemia has been associated with cardiac arrhythmias [123, 124] and various electrocardiographic abnormalities [125].

Normal values of total serum magnesium range from 0.65 to 0.98 mmol/L, while its diffusible fraction is about 55–60% of the total. Commercially available CAPD solutions contain 0.25–0.75 mmol/L of magnesium. In such conditions, when 0.75 mmol/L magnesium and 1.5% glucose solutions are used in CAPD, a slight magnesium uptake from the dialysis solution usually occurs by diffusive gradient [126]. Kwong *et al.*, however, have reported a negative

dialytic balance with the same solution [127]. When ultrafiltration is increased by a 4.25% dextrose solution, convective removal counteracts diffusive uptake, yielding a negative magnesium mass transport in most patients [126]. Peritoneal transport of magnesium is influenced not only by diffusion gradients and ultrafiltration rates, but also by dwell time and peritoneal permeability, because of the large hydrated radius of the molecule [126].

In most papers [128–131] the use of 0.75 mmol/L magnesium solutions resulted in elevated levels of magnesium in the serum. This may lead to an excessive body burden, and potentially inhibits bone remodelling [132, 133]. Other authors pointed out that hypermagnesaemia does not result in any clinical complication; on the contrary, a protective role on soft tissue calcifications has been suggested [134]. Despite such frequent hypermagnesaemia the muscle content of magnesium is generally not altered [118]. Therefore the relationship of serum magnesium to intracellular magnesium concentration and total body magnesium in patients on CAPD is unclear. Dietary magnesium intake is a function of protein intake. On the other hand, magnesium removal with standard 0.75 mmol/L magnesium solutions is negligible. Despite these observations, CAPD patients do not display a continuous increase in serum magnesium levels, and stool magnesium losses may probably have a regulatory function [91].

To achieve a correct balance, Nolph *et al.* suggested lowering dialysate magnesium to 0.25 mmol/L [129]. The use of this solution did not cause hypomagnesaemia, and most patients experienced a normalization of magnesium serum levels [129, 135]. The use of lower or zero magnesium dialysate has also been investigated to permit oral treatment of hyperphosphataemia with magnesium salts as a phosphate binder [136]. This, however, frequently results in a laxative effect, requiring careful monitoring of compliance to therapy and serum magnesium levels [137, 138].

Calcium

CAPD solutions contain 1.175 mmol/L of calcium. Since normal serum concentration of diffusible ionized calcium ranges from 1.15 to 1.29 mmol/L, calcium is absorbed or lost depending on diffusive gradient direction [126]. In CAPD solutions, 30% of calcium is not ionized being 'chelated' by lactate [127]. Ionized calcium probably crosses the peritoneum faster than chelated calcium. As a consequence the ionized calcium gradient is rapidly dissipated. The rapid increase in dialysate pH further contributes to this phenomenon by decreasing calcium ionization in the solution [127].

A significant correlation between a positive calcium balance and the dialysate/serum gradient for ionized calcium has been found by using 1.75 mmol/L calcium solutions [127]. Blumenkrantz *et al.* have also reported that net dialytic calcium uptake inversely correlates with total serum calcium [113]. When ultrafiltration increases in hypertonic exchanges, calcium uptake tend to decrease [126] or even to become negative [127, 139]. Different rates of ultrafiltration may help to explain discrepancies among different studies. Convective removal counterbalances diffusive uptake and decreases the dialysate/serum gradient because of a dilution effect [132].

While a negative balance may result from the use of 1.5 mmol/L dialysate calcium [140], kinetic studies suggest that CAPD solutions with 1.75 mmol/L of calcium (three exchanges with 1.5% glucose and one exchange with 4.25% glucose) generally lead to peritoneal calcium adsorption and rapidly normalize total and ionized calcium serum levels [126–128, 139]. This was suggested to be beneficial in order to prevent progression of osteodystrophy and calcium losses from the bone [131, 141]. However, clinical studies did not confirm such a positive effect [140, 142, 143].

Overall calcium mass-balance is also affected by gastrointestinal adsorption. In CAPD patients an empirical relationship has been found between dietary intake and gastrointestinal adsorption [113]; 720 mg/day of dietary calcium intake resulted in an estimated average gastrointestinal adsorption of 25 mg [113]. If oral calcium supplementations are administered as phosphate binder, significantly greater amounts of calcium are absorbed from the gastrointestinal tract. Assuming a daily phosphate intake of 1000 mg in CAPD patients [144], 70% of this should be bound in the intestinal tract to maintain the balance [139]. This goal can be achieved with 6.25 g of calcium carbonate supplementation (2500 mg of elemental calcium). This leads to an average gastrointestinal calcium adsorption of 700 mg/day [145, 146]. Hence, in a standard patient, total calcium adsorption from the diet and calcium carbonate is approximately 725 mg/day. In such conditions a large number of patients may be subject to an increased risk of hypercalcaemia and soft tissue calcification [147].

On the other hand aluminum-containing phosphate binders are the main source of aluminum in CAPD patients [148] and the dangers of aluminium toxicity in the form of bone disease and encephalopathy are now well recognized [149–151]. A solution to this puzzle has been found in the use of a lower dialysate calcium concentration. This approach has been suggested to avoid the risk of calcium carbonate-related hypercalcaemia [126].

Martis *et al.* [152] have calculated on theoretical bases that a calcium concentration of 1.25 mmol/L in peritoneal fluid would lead to a calcium removal of 160 mg/day when serum ionized calcium is 1.3 mmol/L and to a greater removal in the case of hypercalcaemia.

In a prospective clinical study, Hutchison *et al.* [135] have demonstrated that a 1.25 mmol/L calcium dialysate allowed the administration of larger doses of calcium carbonate with good control of serum phosphate, and maintained serum ionized calcium near to the upper limit of the normal range. Parathyroid hormone was suppressed in the majority of patients and bone histology improved. Similar results have been achieved in a large multicentre study in which 1 mmol/L calcium solution has been used and a low dose of vitamin D and calcium carbonate as phosphate binder has been orally supplemented [153]. However, in the long term a large percentage of patients with low calcium dialysis fluid (23%) showed deterioration of the pre-existing hyperparathyroidism [154]. Low calcium PD fluids have been extensively studied by several investigators and the results confirm the benefit of this approach in uraemic osteodystrophy [155–159].

Long-term usage of lower calcium dialysate by large numbers of patients raises the question of safety in cases of poor compliance to oral calcium carbonate supplementation. In 12 patients treated with a 1.5% glucose and 1.25 mmol/L calcium solution, a net gain of calcium was demonstrated when the serum ionized calcium level was less than 1.25 mmol/L. This observation seems to prove that a very low risk of hypocalcaemia is present in these patients [135]. However, there is a tendency to lose calcium regardless of the serum ionized calcium in those patients treated with 4.25% glucose and low calcium solutions. Since a rapid exacerbation of hyperparathyroidism in some patients converted to low calcium dialysate without adequate oral calcium supplementation has been documented [160] in CAPD patients using two or more hypertonic bags per day and a low calcium solution, a careful surveillance of the mineral metabolism is needed.

The commercially available solutions for intermittent PD treatments are substantially similar to those for CAPD. Adersen [161] reported that a positive calcium transfer from dialysis fluid can be obtained with a 2.16 mmol/L calcium concentration in dialysate both during 1.5% and 4% glucose 30 min dwell-time exchanges, while in automated PD, the low calcium dialysis solution (1.25 mmol/L) could result in a negative calcium balance [162].

In summary, the use of solutions with lower calcium is nowadays common practice in an increased number of dialysis units. This therapeutic approach is further confirmed in patients treated with oral administration of calcium carbonate as a phosphate binder. However, the use of the conventional 1.75 mmol/L calcium solution should not be abandoned, since it is indicated in patients developing a severe hyperparathyroidism with the low calcium solutions and in those with poor compliance with the calcium-based phosphate binders (see also Chapter 19).

Osmotic agents

In PD, net water removal is achieved by adding an osmotic agent to the solution and it is believed to be directly proportional to the dialysate/plasma osmotic gradient (see Chapter 5) [163]. Low molecular weight solutes with high osmotic power (crystalloids) were firstly studied in animals [164]. Only glucose appeared sufficiently safe, effective and readily metabolized. Lately glucose has been used in the solutions for intermittent PD and its reliability was clinically confirmed [165]. However, the peritoneal membrane is not completely impermeable to glucose, and a rapid decline in osmotic gradient, as a consequence of glucose adsorption, is observed during long dwell-time exchanges. This partially limits the osmotic power of glucose and leads to a carbohydrate load in CAPD patients [166].

Several substances have been examined as alternative osmotic agents to glucose. Low molecular weight agents (glycerol, sorbitol, amino acids, xylitol and fructose) have been utilized to overcome some of the metabolic problems caused by glucose. High molecular weight agents (glucose polymers, gelatin, polycations, dextrans and polypeptides) have also been proposed because of their slower absorption, and consequent sustained ultrafiltration in the prolonged dwells [167].

Osmotic power is dependent on the total number of osmotically active molecules in the solution. Therefore, a greater mass of substance is needed to obtain equivalent osmolality gradient, when high molecular weight agents are employed [168].

At high concentration these large molecules are less soluble, hyperviscous, non-physiological and eventually allergenic. Nevertheless, high molar concentrations are not needed in dialysis fluid because these substances may equally provide a sustained slow ultrafiltration due to their lower or absent readsorption. This effect is very similar to that exerted by albumin in biological systems ('colloid' osmotic pressure) (see ref. 169, quoted in ref. 287), and could be exploited in PD to achieve sustained ultrafiltration at low molar concentration using dialysis solutions isosmotic to plasma [170].

The conventional concept that the osmotic flow is proportional to the osmotic gradient may only be applied to an ideal semipermeable membrane. For the biological membranes the direction of osmotic forces is determined by the reflection coefficients of the different molecules and by the molar concentration rather than the total osmolality gradient (see ref. 171 quoted in ref. 287). Consequently an osmotic flow is possible even though the biological membrane separates two solutions with a similar osmolality. It is also possible to induce an osmotic flow towards a hypo-osmolar solution if reflection coefficients of solutes are appropriate [172].

The addition of a low molecular weight agent to a hypo-osmolar solution containing a high molecular weight substance has been proposed to achieve a synergistic effect [173]. In such conditions the crystalloid initiates a rapid phase of ultrafiltration which is then maintained by the slower and prolonged effect of the colloid. By adjusting the proportion of the two agents this bimodal ultrafiltration permits optimization of ultrafiltration kinetics during the exchange. It has been demonstrated that, in a 12 h exchange, a 7.5% glucose polymer plus 0.35% glucose solution may provide greater ultrafiltration (+40%) compared to a 7.5% glucose polymer solution alone [174].

In summary small solutes yield high osmolality, but cross the peritoneal membrane rapidly. Large solutes remain longer in the peritoneal cavity, but attract less water. While the smaller solutes should be favoured for short dwell-time exchanges, the larger solutes are suitable for exchanges with longer dwell-times [168]. Estimated ultrafiltration patterns with several small and large solutes at the same percentage concentration are depicted in Fig. 11.

Low molecular weight osmotic agents

Glucose. Glucose has been the only available osmotic agent in PD solutions for years. The glucose

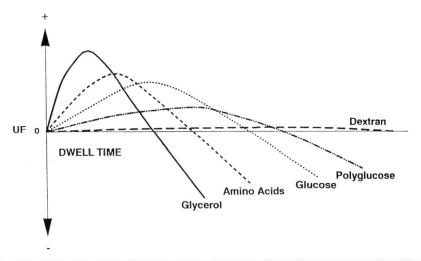

Figure 11. Estimated ultrafiltration patterns with different osmotic agents of various molecular weights at the same percentage concentration (modified from Twardowski *et al.* [168], with permission of Karger AG, Basel).

content of commercial bags is expressed either as dextrose anhydrous or as dextrose monohydrate. Dextrose monohydrate concentrations of 1.5%, 2.5% and 4.25% correspond to 1.36%, 2.26% and 3.86% respectively of dextrose anhydrous. Three basic concentrations of glucose are commonly used, with small differences among the different solution producers: a weak concentration (1.36–1.5%), an intermediate concentration (2.27–2.5%) and a strong concentration, also called hypertonic (3.86–4.25%). In the text the three kinds of solution will be identified as 1.5%, 2.5% and 4.25%.

Since glucose is absorbed during the exchange, a progressive dissipation of osmotic gradient is present [91, 166, 168, 175–179]. This determines the typical curve of the intraperitoneal volume (Fig. 12). Ultrafiltration rate is maximal at the beginning of the exchange and the peritoneal volume reaches the maximal peak after 2–3 h of dwell when the equilibration between dialysate and plasma osmolality occurs. After this point absorption becomes evident with a progressive reduction in the amount of fluid in the peritoneal cavity. The rate of fluid absorption is mainly dependent on the lymphatic flux [180, 181]. In short rapid exchanges, ultrafiltration is maintained throughout the exchange. In CAPD with 4–8 h exchanges a high rate of glucose absorption may result in a final positive fluid balance. Some patients absorb glucose so rapidly that adequate ultrafiltration cannot be achieved even with more concentrated glucose solutions [168].

A significant correlation between the amount of glucose absorbed per day and the glucose concentration in the dialysate has been found in patients on

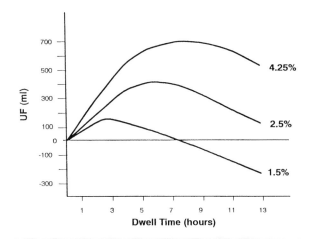

Figure 12. Approximate ultrafiltration volumes related to dwell time with solutions of 1.5%, 2.5% and 4.25% dextrose concentrations (from ref. 168 with permission of Karger AG, Basel).

CAPD. The net daily glucose uptake can therefore be predicted from the empirical equation:

$$Gu \text{ (g/day)} = (11.3 \times [G] - 10.9) \times V$$

where Gu is glucose uptake in grams/day; 11.3 and 10.9 are constants of correlation; $[G]$ is the average dialysate glucose concentration and V is the dialysate inflow volume in litres [182]. This relation has been confirmed by others [183].

Since about 60–80% of the glucose instilled into the peritoneal cavity is absorbed during a 6 h dwell time, 45–60 g of glucose is absorbed from 4.25% solution, 24–40 g from 2.5% and 15–22 g from 1.5% [184]. Consequently a normal glucose uptake in CAPD patients ranges from 100 to 300 g per day

[182–187]. This amount contributes to the total energy intake [20%) in CAPD patients and has been suggested to be beneficial for caloric balance [182]. However, the large amount of absorbed glucose may also result in several metabolic derangements.

A marked hyperglycaemia has been observed in patients undergoing intermittent PD [188, 189]. Although CAPD exchanges with 1.5% glucose dialysate have only a marginal effect on blood glucose and insulin levels [190, 191], a constant tendency towards hyperglycaemia and hyperinsulinaemia has been frequently reported [191, 192]. During hypertonic exchanges, glucose and insulin peak levels occur in patients after 45–90 min while glucagon decreases slightly [183, 190, 191, 193, 194]. These effects are similar to those observed after an oral glucose load [194, 195]. It has been reported that some patients on CAPD developed '*de-novo*' manifest diabetes mellitus due to the continuous hyperglycaemic stress [184]. In addition, since sustained hyperinsulinaemia may possibly increase atherogenesis, the elevated circulating insulin levels represent a potential risk factor for CAPD patients [184]. A hyperlipidaemic effect of CAPD has been demonstrated in several clinical studies. Hypertriglyceridaemia and serum lipoprotein abnormalities were accentuated within the first months of the treatment [185, 186, 196–201] and were attributed to continuous peritoneal absorption of glucose [202]. These changes, however, were at least in part transitory [203], suggesting an adaptation to peritoneal glucose load with a spontaneous reduction of the oral carbohydrate intake [184, 187].

Investigations in the field of peritoneal fluid biocompatibility (see Chapter 16) have raised the question of the long-term toxicity of solutions containing glucose on peritoneal resident cells. To prevent caramelization of glucose during heat sterilization, the pH of the solution is kept low (5–5.5). The high glucose concentration and the low pH of the commercially available solutions have been demonstrated to affect peritoneal cellular host defence mechanisms and peritoneal mesothelial cell viability. In addition, glucose is not entirely stable and some of its breakdown products can be detected in peritoneal dialysate, especially when using fluids stored for a long time [79]. These degradation products, of which 5-hydroxymethylfurfural (5-HMF) is the most easily measurable, have been found significantly elevated after 18 months of storage [204]. A marked reduction of peritoneal ultrafiltration has been associated with the use of solutions which have been stored for more than 18 months. 5-HMF is relatively

atoxic to biological tissues but combines readily with anions including lactate to form Schiff's bases, and this compound may alter the characteristics of many tissue components [80].

The high intraperitoneal glucose concentration has been associated with a non-enzymatic glycosylation of proteins during severe peritonitis. Dobbie *et al.* [205] have demonstrated that repeated and severe episodes of peritonitis can remove the mesothelial layer, exposing the underlying stroma to high concentrated glucose solutions. This condition can result in diabetes-like reduplications of the basement membrane of mesothelium and stromal blood vessels, and in irreversible changes of exposed proteins [206].

Glycerol. Glycerol has been proposed as an alternative osmotic agent for CAPD solutions to overcome some metabolic effects of glucose, mainly in diabetic patients [207, 208].

Glycerol-containing solutions have a higher initial pH; therefore they should be more biocompatible [207]. Glycerol is a small molecular weight alcohol which does not require insulin to be metabolized. It is part of neutral fats and follows the carbohydrate metabolic pathway since it is converted in dihydroxyacetone phosphate, a triose of the glycolitic pathway [209]. From this point glycerol follows the normal metabolic pathways of glucose. In animal studies the infusion of glycerol results in an increased production of glucose, but only when high levels of glycerol are achieved [210].

Glycerol produces greater ultrafiltration than glucose during the early phase of the exchange because of its higher osmotic power. However, due to the low molecular weight, glycerol diffuses very rapidly into the blood, providing lower amounts of total net ultrafiltration throughout the entire exchange [168, 211, 212]. Thus, higher concentrations of glycerol are required to obtain adequate ultrafiltration in CAPD, leading to a caloric load from the solution equivalent to [213], or even higher [211] than, glucose.

In non-diabetics no rise in blood glucose or insulin concentrations over a dialysis cycle was observed [213]. However, in the long run, mean glucose and insulin concentrations rose steadily with the use of glycerol [213]. In diabetic patients the use of glycerol was associated with a decreased insulin requirement, but this favourable effect could not be maintained after 3–4 months [207]. Nevertheless, a better control of glucose homeostasis and a better survival rate have been reported in these patients [209].

The use of glycerol-containing solutions inevitably leads to an accumulation of glycerol in the blood (normal value 0.12 mmol/L) [208, 214]. The mean blood peak values with the 1.4% and 2.5% glycerol solutions have been reported to be 0.62 and 11.65 mmol/L respectively [214]. In a few cases these high glycerol levels have been associated with hyperosmolar symptoms, even though mean plasma osmolality in the studied patients was similar to that observed in CAPD patients treated with standard glucose solution [214].

The long-term studies have shown a dramatic increase in blood fasting triglyceride concentrations after 6 months of treatment [209, 213]. Since glycerol is measured together with triglycerides by the standard methodology, the triglyceride increase appeared to be less dramatic when triglyceride concentrations were corrected for free glycerol concentrations [214].

A further extension of the CAPD treatment with the glycerol-containing solution in diabetics has shown that the glycerol solution was safe and well tolerated if plasma gycerol levels and plasma osmolality are carefully monitored. Particularly excellent diabetic control at relatively low daily doses of insulin, compared with diabetic CAPD patients treated with a glucose dialysate, were achieved [210].

In conclusion, there is a general agreement that glycerol solutions could be used in diabetic patients because of their better control of glucose homeostasis. However, special care should be paid to possible negative effects on other metabolic pathways [213–215].

In non-diabetic CAPD patients the available evidence suggests that glycerol alone has little or no clinical advantage over glucose as an osmotic agent [168, 208, 216, 217].

Xylitol. Xylitol has been suggested as an osmotic agent in diabetic CAPD patients since its metabolism is insulin-independent [218]. A preliminary study in four diabetic patients treated for 6 months showed a marked reduction in insulin requirement; better control of blood glucose levels and normalized levels of triglycerides, cholesterol and HDL-cholesterol. However, an increase of lactic and uric acids was observed [218]. Toxic effects seem to occur at absorption rates greater than 150 g/day [132]. Therefore, patients with fluid excess requiring frequent hyperosmolar exchanges may encounter a high risk of dangerous metabolic abnormalities induced by xylitol [219].

Sorbitol. In the late 1960s sorbitol was tried as a substitute for glucose in dialysis fluid [220], in order to improve blood glucose control and to prevent hyperosmolar symptoms in diabetic patients undergoing intermittent PD. However, since the rate of transperitoneal absorption exceeds the metabolic capacity, this substance accumulates in blood, causing hyperosmolar status with confusion, convulsion and coma [221, 222]. Following these observations, in 1973 the committee on PD solutions did not recommend the use of sorbitol in dialysate [223].

Fructose. Fructose has the same molecular weight as glucose and similar osmotic power, but it is predominantly metabolized in the liver and does not require insulin [224, 225].

Fructose does not appear to provide any advantage over glucose, and it may be more effective than glucose in producing hypertriglyceridaemia [215] and hyperosmolar state [132].

Glycerol and amino acids. As mentioned above, when glycerol was administered in high concentrations a dramatic increase in plasma triglycerides, and in some cases a hyperosmolar syndrome, were recorded. Thus, a mixture with amino acids could be beneficial because a lower concentration of both substances could be administered without losing ultrafiltration capacity [226]. This solution could have several theoretical advantages [227]. In malnourished patients the simultaneous intake of amino acid and carbohydrates could lead to an improved nitrogen balance and to an anabolic state. In this case calories and amino acids could be given in the same bag, since these two substances could be sterilized together. In diabetics the insulin-independent properties of glycerol and of amino acids could improve glycaemic control and reduce the daily glucose load provided by PD. Glucose-containing PD solutions may cause non-enzymatic glycosylation of proteins [205]. The mixture of glycerol and amino acid could potentially avoid this problem since glycerol does not participate in this reaction. In addition a glycerol/amino acid solution could be sterilized with a pH substantially higher than that of glucose [6.7–6.8 vs 5.0–5.5]. Since pH is one of the key factors for solution biocompatibility, the glycerol/amino acid solution could present some advantages in this field.

Different combinations of glycerol/amino acids have been tested in a rat model of single-dwell PD [228] and the formulation containing 1.4% of glycerol and 0.6% of amino acids was selected because of its better ultrafiltration profile, equilibrated nutritional balance and the possibility of being administered twice a day. An evaluation in rats of a single 6-h dwell-time exchange and of a 10-day period showed no differences in net ultrafiltration rate and D/P urea and creatinine between this solution and a 2.5% glucose-containing solution [229]; also no differences were recorded in serum osmolality. A single 6-h exchange was also performed in seven patients with this solution. Again no changes in ultrafiltration or D/P were recorded. A mild increase in blood levels of glycerol after 3 and 6 h was detected [229]. These encouraging results should be validated in larger and long-term studies.

Amino acids. A high percentage of patients treated with PD present with different degrees of malnutrition [230]. Since CAPD patients absorb a substantial amount of glucose from the PD solution, and many of them become obese [231], it seems that protein rather than caloric deficit is the major problem for these patients. Continuous losses of amino acids (3–4 g/day) and proteins (8–15 g/day) contribute greatly to this nutritional derangement [231, 232]. In the late 1960s, Gjessing suggested supplementing PD solutions with a mixture of amino acids to correct serum amino acid abnormalities and to prevent obligate protein losses with dialysate [233]. More than 10 years later Oreopoulos *et al.* proposed an amino acid solution in PD both for nutritional supplementation and as an alternative to glucose as the osmotic agent. Experiments in a uraemic rabbit model [234] and in PD patients [193, 235] underlined the advantages of substituting glucose in the solution and improving nutritional support.

Osmotic efficacy. The molecular weight of different amino acids ranges from 75 to 214 daltons. Since amino acid mixtures for PD usually contain a higher proportion of small molecular weight compounds, the average molecular weight represented in these solutions is approximately 100 daltons [168] and therefore lower than that of glucose. In spite of that, the absorption rate of amino acids is not significantly faster than that of glucose. Since some amino acids are electrically charged, the hydration shell increases the relative Einstein–Stokes radius of the molecules. As a consequence, diffusion coefficients are smaller in comparison to uncharged molecules with equiva-

lent molecular weight, and absorption velocity is reduced. It has been demonstrated that the D/P ratio for creatinine is near to that of glutamine (a near neutrally charged amino acid with almost the same molecular weight), but significantly higher than that of glutamic acid (negatively charged) and of lysine (positively charged), both with the same molecular weight as creatinine [236].

Several studies have been performed to evaluate ultrafiltration capacity of amino acid solutions. A 2% amino acid solution was compared to a 4.25% glucose solution in an acute study on 6 h exchanges [235]. The two solutions induced equivalent amounts of ultrafiltration and similar amounts of urea, creatinine and potassium removal. The initial dialysate osmolality was similar for the two solutions and similar dialysate osmolality changes during dwell-time were observed. At the end of the exchange 90% of the administered amino acids were absorbed. Later, the same group [237] reported a short-term study in which the ultrafiltration obtained with a 1% amino acid solution (osmolality 364 mmOsm/kg) was intermediate between that of 1.5% (osmolality 346 mmOsm/kg) and 2.5% (396 mmOsm/kg) standard glucose solution. Goodship *et al.* confirmed the observation of smaller but not statistically different ultrafiltrate volumes comparing a 1% amino acid solution with a 1.5% glucose solution [238]. A comparison of ultrafiltration profiles and solute mass transfer between a 4.25% glucose (478 mmOsm/kg) and a 2.76% amino acid (501 mmOsm/kg) solutions showed that intraperitoneal volume profiles were equal during the first 180 min of dwell. Later, the volume of amino acid solution tended to decrease more rapidly than that of the glucose solution, leading to a decreased net ultrafiltration at the end of the 6-hour dwell-time exchange [239]. These differences were not statistically significant. Effluent sodium, potassium, urea and total protein levels were similar with the two solutions during the dwell, although D/P values of these solutes after 360 min tended to be higher when using amino acids solutions. This difference was statistically significant for creatinine. In addition, the diffusive mass transport coefficient tended to be higher with amino acid solutions, but the difference was not statistically significant [239]. It was concluded that the peritoneal permeability was not significantly altered by the use of amino acids instead of glucose [240].

Young *et al.* [241] studied ultrafiltration and D/P ratios of several proteins in 8-h dwell-time exchanges using a 1% amino acid solution in comparison with 1.5% glucose standard solution. Volumes of dialysate recovered at the end of the exchanges were significantly less after amino acid exchanges although the osmolality decreased comparably during the dwell time. At the end of the study period (12 weeks) amino acid absorption and protein losses were increased as compared to the beginning of the study. The clearances of the studied proteins expressed as D/P ratios showed 18% and 34% increases respectively at the beginning of amino acid use and after 12 weeks. D/P ratios for creatinine showed 7% and 10% increases respectively, while no differences were observed for urea. The increase in peritoneal permeability during the use of the amino acid-based solution was attributed to an activation of complement by amino acids or their metabolites to produce C5a [242] and the generation of prostaglandin E2 [243]. The peritoneal permeability increase was reversed when standard glucose solutions were resumed [241].

Douma *et al.* [244] have reported a study concerning the peritoneal membrane permeability when a 1.1% amino acid solution is used: the mass transfer area coefficients of low molecular weight solutes (creatinine, urea and urate) were significantly greater with the amino acid solution compared to the glucose solution. The clearances of the macromolecules were also greater with the amino acid solution, but the increase of albumin and IgG clearances was small and not significant. The transcapillary ultrafiltration rate was higher during amino acid treatment, but no significant difference in net ultrafiltration was found. These data indicated a vasoactive effect of the amino acid solution: the increased peritoneal blood flow and the effective peritoneal surface area were probably caused by vasodilation. This was not associated with changes in intrinsic permeability to macromolecules or increased protein loss. This study also demonstrated that these effects were not due to nitric oxide activity (L-arginine contained in the amino acid solution could serve as a substrate for nitric oxide synthesis) nor to the peritoneal release of prostaglandins.

Despite the contradictory results of kinetic studies, in clinical practice amino acid solutions deliver ultrafiltration and small molecule clearances equivalent to those achieved with glucose solutions. The differences among various studies probably reflect differences in concentration and composition of amino acids in the employed solutions. The osmotic power produced by different solutions is not only expressed by the osmolality, calculated or measured, but also depends on the degree of absorption and metabolization of each amino acid [245].

Nutritional efficacy. The nutritional value, the changes in serum amino acid profile, the amino acid absorption and the effects on lipids and glucose metabolism of CAPD amino acid solutions have been evaluated in clinical studies. During the 20-year experiences and attempts to discover the best composition for the amino acid solution, several amino acid formulations of the CAPD solutions have been proposed and tested. Table 8 reports the amino acid composition of some of the most used. Clinical results are often conflicting because different amino acid composition solutions were used, different parameters were taken into account as markers for nutrition, different CAPD populations were studied (malnourished vs. non-malnourished, different caloric intake), different CAPD schedules were used (amino acid solution used in the overnight exchange vs. in exchanges close to a meal).

In the first long-term study [237], a 1% amino acid fluid (solution A in Table 8) was alternated with glucose exchanges for 4 weeks in six patients. A slightly improved nutritional status and an increase of total body nitrogen and serum transferrin were detected. Mean dietary protein intake (0.96–0.93 g/kg/day), energy intake (22–21.2 kcal/kg/day), anthropometric indexes, total body potassium and serum albumin, insulin and glucagon levels did not change during the study. Plasma triglycerides tended to decrease and HDL cholesterol to increase, but after 4 weeks these changes were not statistically significant. BUN levels increased sharply (59%) and blood bicarbonate dropped, although 33 mmol/L of lactate, 7 mmol/L of acetate and 4.5 mmol/L of bicarbonate were present in the solution. The low plasma concentrations of the branched amino acids valine, isoleucine and leucine observed before treatment remained unchanged, while glycine increased and alanine decreased.

Schilling *et al.* [246] found rather discouraging results by using a daily 2% amino acid solution exchange over 5–6 months in three patients, with loss of appetite in two of them.

The same results were obtained in a prospective randomized study [247] in which a 1% amino acid solution was evaluated for its ability to counteract the catabolic effect of peritonitis in CAPD patients. During 4 weeks 12 patients used the amino acid solution twice a day. There was no improvement of nitrogen balance, plasma amino acid pattern or nutritional status. BUN increased by 50% and nine out of twelve patients lost their appetite. The mean dietary protein and energy intakes decreased during peritonitis.

The most recent study with solution A of Table 8 was published by Dombros *et al.* [248]. Five

Table 8. Amino acid composition (mg/dl) of different solutions

		A Ref. 237, 246–8	B Ref. 251	C Ref. 253–7	D Ref. 259–61	E Ref. 263
EBCAA	Valine	46	67	126	139.3	123
EBCAA	Leucine	62	82.6	92	101.9	85
EBCAA	Isoleucine	48	60.8	77	84.9	70
EAA	Threonine	42	46.8	59	64.5	54
EAA	Tyrosine	4	7.8	6	30	27
EAA	Phenylalanine	62		75	57	47
EAA	Lysine	58	60.8	86	76	55
EAA	Hystidine	44	37.4	65	71.4	59
EAA	Tryptophan	18	15.6	25	27	23
EAA	Methionine	58	29.6	77	84.9	36
NEAA	Arginine	104	51.4	97	107.1	68
NEAA	Serine		116.9	46	50.9	55
NEAA	Proline	42	126.3	54	59.5	49
NEAA	Glycine	213	32.7	46	50.9	42
NEAA	Alanine	213	46.8	86	95.1	77
NEAA	Aspartic acid		63.9			65
NEAA	Glutamic acid		140.3			65

EBCAA: essential branch-chained amino acid; EAA: essential amino acid; NEAA: non-essential amino acid.

patients with low daily protein intake (<0.8 g/kg bodyweight) and low serum albumin (<35 g/L) received the 1% amino acid solution during overnight exchange for 6 months. At the end of the study BUN increased slightly and total body nitrogen tended to decrease, while oral total energy and protein intakes, cholesterol, triglycerides, albumin, transferrin, skinfold thickness, total body potassium and plasma amino acid levels remained basically unchanged. The authors concluded that the amino acid formulation, the timing of administration, the patients' low caloric intake and the patients' sufficient nutritional state could be responsible for the ineffectiveness of the amino acid solution.

These studies used solutions not tailored to meet the needs of uraemic patients (large amount of non-essential amino acids) and with an inadequate amount of buffer. Therefore they were not able to normalize the amino acid pattern and contributed to acidosis. Furthermore the energy intake of the patients was low; consequently the intraperitoneal supply of amino acids was probably used as a source of energy [249]. These disadvantages were well recognized by the authors and stimulated the search for an amino acid composition solution more suitable for CAPD patients.

To evaluate the effect of combining amino acids and energy, Okamura et al. [250] studied a solution containing 0.7% of amino acids and 1.5% of glucose in five patients. The solution contained an increased amount of essential amino acids and their plasma concentration increased during the study. Plasma transferrin and BUN also increased.

A new amino acid formulation containing an increased amount of essential amino acids and a decreased concentration of non-essential amino acids, namely glycine and alanine, was used by Pedersen et al. [251] in six patients for 3 months (solution B in Table 8) alternately with a 1.5% glucose solution. Patient protein intake at the beginning of treatment was 1.2–1.5 g/kg/day. During this study no detectable changes in the metabolism of glucose, lipids and proteins occurred. In particular serum triglycerides, cholesterol, albumin and transferrin were not different from the pre-study values. Serum creatinine remained stable while serum BUN increased significantly during the study. Interestingly the serum branched amino acids increased, approaching normal values. The increased amount of branched-chain amino acids in the solution could explain this effect.

Following previous experiences a new 1% amino acid solution was proposed and tested (solution C in Table 8). This solution was designed specifically for patients with renal insufficiency and its related amino acid derangements [252]. Thus, the essential amino acid proportion was increased and the lactate concentration was increased to 35 mmol/L.

Young et al. [253] studied eight hypoalbuminaemic CAPD patients using only a morning exchange for 12 weeks. A modest nutritional benefit was recorded. Transferrin increased significantly and cholesterol and apolipoprotein B tended to decrease. No significant changes occurred in mean dietary protein or energy intakes, fasting amino acid, albumin, prealbumin or apolipoprotein A levels. BUN increased by 36% and bicarbonate decreased by 13% without signs of uraemia or clinical acidosis. As a part of the same study a more detailed analysis [254] showed a significant reduction of total and LDL cholesterol and apolipoprotein B. These parameters returned to baseline 2 weeks after returning the patients to glucose peritoneal fluid.

A more extended observation (6 months) in six non-malnourished patients with one exchange per day of the same solution [255] showed an improved estimated nitrogen balance and serum amino acid profile, an increase of dietary protein and energy intakes and a decrease of serum cholesterol and triglycerides. Plasma protein concentrations remained unchanged, BUN increased by 29%, blood bicarbonate and pH decreased. When this solution was used twice a day in seven patients for 8 weeks [256] the plasma essential amino acid concentrations increased (in particular branched amino acids) as well as serum albumin. However BUN rose by 63% and blood bicarbonate dropped by 31% and a significant acidosis developed in the patients. Other parameters such as anthropometry, total body potassium, dietary protein and caloric intakes, transferrin, insulin, glucagon, and lipids were unchanged.

The longest study available with the 1% amino acid solution describes four diabetic patients followed for more than 12 months [257]. Serum albumin and cholesterol increased as compared with a control group. In addition the amount of insulin administered was reduced in the group receiving amino acids. As expected azotaemia increased by 68% and bicarbonate decreased.

In summary the above-mentioned studies using the improved 1% amino acid solution demonstrated more beneficial effects than the previous solution if patients with signs of protein malnutrition and low dietary protein intake were included. Energy intake should be sufficient to prevent diversion of absorbed amino acids as an energy source [232]. Acidosis remained a common concern. This was most likely due to the acid load delivered by salts of basic amino acids (lysine hydrochloride) and that arising from metabolism of sulphur amino acids to sulphate (methionine) [258].

In order to further improve clinical efficacy, a new formulation of the amino acid solution has been proposed and tested (solution D in Table 8). Essential amino acid concentrations were increased as well as lactate concentration (from 35 to 40 mmol/L). Total amino acid concentration was increased to 1.1% in order to provide the same osmotic effect as the 1.5% standard glucose solution. A multicentre study in CAPD patients with signs of protein malnutrition has been performed [259]. The nitrogen balance, serum transferrin and total protein increased in 19 malnourished patients using one or two 1.1% amino acid solutions for 20 days.

Dietary protein intake of 0.8 g/kg/day and caloric intake of 25–30 kcal/kg/day was prescribed to all patients. Because of the amino acid absorption from dialysis fluid a total protein intake of 1.1–1.3 g/kg/day was achieved in all patients. Protein anabolism was positive, as directly determined from [^{15}N]glycine studies and indirectly from the plasma phosphate and potassium decrease. The amino acid pattern in plasma became more normal during the treatment phase and serum triglycerides and HDL-cholesterol increased. Plasma total CO_2 decreased significantly, showing a tendency towards a metabolic acidosis, mainly in patients treated with two exchanges per day of this solution.

A clinical evaluation of this amino acid solution was performed in a second study [260]. This was a 3-month prospective cross-over study in 15 stable CAPD patients not necessarily malnourished. Only one exchange with amino acid was prescribed at lunch-time to couple amino acid absorption with energy intake. Serum albumin and transferrin improved significantly in patients both with and without malnutrition. Plasma amino acid profile and total proteins did not change. Plasma bicarbonate levels also remained stable.

A prospective randomized study was also performed in order to compare the nutritional effects of the 1.1% amino acid solution with the conventional glucose solution in 54 malnourished patients [261]. After an initial significant increase in serum albumin, transferrin, prealbumin and total protein, after 3 months of treatment the significance of the difference in these parameters was lost compared to the 51 patients in the control group. However, in the tercile with the lowest albumin levels at baseline, serum albumin and prealbumin remained significantly increased. In the tercile with the highest albumin levels at baseline the mid-arm muscle circumference increased significantly after 3 months of treatment. In the whole population treated with the amino acid solution, the circulating insulin-like growth factor 1 increased, while it decreased slightly in the control group.

In a recent acute study the amount of amino acids delivered by the 1% amino acid solution was quantified [262]. It has been shown that the gain of amino acid during one exchange largely exceeded the daily losses of amino acid and proteins. This effect was independent of peritoneal membrane transport type.

In conclusion, in malnourished CAPD patients dialysis solution with a more appropriate and recently introduced amino acid composition may improve protein nutrition and metabolic status. However, increased BUN levels and the tendency towards acidosis remain problems to be solved. The last point was addressed by Jones *et al.* [263]. They tested a modified amino acid solution formulation (solution E in Table 8) in which acidogenetic amino acid concentrations (lysine, arginine and methionine) were reduced in comparison with the 1% amino acid solution (solution C in Table 8). In addition aspartic and glutamic acids, two dicarboxylic acids that generate alkaline equivalents during their metabolism, were added. A substantially better acid–base status was achieved during the treatment with the modified amino acid solution as compared to the conventional amino acid solution.

Amino acids and bicarbonate. Properties of this solution have recently been published by Plum *et al.* [264]. The aim was to combine the nutritional benefit provided by amino acids with the improved biocompatibility achievable with the natural buffer and the physiological pH. Only an acute study with this solution has been published to date. In ten patients three separate 6-h dwell exchanges with solutions containing (a) 1% amino acids and 34 mmol/L bicarbonate, (b) 1.5% glucose and 34 mmol/L bicarbonate, and (c) 1.5% glucose and 35 mmol/L lactate were evaluated. The two bicarbonate-containing solutions were provided in a double-chamber bag for stability reasons. Ultrafiltration rate, creatinine clearance and mass transfer area coefficient (MTAC) were similar in the three solutions. According to earlier reports [241–243] the amino acid solution was accompanied by a small but significant increase of peritoneal membrane permeability to higher-weight molecules since the D/P ratios of β_2-microglobulin, albumin and IgG were increased. Increased concentrations of various cytokines/prostanoids were also recorded in the amino acid-containing solution as compared to those containing glucose. The authors suggested that it was not possible to define whether these levels indicated less suppression of cell functions or were the expression of an underlying inflammatory activity compared to glucose and lactate solution. However, *in-vitro* tests demonstrated that the two bicarbonate buffered fluids were less inhibitory to the studied cell functions than the lactate-buffered solutions. A clearly positive nitrogen balance was also recorded with the amino acid/bicarbonate solution. More extended clinical studies are needed to evaluate the clinical benefit of this solution.

High molecular weight osmotic agents

Albumin. Almost one hundred years ago albumin was shown to delay peritoneal fluid absorption [265]. It is non-toxic systemically and does not cause biochemical or metabolic derangements, thus representing an ideal osmotic agent [266]. Because of its molecular weight (68 kDa) albumin is absorbed slowly from the peritoneal cavity, mainly via lymphatic flow, and exert a sustained oncotic effect as evaluated in a rat model [267]. However it is currently too expensive to be considered as a substitute for glucose in clinical PD, and its use in humans has been restricted to study peritoneal fluid and solute transports [268].

Synthetic polymers. Polyacrylate, polyethylene-amine and dextran sulphate are the synthetic polymers which have been proposed and tried in an 'in-vitro' simulation of PD, in rats and rabbits [269–271]. All obtained results showed high toxicity, and a possible clinical applicability was denied. Nevertheless, slow absorption and high osmotic driving forces in long-dwell exchanges have been observed in animals. Polyacrylate induced intraperitoneal bleeding, peritoneal membrane damage and cardiovascular instability [271]. In addition, despite its high molecular weight (90 kDa) polyacrylate crossed the peritoneal membrane.

Dextran sodium sulphate, with a molecular weight of 500 kDa, exerts the osmotic effect because of sodium trapped in its glycosyl sulphate residue [270]. Dextran was assumed to be non-toxic since, if absorbed, it should be metabolized. However, in animal models intraperitoneal bleeding occurred, leading to the death of animals [271]. Polyethylene-amine was even more toxic, with the death of animals in 1 h [271].

Obviously synthetic polymers are not suitable for clinical use.

Plasma substitutes. Gelatine, neutral dextran and hydroxyethyl starch are widely used in Europe as plasma substitutes to treat severe hypotensive episodes in haemodialysis. Crude gelatine (5%) was first used in the late 1940s as an osmotic agent during acute PD [272]. More recently [271] a 9% gelatine solution was tested in a rat model and it was found to yield a higher and more sustained ultrafiltration during a 7-h dwell time as compared to a 4.25% glucose solution. There were no untoward effects on rats and no alterations of the peritoneal membrane as evaluated by light and scanning electron microscopy. However, high viscosity, gelation at room temperature and difficult sterilization were major problems. To avoid these technical problems a cross-linked gelatin, gelatin isocyanate (Hemaccel 20–35 kDa), was investigated [273]. At 6-h dwell time the ultrafiltration volume of a 5.5% Hemaccel solution was similar to that of 4.25% glucose, while 10% Hemaccel yielded even higher ultrafiltration. Although gelatin is easily metabolized, the half-life of Hemaccel is around 16 h in haemodialysed patients with minimal renal function, and chronic toxicity is unknown [266]. In addition, when used as plasma substitute, Hemaccel has been associated with anaphylactoid reactions in 0.038% of patients [274].

Neutral dextrans as osmotic agents in PD were investigated in the late 1960s [275]. A very low osmotic driving force was exerted by a 6% dextran in saline and little ultrafiltration was achieved. These data were confirmed recently [276], while a 10% dextran solution showed significantly higher ultrafiltration [277]. However, despite its high molecular weight (40 or 70 kDa), 40–60% of dextran was absorbed over a 6-h cycle time [12]. Since accumulation of dextran in patients on maintenance haemodialysis has been demonstrated to yield reticuloendothelial system blockade, dextran does not seem to be a suitable alternative to glucose [278].

Hydroxyethyl starch (HES) is another synthetic substance in which starch has been modified by introducing a hydroxyethyl ether group and then hydrolysed to yield a product with an average molecular weight of 480 kDa. Studies in a rat model with 10% and 6% solutions have reported ultrafiltration profiles and absorption rates similar to those obtained with 6% and 10% dextran solutions [276, 277]. In acute renal failure HES seemed to accumulate in liver, leading to a storage disease [279].

Glucose polymer. Glucose polymers (GP) are a family of polysaccharides consisting of linked glucose residues of varying chain lengths. The way in which glucose molecules are chemically linked determines different characteristics (Fig. 13): in dextrin the linkages are predominantly α 1–4, in dextran α 1–6 and in cellulose β 1–4.

Dextrin is a mixture of polysaccharides with different chain lengths (from one glucose unit to more than 300 glucose units) obtained by the hydrolysis of corn starch. More than 90% of the glucose bonds are 1–4 glucosidic linkages, the remaining 10% are 1–6 linkages [280]. In the human body the amylase present in saliva, pancreatic juice and plasma readily hydrolyses the α 1–4 linkages until disaccharides maltose (α 1–4 linkages) and isomaltose (α 1–6 linkages) are obtained. From these two substances glucose is eventually produced by maltase and isomaltase. Maltase activity is virtually absent in the human circulation but the maltase enzyme is abundant within the intracellular lysosomes and in kidneys [281, 282].

Initial clinical studies used a dextrin preparation with a bimodal distribution of polysaccharides: 67% of molecules with 1 to 12 glucose units and 33% with molecules greater than 12 glucose units. This preparation, with average molecular weight 7000, was studied by Mistry *et al.* [283]. A 5% GP solution was compared to a 1.5% glucose solution, and a 10% GP solution to a 4.25% glucose solution. Both isotonic and hypertonic GP solutions showed a significant increase in net ultrafiltration as compared to the corresponding glucose solutions at 6-h dwell time. Significant increases in creatinine, uric acid and phosphate D/P ratios were observed with GP solutions and similarly, average clearances of solutes were also significantly greater with GP solutions at both concentrations, suggesting that GP solutions may alter peritoneum permeability. The GP absorption from dialysate at 6-h dwell time was 42.5% and 59% respectively for the iso and hyperosmotic GP solutions. However, the caloric load was greater than that provided by the absorption of glucose from the standard solutions. Fractions with 5 to 9 glucose units showed the highest intraperitoneal disappearance without concomitant rise in serum levels, whereas maltose (G2) and maltotriose (G3), with a slightly lower disappearance, produced a substantial rise in serum levels, suggesting considerable breakdown of intermediate molecules to smaller units.

In the United States a preparation of fractioned glucose oligosaccharides with chain lengths ranging from 2 to 15 glucose units (average molecular weight 710 daltons) was used in humans in concentrations ranging from 3% to 8% [284, 285]. When compared to a 4.25% glucose solution, an 8% GP solution produced similar ultrafiltration profile at 8- and 10-h dwell times, despite a markedly lower initial osmol-

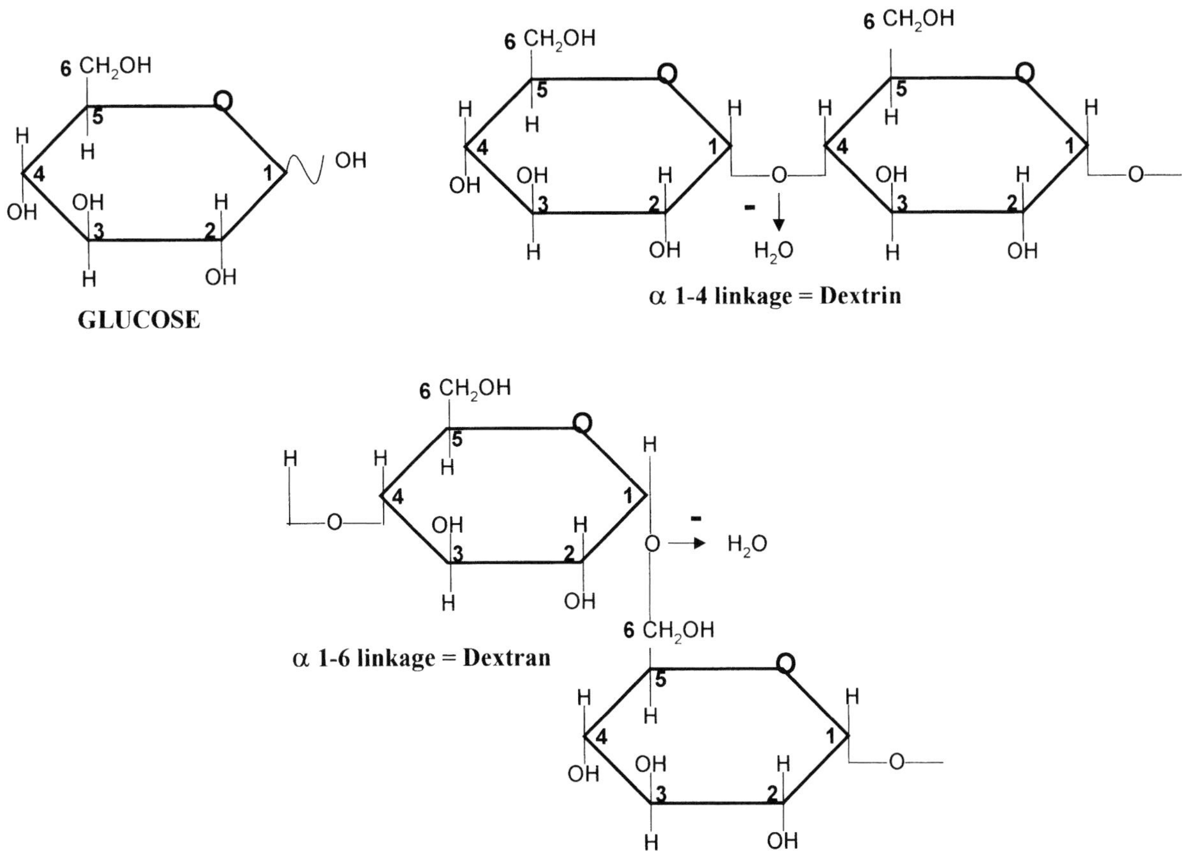

Figure 13. Different glucose linkages in glucose polymers.

ality [357 versus 485 mmOsm/kg). Solute clearances and D/P ratios for urea and creatinine were identical [284]; 57% and 77% of glucose polymers were absorbed at 4 and 10 h respectively. Although the solution was well tolerated by patients, plasma oligosaccharide concentration (in particular G2 and G5) increased sharply during the GP exchange and even higher concentrations were recorded during the subsequent exchange with the standard glucose solution, thus indicating a very slow metabolism and clearance of absorbed oligosaccharides in patients with renal insufficiency. The calculated half-life was about 20 h [284]. Serum free glucose concentrations changed little after the exchanges using the GP solutions. However, the potential energy load from a single exchange of an 8% GP solution was approximately twice that of 4.25% glucose solution. The authors considered the systemic levels of oligosaccharides unacceptably high and the research was abandoned [286].

The potential of glucose polymers was, however, recognized by Mistry and Gokal [287], who realized that the transperitoneal oligosaccharide absorption

is similar to glucose for molecules with chain length less than G12, while those with chain length greater than G12 are poorly absorbed. Thus a modified polymer was prepared (icodextrin, from the Greek *icosa*, meaning twenty) and in subsequent studies [170, 288, 289] a 5% solution of glucose polymer containing polymer fractions of variable chain lengths (ranging from 4 to 300 glucose units with average molecular weight 16 800) was compared with a commercially available 1.5% glucose solution. While the standard glucose solution is slightly hypertonic [332 mmOsm/kg], this GP solution was really isosmotic to uraemic serum [302 mmOsm/kg].

A substantially greater net ultrafiltration was achieved at 6-hour dwell time. For glucose solution the exchange time extended to 12 h led to absorption of fluid with a final drainage volume smaller than that infused. With GP solution, ultrafiltration continued to increase without changes in dialysate osmolality throughout the 12-h exchanges. At 6 and 12 h, 14.4% and 28.1% of glucose polymer had been absorbed, probably via the lymphatic system. Thus in terms of total caloric load there was no difference between the two solutions, but the GP solution provided less than 50% of caloric load of the glucose dialysate per unit of ultrafiltrate. An enhanced peritoneal equilibration for solutes larger than urea was confirmed. A 7–9-fold increase in serum maltose with GP solution was also recorded.

A short-term (7 days) study did not show any side-effects even with continuous use of 5% GP solutions [290]. Later, a 7.5% icodextrin solution was used over a period of 3 months in five non-diabetic patients [291]. GP solution substituted the overnight glucose exchange (12 h) and resulted in 500–1000 ml of net ultrafiltration. Serum biochemistry remained stable during the study period. There was a steady-state accumulation of maltose and maltotriose (30-fold higher than in uraemic serum). No other side-effects were recorded.

A long-term (6 months) randomized multicentre (11 centres) study (MIDAS) in 209 patients (106 with one 7.5% icodextrin solution exchange) was undertaken [292]. Icodextrin produced as much ultrafiltration as 4.25% glucose solution in dwell-times up to 12 h and 3.5 times greater ultrafiltration than 1.5% glucose at 8 h. The transperitoneal transport for small molecules such as potassium, urea, creatinine, calcium, phosphate and uric acid, as well as large molecules, was similar in the two groups, but a small and significant fall in sodium and chloride levels was observed in the icodextrin group compared to controls. The mean level of the maltose rose from 0.04 g/L to a steady-state level of 1.2 g/L, as well as circulating levels of higher molecular weight fractions. A significantly lower carbohydrate absorption during the overnight exchange was observed for the icodextrin solution as compared with the 4.25% glucose solution. No specific side-effects, and similar morbid events, including peritonitis, were found in both groups. A subgroup of 15 diabetics showed no differences in glycaemic control or insulin requirement compared with those in the control group.

Most of the patients enrolled for this 6-month study continued on icodextrin after the end of the study, some of them for 5 years. The treatment remained satisfactory as regards biochemistry and ultrafiltration capacity. No adverse events related to icodextrin occurred [282]. Few patients experienced episodes of a cutaneous hypersensitivity reaction to icodextrin. These episodes were transient and mild in the majority of cases without the need for icodextrin withdrawal [293]. In one patient the skin lesion was classified as severe exfoliative dermatitis and the icodextrin treatment was stopped, with recovery in few days [294]. A subsequent *Staphylo-coccus epidermidis* peritonitis developed, probably in relation to the affected skin around the exit site of the peritoneal catheter. It has been suggested that the allergic mechanism could be similar to that described for dextran, since the molecular structures are similar in the two compounds.

Since icodextrin is partially absorbed via the lymphatic system, and its metabolism is less than complete, increased levels of its breakdown products maltose, maltotriose and high molecular weight molecules occur. Maltose is subsequently partially removed from the circulation by the remaining three CAPD exchanges with conventional glucose solution. It has been calculated that maltose peritoneal clearance is about 3.5 ml/min [170], and this leads to a steady-state level in blood within 2 weeks of starting treatment.

Some concerns have arisen concerning the long-term accumulation of these substances. Long-term effects of these levels are not known. In particular it should be excluded that a storage disease could occur. Since the accumulation within the macrophages leading to impairment of the phagocytic function (defined as reticuloendothelial system blockade) has been documented for dextrans, HES, PVP and gelatin in mice [295], it should be excluded that glucose polymer could exert this effect in the long term. To date there is more than 10 years of clinical experience with icodextrin, several patients being treated for more than 5 years, and none of these effects has been reported.

Davies [296] studied the icodextrin kinetics in 12 patients. After 2 years of icodextrin once-a-day treatment, it was stopped. Maltose and high molecular weight substances fell to pretreatment levels in 7–10 days. When treatment with icodextrin was recommenced after 22 days, plasma levels returned to the previous steady-state levels within 7–10 days. These results suggested that there is no capacity-limited deep compartment for the storage of icodextrin in the human body, and supported the safety in use of icodextrin in CAPD. These studies indicate that the icodextrin solution can be safely used during the overnight exchange as a substitute for the glucose hypertonic solution because of its sustained ultrafiltration over 12 h. The metabolic advantages of the use of icodextrin instead of glucose have been described above. Biocompatibility advantages of icodextrin and iso-osmotic solutions will be discussed in Chapter 16.

Some other clinical indications for icodextrin use have been proposed. One of the most important reasons for the CAPD drop-out is ultrafiltration failure. In patients with a high permeable membrane, fluid balance is often difficult to reach, as well as in patients with peritonitis. Since icodextrin is a large molecule its reabsorption is unaffected by membrane permeability. In high transporter patients icodextrin has been found to produce significantly greater ultrafiltration than hypertonic glucose solution [297]. Also in patients with peritonitis the long overnight dwell with icodextrin resulted in an increased amount of net ultrafiltration [298]. In 33 patients with ultrafiltration failure (85% high or high average transporters) icodextrin extended CAPD technique survival by a median of 22 months [299]. At the time of starting icodextrin treatment these patients were salt and fluid overloaded, and normally they would have required transfer to haemodialysis.

A second clinical indication for icodextrin solution is the long diurnal exchange in patients undergoing CCPD. In large patients adequacy targets are not achieved when residual renal function declines. Automated PD could provide increased clearances if one or two extra exchanges during the day are prescribed. Unfortunately, for these exchanges a long dwell time is required, leading to fluid reabsorption during the dwell, and thus offsetting the net ultrafiltration achieved during rapid nocturnal exchanges. In a randomized study in 38 CCPD patients using either icodextrin or glucose for the daytime dwell (14–15 h), icodextrin significantly increased ultrafiltration in that exchange, while the daily ultrafiltration was also higher, but not statistically different [300]. Creatinine clearance also increased from baseline in the icodextrin group as a consequence of the increased ultrafiltration. These effects permitted a less rigid fluid restriction or an adapted treatment schedule, improving the patients' subjective well-being.

In summary, clinical long-term experience has provided evidence that icodextrin is safe and well tolerated. Its principal attribute is to achieve sustained ultrafiltration in an iso-osmolar solution. This leads to a number of beneficial effects and indications for PD patients thus representing a major advance in the field.

Peptides

Oligopeptides as osmotic agents in PD have been proposed to meet a dual aim: to provide a source of amino acids, thus improving nutrition, and to ameliorate the fluid removal profile as compared with the amino acid solution. Peptides, obtained from hydrolysis of casein and fibrin, have been used in the past for parenteral nutrition [301]. However, hypersensitivity reactions occasionally occurred, mainly related to fractions with higher molecular weight that could be antigenic. When short-chain protein hydrolysates with a maximum of eight to ten amino acids were used anaphylactic reactions were unlikely to occur.

The first use in PD of a mixture of peptides as osmotic agents in a rabbit model was described by Klein *et al.* in 1986 [302]. A 5% solution of milk whey protein was hydrolysed using a combination of trypsin and chymotrypsin in order to prepare a peptide mixture containing three to 10 amino acids. This preparation had an average molecular weight of 857 daltons. The mixture contained approximately 2% free amino acids; 46% of essential amino acids was contained in the peptides. As compared to a 2.5% glucose solution the peptide solution increased net ultrafiltration 2-fold after 1 h of dwell time. Only 3% of the peptide mixture was absorbed from dialysate and no acute toxic effects were recorded. In a subsequent study [303] a 2.5% glucose solution was compared with three peptide-containing solutions with different molecular weights and concentrations in a rat model. Despite the lower osmolality all peptide solutions produced a higher net ultrafiltration than the control solution. The solution containing the 2000 MW peptides was also investigated, to follow the metabolic fate of peptides: the plasma concentration of the amino acids increased after a 6-h dwell, and returned to baseline after 14 h.

In a clinical trial a peptide solution containing 1.5% glucose and 1% peptides (molecular weight 600–700) with 381 mmOsm/kg of osmolality was compared to a standard 2.5% glucose solution (osmolality 404 mmOsm/kg) [304] in 20 patients. The peptide solution was well tolerated in all patients and no differences were found in clearances or mass transfer area coefficient of urea, creatinine and glucose, indicating that no irritating effect of peptide solution was present. Despite the lower osmolality of the peptide solution, no significant changes in ultrafiltration at 4- and 8-h dwell time were recorded. No differences in plasma amino acid profile could be detected. The 57% absorption of oligopeptides after a 4-h dwell was smaller compared to the 67% absorption of glucose.

These preliminary data seem to indicate that peptides could have a potential use as an osmotic agent in PD. A possible effect on nutritional status should be further evaluated [305].

Icodextrin and glucose

Since icodextrin is clinically useful only in long-dwell time, because it produces a slow and sustained ultrafiltration, Mistry and Gokal [306] proposed a mixture of icodextrin and glucose in order to provide an ultrafiltration profile suitable also for the short-term dwell in which rapid ultrafiltration is required. The synergistic combination of a crystalloid osmotic agent (glucose) with a colloid osmotic agent (icodextrin) could result in several advantages. The low levels of glucose reduce the carbohydrate caloric load and the solution is iso-osmotic, thus avoiding one of the principal agents of the bioincompatibility of the PD solution. The reduced levels of icodextrin in the solution result in steady-state levels of maltose and high molecular weight compounds substantially lower than those recorded with the icodextrin-alone solution.

A first clinical study in 11 patients was performed using two solutions, one containing 0.68% of glucose and 2% of icodextrin and the other containing 0.68% of glucose and 2.5% of icodextrin [307]. These solutions were compared with a conventional 1.5% glucose solution in three separate 6-h exchanges in each patient. The mean net ultrafiltration and peritoneal clearances were not significantly different among these three solutions. In a crossover study in 12 patients treated for 2 weeks the same two icodextrin/glucose solutions were tested and compared with the conventional 1.5% glucose solution [308]. The evaluation was performed in the third exchange of the day, often the shortest dwell. The statistical analysis did not demonstrate differences in net ultrafiltration even though the solution containing 2.5% of icodextrin seemed to produce consistently greater ultrafiltration than that containing 2% of icodextrin.

However, in a recent study in rats [309] conflicting results were presented. Three solutions were investigated, one containing 7.5% icodextrin, one containing 7.5% icodextrin plus 0.35% glucose and the last 3.75% icodextrin plus 1.93% glucose. Icodextrin/low glucose and icodextrin/high glucose solutions produced significantly higher net ultrafiltration than icodextrin alone after 2 h of dwell, while after 4 h the net ultrafiltration was significantly lower in the icodextrin/high glucose solution. The authors suggested that the fluid removal induced by the icodextrin was partially due to the lower fluid absorption rate, while by adding glucose to the polyglucose solution, peritoneal fluid absorption may increase. In addition, the net ultrafiltration could be due to the degradation of glucose polymer within the peritoneal cavity, resulting in an increase of the dialysis fluid osmolality.

However, the authors are aware that species differences could have played a key role.

Icodextrin and amino acids

The same rationale for the use of the mixture icodextrin/glucose is applied to the mixture icodextrin/amino acids. In addition some nutritional benefits are expected.

In a clinical study lasting 4 weeks a solution containing 4% of icodextrin and 1% of amino acids was compared to a solution containing icodextrin 7.5% [310]. Twenty patients were enrolled and the two solutions substituted the conventional 4.25% glucose solution for the overnight exchange. The mixed solution was delivered in a double-chamber bag for stability reasons. The osmolalities of the solutions were 485 for glucose, 280 for icodextrin and 344 mOsm/kg H_2O for icodextrin/amino acids. The net ultrafiltration was not different between the two treatment groups, or between the baseline and the study solution for each group. The creatinine clearance evaluated for the overnight exchange was statistically higher in both groups as compared with the baseline but not different between the two study groups, while urea clearance significantly increased only in the icodextrin/amino acid group as compared with the baseline. The mean amino acid absorption in the icodextrin/amino acid group was 86.7% and the plasma total essential amino acid concentration significantly increased in this group. Peritoneal permeability did not change during the study. The plasma high molecular weight substances increased in both groups but in the icodextrin/amino acid group their concentration was half of that recorded in the icodextrin group. No adverse events related to the solution were observed.

Buffers

Derangements of acid–base status are common features in dialysed patients. One of the main tasks for dialysis is to correct these derangements and the target is the normalization of the acid-base parameters. The most frequent alteration is metabolic acidosis that affects several organs and functions, cardiovascular system [311], bone metabolism [312–314] and mainly protein metabolism [315–322], since it has a clear catabolic effect. These untoward effects are related to blood bicarbonate levels [323, 324]; thus, even a mild metabolic acidosis should be corrected.

There are very few data in literature concerning the clinical consequences of alkalosis [325]. They are mainly related to neurological, electrolyte and oxygen transport derangements.

The acids formed in the body during metabolism are neutralized by various buffer systems, bicarbonate being the most important. To maintain the buffering capacity of the body, bicarbonate consumed every day for neutralizing metabolic acid production needs to be regenerated. This function is accomplished by the kidneys.

In end-stage renal failure patients, dialysis replaces the kidney function and the buffer capacity is restored by providing a buffer source in the dialysis fluid. In PD the buffer is included in the fresh dialysis solution daily, infused in the peritoneal cavity.

Bicarbonate was initially used in 1961 by Boen in PD fluid [83], but it was soon replaced by lactate when it was found that calcium carbonate precipitated and the solution became alkaline during autoclaving. However, the sodium salts of several organic oxidizable anions (such as acetate, lactate, citrate malate, pyruvate, succinate, etc.) are able to consume H^+ derived from carbonic acid, causing the regeneration of bicarbonate [326]. Consequently, lactate and acetate were introduced as alkaline agents.

Acetate was first described as buffer substance in PD fluid by Boen et al. in 1962 [327]. Bicarbonate is regenerated when acetate thiokinase activates the reaction between acetate and coenzyme A (CoA) to form acetyl-CoA and one hydrogen ion is captured in this process. Acetyl-CoA may enter different metabolic pathways such as decarboxylation in the Krebs cycle, condensation in ketone bodies or fatty acids and glucose generation via gluconeogenesis [328]. The buffering effect is accomplished and the hydrogen ion is transferred to the respiratory chain only when acetyl-CoA is decarboxylated. Although acetate has been proved to correct uraemic metabolic acidosis even better than lactate, both in CAPD and in intermittent treatment [329], it was quickly abandoned because it seemed to produce vasodilation and alterations of the peritoneal membrane leading to hyperpermeability, loss of ultrafiltration and possibly development of sclerosing peritonitis [330, 331]. Lactate is now the commonly used buffer in PD solution

There is a general conviction that one of the major results achieved by CAPD is the better correction of metabolic acidosis and the maintenance of a satisfactory acid–base status as compared to haemodial-

ysis. This result appears to be stable over time and acid–base fluctuations, typical of intermittent treatments, are not observed. However, more careful analysis [332] has demonstrated that this statement should be at least in part reconsidered. In large series only about 25% of CAPD patients have a normal acid–base status. In intermittent PD, acid–base parameters fluctuate similarly to haemodialysis. At the end of a session blood bicarbonate and pH rise, while a slow decrease in these parameter is observed in the interdialytic period [329].

No data are currently available on modern APD treatments. Acid–base correction in these treatments is probably similar to that achieved in CAPD with small fluctuations depending on the dialytic schedule employed.

Lactate

In nature two stereoisomeric forms of lactate exist: D- and L-lactate. Commercially available PD fluids contain either L-lactate or a mixture of L- and D-lactate.

In humans small quantities of D-lactate are normally generated in the methylglyoxal pathway, while the predominant form is L-lactate. D-lactate is slowly metabolized by an aspecific enzyme (D-2-hydroxyacid-dehydrogenase) NAD-independent [333]. L-lactate, on the contrary, is easily metabolized to pyruvate by lactic dehydrogenase, NAD-dependent.

The buffering effect of lactate is accomplished by its complete metabolization via the Krebs cycle or via gluconeogenesis. With incomplete metabolism of lactate the buffering effect does not take place. Searle et al. [334] demonstrated that 80–85% of the lactate produced in the normal metabolism is oxidized in the Krebs cycle, and only 15–20% is converted to glucose. While the oxidation takes place in all the cells with aerobic metabolism, gluconeogenesis is confined to the liver and renal cortex.

L-lactate turnover in normal subjects ranges from 0.77 to 0.87 mmol/kg/h [334]. In patients with hepatic disease the rate of metabolism may be lower with consequent increase of lactate serum levels. In CAPD patients the lactate infusion rate is about 0.19 mmol/kg/h, that is 25% of endogenous metabolic production [335]. This lactate load does not represent a metabolic problem in patients with normal hepatic function, as demonstrated by some studies reporting normal values of intermediate metabolites [336, 337]. In IPD (5 L/h) the lactate infusion was 1 mmol/kg/h [329] but lactate serum levels only occasionally slightly increased during the session; these data were confirmed more recently [337, 338].

The lactate disappearance rate from dialysate is depicted in Fig. 14 [329, 339, 340]. The rate of absorption is maximal in the first minutes of dwell while it subsequently approaches zero. This behaviour permits adequate buffer transfer even when rapid exchanges are scheduled. It must be noted that D-lactate and L-lactate may have different rates of transport. Rubin *et al.* [340] suggested that the peritoneal membrane could be stereospecific in the process of lactate transport. Other studies have not confirmed different absorption rates between the two stereoisomers of lactate [337, 338]. L-lactate has an higher mass transfer rate and metabolization. D-lactate is very slowly metabolized, but the low mass transfer rate both in IPD and in CAPD seems to enable a complete metabolism [341]. However, high serum levels of D-lactate have been reported in two PD patients and these values were associated with severe neurological impairment (ref. 342 quoted in ref. 343). Increased serum D-lactate concentrations have also been found in a group of patients treated with a solution containing the racemic mixture of D- and L-lactate, while patients treated with the pure L-lactate solution had serum D-lactate levels similar to those of a control population [343]. The D-lactate concentration in these patients (0.6 mmol/L) was close to the level of 0.7 mmol/L reported to be associated with D-lactate encephalopathy [344].

In CAPD, long dwell-times enable an almost complete transfer of buffer from the dialysis solution independently from the initial lactate solution con-

centration that, for this reason, represents the major determinant of base gain.

During dwell-time bicarbonate diffuses back in the dialysate. The major determinant of bicarbonate loss is the blood bicarbonate concentration. Several studies suggest a possible feedback mechanism between blood bicarbonate concentration and the amount of bicarbonate lost in dialysate [336, 337, 339, 345]. An increased blood bicarbonate level yields a parallel increase of bicarbonate loss that, in turn, results in a decrease in blood bicarbonate level. Inversely, in severe metabolic acidosis bicarbonate losses with dialysate are reduced, so yielding a more favourable base balance. Ultrafiltration also plays an important role. When dialysate/plasma equilibration occurs, an increase in drainage volume, due to ultrafiltration, causes a greater loss of bicarbonate [346].

Finally, organic anions that are effective alkaline equivalents are also lost in dialysate. Teehan *et al.* [336] have reported daily losses of 1 mmol of acetoacetate and 4.1 mmol of β-hydroxybutyrate. Other substances are lost in the dialysate, such as tricarboxylic anions, although they have never been quantified; yet a significant anion gap (36 ± 17 mmol/day) was observed in the effluent dialysate [336]. In a more recent paper Uribarri *et al.* [347] have found a significant amount of daily organic acid loss (32.1 ± 10 mmol). The explanation of this discrepancy could be that Teehan's patients were acidotic, while Uribarri's patients were in a normal acid–base status or alkalotic, and consequently with a higher organic acid production.

Despite no major clinical adverse events related to its use have been reported since the introduction of the CAPD treatment, in the past decade some evidence has arisen concerning the ineffectiveness of the lactate CAPD solution in the full correction of uraemic acidosis [332].

Experimental *in-vitro* studies also demonstrated that unphysiologically high lactate concentrations in combination with the low pH of the CAPD solution could have detrimental effects on peritoneal resident cells and their functions (see Chapter 18). In addition some investigators have pointed out other potential metabolic side-effects due to the unphysiologically high lactate flux into the body system [348]. However, these metabolic effects are very difficult to demonstrate in clinical settings, and it was not proven that they have a clinical relevance.

Commercially available CAPD solutions contain 35 or 40 mmol/L lactate. With a dialysis fluid lactate level of 35 mmol/L most patients display a chronic

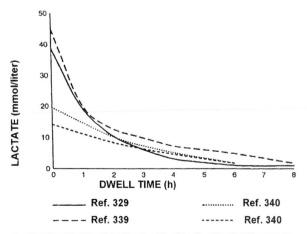

Figure 14. Disappearance of lactate from dialysis fluid during dwell time.

mild metabolic acidosis. Teehan *et al.* [336] demonstrated that lactate uptake from the PD fluid often exceeded bicarbonate loss and metabolic acid production. Out of 10 patients only two had a normal acid–base status defined as a mean arterial blood bicarbonate 20.6 mmol/L and a total CO_2 (T_{CO_2}) 22 mmol/L. Other clinical observations have confirmed these findings [349]. Nolph *et al.* [129] reported a mean venous T_{CO_2} of 23.8 mmol/L in 163 determinations (78 patients) with 38% of values below 22 mmol/L. In a recent multicentre cross-sectional analysis in 75 patients [350], a median arterial blood bicarbonate value of 22.7 mmol/L was recorded and the quartiles were 19.9 and 24.7 mmol/L. About 60% of patients had various degrees of metabolic acidosis (25% with a plasma bicarbonate below 20 mmol/L) and 10% of patients had a metabolic alkalosis. Only about 25% of patients had a normal acid–base status.

In order to correct the negative buffer balance and to improve acid–base status, an increased lactate content to 40 mmol/L in the CAPD solutions has been suggested [129] and significantly better results on blood acid–base status have been reported. Venous T_{CO_2} increased to 27.4 mmol/L after 4 months of treatment (mean baseline value 23.4 mmol/L) while pH and p_{CO_2} did not change. However, since normal venous T_{CO_2} ranges between 26.7 and 30.3 mmol/L (mean value 28.4 mmol/L) [351], in this study [129], 16% of patients had TCO_2 values above the normal range, 52% below the normal range and 32% in the normal range, while the corresponding percentages in patients treated with the 35 mmol/L lactate solution were 3%, 75% and 22%. Moreover a subsequent study [352] in eight stable patients treated with 40 mmol/L of lactate-containing solution showed a mean arterial blood bicarbonate of 21.6 mmol/L and an increased anion gap value (21.4 mmol/L).

In summary, the increased lactate content to 40 mmol/L in the CAPD solution has been shown to improve acid–base status in a remarkable number of CAPD patients. However, a significant proportion of metabolic acidosis still remains, and metabolic alkalosis seems to occur in an increased number of patients. While the deleterious effects of metabolic acidosis on skeletal protein turnover are well demonstrated both in chronic renal failure rats and human patients, the long-term effects of chronic metabolic alkalosis in CAPD patients are unknown.

Some metabolic side-effects of lactate have been suggested, although there is no clear evidence of their clinical relevance. Lactate is a powerful peripheral vasodilator, affects myocardial contractility, reduces blood pressure and could play a role in the blood lipid disorders of the CAPD patients [353, 354]. In addition, the administration of large amounts of L-lactate without proportionate amounts of its redox partner pyruvate results in a lowering of the cellular redox state and the linked phosphorylation potential. This effect could impair many vital cellular functions including the distribution of inorganic ions between intracellular and extracellular fluid [348, 353, 355]. Unbalanced ratios of L-lactate to pyruvate also favour the so-called catabolic state associated with the action of corticosteroid and other hormones potentiating the conversion of muscle protein into glucose [356].

The toxicity of D-lactate differs from that of L-lactate since it is mainly observable in various forms of impaired cerebral function. Patients with blind loop syndrome and abnormal gut flora, producing sufficient of the D-isomer of lactic acid to elevate blood D-lactate to 3 mmol/L, developed clinically manifest encephalopathy [357]. The use of CAPD dialysate containing 40 mmol/L D,L-lactate has been reported to result in repeated episodes of cerebral dysfunction characterized clinically by agitated confusion, depression and hyperventilation, resulting in life-threatening metabolic alkalosis [358].

Bicarbonate

The undesired effects ascribed to lactate-containing solutions have prompted a search for alternative buffering agents. The ideal buffer for PD would be sodium bicarbonate, since this substance is the physiological buffer of the body. However, solutions containing mixtures of bicarbonate, calcium, magnesium and glucose are difficult to prepare, sterilize and store since, during autoclaving, calcium and magnesium precipitate as carbonate salts; glucose also caramelizes, due to the high pH of the solution.

When the double-chamber bag became available (see above), a first preclinical study was performed in one patient treated for 1 week and in three patients treated for few exchanges with a solution containing 35 mmol/L of bicarbonate and 5 mmol/L of acetate as organic acid [345]. The solution was well tolerated and no side-effects occurred. The patient treated for 1 week showed increased blood bicarbonate content until a plateau was achieved at about 29 mmol/L after a few days. In a subsequent study a solution containing 27 mmol/L of bicarbonate and 3 mmol/L of acetate was employed in one patient for 2 months [359]. No biochemical changes were observed but blood bicarbonate remained stable at prestudy level (20 mmol/L).

Contemporaneously, firm evidence of the superior biocompatibility of the bicarbonate solution as compared with the conventional lactate solution was achieved (Chapter 18) and different approaches to provide a stable bicarbonate solution were proposed (Table 9).

A solution containing 34 mmol/L of bicarbonate in the alkaline compartment and a few mmol/L of hydrochloric acid in the acid compartment was tested '*in-vitro*', in an animal model and in clinical conditions. No calcium carbonate precipitation was demonstrated '*in-vitro*' for up to 40 mmol/L of bicarbonate and 2 mmol/L of calcium concentration solutions over a clinical use range of temperatures [360]. In a rat model, repeated intraperitoneal injections of 100 ml/kg were not associated with histological lesions, crystal formation or fibrosis [361].

Kinetic studies demonstrated that changes in dialysate bicarbonate concentration at different dwell times were correlated to bicarbonate blood levels independently of the bicarbonate content of the fresh solution, thus suggesting a self-limited bicarbonate absorption [362, 363]. A short-term clinical evaluation (4 weeks) with this 34 mmol/L bicarbonate solution in six patients showed an increase of blood bicarbonate, a slight but not statistically significant increase of ultrafiltration, and no changes of principal biochemical parameters or dialysis adequacy, thus demonstrating that this solution is safe, well tolerated, does not affect peritoneal dialysis adequacy and is effective in the correction of uraemic acidosis [364].

The results of a large long-term randomized clinical study on this solution have recently been published [365]. Thirty-six patients treated with the bicarbonate-buffered solution completed a 6-month study period, and 15 of them were treated for more than 1 year. During the study the plasma bicarbonate value of those patients with metabolic acidosis at the baseline increased slightly but significantly, while a tendency to decrease was recorded in those

with alkalosis. No changes in acid–base parameters occurred in the lactate control group. The use of the bicarbonate-buffered solution was not associated with any adverse event related to the solution and subjective patient well-being was improved, mainly because of a reduction in abdominal pain induced by the conventional lactate solution.

Although the 34 mmol/L bicarbonate solution was more effective than the conventional 35 mmol/L lactate solution in the acid–base status correction, an alternative formulation with a higher bicarbonate concentration (39 mmol/L) was proposed in order to increase the percentage of the CAPD population with a normal acid–base status. In a pilot study in nine patients treated for 1 month with the new solution, the arterial blood bicarbonate increased significantly in all patients and the normal range was achieved by 6/9 patients [366].

An interventional study in a large population has been reported recently [367]. The aim was to normalize the acid–base status of CAPD patients by using two bicarbonate concentrations in the dialysis fluid. Patients with normal acid–base status at the baseline used the low bicarbonate solution (34 mmol/L), while patients with metabolic acidosis used the high bicarbonate solution (39 mmol/L). During the study the use of the two solutions was modulated according to the blood bicarbonate levels of patients. After 6 months the percentage of patients with normal acid–base status rose from 23% at the baseline to 62%. Since factors affecting acid–base homeostasis are intrinsic characteristics of the individual patient (ultrafiltration, protein catabolic rate, etc.) it is not suprising that only a certain modulation of buffer infusion may ensure a good correction in a large percentage of patients.

Yatzidis [368] proposed a bicarbonate-based PD solution in which bicarbonate (30 mmol/L) is stabilized by the addition of a dipeptide, glycylglycine (10 mmol/L). This solution has been shown to be stable after 18 months in storage and has been tested in rabbits for up to 25 days with no pathological findings in the peritoneum. About 80% of glycylglycine was absorbed. In humans this substance is enzymatically degraded to glycine, which is in turn metabolized to other non-essential amino acids. A first clinical acute study demonstrated that the glycylglycine–bicarbonate solution was well tolerated by patients and significantly increased net ultrafiltration as compared to a standard lactate solution [369]. In addition, since the solution must be cold-sterilized by filtration in order to avoid glucose caramelization, the concentrations of glucose

Table 9. Different bicarbonate based CAPD solutions

Composition	Concentration	Reference
Bicarbonate	34 mmol/L	364, 365
Bicarbonate	39 mmol/L	366, 367
Bicarbonate/glycylglycine	30/10 mmol/L	369
Bicarbonate/lactate	25/15 mmol/L	372

degradation products were considerably reduced [370].

A mixture of several buffers in the same solution was proposed by Veech [348] on theoretical grounds, and was later investigated both *in vitro* and in an animal model [371]. From these studies a solution suitable for clinical practice, containing a mixture of bicarbonate (25 mmol/L) and lactate (15 mmol/L) was prepared. This solution was compared with a conventional solution containing 40 mmol/L of lactate and with a pure bicarbonate solution (38 mmol/L) in a randomized multicentre study involving 45 patients [372]. There was no difference in plasma bicarbonate levels, irrespective of the dialysis solution used, and it could be concluded that the lactate/bicarbonate solution is as effective as lactate solution in treating uraemic acidosis. This solution was also able to reduce the infusion pain experienced by some patients with the lactate solution [373].

All these studies demonstrate that the bicarbonate-buffered CAPD solution is safe, well tolerated and does not present any, even potential, side-effects. In addition some beneficial effects have been suggested; e.g. an improvement of nutritional status and of ultrafiltration (see specific chapters in this book). Furthermore, there is evidence that the bicarbonate PD solution, bicarbonate being the physiological buffer of the body, is more biocompatible in terms of local and systemic effects than the conventional lactate-buffered solution.

Connections

The development of PD as a treatment for chronic renal failure has undergone some major developments. The first dates back to the 1960s, when Tenckhoff and Schechter proposed a bacteriologically safe peritoneal access device [374]. Another one took place about a decade later, with the introduction into clinical practice of the concept of continuous ambulatory peritoneal dialysis (CAPD) by Popovich and Moncrief [375]. This technique in particular has enabled us to obtain some very satisfactory clinical results, also because of the continuous methodological improvements.

Unfortunately, the early experiences with CAPD were burdened by a very high incidence of peritonitis because the connections between the catheter and the glass bottles containing the dialysis solution were unable to prevent the contamination of the peritoneal cavity through the intraluminal way [376].

Many steps were required to perform connections and disconnections from the glass bottles (eleven steps were needed altogether so as to remove the protection cap from the bottle and from the distal end of the transfer set, to connect the bag with the transfer set, and to connect–disconnect the transfer set to catheter of the patient) [377]. This type of disconnect system was necessary in order to give the patient greater freedom to be mobile without the heavy glass solution containers. All the steps illustrated were potentially contaminant and these operative conditions can explain the very high incidence of peritonitis (one episode every few weeks).

Subsequently, the introduction into clinical CAPD practice of collapsible, lightweight plastic bags for solutions led to a substantial fall in peritonitis incidence compared to the previous experiences with glass bottles, and exchange modalities in CAPD became safer [1, 378]. The number of manual interventions for connection/disconnection was reduced to just three per exchange. After solution infusion in the abdominal cavity the empty bag was not disconnected from the catheter, but was folded and carried inside a pocket under the patient's clothes and used to collect the drained effluent at the end of dwell time of each exchange. The wearable bag system has significantly reduced the incidence of peritoneal infection, compared to previous experiences [1], but peritonitis nevertheless remained perhaps the most limiting complication hampering the widespread diffusion of CAPD. Several steps were still potentially contaminant, since they were protected neither by a disinfectant nor by the flush-before-fill effect.

The Italian Y-system

In order to overcome the severe infectious complications of the peritoneal membrane, a critical innovation was proposed by two Italian nephrologists, Buoncristiani and Bazzato, based on the insertion of a Y-shaped device within the dialysate circuit [379, 380] (Fig. 15). The most important was the 'Perugia System' introduced by Buoncristiani [378, 381]. This consists of a Y-shaped short transfer set which is connected permanently to the catheter. The dialysate bag has a long downflow tube. The Y-device is kept constantly connected to the catheter with the lower branch and is filled with a sodium hypochlorite disinfectant solution during dwell time. During the exchange an empty bag and a dialysis fluid-filled bag are connected to the two upper branches of the Y-device. The spent solution dwelling in the peritoneal cavity is drained into the empty

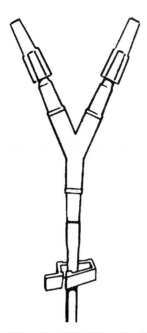

Figure 15. Miniaturized version of the 'Y'-shaped prosthesis (total lenght 8 cm) (from U. Buoncristiani).

bag. This drain serves to discharge the disinfectant out of the Y-set. When the spent dialysis fluid is drained into the empty bag, instillation of fresh dialysate follows. At the end of the exchange the two bags can be disconnected and the Y-set is filled with disinfectant and closed. During the interval between the two consecutive exchanges the patient wears only the very small Y-set device connected to the catheter and thus becomes bag-free.

This transfer technique provides the following advantages: during the interval the Y-device is protected by the disinfectant; after the connection of the empty and filled bags the disinfectant and the flush-before-fill are a combined protection against 'touch' contamination of the connection point; the disinfectant filling the Y seems to inhibit biofilm formation inside the catheter [382, 383].

The Y-set associates the patient convenience of the disconnect system with the advantage of reducing spike-related peritonitis rates [384]. The reason for this occurrence is that a flushing action away from the peritoneal cavity is obtained before any dialysate infusion. On the contrary, in standard spike procedures the infusion occurs immediately after the spike. So any bacterial contamination of the connection can reach the peritoneal cavity. An *in-vitro* study of the flush effect [385] showed that the flush technique used alone in a re-usable CAPD disconnect system may not be sufficient to ensure the removal of touch contaminants. Better peritonitis results can

be obtained by maintaining a disinfectant in the Y-set between exchanges. On the contrary, *in-vivo* experience has shown the importance of the flush effect, as has been pointed out in a French multi-centre study [386] conducted using a single-use or reusable disconnect system without a disinfectant in the transfer lines. The peritonitis rate was identical between the two systems, although in the reusable one it is preferable to spray or soak the connectors in an antiseptic solution before connecting.

Several authors have studied the efficacy of the Y-set in the prevention of peritonitis. The first and most impressive report [387] was a controlled study, performed in two Italian centres, that compared the standard CAPD system described by Oreopoulos *et al.* [116] with a Y-shaped set modified from that proposed by Buoncristiani (Fig. 16) [379, 381]. The amazing results showed a peritonitis incidence of one episode every 11.3 patient-months compared with one episode every 33 patient-months with the two systems, respectively. A similar experience was reported by an Italian group which observed 156 patients during a total follow-up of 4694.4 patient-months [388].

Another study comparing standard spike versus Y-set in CAPD [384] showed a statistically significant reduction in peritonitis rates (1/5.82 episode every patient-months versus 1/30.9). The same group confirmed this huge difference in the peritonitis rate (1/7.57 patient-months versus 1/27.79, respectively) in a further follow-up study [389].

A prospective randomized controlled trial [390] evaluated the efficacy, safety and acceptability of a modified version of the short branch Y-set system compared to the long branch Y-set. The low incidence of peritonitis was very impressive, reaching

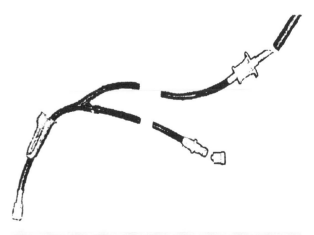

Figure 16. 'Y-solution transfer set'.

the surprising level of one episode in more than 60 patient-months with both systems.

The Canadian CAPD Clinical Trial Group [391] confirmed the efficacy of Y-connector disinfectant compared to standard system in a multi-centre randomized clinical trial, obtaining one episode of peritonitis every 21.5 patient-months and one every 9.9, respectively. It concluded that the Y-set disinfectant system was the gold standard for CAPD treatment and that all new methods should be compared to it.

Another important concept introduced by Bazzato was the 'double-bag system' [380]. In this system the Y is fixed not to the catheter, but to the bag side. Consequently the two bags are permanently connected to the two upper branches of a long Y-set, while the short branch is linked to the catheter only during the exchange. This system allows one to perform the flush-before-fill technique at the exchange start and to disconnect the bags during the interval (Fig. 17).

Despite the system's original concept, it has had not become very widespread, probably because in the original commercial model the connection was performed using a needle connected to the Y-set on the bag side and to one of the rubber caps covering the two ends of the Y-device permanently connected to the catheter (Fig. 18), where there is also an aseptic chamber to prevent touch contamination during needle insertion. The rubber caps were suitable for several needle-pricks.

This particular connection method has encountered several problems: a possible breakdown of the

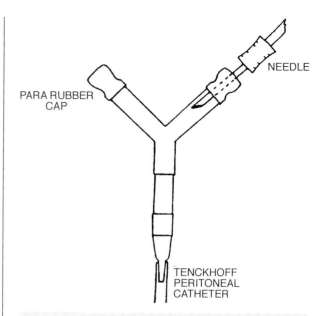

Figure 18. Peritoneal catheter adapter.

needle or the rubber caps, the considerable pressure required to pierce the rubber portions, especially when new [392], the difficulty of obtaining an efficient flow of dialysate to and from the peritoneal cavity, a poor efficiency of the flush action because of the cul-de-sac between the needle and the rubber cap [377]. Another drawback of the system was its insufficient handling in spite of the many efforts to modify its inconveniences [393, 394]. To overcome some of these difficulties a 'closter' was proposed as a new closed sterile connection [393], consisting of a needle mounted on a luer cap and protected by a folding plastic cover. However, the relatively low risk of peritonitis observed by Bazzato et al. [394], has not been confirmed by other authors,.

Clinical experiences with the original system and its modifications have mainly been reported by the Bazzato group which proposed the system. The results show an incidence of peritonitis of one episode every 26.6 patient-months over a long observation period and in a large number of patients (237 patients studied in 13 years) [394].

Another report [395] showed a very significant increase in the peritonitis-free interval in patients on the twin-bag system in comparison with patients using other non-twin-bag systems. The incidence of peritoneal infections was 1/46 patient-months in the first group and 1/9 in the second.

The double-bag concept remains a very important modality in PD exchange, even when substantial innovations in the original connection system

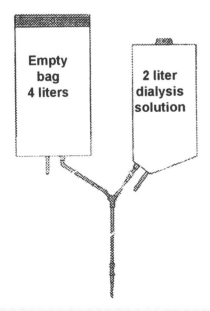

Figure 17. Double-bag system.

between the Y-set on the bag side and catheter have been carried out.

The T-set

This is a system which uses the double-bag with Y-set and a particular device connected to the catheter that remains filled with disinfectant during the dwell-time.

This device, called the T-set, is a small catheter extension for connecting the catheter to the Y of the bags. It has a very short lateral branch, through which the disinfectant (sodium hypochlorite) can be injected at the end of exchange and immediately before disconnection of the bags. The disinfectant stays inside the T-set during the interval between two consecutive exchanges (Fig. 19). The *in-vivo* and *in-vitro* experiences with this device have been reported in a multicentre prospective randomized controlled trial [396]. The results were similar to those obtained with the Y-system and the authors concluded that the T-system represents a further improvement on the Y-set connection.

The Y-set system without disinfectant

The presence of disinfectant inside the catheter extension poses a strong risk for its accidental infusion in the peritoneal cavity, with all its potential clinical effects [397–399]. Thus, some studies have been performed for evaluating whether the use of flushing alone, without on-line disinfectant, can prevent peritonitis [385, 400, 401]. Bazzato *et al.* [380] first proposed and used a Y-set without in-line disinfectant and a double-bag system. In the Bazzato system several technical problems did not allow for a proper evaluation of the capacity to prevent intraluminal contamination of the peritoneum, thanks to the flushing action alone.

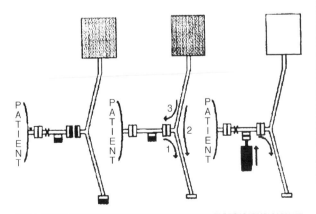

Figure 19. T-set [396].

During the 1980s some studies regarding this subject were performed demonstrating that the flush-before-fill system allows for a reduction in Y-set contamination. The effectiveness of flushing was correlated to the fluid volume used to flush, the number of bacteria colonies, the type of bacteria and the length of contact with the plastic lines [385, 386, 402, 403]. The results showed that the flush was effective in all experiments using *Staphylococcus epidermidis* as contaminant agent (100% of cases), but remarkably less effective with *Staphylococcus aureus* and *Pseudomonas aeruginosa*. For these microorganisms the flush is completely ineffective when the period between contamination and flush is 10 h or longer [386, 402]. In order to improve these results, Verger's group has suggested that an antiseptic agent should be used at least at the level of the connector, providing that it has no side effects on the quality of plastics [386].

This suggestion is accepted differently in most of the systems which do not use the disinfectant in-line. In these systems the end of the connector can be covered by a minicap containing povidone-iodine solution, disinfected using sodium hypochloride or alcohol-based antiseptic or using immersion or spraying. Currently, most if not all centres have stopped using the in-line antiseptic because of the risk of its accidental infusion into the peritoneal cavity.

The O-set

This is a variation of double-bag Y-set system [404]. At the end of infusion the double-bag system is disconnected from the catheter and the filled bag also disconnected from its branch of the Y-set. Then these two connection-free branches (the shorter one, which was linked to the catheter, and the longer one, linked to the drainage bag) are connected to each other, taking on the O configuration that gives its name to the system. The empty bag remains inserted at the third branch of the Y-set. At the next exchange the O-set is opened and the short branch is connected to the catheter and the long one to a new full bag. The O-set can be filled or not filled by disinfectant but, since it is a reusable system, the use of disinfectant is necessary to reduce peritonitis incidence [403].

The first multicentre trial [404] to evaluate the use of the CAPD O-set filled with hypochlorite as disinfectant during the interval period was performed in 76 stable adult CAPD patients retrained using the new device. The peritonitis incidence was

1/12.2 patient-months during the control period and 1/16.6 patient-months while using the O-set. Accidental peritoneal infusion of 0.5% sodium hypochlorite was usually related to poor patient attention during the exchange manoeuvres. This occurred on 22 occasions, usually shortly after the patient had learned the new exchange procedure. No long-term detrimental effects were noted. The authors confirmed that a Y-shaped system using intraluminal disinfectant is useful in CAPD and that the O-set provides an alternative, safe, efficacious CAPD technique, much appreciated by experienced CAPD patients.

Other clinical experiences regarding the comparison of the O-set with different systems have been reported [405–408]. Satisfactory results have been reported in all these trials. In particular the O-set has been considered a more cost-effective CAPD technique than the UVXD (Ultraviolet Irradiation Connector Box), while both are more cost-effective than the conventional spike technique [408].

A.N.D.Y. (A-non-disconnect-Y)

The main characteristic of this system is that at the end of each exchange the distal ending part of the transfer Y-set (connected at the bags) is properly closed with a special irreversible clamp, attached to the catheter, acting as a cup until the next exchange. Thanks to this technique the hazardous opening of the catheter-set circuit is avoided (until the next exchange) and the flush is performed immediately after a new connection. The latter aspect is critical, because it has been demonstrated clearly that the efficacy of the flush is greater if the flushing is performed very early after a possible touch contamination.

The Stay-Safe® *system*

This is the first CAPD system completely manufactured using Biofine®, a new material consisting exclusively of carbon and hydrogen. Previously the material used for PD bags and connections was based on PVC. In the Stay-Safe® system [409] the solution-drainage bag and the fresh-solution bag are connected to the tubing lines by a special disc, which is the real novelty of the system. Turning the disc, all the exchange phases can be performed: outflow, flush, inflow, and automatic closing of the system with a pin. At the last position of the disc a pin is automatically introduced into the lumen of the catheter adapter, which is also protected by a disinfectant

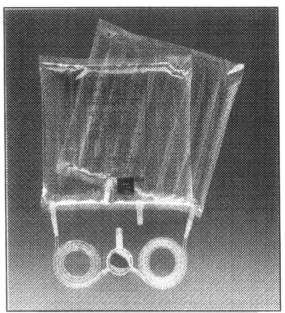

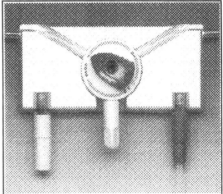

Figure 20. The Stay-Safe system.

cap. At the next exchange the catheter adapter is opened in a disinfected environment (Fig. 20). The sequence of the steps to perform the exchanges is controlled by the turning of the disc and by clamps. The breaking cones are eliminated. This innovative system has not been available for very long so there has not yet been much clinical experience. The new material (Biofine®, the twin-bag concept, the use of the disc for the different phases of the exchange with no disconnection, the automatic sealing of the lumen of the catheter adapter, and the absence of in-line disinfectant, are all elements of great interest, providing that clinical experience is able to confirm the initial information.

The Safe-lock system and Thermoclav

A heat sterilization device, called Thermoclav, was proposed in 1989 [410]. It consists of two parts: a

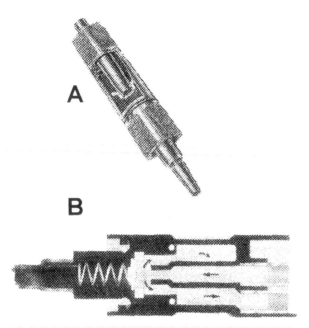

Figure 21. A = Safe-Lock connector; B = Safe-Lock 5F connector in flush position with valve still closed.

unit for temperature control and sterilization time, with a power supply and a thermobox, and an infrared unit as the actual sterilizing device. The system was used to sterilize the special connector 'Safe-Lock' after bag change by heat exposure (Fig. 21).

The Safe-Lock and its later development, the Safe-Lock 5F system [411], were connectors created in order to prevent touch contamination infection. The connector consists of two parts: the cone and the press-fit of the cone in the counterpart which is deeply recessed, so that the fluid path in both connector parts cannot be touched. In the more advanced system, Safe-Lock 5F, a valve inside the catheter ensuring safe sealing towards the peritoneal cavity in the disconnected position was added. The efficacy of the heat sterilization system depends on a temperature above 100°C and a minimum atmospheric pressure of 2.2 inside the Safe-Lock connector [412].

A clinical study has shown the efficacy of the heat sterilization device (Thermoclav) in combination with the Safe-Lock connector [410]. In a one-centre randomized clinical trial the same group evaluated the long-term effects of Thermoclav in comparison to standard systems on peritonitis incidence, and showed a significantly increased likelihood of remaining peritonitis-free using this device, compared to non-heat sterilization devices. The overall peritonitis incidence was 0.29 and 0.34 per patient-year, respectively [413].

Ultraviolet germicidal system

Ultraviolet radiation is considered the method that best fits the criteria for antimicrobial agents (reproducible microbial inactivation without toxic residues, a reasonably rapid effect, portable and with minimum patient involvement) [414]. Ultraviolet radiation is usually generated by passing an electric current between two electrodes in mercury vapour. This radiation significantly alters the DNA molecule, interfering with normal metabolic and reproductive functions. Much higher intensities of light in the ultraviolet spectral range can be obtained utilizing xenon gas instead of mercury vapour, requiring shorter periods of irradiation to reach microbicidal effectiveness. An *in-vitro* evaluation of the efficacy of the ultraviolet germicidal connection system for CAPD proved very encouraging. Using this technique 100% of the touch-contaminated spikes were disinfected [415].

A randomized multicentre clinical trial was performed to evaluate the effects of an ultraviolet germicidal system [416] (Fig. 22). One hundred and sixty-seven patients from 10 centres were followed up during a baseline historical period for a minimum of 4 months; thereafter they were randomized to the control group (93 patients) and to the test group (74 patients), for a trial period lasting 9 months. No significant differences between historical and trial periods in either group or between groups during either period were observed. The authors suggested that the spike contamination may have been an infrequent cause of infection and the peritonitis in patients with a good technique may relate more to other causes than to spike contamination. They concluded that patients with technique problems (motor coordination, compliance, visual or other) or at high risk of such problems could benefit from the ultraviolet germicidal chamber.

An experimental evaluation of a germicidal system using ultraviolet light was performed to test its efficacy by violating the recommended aseptic technique, simulating patient non-compliance [417]. The results were not encouraging, and the conclusions were that well-trained and highly motivated patients with a low incidence of peritonitis might obtain only minor benefits, while poorly trained, poorly motivated patients, with the highest infection rates, would not be protected by this device, with only a small increase in protection using this device.

In-vivo studies on the germicidal efficacy of a xenon-based ultraviolet light device [418] have shown its ability to effectively disinfect the CAPD set to the bag connection. A study comparing

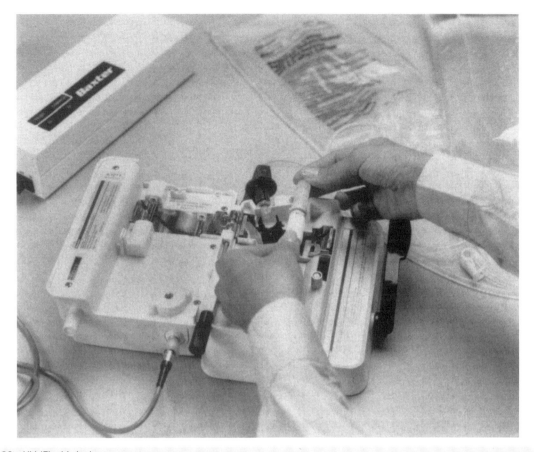

Figure 22. UV 'Flash' device.

different CAPD transfer systems concluded that the ultraviolet irradiation connection box may be reserved for those patients with poor eyesight, and for elderly or diabetic patients [408]. A retrospective study comparing experience using an ultraviolet irradiation system and the O-set system showed no difference in the capacity of the two systems to prevent peritonitis [419].

Other minor devices

Another device is a microwave system used to reduce the incidence of peritonitis. The prototype proposed did not have any further development aimed at regular clinical use, partly because it needed to be significantly reduced in size and weight [420].

The heat-sealing device was used to disconnect the PD tubing. This technique did not become widely used because there was a serious danger of causing burns [421].

References

1. Oreopoulos DG, Robson M, Izatt S, Clayton S, de Veber GA. A simple and safe technique for continuous ambulatory peritoneal dialysis (CAPD). Trans ASAIO 1978; 24: 484.
2. Klatte F. Verfahren zur Hestellung einer auf Hornersatz, Filme, Kunsträden, Lacke und dergleichen verarbeitbaren plastischen Masse. Deutches Reich Patent 231877, 1913.
3. Blass CR. PVC as a biomedical polymer–plasticizer and stabilizer toxicity. Med Device Technol 199; 23: 32.
4. Jaeger RJ, Rubin JR. Plasticizers from plastic devices: extraction, metabolism and accumulation by biomedical systems. Science 1970; 170: 460.
5. Janknegt R, Oldenhof AGJ, Steenhoek A. Is hetomhullen van infuuszzakken zinvol? (effectiveness of wrapping PVC infusion bags). Ziekenhuisfarmacie 1988; 4: 44.
6. D'Arcy PF. Drug interactions with medical plastic. Drug Intell Clin Pharm 1983; 17: 726.
7. Kowaluc EA, Roberts MS, Blackburn HD. Interaction between drugs and polyvinylchloride infusion bags. Am J Hosp Pharm 1978; 35: 541.
8. Jongejan GAM, Smit JCA, Heiling EAM, Hekster YA. De wisselwerking tussen geneesmiddelen en kunststoffen voor medish gebruik (Interaction of drugs with polymer for medical purposes). Pharm Weekbl 1989; 124: 440.
9. Aubuchon JP, Estep TN, Davey RJ. The effect of plasticizers di-2-ethylexylphthalate on the survival of stored RBC's. Blood 1988; 71: 448.
10. Rock G, Tocchi M, Ganz PR, Tackaberry ES. Incorporation of plasticizers into red cells during storage. Transfusion 1984; 4: 24.

11. Arbin A, Ostelius J, Callmer K, Sroka J, Hanninen K, Axelsson S. Migration of chemicals from soft PVC bags into intravenous solutions. Act Pharm Suec 1983; 3: 20.

12. Lemm W, Buknerl ES. Was ist medicinisches no-DOP-PVC? Kardiotechnik 1986; 9: 39.

13. Guess WL, Jacob J, Autian J. A study of polyvinylchloride blood bag assembles. 1. Alteration or contamination of ACD solutions. Drug Intel 1967; 1: 120.

14. Shibiko SI, Blumenthal H. Toxicology of phthalic acid esters used in food packing materials. Envirom Health Perspect 1973; 3: 171.

15. Wendland F. Geologische und Okologische Aspekte des Verhaltens von PVC in Deponien. Julich: Kernforschungsanlage Julichh, 1986 (Interner Bericht KFASTE-1B-8/88)

16. Giam C, Chan H, Neff G. Phthalate ester plasticizers: a new class of marine pollutant Science 1978; 199: 419.

17. EPA, USA. Exposure and risk assessment for phthalate esters. National Technical Information Services. US Dept Commerce, Springfield VA 22161, 1981.

18. Johnson BT, Lulves W. Biodegradation of di-n-butyl phthalate and di-2-ethylexyl phthalate in fresh water hydrosoil. J Fish Res Board Canada 1975; 32: 333.

19. Sein AA, Sluijmers JJ, Verhagen EJH. Onderzooek emissies afvalverbrandingsinstailaties. Eindrapport. (Study into emission by incinerators. Final report). Bilthoven: Rijksinstituut voor Volksgezondheid en Milieuhygiene, 1989.

20. De Leer EWB, Verbeek A. Environmental aspects of waste incineration – possibility for improvement. Toegepaste Wetensch TNO Mag 1990; 7: 6.

21. Reimann DO. PVC als Abfallprodukt. Mull Abfall 1988; 6: 256.

22. Viola PL, Bigotti A, Caputo A. Oncologic response of rat skin, lung and bones to vinylchloride. Cancer Res 1971; 1: 31.

23. Creek JL Jr, Johnson MN. Angiosarcoma of liver in the manufacture of polyvinylchloride. J Occup Med 1974; 16: 150.

24. Nicholson WJ, Henneberger PK, Seidman H. Occupational hazards in the VC–PVC industry. Prog Clin Biol Res 1984; 141: 155.

25. Baser ME, Tockman MS, Kennedy TP. Pulmonary function and respiratory symptoms in polyvinyl chloride fabrication workers. Am Rev Resp Dis 1985; 131: 203.

26. Benfenati E, Natangelo M, Davoli E, Fanelli R. Migration of polyvinylchloride into PVC-bottled drinking water assessed by gas chromatography–mass spectrometry. Food Chem Toxicol 1991; 29: 131.

27. Van Duuren BL. On the possible mechanism of carcinogenic action of vinyl chloride. Ann NY Acad Sci 1975; 246: 258.

28. Estep TN, Pedersen RA, Miller TJ, Stupar KR. Characterization of erythrocyte quality during the refrigerated storage of whole blood containing DEHP. Blood 1984; 64: 1270.

29. Warner WL, Nelson EJ. Container for platelet storage. US patent 4230497, 1981.

30. Jacobson MS, Kevy SV, Grand RJ. Effect of plasticizer leached from polyvinyl chloride on the subhuman primate: a consequence of chronic transfusion therapy. J Lab Clin Med 1977; 89: 1066.

31. Albro PW, Thomas R, Fishbein L. Metabolism of di-ethylhexyl phthalate by rats: isolation and characterization of the urinary metabolites. J Chromatogr 1973; 76: 321

32. Schmid P, Schiatter CH. Excretion and metabolism of (ethylhexyl)phthalate in man. Xenobiotica 1985; 15: 251.

33. Lanina SY, Strakhova NM, Lappo VG. Toxicological estimate of polyvinyl chloride containers for preparation and storage of blood, its components, preservatives and infusion solutions. Med Prog Technol 1982; 18: 19.

34. Pollack GM, Buchanan JF, Slaughter RL, Kohii RK, Shen DD. Circulating concentrations of di(2-ethylhexyl)phthalate and its deesterified phthalic acid products following plasticizer exposure in patients receiving hemodialysis. Toxicol Appl Pharmacol 1985; 79: 257.

35. Gibson TP, Briggs WA, Boone BJ. Delivery of di(2-ethylhexyl)phthalate to patients during hemodialysis. J Lab Clin Med 1976; 87: 519.

36. Mettang T, Fisher FP, Dunst R, Kuhlmann U, Rettenmeier W. Plasticizers in renal failure: aspects of metabolism and toxicity. Perit Dial Int 1997; 17 (Suppl. 2): S31.

37. Peck CC, Albro PW. Toxic potential of the plasticizer DEHP in the content of its deposition and metabolism in primates and man. Environ Health Perspect 1982; 45: 11.

38. Van Dooren AA. PVC as pharmaceutical packing material. Pharmaceutish Weekblag (Scientific edition) 1991; 13: 109.

39. Agarwal DK, Eustin S, Lamb JC IV, Reel JR, Kluwe WM. Effects of DEHP on the gonadal pathophysiology, sperm morphology and reproductive performance in male rats. Environ Health Perspect 1986; 65: 343.

40. Prasad AS. Metabolism of Zinc and its Deficiency in Human Subjects. Springfield, IL: Charles C. Thomas, 1966, p. 250.

41. Wolkowski TR, Jones PC, Marr MC, Kimmel CA. Teratologic evaluation of DEHP in CD-1 mice. Teratology 1983; 3: 27.

42. Moody DE, Reddy JK. Hepatic peroxisome (microbody) proliferation in rats fed plasticizers and related compounds. Toxicol Applied Pharmacol 1975; 45: 497.

43. Reddy JK, Lalwani ND. Carcinogenesis by hepatic peroxisome proliferators: evaluation of the risk of hypolipidemic drugs and industrial plasticizers in humans. CNT Rev Toxicol 1983; 12: 1.

44. Bentley P, Calder I, Elcombe C, Grasso P, Stringer D, Wiegand HJ. Hepatic peroxisome proliferation in rodents and its significance for humans. Food Chem Toxicol 1993; 31: 857.

45. Huber WW, Grasl-Kraupp B, Schulte HR. Hepatocarcinogenic potential of DEHP in rodents and its implications on human risk. Crit Rev Toxicol 1996; 26: 365.

46. Tomita I, Nakamura Y, Aoki N, Inui N. Mutagenic/carcinogenic potential of DEHP and MEHP. Environ Health Perspect 1982; 45: 119.

47. Crocker JFS, Safe SH, Acott P. Effects of chronic phthalate exposure to the kidney. J Toxicol Environ Health 1988; 23: 433.

48. Schultz CO, Rubin RJ, Hutkins GM. Acute lung toxicity and sudden death in rats following the intravenous administration of the plasticizers DEHP, solubilized with twin surfactants. Toxicol Appl Pharmacol 1975; 33: 514.

49. Carilli AD, Ramanamurty MV, Chang YS, Shin D, Sethi V. Non-cardiogenic pulmonary edema following blood transfusion. Chest 1978; 74: 311.

50. Nässberger L, Arbin A, Ostelius J. Exposure of patients to phthalates from polyvinylchloride tubes and bags during dialysis. Nephron 1987; 45: 286.

51. Bommer J, Gemsa D, Waldherr R, Kessler J, Ritz E. Plastic filling from dialysis tubing induces prostanoid release from macrophages. Kidney Int 1984; 26: 331.

52. Mallette FS, von Haam E. Study on the toxicity and skin effects of compounds used in the rubber and plastics industries. Contact Derm Newsl 1972, 308.

53. Mettang T, Thomas S, Kiefer T. Uremic pruritus and the exposure to DEHP in hemodialysis patients. Nephrol Dial Transplant 1996; 11: 2439.

54. Crocker JF, Blecher SR, Safe SH. Chemically induced polycystic kidney disease. Prog Clin Biol Res 1983; 140: 281.

55. Nässberger L, Arbin A. Eosinophilic peritonitis – hypothesis. Nephron 1987; 46: 103.

56. Chen WS, Kerkay J, Pearson KH. Tissue DEHP levels in uremic subjects. Anal Lett 1979; 12: 1517.

57. Sabatini S, Fracasso A, Bazzato G, Kurtzman NA. Effects of phthalate esters on transport in toad bladder membrane. J Pharmacol Exper Ther 1989; 250: 910.

58. Fracasso A, Coli U, Landini S et al. Peritoneal sclerosis: role of plasticizers. Trans ASAIO 1987; 33: 676.

59. Calò L, Fracasso A, Cantaro S et al. Plasticizers induced mononuclear cell Interleukin 1 production: implications with peritoneal sclerosis. Clin Nephrol 1993; 40: 57.

60. Picard C, Brazier M, Bou P, Hary L, Renaux C. Stabilité de quatre solutions de penicillines dans le poches de perfusion multicouches. J Pharm Clin 1993; 13: 45.
61. Jackson A. A comparison of peritoneal dialysis products and their effect on insulin dosage. British Analytical Control, unpublished data, 1994.
62. Verger C, Brunschvic O, Lecharpentier Y. Structural and ultrastructural peritoneal membrane changes and permeability alteration during CAPD. Eur Dial Transplant Assoc 1981; 18: 199.
63. Di Paolo N, Sacchi D, De Mia M. Morphology of the peritoneal membrane during continuous ambulatory peritoneal dialysis. Nephron 1986; 44: 204.
64. Cantù P, Limido A, Caretta E. Influenza del riscaldamento sulla contaminazione particellare delle sacche per CAPD. Atti IV National Meeting on Peritoneal Dialysis. Wichtig Publishers, 1988, p. 213.
65. Chaimovitz C. Peritoneal dialysis. Kidney Int 1994; 45: 1226
66. Fracasso A, Landini S, Morachiello P, Righetto F, Scanferla F, Toffoletto P. Il problema dei plastificanti. In: La Greca G, Petrella E, Cioni A, eds. I Liquidi nella Dialisi. Milan: Ghedini Editore, 1992, p. 85..
67. Carozzi S, Nasini MG, Schelotto C, Caviglia PM, Santoni O, Pietrucci A. A biocompatibility study on peritoneal dialysis solution bags for CAPD. Adv Perit Dial 1990; 13: 55.
68. Darby TD, Johnson AJ, Northup SJ. An evaluation of a polyurethane for use as alcal grade plastic. Toxicol Appl Pharmacol 1978; 446: 449.
69. Anon. 4,4′-Methylendianiline (MDA). US Department of Health and Human Services, Public Health Service, Center for Disease Control, Robert A. Taft Laboratories, 4676 Columbia Parkway, Cincinnati, OH 45266, USA, 25 July 1986, p. 21.
70. Bonk J. REXflexFPO – going beyond polyolefines; presented 27 June at FLEXPO, Huston, Texas, 1996.
71. Lambert P. Packaging of intravenous solutions. Med Dev Technol, September/October 1990, p. 27.
72. Feriani M, Biasioli S, Borin D, Fabris A, Ronco C, La Greca G. Bicarbonate solutions for peritoneal dialysis: a reality. Int J Artif Organs 1985, 8: 57.
73. Ing TS, Quon MJ, Daugirdas JT, Ghandi VC, Epstain MB. Preparation of bicarbonate containing peritoneal dialysate using an automated dialysate delivery system. Int J Artif Organs 1981; 4: 148.
74. Ing TS, Quon MJ, Daugirdas JT, Liu P, Gandhi VC, Reid RR. On line preparation of bicarbonate containing dialysate for use in peritoneal dialysis. Int J Artif Organs 1981; 4: 308.
75. Ing TS, Humayun HM, Daugirdas JT *et al.* Preparation of bicarbonate-containing dialysate for peritoneal dialysis. Int J Artif Organs 1983; 6: 217
76. Ing TS, Ghandi VC, Daugirdas JT, Reid RW, Hunt J, Popli S. Peritoneal dialysis using bicarbonate buffered dialysate. Int J Artif Organs 1984; 7: 166.
77. Maillard LC. Action des acides amines sur le sucres: formation des melanoidines par voie methodique. CR Acad Sci 1912; 154: 66.
78. Dobbie JW. Advanced glycosylation end products in peritoneal dialysis tissue with different solutions. Peri Dial Int 1997; 17 (Suppl. 2): S27.
79. Wieslander A, Linden T. Glucose degradation and cytotoxicity in PD fluids. Perit Dial Int 1996; 16 (Suppl. 1): S114.
80. Henderson IS, Couper IA, Lumsden A. The effect of shelf-life of peritoneal dialysis fluid on ultrafiltration in CAPD. In: La Greca G, Chiaramonte S, Fabris A, Feriani M, Ronco C. eds. Peritoneal Dialysis. Milan: Wichtig Editore, 1986: p. 85.
81. Martinson E, Wieslander A, Kjellestrand P, Boberg U. Toxicity in heat sterilized fluids for peritoneal dialysis derives from degradation of glucose. Trans ASAIO 1992; 38: 370.
82. Rippe B, Simonsen O, Wieslander A, Landgren C. Clinical and physiological effects of a new, less toxic and less acidic fluid for peritoneal dialysis. Perit Dial Int 1997: 17: 27.
83. Boen ST. Kinetics of peritoneal dialysis. Medicine 1961; 40: 243.
84. Henderson LW. Peritoneal ultrafiltration dialysis. Enhanced urea transfer using hypertonic peritoneal dialysis fluid. J Clin Invest 1964; 45: 950.
85. Henderson LW, Nolph KD. Altered permeability of the peritoneal membrane after using hypertonic peritoneal dialysis fluid. J Clin Invest 1969; 48: 992.
86. Nolph KD, Miller FN, Pyle K, Popovich RP, Sorkin MJ. A hypothesis to explain the characteristics of peritoneal ultrafiltration. Kidney Int 1981; 20: 543.
87. Boen ST. History of peritoneal dialysis. In: Nolph KD ed, Peritoneal Dialyis. Dordrecht: Kluwer, 1989: p. 1.
88. Merril JP, Hampers CL. Uremia. N Engl J Med 1970; 282: 953.
89. Lowrie EG, Steinberg SM, Galen MA *et al.* Factors in the dialysis regimen which contribute to alterations in the abnormalities of uremia. Kidney Int 1976; 10: 409.
90. Teschan PE. Electroencephalographic and other neurophysiological abnormalities in uremia. Kidney Int 1975; (Suppl. 2): S210.
91. Nolph KD, Parker A. The composition of dialysis solution for continuous ambulatory peritoneal dialysis. In: Legrain M, ed. Continuous Ambulatory Peritoneal Dialysis. Amsterdam: Excerpta Medica, 1980, p. 341.
92. Nolph KD, Twardowski ZJ, Popovich RP, Rubin J. Equilibration of peritoneal dialysis solutions during long dwell exchanges. J Lab Clin Med 1979; 93: 246.
93. Nolph KD, Sorkin MJ, Moore H. Autoregulation of sodium and potassium removal during continuous ambulatory peritoneal dialysis. Trans ASAIO 1980; 26: 334.
94. Nolph KD, Hano JE, Teschan PE. Peritoneal sodium transport during hypertonic peritoneal dialysis: physiologic mechanisms and clinical implications. Ann Intern Med 1969; 70: 931.
95. Raja RM, Cantor RE, Boreyco C, Bushchri H, Kramer MS, Rosenbaum JL. Sodium transport during ultrafiltration peritoneal dialysis. Trans ASAIO 1972; 18: 429.
96. Raja RM, Kramer MS, Rosenbaum JL, Manchanda R, Lazaro N. Evaluation of hypertonic peritoneal dialysis solutions with low sodium. Nephron 1973; 11: 342.
97. Ahearn DJ, Nolph KD. Controlled sodium removal with peritoneal dialysis. Trans ASAIO 1972; 18: 423.
98. Bosch JP. Permeability characteristics of the peritoneal membrane. In: La Greca G, Chiaramonte S, Fabris A, Feriani M, Ronco C, eds. Peritoneal Dialysis. Milan: Wichtig Editore, 1985: p. 25.
99. Rippe B, Stein G, Haraldsson B. Computer simulations of peritoneal fluid transport in CAPD. Kidney Int 1991; 40: 315.
100. Monquil MCJ, Imholz ALT, Struijk DG, Krediet RT. Does impaired transcellular water transport contribute to net ultrafiltration failure during CAPD? Perit Dial Int 1995; 15: 42.
101. Colombi A. Fluid and electrolyte balance in CAPD patients. In: La Greca G, Chiaramonte S, Fabris A, Feriani M, Ronco C, eds. Peritoneal Dialysis. Milan: Wichtig Editore, 1988, p. 265.
102. De Vecchi A, Paparella M, Scalamogna A, Guerra L, Castelnovo C. Effetti della variazione delle concentrazioni di sodio nel liquido di dialisi peritoneale. In: La Greca G, Petrella E, Cioni A, eds. I liquidi nella dialisi. Milan: Ghedini Editore, 1991, p. 93.
103. Nakayama M, Yokoyama K, Kawaguchi Y, Sakai O. Effect of ultra low sodium concentration dialysate (ULNaD) in patients with UF loss. Perit Dial Int 1991 (Suppl. 1): 187 (abstract).
104. Imholz ALT, Koomen GCM, Struijk DG, Arisz L, Krediet RT. Fluid and solute transport in CAPD patients using ultralow sodium dialysate. Kidney Int 1994; 46: 333.

105. Nakayama M, Yokoyama K, Kubo H *et al.* The effect of ultra-low sodium dialysate in CAPD. A kinetic and clinical analysis. Clin Nephrol 1996; 45: 188.

106. Twardowski ZJ. New approaches to intermittent peritoneal dialysis therapies. In: Nolph KD, ed. Peritoneal Dialysis. Dordrecht: Kluwer,1989, p. 133.

107. Gault MH, Ferguson EL, Sidhu JS, Corbin RP. Fluid and electrolyte complications of peritoneal dialysis. Choice of dialysis solutions. Ann Intern Med 1971; 75: 253.

108. Shen FH, Sherrard DJ, Scollard D, Merrit A, Curtis FK. Thirst, relative hypernatremia and excessive weight gain in maintenance peritoneal dialysis. Trans ASAIO 1978; 24: 142.

109. Twardowski ZJ, Nolph KD, Khanna R, Gluck Z, Prowant BF, Ryan LP. Daily clearances with continuous ambulatory peritoneal dialysis and nightly peritoneal dialysis. Trans ASAIO 1986; 32: 575.

110. Nolph KD. Kinetic of ultrafiltration and electrolyte transport during peritoneal dialysis. In: La Greca G, Chiaramonte S, Fabris A, Feriani M, Ronco C, eds. Peritoneal Dialysis. Milan: Wichtig Editore, 1985, p. 47.

111. Brown ST, Ahearn DJ, Nolph KD. Potassium removal with peritoneal dialysis. Kidney Int 1973; 4: 67.

112. Gokal R. Continuous ambulatory peritoneal dialysis. In: Maher JF, ed. Replacement of Renal Function by Dialysis. Dordrecht: Kluwer, 1989, p. 590.

113. Blumenkrantz MJ, Kopple JD, Moran JK, Coburn JW. Metabolic balance studies and dietary protein requirements in patients undergoing continuous ambulatory peritoneal dialysis. Kidney Int 1982; 21: 849.

114. Sandle GI, Gaiger E, Tapster S, Goodship THJ. Evidence for large intestinal control of potassium homeostasis in uraemic patients undergoing CAPD. Clin Sci 1987; 73: 247.

115. Lameire N, Ringoir S. Introductory remarks: an overview of peritonitis and other complications of continuous ambulatory peritoneal dialysis. In: Legrain M, ed. Continuous Ambulatory Peritoneal Dialysis. Amsterdam: Excerpta Medica, 1980, p. 229.

116. Oreopoulos DG, Khanna R, Williams P. Continuous ambulatory peritoneal dialysis. Nephron 1982; 30: 293.

117. Spital A, Sterns RH. Potassium supplementation via the dialysate in continuous ambulatory peritoneal dialysis. Am J Kidney Dis 1985; 6: 173.

118. Lindholm B, Alvestrand A, Hultman F, Bergstrom J. Muscle water and electrolytes in patients undergoing continuous ambulatory peritoneal dialysis. Acta Med Scand 1986; 219: 323.

119. Heide B, Pierratos A, Khanna R *et al.* Nutritional status of patients undergoing continuous ambulatory peritoneal dialysis. Perit Dial Bull 1983; 3: 138.

120. Rubin J, Kirchner K, Barnes T, Teal N, Ray R, Bower JD. Evaluation of continuous ambulatory peritoneal dialysis. Am J Kidney Dis 1983; 3: 199.

121. Schilling H, Wu G, Petit J *et al.* Nutritional status of patients on long term CAPD. Perit Dial Bull 1985; 5: 12.

122. Randall RE, Cohen MD, Spray CC, Rossmeisl EC. Hypermagnaesemia in renal failure: etiology and toxic manifestation. Ann Intern Med 1964; 61: 73.

123. Whang R. Magnesium deficiency: pathogenesis, prevalence and clinical implications. Am J Med 1987; 82 (Suppl. 3A): 24.

124. Hollifield J. Magnesium depletion, diuretics and arrhythmias. Am J Med 1987; 82 (Suppl. 3A): 30.

125. Selling M. Electrocardiographic patterns of magnesium depletion appearing in alcoholic heart disease. Ann NY Acad Sci 1969; 162: 906.

126. Parker A, Nolph KD. Magnesium and calcium mass transfer during continuous ambulatory peritoneal dialysis. Trans ASAIO 1980; 26: 194.

127. Kwong MBL, Lee JSK, Chan MK. Transperitoneal calcium and magnesium transfer during an 8-hour dialysis. Perit Dial Bull 1987; 7: 85.

128. Gokal R, Fryer R, McHugh M, Ward MK, Kerr DNS. Calcium and phosphate control in patients on continuous ambulatory peritoneal dialysis. In: Legrain M, ed. Continuous Ambulatory Peritoneal Dialysis. Amsterdam: Excerpta Medica, 1980, p. 283.

129. Nolph KD, Prowant B, Serkes KD *et al.* Multicentric evaluation of a new peritoneal dialysis solution with a high lactate and low magnesium concentration. Perit Dial Bull 1983; 3: 63.

130. Kohaut EC, Balfe JW, Potter D, Alexandre S, Lum G. Hypermagnesemia and mild hypocarbia in pediatric patients on CAPD. Perit Dial Bull 1983; 3: 41.

131. Rahman R, Heaton A, Goodship T *et al.* Renal osteodystrophy in patients on CAPD: a five year study. Perit Dial Bull 1987; 7: 1.

132. Rubin J. Comments on dialysis solution, antibiotic transport, poisonings and novel uses of peritoneal dialysis. In: Nolph KD, ed. Peritoneal Dialysis. Dordrecht: Kluwer, 1989, p. 199.

133. Gonella M. Plasma and tissue levels of magnesium in chronically hemodialyzed patients: effects of dialysate magnesium levels. Nephron 1983; 34: 141.

134. Meema HE, Oreopoulos DG, Rapoport A. Serum magnesium level and arterial calcification in end-stage renal disease. Kidney Int 1987; 32: 388.

135. Hutchison AJ, Freemont AJ, Boulton HF, Gokal R. Low-calcium dialysis fluid and oral calcium carbonate in CAPD. A method of controlling hyperphosphataemia whilst minimizing aluminium exposure and hypercalcaemia. Nephrol Dial Transplant 1992; 7: 1219.

136. Hutchison AJ, Gokal R. Improved solutions for peritoneal dialysis: physiological calcium solutions, osmotic agents and buffers. Kidney Int 1992; 42 (Suppl. 38): S153.

137. Breuer J, Moniz C, Baldwin D, Parsons V. The effects of zero magnesium dialysate and magnesium supplements on ionized calcium concentration in patients on regular dialysis treatment. Nephrol Dial Transplant 1987; 2: 347.

138. Shan G. Winer R, Cutler R *et al.* Effects of a magnesium-free dialysate on magnesium metabolism during continuous ambulatory peritoneal dialysis. Am J Kidney Dis 1987; 10: 268.

139. Delmez JA, Slatopolsky E, Martin KJ, Gearing BN, Harter HR. Minerals, vitamin D, and parathyroid hormone in continuous ambulatory peritoneal dialysis. Kidney Int 1982; 21: 862.

140. Digenis G, Khanna R, Pierratos A *et al.* Renal osteodystrophy in patients maintained on CAPD for more than three years. Perit Dial Bull 1983; 3: 81.

141. Gokal R, Ramos JM, Ellis HA *et al.* Histological renal osteodystrophy and 25 hydroxycholecalciferol and aluminum levels in patients on continuous ambulatory peritoneal dialysis. Kidney Int 1983; 23: 15.

142. Delmez JA, Fallon M, Bergfeld M, Gearing BN, Dougan C, Teitelbaum S. Continuous ambulatory peritoneal dialysis and bone. Kidney Int 1986; 30: 379.

143. Bucciante G, Bianchi M, Valenti G. Progress of renal osteodystrophy during CAPD. Clin Nephrol 1984; 6: 279.

144. Lindholm B, Bergstrom J. Nutritional aspects of CAPD. In: Gokal R, ed. Continuous Ambulatory Peritoneal Dialysis. Edinburgh: Churchill Livingstone, 1986, p. 228.

145. Sheikh MS, Maguire JA, Emmett M *et al.* Reduction of dietary phosphorus absorption by phosphorus binders. A theoretical, *in vitro*, and *in vivo* study. J Clin Invest 1989; 83: 66.

146. Ramirez JA, Emmett M, White MG *et al.* The absorption of dietary phosphorus and calcium in hemodialysis patients. Kidney Int 1986; 30: 753.

147. Davenport A, Goel S, MacKenzie JC. Audit of the use of calcium carbonate as phosphate binder in 100 patients treated with continuous ambulatory peritoneal dialysis. Nephrol Dial Transplant 1992; 7: 632.

148. Joffe P, Olsen F, Heaf J, Gammelgaard B, Pondephant J. Aluminium concentrations in serum, dialysate, urine and

bone among patients undergoing continuous ambulatory peritoneal dialysis. Clin Nephrol 1989; 32: 133.

149. Andreoli S, Briggs J, Junior B. Aluminium intoxication from aluminium containing phosphate binders in children with azotemia not undergoing dialysis. N Engl J Med 1984; 310: 1074.

150. Ackrill P, Day J, Ahmed R. Aluminium and iron overload in chronic dialysis. Kidney Int 1988; 33 (Suppl. 24): S163.

151. Altmannn P, Dhanesha U, Hamon C, Cunningham J, Blair J, Marsch F. Disturbance of cerebral function by aluminium in hemodialysis patients without overt aluminium toxicity. Lancet 1989; ii: 7.

152. Martis L, Serkes KD, Nolph KD. Calcium as a phosphate binder: is there a need to adjust peritoneal dialysate calcium concentration for patients using CaCO$_3$. Perit Dial Int 1989; 9: 325.

153. Weinreich T, Passlick-Deetjen J, Ritz E, collaborators of the peritoneal dialysis multicenter study group. Low dialysate calcium in continuous ambulatory peritoneal dialysis: a randomized controlled multicenter trial. Am J Kidney Dis 1995; 25: 452.

154. Weinreich T. Low or high calcium dialysate solutions in peritoneal dialysis? Kidney Int 1996; 50 (Suppl. 56): S92.

155. Cunningham J, Beer J, Coldwell RD, Noonan K, Sawyer N, Makin HLJ. Dialysate calcium reduction in CAPD patients treated with calcium carbonate and alfacalcidol. Nephrol Dial Transplant 1992; 7: 63.

156. Ritz E, Weinreich T, Matthias S. Is it necessary to readjust dialysis calcium concentration? J Nephrol 1992; 5: 70.

157. Brown CB, Hamdy NAT, Boletis J, Kanis JA. Rationale for the use of low calcium solution in CAPD. In: La Greca G, Ronco C, Feriani M, Chiaramonte S, Conz P, eds. Peritoneal Dialysis. Milan: Wichtig Editore, 1991, p. 125.

158. Piraino B, Perlmutter JA, Holley JL, Johnston JR, Bernardini J. The use of dialysate containing 2.5 mEq/l calcium in peritoneal dialysis patients. Perit Dial Int 1992; 12: 75.

159. Hutchison AJ, Gokal R. Towards tailored dialysis fluids in CAPD: the role of reduced calcium and magnesium in dialysis solution. Perit Dial Int 1992; 12: 199.

160. Beer J, Tailor D, Noonan K, Cunningham J. Rapid exacerbation of hyperparathyroidism in patients converted to low calcium dialysate without adequate calcium supplementation. Perit Dial Int 1993; 13 (Suppl. 1): S30.

161. Andersen KEH. Calcium transfer during intermittent peritoneal dialysis. Nephron 1981; 29: 63.

162. Schmitt H, Ittel TH, Schafer L, Sieberth HG. Effect of a low calcium dialysis solution on serum parathyroid hormone in automated peritoneal dialysis. Perit Dial Int 1993; 13 (Suppl. 1): S59.

163. Putman J. The living peritoneum as a dialysis membrane. Am J Physiol 1923; 63: 548.

164. Cunningham RS. Studies on absorption from serious cavities. III. The effect of dextrose upon the peritoneal mesothelium. Am J Physiol 1920; 53: 458.

165. Palmer RA, Quinton WE, Gray JF et al. Prolonged peritoneal dialysis for chronic renal failure. Lancet 1964; 1: 700.

166. Rubin J, Nolph KD, Popovich RP, Moncrief JW. Drainage volumes during continuous ambulatory peritoneal dialysis. ASAIO J 1979; 2: 54.

167. Gokal R, Mistry CD. Glucose polymer as osmotic agent in CAPD. In: La Greca G, Ronco C, Feriani M, Chiaramonte S, Conz P, eds. Peritoneal Dialysis. Milan: Wichtig Editore, 1991, p. 119.

168. Twardowski ZJ, Khanna R, Nolph KD. Osmotic agents and ultrafiltration in peritoneal dialysis. Nephron 1986; 42: 93.

169. Starling EH. On the absorption of fluids from connetive tissue spaces. J Physiol 1895; 19: 312.

170. Mistry CD, Mallick NP, Gokal R. Ultrafiltration with an isosmotic solution during long peritoneal dialysis exchanges. Lancet 1987; 2: 178.

171. Staverman PJ. The theory of measurement of osmotic pressure. Rec Trav Chim Pays-Bas 1951; 70: 344

172. Kiil F. Mechanism of osmosis. Kidney Int 1982; 21: 303.

173. Mistry CD, Gokal R. New osmotic agents for peritoneal dialysis: where we are and where we're going. Semin Dial 1991; 4: 9.

174. Mistry CD, Gokal R. A single daily overnight (12 h dwell) use of 7.5% glucose polymer (Mw 18 700; Mn 7300) + 0.35% glucose solution: a 3-month study. Nephrol Dial Transplant 1993; 8: 443.

175. Ronco C, Feriani M, Chiaramonte S et al. Pathophysiology of ultrafiltration in peritoneal dialysis. Perit Dial Int 1990; 10: 119.

176. Pyle WK, Moncrief JW, Popovich RP. Peritoneal transport evaluation in CAPD. In: Moncrief JW, Popovich RP, eds. CAPD Update. New York: Masson, 1981: p. 35.

177. Maher JF, Bennett RR, Hirszel P, Chakrabarti E. The mechanism of dextrose-enhanced transport rates. Kidney Int 1985; 28: 16.

178. Krediet RT, Boeschoten EW, Zuyderhoudt FMJ, Arisz L. The relationship between peritoneal glucose absorption and body fluid loss by ultrafiltration during continuous ambulatory peritoneal dialysis. Clin Nephrol 1987; 27: 51.

179. Maher JF. Peritoneal transport rate: mechanisms, limitation and methods for augmentation. Kidney Int 1980; 18: S117.

180. Nolph KD, Mactier RA, Khanna R, Twardowski ZJ, Moore H, McGary T. The kinetics of ultrafiltration during peritoneal dialysis: the role of lymphatics. Kidney Int 1987; 32: 219.

181. Mactier RA, Khanna R, Twardowski ZJ, Moore H, Nolph KD. Contribution of lymphatic absorption to loss of ultrafiltration and solute clearances in CAPD. J Clin Invest 1987; 80: 1311.

182. Grodstein GP, Blumenkrantz MJ, Kopple JD, Moran JK, Coburn JW. Glucose absorption during continuous ambulatory peritoneal dialysis. Kidney Int 1981; 19: 564.

183. DeSanto NG, Capodicasa G, Senatore R et al. Glucose utilization from dialysate in patients on continuous ambulatory peritoneal dialysis. Int J Artif Organs 1978; 2: 119.

184. Lindholm B, Bergstrom J. Nutritional management of patients undergoing peritoneal dialysis. In: Nolph KD, ed. Peritoneal Dialysis. Dordrecht: Kluwer, 1989, p. 230.

185. Kreusch G, Bammatter F, Mordasini R, Binswanger U. Serum lipoprotein concentrations during continuous ambulatory peritoneal dialysis. In: Ghal GM, Kessel M, Nolph KD, eds. Advances in Peritoneal Dialysis. Amsterdam: Excerpta Medica, 1981, p. 427.

186. Lindholm B, Karlander SG, Norbek HE, Furst P, Bergstrom J. Carboyhdrate and lipid metabolism in CAPD patients. In: Atkins R, Thomson N, Farrell P. eds. Peritoneal Dialysis. Edimburgh: Churchill Livingstone, 1981, p. 198.

187. Von Baeyer H, Gahl GM, Riedinger H et al. Adaptation of CAPD patients to the continuous peritoneal energy upyake. Kidney Int 1983; 23: 29.

188. Boyer J, Gill GN, Epstein FH. Hyperglycemia and hyperosmolality complicating peritoneal dialysis. Ann Intern Med 1967; 67: 568.

189. Nolph KD, Rosenfeld PS, Powell JT, Danforth JR. Peritoneal glucose transport and hyperglycemia during peritoneal dialysis. Am J Med Sci 1970; 259: 272.

190. Heaton A, Johnston DG, Burrin JM et al. Carbohydrate and lipid metabolism during continuous ambulatory peritoneal dialysis: the effect of a single dialysis cycle. Clin Sci 1983; 65: 539.

191. Amstrong VW, Creutzfeldt W, Ebert R, Fuchs C, Hilgers R, Scheler F. Effect of dialysis glucose load on plasma and glucoregulatory hormones in CAPD patients. Nephron 1985; 39: 141.

192. Amstrong VW, Buschmann U, Ebert R, Fuchs C, Rieger J, Scheler F. Biochemical investigations of CAPD: plasma levels of trace elements and amino acids and impaired glucose tolerance during the course of treatment. Int J Artif Organs 1980; 3: 237.

193. Oreopoulos DG, Marliss E, Anderson *et al.* Nutritional aspects of CAPD and the potential use of amino acid containing dialysis solutions. Perit Dial Bull 1983; 3: 10.

194. Wideroe TE, Smeby LC, Myking OL. Plasma concentrations and transperitoneal transport of native insulin and C-peptide in patients on continuous ambulatory peritoneal dialysis. Kidney Int 1984; 25: 82.

195. Lindholm B, Bergstrom J, Karlander SG. Glucose metabolism in patients on continuous ambulatory peritoneal dialysis. Trans ASAIO 1981; 17: 58.

196. Lindholm B, Bergstrom J, Norbek HE. Lipoprotein (LP) metabolism in patients on continuous ambulatory peritoneal dialysis. In: Gahl GM, Kessel M, Nolph KD. eds. Advances in Peritoneal Dialysis. Amsterdam: Excerpta Medica, 1981, p. 434.

197. Lindholm B, Karlander SG, Norbek HE, Bergstrom J. Glucose and lipid metabolism in peritoneal dialysis. In: La Greca G, Biasioli S, Ronco C. eds. Peritoneal DFialysis. Milan: Wichtig Editore, 1982, p. 219.

198. Gokal R, Ramos JM, McGurk JG, Ward MK, Kerr DNS. Hyperlipidaemia in patients on continuous ambulatory peritoneal dialysis. In: Gahl GM, Kessel M, Nolph KD, eds. Advances in Peritoneal Dialysis. Amsterdam: Excerpta Medica, 1981, p. 430.

199. Roncari DAK, Breckenridge WC, Khanna R, Oreopoulos DG. Rise in high-density lipoprotein-cholesterol in some patients treated with CAPD. Perit Dial Bull 1981; 1: 136.

200. Ramos JM, Heaton A, McGurk JG, Wark MK, Kerr DNS. Sequential changes in serum lipids and their subfractions in patients receiving continuous ambulatory peritoneal dialysis. Nephron 1983; 35: 20.

201. Nolph KD, Ryan KL, Prowant B, Twardowski ZJ. A cross sectional assessment of serum vitamin D and triglyceride concentration in a CAPD population. Perit Dial Bull 1984; 4: 232.

202. Lindholm B, Norbek HE. Serum lipids and lipoproteins during continuous ambulatory peritoneal dialysis. Acta Med Scand 1986; 220: 143.

203. Khanna R, Breckenridge WC, Roncari DAK, Digenis G, Oreopoulos DG. Lipids abnormalities in patients undergoing continuous ambulatory peritoneal dialysis. Perit Dial Bull 1983; 3: S13.

204. Henderson IS, Couper IA, Lumsden A. Potentially irritant glucose in unused CAPD fluid. In: Maher JF, Winchester JF, eds. Frontiers in Peritoneal Dialysis. New York: Field, Rich & Associates, 1986, p. 261.

205. Dobbie JW, Lloyd JK, Gall CA. Categorization of ultrastructural changes in peritoneal mesothelium, stroma and blood vessels in uremia and CAPD patients. In: Khanna R, Nolph KD, Prowant P, Twardowski ZJ, Oreopoulos DG, eds. Advances in Continuous Ambulatory Peritoneal Dialysis. Toronto: Peritoneal Dialysis Bulletin Inc., 1990, p. 3.

206. Dobbie JW. Pathogenesis of peritoneal fibrosis syndromes (sclerosing peritonitis) in peritoneal dialysis. Perit Dial Int 1992; 12: 14.

207. De Paepe M, Matthijs E, Peluso F *et al.* Experience with glycerol as the osmotic agent in peritoneal dialysis in diabetic and non-diabetic patients. In: Keen H, Legrain M, eds. Prevention and Treatment of Diabetic Nephropathy. Boston: MTP Press, 1983, p. 299.

208. Heaton A, Ward MK, Johnston DG, Nicholson DV, Alberti KGMM, Kerr DNS. Short-term studies on the use of glycerol as an osmotic agent in continuous ambulatory peritoneal dialysis. Clin Sci 1984; 67: 121.

209. Matthys E, Dolkart R, Lameire N. Extended use of a glycerol-containing dialysate in diabetic CAPD patients. Perit Dial Bull 1987; 7: 10.

210. Lameire N, Faict D. Peritoneal dialysis solutions containing glycerol and amino acids. Peri Dial Int 1994; 14 (Suppl. 13): S145.

211. Daniels FH, Leonard EF, Cortell S. Glucose and glycerol compared as osmotic agents for peritoneal dialysis. Kidney Int 1984; 25: 20.

212. Lindholm B, Werynski A, Bergstrom J. Kinetic of peritoneal dialysis with glycerol and glucose as osmotic agents. Trans ASAIO 1987; 33: 19.

213. Heaton A, Ward MK, Johnston DG, Alberti KGMM, Kerr DNS. Evaluation of glycerol as an osmotic agent for continuous ambulatory peritoneal dialysis in end-stage renal failure. Clin Sci 1986; 70: 23.

214. Matthys E, Dolkart R, Lameire N. Potential hazards of glycerol dialysate in diabetic CAPD patients. Perit Dial Bull 1987; 7: 16.

215. Hain H, Kessel M. Aspects of new solutions for peritoneal dialysis. Nephrol Dial Transplant 1987; 2: 67.

216. Gokal R, Mistry C. Osmotic agents in continuous ambulatory peritoneal dialysis. In: La Greca G, Chiaramonte S, Fabris A, Feriani M, Ronco C, eds. Peritoneal Dialysis. Milan: Wichtig Editore, 1988, p. 61.

217. Goodship THJ, Heaton A, Wilkinson R, Ward MK. The use of glycerol as an osmotic agent in continuous ambulatory peritoneal dialysis. In: Ota K, Maher J, Winchester J, Hirszel P, eds. Current Concepts in Peritoneal Dialysis. Amsterdam: Excerpta Medica, 1992, p. 143.

218. Bazzato G, Coli U, Landini S *et al.* Xylitol and low dosages of insulin: new perspectives for diabetic uremic patients on CAPD. Perit Dial Bull 1982; 2: 161.

219. Wu G. Osmotic agents for peritoneal dialysis solutions. Perit Dial Bull 1982; 2: 151.

220. Yatuc W, Ward G, Shipetar G, Tenckhoff H. Substitution of sorbitol for dextrose in peritoneal irrigation fluid. A preliminary report. Trans ASAIO 1967; 13: 168.

221. Raja RM, Moros JG, Kramer MS, Rosenbaum JL. Hyperosmolal coma complicating peritoneal dialysis with sorbitol dialysate. Ann Intern Med 1970; 73: 993.

222. Bischel MC, Barbour BH. Peritoneal dialysis with sorbitol versus dextrose dialysate: clinical findings and alterations of blood and cerebrospinal fluid. Nephron 1974; 12: 449.

223. Vidt DG. Recommendations on choice of peritoneal dialysis solutions. Ann Intern Med 1973; 78: 144.

224. Robson MD, Levi J, Rosenfeld JB. Hyperglycemia and hyperosmolality in peritoneal dialysis. Its prevention by the use of fructose. Proc EDTA 1969; 6: 300.

225. Raja RS, Kramer MS, Manchanda R, Lazaro N, Rosenbaum JL. Peritoneal dialysis with fructose dialysate. Prevention of hyperglycemia and hyperosmolality. Ann Intern Med 1973; 79: 511.

226. Faict D, Hartman JP, Lameire N, Kesteloot D, Peluso F. The evaluation of a peritoneal dialysis solution with amino acids and glycerol in a new rat model. Perit Dial Int 1990;10 (Suppl. 1): S60.

227. Lameire N, Faict D. Peritoneal dialysis solutions containing glycerol and amino acids. Perit Dial Int 1994; 14 (Suppl. 3): S145.

228. Faict D, Lameire N, Kesteloot D, Peluso F. Evaluation of peritoneal dialysis solutions with amino acids and glycerol in a rat model. Nephrol Dial Transplant 1991; 6: 120.

229. Van Biesen W, Faict D, Boer W, Lameire N. Further animal and human experience with a 0.6% amino acid/1.4% glycerol peritoneal dialysis solution. Perit Dial Int 1997; 17 (Suppl. 2): S56.

230. Young GA, Kopple JD, Lindholm B *et al.* Nutritional assessment of continuous ambulatory peritoneal dialysis patients: an international study. Am J Kidney Dis 1991; 17: 462.

231. Kopple JD, Blumenkrantz MJ, Jones MR, Moran JK, Coburn JW. Plasma amino acid levels and amino acid losses during continuous ambulatory peritoneal dialysis. Am J Clin Nutr 1982; 36: 395.

232. Lindholm B, Bergstrom J. Nutritional aspects on peritoneal dialysis. Kidney Int 1992; 42 (Suppl. 38): S165.

233. Gjessing J. Addition of amino acids to peritoneal dialysis fluid. Lancet 1968; 2: 812.

234. Oreopoulos DG, Crassweller P, Katirtzoglou A *et al.* Amino acids as an osmotic agent (instead of glucose) in continuous ambulatory peritoneal dialysis. In: Legrain M, ed. Continuous Ambulatory Peritoneal Dialysis. Amsterdam: Excerpta Medica, 1980, p. 335.

235. Williams PF, Marliss EB, Harvey Anderson G *et al.* Amino acid absorption following intraperitoneal administration in CAPD patients. Perit Dial Bull 1982; 2: 124.

236. Nakao T, Ogura M, Takahashi H, Okada T. Charge-affected transperitoneal movement of amino acids in CAPD. Perit Dial Int 1996; 16 (Suppl. 1): S88.

237. Oren A, Wu G, Harvey Anderson G *et al.* Effective use of amino acid dialysate over four weeks in CAPD patients. Perit Dial Bull 1983; 3: 66.

238. Goodship THJ, Lloyd S, McKenzie PW *et al.* Short-term studies on the use of amino acids as an osmotic agent in continuous ambulatory peritoneal dialysis. Clin Sci 1987; 73: 471.

239. Lindholm B, Werynsky A, Bergstrom J. Peritoneal dialysis with amino acid solutions: fluid and solute transport kinetics. Artif Organs 1988; 12: 2.

240. Lindholm B, Traneus A, Werynski A, Osterberg T, Bergstrom J. Amino acids for peritoneal dialysis: technical and metabolic implications. In: La Greca G, Chiaramonte S, Fabris A, Feriani M, Ronco C, eds. Peritoneal Dialysis. Milan: Wichtig Editore, 1986, p. 149.

241. Young GA, Dibble JB, Taylor AE, Kendall S, Brownjohn AM. A longitudinal study of the effects of amino acid-based CAPD fluid on amino acid retention and protein losses. Nephrol Dial Transplant 1989; 4: 900.

242. Young GA, Dibble JB, Brownjohn AM. The use of amino acid based CAPD fluid in chronic renal failure. In: Amino Acids, Chemistry, Biology and Medicine. Lubec and Rosenthal, 1992, p. 850.

243. Steinhauer HB, Lubrich-Birker I, Kluthe R, Baumann G, Schollmeyer P. Effects of amino acid based dialysis solution on peritoneal permeability and prostanoid generation in patients undergoing continuous ambulatory peritoneal dialysis. Am J Nephrol 1992; 12: 61.

244. Douma CE, de Waart DR, Struijk DG, Krediet RT. Effect of amino acid based dialysate on peritoneal blood flow and permeability in stable CAPD patients: a potential role for nitric oxide? Clin Nephrol 1996; 45: 295.

245. Pedersen FB. Alternate use of amino acid and glucose solutions in CAPD. Contr Nephrol 1991; 89: 147.

246. Schilling H, Wu G, Pettit J *et al.* Effects of prolonged CAPD with amino acid containing solutions in three patients. In: Khanna R, Nolph KD, Prowant BF, Twardowski ZJ, Oreopoulos DG, eds. Advances in Continuous Ambulatory Peritoneal Dialysis. Toronto: University of Toronto Press, 1985, p. 49.

247. Schilling H, Wu G, Pettit J *et al.* Use of amino acid containing solutions in continuous ambulatory peritoneal dialysis patients after peritonitis: results of a prospective controlled trial. Proc EDTA-ERA 1985; 22: 421.

248. Dombros NV, Prutis K, Tong M *et al.* Six-month overnight intraperitoneal amino-acid infusion in continuous ambulatory peritoneal dialysis (CAPD) patients. No effect on nutritional status. Perit Dial Int 1990; 10: 79.

249. Lindholm B, Bergstrom J. Amino acids in CAPD solutions: lights and shadows. In: La Greca G, Ronco C, Feriani M, Chiaramonte S, Conz P, eds. Peritoneal Dialysis. Milan: Wichtig Editore, 1991, p. 139.

250. Okamura K, Yamauchi J, Nakahamma H *et al.* The effects of adding essential amino acids to the dialysis solution of continuous ambulatory peritoneal dialysis patients. In: Maekawa M, Nolph KD, Kishimoto T, Moncrief J eds. Machine Free Dialysis for Patient Convenience: The fourth ISAO Official Satellite Symposium on CAPD. Cleveland, ISAO Press, 1984, p. 103.

251. Pedersen FB, Dragsholt C, Laier E *et al.* Alternate use of amino acid and glucose solutions in CAPD. Perit Dial Bull 1985; 5: 215.

252. Alvestrand A, Furst P, Bergstrom J. Plasma and muscle free amino acids in uremia: influence of nutrition with amino acids. Clin Nephrol 1982; 18: 297.

253. Young GA, Dibble JB, Hobson SM *et al.* The use of an amino-acid-based CAPD fluid over 12 weeks. Nephrol Dial Transplant 1989; 4: 285.

254. Dibble JB, Young GA, Hobson SM, Brownjohn AM. Amino-acid-based continuous ambulatory peritoneal dialysis (CAPD) fluid over twelve weeks: effects on carbohydrate and lipid metabolism. Perit Dial Int 1990; 10: 71.

255. Bruno M, Bagnis C, Marangella M *et al.* CAPD with an amino acid solution: a long-term, cross-over study. Kidney Int 1989; 35: 1189.

256. Arfeen S, Goodship THJ, Kirkwood A, Ward MK. The nutritional/metabolic and hormonal effects of 8 weeks of continuous ambulatory peritoneal dialysis with a 1% amino acid solution. Clin Nephrol 1990; 33: 192.

257. Scanziani R, Dozio B, Iacuitti G. CAPD in diabetics: use of amino acids. In: Ota K, Maher J, Winchester J, Hirszel P, eds. Current Concepts in Peritoneal Dialysis. Amsterdam: Excerpta Medica, 1992, p. 628.

258. Jones MR, Martis L, Algrim CE *et al.* Amino acid solutions for CAPD: rationale and clinical experience. Miner Electrolyte Metab 1992; 18: 309.

259. Kopple JD, Bernard D, Messana J *et al.* Treatment of malnourished CAPD patients with an amino acid based dialysate. Kidney Int 1995; 47: 1148

260. Faller B, Aparicio M, Faict D *et al.* Clinical evaluation of an optimized 1.1% amino acid solution for peritoneal dialysis. Nephrol Dial Transplant 1995; 10: 1432.

261. Jones MR, Hagen T, Vonesh E, Moran J, the Nutrineal study group. Use of a 1.1% amino acid solution to treat malnutrition in peritoneal dialysis patients. J Am Soc Nephrol 1995; 6: 580 (abstract).

262. Jones MR, Gehr TW, Burkart JM *et al.* Replacement of amino acid and protein losses with 1.1% amino acid peritoneal dialysis solution. Perit Dial Int 1998; 18: 210.

263. Jones M, Kalil R, Blake P, Martis L, Oreopoulos DG. Modification of an amino acid solution for peritoneal dialysis to reduce risk of acidemia. Perit Dial Int 1997; 17: 66.

264. Plum J, Fussholler A, Schoenicke G *et al.* In vivo and in vitro effects of amino-acid-based and bicarbonate-buffered peritoneal dialysis solutions with regard to peritoneal transport and cytokines/prostanoids dialysate concentration. Nephrol Dial Transplant 1997; 12: 1652.

265. Lazarus-Barlow WS. Observations upon the initial rates of osmosis of certain substances in water and in fluids containing albumen. J Physiol 1895–6; 19: 140.

266. Hain H, Ghal G. Osmotic agent. An update. Contrib Nephrol 1991; 89: 119.

267. Daniels FH, Nedev ND, Cataldo T, Leonard EF, Cortell S. The use of polyelectrolytes as osmotic agent for peritoneal dialysis. Kidney Int 1988; 33: 925.

268. Struijk DG, Bakker JC, Krediet RT, Koomen GCM, Stekkinger P, Arisz L. Effect of intraperitoneal administration of two different batches of albumin solutions on peritoneal solute transport in CAPD patients. Nephrol Dial Transplant 1991; 6: 198.

269. Nolph KD, Hopkins C, Rubin J *et al.* Polymer induced ultrafiltration in dialysis: high osmotic pressure due to impermeant polymer sodium. Trans ASAIO 1978; 24: 162.

270. Rubin J, Nolph KD, McGary TJ. Osmotic ultrafiltration with dextran sodium sulfate: potential for use in peritoneal dialysis. J Dialysis 1979; 3: 251.

271. Twardowski ZJ, Moore HL, McGary TJ, Poskuta M, Stathakis C, Hirszel P. Polymers as osmotic agent for peritoneal dialysis. Perit Dial Bull 1984; 4 (Suppl. 3): S125.

272. Frank HA, Seligman AM, Fine J. Further experiences with peritoneal irrigation for acute renal failure. Ann Surg 1948; 128: 561.

273. Twardowski ZJ, Hain H, McGary TJ, Moore HL, Keller RS. Sustained UF with gelatin dialysis solution during long dwell dialysis exchanges in rats. In: Maher JF, Winchester JF, eds. Frontiers in Peritoneal Dialysis. New York: Field, Rich & Associates, 1986, p. 249.

274. Ring J, Messmer K. Incidence and severity of anaphylactoid reactions to colloid substitutes. Lancet 1977; 2: 466.

275. Gjessing J. The use of dextran as a dialysing fluid in peritoneal dialysis. Acta Med Scand 1969; 185: 237.

276. Hain H, Schutte W, Pustelnik A, Gahl G, Kessel M. Ultrafiltration and absorption characteristics of hydroxyethylstarch and dextran during long dwell peritoneal dialysis exchanges in rat. In: Khanna R, Nolph KD, Prowant BF, Twardowski ZJ, Oreopoulos DG, eds. Advances in Peritoneal Dialysis. Toronto: Peritoneal Dialysis Bulletin Inc., 1989, p. 28.

277. Hain H, Kempf D, Schnell P, Gahl G, Kessel M. Ultrafiltration patterns of dextran and hydroxyethylstarch during long dwell peritoneal dialysis exchanges in nonuremic rats. In: Avram MM, Giordano C, eds. Ambulatory Peritoneal Dialysis. New York: Plenum, 1990, p. 83.

278. Bergonzi G, Paties C, Vassallo G et al. Dextran deposit in tissues of patients undergoing hemodialysis. Nephrol Dial Transplant 1990; 5: 54.

279. Dienes HP, Gerharz CD, Wagner R, Weber M, John HD. Accumulation of hydroxyethyl starch (HES) in the liver of patients with renal failure and portal hypertension. J Hepatol 1986; 3: 223.

280. Alsop RM. History, chemical and pharmaceutical developement of icodextrin. Perit Dial Int 1994; 14 (Suppl. 2): S5.

281. Mistry CD, Fox JE, Mallick NP, Gokal R. Circulating maltose and isomaltose in chronic renal failure. Kidney Int 1987; 32 (Suppl. 22): S210.

282. Peers E, Gokal R. Icodextrin: overview of clinical experience. Perit Dial Int 1997; 17: 22.

283. Mistry CD, Gokal R, Mallick NP. Glucose polymer as an osmotic agent in CAPD. In: Maher JF, Winchester JF, eds. Frontiers in Peritoneal Dialysis. New York: Field, Rich & Associates, 1986, p. 241.

284. Winchester JF, Stegink LD, Ahmad S et al. A comparison of glucose polymer and dextrose as osmotic agents in CAPD. In: Maher JF, Winchester JF, eds. Frontiers in Peritoneal Dialysis. New York: Field, Rich & Associates, 1986, p. 231.

285. Higgins JT, Gross ML, Somani P. Patient tolerance and dialysis effectiveness of a glucose polymer-containing peritoneal dialysis solution. Perit Dial Bull 1984; 4: S131.

286. Winchester JF. Alternative osmotic agents to dextrose for peritoneal dialysis. In: La Greca G, Chiaramonte S, Fabris A, Feriani M, Ronco C, eds. Peritoneal Dialysis: Proceedings of Second International Course on Peritoneal Dialysis. Milan: Wichtig Editore, 1986, p. 135.

287. Mistry CD, Gokal R. Icodextrin in peritoneal dialysis: early development and clinical use. Perit Dial Int 1994; 14 (Suppl. 2): S13.

288. Mistry CD, Mallick NP, Gokal R. The advantage of glucose polymer as an osmotic agent in continuous peritoneal dialysis. Proc EDTA 1985; 22: 415.

289. Mistry CD, Mallick NP, Gokal R. The use of large molecular weight polymer (MW 20 000) as an osmotic agent in continuous ambulatory peritoneal dialysis (CAPD). In: Khanna R, Nolph KD, Prowant BF, Twardowski ZJ, Oreopoulos DG, eds. Advances in Peritoneal Dialysis. Toronto: Peritoneal Dialysis Bulletin Inc., 1986, p. 7.

290. Mistry CD, Gokal R. The use of hyposmolar glucose polymer solution in continuous ambulatory peritoneal dialysis. In: Avram MM, Giordano C, eds. Ambulatory Peritoneal Dialysis. New York: Plenum, 1990, p. 83.

291. Mistry CD, Walker M, Gokal R. Safe use of glucose polymer dialysate over three months in CAPD patients. Nephrol Dial Transplant 1990; 5: 299.

292. Mistry CD, Gokal R, Peers EM, and the MIDAS study group. A randomized multicenter clinical trial comparing isosmolar icodextrin with hyperosmolar glucose solutions in CAPD. Kidney Int 1994; 46: 496.

293. Wilkie Me, Brown CB. Polyglucose solutions in CAPD. Perit Dial Int 1997; 17 (Suppl. 2): S47.

294. Lam Po Tang MKL, Bending MR, Kwan JTC. Icodextrin hypersensitivity in a CAPD patient. Perit Dial Int 1997; 17: 82.

295. Schildt B, Bouveng R, Sollenberg M. Plasma substitute induced impairement of reticuloendothelial system function. Acta Chir Scand 1975; 141: 7.

296. Davies DS. Kinetics of icodextrin. Perit Dial Int. 1994; 14 (Suppl. 2): S45.

297. Krediet RT, Brown CB, Imholz ALT, Koomen GCM. Protein clearance and icodextrin. Perit Dial Int 1994; 14 (Suppl. 2): S39.

298. Gokal R, Mistry CD, Peers EM and the MIDAS study group. Peritonitis occurrence in a multicentre study of icodextrin and glucose in CAPD. Perit Dial Int 1995; 15: S226.

299. Wilkie ME, Plant MJ, Edwards L, Brown C. Icodextrin 7.5% dialysate solution (glucose polymer) in patients with ultrafiltration failure: extension of CAPD technique survival. Perit Dial Int 1997; 17: 84.

300. Posthuma N, ter Wee PM, Verbrugh HA, Oe PL, Peers E, Sayers J, Donker AJ. Icodextrin instead of glucose during the daytime dwell in CCPD increases ultrafiltration and 24-h dialysate creatinine clearance. Nephrol Dial Transplant 1997; 12: 550.

301. Krediet RT, Imholz ALT, Lameire N, Faict D, Koomen GCM, Martis L. The use of peptides in peritoneal dialysis fluid. Perit Dial Int 1994; 14 (Suppl. 3): S152.

302. Klein E, Ward RA, Williams TE, Feldhoff PW. Peptides as substitute osmotic agent for glucose in peritoneal dialysis. Trans ASAIO 1986; 32: 550.

303. Martis L, Burke R, Klein E. Evaluation of a peptide-based solution for peritoneal dialysis. Perit Dial Int 1993; 13 (Suppl. 2): S92.

304. Imholz ALT, Lameire N, Faict D, Koomen GCM, Krediet RT, Martis L. Evaluation of short chain polypeptides as osmotic agent in continuous ambulatory peritoneal dialysis patients. Perit Dial Int 1994; 14: 215.

305. Wang T, Lindholm B. Oligopeptides as osmotic agents in peritoneal dialysis. Perit Dial Int 1997; 17 (Suppl. 2): S75.

306. Mistry CD, Gokal R. Can ultrafiltration occur with a hyposmolar solution in peritoneal dialysis ? The role for 'colloid' osmosis. Clin Sci 1993; 85: 495.

307. Mistry CD, Bhowmick B, Ashman R, Uttley L. Clinical studies of new icodextrin formulations. Perit Dial Int 1994; 14 (Suppl. 2): S55.

308. Peers E. Icodextrin plus glucose combinations for use in CAPD. Perit Dial Int 1997; 17 (Suppl. 2): S68.

309. Wang T, Heimburger O, Cheng HH, Bergstrom J, Lindholm B. Peritoneal fluid and solute transport with different polyglucose formulations. Peri Dial Int 1998; 18: 193.

310. Faller B, Shockley T, Genestier S, Martis l. Polyglucose and amino acids: preliminary results. Perit Dial Int 1997; 17 (Suppl. 2): S63.

311. Marsiglia JC, Cingolani HE, Gonzales NC. Relevance of beta receptor blockade to the negative inotropic effect induced by metabolic acidosis. Cardiovasc Res 1973; 7: 336.

312. Lemann J Jr, Litzow JR, Lennon EJ. The effect of chronic acid loads in normal man: further evidence for the participation of bone mineral in the defence against chronic metabolic acidosis. J Clin Invest 1966; 45: 1608.

313. Bichara M, Mercier O, Borensztein P, Paillard M. Acute metabolic acidosis enhances circulating parathyroid hormone, which contributes to renal response against acidosis in the rat. J Clin Invest 1990; 86: 430.

314. Lefebvre A, de Verneoul MC, Gueris J, Goldfarb B, Graulet AM, Morieux C. Optimal correction of acidosis changes progression of dialysis osteodystrophy. Kidney Int 1989; 36: 1112.

315. Papadoyannakis NJ, Stefanides CJ, Mc Geown M. The effect of the correction of metabolic acidosis on nitrogen and protein balance of patients with chronic renal failure. Am J Clin Nutr 1984; 40: 623.

316. May RC, Kelly RA, Mitch WE. Metabolic acidosis stimulates protein degradation in rat muscle by a glucocorticoid-dependent mechanism. J Clin Invest 1986; 7: 614.

317. Hara Y, May RC, Kelly RA, Mitch WE. Acidosis, not azotemia, stimulates branched-chain amino acid catabolism in uremic rats. Kidney Int 1987; 32: 808.

318. Jenkins D, Burton PR, Bennet SE, Baker F, Walls J. The metabolic consequences of the correction of acidosis in uraemia. Nephrol Dial Transpl 1989; 4: 92.

319. Williams B, Hattersley J, Layward E, Walls J. Metabolic acidosis and skeletal muscle adaptation to low protein diets in chronic uremia. Kidney Int 1991; 40: 779.

320. Stein A, Baker F, Larratt C et al. Correction of metabolic acidosis and protein catabolic rate in PD patients. Perit Dial Int 1994; 14: 187.

321. Graham KA, Reaich D, Channon SM et al. Correction of acidosis in CAPD decreases whole body protein degradation. Kidney Int 1996; 49: 1396.

322. Stein A, Moorhouse J, Iles-Smith H et al. Role of an improvement in acid–base status and nutrition in CAPD patients. Kidney Int 1997; 52: 1089.

323. Garibotto G, Russo R, Sofia A et al. Skeletal muscle protein synthesis and degradation in patients with chronic renal failure. Kidney Int 1994; 45: 1432.

324. Bergstrom J, Alvestrand A, Furst P. Plasma and muscle free amino acids in maintenance hemodialysis patients without protein malnutrition. Kidney Int 1990; 38: 108.

325. Bazilinsky NG, Dunea G, Ing TS. Treatment of metabolic alkalosis in renal failure. Int J Artif Organs 1987; 10: 284.

326. Preuss HG. Biochemistry of bicarbonate, lactate and acetate in man. North Med Proc 1977; 1: 1.

327. Boen ST, Mulinari AS, Dillard DH, Scribner BH. Periodic peritoneal dialysis in the management of chronic uremia. Trans ASAIO 1962; 8: 256.

328. Biasioli S, Feriani M, Chiaramonte S, La Greca G. Buffers in peritoneal dialysis. Int J Artif Organs 1987; 10: 3.

329. La Greca G, Biasioli S, Chiaramonte S et al. Acid–base balance on peritoneal dialysis. Clin Nephrol 1981; 16: 1.

330. Faller B, Marichal JF. Loss of ultrafiltration in CAPD: a role for acetate. Perit Dial Bull 1984; 4: 10–3.

331. Slingeneyer A, Mion C, Mourad G et al. Progressive sclerosing peritonitis. A late and severe complication of maintenance peritoneal dialysis. Trans ASAIO 1983; 29: 633.

332. Feriani M. Adequacy of acid–base correction in continuous ambulatory peritoneal dialysis patients. Perit Dial Int 1994; 14 (Suppl. 3): S133.

333. Brin M. The synthesis and metabolism of lactic acid isomers. Ann NY Acad Sci 1965; 119: 942.

334. Searle GL, Cavalieri RR. Determination of lactate kinetics in the human analysis of data from single injection. Proc Soc Exp Biol Med 1972; 139: 1002.

335. Fabris A, Biasioli S, Chiaramonte S et al. Buffer metabolism in CAPD: relationship with respiratory dynamics. Trans ASAIO 1982; 28: 270.

336. Teehan BP, Schleifer CR, Reichard GA, Cupit MC, Sigler MH, Haff AC. Acid–base studies in continuous ambulatory peritoneal dialysis. In: Moncrief JW, Popovich RP, eds. CAPD Update. New York: Masson, 1981, p. 95.

337. Richardson RMA, Roscoe JM. Bicarboante, L-lactate and D-lactate balance in intermittent peritoneal dialysis. Perit Dial Bull 1986; 6: 178.

338. Nolph KD, Twardowski ZJ, Khanna R et al. Tidal peritoneal dialysis with racemic or L-lactate solutions. Perit Dial Int 1990; 10: 161.

339. Robson MD, Faivoseviz A, Malmoud H. Physiological transfer of acid–base. In: Legrain M, ed. Continuous Ambulatory Peritoneal Dialysis. Amsterdam: Excerpta Medica, 1980, p. 194.

340. Rubin J, Adair C, Johnson B, Bower JD. Stereospecific lactate absorption during peritoneal dialysis. Nephron 1982; 31: 224.

341. Fine A. Metabolism of D-lactate in the dog and in man. Perit Dial Int 1989; 9: 99.

342. Chan L, Slater J, Hasbargen J, Herndon DN, Veech RL, Wolf S. Neurocardiac toxicity of racemic D,L-lactate fluids. Integr Physiol Behav Sci 1994; 29: 383.

343. Anderson YS, Curtis NJ, Hobbs AR et al. High serum D-lactate in patients on continuous ambulatory peritoneal dialysis. Nephrol Dial Transplant 1997; 12: 981.

344. Thurn JR, Pierpont GL, Ludvigsen CW, Eckfeldt JH. D-lactate encephalopathy. Am J Med 1985; 79: 717

345. Feriani M, Biasioli S, Borin D, La Greca G. Bicarbonate buffer for CAPD solution Trans ASAIO, 1985; 31: 668.

346. Feriani M, Ronco C, La Greca G. Acid–base balance with different CAPD solutions. Perit Dial Int 1996; 16 (Suppl. 1): S126.

347. Uribarri J, Buquing J, Oh MS. Acid–base balance in chronic peritoneal dialysis patients. Kidney Int 1995; 47: 269.

348. Veech RL. The untoward effects of the anions of dialysis fluid. Kidney Int 1988; 34: 587.

349. Nissenson AR. Acid–base homeostasis in peritoneal dialysis patients. Int J Artif Organs 1984; 7: 175.

350. Feriani M. Buffers: Bicarbonate, lactate and pyruvate. Kidney Int 1996; 50 (Suppl. 56): S75.

351. Gennari FJ, Cohen JJ, Kassirer JP. Normal acid–base values. In: Cohen JJ, Kassirer JP, eds. Acid/Base. Boston: Little, Brown, 1982, p. 107.

352. Yamamoto T, Sakakura T, Yamakawa M et al. Clinical effects of long-term use of neutralized dialysate for continuous ambulatory peritoneal dialysis. Nephron 1992; 60: 324.

353. Frohlich ED. Vascular effects of the Krebs intermediate metabolites. Am J Physiol 1965; 208: 149.

354. Kirkendol PL, Devia CJ, Bower JD et al. Comparison of the cardiovascular effects of sodium acetate, sodium bicarbonate and other potential sources of fixed base in hemodialysis solutions. Trans ASAIO 1977; 23: 399.

355. Veech RL. The toxic impact of parenteral solutions on the metabolism of cells: a hypothesis for physiological parenteral therapy. Am J Clin Nutr 1986; 44: 519.

356. Sistare FD, Haynes RC. The interaction between the cytosolic pyridine nucleotide redox potential and gluconeogenesis from lactate/pyruvate in isolated rat hepatocytes. J Biol Chem 1985; 23: 12748.

357. Oh MS, Phelpo KR, Traube M et al. D-lactic acidosis in a man with the short bowel syndrome. N Engl J Med 1979; 301: 249.

358. Veech RL, Fowler RC. Cerebral dysfunction and respiratory alkalosis during peritoneal dialysis with D-lactate containing dialysis fluid. Am J Med 1986; 82: 572.

359. Feriani M, La Greca G. CAPD with bicarbonate solution. In: Horl WH, Schollmeyer PJ, eds. New Perspectives in Hemodialysis, Peritoneal Dialysis, Arterovenous Hemofiltration and Plasmaferesis. New York: Plenum, 1989, p. 139.

360. Feriani M, Reinhard B, La Greca G. Calcium carbonate precipitation in oversated bicarbonate containing CAPD solutions. In: La Greca G, Ronco C, Feriani M, Chiaramonte S, Conz P, eds. Peritoneal Dialysis. Milan: Wichtig Editore, 1991, p. 145.

361. Gretz N, Kraft E, Meisinger E, Lasserre J, Strauch M. Calcium deposits due to bicarbonate containing CAPD solutions? In: Khanna R, Nolph KD, Prowant BF, Twardowski ZJ, Oreopoulos DG, eds. Advances in Peritoneal Dialysis. Toronto: Peritoneal Dialysis Bulletin Inc., 1988, p. 220.

362. Feriani M, Biasioli S, Barbacini S *et al*. Acid–base correction in bicarbonate CAPD patients. In: Khanna R, Nolph KD, Prowant BF, Twardowski ZJ, Oreopoulos DG, eds. Advances in Peritoneal Dialysis. Toronto: Peritoneal Dialysis Bulletin Inc., 1989, p. 191.

363. Feriani M, Passlick-Deetjen J, La Greca G. Factors affecting bicarbonate transfer with bicarbonate-containing CAPD solution. Perit Dial Int 1995; 15: 336.

364. Feriani M, Dissegna D, La Greca G, Passlick-Deetjen J. Short term clinical study with bicarbonate containing peritoneal dialysis solution. Perit Dial Int 1993; 13: 296.

365. Feriani M, Kirchgessner J, La Greca G, Passlick-Deetjen J, and the Bicarbonate CAPD Cooperative Group. A randomized multicenter long-term clinical study comparing a bicarbonate buffered CAPD solution with the standard lactate buffered CAPD solution. Kidney Int 1998; 54: 1731.

366. Feriani M, Carobi C, La Greca G, Buoncristiani U, Passlick-Deetjen J. Clinical experiences with a bicarbonate buffered (39 mmol/L) peritoneal dialysis solution. Perit Dial Int 11997; 7: 17.

367. Ryckelynck JP, Feriani M, Passlick-Deetjen J, Jaeckle-Meyer I. Pd patients' need for bicarbonate (Bic): 34 vs 39 mmol/L bic containing PD solutions. Nephrol Dial Transplant 1998; 13: A236 (abstract).

368. Yatzidis H. A new stable bicarbonate dialysis solution for peritoneal dialysis: preliminary report. Perit Dial Int 1991; 11: 224.

369. Slingeneyer A, Faller B, Michel C, Przbylski C, Rolland R, Mion C. Increased ultrafiltration capacity using a new bicarbonate CAPD solution. Perit Dial Int 1993; 13 (Suppl. 1): S57 (abstract).

370. Slingeneyer A, Przybylski C, Rolland R, Mion C. A new bicarbonate buffered solution for CAPD. Perit Dial Int 1993; 13 (Suppl. 1): S57.

371. Schambye HT, Flesner P, Pedersen RB *et al*. Bicarbonate versus lactate-based CAPD fluids: a biocompatibility study in rabbits. Perit Dial Int 1992; 12: 281.

372. Coles GA, Gokal R, Ogg C *et al*. A randomized controlled trial of a bicarbonate and a bicarbonate/lactate containing dialysis solution in CAPD. Perit Dial Int 1997; 17: 48.

373. Mactier RA, Sprosen TS, Gokal R *et al*. Bicarbonate and bicarbonate/lactate peritoneal dialysis solutions for the treatment of infusion pain. Kidney Int 1998; 53: 1061.

374. Tenckhoff H, Schechter H. A bacteriologically safe peritoneal access device. Trans Am Soc Artif Intern Organs 1968; 14: 181.

375. Popovich RP, Moncrief JW, Decherd JF, Bomar JB, Pyle WK. The definition of a novel portable–wearable equilibrium peritoneal dialysis technique. Am Soc Artif Intern Organs 1976; 5: 64 (abstract).

376. Popovich RP, Moncrief JW, Nolph KD, Ghods AJ, Twardowski IJ, Pyle WK. Continuous ambulatory peritoneal dialysis. Ann Intern Med 1978; 88: 449.

377. Buoncristiani U. Continuous ambulatory peritoneal dialysis: connection systems. Perit Dial Int 1993; 13 (Suppl. 2): S139

378. Buoncristiani U. Clinical results of long-term peritoneal dialysis. Proc EDTA 1975; 12: 145.

379. Buoncristiani U, Bianchi P, Cozzari M, Carobi C, Quintaliani G, Barbarossa D. A new safe simple connection system for CAPD. Int J Nephrol Urol Androl 1980; 1: 50.

380. Bazzato G, Coli U, Landini S, Lucatello S, Fracasso A, Moracchiello M. Continuous ambulatory peritoneal dialysis without wearing a bag: complete freedom of patient and significant reduction of peritonitis. Proc EDTA 1980; 17: 266.

381. Buoncristiani U, Cozzari M, Quintaliani G, Carobi C. Abatement of exogenous peritonitis risk using the Perugia CAPD system. Dial Transplant 1983; 12: 14.

382. Dasgupta MK, Lam K, Bettcher KB. Y-set, touch contamination, flush and hypochlorite treatment on the growth of biofilm in Tenckhoff catheter (TC) discs. Perit Dial Bull 1987; 7: S20.

383. Obst G, Gagnon RF, Prentis J. Sterilisation of *Staphylococcus epidermidis* biofilm by Ren New-Pand common disinfecting agents. Adv Perit Dial 1988; 4: 273.

384. Burkart JM. Comparison of peritonitis rates using standard spike versus Y sets in CAPD. Trans ASAIO 1988; 34: 433.

385. Luzar MA, Slingeneyer A, Cantaluppi A, Peluso F. *In vitro* study of the flush effect in two reusable continuous ambulatory peritoneal dialysis (CAPD) disconnect systems. Perit Dial Int 1989; 9: 169.

386. Ryckelynck J-Ph, Verger C, Cam G, Faller B, Pierre D. Importance of the flush effect in disconnect systems. Adv Perit Dial 1988; 4: 282.

387. Maiorca R, Cantaluppi A, Cancarini GC *et al*. Prospective controlled trial of a Y-connector and disinfectant to prevent peritonitis in continuous ambulatory peritoneal dialysis. Lancet 1983; 2: 642.

388. Scalamogna A, De Vecchi A, Castelnuovo C, Guerra L, Ponticelli C. Long-term incidence of peritonitis in CAPD patients treated by Y technique: experience in a single center. Nephron 1990; 55: 24.

389. Burkart JM, Hylander B, Durnell-Figel Th, Roberts D. Comparison of peritonitis rates during long-term use of standard spike versus Ultra-set in continuous ambulatory peritoneal dialysis (CAPD). Perit Dial Int 1990; 10: 41

390. Viglino G, Colombo A, Scalamogna A *et al*. Prospected randomized study of two Y devices in continuous ambulatory peritoneal dialysis (CAPD). Perit Dial Int 1989; 9: 165.

391. Canadian CAPD Clinical Trials Group. Peritonitis in continuous ambulatory peritoneal dialysis (CAPD): a multicentre randomized clinical trial comparing the Y connector disinfectant system to standard system. Perit Dial Int 1989; 9: 159.

392. Salahudeen AK, Cost R, Pingle A. Defects and demerits of the double-bag system. Perit Dial Bull 1987; 7: 106.

393. Bazzato G, Coli U, Landini S *et al*. Closter: a new connection for a double-bag system to prevent exogenous peritonitis. Perit Dial Bull 1986; 6: 138.

394. Bazzato G, Landini S, Fracasso A *et al*. Why the double-bag system still remains the best technique for peritoneal fluid exchanges in continuous ambulatory peritoneal dialysis? Perit Dial Int 1993; 13 (Suppl. 2): S152.

395. Tielens E, Nubé MJ, de Vet JA *et al*. Major reduction of CAPD peritonitis after the introduction of the twin-bag system. Nephrol Dial Transplant 1993; 8: 1237.

396. Viglino G, Colombo A, Cantu P *et al*. *In vitro* and *in vivo* efficacy of a new connector device for continuous ambulatory peritoneal dialysis. Perit Dial Int 1993; 13 (Suppl. 2): S148.

397. Junor BJR, Briggs JD, Forwell MA, Dobbie JW, Hendersen I. Sclerosing peritonitis. The contribution of chlorhexidine in alcohol. Perit Dial Bull 1985; 5: 101.

398. Mackow RC, Argy WP, Winchester JF *et al*. Sclerosing encapsulating peritonitis in rats induced by long-term intraperitoneal administration of antiseptics. J Lab Clin Med 1988; 112: 363

399. Lo W-K, Chan K-T, Leung ACT, Pang S-W, Tse C-Y. Sclerosing peritonitis complicating continuous ambulatory peritoneal dialysis with the use of chlorhexidine in alcohol. Adv Perit Dial 1990; 6: 79.

400. Verger C, Faller B, Ryckelynck J-Ph, Cam G, Pierre D. Efficacy of CAPD Y-line system without disinfectant and standard systems on peritonitis prevention: a multicenter prospective controlled trial. Perit Dial Int 1988; 8: 104.

401. Orange GV, Henderson IS, Marshall EA. Effectiveness of the flush technique in CAPD disconnect systems. Int J Artif Organs 1987 10: 185.

402. Verger C, Luzar M-A. *In vitro* study of CAPD Y-line systems. Adv Perit Dial 1986; 2: 160.

403. Junor BJR. CAPD disconnect systems. Blood Purif 1989; 7: 156.

404. Lempert KD, Kolb JA, Swartz RD *et al.* A multicenter trial to evaluate the use of the CAPD 'O' set. Trans ASAIO 1986; 32: 557.

405. Diaz-Buxo JA. Comparison of peritonitis rates with CCPD, manual CAPD, Y-set, O-set, UV devices and sterile weld. Adv Perit Dial 1989; 5: 223.

406. Swartz R, Reynolds J, Lees P, Rocher L. Disconnect during continuous ambulatory peritoneal dialysis (CAPD): retrospective experience with three different systems. Perit Dial Int 1989; 9: 175.

407. Owen JE, Walker RG, Lemon RG, Brett L, Mitrou D, Becker GJ. Randomized study of peritonitis with conventional versus O-set techniques in continuous ambulatory peritoneal dialysis. Perit Dial Int 1992; 12: 216.

408. Cheng IKP, Chan C-Y, Cheng S-W *et al.* A randomized prospective study of the cost-effectiveness of the conventional spike, O-set, UVXD techniques in continuous ambulatory peritoneal dialysis (CAPD). Perit Dial Int 1994; 14: 255.

409. Van Biesen W, Kirchgessner J, Schilling H, Lage C, Lambert MC, Passlick-Deetjen J. Stay-Safe: a new PVC-free system for peritoneal dialysis: result of the multi-center trial. Int J Artif Organs 1998; 21: 596 (abstract).

410. Steinhauer HB, Lubrich-Birkner I, Keck I, Schollmeyer P. Decreased rate of CAPD-associated peritonitis by using a heat-sterilisation system. Perit Dial Int 1989; 9 (Suppl. 1): S178.

411. Abdel-bary ES, Bartz V. CAPD-System Fresenius. In: La Greca G, Ronco C, Feriani M, Chiaramonte S, Conz P, eds. Peritoneal Dialysis. Milan: Wichtig Editore, 1988, p. 141.

412. Thomae U. Heat sterilization of Safe-Lock connectors using the Thermoclave. Contrib Nephrol 1987; 57: 172.

413. Steinhauer HB, Keck I, Lubrich-Birkner I, Schollmeyer P. Randomized clinical trial comparing a heat sterilization system (Thermoclav) to standard connector systems in prevention of CAPD-associated peritonitis. In: La Greca G, Ronco C, Feriani M, Chiaramonte S, Conz P, eds. Peritoneal Dialysis. Milan: Wichtig Editore, 1991, p. 275.

414. Popovich RP, Moncrief JW, Sorrels-Akar 'P'AJ, Mullins-Blackson C, Pyle WK. The ultraviolet germicidal system: the elimination of distal contamination in CAPD. In: Maher JF, Winchester JF, eds. Frontiers in Peritoneal Dialysis. New York: Field, Rich and Associates, 1986, p. 169.

415. Holmes CJ, Miyake C, Kubey W. *In-vitro* evaluation of an ultraviolet germicidal connection system for CAPD. Perit Dial Bull 1984; 4: 215.

416. Nolph KD, Prowant B, Serkes KD, Morgan LM and a Multicenter Study Group. A randomized multicenter clinical trial to evaluate the effects of an ultraviolet germicidal system on peritonitis rate in continuous ambulatory peritoneal dialysis. Perit Dial Bull 1985; 5: 19.

417. Jensen WM, Ahmad S. Evaluation of a germicidal device for peritoneal dialysis connectors. Perit Dial Bull 1984; 4: 219.

418. Kubey W, Holmes CJ. *In vitro* studies on the microbicidal effectiveness of a Xenon-based ultraviolet light device for continuous ambulatory peritoneal dialysis connections. Blood Purif 1991; 9: 102.

419. Bailic GR, Rasmussen R, Hollister A, Eisele G. Incidence of CAPD peritonitis in patients using UVXD or O-set systems. Clin Nephrol 1990; 33: 252.

420. Bielawa RJ, Carr KL, Bousquet GG. Intraluminal thermosterilization using a microwave autoclave. In: Maher J, Winchester JF, eds. Frontiers in Peritoneal Dialysis. New York: Field, Rich and Associates, 1986, p. 166.

421. Sharp J, Coulthard MG. A heat-sealing device to disconnect peritoneal dialysis lines. Perit Dial Int 1988; 8: 269.

9 | Peritoneal dialysis access and exit-site care including surgical aspects

Z. J. TWARDOWSKI AND W. K. NICHOLS

Introduction

One of the most important components of the peritoneal dialysis system is a permanent and trouble-free access to the peritoneal cavity. The double-cuff Tenckhoff catheter, developed in 1968 for treatment of patients with intermittent peritoneal dialysis [1], is also widely used for continuous ambulatory peritoneal dialysis (CAPD); however, CAPD increases catheter-related complications due to higher intra-abdominal pressure and numerous daily manipulations. These complications, such as catheter-tip migration, dialysate leaks, and exit site infections are frequently encountered and often related to improper insertion and postimplantation care. Catheter exit site and tunnel infections are frequent in CAPD patients, leading to morbidity, prolonged treatment, recurrent peritonitis and catheter failure. Recent improvement in peritonitis rates due to widespread use of the Y-set has shifted the focus of attention to peritoneal access [2–4]. According to the National CAPD Registry, the overall 3-year survival of the various peritoneal catheters was 13–36% in the 1981–87 period [5]. The results have markedly improved in recent years.

Historical perspective

In the early years of peritoneal dialysis the access was not specifically designed for the peritoneal dialysis; rather the available equipment used for other purposes was adapted. Ganter [6] used a metal trochar, Rosenak and Siwon [7] adjusted a glass cannula with multiple side-holes used for surgical drains. Desider Engel [8] from Prague used a glass catheter with a mushroom-like opening inside the peritoneum to maximize fluid distribution and prevent obstruction. Reid, Penfold and Jones [9] used a Foley catheter. Major problems in these years were leakage, infection and catheter occlusion by clot or

omental fat sucked into the catheter lumen. Fine, Frank and Seligman [10] created a subcutaneous tunnel to hamper periluminal bacterial migration into the peritoneal cavity. They adapted a stainless-steel sump drain for dialysate outflow and a rubber mushroom catheter for dialysis solution inflow. Although these innovations showed some improvement in infection rate and drainage, the overall results were not satisfactory and pericatheter leaks were frequent. Some unusual problems that we do not see these days were: rigidity of the tube with resulting pressure on viscera, suction of contaminated air into the peritoneal cavity, and difficulties of proper aseptic fixation of the tube to the abdominal wall.

Stephen Rosenak, a Hungarian physician, who became interested in continuous-flow peritoneal dialysis in his medical student years in the 1920s [7], while working with Oppenheimer at the Mount Sinai Hospital in New York, for the first time developed an access specifically for peritoneal dialysis [11]. Rosenak and Oppenheimer access consisted of a stainless-steel flexible coil attached to a rubber drain. The outer portion of the steel tube was attached to an adjustable tie plate for fixation and prevention of leakage. The access was suitable for continuous-flow dialysis with inflow through the outer tube and outflow through the inner tube. This device did not gain popularity because the major problems were not solved: the rigid tube irritated viscera, dialysate leakage and peritoneal contamination were not eliminated.

A major advance was the introduction of less rigid materials by French physicians. Derot et al. [12] and Marcel Legrain, while working with John Merril [13] in New York, used polyvinyl tube for peritoneal dialysis in acute renal failure. The next major progress was made in late 1950s when Maxwell, Rockney, Kleeman and Twiss [14], from the University of California in Los Angeles, introduced a nylon catheter with multiple tiny distal perforations.

R. Gokal, R. Khanna, R.Th. Krediet and K.D. Nolph (eds.), Textbook of Peritoneal Dialysis, 2nd Edition, 307–361.

The small diameter of perforations prevented the omentum from entering the catheter. At the same time, Doolan and co-workers [15] developed a polyvinyl catheter with multiple ridges to prevent omental wrapping. Both catheters were inserted into the peritoneal cavity with the help of a paracentesis trochar. Smooth, plastic materials were much less irritating to the peritoneum than previously used glass, rubber or steel, thereby omental occlusion became less frequent. The drainage of fluid from the peritoneal cavity was markedly improved, but leakage and pericatheter infections continued to plague the access.

In the early 1960s, Dr Belding Scribner from Seattle invited Dr Boen from the Netherlands to continue his peritoneal dialysis research. With limited capacity for haemodialysis, Scribner expected that peritoneal dialysis would be a good alternative for treating a larger number of patients. Boen implanted a Teflon button in the abdominal wall. Through this button a long catheter was inserted into the peritoneal cavity. After each dialysis the catheter was removed and the button was capped; thus, periodic peritoneal dialysis for chronic renal failure was introduced [16]. Because the method was plagued by frequent peritonitis episodes, Boen *et al.* in 1963 developed the repeated-puncture method [17]. The available catheters which were semirigid and poorly secured with short pericatheter path were not suitable for permanent implantation. For each dialysis a new catheter had to be inserted. The insertion procedure required penetration of the abdominal wall with a paracentesis trochar. The resulting abdominal opening was of greater diameter than the catheter, and pericatheter leaks were frequent.

To circumvent the dialysate leakage problem, Weston and Roberts [18] invented a stylet catheter, which was inserted without a trochar. A sharp stainless-steel stylet inserted through the catheter was used to penetrate the abdominal wall. As a result the abdominal opening fitted snugly around the catheter, thereby preventing leakage. This type of catheter is still being used for acute renal failure.

In another approach to facilitate repeated puncture, Mallette and co-workers [19] implanted a subcutaneous button. Only skin and subcutaneous tissue had to be penetrated for each catheter insertion. Jacob and Deane [20] used a Teflon rod to replace the catheter between dialyses. No puncture was necessary. To decrease the possibility of leakage around the catheter, Barry, Shambaugh and Goler [21] revived the Rosenak and Oppenheimer idea for providing an external seal. They used a Plexiglas

disc and polyvinyl balloon instead of metal plate for the transabdominal cannula. A polyvinyl catheter was inserted through the cannula for each dialysis. The necessity of repeated punctures or catheter insertion through a permanent opening was impractical, and did not gain popularity, especially for home peritoneal dialysis. These catheters were also plagued with infections, dialysate leaks, and obstructions.

A major step forward in creating a permanent peritoneal access was made in 1964. Gutch [22] noticed less irritation of the peritoneum and lower protein losses with silicon rubber catheters as compared to those with polyvinyl ones. About the same time, Russel Palmer, a physician at the Canadian Army Medical Corps, was developing a peritoneal access made of polyethylene, polypropylene, and nylon [23]. These catheters were relatively rigid, and not any better than the others available at that time. Palmer was looking for softer, and more biocompatible material. With the help of Wayne Quinton, a successful manufacturer of silicon rubber shunts for haemodialysis, Palmer developed a catheter which is a prototype of the currently used coiled catheters [24]. The catheter was made of silicon rubber, had a coiled intraperitoneal end, and had numerous perforations extending 23 cm from the tip. A long subcutaneous tunnel on insertion was supposed to hinder periluminal infection. To impede further infection and leakage, a tri-flanged step was created for securing the catheter in the deep abdominal fascia.

In 1965 Henry Tenckhoff, at the University of Washington, was beginning to treat patients on chronic peritoneal dialysis [25]. After an initial few dialyses in the hospital the patients would be trained for home dialysis. At the weekends Tenckhoff would go to a patient's home, insert the catheter and begin dialysis. After the appropriate time on dialysis the patient would remove the catheter and cover the exit wound with a dressing. Although the method was successful in Tenckhoff's hands, the technique was cumbersome, and Tenckhoff recognized its limitations. He was thinking of a more practical solution.

In 1968 McDonald and co-workers [26] developed an external seal composed of polyester (Dacron®) sleeve and polytetrafluoroethylene (Teflon®) skirt. Tissue ingrowth into these elements created a firm external seal to prevent leakage and microorganism migration. No subcutaneous tunnel was created, and the catheter was inserted straight through the abdominal wall.

In the same year Tenckhoff and Schechter published the results of their studies on a new catheter [1]. Their catheter was an improved version of the Palmer catheter. The intra-abdominal flange was replaced by a Dacron® cuff, the subcutaneous tunnel was shortened and a second, external cuff was used to decrease the length of the catheter sinus tract. Ultimately, the coiled intraperitoneal portion was replaced by a straight segment resembling the Gutch catheter. Intraperitoneal segment was kept open-ended and the size of the side holes was optimized to 0.5 mm to prevent tissue suction. A shorter subcutaneous tunnel and straight intraperitoneal segment facilitated catheter implantation at the bedside with the aid of a specially designed trochar (Fig. 1). To avoid excessive bleeding and easy penetration the catheter was inserted through the midline. The Tenckhoff catheter became the gold standard of peritoneal access. Few complications were reported in patients treated by periodic peritoneal dialysis. Even today, more than 30 years later, the Tenckhoff catheter in its original form is the most widely used catheter type. Some of the original recommendations for catheter insertion, such as an arcuate subcutaneous tunnel with downward directions of both intraperitoneal and external exits, are still considered very important elements of catheter implantation.

To prevent exit infection a subcutaneous catheter was developed by the Utah group [27]. The catheter had two tubes in the peritoneal cavity, and a subcutaneous container. The container was to be punctured for each dialysis. Another subcutaneous catheter was developed by Gotloib et al. [28]. Yet another approach to reduce exit site infection rates was to position the subcutaneous cuff at the skin level [29]. Contrary to expectation, such a position increased infection rates [30]. To decrease catheter migration and omental wrapping the intraperitoneal segment of the catheter was provided with a saline inflatable balloon [31] or discs [32]. Valli et al. [33, 34] revived the idea of Goldberg et al. [31] and made a silicone rubber catheter with a balloon-shaped intraperitoneal segment surrounding the catheter tip. Ash et al. [35] replaced the intraperitoneal tubing with a disc located immediately beneath the abdominal wall. Such a catheter cannot migrate but still could be obstructed by clot, bowel or omentum.

Several new or improved catheters have been developed in recent years. Twardowski et al. [36] designed silicone rubber 'swan-neck' catheters that are permanently bent between two cuffs. These catheters may be implanted in an arcuate tunnel with their shape undistorted. A similar principle was applied by Cruz to polyurethane catheters [37]. In 1992, Twardowski et al. [38] described a new catheter that had an exit site on the chest instead of the abdomen. Ash and Janle [39] developed a T-fluted catheter to decrease the rates of outflow obstruction due to omental wrapping. The catheter is composed of a transabdominal tube connecting in a T-shape to a transverse cylinder resting against the parietal peritoneum. Instead of tubing with holes, the intraperitoneal part is provided with eight longitudinal flutes or grooves as fluid conduits. Initial results in dogs and five patients were encouraging. Moncrief et al. [40] described a modified swan-neck catheter with an elongated external cuff. They also substantially changed the technique of catheter insertion by keeping the external part under the skin until the ingrowth of the tissue into the cuff is strong. Only after several weeks (3–6 or more) is the external part exteriorized (see below).

Recently Di Paolo et al. [41] described a self-locating peritoneal catheter, which is a modified Tenckhoff catheter provided with a small 12 g tungsten cylinder incorporated into the silicone rubber at the tip. The role of this weight is to prevent catheter migration out of the true pelvis. The results with 32 self-locating catheters were not different compared to Tenckhoff catheters implanted in the same period, except that none of them dislocated out of the true pelvis, whereas dislocations were significantly ($p = 0.0003$) more frequent in control catheters.

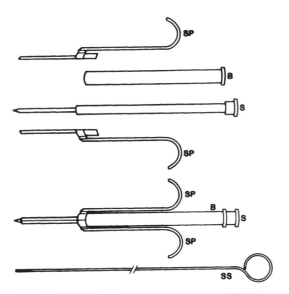

Figure 1. Tenckhoff trochar – assembled (above) and disassesmbled (below). SP, side pieces; S, pointed stylet; B, barrel; SS, stiffening stilette.

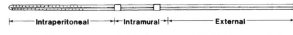

Figure 2. Diagram of double-cuff Tenckhoff catheter showing three segments created after implantation.

Table 1. Catheter-related common complications

Exit/tunnel infection	Pericatheter leak
External cuff extrusion	Peritonitis
Catheter obstruction	Infusion or pressure pain

This chapter will describe in detail some of those catheters which are in current use, their insertion technique, postimplantation care, and long-term results. New, emerging techniques will be briefly reviewed.

Glossary

There are numerous catheter designs and implantation techniques. To avoid confusion I will briefly review terminology pertinent to the currently used peritoneal catheters [42]. After implantation the typical double-cuff Tenckhoff catheter has three segments (Fig. 2): **intraperitoneal**, located intraperitoneally; **intramural**, contained within the abdominal wall tunnel; and **external**, situated outside of the skin exit. The **peritoneal catheter tunnel** is the passageway through the abdominal wall within which the peritoneal catheter is contained. Figure 3 depicts tissue structures in relation to cuff position in healed tunnels. Simple anchorless catheters create peritoneal fistulas and predispose to fluid leaks and peritoneal infections. Such catheters were abandoned after introduction of Tenckhoff catheters in 1968. Tenckhoff catheters consist of a body or tubing and two cuffs which are bands of fabric affixed to the tubing for fibrous tissue ingrowth. After implantation of a single, deep cuff catheter the tunnel is composed of three parts: (1) a sinus tract located between the skin exit and the cuff; (2) a peritoneal tunnel recess,

which is a peritoneal pocket covered with the mesothelium from the internal tunnel exit to the collagen–mesothelial interface at the cuff; and (3) a tunnel proper, comprising the tissue ingrown into the cuff. Another type of single-cuff catheter is provided only with a superficial cuff, has a short sinus tract, but a long peritoneal recess. A properly implanted double-cuff peritoneal catheter, designed by Tenckhoff for treatment of chronic renal failure, creates a tunnel with a short sinus tract, a shallow peritoneal recess, and a 5–7 cm long tunnel proper, which consists of tissue ingrown into the cuffs and a fibrous sheath covering the intercuff tunnel segment. A longer tunnel proper (20–50 cm) is typical for the presternal catheter [38].

Factors influencing catheter complications

The common complications of peritoneal dialysis catheters include (Table 1): exit/tunnel infection, external cuff extrusion, obstruction, which is usually a sequela of catheter-tip migration out of the true pelvis with subsequent omental wrapping or tip entrapment in peritoneal adhesions; dialysate leaks; peritonitis; and infusion or pressure pain. This section of the chapter will describe factors that influence these complications. A video illustrating these factors is available [43].

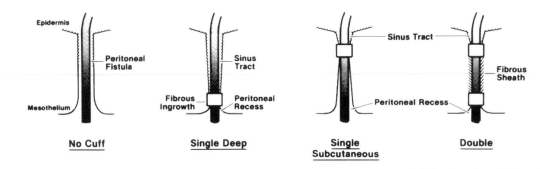

Figure 3. Tissue structures in relation to cuff position in healed tunnels. In catheters without cuffs a peritoneal fistula is formed. A single deep cuff creates a shallow peritoneal recess and a deep sinus tract predisposing to exit infection. A single subcutaneous cuff generates a shallow sinus tract and a deep peritoneal recess predisposing to pseudoherniae. Properly positioned two cuffs limit the depth of both structures. (Reproduced from ref. 57 with permission.)

Tissue reaction to a foreign body penetrating skin

The tissue reaction begins immediately after a break in the integument occurs. Bleeding from capillaries and body fluids forms a coagulum of a hydrophilic fibrin–fibronectin gel and cellular debris. Various cytokines coordinate the subsequent entry of inflammatory cells and fibroblasts and the formation of new blood vessels [44]. Polymorphonuclear neutrophil leukocytes phagocytose local bacteria and, together with the coagulum, form a scab. The polyester cuff is also filled with clotted blood. Gradually neutrophils, macrophages, fibroblasts, and new capillaries penetrate between the polyester fibres. Macrophages coalesce into giant cells which completely or partially surround the polyester fibres. Fibroblasts produce collagen fibres which intertwine with the polyester fibres. The formation of the strong fibrous tissue is completed after approximately 6 weeks. Healing of the sinus starts beneath the scab with the production of granulation tissue composed of new vessels and fibroblasts. A mature granulation tissue is formed when neutrophils are replaced with mononuclear leukocytes, and fibroblasts lay down collagen fibres. Upon this tissue there is a peripheral ingrowth of new epidermal cells.

Epidermal cells spread over the granulation tissue beneath the scab. Based on animal experiments it has been widely accepted that epithelial cells spread over granulation tissue until they meet epithelial cells from the opposite 'shore' or until they encounter dense collagen fibres [45–53]. Winter [53] postulated that, in naturally occurring percutaneous organs such as teeth, the inhibition of epithelial migration is achieved by a periodontal membrane which consists of bundles of collagen fibres embedded in the cementum of the tooth. In his view other situations in which epidermal cell migration is inhibited include macroporous implants and skin autografts. Finally, he theorized that the basement membrane, a collagenous structure, also inhibits basal cell invasion of the dermis.

The hypothesis that collagen fibres play a paramount role in inhibiting epithelial cell spreading [43] led to the development of several devices of porous material to encourage dermal ingrowth and to prevent epithelialization of the tunnel ('marsupialization') [29, 48, 49, 54]. It has been suggested that the epithelium adjacent to a silicone catheter tends to migrate towards and beyond the subcutaneous cuff, creating a sinus between the tubing and the skin that is prone to bacterial colonization with subsequent infection [45].

The development of an epithelialized tract is well supported in animal models [29, 48, 50] and in our previous reviews we cited these data as relevant in human peritoneal catheter sinus tracts [55–57]. However, our observations of catheter tunnels removed from patients showed that in almost all human peritoneal catheter tunnels the epithelium does not reach to the cuff, but stops a few millimetres from the exit in the sinus tract [58]. These observations lead us to believe that granulation tissue *per se* can also inhibit epidermal cell spreading. This observation also has an important influence on catheter design and implantation, particularly the material for the superficial cuff and its distance from the exit.

In humans, unlike experimental animals, the spreading of epidermis is slow. This discrepancy should not be surprising because the epidermal turnover rate in such animals is about six to seven times faster than in humans [59]. We found that in fast-healing catheter exits in humans the epidermis starts entering into the sinus after 2–3 weeks; in slow-healing exits the epidermis starts entering into the sinus after 4–6 weeks [60]. The healing process is complete after about 4–8 weeks, when the epidermis covers approximately half of a visible sinus tract with the remaining half covered with granulation tissue [60].

Tunnel morphology after healing process is completed

A detailed description of peritoneal catheter tunnel morphology has been published elsewhere [58]. A well-healed tunnel of a double-cuff swan-neck Missouri catheter removed electively (Fig. 4) showed four segments: tissue ingrown to the flange and internal cuff, tissue surrounding the intercuff segment, tissue ingrown into the external cuff and the sinus tract. The most external part (0.5–1 cm) of the sinus tract and the skin surrounding the skin exit of the tunnel constitute the exit site. In the majority of humans the epidermal cells penetrate only a few millimetres from the skin exit and may reach the cuff located less than 15 mm from the exit [58, 61]. Although unusual, a single instance of keratinized epithelium penetration all the way to the cuff located 45 mm from the exit has been reported [62]. Close to the exit the surface of the sinus tract is covered with wrinkled epidermis, containing all layers of epidermis including a horny layer. Deeper in the sinus, the epidermis loses the horny layer and becomes similar to the mucosal epithelium, hence the surface becomes glistening and white. The rest

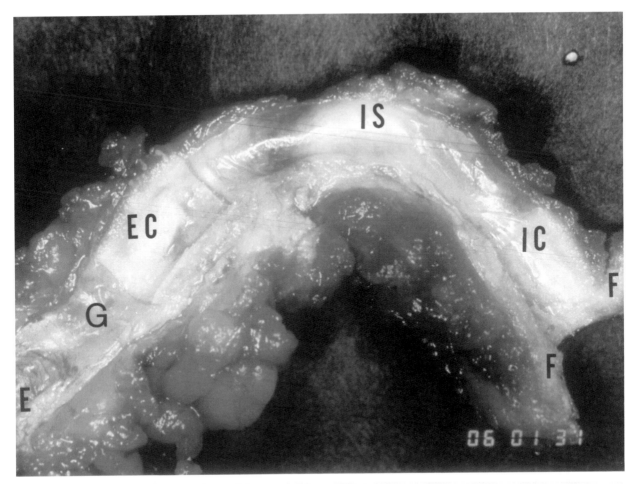

Figure 4. A well-healed tunnel of a double-cuff swan neck Missouri catheter removed electively. From the left: E, epithelium; G, granulation tissue; EC, external cuff; IS, intercuff segment; IC, internal cuff; F, flange.

of the sinus tract is covered with the granulation tissue that is yellowish in appearance. A thick layer of collagen fibres surrounds the sinus. The granulation tissue contains numerous multinucleated giant cells, capillaries, cellular infiltrate composed mostly of mononuclear cells, and scant collagen fibres. The collagen fibres do not attach to the smooth surface of the silicone rubber, the material from which most peritoneal dialysis catheters are made.

The junction between the granulation tissue in the sinus and the cuff is well defined. The cuff is surrounded by a dense fibrous capsule that contains numerous capillaries. About 80% of the polyester fibres are surrounded completely or partially by multinucleated giant cells. Spaces between the polyester fibres are filled with mature collagen and fibroblasts. No neutrophils are seen in an uninfected cuff.

The junction between the cuff and the intercuff segment shows a smooth surface without granulation tissue. The glistening, shiny intercuff tunnel segment resembles a tendon sheath and contains numerous micropits. The absence of any cellular reaction indicates that bacteria do not reach to this part of the tunnel. The surface is covered with an amorphous, mucinous substance on top of a modified layer of fibroblasts forming pseudo-synovium. There are no giant cells in this segment because silicone rubber *per se* does not induce giant cell formation.

The transition between the intercuff segment and the deep cuff is abrupt due to change from an avascular, acellular, fibrous sheath to a highly vascular and cellular tissue ingrown into the cuff. If the deep cuff is implanted into the muscle, the fibrous capsule surrounding the cuff and the cuff tissue itself are highly vascularized, otherwise the tissue ingrown into the cuff is similar to that of the external cuff.

Factors influencing healing and early infection

The most important factors influencing healing process and early infections are (Table 2): tissue perfusion; mechanical factors; sinus bacterial colonization; epithelialization; local cleansing agents; exit direction; and systemic factors.

Tissue perfusion

The coagulum and necrotic tissue are gradually removed from the tunnel. Part of the necrotic tissue is absorbed and part is drained out of the tunnel. The tunnel should not be too tight with reference to catheter circumference, so as to allow free drainage of necrotic tissue and to prevent tissue oedema; both these factors decrease local perfusion and oxygen tension [63], which are critical for the wound-healing process. On the other hand too large an incision prolongs healing by the shear volume of repair needed, and the movement of loose tubing in the tunnel.

Mechanical factors

Mechanical stress slows the healing process [45]; thus the catheter should be relatively tightly anchored in the tunnel and also well immobilized outside the tunnel, especially during the break-in period. Frequent dressing changes involve catheter manipulation, and hence should be avoided during the healing period. Constricting sutures at the exit site can also cause pressure necrosis with skin sloughing, and facilitate bacterial penetration into the tissue [64]; they must not be used.

Microorganisms

The presence of microorganisms in the wound is the major cause of impaired healing [65, 66]. The humoral tissue reaction to the foreign implants is to coat them with various proteins, such as fibronectin, laminin, fibrin, collagen, and immunoglobulins. Some of these substances serve as receptors for colonizing microorganisms. A receptor site for binding *Staphylococcus aureus* has been identified within the 27-kDa aminoterminal fragment of fibronectin [67].

Table 2. Factors influencing healing process and infection

Tissue perfusion	Cleansing agents
Mechanical factors	Exit direction
Microorganisms	Systemic factors
Epithelialization	

Staphylococcus aureus was found to have several receptor sites for soluble and solid-phase fibronectin [68, 69]. *Staphylococcus epidermidis* binding to fibronectin seems to be less extensive than with *Staphylococcus aureus* [70]. Similar receptors to laminin were found in *Staphylococcus aureus* but not in *Staphylococcus epidermidis* [71]. Type IV collagen, vitronectin (S protein), and fibrin may also participate in bacterial adherence, but their role in foreign-body colonization has not been clarified [72, 73].

Bacteria themselves, even without participation of specific protein receptors, may adhere to a foreign body by electrostatic attachment or by London–van der Waal's forces [74]. Adhered bacteria synthesize and excrete a variety of complex polysaccharides (biofilm) which serve to protect them from host mechanisms [75,76]. It is not surprising that almost all peritoneal catheter exits and sinus tracts, even without signs of infection, are colonized by bacteria [77].

Maintaining sterility of the exit and sinus in the initial healing period is of utmost importance. Antibiotic penetration into the coagulum is poor; therefore antibiotics should be present in sufficient concentration in blood and tissue fluids before the coagulum is formed. This may be achieved if antibiotics are given prior to implantation.

These theoretical considerations are supported by recent evidence showing that prophylactic antibiotics given prior to implantation prevent subsequent catheter infections, peritonitis, and wound sepsis [78, 79]; however, the advantage of antibiotics is not universally reported [80].

Epithelialization

Epidermal cells grow over the granulation tissue beneath the scab. If the scab is forcibly removed during cleansing, the epidermal layer is broken, thus prolonging the process of epidermization. Sinus epithelialization is supported by sterile and undisturbed conditions at the exit. Again, frequent dressing changes facilitate exit contamination; on the other hand, liquid serous or sanguineous exudate at the exit promotes bacterial growth. Therefore, the exit should be kept dry, but dressing changes should not be too frequent.

Cleansing agents

Cleansing agents should not only decrease the number of bacteria, but also be harmless to the body defences. Strong oxidants such as povidone-iodine and hydrogen peroxide are cytotoxic to mammalian cells and should not be used [81,82]. If these are used, care should be taken to use them only on the intact skin surrounding the wound or granulation tissue [83]. Non-ionic, amphophilic, non-toxic surfactants, widely used in burn wound care, facilitate necrotic tissue removal without jeopardizing body defence mechanisms [84]. In agreement with the experience of others [85] we found 20% Poloxamer 188 (Shur-Clens®; Calgon Vestal Laboratories, St Louis, MO, USA) to be innocuous, yet excellent in cleansing the exit from contaminants.

Exit direction

Exit direction is also important. Immediate post-implantation drainage of necrotic tissue is facilitated by gravity when the exit is directed downwards.

Systemic factors

During the healing process part of the granulation tissue is gradually resorbed and replaced by fibrous tissue. The fibrous tissue and part of the granulation tissue is covered with the epidermis [58]. Impaired nutrition, diabetes mellitus, uraemia, and corticosteroids are all known factors decreasing wound healing by impeding the process of fibrosis [86]. It is prudent to avoid permanent catheter implantation while the patient is severely uraemic, malnourished or taking glucocorticoids. In Asia, asiatic acid, an extract of *Centella asiatica*, has been used for the treatment of skin wounds. The active ingredient of this extract (which also has mineralocorticoid properties) increases both collagen synthesis in cultured fibroblasts of human skin and tensile strength of skin wounds [87, 88]. Mineralocorticoids may also promote wound healing by promoting fibrosis, though controlled studies on wound healing acceleration in humans have not yet been performed.

Factors influencing infection of healed catheter tunnel

Design of the catheter and its location in the created tunnel influences exit and/or tunnel infection. Other factors which may influence infection rate include (Table 3): bacterial colonization of the sinus; *Staphylococcus aureus* nasal carriage status; catheter skin-exit direction; sinus tract length; number off cuffs; and materials for the external cuff and the tubing in the sinus.

Table 3. Factors influencing infection of healed catheter tunnel

Bacterial colonization of the sinus
Staphylococcus aureus nasal carriage
Catheter skin-exit direction
Sinus tract length
Number of cuffs
External cuff material and tubing in the sinus

Bacterial colonization of the sinus

Almost all healed catheter sinuses are colonized by bacteria [77]. It has been well documented in the surgical literature that wound infection is the result of imbalance between the host defence and bacteria [66]. The number of bacteria as a critical factor in wound infection was already recognized in World War I [65]. Elek [64] demonstrated that it requires 7.5×10^6 staphylococcal organisms to produce a pustule in normal human skin but the number of bacteria necessary to cause infection was reduced 10,000-fold in the presence of a single suture. Bacterial virulence is also important; *Staphylococcus aureus* or *Pseudomonas aeruginosa* are more likely to induce an inflammatory response than is *Staphylococcus epidermidis*.

It appears that there is a constant interaction between the colonizing bacteria and the body defence mechanisms at the sinus tract. The part of the sinus tract covered with epidermis seems to respond to bacteria in the same way as the rest of the body integument but the part covered with granulation tissue appears to respond by constant exudation of serum with white blood cells to suppress bacterial proliferation and curb their penetration deeper into the sinus. If the number of bacteria increases then the amount of exudate increases, granulation tissue proliferates and becomes more vascularized. The number of bacteria entering deeper into the sinus depends on the number and species of bacteria at the exit site, exit direction, as well as sinus tract length, the latter an important contributing factor in the amplitude of catheter movement in the sinus. Optimum defence mechanisms, after the sinus is healed, are observed best in undamaged epidermis and granulation tissue; trauma to these structures may tilt the balance in favour of microorganisms and allow their rapid multiplication.

Staphylococcus aureus *nasal carriage*

The importance of *Staphylococcus aureus* as an aetiological agent of peritoneal catheter exit-site infection has been well established [89, 90]. Nasal carriage of *S. aureus* is reported to be common in patients undergoing haemodialysis [91], and peritoneal dialysis [92, 93]. A recent multicentre study found an increased incidence of exit-site infections in nasal carriers of *S. aureus*; in 85% of these infections the strain from the nares and the strain causing the infection were similar in phage type and antibiotic profile [94]. However, in our study we found that, by antibiotic profile, the strain cultured from exit and the strain cultured from nares were identical only in 21–36% [95]. If cultures were taken from the sinus tract and the periexit skin, the results were congruent in about 50% [95]. Judging by our study there is an increased probability of *S. aureus* exit infection in patients who carry *S. aureus* in nares, but the strain is not the same. In the study of Boelaert *et al.* [96] 15 of 20 haemodialysis patients who carried *S. aureus* in their nares also carried the organism on their hands, but only two of 20 patients who did not carry *S. aureus* in their nares carried *S. aureus* on their hands ($p < 0.001$). Eighty-seven per cent of patients who carried *S. aureus* in their nares and on their hands carried the same strain at both sites. Thus, it is likely that bacteria are carried from the nares to the vicinity of the catheter exit on hands. A large study in 1144 patients receiving continuous ambulatory peritoneal dialysis in nine European centres found *S. aureus* nasal carriage in 267 subjects [97]. The carriers were randomly allocated to treatment or control groups. Members of each group used a nasal ointment twice daily for 5 consecutive days every 4 weeks. The treatment group used calcium mupirocin 2% (Bactroban nasal; Smith Kline Beecham, Welwyn Garden City, United Kingdom) and the control group used placebo ointment. Patients were followed up for a maximum period of 18 months. Nasal carriage fell to 10% in those subjects who received active treatment and 48% in those who used the placebo ointment. Exit infections due to *S. aureus* significantly decreased in the mupirocin group but there were no differences in the rate of tunnel infection or peritonitis and exit infections due to other organisms. There was no evidence of a progressive increase in resistance to mupirocin with time; however, a progressive increase in resistance to mupirocin from 2.7% in 1990 to 65% in 1993 was found in a large teaching hospital, where intranasal mupirocin was used as an adjunct to infection control measures for methicillin-resistant *S. aureus* infections [98].

Catheter skin-exit direction

Tenckhoff's original recommendation of a downward-pointing exit [1] received support in our retrospective analysis which found that, compared to upward-directed exits, the exits directed downwards tended to be infected less frequently and, once infected, were significantly less resistant to treatment [36]. More recent studies in paediatric [99] and adult [100] populations found significantly lower infection rates in patients with catheter exits directed downwards. This should not be surprising since upward-directed tunnels facilitate exit contamination by gravity-aided flow of sweat, water, and dirt (Fig. 5). Once the exit is infected it is resistant to treatment because of poor external drainage; rather the pus tends to penetrate deeper into the tunnel. Also, downward drainage of necrotic tissue immediately postimplantation is easier than drainage against gravity.

The advantage of caudal exit direction in preventing and treating infections has support in several other clinical conditions. Periodontitis, which may be considered as a naturally occurring 'foreign' body exit site infection, most frequently effects the lower incisors ('exits' directed upwards) [101]. The influence of exit position on the frequency and tenacity of paranasal sinus infections was postulated by Zuckerkandl in the nineteenth century. The relatively frequent infections of the maxillary sinus are believed to be due to unfavourable positions for discharge because the *ostium maxillare* (in the upright position of the body) is located at the highest point of the cavity; the cavity must be completely filled with secretions before the discharge may escape [102]. All of the other cavities are more favourably constructed for drainage and less likely to be infected [102]. Exit infections of long-term jugular and/or subclavian catheters are less frequent than those of peritoneal catheters. Using catheters with downward-directed tunnels, So *et al.* [103] reported one exit infection per 998 catheter days, and Raaf [104] reported 16 exit-site infections with 698 catheters in cancer patients.

Sinus tract length

The epidermis covering the sinus tract undergoes a turnover probably similar to the normal epidermis with cell maturation and desquamation; granulation tissue produces exudate. All these contents, if not expelled, create a favourable milieu for bacterial growth. With a long sinus tract the chances of infection are higher [45–47]; therefore the sinus tract

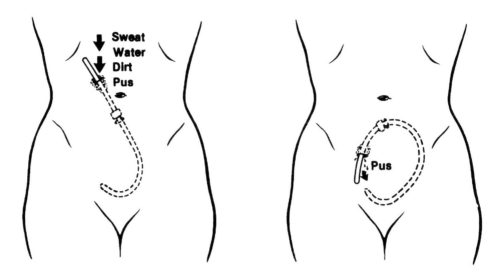

Figure 5. *Left*: Exit easily contaminated with down-flowing sweat, water, and dirt; difficult pus drainage prolongs treatment. *Right*: Good pus drainage facilitates recovery. (Reproduced from ref. 36 with permission.)

should be as short as possible. Tenckhoff recommended that 'the subcutaneous Dacron® felt cuff should be located immediately beneath the skin exit' [105]. Such a localization of the cuff, however, predisposes to its extrusion. Indeed, in some centres the rate of extrusion reached 100% [106]. In other centres the rate, although lower, was high enough to question the wisdom of using the superficial cuff at all. The most recent recommendation is to place the subcutaneous cuff at least 2 cm from the exit site [107].

Number of cuffs

Single (only external) cuff catheters were used by Tenckhoff for treatment of acute renal failure. This type of catheter used in patients undergoing chronic intermittent peritoneal dialysis yielded similar results to those of the double-cuff catheter; however, with continuous ambulatory peritoneal dialysis, double-cuff catheter survival was better than of single-cuff catheters [108]. The complication of a single-cuff catheters was the development of pseudohernias due to high intra-abdominal pressure with constant presence of fluid in the peritoneal cavity.

Another type of single-cuff catheter has only a deep cuff. This type of catheter has been used because of problems with external cuff extrusion and the questionable value of the external cuff. Exit-site infections were found to be similar with single- and double-cuff catheters in some reports [109]; however, in a retrospective survey of catheter results in 395 patients, tunnel infections were almost 3 times

more frequent with single-cuff than with double-cuffs [106]. In our institution we found that exit infections tended to be more frequent and were significantly more resistant to treatment with single-cuff catheters compared to double-cuff ones [36]. Several recently published results on large patient populations revealed an increased risk of peritonitis with single-cuff as compared to double-cuff catheters [99, 110, 111]. In addition, the single-cuff catheter has more exit-site infections and shorter survival times than the double-cuff catheter [112, 113]. It seems that the controversy regarding the number of cuffs is resolved: convincing data exist to indicate that the double-cuff catheter is preferable for chronic peritoneal dialysis [107].

Material for the external cuff and tubing in the sinus

It has been postulated that the external cuff should provide a strong attachment of collagen fibres to limit the epidermal cell spreading [46]. As an example of perfect arrangement the anatomy of the tooth/gingival interface was cited [49]. The periodontal ligament attaches to the cementum, creating an extremely strong bond. The cementum is composed of hydroxyapatite crystals, collagen fibres, proteoglycans and mucopolysaccharides [114]. Such a living material is unlikely to be used for the external cuff.

Dasse *et al.* [49] and Poirier *et al.* [54] evaluated collagen attachment to various materials on their elaborate external seal for the percutaneous energy transmission systems. The seal is composed of a semirigid polyurethane skirt positioned at the sub-dermal level and a hollow collar protruding through the skin. The polyurethane is covered with sintered titanium spheres, porous polytetrafluoroethylene, and Dacron® velour. In experiments on miniature pigs the Dacron® velour, especially wetted with saline before implantation, provided the strongest collagen attachment with an excellent inhibition of epidermal downgrowth. Preliminary experience with this device in CAPD patients was encouraging [49]; however, long-term experience has not yet been published. Others have had very poor results and had to remove all catheters due to exit/tunnel infection (Oreopoulos DG, personal communication).

Favourable experience gained with alumina ceramic in orthopaedic surgery, otorhinolaryngology, and dentistry inspired Amano et al. [115] to use alumina ceramic for a peritoneal catheter. In this catheter the part of the silicone tubing designated to be contained within the sinus tract is replaced by a rigid alumina ceramic connector. Dog experiments with this material revealed only minimal skin downgrowth. Preliminary human experience was encouraging [115], but no long-term results have yet been published

Ogden et al. [30] and Boss et al. [116] found a very high rate of chronic exit-site infections with Right Angle Gore-Tex® catheters. These catheters were provided with a subcutaneous flange covered with expanded polytetrafluoroethylene and a cuff of the same material. Ten of 17 catheters developed chronic exit-site infection and seven of them had to be removed when antibiotics failed to eradicate infections [30].

As mentioned previously, the tissue ingrown into the cuff per se does not seem to constitute a critical barrier for infection spreading [58]. It seems that the basic beneficial role of the external cuff in infection prevention is by anchoring of the catheter resulting in restriction of its piston-like movements, thus decreasing transport of bacteria into the sinus. Favourable results with a 'wing' instead of cuff appear to give clinical support to this hypothesis [117]. This 'wing', however, does not seem to anchor the catheter as well as the cuff. More supportive data are needed to accept a substitute for polyester fabric (Dacron® velour) as a material for the external cuff.

Consistently poor results with cuffs implanted very close to the exit and the results of our study on catheter tunnel morphology [58] lead us to believe that it is not desirable to have epidermis attached to the cuff. The importance of epidermal downgrowth inhibition to prevent exit/tunnel infection with transcutaneous devices based on animal experiments does not seem to be relevant for the transcutaneous devices in humans. One of the important differences between experimental animals and humans is the fact that the epidermis in humans enters only a few millimetres into the sinus tract in majority of patients.

External cuff extrusion

A localization of the cuff close to the exit predisposes to its extrusion. There are at least two forces favouring cuff extrusion (Table 4): (1) the pushing force of catheter resilience and (2) pulling and tugging on the catheter. The resilience of the straight catheter implanted in an arcuate tunnel plays the most important role in cuff extrusion (Fig. 6). Pulling on the catheter with frequent CAPD exchanges contributes to this complication. There is a possibility that the high pressure in the abdomen with the constant presence of fluid in the peritoneal cavity while the patient is ambulatory also tends to extrude the external cuff.

At present we think that the cuff should be implanted approximately 2–3 cm beneath the skin as a compromise between the need of a short sinus tract to prevent infections but not so short as to favour cuff extrusions. Also, resilience forces should be eliminated by creating the tunnel in a shape similar to the shape of the catheter, and tugging on the catheter should be avoided. It is extremely important to avoid resilience forces pushing on the cuff if implanting it relatively close to the skin exit. The catheter should not be implanted in the region with subcutaneous oedema, to avoid cuff extrusion once the oedema is resolved.

Catheter-tip migration

One-way or two-way catheter obstruction is usually the result of catheter wrapping by the omentum. The best conditions for dialysate drainage are created with the catheter tip in the true pelvis because, in the majority of people, the omentum does not reach to the true pelvis. Tenckhoff recommended a caudal direction of the intraperitoneal catheter segment to

Table 4. Causes of cuff extrusion

Catheter resilience
Pulling and tugging
Intra-abdominal pressure?

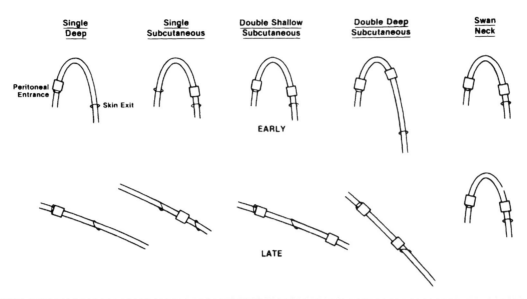

Figure 6. Straight and swan-neck catheters in arcuate tunnels. Upper panel shows catheter configuration immediately after implantation, lower panel portrays catheter shape several months later. Straight catheters forced into arcuate tunnels gradually assume natural, straight configuration. Single-cuff catheters do not extrude cuffs. With long distance between cuffs and shallow subcutaneous tunnel the external cuff extrusion is inevitable (centre), whereas short distance between cuffs and deep position of the subcutaneous cuff precludes its extrusion. Swan-neck catheter maintains its shape. (Reproduced from ref. 57 with permission.)

prevent catheter tip migration out of the true pelvis [105]. If the exit is directed caudally and a straight tunnel points cephalad the catheter must have an intraperitoneal bend to place the tip near the true pelvis, and the tip easily translocates out of the true pelvis due to the silastic 'shape memory'. The internal cuff operates like a fulcrum on which resilience forces turn the catheter tip into the upper abdomen (Fig. 7). If the tip translocates to the left upper abdomen the peristalsis of the descending colon may restore proper position of the tip; however, a tip translocated to the right upper abdomen

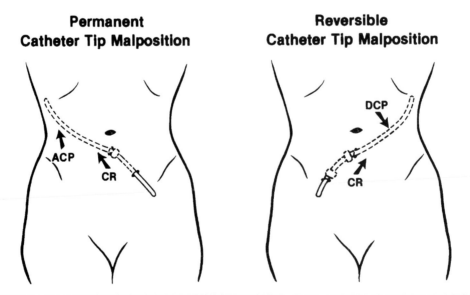

Figure 7. Straight catheter insertion: catheter tip migration out of true pelvis with external exit directed downwards and intraperitoneal entrance directed upwards pointing either to liver or spleen. Note the tendency of catheter to assume its original shape. ACP = ascending colon peristalsis; DCP = descending colon peristalsis; CR = catheter resilience. (Reproduced from ref. 36 with permission.)

usually does not return to the proper position because the forces of both catheter resilience and ascending colon peristalsis push the tip upwards. In support of this hypothesis are observations that, when a catheter is implanted with a straight subcutaneous tunnel, with external exit directed downwards and intraperitoneal entrance directed upwards, even if the catheter tip is placed into the true pelvis during insertion, it migrates out to the upper abdomen significantly more frequently compared to the opposite tunnel direction [36, 118]. Our experience indicates that the dominant factor in catheter-tip position is the resilience force of the catheter. To avoid the unfavourable influence of resilience forces on the intra-abdominal catheter segment, the catheter needs to be moulded in the shape in which it is to be implanted in the tunnel.

The problem of tip migration was approached differently by Oreopoulos et al. [32], who provided the intraperitoneal segment of the catheter with two silicone discs. Once the catheter is in the true pelvis, these discs hinder translocation of the catheter tip. Recently Di Paolo et al. [41] provided the catheter tip with a small, tungsten weight incorporated into the silicone rubber to prevent catheter migration out of the true pelvis. The migration rate of these catheters (no dislocation in 32 catheters over 468 patient-months) was significantly lower than Tenckhoff catheters (nine dislocations in 26 catheters over 415 patient-months). No detrimental effects of these weights were reported. The migration rate of Tenckhoff catheters was rather unusually high in this study.

Pericatheter leak

To avoid excessive bleeding the catheters are frequently inserted through the midline. In patients treated by intermittent peritoneal dialysis, dialysate leaks are rare because the intra-abdominal pressure is low in the supine position. In CAPD patients, pericatheter leaks are frequent due to the continuous presence of dialysate in the upright position where the intra-abdominal pressure is high. Insertion of the deep cuff into the belly of the rectus muscle, as recommended by Helfrich et al. [119], markedly reduces chances of pericatheter leak.

Infusion/pressure pain

Some patients experience pain due to the tip of the catheter with straight intraperitoneal segment. This pain is partly related to a 'jet effect' of the rapidly flowing dialysis solution. Catheters with a coiled intraperitoneal segment are less likely to induce abdominal pain because more of the solution flows shower-like through side-holes, with only part of it through the main lumen that is not in direct contact with the peritoneal membrane. Moreover, the poking force of the coiled catheter is smaller than that of the straight one because the coiled intraperitoneal segment is more flexible. Finally, the larger contact area of the coiled catheter with the parietal peritoneum further reduces the pressure compared to the straight catheter tip.

Currently used chronic peritoneal catheters

The chronic peritoneal catheter is composed of an intraperitoneal and extraperitoneal portion. The latter comprises a tunnel and an external (outside the exit-site) portions. The intraperitoneal and extraperitoneal portions differ in various catheters and there are many combinations of those. Figure 8 shows combinations of intraperitoneal and extraperitoneal designs of currently available chronic peritoneal catheters. Not shown is the catheter of Di Paolo et al. [41], which differs from the Tenckhoff catheter only by the presence of the tungsten cylinder incorporated into the silicone rubber at the tip.

A Computer Interactive Session carried on during the XIV Annual Peritoneal Dialysis Conference in Orlando, Florida, on 24 January, 1994, revealed preferences and practices of 650–690 respondents voting on questions related to peritoneal catheters [120]. Table 5 presents the numbers and percentages of persons who answered positively on a question as to whether they used a particular catheter at least once in 1993. Since the total number of respondents was 660–670 and the number of positive answers was 1552, the programme of each respondent used two or three types of catheter on average. Compared to the surveys conducted in 1987 [5] and 1989 [110], the most striking change was an increase in use of catheters with the bent intramural segment, particularly the swan-neck catheters. Whereas no catheters with bent intraperitoneal segment were included in the 1987 report, and only 12% of these catheters were used in 1989, over 30% of these catheters were used in 1993. An increase in the use of catheters with the coiled intraperitoneal segment was also significant in North America (21.9% in 1987, 40.1% in 1989, and 52.3% in 1993). The Tenckhoff catheter continued to be the most popular, although

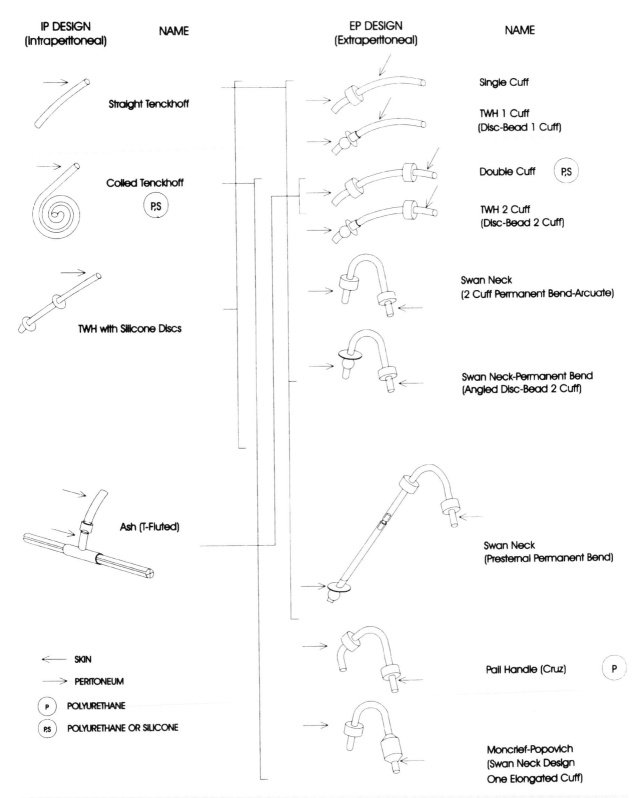

Figure 8. Currently available chronic peritoneal catheters showing combinations of intraperitoneal and extraperitoneal designs. (Reproduced from ref. 107 with permission.)

Table 5. Number and percentages of catheters used in 1993 according to the computer interactive survey, Orlando 1994*

Catheter type	North America		Europe		Rest of the world		Total	
	Number	Percentage	Number	Percentage	Number	Percentage	Number	Percentage
Tenckhoff, double-cuff, coiled	234	23.1	60	24.5	39	13.4	333	21.5
Tenckhoff, double-cuff, straight	144	14.2	61	24.9	80	27.4	285	18.4
Tenckhoff, single-cuff, straight	75	7.4	15	6.1	30	10.3	120	7.7
Tenckhoff, single-cuff, coiled	93	9.2	5	2.0	16	5.5	114	7.3
Total Tenckhoff	*546*	*53.8*	*141*	*57.6*	*165*	*56.5*	*852*	*54.9*
Swan-neck Tenckhoff coiled	98	9.7	13	5.3	21	7.2	132	8.5
Swan-neck Tenckhoff straight	29	2.9	34	13.9	34	11.6	97	6.3
Swan-neck Missouri coiled	44	4.3	8	3.3	7	2.4	59	3.8
Swan-neck Missouri straight	25	2.5	13	5.3	13	4.5	51	3.3
Swan-neck presternal	11	1.1	0	0.0	3	1.0	14	0.9
Swan-neck Moncrief–Popovich	51	5.0	9	3.7	9	3.1	69	4.4
Swan-neck other	34	3.3	6	2.4	8	2.7	48	3.1
Total swan-neck	*292*	*28.8*	*83*	*33.9*	*95*	*32.5*	*470*	*30.3*
Cruz	73	7.2	2	0.8	6	2.1	81	5.2
Toronto Western Hospital	32	3.2	9	3.7	9	3.1	50	3.2
Gore-Tex	16	1.6	0	0.0	2	0.7	18	1.2
Ash	13	1.3	2	0.8	1	0.3	16	1.0
Valli	2	0.2	1	0.4	2	0.7	5	0.3
Other	41	4.0	7	2.9	12	4.1	60	3.9
Other than Tenckhoff/swan neck	*177*	*17.4*	*21*	*8.6*	*32*	*11.0*	*230*	*14.8*
Grand total	*1015*	*100.0*	*245*	*100.0*	*292*	*100.0*	*1552*	*100.0*

* Modified from ref. 120, with permission.

its use was decreasing. The remaining catheters were used in small numbers. A vast majority of nephrologists remained convinced of the superiority of double-cuff catheters over single-cuff ones and the use of the former continued to exceed 70% [120]. The most commonly used catheters are described in detail below.

Straight and coiled Tenckhoff catheters

The catheter consists of silicone rubber tubing with a 2.6 mm internal diameter and a 5 mm external diameter (Fig. 2). The catheter is provided with one or two polyester (Dacron®), 1 cm long cuffs. The overall length of the adult straight double-cuff catheter is about 40 cm. The lengths of segments are: intraperitoneal, about 15 cm; intercuff, 5–7 cm; external, 16 cm. The intraperitoneal segment has an open end and multiple 0.5 mm perforations at a distance of 11 cm from the tip. The coiled Tenckhoff catheter differs from the straight in having a coiled, 18.5 cm long perforated distal end. As mentioned above, the coiled catheter reduces inflow infusion 'jet effect' and pressure discomfort. All Tenckhoff

catheters are provided with a barium-impregnated radiopaque stripe to assist in radiological visualization of the catheter.

Swan-neck catheters

The swan-neck catheter is the second most commonly used catheter at present. Its design is based on a retrospective analysis of complication rates with Tenckhoff and Toronto Western Hospital catheters. This analysis showed that the lowest complication rates were with double-cuff catheters implanted through the belly of the rectus muscle and with both internal and skin exits of the tunnel directed downwards; however, the resulting arcuate tunnel led to frequent external cuff extrusion [36]. Swan-neck catheters feature a permanent bend between cuffs (Table 6) [121]. The catheter was dubbed 'swan-neck' because of its shape. As a result of this design, catheters can be placed in an arcuate tunnel in an unstressed condition with both external and internal segments of the tunnel directed downwards. Downward-directed exit, two cuffs, and an optimal sinus length reduce exit/tunnel infection rates. A perma-

Table 6. Swan-neck catheter features preventing complications

Exit/tunnel infection	Downward exit, double cuff, short sinus
External cuff extrusion	Permanent bend between cuffs
Intraperitoneal tip migration	Downward intraperitoneal entrance
Pericatheter leak	Insertion through the rectus muscle
Peritonitis	Decreased tunnel infections
Infusion/pressure pain	Coiled intraperitoneal tip

nent bend between cuffs eliminates the silastic resilience force or the 'shape memory' which tends to extrude the external cuff. Downwards peritoneal entrance tends to keep the tip in the true pelvis, reducing its migration. Insertion through the rectus muscle decreases pericatheter leaks. Lower exit/tunnel infection rates curtail peritonitis episodes. Finally swan-neck catheters with a coiled intraperitoneal segment minimize infusion and pressure pain.

Swan-neck prototypes (Fig. 9) were designed in 1985 and were used briefly between August 1985 and April 1986. These catheters were made of 80° arc angle tubing and were inserted in a reversed U-shape tunnel with the incision at the top of the tunnel [122]. Only 27 of these catheters were inserted because we noted a tendency to cuff extrusions, which we considered a risk for exit infections [123]. Further observations confirmed our predictions. Cuff extrusion occurred in nine catheters and led to exit infections and finally to catheter removals. Initial excellent results with these catheters because

of elimination of leaks and malfunctions were obviated later by high infection rates. Cuff extrusions resulted from resilience forces pushing on the external cuff due to an insufficient bend of the catheter and too long a distance between cuffs. We considered these catheters as suboptimal and have discontinued their use since April 1986 [123, 124]. Based on this unfavourable observation the catheters were modified; the new catheters, swan-neck 2 and 3 catheters had straight intraperitoneal segments. A major improvement was in the intercuff shape; the distance between cuffs was shortened from 8.5 cm to 5 cm in swan-neck 2 and to 3 cm in swan-neck 3 catheters, and the bend was increased from 80° to 170–180° arc angle. The catheters were provided with short or long intraperitoneal segments, selected according to patient size and insertion site, to secure the catheter-tip position in the true pelvis [121, 123]. Because in several patients infusion pain occurred due to a 'jet effect' and/or tip pressure on the peritoneum, we modified the intraperitoneal segment of the catheters, replacing a straight segment with a coiled one (swan-neck coiled). These catheters were introduced in January 1990 and within a month swan-neck straight catheters were phased out [124].

Swan-neck Tenckhoff straight and coiled

The Tenckhoff type of the swan-neck peritoneal dialysis catheter is provided with two Dacron® cuffs. It differs from the double-cuff Tenckhoff catheter only

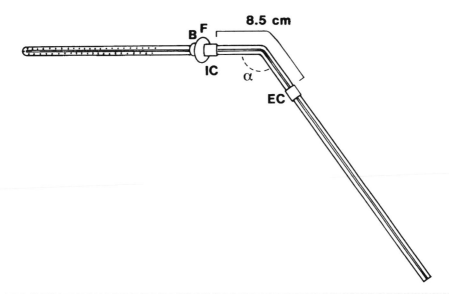

Figure 9. Swan-neck Missouri prototype catheter. Arc angle = 180° − α = 80°. Cuff extrusions were common with these catheters because of insufficient bend and too long a distance between cuffs. We consider these catheters as suboptimal and we have not used them since April 1986.

by being permanently bent between cuffs [121]. This type of catheter may be inserted at the bedside and does not require surgical insertion; however, a subcutaneous tunnel has to be created in the same way as for other swan-neck catheters. The intraperitoneal segment of the swan-neck coiled catheter is identical to that of the Tenckhoff coiled catheter [121]. All swan-neck catheters are manufactured by the Kendall Co. (Bothell, WA, USA).

Swan-neck Missouri straight

The swan-neck Missouri catheter has a flange and bead circumferentially surrounding the catheter just below the internal cuff; the flange and bead are slanted approximately 45° relative to the axis of the catheter. The catheters for left and right tunnels are mirror-images of each other. A swan-neck Missouri 2 catheter with a 5 cm inter-cuff distance is used in average to obese people. The intraperitoneal segment is 21.5 cm long in the swan-neck Missouri 2 long catheters. A swan-neck Missouri 3 catheter with a 3 cm inter-cuff distance is used in lean to average persons [121].

Swan-neck Missouri coiled

The intraperitoneal segment in all swan-neck coiled catheters is 34 cm from the bead to the tip of the coil. Swan-neck Missouri 2 coiled catheters with the 5 cm intercuff distance (Fig. 10) are used in average to obese people. Swan-neck Missouri 3 coiled catheters with 3 cm intercuff distance are used in lean to average persons. The catheters for left and right tunnels are mirror-images of each other [121]. The overall survival values of straight and coiled swan-neck Missouri catheters are not significantly different, but none of the patients experienced infusion or pressure pain with coiled catheters, whereas this complication occurred in several patients who had catheters with straight intraperitoneal segments [124]. Swan-neck catheters are also available in smaller sizes for children and infants.

Swan-neck presternal

Potential advantages of exit location in the chest instead of in the abdomen are shown in Table 7. The chest is a sturdy structure with minimal wall motion; the catheter exit located on the chest wall is subjected to minimal movements, decreasing chances of trauma and contamination. Also, in patients with abdominal ostomies and in children with diapers, a chest exit location reduces the chances of contamination. Moreover, a loose garment is usually worn on the chest and there is less pressure on the exit. Surgical experience indicates that wounds heal better after thoracic surgery than after abdominal surgery; this

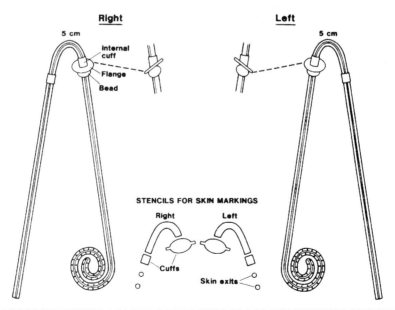

Figure 10. Swan-neck Missouri 2 coiled (curled) catheters and stencils. Swan-neck Missouri 2 catheters have 5 cm intercuff distance and intraperitoneal length of 32 cm from the bead to the tip. The flange and bead are slanted approximately 45° relative to the tubing axis. The catheters for left and right tunnels are mirror-images of each other. The stencil follows exactly the shape of the intramural segment. The stencil can be flipped to be used for right or left catheter. The holes for exit-site markings are located 2 cm and 3 cm from the cuff. A 3 cm mark is used for average or obese persons, a 2 cm mark is suitable for lean or average persons.

Table 7. Potential advantages of the swan-neck presternal catheter compared to the swan-neck Missouri catheter

Attribute	Advantage	Explanation
Exit on the chest	Decreased risk of exit infection	Good immobilization
		Good wound healing
		Loose garment/less pressure
		Easy exit-site care
		Less fat thickness
		Far from ostomies*
		Far from wet diapers†
		Less trauma with creeping†
	Psychosocial	Better body image for some patients
		Easy exit-site care
		May take tub bath without risk of exit contamination
Three cuffs	Decreased risk of peritonitis	Strong (triple) barrier
		Long tunnel, long distance for bacterial penetration

* In patients with ostomies.
† In small children.

may in part be related to less chest mobility. Obese patients have higher exit-site infection rates and a tendency to poor wound healing, particularly after abdominal surgery. The subcutaneous fat layer is several times thinner on the chest than on the abdomen. If fat thickness *per se* is responsible for quality of healing and susceptibility to infection then chest location may be preferred for obese patients. All these favourable factors, together with easy exit-site care using a magnifying mirror, significantly reduce exit-site infections. The catheter chest location of the exit is particularly advantageous in small children because of the greater distance from diapers and is subjected to less trauma during crawling/creeping. The catheter is also advantageous for psychosocial reasons. A chest exit location allows a tub bath without the risk of exit contamination. Although the exit-site can be located in the presternal or parasternal area we will usually refer to this catheter as presternal for simplicity. A long catheter tunnel, combined with three cuffs, may curtail pericatheter bacterial penetration into the peritoneal cavity, thus reducing the incidence of peritonitis [38, 125, 126].

To accommodate these principles we modified the swan-neck peritoneal catheter to have an exit on the chest but preserving all advantages of the swan-neck Missouri coiled catheters; minimizing catheter obstruction, cuff extrusion, pericatheter dialysate leak and infusion pain. A major difference from the swan-neck Missouri catheter is in the length of the subcutaneous tunnel. The catheter (Fig. 11) is composed of two silicone rubber tubes, which are to be connected end to end at the time of implantation [125, 126]. Figure 12 shows the catheter in relation to the torso after implantation. The implanted lower

(abdominal) tube constitutes the intraperitoneal catheter segment and a part of the intramural segment. The upper or chest tube constitutes the remaining part of the intramural segment and the external catheter segment. The lower tube is identical to the swan-neck Missouri catheter, with the exception that it is not bent and does not have a second cuff. The proximal end of the lower tube is straight and with a redundant length to be trimmed to the patient's size at the time of implantation. A titanium connector, provided in a package, is to be coupled with the distal part of the upper or chest part at the time of implantation.

The upper tube carries two porous cuffs, a superficial and a middle or central, spaced 5 cm apart. The tube between the cuffs has a permanently bent section defining an arc angle of 180°. The distal lumen of the upper tube communicates with the proximal lumen of the lower tube through the titanium connector. The tubing grip of the titanium connector is so strong that the two parts of the catheter, especially after connection reinforcement with a prolene suture, in practice cannot separate spontaneously in the tunnel [127]. The swan-neck presternal catheter is available for children and infants [128]. Tubing diameter is smaller for paediatric patients.

Moncrief–Popovich catheter

This catheter is a modified swan-neck Tenckhoff coiled catheter (Fig. 8) with a longer subcutaneous cuff (2.5 cm instead of 1 cm). This catheter is most commonly used in conjunction with the Moncrief–Popovich implantation technique (see below).

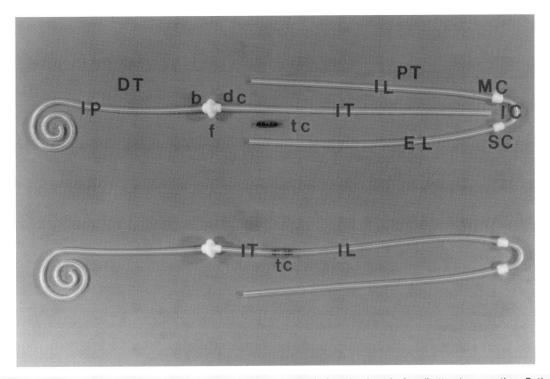

Figure 11. Two tubes of the swan-neck presternal peritoneal catheter before (top) and after (bottom) connection. Both tubes and bead are made of silicone rubber moulded in the shapes as shown. A flange and all cuffs are made of woven polyester fibers. Proximal (upper, chest) tube (PT) consists of an intra-tunnel limb (IL), medial (centre) cuff (MC), inter-cuff segment (IC), superficial cuff (SC), and external limb (EL); 1–2 cm of the external limb adjacent to the superficial cuff is intended to be in the sinus tract of the tunnel (from the cuff to the exit). Distal (abdominal, lower) tube (DT) consists of an intra-tunnel segment (IT), deep (distal, preperitoneal) cuff (dc) flange (f), bead (b), and intraperitoneal segment (IP). After implantation (bottom) the intra-tunnel limb (IL) of the chest tube and the intra-tunnel segment (IT) of the abdominal tube are trimmed to the size of the tunnel and coupled with titanium connector (tc).

Radiopaque stripe

The slanted flange and bead, and bent tunnel segment, require that the swan-neck Missouri and Toronto catheters for right and left tunnels be mirror-images of each other. To facilitate recognition of right and left Toronto and Missouri catheters, each tubing has a radiopaque stripe in front of the catheter (Fig. 10). In a swan-neck presternal catheter the stripe also facilitates proper alignment of the lower and upper tubes. The stripe is also useful during insertion and postimplantation care, facilitating recognition of catheter twisting. Because of this last feature Tenckhoff-type catheters are also provided with the stripe. Right and left swan-neck Tenckhoff catheters differ only with respect to the position of the stripe. Unlike swan-neck Toronto and Missouri catheters the swan-neck Tenckhoff catheter intended for right or left tunnel may be implanted with an opposite tunnel. In this case the stripe should be kept in the back of the catheter. Nevertheless, to retain uniformity of the stripe position it is recommended that swan-neck Tenckhoff catheters be inserted with the corre-

sponding tunnel direction (right tunnel with right catheter, left tunnel with left catheter).

Other catheters

Catheters used in small numbers, such as recently designed catheters with one-centre experience (T-fluted [39], self-locating [41]) and those used in smaller numbers in 1993, as seen in Table 5 (Cruz [37], Toronto Western Hospital [32], Ash (Life-cath, Column disc) [35], Valli [33, 34], and Gore-tex [30]), will not be described in detail. Readers are referred to the original publications.

Accessories for implantation of catheters

Stencils

Stencils have been developed for skin markings to facilitate creation of proper tunnels for swan-neck

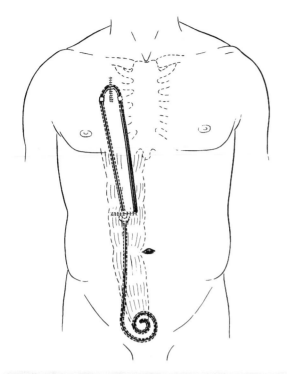

Figure 12. Swan-neck presternal catheter in relation to the torso after implantation. The deep cuff with flange and bead is shown in the rectus muscle, the titanium connector is 2–3 inches (5–7.5 cm) above the deep cuff. The middle and superficial cuffs are in the parasternal area, and the exit is 3 cm below the external cuff. (Reproduced from ref. 126 with permission.)

catheters [121]. Stencils are for swan-neck Missouri 2 (Fig. 10), swan-neck Missouri 3, and swan-neck Tenckhoff catheters. The stencils follow exactly the shape of the intramural segments of the catheters and the catheter tunnels must follow the shape of the catheters exactly as designed to maximize the advantages of this design. The stencils can be flipped to be used for right or left catheters. The holes for exit-site markings are located 2 cm and 3 cm from the cuff. A 3 cm mark is used for average or obese persons, a 2 cm mark is suitable for lean or average persons. Stencils for swan-neck Tenckhoff catheters also reflect precisely the shape of their intramural segments.

Stiffening stilette

A 62 cm long stiffening stilette is used to facilitate catheter insertion into the true pelvis. During insertion about 1 cm of catheter is left beyond the tip of the stilette to protect the bowels. The catheter resumes its natural shape after the stilette is removed [121].

Tunnelling devices

Tenckhoff trochar

Tenckhoff developed a special trochar for bedside insertion of cuffed catheters into the peritoneal cavity (Fig. 1). The trochar (available from Kendall Co., Bothell, WA, USA) consists of: a sharp, stainless-steel stylet; a solid, wide, open-ended barrel; and two side-pieces with handles [105].

Scanlan tunneller

A Scanlan tunneller (Scanlan International, 1 Scanlan Plaza, St Paul, MN 56107, USA) is used during swan-neck presternal catheter implantation to create a tunnel extending from the abdominal wall to the presternal or parasternal area. A tunneller to accommodate vascular grafts up to 8 mm is suitable for presternal catheter implantation. The tunneller, developed for tunnelling vascular grafts, consists of an outside sheath, a blunt tip, and a spring clamp. Depending on the size of the patient either a green (51 cm long) or an orange (30 cm long) tunneller may be used. A stiff metal rod serves to stiffen the tunneller as it is pushed through the subcutaneous tissue and a spring clamp at the tip is used to grasp and pull the upper tubing through the sheath [125].

Exit trochar

The catheter tunnel extending from the cuff to the skin exit should have a diameter close to that of catheter tubing. Thus, the last portion of the tunnel (from external cuff to the exit) should be made with a piercing trochar, e.g. the Faller trochar (Kendall Co, Bothell, WA, USA) or a 3/16 inch (4.76 mm, F 15) trochar for the Hemovac system (Zimmer Mfg Co., 11235 Manchester Road, St Louis, MO 63122, USA) of external diameter similar to that of the catheter tubing [121, 125].

Peritoneoscopic equipment

The basic equipment (Fig. 13) required for this type of insertion (manufactured and distributed by Medigroup, 350 Smoke Tree Plaza, North Aurora, IL 60542-1720, USA) includes a 2.2-mm diameter, 15-cm long Y-TEC peritoneoscope with a 2.5-mm steel cannula with internal trochar and a spiral-wound Quill catheter guide surrounding the cannula [129, 130].

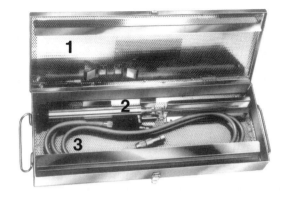

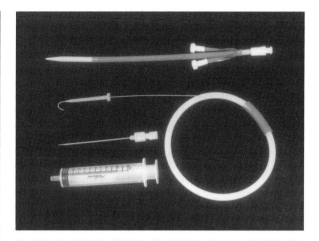

Figure 14. Equipment for guidewire insertion method. From the top: peel-away sheath with dilator, guidewire, needle, and syringe.

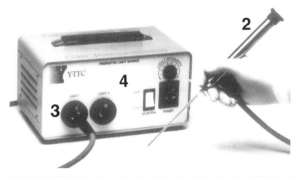

Figure 13. Components for the peritoneoscopic catheter insertion. Above: the sterilization tray (1); the Y-TEC® scope (2); and the light guide (3). Below is the Y-TEC® light source (4), with the scope (2), and light guide (3). (This figure was kindly provided by John Navis, Medigroup, North Aurora, IL, USA.)

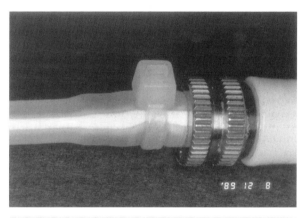

Figure 15. A single-piece titanium adaptor with a barbed connector in the catheter tubing and a male Luer lock connector attached to the female connector of the extension tube. The nylon tie is in place over the catheter/barbed connector junction. The locking segment is over the stripe and will be away from the patient's skin. (Reproduced from ref. 136 with permission.)

Seldinger (guidewire) with peel-away sheath equipment

The essential instruments (Fig. 14) for this technique include a guide needle, attached to a syringe, a Seldinger guidewire, and a tapered dilator with surrounding scored peel-away sheath [131–135]. The necessary equipment and videos can be obtained through Cook Critical Care, Division of Cook Inc., PO Box 489, Bloomington, IN 47402, USA.

Titanium connectors, Tyton ties and a tension tool

The catheter after implantation must be connected to the peritoneal dialysis set. A titanium connector serves this purpose. A single-piece connector shown in Fig. 15 is simply inserted into the end of the external catheter tubing. The external part is equ-

ipped with a female Luer lock adapter and sealing cap. The intracatheter adaptor is barbed and its external diameter is slightly larger than the internal diameter of the tubing to avoid accidental disconnection; however, this titanium connector has been associated with numerous instances of spontaneous separations. Tyton ties and a tension tool (Tyton Corporation, PO Box 23055, 7930 Faulkner Road, Milwaukee, WI 53223, USA) routinely used to secure bundles of electrical wirings, and available in department stores, may be used to prevent disconnection of the titanium adaptor from the tubing. A

4-inch (100 mm) tie is placed around the distal end of the catheter over the adapter. Care is taken to place the tie in the groove between adapter ridges and not over a ridge. Then the tie is tightened with the tension tool which also trims the excess length. The locking segment is located at the stripe which will be positioned at the front of the patient (Fig. 15). This keeps the added bulk away from the patient [121, 125, 136].

A recently introduced two-piece adapter (Baxter Healthcare Corporation, Deerfield IL, USA), shown in Fig. 16, is very safe and no instances of accidental connector disengagements have been reported. The only disadvantage of this design is the markedly higher price.

Rigid catheter

The two most widely used rigid catheters in North America are the Stylocath (Abbott Laboratories, North Chicago, IL 60064, USA) and the Trocath (Baxter Healthcare Corporation, Deerfield, IL 60015, USA).

Pre-insertion patient assessment and preparation

When the need to start peritoneal dialysis is urgent, one may elect to access the peritoneal cavity through a rigid catheter. This catheter can be inserted at the bedside, with minimal preparation. Equipment required for paracentesis is all that is needed.

Bedside insertion should not be offered to patients who are extremely obese, or have had previous abdo-

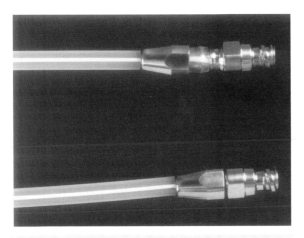

Figure 16. A two-piece adapter (Locking Titanium Adapter – Baxter) with two parts disengaged (upper), with adaptor inserted into the external end of the catheter and after the two pieces are screwed together and tightened (lower).

minal surgery, since abdominal adhesions increase the risk of unintentional viscus perforation. In addition, this approach should be done in children by an experienced paediatric nephrologist or a nephrologist with a paediatrician in attendance. If a nephrologist implants the catheter a surgeon should be on stand-by, in case of complications. The patient should receive preoperative sedation and have nothing to eat or drink at least 12 hours prior to the procedure.

All observers and persons in the immediate area, including the patient, should wear surgical masks. Those patients who experience discomfort while completely supine should raise their heads slightly. In conscious patients it may be useful to familiarize them with the Valsalva manoeuvre. The operator and assistant(s) should 'scrub, gown and glove'. A 'circulating' nurse should be present to assist.

Insertion

Taking all sterile precautions, a small stab wound (2–3 mm) is made in the midline under local anaesthesia, 2–3 cm below the umbilicus. The stab wound should be small so that the abdominal wall holds the catheter firmly, and thus minimizes dialysis solution leak.   With the stylet in place, the catheter is forced through the abdominal wall by a short thrust, or preferably with a rotary motion. The operator will recognize the loss of resistance as a 'pop' as soon as the peritoneal cavity is entered. While the catheter is being thrust through the abdominal wall its tip is directed towards the coccyx. Because successful perforation of the abdominal wall for introduction of the catheter requires a sensitive 'feel' for the pressure applied, infusion of 2–3 litres of dialysate will distend the abdomen, which in turn will facilitate this manoeuvre. Some infuse 2 litres of dialysis fluid via a small-gauge needle prior to stylet puncture. A cooperative patient can also assist successful perforation by voluntarily tightening the abdominal musculature.

Once the peritoneal cavity has been entered the stylet is withdrawn a few centimetres and the catheter is advanced deep into the pelvis. If the operator encounters resistance while the catheter is being advanced, or if the patient complains of pain, the advance in this direction should be stopped and another direction tried. If this is still not possible, the operator may infuse 2–3 litres of dialysis solution into the peritoneal cavity if this has not been done. This can be via the catheter if the holes in the distal end are in the abdominal cavity. This infusion accomplishes two important objectives: first, it facilitates recognition of the 'true' intraperitoneal space; second, dialysis solution in the peritoneal cavity reduces the likelihood of viscus perforation by moving the intra-abdominal contents away from the advancing catheter.

After one or two good in-and-out exchanges, the catheter is firmly secured to the skin with the aid of a metal disc.

Complications

Table 8 shows complications of rigid catheter insertion. After catheter implantation bloody effluent appears after the first exchange in approximately 30% of cases [137, 138]. This bleeding (usually minor) comes from the small vessels in the abdominal wall. After three or four exchanges bleeding usually stops, unless the procedure has damaged a major vessel or the patient has a bleeding disorder. Pressure applied over the catheter insertion site usually controls minor bleeding. Occasionally, a transfusion of fresh blood will stop the bleeding. If the bleeding is copious it may obstruct the catheter; in this event it is a common practice to add 1000 units of heparin to each litre of dialysate to minimize the risk of obstruction. Intraperitoneal heparin is not absorbed in sufficient amount to influence systemic coagulation.

Dialysis solution leak is encountered in 14–36% of patients after rigid catheter insertion [137–139]. Frequent manipulation of the catheter to improve drainage increases the risk of dialysis solution leak from the catheter-exit site. Such leaks may also occur when the catheter is not properly secured to the skin. The risk of external leak is higher in elderly or debilitated patients who have lax abdominal walls. The presence of a large intra-abdominal mass, such as a polycystic kidney(s) may raise the intra-abdominal pressure to high levels and promote dialysis solution leak around the catheter after the standard 2-litre volume has been instilled.

Table 8. Complications of rigid catheter insertion

Bleeding
Dialysis solution leak
Poor drainage
Extraperitoneal space penetration
Viscus perforation
Peritonitis
Abdominal pain
Loss of rigid catheter in the peritoneum

Fluid may extravasate into the abdominal wall, particularly in patients who have had a previous abdominal operation or multiple catheter insertions. This complication usually results from tears in the peritoneum or represents an infusion of dialysate into the potential space between the layers of abdominal wall. Uncommonly dialysis fluid may enter the pleural cavity [140–151]. In such cases peritoneal dialysis is usually discontinued and the patients are switched to haemodialysis. Acute hydrothorax results from either a traumatic or a congenital defect in the diaphragm.

Inadequate drainage is frequent during initial dialysis, and may be due to one or more of the following factors: loss of siphon effect, one-way obstruction, and/or incorrect placement of the catheter. One-way (outflow) catheter obstruction may have multiple causes. Fibrin or blood clots may be trapped in the catheter and block the terminal holes, especially when dialysis is complicated by major haemorrhage or peritonitis. Poor outflow may also reflect extrinsic pressure on the catheter from adjacent organs such as a sigmoid colon full of faeces or a distended bladder. Omental wrapping is likely if the catheter is misplaced into the upper abdomen.

Occasionally, accidental penetration of the extraperitoneal space by the catheter may cause poor drainage. In such a situation continued infusion produces further dissection, and the fluid may become trapped and is no longer available for drainage. Loculation of fluid, another cause of poor drainage, is encountered in patients who have had previous intra-abdominal operations or peritonitis. Such loculation not only diminishes the surface area available for dialysis but may seriously reduce ultrafiltration capacity. The incidence of this complication is low, varying between 0.5% and 1.3% [139, 152, 153].

Perforation or laceration of internal organs during bedside insertion of a catheter has been frequently reported. Lacerated or perforated organs include the bowel, bladder, liver, a polycystic kidney, aorta, mesenteric artery and hernia sac [149, 152–164]. Abdominal distension due to paralytic ileus or bowel obstruction may predispose the patient to bowel perforation. Those who are unconscious, cachectic or heavily sedated are also at high risk. Clinical evidence of bowel perforation includes sudden, sharp or severe abdominal pain followed by watery diarrhoea, and poor drainage of dialysis solution, which may be cloudy, foul-smelling or mixed with faecal material. Such a situation requires prompt removal of the catheter, and allowing the perforation to seal off completely in about 12–24 h.

Abdominal pain may be encountered in as many as 56–75% of patients with the first use of the catheter [137]. There are many causes of abdominal pain, but catheter-related pain occurs when it impinges on any of the viscera. Pain may occur during inflow and outflow of dialysis solution and also when the solution is dwelling. Outflow pain is due to entrapment of omentum in the catheter during the siphoning action of fluid drainage. Constant pain during dialysis indicates pressure effects on intra-abdominal organs and often produces continuous rectal or low-back pain. This complaint calls for an adjustment in catheter position.

Loss of a part or all of the rigid catheter has been reported following its manipulation with the trochar in place [137, 155, 157, 165, 166]. Its distal end may be amputated after intra-abdominal kinking of the catheter, followed by manipulation. However, the presence of broken catheters within the abdominal cavity does not cause symptoms or ill-effects. During laparoscopy, broken catheters have been found lying freely in the peritoneal cavity without causing a peritoneal reaction, or have been found walled off by mesentery without an inflammatory reaction. On routine postmortem examination, Stein [167] discovered such a catheter in a patient who had had previous peritoneal dialysis. Exploration to retrieve the catheter is unnecessary because laparotomy is more hazardous than leaving the catheter in a severely ill patient. The incidence of catheter loss into the peritoneal cavity has been greatly reduced since the introduction of a design which incorporates a metal disc with a central hole; this not only allows the catheter to pass through the wall but also holds the catheter snugly to the skin of the abdominal wall.

The incidence of peritonitis, when the stylet catheter was used, was 2.5% of all the dialyses [165]. The incidence of peritonitis almost doubled when the duration of dialysis was longer than 60 h.

Soft catheter

Because of the high frequency of dialysis solution leak, and poor drainage necessitating frequent catheter manipulation and resultant peritonitis with the use of rigid catheters, some centres prefer to insert a single- or double-cuff Tenckhoff catheter for treatment of acute renal failure. Tenckhoff recommended use of a single-cuff catheter for acute cases [1]. For treatment of chronic renal failure only soft catheters are used.

Patient preparation

Acute dialysis

Patient assessment and preparation before soft catheter implantation for treatment of acute renal failure is the same as that before rigid catheter insertion.

Chronic dialysis

Patient preparation before catheter implantation for treatment of chronic renal failure is more elaborate [107, 121, 125, 168–170]. Prior to surgery, chest and/or abdominal hair should be removed with an electric shaver. Prophylactic antibiotics prior to implantation are recommended [107].

Abdominal exit. The belt line of a patient is identified, preferably in the sitting or standing position, with slacks or pants as usually worn [121]. Depending on the size and shape of the abdomen, presence of previous scars, right- or left-handedness, and patient's preference, the tunnel is marked using the stencil (available with swan-neck catheters) in such a way that the exit hole would be created at least 2 cm from the belt line. Skin markings may be made with any good surgical marker.

Women usually wear a belt above the umbilicus, hence stencils are marked below the belt line in female patients. The catheter should not be subjected to excessive motion with patient activities, and there should not be pressure on the tunnel when the patient bends forward. In obese people, with pendulous abdomens, it is mandatory to insert the catheter above the skin-fold so they can see the exit for its care. Men usually prefer a belt line below the umbilicus and there may not be enough space below the belt line; therefore a stencil is frequently marked above the belt line in male patients. The label of the chosen catheter type is written on the belly of the patient. A band with the catheter label is also attached to the patient's left wrist.

Tap-water enema should be administered and, if feasible, the patient should take a shower. Skin markings may require remarking if they become faint after the shower. Ceftazidime (1.0 g intravenously 1 h preoperatively and repeated 12 h postoperatively) constitutes an appropriate prophylactic therapy [107, 168, 169]. Vancomycin should not be routinely used for perioperative prophylaxis, to avoid development of vancomycin resistant strains, such as *Enterococcus* or *S. aureus.* [107].

Presternal exit. Depending on the size of the patient, the abdominal cuff and flange location is marked over the rectus muscle [125]. To secure the catheter-tip position in the true pelvis, but without an excessive pressure on the pelvic peritoneum, the position of the cuff should be above the umbilicus in small persons and at the level of or slightly below the umbilicus in tall persons. To determine a preferable position of the deep cuff, a coiled catheter tip is placed on the pubic bone and the cuff position is marked. On the chest a superficial cuff is marked at the second or third intercostal spaces and the exit 3 cm from the cuff in the presternal or parasternal area. It is preferable not to cross the midline in patients likely to have heart surgery. Care is taken to avoid an exit site too close to bra lines in females. Prophylactic antibiotics, shower, and enema are used in the same way as for abdominal exit [125].

Catheter preparation

Immediately before implantation the catheter is removed from the sterile peel pack and immersed in sterile saline. Dacron® cuffs and the Dacron® flange are gently squeezed to remove air [121, 125]. Thoroughly wetted cuffs provide markedly better tissue ingrowth compared to unwetted, air-containing cuffs [54].

Implantation method

Blind (Tenckhoff trochar)

While inserting the catheter at the bedside a sterile procedure must be strictly followed. A 2–3 cm incision is made in the skin at the insertion site (e.g. the midline 2 cm inferior to the umbilicus). This places the site of entry at the linea alba, a point of minimal vascularity and tissue resistance [105]. The lateral margins of either rectus muscle are alternative sites because they are also relatively avascular. It should be remembered that the placement through the belly of the rectus muscle using blind insertion may cause injury to the inferior or superior epigastric artery.

Through the skin incision the wound is extended to the linea alba with blunt dissection using a curved haemostat. At this time an 'anchoring' suture is inserted in the fascia. The peritoneal cavity is entered with a 'priming needle' (a 'catheter over a needle', venicath-type needle or a stylet peritoneal catheter) into the superior aspect of the wound and through the linea alba. One must take care to ensure 'intraperitoneal' placement of all hole outlets of the priming device. If the parietal peritoneal membrane is separated from the preperitoneal tissue this will result in

'preperitoneal' infusion of dialysis fluid and make impossible any further intraperitoneal infusion of dialysis fluid by this method. Furthermore the expansion of the preperitoneal 'pocket' is extremely painful. When dialysis solution infusion produces pain, the operator should suspect preperitoneal instillation; however, the heavily sedated patient may not be able to voice an objection. At this time poor dialysis solution inflow may also indicate that hole outlets are lodged in a preperitoneal position, although one might also expect a moderate restriction of flow in any case, given the relatively small lumen of the access catheter.

Following sterile connection of the administration tubing, 2–3 litres of dialysis solution are infused into the peritoneal cavity, until the patient feels distended. While dialysate is being instilled to the desired volume the Tenckhoff catheter should be 'prepared' by wetting it with a small volume of normal saline. Air from the cuffs is removed by squeezing. A wetted stiffening stilette is inserted into the catheter, thus straightening and 'stiffening' it to permit introduction of the catheter into the Tenckhoff trochar, and beyond it into its correct intraabdominal position.

It is useful to start perforation of the linea alba with a smaller trochar or dilator rather than a needle, thereby facilitating introduction of the larger Tenckhoff trochar. With firm but gentle pressure, and a twisting action, the trochar with its pointed stylet in place (Fig. 1) is pushed into the peritoneal cavity via the small perforation. Immediately after the resistance ceases (indicating entrance into the peritoneal cavity), the obturator is removed. Then the true intraperitoneal placement should be recognized by the 'welling-up' of dialysis solution into the barrel of the trochar. If the operator has instilled enough dialysis solution during the priming procedure, he/she should insert the trochar until its wider portion comes to rest on the linea alba. This portion should not enter the peritoneal cavity, thus keeping the perforation at the desired diameter. This larger barrel is designed not only to accept the Tenckhoff catheter, but it also allows for the passage of the Dacron® cuffs.

The catheter is threaded on a stiffening stilette. About 1 cm of catheter is left beyond the tip of the stilette to protect the bowels. Proper placement of the catheter in the pelvis will greatly facilitate siphon drainage. During this phase of insertion certain details, although they may seem trivial, if not attended to with care, may produce unfavourable results. For example, as the catheter is introduced into the trochar on its way to the abdominal cavity, the tip should be passed smoothly beyond the trochar. Careful, gentle, and angular movement of the trochar and stiffened catheter (adjusting its intra-abdominal position and relationship to abdominal contents) may be needed to achieve easy passage of the catheter deep into pelvis.

Once the catheter has completed its 'internal' course, the detachable trochar barrel should be removed, leaving the split side-pieces *in situ* for easier manipulation until the final positioning is satisfactory. At this point the stiffening stilette should be removed while the operator holds the catheter firmly in place. Once the desired depth of placement is achieved, the remaining catheter is 'fed' into the peritoneal cavity while slowly withdrawing the stiffening stilette until the preperitoneal (inner or deep) Dacron® cuff comes to rest on the linea alba. Then the trochar is separated into its two longitudinal sections and withdrawn, leaving the catheter cuff in proper position. The ideal location for the internal cuff is at the preperitoneal level. However, if the catheter is intended for a short-term use until the patient recovers from an acute renal failure event, the location of deep cuff at the preperitoneal level is not as critical as in the case of long-term use.

Catheter patency is tested in the same manner described in the surgical procedure. When the function is deemed satisfactory the catheter is secured in place to the linea alba with an anchoring suture before preparing for the creation of the subcutaneous tunnel towards the proposed exit site.

After choosing the catheter exit site, a stab wound (not an incision) is made using a blade, taking care to penetrate only the skin. The opening should be just the size of the catheter. Choose a site that will permit the creation of a tunnel of an appropriate length and shape of the catheter. A subcutaneous tunnel is created using a malleable uterine sound or the Faller trochar, being careful to manipulate the catheter gently. For the swan-neck Tenckhoff catheter the tunnel must follow the skin marking made prior to the insertion. The outer cuff should be positioned approximately 2 cm from the skin exit. The recommended method for tunnel creation for the swan-neck Tenckhoff catheter is to make a superior subcutaneous pocket as described for surgical insertion (see below) and penetrate the exit with the piercing trochar. The titanium connector is then inserted into the end of the catheter. The skin of the insertion wound is sutured, and appropriate surgical dressings applied. Dressings are applied for at least 1 week while leaving an accessible length of catheter to permit the catheter to be handled without disturbing the dressings.

Peritoneoscopic

The use of peritoneoscopy for peritoneal catheter placement was developed by Ash at Lafayette, Indiana [129, 130, 171]. Tenckhoff and swan-neck Tenckhoff (straight and coiled) catheters may be implanted with this technique. Like blind insertion, it is performed through a single abdominal puncture. No fluid is instilled before insertion of the cannula and the trochar into the abdomen (through the medial or lateral border of the rectus). The trochar is removed, and the scope is inserted through the cannula. After assuring the intraperitoneal location by observing motion of glistening surfaces, the scope is removed and 600 cm³ of air placed in the peritoneal cavity with the patient in the Trendelenburg position. The scope is reinserted and, during continuous observation, scope, Quill, and cannula are advanced into the clearest space and most open direction between the parietal and visceral peritoneum. Following this, the scope and cannula are removed and the Quill catheter guide is left in place. The next step in the procedure involves the dilation of the Quill and musculature to approximately 0.5 cm. This is large enough to allow the catheter to be easily inserted through the rectus muscle and the cuff to be advanced into the muscle. The catheter follows the path previously viewed by the peritoneoscope as directed by the Quill guide. As long as the Quill guide stays in position the catheter will advance into the desired place. The catheter is advanced on a stylet and is actually 'dilating' its way until the cuff arrives and stops at the muscular layer. Placing the cuff in the musculature can be accomplished using a pair of haemostats advancing the cuff within the Quill guide. Thereafter, the Quill guide is removed, hydraulic function of the catheter checked, the tunnel made subcutaneously using a trochar, and the catheter brought out through the exit site – similar to the surgical insertion technique.

Excellent results with this technique were reported by its originator. More recently Copley *et al.* [172] reported 1183 patient-months experience with 135 double-cuff swan-neck coiled catheters inserted peritoneoscopically over 40-month period. Complications were few and the overall 40-month survival probability was 62%. Nine catheters were removed because of obstruction and 16 for catheter-related infections.

Seldinger (guidewire) and peel-away sheath

This technique may be used for insertion of a straight and coiled Tenckhoff catheters as well as of swan-neck Tenckhoff straight and coiled catheters. The pre-insertion patient preparation is similar to the preparation described for rigid catheter insertion. The procedure may be done with [131] or without [132–135] prefilling the abdomen with dialysis solution. Prefilling of the abdomen is accomplished through a temporary peritoneal catheter.

In the 'dry' method a 2 cm incision is made and the 'dry' abdomen is entered with an 18-gauge needle (e.g. the Verres needle as used for laparoscopy). A guidewire is passed through the needle and the needle is withdrawn. The introducer (dilator) with sheath is passed over the guidewire. After the dilator-sheath is inserted, the dilator is removed, leaving the sheath in place. The Tenckhoff or swan-neck Tenckhoff catheter, stiffened by a partially inserted blunt stiffening stilette, is then directed down into the sheath [134, 135]. The catheter may also be introduced without stiffening [132, 133]. As the cuff advances, the sheath is split by pulling tabs on its opposing sides. Splitting the sheath allows the cuff to advance to a position next to the abdominal wall. By further splitting and retraction the sheath is removed from its position around the catheter. The subcutaneous tunnel is then created as in surgical placement. With this technique the incidence of early leak is very low. However, the risk of viscus perforation and improper placement of catheter are the drawbacks of this technique.

Surgical (by dissection)

Surgeons perform 87% of catheter implantations, and the majority of the procedures (73%) are done by surgical dissection [120]. Dissective placement is mandatory for catheters with stabilizing devices (e.g. flanges) at the parietal surfaces (Toronto Western Hospital, swan-neck Missouri, and swan-neck presternal). The paramedian approach through the rectus muscle, currently used in our centre, will be described [57, 121, 125].

General anaesthesia is avoided, if possible, because it predisposes patients to vomiting and constipation, and requires voluntary coughing during the postoperative period as a part of pulmonary atelectasis prevention; coughing, vomiting and straining markedly increase intra-abdominal pressures and predispose patients to abdominal leaks [173]. The patient frequently receives propofol 100 µg/kg/min intravenously for 6 min to initiate

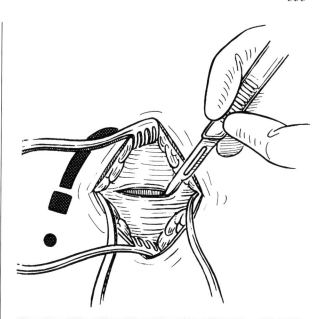

Figure 17. An incision through the anterior rectus sheath. (Figs 17–24 are reproduced from ref. 130 with permission.)

monitored anaesthesia care (MAC) sedation prior to catheter placement and a maintenance dose of 25–50 µg/kg/min thereafter.

The surgical preparation of the abdominal wall consists of a threefold scrub with Betadine soap, pat-drying and painting with Betadine paint solutions and again pat-drying. Skin markings are usually very faint after surgical preparation and require remarking with a sterile surgical pen. Finally the abdomen is covered with a sterile, transparent surgical drape. The skin and surrounding tissues of the tunnel are anaesthetized with 1% lidocaine.

A 3–4 cm transverse incision is made through the skin and the subcutaneous tissue. Perfect haemostasis, preferably using electrocautery, is mandatory. The anterior rectus sheath is exposed and infiltrated with 1% lidocaine. A transverse incision is made in the anterior rectus sheath (Fig. 17). The rectus muscle fibres are separated bluntly in the direction of the fibres down to the posterior rectus sheath. Self-retaining retractors are helpful to hold muscle fibres away from the operative field. The sheath is infiltrated with 1% lidocaine. A purse-string non-absorbable suture of 2-O monofilament is placed through the posterior rectus sheath, transversalis fascia and the peritoneum. A 5 mm incision, reaching the peritoneal cavity, is made with a scalpel and stretched slightly (Fig. 18).

The catheter is threaded on a long, blunt stiffening stilette. About 1 cm of catheter is left beyond the tip of the stilette to protect the bowels. The edges of the

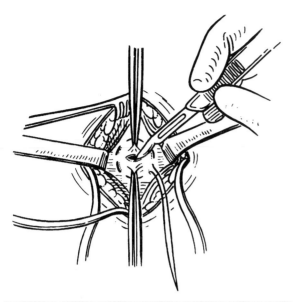

Figure 18. The posterior rectus sheath has been exposed, a purse-string suture has been made, and a 5 mm incision reaching the peritoneal cavity is being created with a scalpel.

opening are lifted. The catheter is inserted through the opening and introduced into the opposite deep pelvis if there is no resistance. The patient may feel some pressure on the bladder or rectum. When the catheter with stilette is about half to three-quarters inserted, the stilette is removed and the catheter continues to be pushed into the pelvis.

Using a combination of retraction on the peritoneal edge and pushing, the bead is introduced into the peritoneal cavity. The flange is placed flat on the posterior rectus sheath and the purse-string suture is tied securely between the bead and the flange (Fig. 19). The stripe must be positioned anteriorly and the flange is anchored with four 2-O monofila-

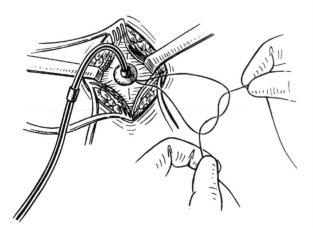

Figure 19. A purse-string suture of peritoneum and rectus fascia is tied securely between the bead and the flange.

ment, non-absorbable sutures into the posterior rectus sheath at the 6, 9, 12, and 3 o'clock positions (Fig. 20). The self-retaining retractors are removed and the deep or internal cuff is buried among the muscle fibres. A small stab wound is made in the anterior rectus sheath above the transverse incision. The catheter is grasped with a haemostat and pulled through the stab incision (Fig. 21). The stripe is positioned anteriorly. The remaining procedure differs for the swan-neck Missouri and swan-neck presternal catheter. The relationship of the catheter

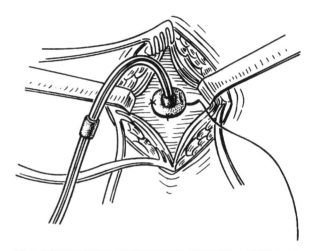

Figure 20. The flange is anchored with four 2-O monofilament, non-absorbable sutures into the posterior rectus sheath at the 6, 9, 12, and 3 o'clock positions.

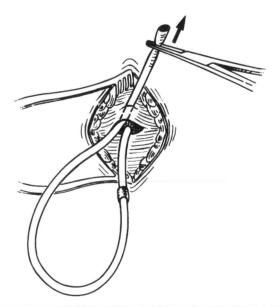

Figure 21. The catheter is passed through the incision centred above the transverse incision.

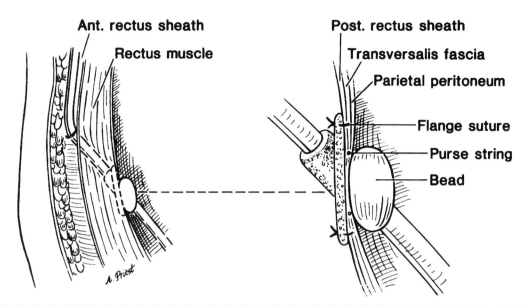

Figure 22. The relationship of the catheter to the tissue structures of the abdominal wall. The bead is in the peritoneal cavity, the flange is flat on the posterior rectus sheath, the purse-string is between the bead and the flange, the deep cuff is in the rectus muscle.

to the tissue structures of the abdominal wall is shown in Fig. 22.

Swan-neck Missouri. A superior subcutaneous pocket is made to the level of skin marking to accommodate the bent portion of the catheter and the external cuff (Fig. 23). The catheter tunnel extending from the cuff to the skin exit should have a diameter

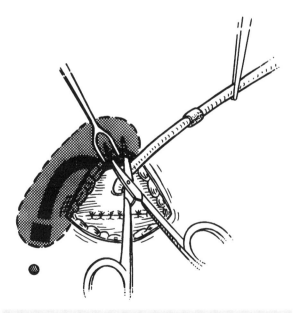

Figure 23. A subcutaneous pocket is made to the level of skin marking to accommodate the bent portion of the catheter and the external cuff.

close to that of catheter tubing. Thus, the last portion of the tunnel (from external cuff to the exit) should be made with a piercing trochar, e.g., the Faller trochar (Kendall Co, Bothell, WA, USA) or a 3/16-inch (4.76 mm, F 15) trochar for Hemovac system (Zimmer Mfg. Co., 11235 Manchester Road, St Louis, MO 63122, USA) of external diameter similar to that of the catheter tubing [121, 125]. A trochar is attached and carefully passed through the pocket and the external exit indicated by the stencil mark (Fig. 24). The bent portion of the catheter is positioned carefully in the subcutaneous pocket. Care is taken to keep the stripe facing frontwards. The external cuff is positioned 2–3 cm from the skin exit. A titanium adapter is attached to the catheter and an extension tube is connected to the adapter [57, 121]. A 1-litre bag of sterile saline or dialysis solution containing 1000 units of heparin is spiked via the extension tubing and the solution is infused. The fluid should all run in 5 min. The wound is checked for leaks and inspected for haemostasis. The transverse incision in the anterior rectus sheath is sewn with a 2–O monofilament non-absorbable suture. After filling the abdomen the bag should be lowered and at least 200 ml of solution should drain within 1 min. If good flow is obtained the wound is irrigated and the skin incision is closed with absorbable subcuticular sutures. The catheter is never sutured at the exit-site. The position of the catheter is confirmed while still in the operating room on abdominal X-ray. The incision is covered with Steri-

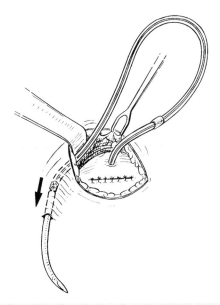

Figure 24. A trochar is attached and passed through the pocket and the external exit indicated by the stencil mark. The piercing trochar is the same diameter as the tubing.

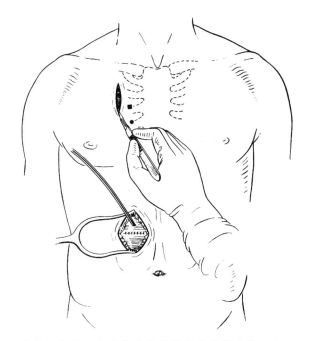

Figure 25. Vertical incision in the parasternal area. (Figs 25–29 are modified from ref. 38 with permission.)

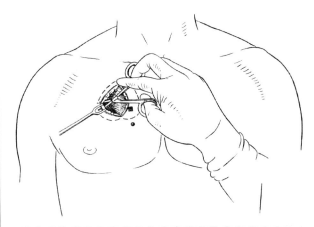

Figure 26. Two small subcutaneous pockets are made on both sides of the chest incision to accommodate the bent section of the upper tube of the catheter.

strips, several layers of high-absorbency gauze dressings and secured with Tegaderm®, which also immobilizes the catheter. The dressing is to be left in place for a week. In cases with bleeding or large drainage from the incision or exit the dressing should be changed earlier.

Swan-neck presternal. A vertical 3–4 cm incision is made in the parasternal area (Fig. 25) or over the sternum at the level of the second and third rib [38, 125]. Using a combination of sharp and blunt dissection, two small subcutaneous pockets are made on both sides of the incision to accommodate the bent section of the upper (chest) tube of the catheter. The pockets are dissected enough to accommodate the middle and superficial cuffs (Fig. 26). Careful haemostasis is essential.

A Scanlan tunneller (Scanlan International, 1 Scanlan Plaza, St Paul, MN 56107, USA) is used to create a tunnel extending from the abdominal incision to the presternal or parasternal area to permit joining the upper and lower tube. The tunneller, developed for tunneling vascular grafts, consists of an outside disposable sheath, blunt tip, and an inner rod with a spring clamp. Depending on the size of the patient either a green (51 cm long) or an orange (30 cm long) tunneller may be used. The metal rod serves to stiffen the tunneller as it is pushed through the subcutaneous tissue and the spring clamp is used to grasp and pull the upper tube through the sheath

[125]. The tunneller is pushed from the abdominal incision to the chest incision (Fig. 27) using great care. The blunt tip of the outside sheath is removed. Keeping the stripe in front as a guide, the abdominal end of the upper tube is grasped with the spring clamp and pulled caudally through the sheath, and the sheath is removed by pulling in the caudal direction.

The middle cuff of the upper tube is carefully placed on the stencil mark. When the catheter is appropriately positioned the lengths of the two tubes are measured and the tubes are trimmed to an

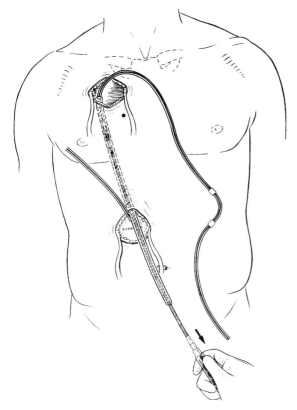

Figure 27. A tunnel between the abdominal and chest incisions is made with a Scanlan tunneller, the upper tube is pulled caudally through the sheath.

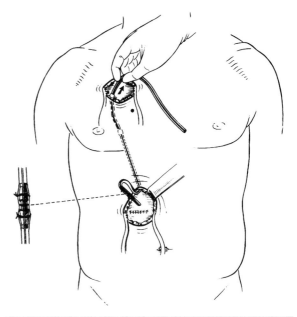

Figure 28. Both parts of the catheter are tied over the titanium connector and the catheter is pulled cephalad.

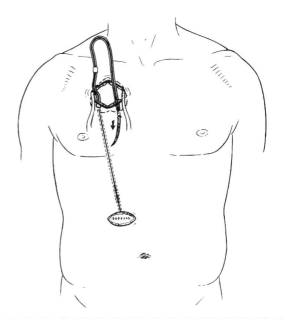

Figure 29. A trochar of the same size as the catheter tubing is attached and carefully passed through the pocket, and the external exit is indicated by the stencil mark.

appropriate length. Sufficient length on each tube should be left to facilitate connection. A titanium connector is inserted into the upper tube and then the connector is inserted into the lower tube. The stripes on both tubes are placed facing up. A 1-O Ticron® tie is now placed and tied on both tubes over the appropriate groove of the titanium connector. The two sutures are tied together (Fig. 28) and the titanium connector is positioned in the subcutaneous tissue approximately 5–8 cm above the abdominal incision.

A trochar of the same size as the catheter tubing is attached and carefully passed through the pocket and the external exit indicated by the stencil mark (Fig. 29). The stripe should be facing front. The trochar is disconnected. The bent portion of the catheter is carefully positioned in the subcutaneous pocket. The titanium Luer lock connector is attached. One litre of normal saline is infused through the infusion set and drained immediately. Outflow should be approximately 200 ml in 1 min. The wounds are checked for leaks, irrigated, and inspected for haemostasis. The transverse incision in

the anterior rectus sheath is closed with a 2-O monofilament non-absorbable suture. Skin incisions are again inspected for haemostasis. Any bleeding vessels are controlled with electrocautery cauterized and the incisions are closed with absorbable subcuticular sutures. The operative site is covered with several layers of high-absorbency gauze dressings and secured with Tegaderm®, which also immobilizes the catheter. The dressing is to be left in place for a week.

Tenckhoff. This technique is similar to that of the swan-neck Missouri catheter; however, because there is no inter-cuff bend, the anterior stripe position is not essential and the subcutaneous pocket is not needed. Instead a straight upward or laterally curved tunnel is made with the help of a piercing trochar. The subcutaneous cuff is positioned 2–3 cm from the exit. As there is no flange the deep cuff is positioned longitudinally, parallel to the rectus muscle fibres, on the posterior rectus fascia.

Swan-neck Tenckhoff. A combination of techniques for the Tenckhoff and swan-neck Missouri catheters is used. Deep (inner cuff) is positioned longitudinally on the posterior rectus sheath with the stripe facing front. As explained earlier, in the section entitled 'Radiopaque stripe', if the left catheter is used for the right tunnel and vice-versa, the stripe must be positioned posteriorly. The subcutaneous pocket is made in the same way as with swan-neck Missouri catheter.

Moncrief–Popovich technique. This is a new technique which allows tissue ingrowth into the cuff material without exposure to the skin surface area. Unlike other techniques the distal (external segment) of the catheter is completely buried and remains in the subcutaneous tunnel until exteriorized after 3–8 weeks post-catheter insertion [40]. A video [174] demonstrating the technique is available from the Austin Biomedical Research Institute, 4211 Medical Parkway, Austin, TX 78756, USA. Using swan-neck catheters with this technique Moncrief and co-workers reported a significant reduction in peritonitis incidence [40].

Laparoscopic technique

Nijhuis, Smulders, and Jakimowicz [175] have described a unique peritoneoscopic technique using a two-puncture technique for the placement of a continuous ambulatory peritoneal dialysis catheter. A pneumoperitoneum is created using a combination 4.5 mm trochar/veress needle introduced into the contralateral upper abdominal quadrant. A 3.5 mm zero-degree telescope is inserted through this trochar and an abdominal exploration is carried out. A 1.5–2 cm long incision is made in a perimedian site on the ipsilateral side of the abdomen. The sub-

cutaneous tissues are dissected and the anterior rectus sheath is transversely incised. Using blunt dissection a pathway is created between and beneath the muscle. A 10 mm trochar is passed under visual control above of the transversalis fascia and peritoneum. The trochar is then introduced into the abdominal cavity under direct vision and the peritoneal catheter is positioned in the pouch of Douglas. The cannula is removed and the catheter withdrawn so that the deep cuff is situated within the rectus muscle. The incisions are closed in standard fashion. This technique allows visual control and correct placement of the catheter in the pelvis. By placing the catheter in this fashion the authors have reduced their catheter-related problems and established a functioning catheter in about three-quarters of the cases.

The laparoscope can also be used for other purposes in patients on chronic peritoneal dialysis. Specifically, catheter malposition and intra-abdominal adhesions are two conditions in which the laparoscope may be of considerable help. Entry to the abdominal cavity is established by direct cut down in one of the upper abdominal quadrants. A purse-string suture is placed in the peritoneum and posterior fascia so that a snug fit around the trochar will be obtained. The trochar is inserted under direct vision and the purse-string tied, a pneumoperitoneum is created by connecting to a CO_2 source. Visual inspection will then demonstrate the problem of either adhesions and/or catheter malposition. Clinical judgement is used to place a second port, which is done under direct vision. Using grasping forceps or an electrocautery hook or scissors, the catheter can be repositioned, or the adhesions may be taken down. These techniques are of great help in salvaging an otherwise unworkable catheter.

Catheter break-in and catheter care

Immediate intraperitoneal segment care

In the operating room the position of the catheter is checked by a plain X-ray of the abdomen. Absence of catheter kink in the tunnel and the catheter-tip location in the true pelvis usually predict excellent catheter function.

Peritoneal dialysis

Postoperatively, the patient is attached to a cycler to perform additional exchanges. Each litre of dialysis solution contains 1000 units of heparin. One-half or 1 litre volumes of dialysis solutions are used for the first supine peritoneal dialysis. Usual cycler settings are: 10 min fill time, 0 min dwell, and 12 min outflow. In spite of clear dialysate in the first post-implantation washout, the dialysate is usually blood-tinged during the first cycler exchange. No dwell exchanges are continued until the dialysate is clear. If immediate peritoneal dialysis is needed the patient continues on a cycler in the strict supine position with dwell time prolonged to 30–40 min. We do not commence peritoneal dialysis in the vertical position sooner than 10 days postimplantation; thus CAPD or a last bag CCPD are not used for 10 days. The patient may be maintained on haemodialysis through the temporary access for logistical reasons before peritoneal dialysis training can be started, or may require haemodialysis because of catheter malfunction (see below).

Exit-site care

Exit-site care in the immediate postimplantation period seems to be crucial for long-term results regarding infectious complications. The exit should be carefully evaluated every week for quality of healing.

Exit-site appearance postimplantation

Unless a large haematoma in the wound is present, all exits look the same a week after implantation [60]. The exit is painless or minimally tender with light pink colour of less than 13 mm in diameter from border to border (including the width of the catheter). Blood clot or serosanguineous drainage is visible in the sinus. No epidermis is visible in the sinus and the sinus lining is white and plain. Signs of good healing include a decrease in colour saturation and diameter around the exit, change of drainage to serous, decreased drainage amount, decreased tenderness, and progression of epidermis into the sinus. An increase in colour diameter or saturation around the exit, change of drainage to yellow, change of granulation tissue colour to mottled, pink or red, change of granulation tissue texture into slightly exuberant or exuberant are signs of poor healing.

Our exit site study [60, 176] revealed four types of healing exits. (1) Fast healing exits had no drainage or minimal moisture deep inside by the third week; epidermis started to enter into the sinus within 2–3 weeks, progressed steadily, and covered at least half the visible sinus tract 4–6 weeks after implant-ation. (2) In slow-healing exits without infection, epidermis started to enter into the sinus after 3 weeks or progressed slowly and did not cover half the visible sinus by 5 weeks; the sinus might have had serous or serosanguineous, but never purulent, drainage persistent up to 4 weeks. (3) Healing interrupted by infection initially looked identical to the fast-healing exit, but within 6 weeks the epidermis had not progressed, or had regressed, granulation tissue became soft or frankly fleshy; drainage increased and/or became purulent. (4) In slow-healing exits due to early infection, granulation tissue became soft or fleshy and/or drainage became purulent by 2–3 weeks; sinus epidermization was delayed or progressed slowly, only after infection was appropriately treated.

Early colonization of the exit was the most significant factor in determining the healing pattern; the later the colonization, the better healing [60]. Positive culture from either sinus washout or peri-exit smear 1 week after implantation was associated with early exit infection, a higher peritonitis rate, and a high probability of catheter loss due to an exit/tunnel infection, and higher peritonitis rate; however, the time to the first peritonitis episode was not shorter than in the groups with later exit colonization [60].

Early care

To delay bacterial colonization of the exit site and to minimize trauma, dressings should not be changed frequently [177]. It is generally agreed that postoperative dressing changes should be restricted to specially trained staff [178]. We do weekly dressing changes for the first few weeks post-catheter implantation if there is no excessive drainage. Once the exit is colonized, by week 3 in the majority of cases [60], more frequent dressing changes are indicated, because the major rationale for infrequent dressing changes, avoidance of exit colonization, no longer exists. Moreover, more frequent cleansing of the exit will decrease the number of bacteria at the exit. Aseptic technique, including both masking and wearing sterile gloves, should be used for postoperative dressing changes. Non-ionic surfactant is used to help gauze removal if it is attached to the scab. If the scab is forcibly removed the epidermal layer is broken, a new scab has to be made and the epidermization is prolonged. Care is taken to avoid catheter pulling or twisting. The exit and skin surrounding the catheter are cleansed with non-ionic surfactant (e.g. Poloxamer 188), patted dry with sterile gauze, covered with several layers of gauze dressings, and secured with air-permeable tape.

The exit and visible sinus should be evaluated for quality of healing at each dressing change throughout the 6-week healing period. If healing does not progress, if there are signs of deterioration or infection, the exit is probably already colonized [60]. A clinical culture of the exudate should be taken, and an appropriate systemic antibiotic should be given.

We recommend that our patients do not shower or take tub baths post-catheter implantation, to avoid colonization with waterborne organisms, and to prevent skin maceration. Once more frequent dressing changes are started (after approximately 2 weeks) the patient may take a shower, but only before the dressing change, otherwise he/she must take sponge baths and avoid exit wetting.

Protecting the catheter from mechanical stress seems to be extremely important, especially during break-in. Catheters should be anchored in such a way that the patient's movements are only minimally transmitted to the exit. The method of catheter immobilization is individualized, depending on exit location and shape of the abdomen. We believe that better exit protection prevents infections in most patients.

Extended prophylactic antibiotics

Our findings of the detrimental effect of the early exit colonization on the quality of healing and long term infectious complications led us to postulate that exit infections and peritonitis rates might be decreased by delaying exit colonization using prophylactic antibiotics for at least 2 weeks after implantation [60]. Such an approach has not been evaluated in patients in prospective randomized studies; however, a study in rats showed that intraperitoneal antibiotic prophylaxis for 3 weeks after catheter implantation was an effective way to prevent early colonization of exit-sites, provided a better healing quality and lower incidence of catheter-related infections [179]. Based on these premises, our current approach is to use a systemic antibiotic against Gram-positive bacteria (usually cephalothin or trimethoprim-sulphamethoxazole) for 2 weeks after implantation, and a local antibiotic (usually mupirocin ointment or cream) for at least 6 weeks.

Late care

Traditional approach. Late care, after the healing process is completed, is simpler. The results of a prospective study indicate that cleaning with soap and water is the least expensive and tends to prevent infections better than povidone-iodine painting and hydrogen peroxide cleaning [180]. After cleansing, the exit has to be patted dry with sterile gauze and well immobilized. Most of our patients use a dressing cover for 6–12 months after implantation. One year after implantation patients are allowed to omit use of a cover dressing, if desired. We could not find any reason why in some patients an uncovered exit seems to do better, in others worse.

We recommend that our patients use only a shower, and avoid submersion in water, particularly in a Jacuzzi, hot tub, or public pool, unless watertight exit protection can be implemented. Prolonged submersion in water containing high concentrations of bacteria frequently leads to severe infection with consequent loss of catheter. Swimming in the ocean, and well-sterilized private pools, is less dangerous. Exit care must be performed immediately after a shower or water submersion, with particular attention to obtaining a well-dried exit. The surrounding skin is coated with a skin protector and secured with Tegaderm. Patients with the swan-neck presternal catheter may take a hot tub bath without exit-site submersion. Because of this feature this catheter was dubbed the 'bath-tub' catheter [108].

Emerging approach. Excellent results observed with mupirocin ointment in healing exits, in prevention of infections in *S. aureus* nasal carriers, and in treatment of equivocal exits and recurrent exit-site (see below) infections inclined us to extend indefinitely the use of mupirocin ointment on the exit, with excellent results. Patients report that the epidermis around the exit is less dry and chafed as the catheter 'glides' better over the sinus epidermis. It is possible that the good results of mupirocin and other ointments applied on the exits are, at least partly, related to the moisturizing/lubricating action of the ointment base.

Early soft catheter complications

Early complications post-soft catheter insertion are similar to those after implantation of the rigid catheter (Table 9), but their frequency is lower, particularly with surgical, peritoneoscopic, or laparoscopic insertion. Blood-tinged dialysate is common post-implantation but severe bleeding occurs very rarely with surgical insertion. Dialysate leaks are unlikely if ambulatory peritoneal dialysis is postponed for at least 10 days after implantation [181]. This compli-

Table 9. Early catheter obstruction

Cause	Prevention/treatment
Occlusion by bowel	Laxatives
Occlusion by bladder	Empty bladder
Clot	Rinse out blood, heparin, urokinase, dislodge
Omental wrap	Partial omentectomy
Multiple adhesions	Adhesiolysis
Kink in the tunnel	Surgical correction

cation is particularly rare with the Toronto Western Hospital, swan-neck Missouri, swan-neck presternal, and Lifecath® column disc catheters. Early leak is usually external and may be confused with serous drainage from the exit. A diagnosis of a leak is supported by a higher glucose concentration in the drainage compared to the simultaneously measured blood glucose concentration.

Poor dialysate return is usually due to catheter obstruction if loss of siphon or tubing occlusion is ruled out. The most common reason of catheter obstruction is occlusion of the tip by bowel and/or bladder or intraluminal formation of clot (Table 9). Emptying the bladder and using laxatives may restore catheter function if there is occlusion by bladder or bowel. Clot may be prevented by rinsing out blood from the peritoneal cavity and using heparin and/or can be dislodged by pushing into the peritoneal cavity or pulling by suction using a syringe filled with heparinized saline. If these manoeuvres are unsuccessful the catheter may be filled with urokinase (Abbokinase) 5000 IU, diluted in normal saline. Urokinase may open the obstruction in 10–15% of cases [182]. Using high pressure during fluid infusion, Hashimoto *et al.* [183] were able to open six catheters occluded by clots. Catheter kinking in the tunnel is usually associated with two-way obstruction, is recognizable on abdominal X-ray in two views, and requires surgical correction as soon as diagnosis is made. If the catheter is not kinked, but does not function for 2 weeks, omental wrapping or multiple adhesions are most likely and omentectomy or adhesiolysis using laparoscopy may be required.

A reversed one-way peritoneal catheter obstruction, in which the fluid can be drained but the next infusion cannot be performed, is extremely rare. Recently we have observed such a case [184]. The catheter tip was obstructed with a clot, which caused inflow obstruction. This clot was removed by suction with a syringe. We speculated that the clot was firmly anchored in the catheter tip, and that only a few proximal side-holes were opened. The outflow was not obstructed because the catheter tip must have been located in a large pocket of free space. The clot behaved like an accordion. During drainage the clot became stretched and narrowed (like an accordion bellow in extension) and fluid was able to flow through some of the side-holes. During infusion the clot buckled up and widened (like a compressed accordion bellow), completely occluding the central lumen and side-holes.

Another reason for obstruction may be catheter adherence to the peritoneum. This complication was found in children who have undergone partial omentectomy at the time of insertion of a single-cuff, straight Tenckhoff catheter. Relocation of such catheters may be attempted with a so-called 'whiplash' technique [185]. After localization of the catheter adherence site, using a strict sterile technique, a blunted steel trochar is inserted into the catheter and gently advanced until the trochar tip is 5–7 cm proximal to the tip of the catheter. Using a deep cuff as a fulcrum, and using short and rapid whiplash motions, the catheter is then freed from the adherence point. The catheter tip is then, under fluoroscopy, relocated to a new site. A modification of this method using a pliable copper thread was successfully used in adults [186]. A catheter migrated to the upper abdomen may be relocated using a guidewire [118, 187, 188]. Although these methods may obviate the need for surgery, they are not without risk. The guidewire may break during manipulations, perforate the catheter and lead to recurrent peritonitis.

Catheter migration out of the true pelvis is seen frequently on abdominal X-rays done for various reasons in patients with functioning catheters [189]. While about 20% of X-rays showed the catheter tip translocated to the upper abdomen, only 20% of these translocated catheters (4% of the total) were obstructed. The remaining functioning malpositioned catheters were either permanently translocated or repositioned spontaneously to the true pelvis. About 3% of catheters in our series were obstructed with the tip in the true pelvis [190].

While the great majority of malpositioned catheters are not obstructed, a catheter with its tip in the upper abdomen is still about six times more likely to be obstructed than a normally positioned catheter. The migration of the catheter tip may, however, be the result of the obstruction rather than its cause; omentum entangling the catheter tip may be responsible for its translocation.

Repositioning of the internal catheter segment is best done surgically using a laparoscopic method.

In our experience, if this method fails to restore catheter function because the peritoneum is not usable for peritoneal dialysis because of massive adhesions, catheter relocation or replacement in such a situation is worthless. The patient has to be transferred to haemodialysis.

Viscus perforation is unlikely with surgical catheter insertion. Early peritonitis with a soft catheter is half of that reported with a rigid catheter, even in treatment of acute renal failure [165]. Abdominal pain is more likely with straight catheters due to 'jet effect' and tip pressure, as discussed in the section on infusion/pressure pain.

Late soft catheter complications

Factors influencing catheter complications have been discussed earlier (see Table 1). Complications are not randomly distributed throughout the life of the catheter. Whereas leaks and malfunctions occur shortly after catheter implantation, infectious complications lead to catheter failure later [124].

Exit-site infection

There is no single definition of exit-site infection that has achieved universal approval. The most widely accepted is that published by Pierratos in 1984 [191], which was agreed upon by the vast majority of *Peritoneal Dialysis Bulletin* Editorial Board members. Pierratos defined exit-site infection as: 'Redness or skin induration or purulent discharge from the exit site. Formation of crust around the exit may not indicate infection. Positive cultures from the exit site in the absence of inflammation do not indicate infection'. This definition implies the presence of infection in the instance in which laboratory cultures are negative, and rejects the existence of infection based on a positive culture without inflammation.

Several publications used similar criteria [192–194]. This definition, however, is not sufficiently precise to differentiate infected from non-infected exits in many instances. It is inferred that an exit without signs of infection is healthy, thus only two categories (infected or not infected) are assumed. We have found only one description of a normal exit-site and various degrees of infection in the 1980s [195]. The rates of exit infections and the outcome of treatment are astonishingly discrepant in the literature. Rates as low as 0.05 or 0.1 per patient per year [196, 197], or as high as 1.02 per patient per year [193], have been reported. It is

likely that this discrepancy in infection rates does not reveal a real variation but reflects disagreement regarding exit-site infection definition [195, 198].

There is no difficulty in the diagnosis of peritonitis; the dialysate contains either a small number of cells when uninfected or a large number of cells, mostly granulocytes, when infected. Normal dialysate does not contain microorganisms; a correctly performed culture is usually positive in peritonitis. Bacterial peritonitis cannot be cured without antibiotics. Attempts to classify exit appearance into two categories (infected and not infected) is difficult, if not impossible, because infected and uninfected exit appearances overlap. This overlap is due to the peculiarity of tissue reaction to the foreign body penetrating the skin, and stems from the delicate balance between bacteria in the sinus and host defences as described above. The presence of a small amount of exudate causing crust formation does not indicate infection, but if the bacterial attack is more severe, or the host defences are weakened, then the amount of exudate increases; granulation tissue proliferates, becomes more vascularized, epithelium regresses and signs of infection become obvious. Low-grade exit infection may abate without systemic antibiotics.

Classification of exit-site appearance

For 8 years we evaluated exit-site appearance in the immediate postimplantation period and later, after the exit is healed [60, 77]. From the 565 evaluations of 61 healed exit-sites in 56 patients evolved a new classification [199]. The classification is based on the cardinal signs of inflammation as proposed by Aulus Cornelius Celsus in his treatise, *De Medicina*, written in the first century AD. These are well known: *calor* (heat), *rubor* (redness), *turgor* (swelling), and *dolor* (pain). Additional features, specific for an exit of any skin-penetrating foreign body, are: drainage, regression of epidermis, and exuberance (profuse overgrowth) of granulation tissue ('proud flesh'). Granulation tissue is defined as exuberant if it is significantly elevated above the epidermis level. Culture results did not influence exit classification. Positive cultures in exits not inflamed indicate colonization, not infection. Cultures were commonly negative from infected exits on antibiotic therapy. However, inflammation in almost all cases is caused by infection, regardless of culture results. Inflammatory responses to tubing itself or local irritants are rare.

Improvement or deterioration of inflammation is associated with respective decreases or increases of pain, induration, drainage, and/or exuberant granulation tissue, and/or regression or progression of epithelium in the sinus. Increased lightness (pink, pale pink) or darkness (deep black, brown) and decrease in colour diameter indicate improvement, increase in red colour saturation and diameter indicate deterioration. Ultimately a new classification with five distinct categories of exit appearances has been established: acute infection, chronic infection, equivocal, good and perfect. Finally, two special categories were identified: external cuff infection and traumatized exit. Trauma may result in various appearances. Cuff infection may not be associated with exit infection. Detailed descriptions of the various exit appearances illustrated by over 200 colour photographs have already been published [60, 77, 176, 199]. The characteristics for each category of catheter exit site are summarized in Table 10 .

Acute catheter exit-site infection.   This involves purulent and/or bloody drainage from the exit-site, spontaneous or after pressure on the sinus; and/or swelling; and/or erythema with diameter 13 mm or more from border to border; and regression of epithelium in the sinus. Acute catheter inflammation lasts less than 4 weeks and may be accompanied by pain, exuberant granulation tissue around the exit or in the sinus and the presence of a scab or crust. Exit culture may be negative in patients receiving antibiotics.

Chronic catheter exit site infection.   There is purulent and/or bloody drainage from the exit-site, spontaneous or after pressure on the sinus; and/or exuberant granulation tissue around the exit and/or in the sinus; and regression of epithelium in the sinus. Chronic infection persists for more than 4 weeks and crust or scab is frequently present. Swelling, erythema, and/or pain indicate exacerbation, otherwise they are absent. Exit culture may be negative in patients receiving antibiotics.

Equivocally infected catheter exit site.   There is purulent and/or bloody drainage that cannot be expressed outside the sinus, accompanied by the regression of epithelium, and occurrence of slightly exuberant granulation tissue around the exit and/or in the sinus. Erythema with a diameter less than 13 mm from border to border may be present, but pain, swelling, and external drainage are absent. Exit culture may be negative in patients receiving antibiotics.

Good catheter exit.   Exit colour is natural, pale pink, purplish or dark and there is no purulent or bloody drainage. Clear or thick exudate may be visible in the sinus. Mature epithelium covers only part of the sinus; the rest is covered by fragile epithelium or plain granulation tissue. Pain, swelling, and erythema are absent. Positive peri-exit smear culture, if present, indicates colonization not infection.

Perfect catheter exit.   This is at least 6 months old with its entire visible length of sinus tract covered with the keratinized (mature) epithelium. Exit colour is natural or dark and there is no drainage. A small, easily detachable crust may be present in the sinus or around the exit. Positive peri-exit smear culture, if present, indicates colonization not infection.

External cuff infection without exit infection.   This involves intermittent or chronic, purulent, bloody or gooey drainage, spontaneous or after pressure on the cuff, and induration of the tissue around the cuff. Exuberant granulation tissue may be seen deep in the sinus; sinus epithelium may be chronically or intermittently macerated. Exit site may look normal on external examination. Ultrasound may show fluid collection around the cuff, but negative ultrasound does not rule out cuff infection. Exit culture may be negative in patients receiving antibiotics.

Traumatized exit.   Features of traumatized exit depend on the intensity of trauma and the time interval until examination. Common features of trauma are: pain, bleeding, scab and deterioration of exit appearance (e.g. perfect exit transforms to good or equivocal or acutely infected).

Care and treatment recommendations

The use of the classification system facilitates early diagnosis of exit problems, and treatment can be more specific. Exit-site care and treatment for each appearance category are summarized in Table 11.

Acute exit-site infection.   A culture of exit-site exudate or, if there is swelling/erythema without expressible exudate, a smear culture of the skin surrounding the exit should be taken as soon as a clinical diagnosis of an acute exit-site infection is made. Systemic antibiotics should be started before culture results are available. Gram-positive organisms are frequently the cause of exit-site infections. Accordingly, oral cephalosporin or trimethoprim-sulphamethoxazole may be selected as the initial

Table 10. Characteristics of each category of exit-site appearance

	Perfect	Good	Equivocal	Acute infection <4 weeks	Chronic infection >4 weeks	Cuff infection without exit infection
Exit						
Pain/tenderness	None	None	None	May be present	Only if exacerbation	May be present over cuff
Colour	Natural, pale pink or dark	Natural, pale pink, purplish or dark, bright pink <13 mm	Bright pink or red <13 mm	Bright pink or red >13 mm	Bright pink or red >13 mm only if exacerbation	Natural, pale pink, purplish or dark, bright pink <13 mm
Crust	None or small, easily detached or specks of crust on dressing	None or small, easily detached or specks of cust on dressing	Present, may be large and difficult to detach	Present	Present, may be difficult to detach	Typically absent
Scab	None	None	None	May be present	May be present	Absent
Drainage	None	None	None even with pressure on sinus; dried exudate on dressing	Purulent or bloody, spontaneous or after pressure on sinus; wet exudate on dressing	Purulent or bloody, wet exudate on dressing	Chronic or intermittent; purulent, bloody, tenacious or 'gluey'
Swelling	None	None	None	May be present	Occurs only if exacerbation	Cuff induration may be felt on palpation; negative ultrasound does not rule out the diagnosis
Granulation tissue	None	None	Plain or slightly exuberant	Slightly exuberant or 'proud flesh' may be present	'Proud flesh' or slightly exuberant typically visible	None
Sinus						
Epithelium	Strong, mature; covers visible sinus	Strong, mature at rim; fragile or mucosal deeper	Absent or covers part of sinus	Absent or covers part of sinus	Absent or covers only part of sinus	Covers most or all of sinus; may be macerated
Granulation tissue	None	Plain beyond epithelium	Slightly exuberant	Slightly exuberant or 'proud flesh'	'Proud flesh' or slightly exuberant	None or exuberant deep in sinus
Drainage	None or barely visible; clear or thick	None or barely visible clear or thick	Purulent or bloody, sometimes clear	Purulent or bloody	Purulent or bloody	Purulent, bloody, gluey; may be seen only after pressure on cuff; clot or dried blood in sinus

Trauma may result in pain, bleeding, scab, and deterioration of exit appearance. Exit appearance depends on intensity of trauma and time of evaluation.
Reprinted from ref. 200 with permission.

Table 11. Exit-site treatment and care for each category of exit-site appearance

	Equivocal infection	Acute infection	Chronic infection	Cuff infection
Evaluation	Culture and sensitivities on peri-exit smear; Gram stain	Culture and sensitivities on exudate; Gram stain	Culture and sensitivities on exudate; Gram stain	Palpation of cuff and tunnel; culture and sensitivities and Gram stain of exudate (spontaneous or after pressure on cuff); ultrasound or cuff/tunnel
Initial therapy	Cauterize slightly exuberant granulation tissue. Topical mupirocin. Exit care daily; clean with mild disinfectant soap; do not use strong oxidants on granulation tissue; use a sterile absorbent dressing.	Cauterize slightly exuberant and exuberant granulation tissue. First-generation cephalosporin for Gram-positive organisms; Quinolone for Gram-negative organisms; vancomycin for methicillin-resistant S. aureus. Exit care daily or b.i.d.; clean with mild disinfectant liquid soap or nonionic surfactant agent; do not use strong oxidants on granulation tissue; use a sterile, absorbent dressing.	Cauterize slightly exuberant and exuberant granulation tissue. First-generation cephalosporin for Gram-positive organisms; Quinolone for Gram-negative organisms; vancomycin for methicillin-resistant S. aureus. Exit care daily or b.i.d.; clean with mild disinfectant liquid soap or nonionic surfactant agent; do not use strong oxidants on granulation tissue; use a sterile, absorbent dressing.	Cauterize proud flesh. Initial antibiotic therapy based on Gram stain results.
48 hours	Change to neosporin, gentamicin, or chloramphenicol ointment if Gram-negative organisms on culture.	Adust therapy according to culture and sensitivities.	Adjust therapy according to culture and sensitivities.	Adjust antibiotic according to culture and sensitivities.
Follow-up	If no improvement in 2 weeks, change to systemic antibiotic based on initial culture and sensitivities. Continue therapy 7 days past achieving a good appearance.	Evaluate weekly; reculture if no improvement. Continue to treat for 7 days after achieving a good appearance.	Evaluate every 2 weeks; reculture every 2 weeks if no improvement on appropriate therapy. Add synergistic drug or change antibiotic according to culture and sensitivities. If infection recurs repeatedly after achieving a good appearance: (a) consider chronic antibiotic suppression; (b) if no improvement after a month of treatment, suspect cuff infection and treat as such. If accompanying peritonitis, remove catheter.	Re-evaluate every 2 weeks; reculture monthly. If no remission: (a) consider catheter shaving; (b) consider catheter replacement. If accompanying peritonitis, remove catheter.

Modified from ref. 200 with permission.

antibiotic. The antibiotic prescription should be adjusted after the organism is identified and the antibiotic sensitivity results are available. The antibiotic is initially prescribed for a period of 7–10 days, the time required for an uncomplicated acute infection to heal (achieve a good appearance). If there is no improvement after this period, another appropriate antibiotic is substituted or a second synergistic antibiotic is added. Rifampin is frequently used as a second antibiotic for Staphylococcal infections. Antibiotic therapy is continued for 7 days after achieving the healthy appearance of an exit.

Conditions that delay healing or make therapy ineffective are: cuff and/or tunnel infection, infection due to a resistant organism or virulent pathogens (such as *Staphylococcus aureus*, *Pseudomonas* sp., *Candida*, etc.), and patient non-compliance.

Exuberant granulation tissue (proud flesh) is cauterized with a silver nitrate stick, a procedure widely used in surgical practice, veterinary and human [198, 201]. No more than one or two applications may be necessary in acute infection. This procedure speeds up the healing process and facilitates epithelialization. Cauterization should be restricted to granulation tissue only, and accidental touching of the adjacent epithelium should be avoided. Use of a magnifying glass aids in precise cauterization. This can be done safely by a physician or nurse [202].

Recommendations for the care of infected exit-sites are based on sound surgical practices, and anecdotal experiences. Increasing the frequency of dressing changes to once or twice a day helps the healing process, especially in those with copious drainage. Non-irritating solution (e.g. non-ionic surfactant) is our preferred cleanser to remove drainage and reduce the number of microorganisms. An infected exit should be covered with a sterile dressing to absorb drainage, protect against trauma, and shield against superinfection.

Topical treatments include application of soaks to the exit twice to four times daily, as well as the application of dry heat [107, 178, 203]. Soaking solutions include normal saline, hypertonic saline, sodium hypochlorite, dilute hydrogen peroxide, povidone-iodine and 70% alcohol. Local applications of povidone-iodine ointment, mupirocin, and Neosporin® cream, ointment or ophthalmic solutions have been recommended [178]. In our opinion, strong oxidants and other irritating solutions should not be used. It is our belief that topical antibiotics are of limited value in treating acute or chronic infection with copious drainage, because of the inability to achieve sufficiently high local concentrations [198]; however, topical antibiotics are helpful once drainage diminishes.

Catheter immobilization is a sound practice. Immobilizing a catheter protects it from accidental trauma. Trauma leads to bleeding, and blood is a good medium for microorganisms to multiply in. Catheter immobilization should be continued or implemented during the acute infection stage.

Most acute infections respond favourably to therapy [90]. An exit-site with an acute infection in association with proud flesh and bleeding requires prolonged antibiotic therapy. Association with a positive nasal culture had no influence on the outcome. Recurrent infections that progress to chronic infection and/or cuff infection are associated with a poor prognosis. Catheter removal is indicated when acute exit-site infection leads to tunnel infection and peritonitis.

Chronically infected exit site. The work-up leading to the proper diagnosis of a chronically infected exit-site is similar to that performed to diagnose acute infection. An antibiotic is started immediately after diagnosis, if the patient has not already been on antibiotic. Once the culture and antibiotic sensitivity results are available, an appropriate antibiotic is chosen. A combination of synergistic antibiotics is preferred to a single agent, to avoid emergence of resistant organisms, since the therapy is given over a prolonged period. In chronic infection the bacterial flora or the antibiotic sensitivity may change during the course of treatment. Therefore, an unresponsive exit site may have to be cultured repeatedly for timely diagnosis. The response to treatment is usually slow. The features of the chronic infection change very slowly to those of an equivocal exit and then eventually to those of a good exit site.

The antibiotic therapy and local care of the exit site are continued until the desired features of a good exit are achieved. In some cases exit features change to equivocal and remain as such for a long time. In such cases the systemic antibiotic may be discontinued and replaced with a topical antibiotic. Chronic infection requires repeated cauterization of exuberant granulation tissue. Typically, weekly cauterization for several weeks is necessary. The cauterization is continued as long as the proud flesh persists. The cauterization will discolour the proud flesh from red to grey. Some cases of chronic infection may require long-term (6 months to several years) suppressive doses of a systemic antibiotic. Typically, these cases show reinfection on discontinuing the systemic antibiotic. It is likely that such cases represent undiagnosed cuff infection.

Local care is similar to that used in treating acute infection. After achieving the features of an equivocal exit, the frequency of local care may be reduced to once a day.

Equivocal exit. The equivocal exit site is a subclinical form of infection. If left untreated, most equivocal exits will progress to acute infection. Therefore, aggressive management of equivocal exits assumes great importance. Aggressive local care with a topical antibiotic may cure most equivocal exit sites. Exits with external, slightly exuberant granulation tissue, which usually progress to acute infection, require systemic antibiotics.

Cauterization of the slightly exuberant granulation tissue in the sinus may be necessary. An acute infection may acquire equivocal features during the recovery phase. Such an exit site warrants less aggressive therapy compared to one with acute infection; discontinuation of the systemic antibiotic and daily local care is continued in such a situation.

Local therapy with topical antibiotics is the mainstay of treatment for such an equivocal exit site. A topical antibiotic is chosen based on the exit swab culture results. The topical antibiotics that we have successfully used include mupirocin, Neosporin®, gentamicin, chloramphenicol, and tobramycin. This effectiveness is due to the absence of copious drainage from the sinus tract. Systemic antibiotic may be used in cases unresponsive to topical therapy. Response to therapy is excellent, with cure occurring in almost all instances

Good and perfect exit. Catheter immobilization, protection from trauma, use of liquid soap and water for daily care, and use of Shur-Clens® to remove large, irritating crust are appropriate measures to prevent infection. In our experience a perfect exit is unlikely to become infected unless severely traumatized or grossly contaminated after submersion in water loaded with bacteria.

Traumatized exit. Bleeding is a common sequela of trauma. Extravasated blood is a good medium for bacterial growth. Bacteria that have colonized the exit multiply rapidly in the presence of decomposing blood and infect the disrupted tissue. Infection may occur as early as 24–48 h after trauma. The prompt administration of an antibiotic, chosen based on the past history of skin colonization, may prevent acute infection. In the absence of the information about

previous skin colonies, an antimicrobial agent sensitive to Gram-positive organisms, such as a cephalosporin or a quinolone, may be chosen. Therapy may have to be continued for about 7 days after achieving a good appearance. Aggressive treatment is necessary in every instance of trauma reported by the patient. Local care requires gentle cleansing of all blood from the exit site.

External cuff infection with or without exit infection. Ultrasound examination of the tunnel is a valuable tool in the diagnosis of cuff infection. While positive findings with ultrasound examination help to establish a diagnosis of tunnel infection, a negative examination does not rule out the existence of an infection. Cuff infection responds to therapy slowly, if at all, and a complete cure is unlikely. As mentioned above, ultrasound may show fluid collection around the cuff, but a negative ultrasound result does not rule out cuff infection. Local care has to be given aggressively. Deroofing the sinus tract and cuff shaving have been practised with some success [204]. Others find these measures ineffective [205]. In our experience cuff shaving prolonged catheter life for approximately 6–12 months [77]. These temporary measures may be suitable for patients who are expected to stay on therapy for a short period, e.g. patients awaiting transplant; however, cuff infection is a strong indicator for catheter removal in long-term peritoneal dialysis patients. Lately, catheter replacement and removal are being done in one procedure if there is no active peritonitis. The preliminary experience of combining the two procedures is promising.

Anecdotal reports suggest that cuff shaving may provide better results in presternal catheters [127, 206]. This may be related to the presence of three cuffs and a long tunnel in the presternal catheter. Shaving of the subcutaneous cuff leaves two cuffs as a double barrier against peri-luminal bacterial penetration.

Local and systemic use of antibiotics for prophylaxis and treatment of exit infection. There is no evidence to support the use of prophylactic antibiotics to reduce the incidence or frequency of infections in healed exit sites and tunnels [207, 208]. Healthy exit sites usually do not become infected unless traumatized; therefore, a prophylactic antibiotic is not recommended for good or perfect exit sites in the absence of trauma. A prophylactic antibiotic is indicated for the management of accidentally traumatized exits. In most cases of trauma this may be considered a treatment, not prophylaxis, since in most reported trauma cases the exit deteriorates to equivocal, which is a subclinical form of exit infection. The other indication for prophylaxis is the chronic infection where discontinuation of systemic antibiotics results in reappearance of the infection [209]. In such a case long-term prophylaxis with a suppressive dose of an antibiotic is useful. As mentioned above, these are probably cases of undiagnosed low-grade external cuff infection.

In nasal carriers of *Staphylococcus aureus*, randomized trials showed decreased infectious complication in patients treated with prophylactic systemic trimethoprim-sulphamethoxasole [210] or rifampin [211]. Topical intranasal application of antibiotics against *Staphylococcus aureus* is less likely to prevent exit infection, unless there is a high probability of microorganism transfer from the nares to the exit on fingers or by other means. As mentioned above, in our studies the strains are usually different in the nares and at the exit. Even if the strains were the same, it seems preferable to use topical antimicrobial agents on the exit, where the bacteria are harmful, instead of using it in nares. In a prospective, randomized study, Bernardini *et al.* [212] found mupirocin ointment at the exit site equally effective to oral rifampicin in reducing infections in *S. aureus* nasal carriers.

Local antibiotics in acute or chronic infection are of little value because they cannot achieve proper local concentrations before being washed away with large drainage; antibiotics administered systemically can provide therapeutic concentrations locally by being excreted into the drainage. Local antibiotics can achieve high concentrations in the sinus in equivocal, good, or perfect exits but are most useful for equivocal exits. As mentioned above, many patients use local ointments (mostly mupirocin) indefinitely to moisturize, lubricate, and decrease or eradicate bacterial colonization of the sinus and exit site. We have not observed any change in physical properties, such as colour or texture, of silicone rubber catheters in patients using ointments for up to 5 years.

External cuff extrusion

As discussed in the section entitled 'External cuff extrusion', the main cause of cuff extrusion is placement of the external segment of the catheter in any shape other than its natural design with the cuff too close to the exit. Due to the resilience force of the silicone rubber, the catheter tends to slowly assume its original shape, and may push the cuff out of the sinus. If the cuff is not infected it is left alone; however, the cuff usually becomes infected during this process and requires systemic antibiotics or even surgical intervention. If there is no peritonitis or deep cuff infection then the catheter may be saved, at least for some time, by shaving off the infected cuff [213]. Infection is another cause of cuff extrusion. In this instance the cuff becomes infected while still in the sinus, and is extruded by tissue retraction around the cuff. Two such extrusions were observed with swan-neck Missouri catheters [124].

Catheter obstruction

'Capture' of the catheter by active omentum may cause outflow obstruction. Obstruction from this cause, in the absence of peritonitis, when it occurs is usually a postoperative event (related to a new catheter). We have never seen an obstruction (in the absence of peritonitis) due to omental 'capture' as a late event. We believe that Silastic® is more prone to attract omentum very early. In due course of time, with or without use, a proteinaceous (not bacterial) biofilm catheter coating may make the Silastic® less 'foreign' to omental tissue. Slow drainage due to catheter translocation, occlusion by bowel or fibrin clot formation occurs from time to time in some patients. Laxatives and/or addition of heparin 500 U/L of dialysis solution are usually successful in restoring good catheter function. Some patients have permanently translocated catheter out of the true pelvis. If the catheter functions (even with slower drainage) we do not attempt to reposition the catheter. If catheter does not function after implementing simple manoeuvres, a more aggressive measures, similar to those described in the section on early soft catheter complications should be tried.

An unusual cause of Cruz catheter blockage, which occurred 4 weeks after initiation of dialysis as a result of the tip wrapping by a fallopian tube, was recently reported [214]. The fimbriae of the oviduct penetrated through the side-holes of the catheter and occluded the central lumen. Catheter function was restored surgically. A high dialysate flow and bigger side-holes of the polyurethane device (the Cruz™ catheter) as compared to silicone rubber catheters might have contributed to this complication.

Pericatheter leak

Dialysis solution leaks may occur months or even years after starting CAPD. Management of late leak

Table 12. Late dialysate leak

Acute	Chronic
After heavy lifting, coughing, or straining	Usually a sequela of acute leak
Sudden drop of ultrafiltration	Poor ultrafiltration
May be mild and intermittent	Fluid overload
Abdominal wall oedema	Localized abdominal oedema
Peau d'orange	Usually without thigh oedema
Spongy feeling	

is similar to that described for early leak. However, most cases of late leak are refractory to conservative therapy and require surgical repair. As discussed earlier, pericatheter leaks are more likely with the midline catheter insertion than with the insertion through the rectus muscle [36, 119]. Similar to the acute leak, this complication is rarely seen with the catheters provided with a bead and polyester flange at the deep cuff (Toronto Western Hospital, swan-neck Missouri, swan-neck presternal). We have not observed a single late pericatheter leak with 181 swan-neck Missouri catheters [124].

Contrary to the early leaks, which are usually external, the late leaks infiltrate the abdominal wall (Table 12). The acute leak causes a sudden drop of ultrafiltration and usually occurs after a sudden increase in intra-abdominal pressure (heavy lifting, coughing or straining). The leak may be mild and intermittent. Such a leak may be difficult to localize. Immediately after leak occurrence the patient may be in good fluid balance without oedema on lower extremities. Abdominal wall oedema reveals a dimpling of the skin that gives it the appearance of the skin of an orange (*peau d'orange*) and spongy feeling on palpation. Chronic leak is usually a sequela of an acute leak but may occur gradually. The patient is usually fluid overloaded due to poor ultrafiltration. A repeated peritoneal equilibration test shows unchanged solute transport characteristics but drain volume is lower [215].

The best method of leak localization is a computerized tomography (CT) scan with intraperitoneal contrast [216, 217]. Prior to the study the peritoneal cavity is drained completely. A fresh bag of 2 litres 2.5% dextrose dialysis solution is prepared, 100 ml of 60% diatriazoate meglumine is injected into the dialysis solution bag through the injection port, the solution is mixed and infused into the peritoneal cavity. No oral or intravenous contrast material is needed. To increase intra-abdominal pressure [173] the patient should stand up, walk, strain, cough and bend over for at least 30 min, then assume the supine

position on the CT table. The images are taken every 6 mm with 6 mm slice thickness in the region of suspected leak; in other regions 12 mm slice thickness every 12 or 24 mm are used. An example of a leak in the periumbilical area without relation to the catheter is shown in Figs 30 and 31 . A leak around

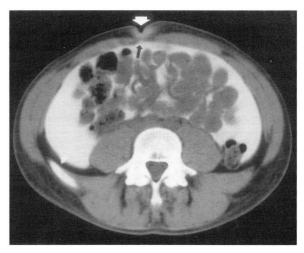

Figure 30. In a CAPD patient a small area of swelling around the umbilicus occurred after lifting a 100 lb weight. CT scan of the abdomen after infusion of 2 litres of contrasted dialysate shows a small amount of extravasated contrast containing dialysate in the umbilical area (white arrow). (Figs 30–32 are reproduced from ref. 217 with permission.)

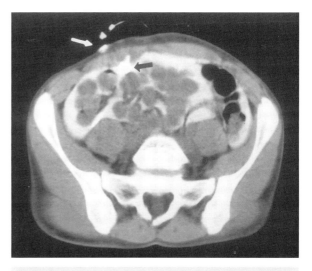

Figure 31. Swan-neck Missouri catheter entering the peritoneal cavity in the vicinity of the extravasated fluid. The intraperitoneal bead (black arrow) and intramural segment leaving the subcutaneous tunnel (white arrow) are clearly recognizable. No extravasated fluid is seen around the catheter entrance into the peritoneum. Pericatheter leak is ruled out.

the Tenckhoff catheter implanted through the midline is shown in Figure 32 .

Peritonitis

Bacteria causing peritonitis, or migrating along the catheter tunnel, may colonize the intraperitoneal segment. As discussed in the section on microorganisms, these bacteria synthesize biofilm, which protects them from host mechanisms and antibiotics. It is believed that such colonization may lead to recurrent peritonitis with the same organism [76].

Recurrent peritonitis may also be the result of deep cuff infection with formation of microabscesses [218]. Korzets *et al.* [219], using ultrasound examination of double-cuff Tenckhoff catheters, found frequent involvement of the deep cuff in peritonitis and exit site infection episodes. In cases of exit-site infection, an apparent downward extension of the infection into the deep cuff led the authors to the conclusion that the peritoneal catheter exit site should be pointing down or have a swan-neck configuration. Finally, bowel trauma by the catheter may lead to peritonitis [220]. This mechanism may explain higher removal rates due to peritonitis of the Toronto Western Hospital catheters found in the CAPD Registry Special Survey [5].

Infusion or pressure pain

The mechanism of this complication was discussed in the section on infusion/pressure pain. Coiled cath-

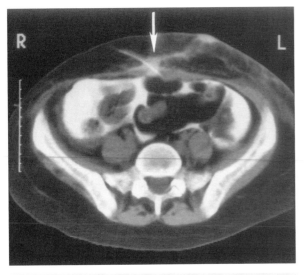

Figure 32. Contrast-enhanced dialysate extravasating around the Tenckhoff catheter (arrow) implanted through the midline.

eters are less likely than the straight ones to induce infusion pain. The pain is usually most intense at the beginning of infusion and at the end of drainage. In the majority of cases the pain is transient and disappears within a few weeks. Table 13 shows the manoeuvres, which we use to alleviate the pain. Decreased infusion rate is frequently helpful. If pain occurs only at the beginning of inflow and the end of outflow, incomplete drainage and/or tidal mode for nightly peritoneal dialysis may be successful. Alkalization of fluid with sodium bicarbonate or use of lidocaine is sometimes effective. If all these manoeuvres are ineffective the catheter has to be replaced. The replacement catheter should be a coiled one and the catheter should be implanted in such a way that no undue pressure is exerted at the tip. Outflow pain is usually secondary to a negative pressure exerted on the peritoneum.

Unusual complications

Organ erosion

Damage of the internal organ leading to intra-abdominal bleeding and/or peritonitis, as well as genital oedema due to peritoneal laceration, have been reported as late catheter complications of straight Tenckhoff and Toronto Western Hospital catheters [220–230]. These complications most likely are due to the pressure exerted by 'soft' but resilient tubing with a pointed tubing end of the straight Tenckhoff catheter or the relatively sharp silastic discs of the Toronto Western Hospital catheter. In most instances the catheters had not been used for 1–12 weeks before the complication was diagnosed [221, 226–230]. We are not aware of such complications being reported with coiled (curled) catheters.

A catheter in the abdomen without dialysate is more likely to cause organ erosion or bowel obstruction than is a catheter used for fluid delivery to and drainage from the peritoneal cavity. A series of serious and/or unusual complications with ventriculoperitoneal shunts were reported. In two cases

Table 13. Manoeuvres to alleviate infusion pain

Slower infusion rate
Incomplete drainage
Tidal mode for nightly peritoneal dialysis
Solution alkalization (sodium bicarbonate: 2–5 mEq/L)
1% lidocaine – 2.5 ml/L (50 mg/exchange)
Catheter replacement

ventriculoperitoneal catheters knotted around the bowel loops, causing obstruction [231]; a catheter extruded through the urethra [232], per rectum [233], or per mouth [234], invaded into the inferior vena cava [235], or migrated into the pleural space [236].

Mechanical accidents

Golper and Carpenter [237] reported two instances of catheters being accidentally cut with scissors. We have observed several such instances despite our teaching that scissors should not be used during dressing changes. Silicone rubber will not self-seal if punctured and such instances occur during implantation procedure and shaving of the cuff.

To avoid system contamination the catheter should be clamped immediately. If the damage is at least 15 mm from the exit the catheter may be saved using a peritoneal catheter Peri-Patch® repair kit, available from the Kendall Co. While repairing the catheter a sterile procedure must be strictly followed. The operator should 'scrub, mask, and glove'. A 'circulating' nurse should be present to assist. The operating field has to be well protected with sterile towels, the catheter should be wrapped with Betadine® soaked gauze for 5 min. The catheter is transversely cut with a sterile blade proximal to the damaged site. The catheter clamp is released and the catheter is squeezed with fingers. The patient is asked to strain, to allow dialysate flow from the peritoneal cavity. The flowing dialysate will flush eventual contaminant. While the fluid is still flowing the Teflon® tubing of the repair kit is inserted into the catheter as far as possible. Then the silicone rubber tubing of the repair kit is clamped to stop dialysate flow. The connection is dried with gauze. A mould is positioned over the connection and filled with sterile silicone glue. The extension tubing is connected to the catheter in the usual way. The glue cures for 72 h. Using this method we have been able to extend the life of seven peritoneal catheters by a mean of 26 months (range 1–87 months) [238].

Material breakdown

There are reports of problems arising from the physical properties of the catheter material. The inclusion of barium sulphate throughout the entire catheter to render it radiopaque has been reported to make the catheter brittle [239]. Currently the catheters contain only a stripe of barium sulphate and seem to be less prone to this mode of failure. Silicone rubber catheters have been observed to stretch, crack or become brittle with age or after repeated exposure to Betadine® [239]. We have observed four such instances [238]. One 9-year catheter broke at skin level and had to be replaced. This catheter, subjected to 5 years of Betadine® exposure, became discoloured and brittle. Another catheter, 6 years old, became stretched approximately 6 cm from the exit. This catheter, never subjected to Betadine®, did not break and could be repaired. The third catheter broke twice at the ages of 7 and 9 years; this catheter was repaired successfully twice and functioned 127 months after implantation until the patient was successfully transplanted. The fourth catheter broke twice in the proximity of the stripe at the age of 3 and 5 years and was also successfully repaired.

Polyurethane is even more likely to be damaged with ageing because of so-called *environmental stress cracking (ESC)*. As its name suggests, ESC leads to microcracks in the surface materials of a device, the result of corrosive forces of the living organism. Once the process begins, ultimate failure is inevitable [240].

As mentioned above, the use of ointments on silicone rubber has not been associated with changes in its physical properties. We do not know whether polyurethane tubing may be subjected to long-term ointment exposure.

Allergic reaction

Eosinophilic peritonitis occurs most frequently in the postimplantation period. Although there are many possible causes of this entity, such as blood, air or antibiotics, one cannot exclude reaction to Silastic® tubing. As discussed in the section on catheter obstruction, gradually the Silastic® tubing is covered with proteinaceous biofilm. The coated catheter is less likely to cause an allergic reaction. Allergic eosinophilic dermatitis due to silicone rubber has been reported [241, 242].

Catheter removal

Indications

The need for catheter removal occurs under various conditions. These may be broadly categorized under two headings: catheter malfunction and complicating medical conditions with a functioning catheter. Finally the catheter may be removed electively because it is not needed.

Malfunction

The decision to remove the catheter is usually made only when conservative measures (described in the sections on early soft catheter complications and catheter obstruction, and in Table 9) to restore function have failed. Catheter malfunction requiring catheter removal may be seen in the following conditions: (1) intraluminal obstruction with blood or fibrin clot or omental tissue incarceration, (2) catheter tip migration out of the pelvis with poor drainage, (3) a catheter kink along its course, (4) catheter tip caught in adhesions following severe peritonitis, and (5) accidental break in the continuity of the catheter.

Functioning catheter with a complication

Under the following conditions catheters may have to removed: (1) recurrent peritonitis with no identifiable cause; (2) peritonitis due to exit-site and/or tunnel infection; (3) catheter with persistent exit-site infection; (4) tunnel infection and abscess; (5) late recurrent dialysate leak through the exit site or into the layers of the abdominal wall; (6) unusual peritonitis, i.e. tuberculosis, fungal, etc.; (7) bowel perforation with multiple organism peritonitis; (8) refractory peritonitis of other causes; (9) severe abdominal pain either due to catheter impinging on internal organs or during solution inflow; and (10) catheter cuff extrusion with infection.

Functioning catheter that is no longer needed

This situation is encountered after a successful renal transplantation or peritoneal dialysis is discontinued because dialysis is no longer needed, or the patient transfers to another form of dialysis.

Removal methods

Uncuffed catheter

Removal of the uncuffed catheter is a simple procedure. After cutting an anchoring suture the catheter is simply pulled out and the opening is covered with a sterile dressing.

Cuffed catheters

A Tenckhoff catheter inserted through the midline may be removed at the bedside. After preparation of the operating field local anaesthesia is applied around the cuffs, the incisions are reopened, the cuffs are excised, and the catheter is pulled. The incisions

of catheters removed for cuff/tunnel infection should be packed open and allowed to heal by second intention. In our experience calcium–sodium alginate fibres (Kaltostat Wound Dressing) are excellent for wound packing. The fibres absorb exudate very efficiently, control minor bleeding, and protect the wound from contamination. Once-daily dressing change is usually sufficient for wound packing with the fibres.

The catheters inserted through the belly of the rectus muscle require surgical dissection in the operating room to remove. Although the catheter can be removed using a local anaesthetic, patient comfort usually dictates a general anaesthetic, particularly for the Toronto Western Hospital, swan-neck Missouri and presternal catheters. After an appropriate surgical scrub and routine draping the incision is re-opened. The anterior rectus fascia is re-opened along the site of the previous incision and the catheter/cuff/flange are sharply dissected free of the ingrown rectus muscle. The previously placed four quadrant sutures in the flange and the purse-string sutures are cut and, with traction and continued sharp dissection, the abdominal portion of the catheter is removed. Care must be taken to protect the underlying viscera. The remaining small opening into the abdomen is closed with O or OO Prolene™ sutures. The anterior fascia is re-approximated in a similar fashion. Depending on the clinical indication for removal, the incision may either be closed or packed open and allowed to heal by second intention.

Swan-neck presternal catheter

Removal of a swan-neck presternal peritoneal dialysis catheter is a surgical procedure performed in the operating room, preferably with general anaesthesia. After an appropriate surgical scrub and routine draping of both the chest and abdomen, both the chest and abdominal incisions are re-opened. Bleeding is controlled with electrocautery. Using blunt and sharp dissection, the two cuffs at the bent portion of the catheter are freed from the adjacent subcutaneous tissue. Working from the abdominal incision, the catheter is divided between sutures *above* the titanium connector. The chest portion of the catheter is pulled out in a cephalad direction through the chest (parasternal) incision. The abdominal part of the catheter is then removed in an identical way as described for the swan-neck Missouri and Toronto Western Hospital catheters. Depending on the clinical indication for removal, the two incisions may either be closed or packed open and allowed to heal by second intention.

Operations in peritoneal dialysis patients

Extra-abdominal

A number of operative procedures may be carried out in the dialysis patient. The patients may undergo a variety of extra-abdominal operations such as coronary artery bypass, lower extremity revascularization, carotid endarterectomy and on occasion the creation of a haemodialysis access. Prior to the operative procedure the dialysis fluid should be drained. Since the abdominal cavity has not been violated, dialysis may be started immediately following the patient's return to the surgical floor. Special caution is required in patients who have presternal catheters. Patients undergoing coronary artery bypass surgery or thoracotomy require particular attention to the location of the presternal catheter to avoid damage to the catheter. In three of our patients open-heart operations were performed without any harm to the catheter located in the parasternal region. Peritoneal dialysis was restarted on the day of surgery in the supine position in each of these patients.

Abdominal

A whole series of abdominal operations may be contemplated and carried out in patients on chronic ambulatory peritoneal dialysis. The operations range from cholecystectomy to colectomy to hernia repairs. Operations on the abdominal wall carry less risk to the patient from the standpoint of developing peritonitis or catheter loss. These operations include all abdominal wall hernias and they can be carried out with some ease and a high degree of safety.

Intra-abdominal procedures on the intestine or the gallbladder for acute or chronic disease may predispose to a risk of infection or loss of the catheter secondary to infectious complications. Procedures such as laparoscopic cholecystectomy can be carried out with minimal risk of spillage of bile or contaminated contents, and after rinsing the abdominal cavity the catheter can be rested and dialysis begun in a few weeks time. In the case of a perforated viscus such as a perforated sigmoid diverticulum or a perforated peptic ulcer with peritoneal soilage the catheter will undoubtedly be lost at that setting. It is safer to remove the peritoneal catheter with massive abdominal soilage because the presence of a foreign body will often prolong or potentiate the risk of persisting infection. Once the patient is recovered from the acute intra-abdominal process consideration can be given to restarting peritoneal dialysis. Depending upon the extent of peritonitis and intra-abdominal adhesion formation, peritoneal dialysis may or may not be possible.

In general, prior to abdominal procedures the abdomen should be drained prior to operation. In our institution we use a first-generation cephalosporin as a prophylactic antibiotic for elective operations and therapeutic antibiotics based on culture for operations associated with significant intra-abdominal soilage. As mentioned, those patients having significant intra-abdominal peritonitis are better served by removal of their catheter at the time of their initial operation with a re-establishment of peritoneal dialysis at a future date. After an elective operation such as cholecystectomy in-and-out exchanges in the supine position are started immediately after the patient reaches the floor. We limit the volume of exchanges to 1 litre and heparin 1000 units per litre is added to the fluid. These exchanges continue until the dialysate is clear. Ceftazidime 500 mg is added to the last exchange and that exchange is not drained. Metronidazole 500 mg *per os*/intravenous/rectal is used for 5 days following elective procedures. The day following the operation, in-and-out exchanges are repeated until the dialysate is clear and again 500 mg of ceftazidime is added to the last exchange, which is not drained for 12 h.

To prevent incisional hernia/leak ambulatory peritoneal dialysis is delayed for 2–6 weeks depending upon the type of operation and the general condition of the patient. Collagen maturation is slower in diabetic, immunosuppressed, and undernourished patients. Restart of peritoneal dialysis should be delayed in such patients.

Long term results

National CAPD Registry survey

In 1987 the National CAPD Registry of the National Institutes of Health reported the results of a survey that attempted to determine the natural history of implanted peritoneal catheters and to estimate the survival distribution of different types of catheters [5]. The survey also estimated frequency of catheter complications as well as reasons for catheter removal. Standard straight ($n = 957$; 64%) and curled ($n = 330$; 22%) Tenckhoff catheters, and Toronto Western Hospital catheters ($n = 94$; 6%), Column-disc or Ash ($n = 49$; 3%), Gore-tex ($n = 28$; 2%), and others ($n = 2$; 0.1%) comprised the catheters reported for the survey. The survey did not clearly show major differences in catheter survival among various types of catheters. The probability of catheter survival at 6, 12, 18, 24, and 36 months for double-cuff standard straight Tenckhoff catheter was 80%, 70%, 60%, 51% and 33%; for standard curled Tenckhoff catheters the survival rate was 85%, 69%, 51%, 43%, and 34%; and for double-cuff Toronto Western catheter the survival rate was 80%, 69%, 52%, 35% and 22%, respectively. The probability of survival at 6, 12, 18 and 24 months for the column-disc catheter was 81%, 71%, 59% and 47%, respectively. None of the Toronto Western Hospital catheters was removed because of a drainage problem; however, they were most likely to be removed due to peritonitis. The reason for the high failure rate due to peritonitis is unclear, but is probably related to the presence of intraperitoneal discs. Column-disc catheters had a high rate of failure due to peritonitis and obstruction, but the lowest rate of failure due to exit/tunnel infections. This survey also found exit-site infection and peritonitis to be disproportionately distributed among the cuff types. Exit-site infections were reported in proportionately more patients using a single subcutaneously placed cuff (13%) than in patients using a double-cuff (7%). Gore-tex catheters, which were designed to reduce exit-site infections, had an extremely high failure rate due to infections.

Swan-neck catheters

At the University of Missouri, Columbia, between August 1985 and September 1991, 181 swan-neck catheters were implanted in three Columbia hospitals and cared for by the technique described above. Survival and complications were monitored prospectively. The prospectively collected data with the swan-neck catheters, and retrospectively collected data with Tenckhoff and Toronto Western Hospital catheters, were compared [123, 124].

There were 148 Tenckhoff and Toronto Western Hospital catheters, 27 swan-neck prototypes, 105 swan-neck Missouri 2 and 3 straight, and 49 swan-neck Missouri 2 and 3 coiled (curled). The overall observation periods of Tenckhoff and Toronto Western Hospital catheters, swan-neck prototypes, swan-neck Missouri 2 and 3 straight, and swan-neck Mis-

souri 2 and 3 coiled were 1859, 427, 1487 and 305 catheter-months. The probability of catheter survival at 6, 12, 18, 24 and 36 months for Tenckhoff and Toronto Western Hospital catheters was 75%, 61%, 52%, 48% and 29%, similar to that reported by the CAPD Registry Special Survey [5], for swan-neck Missouri 2 and 3 straight the probability was 93%, 85%, 79%, 68% and 61%, and for swan-neck Missouri 2 and 3 curled it was 88% and 88% at 6 and 12 months, respectively. The survival probability of swan-neck Missouri straight and coiled catheters was significantly higher than that of Tenckhoff and Toronto Western Hospital catheters. Compared to the CAPD Registry Special Survey [5], in our series more Tenckhoff and Toronto Western catheters were removed due to obstruction, but fewer due to peritonitis. The overall removal percentage was similar.

Swan-neck Missouri 2 and 3 with straight intraperitoneal segments yielded markedly better results. The estimated survival probability at 3 years doubled compared to previously used Tenckhoff and Toronto Western Hospital catheters. Improvement was noted in malfunctions, leaks, cuff extrusions, and exit/tunnel infections. Cuff extrusion occurred only in two swan-neck straight catheters, in both instances after exit-site infection, not due to catheter resilience. This was a notable reversal of the event sequence compared to previously used catheters, in which cuff extrusion usually preceded exit/tunnel infection.

The results regarding survival and removal rates with swan-neck coiled catheters were not significantly different from those of the swan-neck Missouri 2 and 3 straight catheters. Nevertheless, there are two major advantages with these catheters, the same as with other coiled catheters: a reduction in the incidence of infusion pain due to a 'jet effect' and pain related to straight catheter tip pressure on the peritoneum experienced by some patients.

Low complication rates and higher probability of survival with swan-neck catheters compared to other catheters have also been reported by others [243, 244]. A prospective comparison by life-table analysis of 25 double-cuff Tenckhoff and 25 swan-neck catheters showed patient survival of 75% and 79%, respectively at 12 months, and dialysis technique survival of 80% and 82%, respectively [242]. The groups were too small to reveal the statistical significance of differences; also catheter-related complications were not statistically significantly different [245]. Preliminary experiences with swan-neck presternal catheters in adults and in children were very encouraging [39, 126, 127, 128]. These preliminary results were confirmed on a larger group with 6 years of experience [246, 247]. All complication rates were lower than with other catheters and the catheter survival probabilities of 95% and 86% at 2 and 3 years respectively are the best results ever reported. Lye *et al.* [248] reported significantly lower exit-site infection rates with swan-neck catheters, and insignificantly worse catheter survival and tip migrations with Tenckhoff catheters.

United States Renal Data System report 1992

In a national study of all patients starting CAPD therapy in the United States during January through June 1989 the prevailing catheter practices were appraised and the peritonitis risk was assessed by catheter-related factors in 2807 patients followed for up to 21 months [110]. Of these patients, 44% used a straight intraperitoneal segment with no bend, 40% used a curled (coiled) catheter with no bend, 12% used a catheter with 'a preformed bend' [swan neck] with either straight or curled intraperitoneal segment. Four per cent of patients used 'other' (Life-cath and unspecified) catheters. Double-cuff catheters were used in 78%, single deep-cuff in 13%, single superficial in 5%, and data were not available in 10% of patients. Surgeons and nephrologists implanted 88% and 10% of these catheters respectively (data for 2% unavailable). Surgical dissection was used in 74% of cases, peritoneoscopy in 6%, and blind (trochar or guidewire) in 8%. Midline insertion was used in 20%, paramedian in 33% and lateral in 14% of these cases. Prophylactic antibiotics were used in 43% of insertions; data were not available in 28% and the antibiotics were not used in 29% of cases. This study did not assess catheter survival and all complications; only the relative risk of a first peritonitis episode was analysed using Cox proportional hazards model. The relative risk of peritonitis was essentially identical for straight, curled, and bent catheters; the risk was significantly higher for 'other' catheters. When the analysis was repeated with adjustment for possible centre effect the peritonitis risk was significantly (40%) lower among patients having catheters with 'a permanent bend' (swan neck). (Port, F., oral communication during the XV Annual PD Conference, Orlando, FL, 25 January 1994). Compared to double-cuff catheter the risk of peritonitis was 16% and 31% higher for single deep-cuff and single superficial-cuff catheters respectively. Insertion by a nephrologist was associated with a 15% higher peritonitis risk as compared to insertion by a surgeon.

Concluding remarks

Peritoneal catheters are lifelines for peritoneal dialysis patients. Soft catheters are gradually replacing rigid catheters in the treatment of acute renal failure. Soft catheters are used exclusively for the treatment of chronic renal failure. The Tenckhoff catheter continues to be the most widely used catheter although its use is decreasing in favour of swan-neck catheters. Surgical implantation virtually eliminated such early complications as bowel perforation or massive bleeding. Other complications, such as obstruction, pericatheter leaks, and superficial cuff extrusions have been markedly reduced in recent years, particularly with the use of swan-neck catheters and insertion through the rectus muscle instead of the midline.

The exit should be located in a place only minimally subjected to pressure and movement. Prophylactic antibiotics and a meticulous sterile surgical technique with perfect haemostasis prevent early infection. Healing of the exit takes 4–8 weeks. During this time a non-occlusive (air-permeable) dressing is recommended. After the exit is healed the simplest and best method of care is protection from trauma, cleansing with water and liquid soap containing mild disinfectant, and avoidance of gross exit contamination. Continuous use of local antibiotic ointments is effective in decreasing infectious complications. Early systemic antibiotics for mild infections prevent severe infections leading to catheter loss. Whereas supine peritoneal dialysis may be started immediately postimplantation, ambulatory peritoneal dialysis should be postponed for at least 10 days after implantation, to avoid early leaks. The success of the catheter depends on meticulous adherence to the details of catheter insertion and post-implantation care.

References

1. Tenckhoff J, Schechter H. A bacteriologically safe peritoneal access device. Trans Am Soc Artif Intern Organs 1968; 14: 181–7.
2. Buoncristiani U, Cozzari M, Quintaliani G, Carobi C. Abatement of exogenous peritonitis risk using the Perugia system. Dial Transplant 1983; 12: 14–25.
3. Maiorca R, Cantaluppi A, Cancarini GC *et al.* Prospective controlled trial of a Y connector and disinfectant to prevent peritonitis in continuous ambulatory peritoneal dialysis. Lancet 1983; 2: 642–4.
4. Churchill DN, Taylor DW, Vas SI *et al.* Peritonitis in continuous ambulatory peritoneal dialysis (CAPD): a multi-

center randomized clinical trial comparing the Y connector disinfectant system to standard system. Perit Dial Int 1989; 9: 159–63.

5. Lindblad AS, Hamilton RW, Novak JW. Complications of peritoneal catheters. In: Lindblad AS, Novak JW, Nolph KD, eds. Continuous Ambulatory Peritoneal Dialysis in the USA – Final Report of the National CAPD Registry. Dordrecht: Kluwer, 1989, pp. 157–66.

6. Ganter G. Ueber die Beseitigung giftiger Stoffe aus dem Blute durch Dialyse. Munch Med Wochenschr 1923; 70: 1478–80.

7. Rosenak S, Siwon P. Experimentelle Untersuchungen über die peritoneale Ausscheidung harnpflichtiger Substanzen aus dem Blute. Mitt Grenzgeb Med Chir 1925; 39: 391–408.

8. Engel D, Kerkes A. Beitrage zum permeabilitats Problem: Entgiftungsstudien mittels des lebenden Peritoneums als 'Dialysator'. Z Gesamte Exp Med 1927; 55: 574–601.

9. Reid R, Penfold JB, Jones RN. Anuria treated by renal decapsulation and peritoneal dialysis. Lancet 1946; 2: 749–53.

10. Fine J, Frank HA, Seligman AM. The treatment of acute renal failure by peritoneal irrigation. Ann Surg 1946; 124: 857–78.

11. Rosenak SS, Oppenheimer GD. An improved drain for peritoneal lavage. Surgery 1948; 23: 832–3.

12. Derot M, Tanzet P, Roussilon J, Bernier JJ. La dialyse peritoneale dans le traitement de l'uremie aigue. J Urol 1949; 55: 113–21.

13. Legrain M, Merril JP. Short term continuous peritoneal dialysis. N Engl J Med 1953; 248: 125–9.

14. Maxwell MH, Rockney RE, Kleeman CR, Twiss MR. Peritoneal dialysis. JAMA 1959; 170: 917–24.

15. Doolan PD, Murphy WP, Wiggins RA *et al.* An evaluation of intermittent peritoneal lavage. Am J Med 1959; 26: 831–44.

16. Boen ST, Mulinari AS, Dillard DH, Scribner BH. Periodic peritoneal dialysis in the management of chronic uremia. Trans Am Soc Artif Intern Organs 1962; 8: 256–65.

17. Boen ST, Mion CM, Curtis FK, Shilipetar G. Periodic peritoneal dialysis using the repeated puncture technique and an automated cycling machine. Trans Am Soc Artif Intern Organs 1964; 10: 409–13.

18. Weston RE, Roberts M. Clinical use of stylet catheter for peritoneal dialysis. Arch Intern Med 1965; 115: 659–62.

19. Mallette WG, McPhaul JJ, Bledsoe F, McIntosh DA, Koegel E. A clinically successful subcutaneous peritoneal access button for repeated peritoneal dialysis. Trans Amer Soc Artif Intern Organs 1964; 10: 396–8.

20. Jacob GB, Deane N. Repeated peritoneal dialysis by the catheter replacement method: description of technique and a replaceable prosthesis for chronic access to the peritoneal cavity. Proc Eur Dial Transplant Assoc 1967; 4: 136–40.

21. Barry KG, Shambaugh GE, Goler D. A new flexible cannula and seal to provide prolonged access for peritoneal drainage and other procedures. J Urol 1963; 90: 125–8.

22. Gutch CF. Peritoneal dialysis. Trans Am Soc Artif Intern Organs 1964; 10: 406–7.

23. Palmer RA, Maybee TK, Henry EW, Eden J. Peritoneal dialysis in acute and chronic renal failure. Can Med Assoc J 1963; 88: 920–7.

24. Palmer RA, Quinton WE, Gray JE. Prolonged peritoneal dialysis for chronic renal failure. Lancet 1964; 1: 700–2.

25. Tenckhoff H, Schechter H, Boen ST. One year experience with home peritoneal dialysis. Trans Am Soc Artif Intern Organs 1965; 11: 11–14.

26. McDonald HP Jr, Gerber N, Mischra D, Wolm L, Peng B, Waterhouse K. Subcutaneous Dacron® and Teflon® cloth adjuncts for silastic arteriovenous shunts and peritoneal dialysis catheters. Trans Am Soc Artif Intern Organs 1968; 14: 176–80.

27. Stephen RI, Atkin-Thor E, Kolff WJ. Recirculating peritoneal dialysis with subcutaneous catheter. Trans Am Soc Artif Intern Organs 1976; 22: 575–84.

28. Gotloib L, Nisencorn I, Garmizo AL, Galili N, Servadio C, Sudarsky M. Subcutaneous intraperitoneal prosthesis for maintenance of peritoneal dialysis. Lancet 1975; 1: 1318–20.

29. Daly BDT, Dasse KA, Haudenschild CC *et al.* Percutaneous energy transmission systems: long-term survival. Trans Am Soc Artif Intern Organs 1983; 29: 526–30.

30. Ogden DA, Benavente G, Wheeler D, Zukoski CF. Experience with the right angle Gore-Tex® peritoneal dialysis catheter. Advances in Continuous Ambulatory Peritoneal Dialysis. Selected papers from the Sixth Annual CAPD Conference, Kansas City, Missouri, February 1986. Toronto: Peritoneal Dialysis Bulletin, Inc., 1986, pp. 155–9.

31. Goldberg EM, Hill W. A new peritoneal access prosthesis. Proc Clin Dial Transplant Forum 1973; 3: 122–5.

32. Oreopoulos DG, Izatt S, Zellerman G, Karanicolas S, Mathews RE. A prospective study of the effectiveness of three permanent peritoneal catheters. Proc Clin Dial Transplant Forum 1976; 6: 96–100.

33. Valli A, Comotti C, Torelli D *et al.* A new catheter for peritoneal dialysis. Trans Am Soc Artif Intern Organs 1983; 29: 629–32.

34. Valli A, Andreotti C, Degetto P *et al.* 48-months' experience with Valli-2 catheter. In: Khanna R, Nolph KD, Prowant BF, Twardowski ZJ, Oreopoulos DG, eds. Advances in Continuous Ambulatory Peritoneal Dialysis. Selected papers from the Eighth Annual CAPD Conference, Kansas City, Missouri, February 1988. Toronto: Peritoneal Dialysis Bulletin, Inc., 1988, Vol. 4, pp. 292–7.

35. Ash SR, Johnson H, Hartman J *et al.* The column disc peritoneal catheter. A peritoneal access device with improved drainage. ASAIO J 1980; 3: 109–15.

36. Twardowski ZJ, Nolph KD, Khanna R, Prowant BF, Ryan LP. The need for a 'Swan Neck' permanently bent, arcuate peritoneal dialysis catheter. Perit Dial Bull 1985; 5: 219–23.

37. Cruz C. Clinical experience with a new peritoneal access device (the Cruz™ catheter). In: Ota K, Maher J, Winchester J, Hirszel P, Ito, K, Suzuki T, eds. Current Concepts in Peritoneal Dialysis: Proceedings of the Fifth Congress of the International Society for Peritoneal Dialysis, Kyoto, 21–24 July 1990. Amsterdam: Excerpta Medica, 1992, pp. 164–9.

38. Twardowski ZJ, Nichols WK, Nolph KD, Khanna R. Swan neck presternal ('bath tub') catheter for peritoneal dialysis. Adv Perit Dial 1992; 8: 316–24.

39. Ash SR, Janle EM. T-fluted peritoneal dialysis catheter. Adv Perit Dial 1993; 9: 223–6.

40. Moncrief JW, Popovich RP, Broadrick LJ, He ZZ, Simmons EE, Tate RA. Moncrief–Popovich catheter: a new peritoneal access technique for patients on peritoneal dialysis. ASAIO J 1993; 39: 62–5.

41. Di Paolo N, Petrini G, Garosi G, Buoncristiani U, Brardi S, Monaci G. A new self-locating peritoneal catheter. Perit Dial Int 1996; 16: 623–7.

42. Twardowski ZJ. Peritoneal dialysis glossary. II. Perit Dial Int 1988; 8: 15–17.

43. Twardowski ZJ, Khanna R, Nolph KD, Nichols WK. Peritoneal dialysis catheter: principles of design, implantation, and early care. Video produced by the Academic Support Center, University of Missouri, Columbia, MO, USA, 1993.

44. Blistein-Willinger E. The role of growth factors in wound healing. Skin Pharmacol 1991; 4: 175–82.

45. Kantrowitz A, Freed PS, Ciarkowski AA *et al.* Development of a percutaneous access device. Trans Am Soc Artif Intern Organs 1980; 26: 444–9.

46. Hall CW, Adams LM, Ghidoni JJ. Development of skin interfacing cannula. Trans Am Soc Artif Intern Organs 1975; 21: 281–7.

47. Yaffe A, Ahoshan S. Cessation of epithelial cell movement at native type I collagen–epithelial interface *in vitro*. Collagen Res Rel 1985; 5: 533–40.

48. Bar-Lev A, Freed PS, Mandell G *et al.* Long-term percutaneous access device. In: Khanna R, Nolph KD, Prowant BF, Twardowski ZJ, and Oreopoulos GD, eds. Advances in Continuous Ambulatory Peritoneal Dialysis. Selected papers from

the Seventh Annual CAPD Conference, Kansas City, Missouri, February 1987. Toronto: Peritoneal Dialysis Bulletin, Inc., 1987, pp. 81–7.

49. Dasse KA, Daly BDT, Bousquet G, King D, Smith T, Mondou R, Poirier VL. A polyurethane percutaneous access device for peritoneal dialysis. In: Khanna R, Nolph KD, Prowant BF, Twardowski ZJ, Oreopoulos GD, eds. Advances in Continuous Ambulatory Peritoneal Dialysis. Selected papers from the Eighth Annual CAPD Conference, Kansas City, Missouri, February 1988. Toronto: Peritoneal Dialysis Bulletin, Inc., 1988, pp. 245–52.

50. Krawczyk WS. Some ultrastructural aspects of epidermal repair in two model wound healing systems. In: Maibach HI, Rovee DT, eds. Epidermal Wound Healing. Chicago: Year Book Medical, 1972, pp. 123–31.

51. Winter GD. Movement of epidermal cells over the wound surface. In: Montagna W, Billingham RE, eds. Advances in Biology of Skin, Vol. 5: Wound Healing. Oxford: Pergamon Press, 1964, pp. 113–27.

52. Winter GD. Epidermal regeneration studied in the domestic pig. In: Maibach HI, Rovee DT, eds. Epidermal Wound Healing. Chicago: Year Book Medical, 1972, pp. 71–112.

53. Winter GD. Transcutaneous implants: reactions of the skin-implant interface. J Biomed Mater Res 1974; 8: 99–113.

54. Poirier VL, Daly BDT, Dasse KA, Haudenschild CC, Fine RE. Elimination of tunnel infection. In: Maher JF, Winchester JF, eds. Frontiers in Peritoneal Dialysis. Proceedings of the III International Symposium on Peritoneal Dialysis. Washington, D.C., 1984. New York: Field, Rich, 1986, pp. 210–17.

55. Twardowski ZJ, Prowant BF. Can new catheter design eliminate exit site and tunnel infections? Perspect Periton Dial 1986; 4: 5–9.

56. Khanna R, Twardowski ZJ. Peritoneal catheter exit site. Perit Dial Int 1988; 8: 119–23.

57. Twardowski ZJ, Khanna R. Swan neck peritoneal dialysis catheter. In: Andreucci VE, ed. Vascular and Peritoneal Access for Dialysis. Boston: Kluwer, 1989, pp. 271–89.

58. Twardowski ZJ, Dobbie JW, Moore HL et al. Morphology of peritoneal dialysis catheter tunnels. Macroscopy and light microscopy. Perit Dial Int 1991; 11: 237–51.

59. Wright NA. The cell proliferation kinetics of the epidermis. In: Goldsmith LA, ed. Biochemistry and Physiology of the Skin. New York: Oxford University Press, 1983, pp. 203–29.

60. Twardowski ZJ, Prowant BF. Exit-site post catheter implantation. Perit Dial Int 1996; 16 (suppl. 3): S51–70.

61. Stricker GE, Tenckhoff HAM. A transcutaneous prosthesis for prolonged access to the peritoneal cavity. Surgery 1971; 69: 70–4.

62. Pru CP, Barriola JA, Garcia V. Pathological evaluation of one cuff peritoneal dialysis catheter tunnel (OCPDCT). Perit Dial Int 1993; 13 (suppl. 1): S24 (abstract).

63. Heppenstall RB, Littooy FN, Fuchs R, Sheldon GF, Hunt TK. Gas tensions in healing tissues of traumatized patients. Surgery 1974; 75: 874–80.

64. Elek SD. Experimental staphylococcal infections in the skin of man. Ann NY Acad Sci 1956; 54: 85–90.

65. Hepburn H. Delayed primary suture of wounds. Br Med J 1919; 1: 181–3.

66. Krizek TJ, Robson MC. Biology of surgical infection. Surg Clin N Am 1975; 55: 1261–7.

67. Mosher DF, Proctor RA. Binding and factor XIIIa-mediated cross-linking of a 27 kilodalton fragment of fibronectin to Staphylococcus aureus. Science 1980; 209: 927–9.

68. Maxe I, Rydén C, Wadström T, Rubin K. Specific attachment of Staphylococcus aureus to immobilized fibronectin. Infect Immun 1986; 54: 695–704.

69. Proctor RA. The staphylococcal fibronectin receptor: evidence for its importance in invasive infections. Rev Infect Dis 1987; 9 (suppl.): S335–40.

70. Russel PB, Kline J, Yoder MC, Polin RA. Staphylococcal adherence to polyvinyl chloride and heparin-bonded polyure-

thane catheters is species dependent and enhanced by fibronectin. J Clin Microbiol 1987; 25: 1083–7.

71. Lopes JD, dos Reis M, Brentani RR. Presence of laminin receptors in Staphylococcus aureus. Science 1985; 229: 275–7.

72. Vercelotti GM, McCarthy JB, Lindholm P, Peterson PK, Jacob HS, Furcht LT. Extracellular matrix proteins (fibronectin, laminin, and type IV collagen) bind and aggregate bacteria. Am J Pathol 1985; 120: 13–21.

73. Dickinson GM, Bisno AL. Infections associated with indwelling devices: concepts of pathogenesis; infections associated with intravascular devices. Antimicrob Agents Chemother 1989; 33: 597–601.

74. Marshall KC. Mechanism of bacterial adhesion at solid water interfaces. In: Savage DC, Fletcher M, eds. Bacterial Adhesion: mechanisms and physiological significance. New York: Plenum, 1985, pp. 133–61.

75. Costerton JW, Watkins L. Adherence of bacteria to foreign bodies: the role of biofilm. In: Root RK, Trunkey DD, Sande MA, eds. New Surgical and Medical Approaches in Infectious Diseases. New York: Churchill Livingstone, 1987, pp. 17–30.

76. Dasgupta MK, Bettcher KB, Ulan RA et al. Relationship of adherent bacterial biofilms to peritonitis in chronic ambulatory peritoneal dialysis. Perit Dial Bull 1987; 7: 168–73.

77. Twardowski ZJ, Prowant BF. Exit-site study methods and results. Perit Dial Int 1996; 16 (suppl. 3): S6–31.

78. Golper TA, Transæus A. Vancomycin revisited. Perit Dial Int 1996; 16: 116–17.

79. Wikdahl AM, Engman U, Stegmayr B, Sorenson JG. One dose cefuroxime i.v. and i.p. reduces microbial growth in PD patients after catheter insertion. Nephrol Dial Transplant 1997; 12: 157–60.

80. Lye WC, Lee EJ, Tan CC. Prophylactic antibiotics in the insertion of Tenckhoff catheters. Scand J Urol Nephrol 1992; 26: 177–80.

81. Van den Broek PJ, Buys LF, Van Furth R. Interaction of povidone-iodine compounds, phagocytic cells, and macroorganisms. Antimiocrob Agents Chemother 1982; 22: 593–7.

82. Iwasaki N, Kamoi K, Bae RD, Tsutsui T. Cytotoxicity of povidone-iodine on cultured mammalian cells. J Jap Assoc Periodont 1989; 31: 836–42.

83. Oberg MS, Lindsey D. Do not put hydrogen peroxide or povidone iodine into wounds! Am J Dis Child 1987; 141: 27–8.

84. Laufman H. Current use of skin and wound cleansers and antiseptics. Amer J Surg 1989; 157: 359–65.

85. Bryant CA, Rodeheaver GT, Reem EM, Nitcher LS, Kennedy JC, Edlich RF. Search for a nontoxic surgical scrub solution for periorbital lacerations. Ann Emerg Med 1984; 13: 317–19.

86. Orgill D, Demling R. Current concepts and approaches to wound healing. Crit Care Med 1988; 16: 899–908.

87. Rosen H, Blumenthal A, McCallum J. Effect of asiaticoside on wound healing in the rat. Proc Soc Exp Biol Med 1967; 125: 279–80.

88. Maquart FX, Bellon G, Gillery P, Wegrowski Y, Borel JP. Stimulation of collagen synthesis in fibroblast cultures by a triterpene extracted from Centella asiatica. Connect Tissue Res 1990; 24: 107–20.

89. Zimmerman SW, O'Brien M, Wiedenhoeft FA, Johnson CA. Staphylococcus aureus peritoneal catheter-related infections: a cause of catheter loss and peritonitis. Perit Dial Int 1988; 8: 191–4.

90. Abraham G, Savin E, Ayiomamitis A et al. Natural history of exit-site infection (ESI) in patients on continuous ambulatory peritoneal dialysis (CAPD). Perit Dial Int 1988; 8: 211–16.

91. Yu VL, Goetz A, Wagener M et al. Staphylococcus aureus nasal carriage and infection in patients on hemodialysis. N Engl J Med 1986; 315: 91–6.

92. Davies SJ, Ogg CS, Cameron JS, Poston S, Nobble WC. Staphylococcus aureus nasal carriage, exit-site infection and catheter loss in patients treated with continuous ambulatory peritoneal dialysis. Perit Dial Int 1989; 9: 61–4.

93. Sewell CM, Clarrige J, Lacke C, Weinman EJ, Young EJ. Staphylococcal nasal carriage and subsequent infection in peritoneal dialysis patients. JAMA 1982; 248: 1493–5.

94. Luzar MA, Coles GA, Faller B *et al. Staphylococcus aureus* nasal carriage and infection in patients on continuous ambulatory peritoneal dialysis. N Engl J Med 1990; 322: 505–9.

95. Twardowski ZJ, Prowant BF. *Staphylococcus aureus* nasal carriage is not associated with an increased incidence of exit site infection with the same organism. Proceedings of the ISPD Meeting, Thessaloniki, Greece, 1–4 October 1992. Perit Dial Int 1993; 13 (suppl. 2): S306–9.

96. Boelaert JR, Van Landuyt HW, Gordts BZ, De Baere YA, Messer SA, Herwaldt LA. Nasal and cutaneous carriage of *Staphylococcus aureus* in hemodialysis patients: the effect of nasal mupirocin. Infect Control Hosp Epidemiol 1996; 17: 809–11.

97. Anonymous. Nasal mupirocin prevents *Staphylococcus aureus* exit-site infection during peritoneal dialysis. Mupirocin Study Group. J Am Soc Nephrol 1996; 7: 2403–8.

98. Miller MA, Dascal A, Portnoy J, Mendelson J. Development of mupirocin resistance among methicillin-resistant *Staphylococcus aureus* after widespread use of nasal mupirocin ointment. Infect Control Hosp Epidemiol 1996; 17: 811–13.

99. Warady BA, Sullivan EK, Alexander SR. Lessons from the peritoneal dialysis patient database: a report of the North American Pediatric Renal Transplant Cooperative Study. Kidney Int 1996; 49 (suppl. 53): S68–71.

100. Golper TA, Brier ME, Bunke M. Risk factors for peritonitis in long-term peritoneal dialysis: the Network 9 Peritonitis and Catheter Survival Studies. Am J Kidney Dis 1996; 28: 415–19.

101. Bossert WA, Marks HH. Prevalence and characteristics of periodontal disease on 12,800 persons under periodic dental observation. J Am Dent Assoc 1956; 52: 429–42.

102. Hajek M. Pathology and Treatment of the Inflammatory Diseases of the Nasal Accessory Sinuses, transl. and ed. by Heitger JD, Hansel FK, 5th edn. St. Louis: Mosby, 1926, p. 100.

103. So SKS, Mahan JD Jr, Mauer SM, Sutherland DER, Nevins TE. Hickman catheter for pediatric hemodialysis: a 3-year experience. Trans Am Soc Artif Intern Organs 1984; 30: 619–23.

104. Raaf JH. Results from use of 826 vascular access devices in cancer patients. Cancer 1985; 55: 1312–21.

105. Tenckhoff H. Home peritoneal dialysis. In: Massry SG, Sellers AL, eds. Clinical Aspects of Uremia and Dialysis. Springfield: Charles C Thomas, 1976, pp. 583–615.

106. Smith C. CAPD: one cuff vs two cuff catheters in reference to incidence of infection. In: Maher JF, Winchester JF, eds. Frontiers in Peritoneal Dialysis. Proceedings of the III International Symposium on Peritoneal Dialysis. Washington, D.C., 1984. New York: Field, Rich, 1986, pp. 181–2.

107. Gokal R, Alexander S, Ash S *et al.* Peritoneal catheters and exit-site practices toward optimum peritoneal access: 1998 update (Official report from the International Society for Peritoneal Dialysis). Perit Dial Int 1998; 18: 11–33.

108. Diaz-Buxo JA, Geissinger WT. Single cuff versus double cuff Tenckhoff catheter. Perit Dial Bull 1984; 4 (suppl. 3): S100–2.

109. Kim D, Burke D, Izatt S *et al.* Single – or double cuff peritoneal catheters? A prospective comparison. Trans Am Soc Artif Intern Organs 1984; 30: 232–5.

110. US Renal Data System, USRDS 1992 Annual Data Report, VI. Catheter-Related Factors and Peritonitis Risk in CAPD Patients. Am J Kidney Dis 1992; 5 (suppl. 2): 48–54.

111. Honda M, Iitaka K, Kawaguchi H *et al.* The Japanese National Registry data on pediatric CAPD patients: a ten-year experience. A report of the Study Group of Pediatric PD Conference. Perit Dial Int 1996; 16: 269–75.

112. Lindblad AS, Hamilton RW, Nokph KD, Novak JW. A retrospective analysis of catheter configuration and cuff type: a National CAPD Registry report. Perit Dial Int 1988; 8: 129–33.

113. Favazza A, Petri R, Montanaro D, Boscutti G, Bresacola F, Mioni G. Insertion of straight peritoneal catheter in an arcuate subcutaneous tunnel by a tunneler: long-term experience. Perit Dial Int 1995; 15: 357–62.

114. Schroeder HE, Page RC. The normal periodontium. In: Schluger S, Youdelis RA, Page RC, eds. Periodontal Disease. Philadelphia: Lea & Febiger, 1978, pp. 7–55.

115. Amano I, Katoh T, Inagaki Y. Clinical experience with alumina ceramic transcutaneous connector to prevent skin-exit infection around CAPD catheter. Adv Perit Dial 1990; 6: 150–4.

116. Boss HP, Ganger KH, Gluck Z. Gore-tex versus Oreopoulos peritoneal catheters: a clinical evaluation and comparison (letter). Perit Dial Bull 1987; 7: 209.

117. Rottembourg J, Quinton W, Durande JP, Brouard R. Wings as subcutaneous cuff in prevention of exit-site infection in CAPD patients. Abstracts of the IV International Symposium on Peritoneal Dialysis, Vicenza, Italy, 29 June–2 July 1987. Perit Dial Bull 1987; 7 (suppl.): S63.

118. Schleifer CR, Ziemek H, Teehan BP, Benz RL, Sigler MH, Gilgore GS. Migration of peritoneal catheters: personal experience and a survey of 72 other units. Perit Dial Bull 1987; 7: 189–93.

119. Helfrich GB, Pechan BW, Alijani MR, Bernard WF, Rakowski TA, Winchester JF. Reduced catheter complications with lateral placement. Perit Dial Bull 1983; 3 (suppl. 4): S2–4.

120. Twardowski ZJ, Nolph KD, Khanna R, Prowant BF. Computer interaction: catheters. Adv Perit Dialysis. 1994; 10: 11–18.

121. Twardowski ZJ, Nichols WK, Khanna R, Nolph KD. Swan neck Missouri peritoneal dialysis catheters: design, insertion, and break-in. Video produced by the Academic Support Center, University of Missouri, Columbia, MO, USA, 1993.

122. Twardowski ZJ, Khanna R, Nolph KD, Nichols WK, Ryan LP. Preliminary experience with the Swan Neck peritoneal dialysis catheter. Trans Am Soc Artif Intern Organs 1986; 32: 64–7.

123. Twardowski ZJ, Prowant BF, Khanna R, Nichols WK, Nolph KD. Long-term experience with Swan Neck Missouri catheters. ASAIO Trans 1990; 36: M491–4.

124. Twardowski ZJ, Prowant BF, Nichols WK, Nolph KD, Khanna R. Six year experience with swan neck catheter. Perit Dial Int 1992; 12: 384–9.

125. Twardowski ZJ, Nichols WK, Khanna R, Nolph KD. Swan neck presternal peritoneal dialysis catheter: design, insertion, and break-in. Video produced by the Academic Support Center, University of Missouri, Columbia, MO, USA, 1993.

126. Twardowski ZJ, Prowant BF, Pickett B, Nichols WK, Nolph KD, Khanna R. Four-year experience with swan neck presternal peritoneal dialysis catheter. Am J Kidney Dis 1996; 27: 99–105.

127. Twardowski ZJ, Nichols WK, Nolph KD, Khanna R. Swan neck presternal peritoneal dialysis catheter. Proceedings of the ISPD Meeting, Thessaloniki, Greece, 1–4 October 1992. Perit Dial Int 1993; 13 (suppl. 2): S130–2.

128. Sieniawska M, Blaim M, Warchol S. Swan-neck presternal catheter (SNPC) for CAPD in children. Perit Dial Int 1993; 13 (suppl. 1): S22.

129. Ash SR, Daugirdas JT. Peritoneal Access devices. In: Daugirdas JT, Ing TS, eds. Handbook of Dialysis. Boston: Little Brown, 1994, pp. 275–300.

130. Ash SR, Nichols WK. Placement, repair, and removal of chronic peritoneal catheters. In: Gokal R, Nolph KD, eds. Textbook of Peritoneal Dialysis. Dordrecht: Kluwer, 1994, pp. 315–33.

131. Gonzales AR, Goltz GM, Eaton CL, Ratajeski G, Olin JW. The peel away method for insertion of Tenckhoff catheter. Am Soc Nephrol 1983; 16: 119A (abstract).

132. Updike S, O'Brien M, Peterson W, Zimmerman S. Placement of catheter using pacemaker-like introducer with peel-away sleeve. Am Soc Nephrol 1984; 17: 87A (abstract).

133. Updike S, Zimmerman S, O'Brien M, Peterson W. Peel-Away® sheath technique for placing peritoneal dialysis catheters. Video produced by Television Studio, School of Nursing, Univerity of Wisconsin, Madison, WI, USA, 1984.

134. Zappacosta AR, Perras ST, Closkey GM. Seldinger technique for Tenckhoff catheter placement. ASAIO Trans 1991; 37: 13–15.

135. Zappacosta AR. Seldinger technique for placement of the Tenckhoff catheter. Video produced by the Bryn Mawr Hospital, 1984.

136. Schmidt LM, Craig PC, Prowant BF, Twardowski ZJ. A simple method of preventing accidental disconnection at the peritoneal catheter adapter junction. Perit Dial Int 1990; 10: 309–10.

137. Vaamonde CA, Michael VF, Metzger RA, Carrol KE. Complications of acute peritoneal dialysis. J Chron Dis 1975; 28: 637–59.

138. Valk TW, Swartz RD, Hsu CH. Peritoneal dialysis in acute renal failure: analysis of outcome and complications. Dial Transplant 1980; 9: 48–54.

139. Maher JF, Schreiner GE. Hazards and complications of dialysis. N Engl J Med 1965; 273: 370–7.

140. Anderson G, Bergquist-Poppen M, Bergstrom J, Collste LG, Huttman E. Glucose absorption from the dialysis fluid during peritoneal dialysis. Scand J Urol Nephrol 1971; 5: 77.

141. Firmat J, Zucchini A. Peritoneal dialysis in acute renal failure. Contrib Nephrol 1979; 17: 33–8.

142. Edward SR, Unger AM. Acute hydrothorax a new complication of peritoneal dialysis. JAMA 1967; 199: 853–5.

143. Finn R, Jowett EW. Acute hydrothorax: complication of peritoneal dialysis. Br Med J 1970; 2: 94.

144. Holm J, Lieden B, Lindgrist B. Unilateral effusion – a rare complication of peritoneal dialysis. Scand J Urol Nephrol 1971; 5: 84–5.

145. Haberli R, Stucki P. Akuter hydro-thorax als komplikation bei peritonealdialyse. Praxis 1971; 60: 13–14.

146. Fehmirling E, Christensen E. Hydrothorax under peritonealdialyse. Ugeskr Laeg 1975; 137: 1650–1.

147. Alquier Ph, Achard J, Bonhomme R. Hydrothorax aign au loure de dialyses péritonealés. A propos de 5 cas. Nouv Presse Med 1975; 4: 192.

148. Rudnick MR, Coyle JF, Beck H, McCurdy DK. Acute massive hydrothorax complicating peritoneal dialysis, report of 2 cases and a review of the literature. Clin Nephrol 1980; 12: 38–44.

149. Milutinovic J, Wu W-S, Lindholm DD, LeRoy Lapp N. Acute massive unilateral hydrothorax: a rare complication of chronic peritoneal dialysis. South Med J 1980: 73: 827–8.

150. Grefberg N, Danielson BG, Benson L, Pitkanen P. Right sided hydrothorax complicating peritoneal dialysis. Nephron 1983; 34: 130–4.

151. Kennedy JM. Procedures used to demonstrate a pleuroperitoneal communication: a review. Perit Dial Bull 1985; 5: 168–70.

152. Ribot S, Jacobs MG, Frankel HJ, Bernstein A. Complications of peritoneal dialysis. Am J Med Sci 1966; 252: 505–17.

153. Mion CM, Boen ST. Analysis of factors responsible for the formation of adhesions during chronic peritoneal dialysis. Am J Med Sci 1965; 250: 675–9.

154. Matalon R, Levine S, Eisinger RP. Hazards in routine use of peritoneal dialysis. NY State J Med 1971; 71: 219–24 .

155. Henderson LW. Peritoneal dialysis. In: Massry SG, Sellers AL, eds. Clinical Aspects of Uraemia and Dialysis. Springfield: Charles C. Thomas, 1976, p. 574.

156. Simkin EP, Wright FK. Perforating injuries of the bowel complicating peritoneal catheter insertion. Lancet 1968; 1: 61–7.

157. Chugh KS, Bhattacharya K, Amaresan MS, Sharma BK, Bansal VK. Peritoneal dialysis our experience based on 550 dialyses. J Assoc Phys India 1972; 20: 215–21.

158. Nienhuis LI. Clinical peritoneal dialysis. Arch Surg 1966; 93: 643–53.

159. Pauli HG, Billikofer E, Vorburger C. Clinical experience with peritoneal dialysis. Helv Med Acta 1966; 33: 51–8.

160. Krebs RA, Burtiss BB. Bowel perforation. JAMA 1966; 198: 486–7.

161. Denovales EL, Avendano LN. Risks of peritoneal catheter insertion (letter). Lancet 1968; 1: 473.

162. Dunea G. Peritoneal dialysis and hemodialysis. Med Clin N Am 1971; 55: 155–75.

163. Rigalosi RS, Maher JF, Schreiner GE. Intestinal perforation during peritoneal dialysis. Ann Intern Med 1964; 70: 1013–15.

164. Edwards DH, Gardner RD, Williams DG. Rupture of a hernial sac: a complication of peritoneal dialysis. J Urol 1972; 108: 255–6.

165. Smith E, Chamberlain MJ. Complications of peritoneal dialysis. Br Med J 1965; 1: 126–7.

166. Goldsmith HJ, Edwards EC, Moorhead PJ, Wright FK. Difficulties encountered in intermittent dialysis for chronic renal failure. Br J Urol 1966; 38: 625–34.

167. Stein MF Jr. Intraperitoneal loss of dialysis catheter. Ann Intern Med 1969; 71: 869–70.

168. Oreopoulos DG, Helfrich GB, Khanna R et al. Peritoneal dialysis catheter implantation. Video developed by Baxter's Catheter and Exit Site Advisory Committee, Baxter Healthcare Corporation, 1988.

169. Oreopoulos DG, Helfrich GB, Khanna R et al. Peritoneal catheters and exit-site practices: current recommendations. Perit Dial Bull 1987; 7: 130–8.

170. Gokal R, Ash SR, Helfrich GB et al. Peritoneal catheters and exit-site practices: toward optimum peritoneal access. Perit Dial Int 1992; 13: 29–39.

171. Ash S. Y-TEC peritoneoscopic implantation of the peritoneal dialysis catheter. Video produced by Medigroup Inc., North Aurora, IL, USA, 1993.

172. Copley JB, Lindberg JS, Back SN, Tapia NP. Peritoneoscopic placement of Swan neck peritoneal dialysis catheters. Perit Dial Int 1996 (suppl. 1): S330–2.

173. Twardowski ZJ, Khanna R, Nolph KD et al. Intraabdominal pressure during natural activities in patients treated with continuous ambulatory peritoneal dialysis. Nephron 1986; 44: 129–35.

174. Moncrief–Popovich catheter. A video produced by Austin Biomedical Research Institute, Austin, TX, USA.

175. Nijhuis PHA, Smulders JF, Jakimowicz JJ. Laparoscopic introduction of a continuous ambulatory peritoneal dialysis (capd) catheter by a two puncture technique. Surg Endosc 1996; 10: 676–9.

176. Twardowski ZJ, Prowant BF. Appearance and classification of healing peritoneal catheter exit sites. Perit Dial Int 1996; 16 (suppl. 3): S71–93.

177. Prowant BF, Twardowski ZJ. Recommendations for exit care. Perit Dial Int 1996; 16: S94–9.

178. Prowant BF, Warady BA, Nolph KD. Peritoneal dialysis catheter exit-site care: results of an international survey. Perit Dial Int 1993; 13: 149–54.

179. Pecoits-Filho RFS, Twardowski ZJ, Khanna R, Kim YL, Goel S, Moore H. The effect of antibiotic prophylaxis on the healing of exit-sites of peritoneal dialysis catheters in rats. Perit Dial Int 1998; 18: 60–3.

180. Prowant BF, Schmidt LM, Twardowski ZJ et al. Peritoneal dialysis catheter exit site care. Am Nephr Nurs Assoc J 1988; 15: 219–22.

181. Twardowski ZJ, Ryan LP, Kennedy JM. Catheter break-in for continuous ambulatory peritoneal dialysis – University of Missouri experience. Perit Dial Bull 1984; 4 (suppl. 3): S110–11.

182. Ash SR, Carr DJ, Diaz-Buxo JA. Peritoneal access devices: hydraulic function and compatibility. In: Nissenson AR, Fine RN, Gentile DE, eds. Clinical Dialysis, 2nd edn. Norwalk: Appleton & Lange, 1990, pp. 212–39.

183. Hashimoto Y, Yano S, Nakanishi Y, Suzuki S, Tsutsumi M. A simple method for opening an obstructed peritoneal cath-

eter using an infusion accelerator. Adv Perit Dial 1996; 12: 227–30.

184. Twardowski ZJ, Pasley K. Reversed one-way obstruction of the peritoneal catheter (the accordion clot). Perit Dial Int 1994; 14: 296–7.

185. O'Regan S, Garel L, Patriquin H, Yazbeck S. Outflow obstruction: whiplash technique for catheter mobilization. Perit Dial Int 1988; 8: 265–8.

186. Honkanen E, Eklund B, Laasonen L, Ylinen K, Grönhagen-Riska C. Reposition of a displaced peritoneal catheter: the Helsinki whiplash method. Adv Perit Dial 1990; 6: 159–64.

187. Diaz-Buxo JA, Turner MW, Nelms M. Fluoroscopic manipulation of Tenckhoff catheters: outcome analysis. Clin Nephrol 1997; 47: 384–8.

188. Yoshihara K, Yoshi S, Miyagi S. Alpha replacement method for the displaced swan neck catheter. Adv Perit Dial 1993; 19: 227–30.

189. Ersoy FF, Twardowski ZJ, Satalowich RJ, Ketchersid T. A retrospective analysis of catheter position and function in 91 CAPD patients. Perit Dial Int 1994; 14: 409–10.

190. Twardowski ZJ. Malposition and poor drainage of peritoneal catheters. Semin Dial (Dial Clin section) 1990; 3: 57.

191. Pierratos A. Peritoneal dialysis glossary. Perit Dial Bull 1984; 4: 2–3.

192. Keane WF, Everett ED, Fine RN, Golper TA, Vas SI, Peterson PK. CAPD related peritonitis management and antibiotic therapy recommendations. Perit Dial Bull 1987; 7: 55–68.

193. Piraino B, Bernardini J, Sorkin M. Catheter infections as a factor in the transfer of continuous ambulatory peritoneal dialysis patients to hemodialysis. Am J Kidney Dis 1989; 13: 365–9.

194. Luzar MA, Brown CB, Balf D et al. Exit-site care and exit-site infection in continuous ambulatory peritoneal dialysis (CAPD): results of a randomized multicenter trial. Perit Dial Int 1990; 10: 25–9.

195. Copley JB. Prevention of peritoneal dialysis catheter-related infections. Am J Kidney Dis 1987; 10: 401–7.

196. Gloor HJ, Nichols WK, Sorkin MI et al. Peritoneal access and related complications in continuous ambulatory peritoneal dialysis. Am J Med 1983; 74: 593–8.

197. Vogt K, Binswanger U, Buchmann P, Baumgartner D, Keusch G, Largiadèr F. Catheter-related complications during continuous ambulatory peritoneal dialysis (CAPD): a retrospective study on sixty-two double cuff Tenckhoff catheters. Am J Kidney Dis 1987; 10: 47–51.

198. Twardowski ZJ. Peritoneal catheter exit site infections: prevention, diagnosis, treatment, and future directions. Semin Dial 1992; 5: 305–15.

199. Twardowski ZJ, Prowant BF. Classification of normal and diseased exit sites. Perit Dial Int 1996; 16 (suppl. 3): S32–50.

200. Twardowski ZJ, Prowant BF. Current approach to exit site infections in patients on peritoneal dialysis. Nephrol Dial Transplant 1997; 12: 1284–95.

201. Bertone AL. Management of exuberant granulation tissue. Vet Clin N Am: Equine Pract 1989; 5: 551–62.

202. Khanna R, Twardowski ZJ. Recommendations for treatment of exit-site pathology. Perit Dial Int 1996; 16: S100–4.

203. Strauss FG, Holmes D, Nortman DF, Friedman S. Hypertonic saline compresses: therapy for complicated exit site infections. Adv Perit Dial 1993; 9: 248–50.

204. Scalamogna A, Castelnovo C, De Vecchi A, Ponticelli C. Exit-site and tunnel infections in continuous ambulatory peritoneal dialysis. Am J Kidney Dis 1991; 28: 674–7.

205. Piraino B, Bernardini J, Peitzman A, Sorkin M. Failure of peritoneal catheter cuff shaving to eradicate infection. Perit Dial Bull 1987; 7:179–82.

206. Prowant BF, Khanna R, Twardowski ZJ. Case reports for independent study. Perit Dial Int 1996; 16: S105–14.

207. Low DE, Bas SI, Oreopoulos DG et al. Randomized clinical trial of prophylactic cephalexin in CAPD. Lancet 1980; 2: 753–4.

208. Churchill DN, Oreopoulos DG, Taylor DW, Vas SI, Manuel MA, Wu G. Peritonitis in CAPD patients – a randomized clinical trial of trimethoprim-sulfamethoxazole prophylaxis. Am Soc Nephrol 1987; 20: 97A (abstract).

209. Twardowski ZJ. Recurrent peritoneal catheter exit-site infection: II. Semin Dial 1993; 6: 406–8.

210. Swartz R, Messana J, Starmann B, Weber M, Reynolds J. Preventing *Staphylococcus aureus* infection during chronic peritoneal dialysis. J Am Soc Nephrol 1991; 2: 1085–91.

211. Zimmerman SW, Ahrens E, Johnson CA et al. Randomized controlled trial of prophylactic rifampin for peritoneal dialysis-related infections. Am J Kidney Dis 1991; 18: 225–31.

212. Bernardini J, Piraino B, Holley J, Johnston JR, Lutes R. A randomized trial of *Staphylococcus aureus* prophylaxis in peritoneal dialysis patients: mupirocin calcium ointment 2% applied to the exit site versus cyclic oral rifampin. Am J Kidney Dis 1996; 27: 695–700.

213. Nichols WK, Nolph KD. A technique for managing exit site and cuff infection in Tenckhoff catheters. Perit Dial Bull 1983; 3 (suppl. 4): S4–5.

214. Abouljoud MS, Cruz C, Dow RD, Mozes MF. Peritoneal catheter obstruction by a fallopian tube: a case report. Perit Dial Int 1992; 12: 257–8.

215. Twardowski ZJ. Clinical value of standardized equilibration tests in CAPD patients. Blood Purif 1989; 7: 95–108.

216. Twardowski ZJ, Tully RJ, Nichols WK, Sunderrajan S. Computerized tomography in the diagnosis of subcutaneous leak sites during continuous ambulatory peritoneal dialysis (CAPD). Perit Dial Bull 1984; 4: 163–6.

217. Twardowski ZJ, Tully RJ, Ersoy FF, Dedhia NM. Computerized tomography with and without intraperitoneal contrast for determination of intraabdominal fluid distribution and diagnosis of complications in peritoneal dialysis patients. ASAIO Trans 1990; 36: 95–103.

218. Dimitriadis A, Antoniou S, Toliou T, Papadopoulos C. Tissue reaction to deep cuff of Tenckhoff catheter and peritonitis. Adv Perit Dial 1990; 6: 155–8.

219. Korzets Z, Erdberg A, Golan E et al. Frequent involvement of the internal cuff segment in CAPD peritonitis and exit-site infection – an ultrasound study. Nephrol Dial Transplant 1996; 11: 336–9.

220. Grefberg N, Danielson BG, Nilsson P, Wahlberg J. An unusual complication of the Toronto Western Hospital catheter (letter). Perit Dial Bull 1983; 3: 219.

221. della Volpe M, Iberti M, Ortensia A, Veronesi GV. Erosion of the sigmoid by a permanent peritoneal catheter (letter). Perit Dial Bull 1984; 4: 108.

222. Watson LC, Thompson JC. Erosion of the colon by a long dwelling peritoneal catheter. JAMA 1980; 243: 2156–7.

223. Valles M, Cantarell C, Vila J, Tovar JL. Delayed perforation of the colon by a Tenckhoff catheter. Perit Dial Bull 1982; 2: 190.

224. Shohat J, Shapira Z, Yussim A, Boner G. An unusual cause of massive intraperitoneal bleeding in CAPD (letter). Perit Dial Bull 1984; 4: 257–8.

225. de los Santos AC, von Eye O, d'Avila D, Mottin CC. Rupture of the spleen: a complication of continuous ambulatory peritoneal dialysis. Perit Dial Bull 1986; 6: 203–4.

226. Braden GL, Germain MJ, Guardione VA, Fitzgibbons JP. Infected intra-abdominal hematoma associated with an indwelling Tenckhoff catheter. Perit Dial Bull 1984; 4: 248–50.

227. Jamison MH, Fleming SJ, Ackrill P, Schofield PF. Erosion of rectum by Tenckhoff catheter. Br J Surg 1988; 75: 360.

228. Brady HR, Abraham G, Oreopoulos DG, Cardella CJ. Bowel erosion due to a dormant peritoneal catheter in immunosupressed renal transplant recipients. Perit Dial Int 1988; 8: 163–5.

229. Kourie TB, Botha JR. Erosion of caecum by a Tenckhoff catheter. A case report. S Afr J Surg 1985; 23: 117–18.

230. Schröder CH, Rieu P, De Jong MCWJ, Monnens LAH. Peritoneal laceration: a rare cause of scrotal edema in a 2-year old boy. Perit Dial Int 1993; 13: S27 (abstract).

231. Sanan A, Haines SJ, Nyberg SL, Leonard AS. Knotted bowel: small-bowel obstruction from coiled peritoneal shunt catheters. Report of two cases. J Neurosurg 1995; 82: 1062–4.

232. Prasad VS, Krishna AM, Gupta PK. Extrusion of peritoneal catheter of ventriculoperitoneal shunt through the urethr. Br J Neurosurg 1995; 9: 209–10.

233. Ashpole R, Boulton R, Holmes AE. A case of asymptomatic passage per-rectum of a fractured redundant peritoneal catheter from a ventriculo-peritoneal shunt. Eur J Pediatr Surg 1995; 5: 280–1.

234. Fermin S, Fernandez-Guerra RA, Sureda PJ. Extrusion of peritoneal catheter through the mouth. Child Nerv Syst 1996; 12: 553–5.

235. Haralampopoulos F, Iliadis H, Karniadakis S, Koutentakis D. Invasion of a peritoneal catheter into the inferior vena cava: report of a unique case. Surg Neurol 1996; 46: 21–2.

236. Johnson MC, Maxwell MS. Delayed intrapleural migration of a ventriculoperitoneal shunt. Child Nerv Syst 1995; 11: 348–50.

237. Golper TA, Carpenter J. Accidents with Tenckhoff catheters. Ann Intern Med 1981; 95: 121–2.

238. Usha K, Ponferrada L, Prowant BF, Twardowski ZJ. Repair of chronic peritoneal dialysis catheter. Perit Dial Int 1998; 18: 419–23.

239. Ward RA, Klein E, Wathen RL (eds). Peritoneal catheters. In: Investigation of the risks and hazards with devices associated with peritoneal dialysis and sorbent regenerated dialysate delivery systems. Perit Dial Bull 1983; 3 (suppl. 3): S9–17.

240. Szycher M, Siciliano AA, Reed AM. Polyurethane in medical devices. Med Design Mat 1991: pp. 18–25.

241. Kurihara S, Tani Y, Tateishi K *et al.* Allergic eosinophilic dermatitis due to silicone rubber: a rare but troublesome complication of the Tenckhoff catheter. Perit Dial Bull 1985; 5: 65–7.

242. Prowant BF, Schmidt LM, Twardowski ZJ *et al.* Use of exudate smears for diagnosis of peritoneal catheter exit site infection. In: Avram MM, Giordano C, eds. Ambulatory Peritoneal Dialysis – Proceedings of the IV Congress of the International Society for Peritoneal Dialysis, Venice, Italy, 29 June–2 July 1987. New York: Plenum, 1990, pp. 220–2.

243. Bozkurt F, Keller E, Schollmeyer P. Swan neck peritoneal dialysis catheter can reduce complications in CAPD patients. Abstracts of the IV Congress of the International Society for Peritoneal Dialysis. Venice, Italy, 29 June–2 July 1987. Perit Dial Bull (suppl.) 1987; 7 (suppl. 2): S9.

244. Gucek A, Bren FA, Lindic J, Premru V, Kveder R. CAPD catheter survival: our 9-year experience. Perit Dial Int 1992; 12 (suppl. 2): S49 (abstract).

245. Ahlmén J, Brunes L, Schönborg C. A randomized comparison of two peritoneal dialysis catheters. ASAIO 1993 Abstracts. 39th Annual Meeting, New Orleans Hilton Hotel, New Orleans, Louisiana, 29–30 April and 1 May 1993, p. 110.

246. Twardowski ZJ, Prowant BF, Nichols WK, Nolph KD, Khanna R. Six-year experience with swan neck presternal peritoneal dialysis catheter. Abstracts of the XXXth Annual Meeting, San Antonio, Texas, 2–5 November 1997. J Am Soc Nephrol 1997; 8: 183A.

247. Twardowski ZJ, Prowant BF, Nichols WK, Nolph KD, Khanna R. Six-year experience with swan neck presternal peritoneal dialysis catheter. Perit Dial Int 1998; 18: 598–602.

248. Lye WC, Kour NW, van der Straaten JC, Leong SO, Lee EJ. A prospective randomized comparison of the swan neck, coiled, and straight Tenckhoff catheters in patients on CAPD. Perit Dial Int 1996; 16: (suppl. 1): S333–5.

10 Organization of a peritoneal dialysis programme – the nurses' role

L. UTTLEY AND B. PROWANT

Introduction

Over the past decade the use of peritoneal dialysis (PD) in the treatment of end-stage renal disease has escalated due to the use of improved technology (Y sets, cycler dialysis) and new dialysis solutions (icodextrin, bicarbonate) all of which have enhanced clinical outcome.

More patients are selecting PD as a first-line treatment and currently there are more than 120 000 patients worldwide. Credit for the continuing success of PD therapy must in part be given to the PD nurses who have mastered the technology, improved patient training and follow-up care and now have a solid framework for the organization of a PD unit. Indeed it is now agreed that PD units could not function without these highly motivated and loyal nurses [1]. The organization of the PD programme requires time, thought and careful planning. Managing a patient on PD combines thorough technical instruction with moral support to promote self-motivation. This chapter reviews the essential elements required, the role and qualities of a PD nurse, protocols and teaching plans, all of which are crucial to the success of a PD programme.

Requirements of a PD programme

Although PD is a simple technique, it is now generally accepted that it should ideally be performed in the right setting, with appropriate staff and facilities, and be integrated into a renal replacement programme [2, 3]. Doctors, nurses and paramedical staff need to work together to form a cohesive multidisciplinary team. A teaching plan needs to be established and step-by-step protocols formulated, prior to the admittance of any patient. The temptation to open a PD unit without guidelines or experienced personnel should be avoided. In developing coun-

tries it may be possible, with the help of grants from societies such as the International Society of Peritoneal Dialysis (ISPD), to second nurses and physicians to established PD units for training. The major requirements are outlined in Table 1. Using these broad guidelines it is possible to deliver to the patient the care required for his/her continued long-term well-being.

Establishing a PD programme

If PD is to be a success it is essential that it be integrated with haemodialysis and transplantation [4, 5]. Temporary haemodialysis is often necessary due to catheter removal, peritonitis, hernia repair or other medical and surgical-related problems [6]. In an integrated programme patients can transfer back and forth between therapies with ease and continuity of care can be achieved over many years.

Table 1. Essential requirement for PD programmes

Place	Suitable location
	Single rooms or purpose-built PD area for training
	Outpatient follow-up care facilities
	Back up haemodialysis; inpatient beds
Staff	Adequate experienced medical and nursing staff 24 h on-call
	Multidisciplinary team approach
	Staff orientation
Training	Teaching plan and training manual
	Established protocols
	Continuing education
	Commitment to teaching PD
Equipment	Reliable equipment suitable for all patients
	Storage space
	Home delivery system
Finance	Adequate funding for patient population
	Billing procedures
	Compliance with statutory regulations

R. Gokal, R. Khanna, R.Th. Krediet and K.D. Nolph (eds.), Textbook of Peritoneal Dialysis, 2nd Edition, 363–386.
© 2000 Kluwer Academic Publishers. Printed in Great Britain.

A PD head nurse should be appointed to spearhead the programme [7]. It is imperative that she has total commitment to the treatment and believes that patients can dialyse safely and effectively at home; indeed this should be the philosophy for all PD personnel including the medical director whose main task is to monitor both patients and dialysis process [8]. If a PD programme is to obtain adequate space, personnel and equipment it is crucial that the finance to support the programme and allow it to flourish is agreed at the outset. Little will be achieved if there are staffing shortages, inflexibility with dialysis systems and inadequate space for training and follow-up care [9]. PD can be a revenue-producing treatment, but in order to profit one has to invest. Severe budget restrictions can lead to inadequate patient care and low staff morale, 'a noose around the neck' in the running of any PD programme.

The effectiveness of the PD programme as a whole should be monitored [10]. Evaluation of rates of infection, hospitalization, dropout and technique failure should take place annually and such quality assurance reviews can ensure periodic revision to protocols and procedures. Keeping the multidisciplinary team enthusiastic and creative about programme innovations can ensure that the patients receive the highest standard of dialysis and rehabilitation.

Training area

All PD programmes should have an area that is conducive to learning and free from through traffic. The training area should be calm and peaceful, providing the privacy necessary for learning whilst reducing the risk of cross-infection. Depending on the catchment population a programme may be training two or three patients at any one time. Whilst some of the teaching sessions will need to be on an individual basis, some group sessions may be appropriate and the accommodation should befit both types. It is desirable that part of the training area should mimic closely the conditions the patients would have in their own homes, to avoid confusion and disorientation after discharge. The area needs to be light and airy with ample space for free movement. Good artificial lighting, especially for the poorly sighted, is essential. A resource area with comfortable seating, where patients can make use of visual aids, computers and practice equipment, can double as a rest area for patients training on an

Table 2. Rooms required in PD unit

Resource room: group training area; visual aids, teaching equipment; rest area
Single rooms: CCPD; exchange, CAPD
Store room
Toilet/showers
Nurses' office
Doctors' office
Clean utility room
Dirty utility room
Clerical and administration offices – computer base
Access to emergency beds and haemodialysis
Clinic area
Supply storage

Table 3. Equipment requirements in PD training rooms

Comfortable chair/bed	Shelving for consumables
Washbasin	Bag-warming equipment
Surface/trolley	Ambulatory PD machine
Weighing scales	Clock
Drip stand/hook	Sphygmomanometer

outpatient basis. It may be necessary in some cases for patients to be admitted whilst training, therefore bedroom and en-suite facilities should be provided. The overall area will accommodate all procedures and personnel (Table 2) whilst the individual training rooms require essential equipment (Table 3).

For patients who are severely disabled or blind it is often a good idea to perform whole or part of the training programme in the patient's own home. Adaptations may already have been made to accommodate the disability and the patient will inevitably feel more at ease [11]. The patient will then avoid the unnecessary upheaval of learning the procedures in hospital and adapting them to the home situation, which may be quite different.

Team interactions

The necessity of interdisciplinary collaboration and a team approach to PD patient care has been emphasized [12, 13]. The team typically includes physicians, nurses, dietician and social worker, but is often expanded to include others such as the surgeon responsible for catheter placement, a microbiologist, a psychologist, a physiotherapist, or rehabilitation specialist. PD programmes may also encourage the patient and family to participate in the team's discussion and decision-making processes.

At least some formal structure is required to promote optimal function of the team. Definition of roles and job responsibilities is essential. Shared goals and philosophy regarding home PD therapy will promote cohesion and reduce conflict among members. Regularly scheduled team meetings such as patient-care conferences and quality improvement meetings give the entire team opportunity for inter-action and collaborative decision-making. PD clinics that are structured so two or three team members see the patient together also facilitate communica-tion among the team.

Head nurse/senior clinical manager

When planning a PD programme a senior nurse should be appointed before the unit is opened for patient care. She should have a broad background in dialysis theory and be familiar and experienced in dealing with all types of dialysis and compli-cations. She should have leadership potential, be an independent worker, innovative, creative and empathic [14]. It is very desirable that the nurse should possess a recognized qualification in nephrol-ogy nursing such as the English National Board 136 Certificate (United Kingdom) or the Certified Nephrology Nurse credential (CNN) (United States). A survey undertaken by Brennan for the American Association of Nephrology Nurses (ANNA) showed that 68% of head nurses ($n = 625$) had 6–15 years experience in nephrology nursing practice with 19% holding associate degrees, 36% bachelor's degrees and 40% were diploma graduates [15]. The senior nurse becomes the key member of the nursing staff and will liaise with other members of the team, coordinate nursing duties and ensure continuing nursing care (Table 4).

Qualities of a PD nurse

A PD nurse must have total commitment and belief in the treatment, and possess several important qual-ities [16].

Broad renal and nursing background

The nurse should be familiar with other forms of renal replacement therapies, especially since PD patients may have had, or are likely to have; haemo-dialysis or transplantation. She should also have a broad background in general medical and surgical nursing.

Table 4. Duties of the senior nurse

Patient care
1. Accountable for basic nursing practice
2. Responsible for continuity of care in the home
3. Assessment of patients – predialysis
4. Communication with physicians and other team members regarding patient problems
5. Collaboration with ward/floor staff for inpatient care
6. Responsible for control of infection
7. Communication with patient's family, assessment of coping strategies
8. Recognition and management of peritonitis and other PD complications

Administration
1. Organization and administration of nursing services
2. Responsibility for nursing budget and compliance with reimbursement regulations
3. Organization of follow-up clinics
4. Evaluation of new equipment
5. Participation in renal committees, multidisciplinary team meetings
6. Coordination of teaching including securing resources and teaching aids
7. Responsible for data-collection and computing services
8. Implementation of quality assurance programme
9. Documentation of care and medical records

Educator
1. Development and implementation of a patient-training programme
2. Assessor and teacher of nurses in training licensed, practical nurses (LPNs) and technicians
3. Assists in patient teaching
4. Teaches at in-service sessions
5. Presents papers at local, regional, national and international meetings

Staff care
1. Responsible for staff well-being and morale
2. Duty rotas and holiday administration
3. Counselling of staff – to prevent 'burn-out'
4. Responsible for continuing education programmes
5. Attends and encourages staff to participate in professional organizations

Research
1. Implementation of research projects into PD
2. Evaluation of nursing practice
3. Collaboration with physicians and research fellows in PD research

Teaching skills

It is a common but erroneous belief that anyone can teach PD, but it requires special skills and the suc-cess depends upon the approach adopted. Many nurses are not familiar with self-care and do not believe that patients can perform nursing duties with the same accuracy. The nurse must want the patient to succeed, and be able to impart her knowledge to make the patient independent and confident at home. The ability to communicate with people of all walks of life and backgrounds is crucial.

Patience

This must be in evidence at all times, particularly during teaching sessions. It is of no value to speed up the training unnecessarily. Procedures may have to be repeated many times until the patient is able to perform them correctly. A patient should not be belittled for making mistakes. Encouragement at all times is highly desirable.

Consistency

The nurse needs to remember that a less than rigid technique may lead to an episode of infection. Therefore consistency in teaching various procedures must be of prime importance to avoid patient confusion. Consistency is akin to a life-support system for a PD patient and all members of the nursing team should work together to avoid disaster.

Flexibility

Every patient is different and each is his or her own person. Therefore a degree of flexibility is called for in the approach to patient training and follow up. Using innovation and ingenuity the nurse needs to cover every aspect of patient care without jeopardizing the consistency and routine that PD requires.

Sense of humour

This is an essential component of the PD nurse's make-up. Stress is a common factor among staff and patients [17] and a sense of humour can diffuse a difficult and tense situation [18]. This is particularly important when dealing with patients and families in their own homes.

Ability to communicate

Better patient care and training will result only with good communication. The PD nurse must establish a rapport with patients and families, as well as other members of the multidisciplinary team.

Judgement

Good judgement, the ability to lead and make decisions, are desirable attributes for any PD nurse.

Nursing staff numbers and recruitment

It is the head nurse who will assess the projected workload based on patient population increases and give advice to higher authorities on the staffing levels required. The most important changes and developments affecting nephrology nursing during the 1980s were the switch from task-orientated to primary nursing, the increase in the number of patients, and changing case mix to include more elderly and diabetic patients [19]. The high-risk patient requires more nursing supervision and this will inevitably affect staffing levels [20]. Other important factors to consider when determining adequate staffing levels are the amount of non-nursing duties performed by nurses, extensive haemodialysis and/or transplantation responsibilities, inpatient peritoneal dialysis responsibilities and follow-up care including home visiting.

Studies suggest that the desirable staff–patient ratio for adequate cover does not exceed 1–25 [8, 20, 21]. However, during the 1990s this ratio is becoming increasingly more difficult to achieve and there are various reasons for this. Firstly, financial restrictions brought about by changes in the health service in the UK [22] and the reduction in the reimbursement regulations in the USA [23] have had a serious effect on the staffing of dialysis units. Staff salaries usually represent the largest portion of operating expenses, and have had to be reduced. More units are replacing registered nurses with licensed practical nurses (LPN), licensed vocational nurses (LVN) and technicians [24]. Salaries in some units have been frozen and on call and overtime payment reduced or eliminated. Staff education programmes have also been decreased.

These cutbacks have resulted in low staff morale, increased sickness, rapid staff turnover and burnout [25]. This is on top of an already established shortage of nurses throughout the western world. Renal units will in the future have to look closely at the effectiveness of direct patient care by professional registered nurses versus LPN/LVN [26]. However, organizational outcomes such as job satisfaction of the professional nurse should also be taken into consideration [27]. Many nurses are now leaving the hospital environment to work in industry, where they are offered better working conditions and higher salaries, and the recruitment and retention of professional nurses for PD units has become a formidable task [28, 29].

Table 5. Staff orientation topics specific to peritoneal dialysis

1. Programme philosophy
2. Brief history of PD
3. Anatomy of the peritoneum
4. PD kinetics
5. Factors affecting PD efficiency
6. Types of PD
7. PD catheters
8. Catheter insertion: preoperative nursing care, postoperative catheter care
9. Catheter break-in
10. Catheter exit-site care: postoperative care; chronic care; care of the inflamed/infected exit
11. Dialysis prescriptions: solutions; exchange volumes; dextrose concentrations; evaluation of membrane characteristics; assessment of adequacy
12. Procedure: CAPD exchanges; intraperitoneal medications; cycler dialysis; tubing changes; catheter repair
13. Patient education
14. Nursing follow-up and management
15. Dietary recommendations for PD patients
16. Routine medications
17. Acceptable blood chemistries
18. Infectious complications of PD
19. Non-infectious complications of PD: early complications (post catheter insertion); late complications
20. Technical problems
21. Options for back-up dialysis

Staff recruitment

Peritoneal dialysis is a home therapy that requires the patient and family to accept the responsibility for self-care. The focus of nursing care is initially to teach the patient to perform dialysis and manage renal disease at home, and subsequently to provide ongoing guidance and support. It is therefore important to recruit nurses who not only believe in the concept that patients can care for themselves effectively but who are also willing to assist patients to become independent; nurses should also enjoy teaching and chronic care. It is often very difficult for acute-care nurses, used to working with high technology and a fast pace, to adjust to a position in home dialysis therapy.

Some units in the western world are training nurses to become 'specialists' [30]. These nurses undertake duties normally done by junior doctors, such as clinical assessment and insertion of lines and catheters. Although highly competent and invariably saving valuable resources, doctors' time and money, it may be rather short-sighted to take nurses away from standard nursing duties at a time when there is a recruitment crisis in the nursing profession, and nephrology in particular.

Staff training and orientation

Over the past 10 years, with the increasing number of patients on PD, the need for a specialized post-basic training has become obvious. Recognized courses in the UK, USA and Canada have been emulated throughout Europe [31–35] and other continents [36]. Even in developing countries nurses caring for the patients on PD are showing an interest in specialization, and recognize the need for training. If a formal education programme is unavailable,

on-the-job orientation, in-service and continuing education are critical prerequisites to quality care. Peritoneal dialysis orientation is extensive and may last 6–8 weeks. Topics unique to peritoneal dialysis are listed in Table 5.

Nurses with haemodialysis or other nephrology nursing experience may complete orientation more quickly because they already have knowledge of renal anatomy and physiology, renal diseases, and chronic renal failure. It is imperative that all nurses review principles of patient and adult education. The nurse orientee is frequently assigned a mentor to work with, to observe procedures, patient education, and clinical care. The mentor then serves as a consultant to advise and assist the new nurse as she begins providing direct patient care. Because the emphasis is on understanding the dialysis process and nursing management of PD patients, it may be several months before new staff members are entirely comfortable with the role.

In-service education can be used to update staff on new products, drugs, policies and procedures, and essentials such as cardiopulmonary resuscitation and disaster drills. In-service education meetings can also be used to review various nephrology nursing topics in preparation for certification examinations, to present data from clinical research projects, and as a forum for nurses to share what they have learned at national or international meetings.

Staff stress

Burnout has been described as a syndrome of emotion, exhaustion, depersonalization, and reduced personal accomplishment. A survey of nephrology nurses in the USA found that scores for burnout were higher than in previously reported studies of nurses and physicians [37]. The same study identifies the workload, patient interactions, death and dying issues, and a lack of staff support as the most frequent work-related stresses. Another survey supports the concept that patient interactions are stressful, indicating that nephrology nurses view the typical patient as old, chronically ill, dependent, non-compliant and often in a negative mood [38]. Nurses working more than 40 hours per week had significantly higher levels of burnout than their counterparts. Strategies to reduce job-related stress include maintaining adequate staffing, flexible scheduling and providing assistance and emotional support for nurses with a heavy caseload. A more global and proactive strategy is to encourage staff members to recognize and appreciate the expertise and talents of their colleagues and to develop an environment where they support and complement one another [39].

A focused plan for job enrichment and professional enhancement can contribute to improved morale, motivation, job satisfaction and reduced staff turnover. Nurses may be assigned specific projects that will challenge them to learn new information or enable them to develop new skills. Such projects could include developing patient education modules or materials, responsibility for peritonitis data, participation in quality-improvement projects, reviewing and revising policies and procedures, and responsibility for an in-service education programme. Clinical nurses should also be encouraged to develop clinical expertise in relevant specialities such as geriatric nursing and management of diabetic patients.

Opportunities to attend continuing education meetings outside the institution will give staff members a broader perspective of nephrology nursing and state-of-the-art information. These meetings also help develop a network with other nurse colleagues, to discuss problems and impart information. Participation in continuing education meetings often stimulates staff members to try new approaches in clinical care, to initiate new projects, to become involved in research, or to learn more about a particular area of interest.

Nurses and managers alike can achieve intellectual and professional advancement by participating in research projects, presenting at professional meetings and serving on institutional committees.

Method of nursing

The head nurse and higher nursing authorities will be responsible for establishing the method of nursing that will best suit patient needs. PD is a continuous process, leading from hospital to home, and lends itself to assigned patient care or the primary nursing system [40]. A primary nurse is assigned specific patients and assumes the responsibility for providing total nursing care. According to Marram *et al.* [41], there are five components to this: continuity, accountability, autonomy, authority and personalized patient-centred care. These can be simplified into the nurse's role, nurse–patient relationships and the structure in which the nurse works [42]. In this type of care assigned patients will be trained and looked after following discharge by the same nurse. The nurse teaches the patient on a one-to-one basis, giving general nursing care, assessing progress and discussing problems. Following discharge the same nurse will follow patients at the outpatient clinic and visit them in their homes. In this way a good relationship and rapport is established with patients and their families. The nursing process then becomes complete and continuous. During 'off-duty' and holidays, patient care is handed over to a deputy or associate nurse. This method of nursing is common throughout the USA, Van Waeleghem *et al.* [19] state that 50% of units throughout Europe now employ primary nursing and other countries are introducing this type of care [43].

Home PD nurse

The home PD nurse is an invaluable member of the team, whose aim is to reduce morbidity, increase support, and help in achieving rehabilitation, especially in the high-risk group of patients such as the elderly and diabetics [44]. Starmann *et al.* [20] noted that 93% of nurses stated that the high-risk groups of patients required 2–3 h per week per patient post-training nursing care. One may then conclude that having separate home-visiting nurses to deliver care will reduce the workload and responsibilities on the already overstretched unit staff while giving home patients, of both modalities, quality care in their own homes. In the UK, where home visiting is more extensive, the home dialysis nurse will also visit home haemodialysis patients. The aim and role of a home visiting nurse are outlined in Table 6.

Call systems

Most PD programmes provide both physician and nursing back-up support for home patients. In our

Table 6. Aims and roles of home visiting nurse

Aims
1. To reduce hospital visits and inpatient stays to a minimum
2. Prevent peritonitis
3. Continue and reinforce learning process
4. Encourage a return to previous or improved social status
5. Nurturing a close link between home and hospital
6. Giving moral support to the patient and his/her family

Roles
1. Assessing patient's home
2. Establishing home PD in new discharged patients
3. Observations of exchange procedures at home
4. Performing transfer set changes at home
5. Routine visits
6. Initiation of therapy for peritonitis and other infections
7. Record keeping
8. Trouble shooting re problems connected with employment, holidays, etc.
9. Counselling and support of both family and patient

experience patients rarely abuse the call system and most calls are made to report a new problem or complication.

The primary disincentive for a nursing on-call system is the expense. The assumption has been made that the on-call physician can and will intervene appropriately for all types of problem. Yet nurses working in PD programmes without continuous back-up nursing support report that patients are much more reluctant to call physicians, and that physicians are not always effective in assisting patients with nursing-related problems. Therefore, these problems often worsen over the weekend and ultimately require excessive nursing time on Monday or even result in emergency room visits or hospitalization.

Legal issues

Expanded nursing practice has resulted in part from increasing nursing knowledge and specialization. Many PD nurses operate in expanded roles. Key issues to consider are whether the functions performed by the PD nursing staff are within the legal definition of nursing and whether the dialysis unit policies and procedures are specific as to the role of the PD nurse. Policies and procedures must be periodically reviewed to ensure that they are complete, accurate and current. Medication procedures should specifically address antibiotic administration. Job descriptions and responsibilities of unlicensed nurses and technicians must not place either these individuals or the supervising professional nurses in legal

jeopardy. Rosario [45] has recommended a number of strategies that can reduce the risk of legal complications (Table 7).

Cost-effectiveness

Nursing time and supplies are the most costly components of a chronic PD programme. Appropriate use of non-nursing personnel can greatly enhance the efficiency of a PD programme with significant cost savings [46]. Secretarial/clerical personnel or technicians can be used for scheduling, inventory, ordering, and stocking supplies, assembling medical records, transient patient arrangements, medical record requests, monthly charges, routine computer entry and data collection, machine set-up and teardown, machine maintenance, blood sampling, dialysate sampling, and other technical procedures [46]. It is critical, however, that the delegation of responsibilities complies with professional criteria for delegation to unlicensed personnel, that the activities of unlicensed personnel are supervised by professional nurses and that documentation is appropriate [47].

Inventory control for the outpatient clinic, inpatient unit and home-patient supplies is also a very effective method of controlling costs. Anticipating an appropriate distribution of dialysis solution volumes and dextrose concentrations, and avoiding excessive waste associated with prescription changes, can dramatically reduce the amount of unused and outdated dialysis solution in the patient's home and in the clinic. Reuse of cycler tubing has been demonstrated to be both safe and cost-effective with gravity

Table 7. Strategies to reduce legal complications

1. Obtain voluntary consent for dialysis treatment from a competent person
2. Document that recommedations for treatment were made without pressure and that consent was not coerced
3. Do not treat any patient without physician orders
4. Do not dispense prescription medications to the patient for home use
5. Document the client's response to education. (Training or education checklists do not serve as documentation of the patient's response)
6. Update patient education materials periodically
7. Review dialysis procedures with the patient at specific intervals
8. Review discharge instructions with the patient and give a written copy of instructions
9. Each nurse should stay well within the area of individual competence
10. Communicate with the client in a caring and professional manner and foster a good nurse–patient relationship

flow cyclers [48, 49]; however, reuse may be problematic with other types of cyclers [50]. The impact of reuse must be evaluated for each new system. If a reuse programme is initiated it is appropriate to re-evaluate the cycler system and procedures, to seek legal counsel regarding liability, and to obtain informed consent for reuse.

Quality improvement

A continuing evaluation of quality is recommended, and in many countries is mandated by accrediting agencies. The overall goals of a quality improvement programme are to enhance the effectiveness of care and to improve clinical outcomes. There are several aspects of peritoneal dialysis which should be reviewed annually. These include adequacy of dialysis, infection rates, catheter complications, and technique survival. Other areas for quality assessment in chronic peritoneal dialysis programmes are listed in Table 8.

As more data become available from large, national samples, it is possible for individual dialysis programmes to use this information as benchmarks against which to compare their data. For example, the US Health Care Financing Administration's Core Indicators Project has collected and published data regarding PD dialysis prescription, adequacy of dialysis, haematocrit,

Table 8. Areas for quality-improvement projects in peritoneal dialysis

Adequacy of dialysis
Catheters
   Reduction of catheter complications
   Improvement in catheter survival
Dialysis policies, procedure and protocols
Documentation of patient education and follow-up
Fluid balance and blood pressure control
Glucose control in diabetic patients
Haematocrit levels, iron supplementation and Erythropoietin use
Hospitalization for dialysis-related problems
Infectious complications
   Reduction in the incidence of peritonitis
   Decrease in the proportion of recurrent peritonitis episodes
   Reduction in the incidence of exit site and tunnel infections
Management of dialysis during hospital admission
Nutrition
   Routine monitoring of nutritional status
   Prevention of malnutrition
   Treatment of malnourished patients
Patient satisfaction
Phosphorus and calcium balance, bone disease
Technique survival
   Evaluate the reasons for transfer to haemodialysis

erythropoietin dose, albumin levels and blood pressure since 1995 [51–55]. Once problems are identified, efforts are directed at determining the source and contributing factors. Then an action plan can be developed and implemented. Continued monitoring or re-evaluation documents the effectiveness of the intervention(s).

The incidence of peritonitis can be calculated using a simple ratio of the number of peritonitis episodes over the patient-months of exposure, or life-table analysis may be used to determine the probability of the first (or subsequent) peritonitis episodes [56–58]. A comparison of infection rates for each PD modality and each type of PD system may also be of value [59]. Identifying the presumed aetiology of each infection may help in identifying trends and developing strategies to reduce the incidence of peritonitis. Similarly, determining the incidence and presumed aetiology of catheter exit site and tunnel infections assists the Continuous Quality Improvement team in developing effective strategies to prevent infections. CQI projects have resulted in reduced infection rates through improved patient education, prophylactic therapy for known contamination, changes in procedures for exit-site care, and changing the dialysis system for individual patients, either alone or in combination with other interventions [60–69].

Standards

A set of standards of clinical practice is a basic requirement to ensure quality care and successfully trained patients. Mason states that nursing standards define unequivocally what quality care is, and provides specific criteria that can be used to determine whether quality care has been provided [70]. A standard describes what should be done and how the patient will benefit from the care. The American Nephrology Nurses Association and the European Dialysis Transplant Nurses Association have published standards of clinical practice for nephrology nurses [71, 72]. These standards can be adapted to suit any dialysis unit.

Protocols

Each unit needs to have protocols for various procedures, to ensure safe consistent care. It is essential that all members of the team are aware of those, and any amendments that are made. Protocols are developed by the nursing staff and the medical direc-

Table 9. Protocols

1. CAPD exchange procedure (for each system)
2. Cycler set-up procedure (for each cycler)
3. Dialysate and urine collections for adequacy assessment
4. Intermittent PD regimes, e.g. IPD, CCPD
5. Exit-site care (postimplantation and chronic)
6. Administration of intraperitoneal medication
7. Transfer set change procedure
8. Peritoneal equilibration test
9. Treatment of infections: peritonitis, exit site
10. Managing complications, e.g. poor inflow–outflow crack in catheter
11. Holiday dialysis
12. Discharge to home
13. Erythropoietin usage

tor and should be reviewed on a regular basis. Protocols should be based on sound scientific principles and research findings, thus contributing to a research-based practice. Table 9 outlines the protocols required for a peritoneal dialysis programme.

Predialysis assessment and education

Early education for the predialysis patient has the potential to improve patient satisfaction, delay the onset of dialytic treatment and increase cost-effectiveness [73]. Patients are anxious and have fears about the unknown. Predialysis counselling and education can allay such fears and help patients to adjust. However, education programme content should be judiciously evaluated to provide information that is unbiased and realistic, and should be evaluated by members of each discipline to provide a collaborative approach to patient education [74]. Such education can assist patients to choose appropriate treatment options and also help nurses to plan in advance. However, currently there are no specific referral criteria to predialysis programmes, and in some countries lack of reimbursement is a significant barrier to establishing early education. The objectives of the programme are outlined in Table 12. The times of the education sessions should be flexible to occur in the day or evening to accommodate patient and family schedules as much as possible. Initial meetings will identify the learning needs, and dispel rumours and preconceived notions about renal failure and dialysis. Following assessment, an initial package and counselling can be arranged and both the patient and the family should be encouraged to keep in contact if further information or assistance is required.

Teaching

Initial learning is only part of the process of patient education. The second part is that of retaining the information and the ability to adapt techniques and procedures to the home environment. The PD nurse must remember that renal failure patients may be uraemic at the beginning of a training period. They have short attention spans and decreased levels of concentration, thus requiring more repetition of information, clarification, and positive reinforcement and reassurance [75]. The planning phase of the teaching process is critical to achieving a successful outcome. Unless an individual is ready to learn, learning will not take place despite the fact that teaching occurs. Therefore the patient's ability and readiness to learn should be assessed and the equipment and teaching tools best suited to that patient selected. Each patient will be different and will require varying teaching strategies. The PD system and teaching aids used will depend upon the patient's age, intelligence, disability and cognitive state.

A teaching plan (Table 11) will encourage consistency but needs to be flexible and adaptable to patient needs. The plan is set in separate stages, each stage having several modules. These modules will define the objectives and discuss teaching methods. The primary nurse will follow these modules, utiliz-

Table 10. Predialysis education

Session	Approx length and place
Initial interview Meet nephrologist, dietician, social worker PD nurse Patient/family learning needs assessed Allay fears Provide written information	½–2 h at clinic
Basic anatomy – physiology Kidney failure – signs, symptoms Overview of treatment	1 h at clinic
Tour of renal unit	½ h

Home visit
  More detailed information PD/HD, verbally written
  Discuss options
  Assess home – discuss alterations, storage
  Meet the family/carers
Educational evening
  Meet the multidisciplinary team
  Meet patient peer HD/PD
  Short presentations, kidney disease, treatments
  Patient organizations in attendance	

Table 11. Example of teaching plan

Stage 1
(a) Acceptance of need for treatment
(b) Introduction to renal disease
(c) Principles of PD
(d) Introduction to CAPD, APD
(e) Personal hygiene

Stage 2
(a) Aseptic technique – hand-washing
(b) Steps in exchange procedure – setting up cycler

Stage 3
(a) Emergency procedures for contamination
(b) Exit-site care

Stage 4
(a) Addition of medication to bags

Stage 5
(a) Complications: (1) peritonitis; (2) exit-site infection, (3) fluid
    balance, (4) fibrin, (5) drainage–inflow, (6) leaks, (7) pain,
    (8) bleeding, (9) machine faults, (10) constipation, (11) itching.

Stage 6
(a) Record keeping
(b) Weight, blood pressure control
(c) Diet

Stage 7
(a) Home adaptations
(b) Bag-warming
(c) Supplies of equipment

Stage 7
(a) Clinic
(b) Home visiting
(c) Communication with hospital
(d) Employment, hobbies, sports
(e) Psychosocial, counselling
(f) Holidays
(g) Patient association
(h) Transplantation

Stage 9
(a) Overall evaluation

ing such aids as videos, practice equipment, dummy torso, books and computer-assisted learning packages [76]. Lecture and discussion are the primary modes of patient teaching along with demonstration and simulation problem-solving.

A training manual should be available for patient use. This manual encompasses all the information a patient is likely to need, e.g. information regarding supplies, record keeping, patient support groups, holidays, together with an outline of all essential procedures and protocols. These need to be written in a simple form and be easy to follow and read [77]. The manual should be translated into other languages if there are significant ethnic patient groups. Illiterate patients should be provided with step-by-step photographs or videos where possible, while blind patients may be given audiotapes or information in Braille.

Evaluation is an integral part of patient training and should take place throughout the teaching process. Refresher classes are required regularly once the patient is home, particularly if patients develop a problem such as peritonitis, or if procedures are changed [78]. The training period varies in length depending upon the patient's ability to learn, but on average takes between 5 and 10 days. However, the greatest challenge in teaching PD is the relatively short time available for staff to facilitate a patient's positive adjustment to what may be a lifelong treatment. It may be necessary for the training period to be lengthened beyond the necessary mastery of dialysis procedures because the patient may need additional support [79]. A patient should not be discharged to self-care until everyone, including the patient, feels ready.

Problem solving

Problem solving is an integral and important part of any home PD programme. Patients must be able to recognize, assess and correct common PD problems. A problem-solving guide (Table 12) should be included in the patient manual or the patient should receive information, which is now available, some of which is from commercial sources [80].

Follow-up care

PD patients require frequent monitoring, guidance and support after discharge home.

Clinics

Clinic visits are required on a regular basis; the first visit is typically scheduled a week post-discharge. Thereafter the frequency is adjusted depending on how well the patient is coping and how often he or she is visited by the nursing team. Most units require the patient to attend clinic at least every 8–12 weeks once home dialysis is established. A clinic visit will allow the patient to query problems that have arisen and also express any anxieties. The medical team will assess blood pressure control, fluid balance, exit-site status, blood chemistry, medication and dietary control. X-rays, electrocardiogram, lipids and parathormone levels may be done as appropriate. The visit will give the nursing team an opportunity to

Table 12. Problem-solving guide

Problem	Treatment
Difficulty with draining in	
Bag snap seal broken	Break snap seal
Twisted or kinked tube	Attempt to untwist or remove kink
Blockage caused by air or fibrin	Squeeze bag. Add heparin to next bag of fibrin
If these measures fail to produce inflow, call the hospital	
Difficulty with draining out	
Bag lower than abdomen	
Twisted or kinked tube	Attempt to untwist or remove kink
Blockage caused by fibrin	Milk tubing to remove fibrin
	Add heparin to next bag
Constipation	Take laxative
Disconnection of tubing	
Disconnection at catheter	Clamp catheter
	Go to hospital
	Do not reconnect and drain in
When a disconnection occurs it is important to commence antibiotic therapy as soon as possible	
Fluid-related	
Cloudy efifluent – peritonitis	Inform hospital immediately
Blood in effluent – periods – vigorous exercise	Do an exchange. If it does not clear, inform hospital
Deep yellow or orange effluent	Ensure it is not cloudy
	Colour may be caused by antibiotics, excessive dwell time, jaundice
Equipment-related	
Breakage of roller clamp	Clamp line, will require line change
Hole in line or bag	Clamp at junction with catheter, will require line change and antibiotics
	Go to hospital
Accidental contamination of line or minicap	Inform hospital
Symptom-related	
Abdominal pain	
Constipation	Take mild laxative
Dialysis fluid cold or hot	Check bag temperature
Hypertonic bags	
Peritonitis	Drain out, if cloudy
	Inform hospital
Inflow–outflow	Slow down rate of inflow–outflow
Dragging cramp-like pain on complete drainage	Stop drainage towards the end of drain phase
Shoulder pain	
Caused by pressure in addomen or air under diaphragm	Take analgesic
	Drain in knee–chest position
Headaches	
High blood pressure	Check blood pressure
	Inform hospital
Cramps	
Dehydration	Replace fluid and salt as instructed
Itching	Comply with medication regimes
	Inform hospital
Dizziness	
Low blood pressure	Check blood pressure, weight
	Inform hospital
Swollen ankles	
Fluid overload	Check weight. Reduce fluid, salt, intake
	Use stronger solution
Shortness of breath	
Fluid overload	Check weight
	Inform hospital
High temperature	
Infection	Check clarity of effluent
	Check exit site
	Inform hospital
Diarrhoea, vomiting	
Peritonitis or other infection	Check density of bags, weight, temperature
	Inform doctor
Exit-site related	
Leakge, redness, pain	
Infection	Inform hospital

reinforce procedures and perform transfer set changes. Dieticians and social workers should be made available to the patient when necessary [14].

Home visits

Regular home visits are an important part of follow-up care, as the family and patient need to realize that continuing support is available. Visiting the patient at home provides valuable insight about family interactions. Often problems regarding the patient's health are of a personal nature, e.g. psychosexual problems, and a couple may be too embarrassed to discuss these issues at the hospital. In familiar surroundings, when there is an atmosphere of rapport and trust, these topics can be more easily aired.

It is advisable that the first exchange after discharge from hospital is in the presence of a nurse. She can reassure the patient and help him/her to adapt the procedure to the home environment. Thereafter the home visiting nurse will continue to make routine calls to those patients with perceived problems (e.g. high-risk groups), as well as to those doing well. Dialysis problems, medical, social and supply problems will all need discussion [81]. Close liaison will be kept with other members of the multidisciplinary team including local community nurses, social workers and family doctors. Early recognition and management of problems will assist in keeping the patient healthy and well rehabilitated, and will hopefully reduce hospital visits and inpatient stays.

Rehabilitation

Rehabilitation of patients on PD should encompass all aspects of the patient's well-being and include vocational, physical and medical therapies. This is best achieved by careful management of the patient before the start of dialysis, as well as by provision of adequate dialysis [82]. The desires and expectations of PD patients are the same as those without renal failure. They wish to live full productive lives, the kidney disease does not decrease their desire to realize their dreams. However, the disease may place barriers and limitations on their ability to do what they desire, therefore the PD nurse should help her patients to maximize their strengths through encouragement and assistance. Firstly patients should be in optimal health. Adequate dialysis meeting standard ranges, target haemoglobin (using recombinant human erythropoietin – EPO, if necessary) controlled blood pressure and blood glucose and ideal

dry weight. If the guidelines were met the patient would then be a suitable candidate for employment, able to exercise, take holidays and enjoy family life.

Employment

Purpose, status, income, social contact, a structure to our days and lives and a sense of belonging all come from employment [83]. For patients who are employed, efforts should be made to maintain that employment with early assessment of the work environment and necessary alterations of job characteristics. Providing education and liaison with employers is also beneficial. Early initiation of dialysis to prevent severe uraemic symptoms, and strong consideration for flexibility in PD therapies may assist patients to retain employment. Vocational counselling from specialist disabled rehabilitation officers should be sought for the unemployed capable of work or retraining. Patients who remain in the workforce report lower anxiety and fatigue levels and have higher self-esteem. Conversely, unemployment is linked to physical, mental and social morbidity.

Exercise

PD patients may have unique problems from exercise such as catheter-related problems or herniation. However, the benefits of exercise, decreased risk factors for cardiovascular disease, improved blood pressure control and improved psychological status should be weighed against possible stress fracture, hypoglycaemia and muscle or joint problems. Careful consideration for each patient should be given before recommending sport and exercise; however, in the vast majority of cases exercise is thought beneficial. Only sports which involve very heavy lifting, or present a risk of severe strain, should be avoided. Patients may feel better when running or jumping if the peritoneal cavity is empty, and although this entails loss of dialysis time, the psychological benefit may more than compensate [84].

Swimming

Submersion of exit sites which have not completely healed, or have recently been, traumatized or infected, may be a risk factor for infection. Yet many patients find swimming beneficial both physically and psychologically, and PD should not be an absolute contraindication [80, 85]; however, swimming in dirty water should be avoided. To ensure that the water does not contaminate the PD equipment the following procedure should be carried out.

1. Completely cover catheter with large waterproof dressing.
2. After swimming the exit site should be cleansed and redressed and the disconnect cap should be replaced.

Holidays

The ability to perform exchanges almost anywhere has always been one of the big advantages of CAPD, and cycler machines can be dismantled and be transported, allowing APD patients the same flexibility with holiday arrangements. Certain steps must be taken to ensure the procedure remains consistent and all eventualities are covered if a crisis occurs.

First the patient should inform the unit when and where the holiday will take place. If the holiday is of short duration, and within a short distance, the patient may transport the dialysis equipment. If the holiday is abroad, or some distance away, arrangements should be made for delivery of the equipment to the holiday destination. Most manufacturers are happy to make these arrangements. Several weeks' notice is often necessary and it is helpful if the nursing staff at clinics or home visits reminds patients of this.

Holiday insurance should be arranged by the patient, who should be aware that pre-existing medical conditions and cycler equipment might not be covered. Certain countries have reciprocal arrangements, as for example countries within the European Community. Before departure the patient should receive from the unit:

1. A letter giving medical and dialysis details.
2. Name and address of dialysis facility nearest to holiday accommodation.
3. Antibiotic therapy for use in the event of peritonitis if this cannot be obtained at the holiday destination.

At Manchester Royal Infirmary the patients now benefit from an annual holiday organized and accompanied by two experienced PD nursing staff. This gives elderly, disabled patients, patients who live alone and new patients who are not yet confident, a chance to take a holiday without the worry of organization and fear of inability to cope with a crisis while away from home. Families and spouses are also encouraged to take a holiday with the patient group, or are given this opportunity to take a break separately. The accompanying nurses organize the travel arrangements, accommodation and social activities, and will perform the dialysis for patients who normally require help. The benefits of this holiday to the patients outweigh the obvious hard work involved for the nurses, and such holidays can only be recommended.

Telephone calls

After discharge to home, telephone communication becomes an important part of follow-up care. Patients should be given telephone numbers where PD-trained nurses can be contacted 24 hours a day. Patients should be encouraged to contact the staff with problems, and should not be made to feel a nuisance when doing so. Any instructions or information given over the telephone should be clear and precise, if possible in the patient's own language, and should be given only by experienced nurses. Telephone calls can be extremely time-consuming for the nursing staff and this factor should be taken into account when staffing levels are negotiated.

Nursing-home follow-up

Nursing-homes can provide a much-needed haven for some PD patients, particularly the elderly and disabled [86]. Care must be taken by the training nurse to coordinate with the nursing home staff all that is entailed in managing PD therapy [87]. PD nurses have successfully taught the staff at nursing-homes in a similar way to that used for a patient and the family. It is important at the initial contact to address all patients' problems and encourage a mutually cooperative relationship. Education and in-servicing of staff is initiated before the patient is placed, and regular refresher courses, visits and telephone contact help to foster a team approach [88].

Limited follow-up at general hospital

PD programmes can share follow-up care successfully with affiliated hospitals, particularly when patients live a long distance away from the main centre [89]. This has the advantage of reducing not only travel, but also cost. Clinics can be held and will follow the same practices and protocols as the parent clinic. Infections and minor problems can also be treated on an on-call basis. Nursing staff may require some training into PD procedures and it is imperative that the hospital has supplies and follows procedures compatible with those the patients use at home. Both parties will require good-will and cooperation but the patient would welcome expert local care.

Hospitalized patients

Patients may have to be admitted for dialysis or other problems into a hospital ward. During this time it is possible that exchanges may have to be performed by nursing staff. It is essential that only trained staff be involved in any PD procedures, to avoid contamination and infection. If the hospital cannot provide such nurses then nurses from the parent unit must perform the PD procedures until members of staff can be trained. If this is impossible the patient will have to be transferred to a hospital with a PD programme. In any event liaison should be maintained between staff at both nursing and medical levels.

Catheter break-in

Increased intra-abdominal pressure (IAP) in patients on PD has been implicated as a cause of dialysate leaks, which interferes with tissue ingrowth after catheter insertion and increases the risk of infection [90]. The goal of catheter break-in protocols is to keep IAP as low as possible. One way to do this is to delay using the catheter for PD for 10–14 days. The catheter is rinsed with heparinized saline postoperatively until the drainage is no longer blood-tinged. Following complete drainage of the peritoneal cavity, 50–100 ml of heparinized solution may be infused to cushion the catheter. The Moncrief–Popovich catheter [91] is implanted with the distal or external segment completely buried in the subcutaneous tunnel for several weeks. This allows healing at the catheter cuffs without increased IAP.

If PD is initiated shortly after catheter insertion, dialysing with small exchange volumes with the patient supine will reduce IAP. It is also important to avoid constipation and straining, and control coughing or vomiting, as these activities have been shown to dramatically increase IAP in patients receiving PD [92].

Exit-site care

Exit-site and tunnel infections are all-too-frequent complications of PD and may necessitate catheter removal. Exit-site care is primarily a nursing responsibility, but requires the commitment and coopera-

tion of the physician as well. There is no clear consensus as to what is the optimal care for peritoneal catheter exit sites. There have not been enough well-designed research studies to develop a research-based practice, so the recommendations for exit-site care are based on broad principles of wound healing and clinical experience as well as PD exit-site care research.

Goals of exit-site care post-catheter implantation are to prevent colonization during the early healing period, to reduce bacteria at the exit during later healing, to prevent trauma to the exit and cuffs, and to promptly diagnose complications [93]. Principles of postimplantation exit-site care are shown in Table 13 [93–104].

It is generally agreed that postoperative dressing changes should be restricted to specially trained staff [94, 103, 104]. Daily dressing changes postimplantation are not required, for two reasons: first, there is the risk that each dressing change may contaminate the exit with bacteria even though aseptic technique is used; secondly, catheter movement during the dressing change increases the risk of trauma to the wound [93, 102].

Aseptic technique should be used for postoperative dressing changes [93]. The skin surrounding the exit should be cleansed with a non-irritating agent. If strong oxidants such as povidone-iodine and hydrogen peroxide are used, care should be taken to use only on the intact skin surrounding the wound or granulation tissue [98]. Sterile water or sterile normal saline should be used to rinse the exit, and it should be gently patted dry. The exit should be covered with absorbent dressings. Semipermeable dressings should not be applied directly to the wound, because they trap drainage around the exit, and the drainage is an excellent medium for bacterial growth [102]. The catheter should be immobilized

Table 13. Principles of postimplantation catheter care procedures

Prophylactic antibiotic therapy at catheter insertion
Restrict postoperative dressing changes to trained staff
Frequent dressing changes during the first 2 weeks are not
    necessary unless dressings are wet
Aseptic technique using both masks and gloves
A mild, non-irritating agent should be used to clean the exit and
    surrounding skin
Sterile water or saline should be used to rinse the exit
The exit should be dried
An absorbent, sterile dressing should be placed over the exit site
The catheter must be immobilized
Exit site should be evaluated at each dressing change

to prevent accidental trauma to the healing exit [94, 99, 102]. The exit site should not be submerged immediately postimplantation, in order to avoid early colonization with water-borne organisms [93]. There is no consensus when patients may begin to shower or change to chronic exit-care procedures.

Goals of chronic exit-site care are to prevent infection and to assess exit site for signs of infection and other complications. Principles of chronic exit-site care are listed in Table 14.

The choice of a cleansing agent may need to be individualized because of skin sensitivities or allergies. A clean wash-cloth and towel are recommended; sterile supplies are not necessary for chronic care. Mupirocin calcium 2% may be applied after cleansing as prophylaxis in *Staphylococcus aureus* carriers [106]. Topical antibiotics may also be applied as therapy for equivocally infected exits [102, 107]. Adequate immobilization of the catheter is recommended to minimize catheter movement, to prevent tension or tugging on the catheter during procedures, and to prevent accidental trauma. Tape, semipermeable dressings, or immobilizing devices have been used, but there are no data to suggest that any device or method is superior [108]. The method of stabilizing the catheter may need to be individualized.

Although there are no studies indicating that use of dressings reduces the incidence of exit-site infections or improves outcomes of healthy exit sites, there are some theoretical advantages of exit-site dressings. They may protect from dirt and gross contamination, help secure the catheter, and protect from trauma. Dressings are recommended for paediatric patients [109, 110] and for infected exit sites [93, 102].

The patient or a partner should inspect and assess the exit site and tunnel prior to exit care. Patients should be taught the signs and symptoms of exit infection and should be encouraged to notify the PD unit staff promptly when signs of exit-site deterioration develop.

Exit-site assessment should be done by PD staff site at routine visits. Twardowski and Prowant recommend that this assessment include visual inspection of the exit site and sinus using magnification and good lighting [111]. The tunnel, and especially the cuff, should be palpated for tenderness and induration. Exit characteristics should be documented and can be used to classify the exit site.

The nurse and peritonitis

Peritonitis continues to be the major cause of morbidity in PD patients. Although there is a multitude of factors directly or indirectly related in the causation, prevention to some extent depends upon the compliance of the patient and his/her ability to adhere to a strict routine [112]. The tedium and monotony of repeated exchanges day in day out can easily lead to mistakes.

A strict, aseptic exchange technique remains the cornerstone of prevention of peritonitis in the majority of patients; however, since the introduction of the Y disconnect systems infection rates have decreased [113]. Infection rates of patients utilizing cyclers and ultraviolet light are also less than those using standard PD systems [114, 115].

To prevent peritonitis the nurses should ensure that the dialysis system chosen matches the patient's abilities. Regular re-evaluation of the technique procedure can help in identifying and eliminating problem areas; however, it may be prudent to change a patient's system to a Y set or UV system if peritonitis occurs frequently.

Effective teaching to identify and treat contamination and disconnection will reduce the incidence of infection. Prophylactic antibiotics for such calamities are recommended [116].

Nursing procedure following diagnosis of peritonitis

1. The patient must attend a PD unit, or an associated centre, versed in the handling of PD fluid and culture technique.
2. The diagnosis is confirmed from a freshly drained effluent, which is sent for cell count and a full bacteriological analysis.
3. Appropriate first-line antibiotics [117] are injected into the next bag. The procedure for drawing up the antibiotics, dose and injection

Table 14. Principles of chronic PD exit-site care [93, 102, 103, 105]

Good handwashing prior to exit-site care
Inspect the exit and tunnel prior to cleansing
Clean with an antibacterial soap or medical disinfectant
Use liquid soap to reduce the risk of cross-contamination
Be gentle to avoid trauma (do not forcibly remove cuticle, crust or scab)
Rinse with clean, chlorinated water
Dry
Secure the cathether

into the bag should be reviewed with the patient, if he or she has to administer antibiotics at home.

4. It is advisable to give heparin with the antibiotic to prevent fibrin clots.

5. There is usually a need to review fluid balance, as there is invariably a loss of ultrafiltration during a peritonitis episode.

6. Following the cure of the infection the nurse needs to review the exchange or connection procedure and elicit a cause if possible. The nurse can take this opportunity to reassure the patient and the family, while ensuring that short cuts in procedures are not being taken. Patients and relatives will require help and understanding during an infection, to overcome the guilt and depression that may result.

Adequacy and prescription

Membrane characterization

Several tests can be used to characterize an individual patient's peritoneal membrane. These include determination of the mass transfer area coefficient [118–126], the peritoneal equilibration test (PET) [127, 128], the peritoneal function test [129], and the personal dialysis capacity test (PDC) [130, 131].

The PET is perhaps the most widely used standardized diagnostic procedure to assess an individual patient's peritoneal membrane characteristics. In haemodialysis therapy the characteristics of each type of dialyser are well defined and are used to determine the dialysis prescription. Data from the PET are analogous to the package insert, which gives the performance characteristics of a dialyser. An initial PET done shortly after initiating PD gives the physician information upon which to determine the optimal type of PD regimen and to develop an appropriate dialysis prescription.

Patients with average transport rates do well on continuous PD therapies. Patients with low transport rates have slow solute transport and relatively slow glucose absorption [132–134]. This results in excellent ultrafiltration, but often solute removal is inadequate. These patients do best on a continuous therapy with larger exchange volumes and may require more than four daily exchanges.

Patients with high transport rates have rapid glucose absorption with poor ultrafiltration and are likely to have problems with inadequate fluid removal [132, 133]. These patients have good solute removal, so may benefit from shorter dialysis exchanges that are drained at or before the peak ultrafiltration volume. Cycler dialysis is often prescribed for these patients.

Repeat equilibration tests may be used to document changes in membrane characteristics, to aid in the diagnosis of internal leaks, to confirm or rule out the likelihood that a patient is not performing exchanges as prescribed, to evaluate ultrafiltration failure and/or membrane failure.

The abridged PET consists of one dialysis exchange using a standardized preceding exchange (8–12 h), volume (2 L), dextrose concentration (2.5%), and dwell time (4 h), with dialysate samples at 2 and 4 h and a single blood sample [135]. Results are presented as dialysate to plasma ratios of creatinine and the ratio of glucose to the glucose at time 0. These data can be compared to values from large-scale studies to determine how the patient's characteristics compare to the 'average'. It is critical that the PET be performed accurately for results to be meaningful. Each unit must have a detailed procedure for the PET to maintain consistency from one test to the next, so that data can be analysed for trends and changes. If an individual patient has the PET done with a volume other than 2 L this should be clearly documented so that subsequent tests for the same patient will be performed in the same manner. Common errors in performing the PET are listed in Table 15.

Assessment of dialysis adequacy

The National Kidney Foundation Dialysis Outcomes Quality Initiative (DOQI) Clinical Practice Guideline for Peritoneal Dialysis Adequacy recommend that both weekly Kt/V urea and weekly creatinine clearance be routinely used to measure dialysis adequacy [136]. Twenty-four-hour dialysate and urine collections are recommended because abbreviated collections and other sampling techniques may be inaccurate [137, 138]. The accuracy of 24-h collections depends on the patient's ability to comply with instructions. We have found that providing

Table 15. Common PET errors

Preceding exchange is incompletely drained
Inadequate dialysate is drained for 2 h sample
Timing errors
Inadequate mixing of dialysate prior to 2 or 4 h sampling
Improper labelling of dialysate samples
Fresh dialysis solution is allowed to mix with dialysate when
  sampling from Y-sets
Mathematical errors

Table 16. Common problems with 24-h dialysate and urine collections

Dialysis done during the collection period is not representative of routine dialysis
The patient saves too many or too few exchanges
Urine and dialysate are not collected on the same day
Not all urine is saved
Actual times are not recorded
Collection time is greater than or less than 24 h

For patients who obtain the dialysate sample at home
Not all dialysate is included in the sample
Inadequate mixing of sample
Incorrect volume determination

both detailed verbal and written instructions and a form to record exchange times and voiding reduces errors and improves the reliability of dialysis adequacy measurements [139]. Common errors in 24-h urine and dialysate collections are listed in Table 16.

Prescription adjustments to improve dialysis adequacy

The adequacy of dialysis can be quantitatively improved by increasing the daily dialysate drainage volume and/or maximizing dwell times [140, 141]. Increasing the dialysate volume can be accomplished by the use of larger fill volumes or an increase in the number of exchanges. Overnight cycler patients may require a daytime dwell, and CAPD patients may need an additional night-time exchange using an automated exchange device [142]. Blake *et al.* state that, with the exception of patients with high transport rates, all cycler patients will require daytime exchange(s) in the absence of residual renal function [141]. Whereas increasing the number of exchanges will improve adequacy in patients with high peritoneal transport rates, patients with low peritoneal transport may benefit most from increased exchange volume and a more even distribution of dwell times [140, 141, 143].

Tidal peritoneal dialysis (TPD)

Tidal peritoneal dialysis has been shown to improve clearances in intermittent peritoneal dialysis [144]. Prior to initiating TPD Craig and Kuharcik recommended that (a) a peritoneal equilibration test be performed, (b) residual renal clearance be determined, (c) body surface area be estimated and the amount of required creatinine clearance and ultrafiltration be estimated and (d) the dialysate volume (L) per treatment be determined [145]. The tidal

volume is approximately half of the total exchange volume tolerated in a supine position. When determining the amount of solution to hang, add the initial fill volume, plus the tidal fill volume × number of exchanges minus one, and add an additional 300–500 ml to prime and purge tubing. Cycle time is determined by subtracting the initial fill and final drain times and the length of one dwell from the total dialysis time and dividing the remaining time by the total number of exchanges minus one. The tidal ultrafiltration volume is determined by dividing the total UF by the number of cycles. If the final drain volume is less than the initial fill plus cycle UF, the cycle UF should be reduced; if it is higher, the cycle UF should be increased accordingly. The patient will need to change the cycle UF setting depending on the dialysis solution dextrose concentration. Written instructions for the tidal UF volume for each prescribed combination of dextrose dialysis solutions provides the patient with a reference and reduces errors. Tidal dialysis is somewhat more complex than regular IPD, and patients may require somewhat longer training time and more detailed home records. TPD is also relatively more expensive because of the larger volume of dialysis solution that is used.

Administration of erythropoietin

The ability of recombinant human erythropoietin (EPO) to correct the anaemia of renal failure has dramatically improved the lives of patients with end-stage renal disease [146, 147]. As its use becomes more widespread, PD nurses will need to know how to administer the drug and monitor the patients receiving it for progress and side-effects. Various studies have taken place to discuss the feasibility of giving EPO either by subcutaneous injection or intraperitoneally in the dialysis solution [148, 149]. Intraperitoneal administration limits drug absorption and the higher cost of achieving adequate haemoglobin level rules out this method [150]. Subcutaneous administration has proven to be effective using low doses, and the slower absorption produced by this method of injection mimics the production of endogenous EPO more closely than the peaks and troughs that result from intravenous administration [149]. PD patients are uniquely suited to self-administration of EPO because they are experienced with home procedures and can usually be taught the injection procedure in one session [151].

Most PD patients will already be familiar with injection techniques but will require further education in aseptic technique, selection of injection site, storage of EPO and potential problems. Nursing and patient education care plans such as the one in ref. 152 should be used so that both nurses and patients understand the rationale for EPO usage, can identify the side-effects and make appropriate interventions.

Regular clinic attendance is necessary and nurses should be alert for causes of reduced response to EPO such as infection, bleeding, iron deficiency, aluminium overload and severe hyperparathyroidism [153]. Monthly monitoring of blood counts and serum ferritin should take place, and in addition nurses should monitor the blood pressure, vascular access and the patient's well-being to minimize side-effects [154].

Special problems for patients with diabetes mellitus

The number of patients with diabetes treated by PD continues to grow. The advantages of PD for this group of patients include the maintenance of a residual renal function, use of intraperitoneal insulin, better blood pressure control and a less rigid fluid and dietary regimen [155]. Unfortunately, most dialysis patients with diabetes have other complications including retinopathy, coronary artery and peripheral vascular disease, autonomic neuropathy, and in addition suffer from malnutrition [156]. It is a challenge to all PD nurses to assist these patients to manage and adapt to two chronic illnesses and hopefully to enhance their quality of life.

Training

When selecting the type of equipment best suited to the patient's needs visual acuity, mobility, manual dexterity and the use of a partner should be taken into account. For blind patients devices such as exchange and UV devices can assist the patient with the exchange procedure while click syringes, injection aids and Novopens® can help with the insulin injections. If a partner is needed it may be less tedious to have the patient dialysed overnight using a cycler.

The PD training nurse may have to displace bad habits that have accumulated over a number of years [157]. Careless regard for insulin dose, diet and foot care must now be replaced with good technique and careful monitoring. Sterile technique is now vital if insulin is to be injected into dialysis bags, and the

nurse must motivate the patient to high standards. A change from subcutaneous injection to intraperitoneal injection may aid compliance. Initially the patient may have to monitor blood glucose levels several times a day and make adjustments to insulin dosage when using hypertonic solutions.

Follow-up care

A multidisciplinary approach to care is used to the best advantage when treating patients with diabetes and renal failure. Specialist help from dieticians, ophthalmologists, diabetologists and foot-care nurses will assist the patient to achieve good rehabilitation. At Manchester Royal Infirmary PD patients with diabetes attend a joint Renal/Diabetic clinic where access to all these specialities is to be found under one roof. This not only reduces the number of clinics the patient has to visit but also ensures that all possible complications are seen at an early stage and are monitored thoroughly [158]. The importance of support from the patient's family cannot be over-emphasized. Anderson *et al.* observed that when the courage and strength of family members has been drained the patient might be unable to continue alone [159]. The family burden is often beyond the limits of tolerance; therefore when necessary families should be offered respite care, support and encouragement so that they do not surrender their own optimism and determination [160].

Special problems of the elderly

Among the most common problems of elderly populations are visual and hearing losses. Compensating for these losses is important, especially during patient education. Working in an environment free from background noise is recommended for the hearing-impaired. Sitting at the same level; establishing eye contact; speaking slowly, clearly and not too loudly all improve comprehension.

Good vision in elderly patients is dependent on good light, good contrast and adequate size [161]. Written instructions for the elderly should be in large print in a simple, bold typeface. Good lighting and a contrasting background are essential for the work area where PD exchanges or cycler connections will be done.

A number of factors contribute to poor nutrition in the elderly PD population. Taste and smell perception diminishes with age, and dysgeusia is a common symptom of uraemia and inadequate dialysis. Elderly patients with lack of dentition or poorly fitting dentures may compensate by changing to soft foods, which limits protein intake. Furthermore, individuals on a limited income may not be able to afford protein-rich foods. Finally, the added anorexia of end-stage real disease compounds the problem of obtaining adequate protein, and calories from dialysis glucose absorption may blunt the appetite. Correcting dental problems, liberalizing the dietary recommendations and identifying sources of supplemental income may improve both caloric and protein intake.

Safety is also a major concern for elderly patients. A list of ageing changes that predispose to falls includes 10 items [162]. Six of the 10 conditions are common in the elderly end-stage renal disease population: diabetes mellitus, visual impairment, gait changes, reduced postural control, postural hypotension and reduced cerebral functioning. Excessive fluid removal and resulting dehydration further increase the risk of falls in PD patients. Because tripping causes many falls, it is important that both the clinic and patient's home do not have loose mats or slippery floors. Good lighting also reduces the risk of falls. The temperature of dialysis solutions should also be carefully monitored in elderly patients.

Miscellaneous information

Showering, bathing

PD patients must be encouraged to have high standards of personal hygiene. It is preferable that they take a shower every day; however, if desirable they can take a bath. Bath water should be shallow and should not cover the exit site. Following bathing the exit site should be inspected, cleansed, dried and re-dressed.

Warming of solutions

It is not essential to warm PD fluid but some patients experience discomfort when infusing cold solutions. APD machines have an in-built warming mechanism, which is temperature controlled. CAPD patients have various ways of warming the fluid in the home, the most common ones are:

1. Airing cupboards.
2. Hot-water bottles – used in conjunction with insulated bags.
3. Heating pads specially manufactured for this purpose.
4. Radiators.
5. Microwave ovens.

Microwave warming of solutions is not acceptable in all countries due to legal safety measures brought about by the potential risk for patient burns, resulting from hot-spots within the dialysis fluid when warmed by this method. A recent study by Armstrong and Zalatan [163] in the USA suggests microwave warming is a safe procedure in the hospital setting. Following warming, the dialysis fluid should be agitated to even out the temperature of the fluid in the bag; however, it should be noted that microwave ovens vary in wattage and size and this could produce a difference in heating factors.

Body image

The specific changes brought about to introduce peritoneal dialysis are essential and necessary evils to sustain life, yet patient acceptance of these intrusions can take a considerable period of time. Not surprisingly PD patients are often shocked when told that the insertion of a Tenckhoff catheter into the abdomen will be necessary to facilitate the exchange procedure. They fear that they may look different and more noticeable even though the catheter can be concealed under the clothing [164]. Paris states that 76% of female CAPD patients and 47% males are worried about their body image [165]. She also reported that 50% of patients expressed negative changes regarding body image and sex life. The large volumes of fluid in the abdomen plus obesity due to absorption of glucose from dialysis fluids can also cause negative feelings and anxiety.

Predialysis counselling and careful psychological preparation can often alleviate the stress and tensions associated with body-image misconceptions. The exit-site placement and patient lifestyle should be discussed between surgeon and patient before operation. Practical issues such as concealment of the catheter and reassurance regarding attractive clothing should be discussed early, as disillusionment at this stage could mean total rejection of the procedure. Patients could be introduced to others who are established on PD and who can discuss problems at first hand. With the advent of disconnect systems body-image problems have been greatly improved [166]. Patients now report that they have more freedom of movement, are no longer afraid the catheter will be displaced and are more confident. The nurse should try to understand the needs of her patients whose lives and psyche are affected by body-image problems, and time should be spent helping the patients come to terms and explore their feelings.

Compliance/non-compliance

Non-compliance is an age-old problem dating back to the time of Hippocrates, but still remains a significant threat to morbidity and mortality in the PD population [167]. There are several factors which lead to the patient's inability to follow dietary, fluid and medication regimes, and which should be considered by the health-care team when trying to convince patients to comply.

Culture

Culturally related habits may affect a patient's beliefs and behaviour about his/her illness and treatment. Dietary restrictions, which tear apart traditional eating habits, may simply impose too great a strain to be followed [168].

Depression

Depression with symptoms of loss of interest and motivation, feelings of helplessness and loss of control may result in patients ignoring restrictions.

Social support

Health-care teams often underestimate the part that a stable relationship, employment and an active social life has on compliance with tedious regimes. Hartman and Becker found less compliance when patients had little social support; however, increased compliance was associated with marriage [169].

Amount of treatment

The compliance rate declines with an increase in the treatment and procedures. PD patients have several strict regimens to follow at any one time and may find the burden of compliance too great.

Knowledge

It is essential that PD patients understand their illness and treatment regimes. Sadly, it is not always the case that adequate knowledge will enhance patient compliance. In a study of 136 home dialysis patients Uttley *et al.* [170] showed that 87% of patients studied ($n = 120$) had adequate knowledge of bone disease and phosphate control; however, 79% admitted to non-compliance with drug regimens.

The health-care team should always assess a patient's psychological, social and medical situation when determining possible causes for non-compliance. Practical reasons such as finance and ability to shop and cook should also be explored, and assistance given where necessary. Ongoing educational programmes will be more productive and encouragement should be given when compliance is achieved. The patient has a right to know everything about the treatment regime including what will happen if the plan is not followed. When the team has ascertained that the patient is neither ignorant nor misinformed, the responsibility of complying with therapy then rests with the patient. It is unrealistic for the team to assume that they can control patient behaviour, as most of the events that determine compliance are connected with ordinary everyday living, which ultimately is most subject to influence by the patient alone.

Infection control procedures

Universal body substance precautions recommended in 1987 treat all body substances from all patients as potentially infectious [171]. Infection control procedures specific to dialysis [172] and PD have also been recommended [173]. Staff are required to wear gloves to handle and transport dialysate bags. Bags are to be kept in a covered container in the disposal area until the end of each day. The individual disposing the dialysate must wear gloves, a plastic apron and face shield and avoid splashing when emptying bags. Empty bags and tubing must be disposed of in plastic rubbish bags labelled 'infectious waste'. A 1:10 bleach solution is poured into the disposal sinks and allowed to remain for 30 min.

Guidelines for home patients specify that the patient should dispose of dialysate in the toilet and empty bags should be placed in a plastic bag, secured with a knot and placed in the refuse. If another person disposes of the dialysate that person should wear gloves and avoid splashing [171–174].

Disaster preparedness

Disaster plans recommend that home-dialysis patients keep a 2-week supply of medications and 2–4 weeks of dialysis supplies. Alternative methods of warming solutions should be reviewed in preparation for power shortages. Patients using electric or battery-operated devices for dialysis exchanges need to keep batteries charged and/or be prepared to switch to a manual system. Likewise, cycler patients may be cross-trained to perform manual CAPD exchanges, but need to have appropriate solution volumes for CAPD exchanges. Patients should wear medical information emblems, which identify them as dialysis recipients at all times. Patients should also receive information regarding the length of time they can safely go without dialysis exchanges, an emergency diet plan, and emergency communications with the dialysis unit.

Research

Stetler, a nurse researcher, identified several levels of nursing involvement [175]. The most basic level is using the scientific process for clinical problem solving. A second level is research utilization incorporating pertinent research findings in clinical practice. The next level is to facilitate and/or participate in the research projects directed by others. All PD nurses can participate in research at these three levels.

Because continuous PD is a relatively new form of therapy, clinical research provides information, regarding intervention strategies and outcomes. Research activities, like clinical care, are often undertaken by the interdisciplinary team, and this provides nurses with opportunities to participate in clinical research directed by others and to learn research-related skills.

Well-defined clinical research inevitably improves the quality of care in chronic dialysis programmes. Enhanced care may result from: (a) increased knowledge, (b) improved assessment skills, (c) more effective patient education, (d) improved documentation and communication among team members, (e) alternative methods of managing problems, (f) identification for risk factors for specific complications and (g) development of new procedures, dialysis regimes or delivery systems.

Patient support groups

There are several elements which influence a patient to comply and achieve well-being whilst on dialysis. One of these is the patient support group. These organizations are in the main run by patients for the support of other patients. One of their most important tasks is to distribute information to enhance the knowledge of patients and their families. Other responsibilities include helping patients to make contact with others undergoing dialysis, coun-

selling, arranging social and fund-raising events, financing patients in need and, last but not least, campaigning on behalf of kidney patients to improve facilities and increase public awareness [176]. Many of these organizations are registered charities, and publish magazines or newsletters regularly. The benefit of such groups is legend, and nursing staff should inform patients and their families about the existence of such groups either locally or nationally.

References

1. Oreopoulos DG. Nurses from yesterday's handmaidens to today's knowledgeable colleagues. Perit Dial Bull 1983; 4: 171–2.
2. Clayton S. The organization and implementation of a peritoneal dialysis program. Perit Dial Bull 1981; 1: 134–6.
3. Marsden A, Uttley L, Moon J. A successful CAPD program – what are the essential requirements? Proc EDTNA 1985; 14: 80–5.
4. Boen ST. Integration of CAPD into endstage renal failure programs – present and future. In: Atkins RC, Thomson NM, Farrell PC, eds. Peritoneal Dialysis. Edinburgh: Churchill Livingstone, 1981, pp. 42–9.
5. Gokal R. CAPD – current status in the UK. In: Parson FM, Ogg CS, eds. Renal Failure – Who Cares? Lancaster: MTP Press, 1982, pp. 137–50.
6. Eaton A, Penn A, Bungey M, Ogg LSHD. Support for a CAPD program. In: Monkhouse P, Stevens E, eds. Aspects of Renal Care. Eastbourne: Bailliere, Tindall, 1986, pp. 87–92.
7. Oreopoulos DG. Requirements for the organization of a continuous ambulatory peritoneal dialysis program. Nephron 1979; 24: 261–3.
8. Holley J, Piraino B. Initiating a PD program: personnel administrative requirements. Patient Recruitment and Training. Semin Dial 1990; 3: 123–6.
9. Hebelman FP. A framework for organizing a CAPD training program. J Nephrol Nurs 1985; 2: 56–60.
10. Holley JL, Piraino BM. Operating a peritoneal dialysis program, patient and program monitoring. Semin Dial 1990; 3: 182–6.
11. Jerrum C. CAPD: the state of the art. Nursing 1991; 4: 28–30.
12. Lambert MC. Peritoneal dialysis in Europe: nursing issues. Perit Dial Int 1996; 16 (suppl. 1): S443–7.
13. McShane M. Multidisciplinary teams; reality or myth. EDTNA/ERCA J 1994; 20: 29–31.
14. Green M. The nuts and bolts of establishing a home training program. AANNT J 1983; 10: 42–5.
15. Brennan DT. Impact of prospective payment regulations. Results of head nurse survey. ANNA J 1984; 11: 49–52.
16. Oreopoulos DG. The peritoneal dialysis nurse. The key to success. Perit Dial Bull 1981; 1: 113–14.
17. Morris B. Nursing intervention to prevent CAPD burnout. Contemp Dial Nephrol 1990; July: 23–4.
18. Leibovitz Z Humour and dialysis. EDTNA/ERCA J 1998; 24: 17–18.
19. Van Waeleghem JP, Gammer N, Lambert MC, Larno L, Verschoot M. Development of nephrology nursing care in Europe 1978–1988. ANNA J 1989; 16: 23–35.
20. Starmann B, Lees P, Reynolds J. University of Michigan national CAPD survey. Dial Transplant 1988; 17: 47–57.
21. Ray R, Samar D. CAPD nursing follow-up: How much time does it take? J Am Assoc Nephrol Nurses Techn 1981; 8: 26–7.
22. Gokal R. Who's for CAPD? Br Med J 1993; 306; 155–60.
23. Public Law (PL) October 1972, 92–603. Public Law (PL) June 1978, 95–292. Omnibus Budget Reconciliation Act (PL) 1981; 97–135.

24. Jordon P. 1988 nursing shortage survey. ANNA J 1988; 15: 253–5.

25. Muthny FA. Job strains and job satisfaction of dialysis nurses. Psychother Psychosom 1989; 51: 150–5.

26. Meldrum J. Implications of health care assistants in nephrology units. EDTNA/ERCA J 1994; 20: 38–40.

27. Parker J. Reduction in ESRD reimbursement rate: Identifying research priorities and quality indicators. ANNA J 1990; 17: 147–50.

28. Lester M. Staffing the renal unit effectively; quality Vs quantity. EDTNA/ERCA J 1994; 20: 32–9.

29. Price R, Thomas N, Tibbles R. Bridging the gap, spreading the load, and mixing the skills, a training for junior staff nurses. EDTNA/ERCA J 1996; 22: 25–6.

30. Bolton WK. Nephrology nurse practitioners in a collaborative care model. Am J Kidney Dis 1998; 31: 786–93.

31. Balhorn J. Patient classification used as a tool for assessment of staff patient ratios. EDTNA/ERCA J 1998; 24: 13–16.

32. Bergstrom K. Education for nephrology nurses. EDTNA/ERCA J 1994; 20: 12–13.

33. Ritt H. Clinical training; an important skill for nephrology nurses. EDTNA/ERCA J 1994; 20: 14–16.

34. Balhorn J. Implementation of the European Core Curriculum. EDTNA/ERCA J 1997; 23: 25–30.

35. Kuntzle W. Job description for the certified nephrology nurse; professional and legal aspects. EDTNA/ERCA J 1998; 24: 9–11.

36. Stewart G. Specialization in nursing – implications in Australia. EDTNA/ERCA J 1997; 23: 38–9.

37. Lewis SL, Campbell MA, Becktell PJ *et al.* Work stress, burn-out, and sense of coherence among dialysis nurses. ANNA J 1992; 19: 545–53.

38. Taylor S, Breckenridge D, Butera E. Images of nephrology nursing practice: report of a survey. ANNA J 1992; 19: 361–6.

39. Winder E. The role of education in developing specialist practice. EDTNA/ERCA J 1996; 22: 21–4.

40. Zappacosta AR, Perras ST. Primary Nursing in CAPD. Philadelphia, PA: Lippincott, 1984, pp. 35–9.

41. Marram GD, Barrett MW, Brevis EO. Primary Nursing: a model for individualized care. St Louis, Mosby, 1979.

42. Perras S, Mattern M, Hugues C *et al.* Primary nursing is the key to success in an out-patient CAPD teaching program. Nephrol Nurse 1983; 5: 8–11.

43. Flett A. Introducing primary nursing to a satellite dialysis setting in Singapore. EDTNA/ERCA J 1997; 23: 41–3.

44. Moon J, Uttley L, Manos J, Gokal R. Home CAPD nurse, an asset to a CAPD program. In: Maher JF, Winchester JF, eds. Frontiers in Peritoneal Dialysis, New York: Field, Rich, 1986, pp. 360–3.

45. Rosario M. Nursing management of a PD program: legal issues. Syllabus, 11th annual conference on peritoneal dialysis, Nashville, Tennessee, 1991, pp. 179–201.

46. Burrows L. Peritoneal dialysis technician: a process for role definition. ANNA J 1995; 22: 319–22.

47. Bednar B. Delegation of nursing tasks to licensed and unlicensed personnel: a guide for ESRD facilities (editorial). ANNA J 1992; 19: 337–8.

48. Frederick GA. Reuse with continuous cyclic peritoneal dialysis. ANNA J 1986; 13: 80–2.

49. Wadhwa NK, Cabralda T, Suh H *et al.* Multiple use of cycler set in cycler peritoneal dialysis. Adv Perit Dial 1992; 8: 192–4.

50. Ponferrada LP, Prowant BF, Rackers JA *et al.* A cluster of gram-negative peritonitis episodes associated with reuse of Home Choice cycler cassettes and drain lines. Perit Dial Int 1996; 16: 636–8.

51. Health Care Financing Administration. Highlights from the 1995 ESRD core indicators project for peritoneal dialysis patients. Baltimore: Department of Health and Human Services, Health Care Financing Administration, Office of Clinical Standards and Quality, May 1996.

52. Health Care Financing Administration. Highlights from the 1996 ESRD core indicators project for peritoneal dialysis

patients. Baltimore: Department of Health and Human Services, Health Care Financing Administration, Office of Clinical Standards and Quality, January 1997.

53. Health Care Financing Administration. Highlights from the 1997 ESRD core indicators project for peritoneal dialysis patients. Baltimore: Department of Health and Human Services, Health Care Financing Administration, Office of Clinical Standards and Quality, October 1997.

54. Rocco MV, Flanigan MJ, Beaver S *et al.* Report from the 1995 core indicators for peritoneal dialysis study group. Am J Kidney Dis 1997; 30: 165–73.

55. Health Care Financing Administration. 1998 annual report ESRD core indicators project. Baltimore: Department of Health and Human Services, Health Care Financing Administration, Office of Clinical Standards and Quality, December 1998.

56. D'Apice AJF, Atkins RC. Analysis of peritoneal dialysis data. In: Atkins RC, Thomson NM, Farrell PC, eds. Peritoneal Dialysis. Edinburgh: Churchill Livingstone, 1981, pp. 440–4.

57. Corey P. An approach to the statistical analysis of peritonitis data from patients on CAPD. Perit Dial Bull 1981; 1: S29–32.

58. Pierratos A, Amair P, Corey P, Vas SI, Khanna R, Oreopoulos DG. Statistical analysis of the incidence of peritonitis on continuous ambulatory peritoneal dialysis. Perit Dial Bull 1982; 2: 32–6.

59. Sims TW. Quality assurance works (case study). ANNA J 1990; 17: 258.

60. Gray JS, Nickles JR. Improving infection control in a PD unit. Nephrol News Issues 1995; 9: 14–18.

61. Benson B, Lutz N. CQI process helps identify patient training as a requirement for improving peritonitis management. Perit Dial Int 1997; 17 (suppl. 1): S42 (abstract).

62. Pagnotta-Lee R, Hershfeld S, Fitzsimmmons D, Manners D. Implementing changes in a PD program to improve peritonitis rates. Perit Dial Int 1998; 18 (suppl. 1): S33 (abstract).

63. Hall G, Lee S, Davachi F *et al.* Continuous quality improvement (CQI) process helps to improve peritonitis rates. Perit Dial Int 1998; 18 (suppl. 1): S58 (abstract).

64. Holland LP. Implementation of a quality improvement (QI) audit to improve episodes of peritonitis (EOP). Perit Dial Int 1998; 18 (suppl. 1): S58 (abstract).

65. Street JK, Krupka DL, Broda L *et al.* Utilizing the CQI process to decrease episodes of peritonitis. Perit Dial Int 1998; 18 (suppl. 1): S59 (abstract).

66. Chemleski B, Enrico R, Montes P *et al.* Continuous quality improvement (CQI) demonstration project: peritonitis rate in the home dialysis unit. Perit Dial Int 1996; 16 (suppl. 2): S84 (abstract).

67. Thompson MC, Speaks DD. Exit site infections reduced through CQI exit site care study. Perit Dial Int 1997; 17: (suppl. 1): S46 (abstract).

68. Boorgu NR, Liles V. CQI initiated focusing on exit-site infection. Perit Dial Int 1998; 18 (suppl. 1): S59 (abstract).

69. Martin P, McGauvran J, Reimer L. CQI impacts exit-site infection. Perit Dial Int 1998; 18 (suppl. 1): S59 (abstract).

70. Mason EJ. How to Write Meaningful Nursing Standards, 2nd edn. New York: John Wiley, 1984.

71. Brennan DT, Burrows-Hudson S, Day C, Libonate J. Standards of Practice for Nephrology Nursing. New Jersey: A.J. Jannetti Inc., Pitman, 1988.

72. EDTNA – Standards of Nephrology Nursing Practice. EDTNA/ERCA Switzerland, 1996.

73. Hayslip DM, Suttle CD. Pre-ESRD patient education. A review of the literature. Adv Renal Replac Therap 1995; 2: 217–26.

74. Uttley L, Gokal R. What I tell my patients about CAPD. Br J Renal Med 1998; 3: 13–15.

75. Lancaster LE. Core Curriculum for Nephrology Nursing. New Jersey: A.J. Jannetti Inc., Pitman, 1995.

76. Luker KA, Caress AL. Rethinking patient education. J Adv Nurs 1989; 14: 711–18.

77. Jeffrey JE, Burton HJ, Meidenheim AP, Lindsay RM. A comparison of home training and problems encountered with initial home dialysis. Hemodialysis versus CAPD. ANNT J 1982; 9: 56–62.

78. Hanson PC. Teaching CAPD. Nephrology Nurse. May/June, 1980; 41–2.

79. Lauder SM, Zappacosta AR. Components of a successful CAPD education programme. ANNA J 1988; 15: 243–47.

80. Coles GA. Manual of Peritoneal Dialysis. Practical procedures for medical and nursing staff. Lancaster: Kluwer, 1990.

81. Bernadini J, Dacko C. A survey of home visits at peritoneal dialysis centers in the United States. Perit Dial Int 1998; 18: 528–31.

82. Blagg CR. The socioeconomic impact of rehabilitation. Am J Kidney Dis 1994; 24 (suppl.): S17–21.

83. Jerrum CD, Blundell L. Employment and dialysis: investigations study of patients and employers. EDTNA/ERCA J 1995; 21: 33–6.

84. Abse BJ. Precautions for sports-minded patients on PD. ANNA J 1995; 22: 332–3.

85. Vigneux A, Steele B. CAPD is not a contraindication for swimming in children. Perit Dial Bull 1982; 2: 99.

86. Uttley L. CAPD in the elderly, follow up care. In: Ota K, ed. Current Concepts in Peritoneal Dialysis. Amsterdam: Excerpta Medica, 1992, pp. 145–52.

87. Anderson JE. Ten years experience with CAPD in a nursing home setting. Perit Dial Int 1997; 17: 255–61.

88. Jorden L. Establishing a peritoneal dialysis programme in a nursing home. Adv Renal Replac Therap 1996; 3: 266–8.

89. Manos J, Uttley L, Moon J et al. Successful joint care of CAPD patients with two district general hospitals. In: Avram M, ed. Ambulatory Peritoneal Dialysis. New York: Plenum, 1990, pp. 272–3.

90. Tenckhoff H. Chronic Peritoneal Dialysis. A manual for patients, dialysis personnel and physicians. University of Washington, Seattle 1974.

91. Moncrief J, Popovich R, Broadrick LJ et al. The Moncrief–Popovich catheter: a new peritoneal access technique for patients on peritoneal dialysis. ASAIO J 1993; 39: 62–5.

92. Twardowski ZJ, Khanna R, Nolph KD et al. Intra abdominal pressure during natural activities in patients treated with continuous ambulatory peritoneal dialysis. Nephron 1986; 44: 129–35.

93. Prowant BF, Twardowski ZJ. Recommendations for exit care. Perit Dial Int 1996; 16 (suppl. 3): S94–9.

94. Copley JB, Smith BJ, Koger DM et al. Prevention of postoperative peritoneal dialysis catheter-related infections. Perit Dial Int 1988; 8: 195–7.

95. Jenson SR, Davidson M, Pomeroy M et al. Evaluation of dressing protocols that reduces peritoneal dialysis catheter exit site infections. ANNA J 1989; 16: 425–31.

96. Schmidt L, Prowant B, Schaefer R et al. An evaluation of nursing intervention for prevention of postoperative peritoneal catheter exit site infections. ANNA J 1986; 13: 98 (abstract).

97. Twardowski ZJ, Prowant BF. Exit-site healing post catheter implantation. Perit Dial Int 1996; 16 (suppl. 3): S51–70.

98. Oberg MS, Lindsey D. Do not put hydrogen peroxide or povidone iodine into wounds! Am J Dis Child 1987; 141: 27–8.

99. Gokal R, Ash SR, Helfrich GB et al. Peritoneal catheters and exit-site practices: toward optimum peritoneal access. Perit Dial Int 1993; 13: 29–39.

100. Prowant BF. Nursing interventions related to peritoneal catheter exit-site infections. Adv Renal Replace Ther 1996; 3: 228–31.

101. Twardowski ZJ, Prowant BF. Current approach to exit-site infections in patients on peritoneal dialysis. Nephrol Dial Transplant 1997; 12: 1284–95.

102. Gokal R, Alexander S, Ash S et al. Peritoneal catheters and exit site practices toward optimum peritoneal access: 1998 update. Perit Dial Int 1998; 18: 11–33.

103. Prowant BF, Warady BA, Nolph KD. Peritoneal dialysis catheter exit-site care: results of an international survey. Perit Dial Int 1993; 13: 149–54.

104. Lewis SL, Prowant BF, Douglas C, Cooper CL. Nursing practice related to peritoneal catheter exit site care and infections. ANNA J 1996; 23: 609–15.

105. Piraino B. Exit-site care. Perit Dial Int 1996; 16 (suppl. 1): S336–9.

106. Bernardini J, Piraino B, Holley J et al. A randomized trial of Staphylococcus aureus prophylaxis in peritoneal dialysis patients: Mupirocin calcium ointment 2% applied to the exit site versus cyclic oral rifampin. Am J Kidney Dis 1996; 27: 695–700.

107. Khanna R, Twardowski ZJ. Recommendations for treatment of exit-site pathology. Perit Dial Int 1996; 16 (suppl. 3): S100–4.

108. Turner K, Edgar D, Hair M, Uttley L. Does catheter immobilization reduce exit-site infections in CAPD patients? Adv Perit Dial 1992; 8: 265–8.

109. Watson AR, Vigneux A, Hardy BE, Balfe JW. Six-year experience with CAPD catheters in children. Perit Dial Bull 1985; 5: 119–22.

110. Warady BA, Jackson MA, Millspaugh J et al. Prevention and treatment of catheter-related infections in children. Perit Dial Bull 1987; 7: 34–6.

111. Twardowski ZJ, Prowant BF. Classification of normal and diseased exit sites. Perit Dial Intl 1996; 16 (suppl. 3): S32–50.

112. Oreopoulos DG, Vas S, Khanna R. Prevention of peritonitis during CAPD. Perit Dial Bull 1985; 5: 518–20.

113. Maiorca R, Cantaluppi A, Cancarini GC et al. Prospective controlled trial of a Y-connector and disinfectant to prevent peritonitis in continuous ambulatory peritoneal dialysis. Lancet 1983; 2: 642–4.

114. Diaz-Buxo JA. Does CCPD lower the peritonitis rate? Contrib Nephrol 1987; 57: 191–6.

115. Zappacosta AR, Perras ST. Reduction of CAPD peritonitis rate by ultraviolet light with dialysate exchange assist device. Dial Transplant 1988; 17: 483–5.

116. Baxter Health Care Corporation. The Best Demonstrated Practices Program. Peritonitis management and antibiotic therapy practices. Deerfield, IL, 1987.

117. Keane WF, Everett ED, Golper TA et al. PD related peritonitis treatment recommendations 1993 update. Perit Dial Int 1996; 16: 557–73.

118. Henderson LW, Nolph KD. Altered permeability of the peritoneal membrane after using hypertonic peritoneal dialysis fluid. J Clin Invest 1969; 48: 992–1001.

119. Garred LJ, Canaud B, Farrell PC. A simple kinetic model for assessing peritoneal mass transfer in chronic ambulatory peritoneal dialysis. ASAIO J 1983; 6: 131–7.

120. Randerson DH, Farrell PC. Mass transfer properties of the human peritoneum. ASAIO J 1980; 3: 140–6.

121. Pyle WK. Mass transfer in peritoneal dialysis (dissertation). Austin, TX: University of Texas, 1981.

122. Pyle WK, Moncrief JW, Popovich RP. Peritoneal transport evaluation in CAPD. In: Moncrief JW, Popovich RP, eds. CAPD Update: Continuous ambulatory peritoneal dialysis. New York: Masson, 1981, pp. 35–52.

123. Popovich RP, Moncrief JW, Pyle WK. Transport kinetics. In: Nolph KD, ed. Peritoneal Dialysis, 3rd edn. Dordrecht: Kluwer, 1989, pp. 96–116.

124. Rippe B, Stelin G. Simulations of peritoneal solute transport during CAPD. Application of two-pore formalism. Kidney Int 1989; 35: 1234–44.

125. Rippe B. A three-pore model of peritoneal transport. Perit Dial Int 1993; 13 (suppl. 2): S35–38.

126. Rippe B, Krediet RT. Peritoneal physiology – transport of solutes. In: Gokal R, Nolph KD, eds. The Textbook of Peritoneal Dialysis. Dordrecht: Kluwer, 1994, pp. 69–113.

127. Verger C, Larpent L, Dumontet M. Prognostic value of peritoneal equilibration curves in CAPD patients. In: Maher JF, Winchester JF, eds. Frontiers in Peritoneal Dialysis. New York: Field, Rich, 1986, pp. 88–93.

128. Twardowski ZJ, Nolph KD, Khanna R *et al*. Peritoneal equilibration test. Perit Dial Bull 1987; 7: 138–47.

129. Gotch FA, Keen ML. Kinetic modeling in peritoneal dialysis. In: Nissenson AR, Fine RN, Gentile DE, eds. Clinical Dialysis, 3rd edn. Norwalk, CT: Appleton & Lange, 1995, pp. 343–75.

130. Haraldsson B. Assessing the peritoneal dialysis capacities of individual patients. Kidney Int 1995; 47: 1187–98.

131. Imai H, Satoh K, Ohtani H *et al*. Clinical application of the personal dialysis capacity (PDC) test: serial analysis of peritoneal function in CAPD patients. Kidney Int 1998; 54: 546–53.

132. Diaz-Buxo JA. Peritoneal permeability in selecting peritoneal dialysis modalities. Perspect Perit Dial 1988; 5: 6–10.

133. Twardowski ZJ. Clinical value of standardized equilibration tests in CAPD patients. Blood Purif 1989; 7: 95–108.

134. Twardowski ZJ. New approaches to intermittent peritoneal dialysis therapies. In: Nolph KD, ed. Peritoneal Dialysis, 3rd edn. Dordrecht: Kluwer, 1989, pp. 133–51.

135. Schmidt LM, Prowant BF. How to do a peritoneal equilibration test. ANNA J 1991; 18: 368–70.

136. NKF-DOQI clinical practice guidelines for peritoneal dialysis adequacy. Am J Kidney Dis 1997; 30 (suppl. 2): S67–136.

137. Burkart JM, Jordan JR, Rocco MV. Assessment of dialysis dose by measured clearance versus extrapolated data. Perit Dial Int 1993; 13: 184–8.

138. Ponferrada L, Moore H, Van Stone J, Prowant B. Is there an alternative dialysate sampling method for *Kt/V* determination in CAPD patients? ANNA J 1993; 20: 281 (abstract).

139. Uttley L, Prowant B. Organization of the peritoneal dialysis program – the nurses' role. In: Gokal R, Nolph KD, eds. The Textbook of Peritoneal Dialysis. Dordrecht: Kluwer, 1994, pp. 335–56.

140. Burkart JM, Schreiber M, Korbet SM *et al*. Solute clearance approach to adequacy of peritoneal dialysis. Perit Dial Int 1996; 16: 457–70.

141. Blake P, Burkart JM, Churchill DN *et al*. Recommended clinical practices for maximizing peritoneal dialysis clearances. Perit Dial Int 1996; 16: 448–56.

142. Diaz-Buxo JA. Enhancement of peritoneal dialysis: the PD plus concept. Am J Kidney Dis 1996; 27: 92–8.

143. Keshaviah P. Establishing kinetic guidelines for peritoneal dialysis modality selection. Perit Dial Int 1997; 17 (suppl. 3): S53–7.

144. Twardowski ZJ, Nolph KD, Khanna R *et al*. Daily clearances with continuous ambulatory peritoneal dialysis and nightly peritoneal dialysis. Trans Am Soc Artif Intern Organs 1986; 32: 575–80.

145. Craig C, Kuharcik C. Tidal peritoneal dialysis. Syllabus, 13th annual conference on peritoneal dialysis, San Diego, California, 1993, pp. 186–99.

146. Winearls CG, Oliver DO, Pippard MJ *et al*. Effect of human erythropoietin derived from recombinant DNA on the anaemia of patients maintained by chronic haemodialysis. Lancet 1986; 2: 1175–8.

147. Cotton SL, Holechek MJ. Management of anemia using RHuEPO in patients on chronic haemodialysis. ANNA J 1989; 16: 463–8.

148. Boelaert JR, Schurgers ML, Matthys EG *et al*. Comparative pharmacokinetics of RHuEPO administered by IV SC IP routes in CAPD patients. Perit Dial Int 1989; 9: 95–8.

149. Lui SF, Chung WW, Leung CB *et al*. Pharmacokinetics and pharmacodynamics of SC and IP administration of RHuEPO in patients on CAPD. Clin Nephrol 1990; 33: 47–51.

150. Frenken LA, Coppens PJ. Intraperitoneal erythropoeitin. Lancet 1988; 2: 1495.

151. York S, Kinney R, Taber T. Self-administration of epoetin beta by PD patients. ANNA J 1991; 18: 549–52.

152. Prowant BF, Gallagher NM, Binkley LS *et al*. Nephrology nursing care plan and patient education plan for the patient receiving Epogen. ANNA J 1991; 18: 188–94.

153. Sujkova S. Erythropoietin: an update and where to in the future. EDTNA/ERCA J 1998; 24: 30–2.

154. Bennet L. The anaemia research nurse in an effective multidisciplinary management of patients on erythropoietin. RDTNA/ERCA J 1998; 24: 38–9.

155. Gokal R, Friedman EA, Rottembourg J *et al*. PD in diabetic ESRD patients. Dial Transplant 1991; 20: 59, 63, 66, 88.

156. Haas LB. Chronic complications of diabetes mellitus: peritoneal dialysis. ANNA J 1992; 19: 439–46.

157. Clayton S. Training the diabetic patient on CAPD. Perit Dial Bull 1982; 2 (suppl.): S38–9.

158. Boulton AJM, Gokal R, Masson EA. The formation of a diabetic nephropathy clinic. Report of the first six months experience. Postgrad Med J 1988; 64 (suppl. 3): 84–5.

159. Anderson RB, Conway PA, Piening S *et al*. Was it worth it? Significant others' view of diabetic renal failure. Dial Transplant 1986; 15: 315–20.

160. Piening S. Family stress in diabetic renal failure. Health and Social Work 1984; 9: 134–41.

161. Cullinan TR, Redfern SJ, Sight P. Nursing Elderly People, 2nd edn. Edinburgh: Churchill Livingstone, 1991, pp. 91–8

162. Ham RJ, Pattee J, Marcy ML. Accidents in the elderly. In: Hamm RJ, Holtzman JM, Marcy ML, Smith RM, eds. Primary Care Geriatrics. Boston, MA: John Wright, 1983, pp. 235–57.

163. Armstong S, Zalatan SJ. Microwave warming of PD fluid. ANNA J 1992; 19: 535–40.

164. Uttley L, Gokal R. Organisation of a CAPD program: the nurse's role in CAPD. In: Gokal R, ed. CAPD. Edinburgh: Churchill Livingstone, 1986, pp. 145–62.

165. Paris V. CAPD body image and sexuality, are they compatible? EDTNA/ERCA J 1992; 28: 33–4.

166. Verger C, Dumont M, Misrahi B *et al*. CAPD without wearing bags, less peritonitis more freedom. EDTNA J 1983; 12: 38–43.

167. King K. Noncompliance in the chronic dialysis population. Dial Transplant 1991; 20: 67–8.

168. Braybrooke ME. Understanding other cultures; the need for training. EDTNA/ERCA J 1988; 24: 19–21.

169. Hartman PE, Becker MH. Non-compliance with prescribed regimen among chronic hemodialysis patients. Dial Transplant 1978; 7: 978–89.

170. Uttley L, Fawcett J, Hutchinson A. Phosphate control – what do our patients know? EDTNA/ERCA J 1993; 1: 7–8.

171. Recommendations for prevention of HIV transmission in health-care settings. MMWR 1987; 36 (suppl. 2): 3S–18S.

172. Recommendations for providing dialysis treatment to patients infected with human T-lymphotrophic virus type III/lymphadenopathy-associated virus. MMWR 1986; 35: 376–8, 383

173. Schoenfeld P. Renal disease and HIV infection: clinical course, treatment outcome, and infection control. ANNA J 1990; 17: 212–18.

174. Baldasseroni A. The HIV positive patient on peritoneal dialysis: nursing issues. Syllabus, 12th annual conference on peritoneal dialysis, Seattle, Washington, 1992, pp. 361–7.

175. Stetler CB. Nurses and research, responsibility and involvement. NITA 1983; 207.

176. Hedman H. Patient compliance in the renal replacement therapy, whose problem is it? The patient's perspective. EDTNA/ERCA J 1998; 24: 15–16.

11 | Continuous ambulatory peritoneal dialysis

E. W. Boeschoten

Introduction

Continuous ambulatory peritoneal dialysis (CAPD) was introduced as a new technique for dialysis in 1976 [1]. Until that time intermittent peritoneal dialysis (IPD) was the only alternative to chronic intermittent haemodialysis. Despite safe indwelling catheters and the development of more or less sophisticated machines for automatic peritoneal dialysis, favouring IPD as a treatment at home, peritoneal dialysis remained far behind haemodialysis in the treatment of chronic renal failure. Under usual operating conditions (one or two 2-litre exchanges per hour) the urea clearance is only 20 ml/min or less. Because of this low clearance, on a weekly basis 30–50 dialysis hours were necessary to equal 12 h per week of haemodialysis [2]. Furthermore, protein loss during dialysis and peritonitis were regarded as a major drawback of IPD. In 1977 all over the world a total of 789 patients on IPD could be traced [3]. A publication of the National Institutes of Health in 1978 showed that less than 3% of patients with dialysis were managed on IPD [4].

In 1976 Popovich, Moncrief and co-workers submitted an abstract to the American Society for Artificial Internal Organs which was entitled 'The definition of a novel portable–wearable equilibrium peritoneal technique' [1]. They described a method for permanent peritoneal dialysis during which the patient performed normal activities. Except for five daily periods of drainage and instillation of a fresh dialysis solution, 2 L dialysate was continuously present in the abdominal cavity. In 1978 they published the promising results of this new treatment in nine patients [5]. The name of the procedure was changed and continuous ambulatory peritoneal dialysis was born. In the same year Moncrief reported the results in even more patients and summed up the desirable features of CAPD [6, 7]. Nolph discussed the theoretical and practical impli-

cations of CAPD [8] and in the Toronto Western Hospital the CAPD technique was improved by the introduction of plastic bags instead of cumbersome bottles [9]. As the empty bags remained connected to the abdominal catheter until the next exchange, the number of disconnections could be minimized and this resulted in a reduction in the incidence of peritonitis. A questionnaire showed that in July 1978 in Canada already 165 patients were being treated with CAPD [10]. In 1979 other promising reports were published. Moncrief and co-workers discussed the combined clinical experience of 75 CAPD patients from three centres [11]. The first studies concerning peritoneal clearances during CAPD were published [12, 13]. Oreopoulos and co-workers presented the results of CAPD in the Toronto Western Hospital [14, 15]. Because of technical improvements the infection rate could be reduced to one peritonitis episode every 10.5 patient-months. Their experience indicated that 'CAPD was superior to IPD in controlling the biochemical abnormalities'. In June 1979 the 16th EDTA meeting was held in Amsterdam. Several investigators reported the results of CAPD in the treatment of end-stage renal failure. These results were very encouraging. The same conclusion could be drawn from symposia on peritoneal dialysis which were held in the autumn of 1979 in New York and Paris. From 1980 on the numbers of patients treated with CAPD increased rapidly all over the world.

In 1997 worldwide 115,000 patients were being treated with chronic peritoneal dialysis. Between 1993 and 1997 the annual growth rate was 7.4%. The difference between countries with regard to the utilization of peritoneal dialysis is substantial (Fig. 1). In most countries where dialysis is performed this modality is still a minority, whereas in other countries the majority is treated by peritoneal dialysis.

At the introduction of CAPD, more than 20 years ago, it could not be expected that this new dialysis

R. Gokal, R. Khanna, R.Th. Krediet and K.D. Nolph (eds.), Textbook of Peritoneal Dialysis, 2nd Edition, 387–417.
© 2000 Kluwer Academic Publishers. Printed in Great Britain.

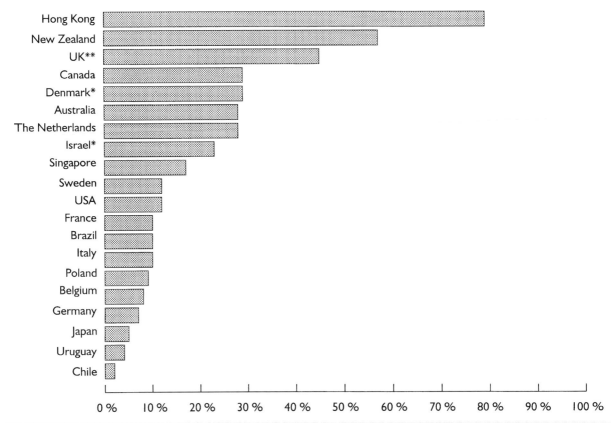

Figure 1. Global peritoneal dialysis utilization. Percentage of all prevalent dialysis patients receiving CAPD or CCPD for selected countries on December 31, 1997. Data from USRDS 1999 (* 1996, ** 1994).

modality would spawn an entirely new industry to manufacture and distribute the materials required to safely deliver this form of home dialysis. The International Society for Peritoneal Dialysis has been organized and a new international journal, *Peritoneal Dialysis International*, has been developed for the dissemination of scientific information. Worldwide many symposia are dedicated to the research projects associated with this broad, expanding therapeutic system.

Principles of CAPD

The concept of CAPD

In peritoneal dialysis the peritoneal membrane is used like a capillary kidney in haemodialysis. Transport of water and solutes occurs between capillaries in the peritoneal membrane and dialysis fluid in the peritoneal cavity. For low clearance systems such as urea removal in CAPD, Popovich and Moncrief have demonstrated that body fluids can be consid-

ered as a single well-mixed pool [16]. For peritoneal dialysis they defined the clearance as

$$K_D = \frac{V_D}{t} \frac{C_D}{C_B} \qquad (1)$$

where V_D is the drained dialysate volume with a mean BUN concentration C_D over a total time period t and a blood urea concentration C_B. With prolonged dwell periods as used in CAPD, for urea an equilibrium can be assumed for the urea concentration in blood and dialysate, resulting in $C_B = C_D$. In this situation equation (1) is reduced to

$$K_D = \frac{V_D}{t} = Q_D \qquad \text{dialysate flow rate} \qquad (2)$$

This simplified model has directly led to the clinical CAPD protocol. This theory predicted that an anephric patient will maintain a steady BUN concentration of approximately 80 mg/L if 10 L of dialysis fluid were allowed to equilibrate with body fluids on a daily basis. With an usual infusion volume of

2 L, four infusions will results in a total of 8 L. To remove fluid from the body, approximately 2 L per day are ultrafiltrated. This will result in a total volume of 10 L per day, which was considered sufficient to maintain acceptable BUN levels.

In 1985 Gotch and Sargent published a mechanistic analysis of the National Cooperative Dialysis Study [17]. In that study they described the adequacy of haemodialysis as a function of protein catabolic rate (PCR) and the magnitude of dialysis. The PCR can be calculated directly from the net urea generation rate and is strongly related to the daily intake of proteins. To describe the magnitude of dialysis the concept of Kt/V was developed, where K was the dialyse urea clearance (ml/min), t the treatment time (min) and V the urea distribution volume (ml). V can be estimated as a fixed percentage of body weight (usually 60%) or from an anthropometric formula such as the Watson equation [18]. Large patients need a greater Kt than small patients to obtain the same Kt/V. This means that large patients need more dialysis than small patients. Analysis of the statistical model showed that all patients in the National Cooperative Dialysis Study with PCR < 0.80 received a small quantity of dialysis ($Kt/V < 0.70$). It was concluded that there is a higher probability of treatment failure related to hospitalizations, withdrawal for medical reasons and death with $Kt/V < 0.70$.

The concept of Kt/V has also been used in CAPD [19–25]. In CAPD Kt/V is defined as

$$\frac{Kt}{V} = \frac{K_D t}{V} \tag{3}$$

where $K_D = V_D/t$ and V is the volume of distribution. This means that

$$\frac{Kt}{V} = \frac{V_D}{t}\frac{t}{V} = \frac{V_D}{V} \tag{4}$$

In the absence of residual renal function, Kt/V in CAPD is entirely determined by dialysate volume (L) and volume of distribution (L). Usually Kt/V, calculated from 24-h dialysate, is given as Kt/V per week. Based on the available evidence, the Dialysis Outcomes Quality Initiative (DOQI) defined a Kt/V of 2.0 per week as the minimum dose target in CAPD [26].

Solute removal

Small solutes are removed from the peritoneal capillaries by diffusion and convection. Diffusion is the most important mechanism. It is evident that clearance is not a good concept to characterize the function of a membrane when long dwells are used. The clearance is the greatest at the start and then diminishes gradually until an equilibrium between blood and dialysate is reached. The smaller the solute, the earlier an equilibrium (Fig. 2). Therefore for the characterization of small solute transport in CAPD other methods are developed. Most commonly the dialysate/plasma (D/P) ratio is used for this purpose [27, 28]. D/P ratios, mostly for urea and creatinine, are used in the peritoneal equilibrium test (PET). The PET test is a simple technique for semiquantitative measurement of peritoneal transport properties. It is, however, an indirect method and not an accurate model to describe transport characteristics in peritoneal dialysis. The best way to measure the clearance of small solutes in CAPD is the calculation of the mass transfer area coefficient (MTAC) [29–31]. The MTAC is the maximal theoretical clearance at time zero, before diffusion is started. Good correlations have been reported between MTAC and D/P ratios [32, 33].

In contrast to small solutes, macromolecules are transported from blood to the dialysate very slowly, and the decrease in concentration gradient is neglectable. In this situation the MTAC equals peritoneal clearance. Therefore, for large molecules peritoneal clearance is calculated to estimate peritoneal permeability [31].

The permeability characteristics of the peritoneal membrane and the continuous nature of the dialytic

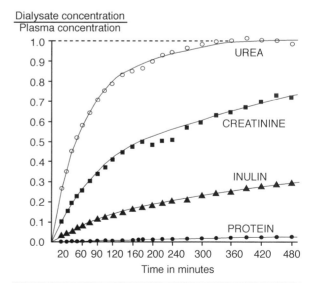

Figure 2. Solute concentration–time profiles for a typical long dwell time exchange. (From ref. 5 with permission.)

procedure result in a better removal of macro-molecules in CAPD than in haemodialysis [34]. This applies also to the removal of 'middle molecules' such as vitamin B12 (1355 Da) and inulin (5200 Da). Various beneficial effects of CAPD, for example better control of anaemia [35] and improved platelet function [36], have been ascribed to the better removal of middle molecules in CAPD. However, this middle molecules hypothesis was never clinically validated.

Fluid removal

Transperitoneal fluid transport is determined by structural characteristics of the peritoneal membrane and physiological forces across it. Structural characteristics of importance are the anatomical surface area, the thickness and composition of the peritoneal membrane and the peritoneal capillaries. Vasoconstriction and vasodilation may influence the blood supply to the peritoneum. Physiological forces are the crystalloid osmotic pressure gradient, the colloid osmotic pressure gradient, the hydrostatic pressure gradient and the lymphatic absorption. Of practical clinical importance are the crystalloid osmotic pressure gradient and the lymphatic drainage.

Fluid removal in peritoneal dialysis depends upon the tonicity of the dialysate [37]. The higher the tonicity the higher the ultrafiltration rate (Fig. 3). Glucose is the osmotic agent commonly used in commercially available solutions, with a glucose concentration varying from 1.5% (70 mmol/L) to 4.25% (198 mmol/L). The osmolality of these solutions is 344 mosmol/L and 483 mosmol/L respectively.

Because glucose is absorbed from the dialysate, the concentration gradient of glucose is maximal at the start of a dialysis dwell and decreases thereafter. During a 6-h dwell about two-thirds of the total instilled amount of glucose is absorbed [38]. This means that the transcapillary ultrafiltration reaches its maximum at the start of a dialysis dwell. For the 1.5% and 4.25% glucose solutions maximal transcapillary ultrafiltration rates of respectively 10 ml/min and 15 ml/min were found [39].

Fluid can be absorbed from the peritoneal cavity by two mechanisms: reabsorption of fluid into the capillaries due to the colloid osmotic pressure gradient (transcapillary absorption) and uptake via the, mainly subdiaphragmatic, lymphatics in the peritoneal cavity: lymphatic absorption [40]. The peritoneal lymphatics continuously absorb fluid and solutes from the peritoneal cavity [41, 42]. In CAPD patients lymphatic disappearance rates of 1.0–1.5 ml/min have been found [42, 43]. The absorption by lymphatics is influenced by the intraperitoneal pressure. An increase in intraperitoneal dialysate volume increases lymphatic flow rate [44]. This results in a reduced net ultrafiltration rate.

Regarding the complex nature of fluid and solute transport in CAPD it is not surprising that large interindividual differences are present among CAPD patients [31]. These differences have consequences for the dialysis prescription in individual patients. Patients with a high solute transport rate have a rapid absorption of glucose, which results in poor ultrafiltration. These patients benefit from short exchanges, usually performed with cycler dialysis. In patients with a low solute transport rate the absorption of glucose is slow and an osmotic concentration gradient persists for a longer period of time. These patients benefit from continuous treatment with long dwell times and volumes of more than 2 L.

Besides inter-individual differences, intra-individual differences exist for the removal of solutes and fluid. These differences are unlikely to be caused by body posture [45]. On the other hand, the residual volume after drainage of a dialysate bag can show marked intra- and interpatient variations [42]. Furthermore several drugs have been shown to alter peritoneal transport rates [46]. Effects of locally produced vasoactive substances have also been assumed to cause alterations of peritoneal transport,

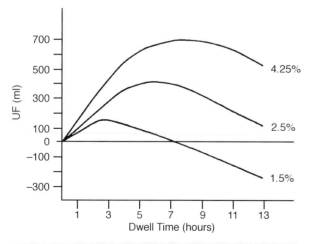

Figure 3. Approximate ultrafiltration volumes related to dwell time with solutions of 1.5%, 2.5%, and 4.25% dextrose concentration. (From ref. 37 with permission.)

but this has been established only during peritonitis [47]. Further understanding of the physiology of the peritoneal membrane is necessary to make active intervention in peritoneal solute and fluid transport clinically feasible.

Peritoneal access

For chronic peritoneal dialysis a soft indwelling catheter is required. In 1968 Tenckhoff and Schechter introduced the 'Tenckhoff catheter' [48] which is still the most commonly used catheter in CAPD. This catheter is made of silicone rubber and has one or two Dacron cuffs. The intraperitoneal segment has multiple 0.5 mm perforations in the 3–9 cm terminal part. The variety of catheter length permits to choosing an appropriate catheter for every patient size.

In order to eliminate the 'shape memory' which tends to extrude the external cuff if a straight catheter is forced to an accurate tunnel, the 'swan-neck catheter' was designed [49]. This catheter has a permanent bend between the cuffs and is placed with both the internal and external part directed downwards. The intra-abdominal part of the catheter may be straight or curled. Curled or coil catheters are designed to reduce discomfort by minimizing the 'jet effect' caused by the high flow of dialysate, and are potentially less prone to migration [50]. Several other catheters, designed to prevent obstruction and migration, e.g. the 'Column disk catheter' and the 'Ash catheter' [51] are less frequently used. The Cruz catheter has a larger inner diameter allowing high flow rates and faster bag exchange procedures [52]. This catheter, in contrast to most other catheters, is made of polyurethane, a material with greater strength, allowing thinner walls. Like silicone, polyurethane is degraded by alcohol and iodine. Repeated exposure of the catheter to these agents may result in crack development [53]. The Gore-tex catheter, developed to prevent exit-site infection, did not fulfil this expectation [54]. Likewise the results of silver-impregnated catheters have been disappointing in patients [55].

There are no long-term controlled studies to suggest the superiority of one catheter over the other. Any new catheter must compete with the long-term experience of the Tenckhoff catheter.

Whatever the type of catheter chosen, at best a 3-year catheter survival rate of 80% should be expected. The minimum acceptable catheter survival rate is regarded as 50% at 12 months [53]. A good survival rate seems more dependent on a good insertion technique and meticulous care than on the catheter device chosen. The implantation should be performed by a competent experienced operator under strict sterile conditions. Exit-site care and attention to detail is of paramount importance.

In general there are three types of insertion technique:

Blind placement: this technique can be performed at the bedside under local anaesthesia. For the introduction of the catheter several devices have been developed.

Peritoneoscopic placement: this technique allows intra-abdominal visualization during the insertion procedure. As in the blind procedure local anaesthesia can be used.

Surgical placement: this is the most prevalent method of insertion. Under general anaesthesia the surgeon dissects through the rectus muscle or through the midline and opens the peritoneum. The catheter is placed under direct vision in the pouch of Douglas.

Before the operation the bowel should be prepared to avoid obstipation, and the bladder should be emptied. Antibiotic prophylaxis with cephalosporins, penicillinase-resistant penicillins or vancomycin is usually recommended. There is, however, no hard evidence indicating that subsequent exit-site infections, tunnel infections or peritonitis are prevented with perioperative antibiotic treatment [56, 57]. Postoperatively the catheter should be flushed with small volumes (500 ml) until the effluent is clear. In general for about 2 weeks a break-in period with an empty abdomen is recommended. Trauma to the exit site should be prevented by immobilization of the catheter. Showering and bathing is usually allowed after 4–8 weeks when the wound is healed [53].

Systems and solutions

In 1976, when CAPD was introduced, the dialysis solutions were delivered in glass containers. The bottles were connected to the catheter by an infusion set. In contrast to peritoneal catheters, many important developments have occurred in the connection technique. Early modifications included the replacement of glass bottles by plastic bags and the addition of an adaptor between the catheter and the administration set. This adaptor lessened the risk of accidental disconnection. The administration set remained attached to the catheter and the dialysate bags were connected to the administration set by a spike or screw connector. In most centres these straight-line connect systems were used for many years. With these systems the empty dialysate bag remained connected to the administration set in between the exchanges and was used for drainage of the peritoneal cavity.

The most important improvements until now are the Y-systems based on the 'drain-before-fill' concept which was developed in Italy [58]. With these systems the catheter is connected to a Y-set tubing attached to a full and an empty dialysate bag. In between the dialysate exchanges the Y-set is disconnected from the catheter. These disconnect Y-systems have gradually replaced the straight-line connect systems.

For CAPD several types of dialysate solutions are available for clinical practice. The sterile fluids are available in varying volumes and various glucose concentrations. The composition of the dialysate solutions used today are remarkably similar to the solutions used by Boen in the 1950s [59, 60]. Nowadays commercial CAPD solutions contain Na (132–134 mmol/L), Ca (1.25–1.75 mmol/L), Mg (0.25–0.75 mmol/L), Cl (95–106 mmol/L), lactate (35–40 mmol/L) and glucose 1.5%, 2.5% or 4.25%.

Clinical studies suggesting an adverse effect of hypertonic glucose-containing solutions on peritoneal morphology and function [61–63] have promoted studies on alternative solutions for peritoneal dialysis. Until now the most promising alternatives were amino acid solutions, glycerol and icodextrin.

One of the disadvantages of amino acid solutions such as Nutrineal® is their rapid absorption from the peritoneal cavity due to their low molecular weight. Therefore their use as osmotic agents is limited. On the other hand, due to this resorption, amino acid solutions lead to a positive nitrogen balance and can be used as an intraperitoneal nutritional supplement [64, 65].

Glycerol-based solutions have been used in a limited number of CAPD patients for more than 10 years [66]. Because of a relatively low molecular weight, being about half that of glucose, the osmolality per gram of the solution is higher. With respect to ultrafiltration rates, a 2.5% glycerol solution has been regarded as equal to a 4.25% glucose solution. Due to the high absorption rates of glycerol, plasma glycerol concentrations increase. Occasionally this has resulted in a hyperosmolar syndrome [67].

In contrast to low-molecular weight solutes the use of high-molecular solutes is not restricted by peritoneal absorption. The most widely used macromolecules in CAPD are glucose polymers. Of these solutes, 7.5% icodextrin (a mixture of glucose polymers with an average molecular weight of 20 kDa) is commercially available. Because icodextrin is removed from the peritoneal cavity not by diffusion but by lymphatic absorption, the osmotic gradient is better preserved than with glucose. The mechanism of ultrafiltration with icodextrin resembles colloid osmosis [68, 69]. Therefore icodextrin is especially effective during long dwells, and has been used successfully in patients with ultrafiltration failure [70]. A drawback of icodextrin is the presence of icodextrin and its metabolites in plasma. With one daily exchange icodextrin and maltose levels stabilized at respectively 4.7 and 1.1 mg/L. After discontinuation of icodextrin these levels dropped to pretreatment concentrations in 7–10 days [71].

Until now no solution has enough advantages to replace glucose as osmotic agent in long-term treatment of CAPD patients. For the future the development of combinations with low-molecular solutes and macromolecules is probably the best approach.

The bag exchange procedure

As nowadays the disconnect Y-set is the most widely used system in CAPD only the bag exchange procedure with this system is described (Fig. 4). This system includes a lengthening of the catheter with an extension line. This line is connected to the adaptor on the catheter and is replaced every half-year.

A Y-set tubing, attached to a full and empty bag, is connected to the extension line. The patient drains the effluent from the peritoneal cavity in the empty bag. Next the patient flushes a small volume of dialysate from the bag with fresh dialysate through the tubing into the drain bag. Finally fresh dialysate is infused and the Y-set is disconnected from the extension line, which is capped by an iodine-containing cap.

Complications

Infectious complications

During recent decades important knowledge has been gained concerning the applicability of peritoneal dialysis. Systems and solutions have significantly improved. However, the continuous introduction of fluid into the peritoneal cavity

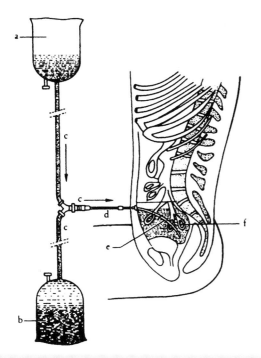

Figure 4. The bag exchange procedure: (a) full bag with fresh dialysate, (b) empty drainage bag, (c) tubing with connector, (d) extension line, (e) intraperitoneal segment of the catheter, (f) bowel loops.

always implies a risk for contamination of the dialysate, resulting in peritonitis. Besides this, peritoneal dialysis alters the normal defence mechanisms of the peritoneum. The function of mesothelial cells and peritoneal macrophages is significantly influenced by the hyperosmolarity, the low pH and the high glucose and lactate concentrations of the dialysate [72]. Humoral and cellular factors, important for the normal regeneration of the peritoneum, are washed out with the dialysate. The importance of these defence mechanisms has been reviewed by Lewis and Holmes [73, 74]. However, the clinical consequences of the impairment of these natural defence mechanisms are still unclear, and it is yet unknown how these mechanisms can be improved.

Peritonitis

The diagnosis of peritonitis is based on the following criteria: (1) presence of organisms on Gram stain or culture of dialysis fluid; (2) cloudy fluid (cell count > 100 leukocytes/mm^3 with predominantly polymorphonuclear cells); (3) symptoms of peritoneal inflammation. Peritonitis is defined as the presence of any two of these three criteria [75].

Usually CAPD peritontitis is diagnosed in an early phase because the patient is alerted by visible changes in the dialysate and/or abdominal pain. The presenting symptoms of peritonitis have been reviewed by Tranaeus *et al.* [76] and classified according to the degree of severity. Subclinical peritonitis (cloudy dialysate without clinical symptoms) was present in 27% of patients. Mild peritonitis (cloudy dialysate and/or subfebrility and/or mild abdominal pain) was found in 31%, severe peritonitis (severe abdominal pain, febrility, prominent turbidity) in 11%, and in 31% of patients the clinical symptoms were classified as moderate (between mild and severe).

In many episodes of peritonitis the reason for the development of the infection is not known [76]. As the causative microorganisms are usually part of the Gram-positive skin flora of patients, external contamination, either through or along the catheter, seems to be the most frequent route.

Penetration of bacteria along the external surface or the catheter is very likely when peritonitis episodes are preceded by an exit-site or tunnel infection.

Tranaeus *et al.* [76] reported 8% of the peritonitis episodes being preceded by either exit-site or tunnel infections, whereas Prowant *et al.* [77] found a relationship with exit-site or tunnel infections in 20% and Bernardini *et al.* [78] in 13–20% of cases.

Contamination of dialysate by bacteria during bag exchange is probably the most common cause of peritonitis. This is supported by the observation that the incidence of peritontitis decreases when CAPD is done for a longer period of time, reflecting increasing patient and centre experience [76]. Furthermore, several devices designed to prevent contamination during bag exchange have been reported to be effective in reducing the incidence of peritonitis [58, 78–81].

Penetration of bacteria through the intestinal wall is possible [82] and this may be the route of contamination in peritonitis episodes caused by Enterobacteraceae.

In a prospective study in CAPD patients with and without diverticulosis, Wu *et al.* [83] found a higher incidence of faecal peritonitis in patients with this abnormality. This finding was not confirmed by Tranaeus *et al.* [84], who identified neither diverticula in the sigmoid colon, nor diverticulitis, as assessed by radiological findings, as risk factors. However, they found diverticular disease of the non-sigmoid colon being associated with enteral episodes of peritonitis. Transmural migration is also probable in peritonitis episodes caused by *Campylobacter jejuni*, a microorganism known for its invasive capacity [85].

Haematogenous spread should be considered in episodes caused by streptococci. Vas [75] reported peritonitis with *Streptococcus viridans* in CAPD patients who had acute upper respiratory infections. A haematogenous route is also likely in peritonitis caused by *Mycobacterium tuberculosis* [86].

The statement of Williams *et al.* [87]: 'Treatment of peritonitis in patients on CAPD: no longer a controversy' has proven to be a little too optimistic. Many treatment regimens are being used and many questions concerning optimal treatment of peritonitis still await an answer.

Millikin *et al.* reviewed the published data concerning therapeutic regimens which have been proposed for the management of CAPD-associated peritonitis [88]. The highest cure rate with empiric antibiotic treatment was reported with the use of vancomycin in combination with ceftazidime or aminoglycosides as initial antimicrobial agents. Based upon these data, in 1993 the *ad-hoc* advisory committee on peritonitis management advised using either the combination of vancomycin/ceftazidime or vancomycin/aminoglycoside as first-line treatment [89].

A disadvantage of the abundant use of vancomycin, however, is the emergence of vancomycin resistance. Vancomycin-resistant enterococci (VRE) have become a serious problem in the United States [90, 91]. Troidle *et al.* [92] described nine episodes of peritoneal dialysis-associated peritonitis with VRE. Transfer of vancomycin resistance from enterococci to *S. aureus* has been demonstrated *in vitro* [93]. Methicillin-resistant *S. aureus* (MRSA) strains with reduced susceptibility to vancomycin have emerged in Japan and the United States [94, 95]. Vancomycin-resistant MRSA is still not present in Europe and VRE are rare in European countries [96, 97]. However, as glycopeptides are the only antibiotics suitable for the treatment of MRSA, the emerging vancomycin resistance could create an important problem in the future. Therefore, frequent use of glycopeptides should be avoided as much as possible, even in European countries.

The emergence of vancomycin resistance was the principal motive for revision of the 1993 treatment recommendations [98]. In this 1996 update the use of vancomycin is discouraged. For empiric treatment the combination first-generation cephalosporin/aminglycoside is advocated. According to these recommendations aminoglycosides can be administered continuously or intermittently in a single daily dose. However, experience with intermittent dosing in CAPD patients is limited, and serum and peritoneal aminoglycoside concentrations are shown to vary widely among patients [99]. The use of aminoglycosides in the treatment of CAPD peritonitis may cause ototoxicity and vestibulotoxicity [100] and impairment of residual renal function. Therefore, intermittent treatment with aminoglycosides is suitable only if the dose is adapted to serum levels.

For optimal treatment of CAPD peritonitis adequate diagnostic procedures are essential. The incidence of culture-negative peritonitis varies from 2% to 40% [80, 101–104], depending on the culture technique used. Only a very small portion of the culture-negative peritonitis episodes can be ascribed to the peritoneal eosinophilia syndrome, which rarely occurs in early stages of CAPD [105]. For an optimal outcome of culture results aseptic sampling of large volumes (50–200 ml), subsequent concentration of the dialysate (either by centrifugation or filtration) and culturing under aerobic and anaerobic conditions seems essential [98, 101, 106–108].

Mortality associated with CAPD peritonitis varies between 0.8% and 12.2% [109–111]. However, sometimes these deaths are due not to the infection itself but to a complication such as myocardial infarction occurring during the peritonitis episode. Peritonitis associated with gastrointestinal perforation is notorious for a high mortality rate of about 40% [111–113].

Prevention of peritonitis has been one of the most important issues in CAPD. In 1978 the incidence of peritonitis was reported to be 4.6 episodes per patient per year [5]. Improvement of the technique and training programmes in the centres resulted in a reduction of the peritonitis rates to 1.0–1.5 episodes per patient per year [75]. As early as the early 1980s Italian investigators reported excellent results with a Y-connector set filled with disinfectant during dwell time [58, 114, 115]. With this system a peritonitis incidence as low as one episode in 57 patient-months was reported [116]. Even without the use of a disinfectant these good results have been confirmed in other studies [79, 80, 117].

Exit-site infection

With the significant reduction in the incidence of peritonitis, exit-site and tunnel infections have now gained relatively more importance than in earlier years. Unlike peritonitis, however, exit-site infections have no singular precise definition. Definitions may vary from unspecified clinical signs of infection confirmed with a positive culture [118, 119] to a description of marked redness around the exit site accompanied by pain, induration, drainage or granulation tissue [53, 120–122]. The presence of a causative microorganism in the culture of the exit site may facilitate the diagnosis. Based upon an extensive, 30-year experience, Twardowski *et al.* classified normal, diseased, immature and healing exit sites [123].

An exit site is healed approximately 6 weeks post-catheter implantation and is usually dry. A slight crust formation around the exit is generally not an indication of infection. A positive culture from the exit without any sign of inflammation does not indicate infection and should better be termed 'colonization'.

Tunnel infections can be diagnosed by erythema, oedema and/or tenderness of the subcutaneous catheter pathway [53]. Usually purulent drainage is present at the exit site or can be made visible by gentle massage of the tunnel.

Sometimes ultrasound examination is useful in establishing the diagnosis [124, 125]. Often infection of the deep cuff is involved in an infection of the tunnel, which is rarely cured by (repeated) courses of antibiotic treatment. In most cases with deep cuff infection catheter removal is inevitable. The majority of exit-site infections is caused by *S. aureus* [53, 123, 126–128]. Although the incidence of exit-site infections caused by *Pseudomonas* spp. is reported to be low, infection with this microorganism often results in catheter loss [129].

Exit-site infections are usually treated with oral antibiotics, penicillinase-resistant penicillin or first-generation cephalosporins [98]. Ciprofloxacin is used in Gram-negative infections. *Pseudomonas* infections may require the addition of other antipseudomonal agents such as ceftazidime. Besides a perfect catheter insertion technique, the cornerstone for prevention of exit-site infections is proper exit-site care with immobilization of the catheter [130]. Prophylaxis with intranasal mupirocin can be considered in *S. aureus* nasal carriage [98].

Despite all these technical improvements during recent decades peritonitis and exit-site infections are still the major complication of CAPD [109, 131–133]. Further improvements are essential. An international multicentre infection study project under the auspices of the International Society of Peritoneal Dialysis offers new possibilities for the development of new treatment guidelines [98]. For optimizing results in individual centres epidemiological monitoring of the incidence of peritonitis, exit-site and tunnel infections is essential.

Non-infectious catheter-related complications and complications related to increased intra-abdominal pressure

Insertion of the peritoneal dialysis catheter requires a good placement technique by a dedicated team [53]. In patients having had previous intra-abdominal surgery usually the feasibility of catheter implantation and subsequent use for CAPD is not influenced [134].

Bleeding

Following catheter insertion minor intra-abdominal bleeding may occur, which will stop after the first dialysate exchanges. Laceration of medium-sized or large blood vessels in the anterior abdominal wall, resulting in intensifying bleeding in the dialysate, requires surgical intervention. Bleeding in the exit site can usually be stopped by bandages. Sometimes persistent bleeding from an artery in the subcutaneous tunnel has to be stopped surgically under local anaesthesia.

Pain

Postoperative shoulder pain, which is interpreted as reference pain from the diaphragm, is present in about 25% of patients and disappears spontaneously within a few days. After the start of CAPD patients may complain of abdominal pain, usually localized in the pouch of Douglas. The pain is most prominent with empty abdomen or during rapid inflow of the dialysate, and can be decreased by diminishing the inflow rate. Usually this pain lessens or disappears within a few months after the start of CAPD. In patients with persisting intra-abdominal pain the addition of sodium bicarbonate (2–5 mEq/L) or lidocaine 1% (2.5 ml/L) to the dialysate may give some relief [135].

Perforation

During catheter insertion perforation of viscera may occur. To avoid this, patients must have an empty bladder when they are operated. The risk for perforation of the bowel is increased when intra-abdominal adhesions are present from previous surgical procedures or peritonitis. The risk for perforation is also increased in the presence of paralytic ileus. In case of a small bowel-perforation a new catheter can be inserted at the same operation. In case of large perforations, with spilling of intestinal contents, an exploratory laparotomy should be performed. Perforation of viscera by erosion of the peritoneal catheter is rare but well recognized [136]. This complication is facilitated by peritonitis, an empty peritoneal cavity, the use of steroids or the presence of vasculitis.

Leakage

Pericatheter leakage occurs most frequently in the immediate postoperative period. This complication is seen in 7–24% of patients [136]. Postoperative catheter leakage can largely be prevented by a break-in period of about 2 weeks, during which the wound can heal and ingrowth of fibrous tissue can anchor the Dacron cuffs. When peritoneal dialysis is started without a break-in period a reduction of the dialysate volume (500–1000 ml in adults) is recommended for the initial period. Leakage can usually be managed by cessation of peritoneal dialysis for about 2 weeks.

Dialysate leaks may also occur as a late complication of CAPD. The treatment is similar to the treatment in early leakage. Late leakage is usually provoked by a sudden increase in intra-abdominal pressure, for example during coughing or heavy lifting.

Under influence of the increased intra-abdominal pressure, dialysate can also dissect through peritoneal discontinuities into the soft tissues of the anterior abdominal wall. This can occur along the catheter insertion site or through defects in the peritoneum. The extraperitoneal dialysate can cause oedema in the abdominal wall and the genitals. Abdominal wall oedema is often difficult to diagnose. The abdomen may look asymmetrical, or the imprint of clothing seems to be deeper than usual. Sometimes the patient notices a decreasing dialysate return together with an increasing abdominal girth. Genital oedema can easily be confused with genital hernias.

The diagnosis of fluid dissection can be facilitated by nuclear medicine and radiological imaging [137, 138].

Dislocation

Dislocation of the catheter is suspected when one-way obstruction occurs; inflow is easy, but outflow is absent or impaired because the tip of the catheter is not positioned at the lowest level in the peritoneal cavity. Furthermore, malpositioned catheters can be obstructed by omentum, which is absent in the pouch of Douglas. Malposition can easily be diagnosed with a plain straight abdominal X-ray when common radiopaque peritoneal catheters are used.

In non-radiopaque catheters catheterography after infusion of sterile radiopaque material into the catheter may be useful [139]. One-way obstruction due to malposition is usually an early complication occuring in 1–28% of CAPD patients [136]. Usually the problem can be solved with patience, observation, mobilization of the patient and the administration of enemas to stimulate peristaltic forces. In the few cases with persisting outflow problems manipulation of the catheter with a semiflexible probe under fluoroscopic guidance is reported to be useful [53, 136].

Total obstruction

Total catheter obstruction occurs when fibrin, cellular debris or blood clots are present in the catheter. Forcing 20–50 ml of dialysate with a syringe into the catheter lumen can relieve the obstruction. Sometimes intraluminal heparin is useful and finally, fibrinolytic agents such as urokinase can be used to dissolve the clot [136].

Hernias

The increased intra-abdominal pressure during CAPD not only results in a risk for dialysate leaks. The elevated pressure can also provoke hernia formation and hydrothorax. Normally the intra-abdominal pressure in CAPD patients ranges from 3 to 15 mmHg, being an average 6 mmHg higher in the upright than in the recumbent position [45]. Transiently, during coughing or straining, the intra-abdominal pressure can reach values as high as $300 \ cmH_2O$ [140].

Hernias of the abdominal wall occur in 10–25% of CAPD patients [137, 141]. A lesser incidence has been reported in intermittent peritoneal dialysis [141]. A variety of hernias have been reported in the literature [137], but most common are umbilical, inguinal and incisional hernias. Predisposing factors for the development of hernias are a weak anterior abdominal wall (multiparicy), congenital defects of the abdominal wall and polycystic disease. Small hernias have a risk for bowel incarceration. Large hernias do not carry as great a risk but may be troublesome for the patient. Hernias should be repaired surgically. Usually, after a period of haemodialysis, CAPD can be restarted 2–4 weeks after the operation.

Hydrothorax

Hydrothorax secondary to leakage of peritoneal dialysate occurs in 1.6–10% of CAPD patients and is caused by anatomical defects of the diaphragm in the presence of increased intra-abdominal pressure [142]. This complication is more common in females than in males. Previous stretching of the diaphragm during pregnancy may be a promoting factor. Like hydrothorax complicating ascites in hepatic cirrhosis or ascites in Meigs's syndrome, hydrothorax complicating CAPD is almost always right-sided. As an explanation for this finding it can be hypothesized that left-sided defects in the diaphragm are largely covered by the heart and pericardium. Hydrothorax can be treated with the use of smaller volumes or by keeping the peritoneal cavity temporarily dry. When these measures are not successful, either pleurodesis (with either talc, tetracycline, antologous blood or Tissucol®), or surgical closure of the diaphragmatic defects can be considered in patients strongly motivated to continue CAPD.

Ultrafiltration failure

Ultrafiltration failure is clinically defined as the inability to achieve an adequate fluid balance despite the use of three or more hypertonic (4.25% glucose) exchanges per day [43]. This definition is not very precise as fluid balance is determined not only by ultrafiltration, but also by fluid intake. Therefore, the definition ultrafiltration failure should preferably be based on the net ultrafiltration obtained after a standardized dialysis dwell. With a 4-h 2.5% glucose PET a net ultrafiltration of less than 100 ml is considered abnormal [144, 145]. Using a 1.5% glucose solution ultrafiltration failure is indicated by a negative net ultrafiltration after 4 h [146]. Studies using 4-h 4.25% glucose dwells suggest ultrafiltration failure when the net ultrafiltration volume is less than 400 ml [39, 143, 147, 148]. As standarized dwells with lower glucose concentrations have been shown to overestimate ultrafiltration failure [149], 4.25% glucose should be used for identification of patients with this complication. In the literature the prevalence of ultrafiltration failure in patients on CAPD has been reported as being between 3% and 31% [149], depending on the duration of CAPD treatment. Currently three types of ultrafiltration failure are being distinguished: ultrafiltration failure due to rapid solute transport (type I membrane failure), ultrafiltration failure associated with impaired solute transport (type II membrane failure) and ultrafiltration failure due to excessive lymphatic absorption (type III membrane failure).

Ultrafiltration failure due to rapid solute transport

Increased transperitoneal transport of low molecular weight solutes, resulting in a rapid absorption of glucose and loss of the osmotic gradient, is the most common cause of chronic ultrafiltration failure in CAPD patients. Longitudinal studies have shown a decrease of ultrafiltration with time on CAPD [150–152], suggesting an increase of effective peritoneal surface area due to an increase in the number of microvessels in the peritoneum of long-term CAPD patients. Also impaired aquaporin-mediated water transport can be responsible for loss of ultrafiltration in CAPD patients [153]. This condition is also present in most patients presenting with sclerosing peritonitis (see later).

Ultrafiltration failure caused by increase in the transport of low-molecular weight solutes can also occur during peritonitis [154, 155]. This can be ascribed to an increased number of perfused capillaries during the inflammation. In contrast to chronic ultrafiltration failure, during the acute phase of peritonitis the large pore size is also increased, resulting in an increased loss of proteins [155]. This is possibly related to the release of inflammatory mediators during peritonitis [47]. Loss of ultrafiltration during peritonitis is usually reversible.

Ultrafiltration failure associated with impaired solute transport

The combination of poor ultrafiltration and small solute transport failure is rare and has been reported in a minority of patients with peritoneal sclerosis [156, 157]. Extensive adhesion-formation after severe episodes of peritonitis or intraperitoneal bleeding can present as this type of ultrafiltration failure. Although in this situation solute transport is usually intact, the decrease in the amount of peritoneal surface area can result in an overall decrease in fluid and solute removal.

Ultrafiltration failure with normal solute transport

Ultrafiltration failure with normal solute transport can occur in catheter malfunction or leakage of dialysate. These causes should be distinguished from extensive lymphatic absorption. The lymphatic absorption rate can be measured by calculating the disappearance rate of a macromolecular marker. For this purpose a marker such as dextran 70 can be added to the dialysate [31]. Loss of ultrafiltration due to a high effective lymphatic absorption rate is relatively rare [43].

Peritoneal sclerosis

Peritoneal sclerosis should be defined as the presence of two clinical symptoms, either abdominal complications (bowel obstruction, bloodstained effluent, severe ascites after discontinuation of peritoneal dialysis) or ultrafiltration failure, in combination with confirmation of the diagnosis by macroscopic examination of the abdominal viscera either at laparotomy or autopsy [158]. The peritoneal membrane shows a sclerotic thickening with or without adhesions. Sometimes sclerosing encapsulating peritonitis is present with encasement of the bowel by a new membrane. On microscopic examination dense fibrous tissue permeated with chronic inflammatory infiltrate is seen [159]. Computerized tomography (CT) scanning of the abdomen, showing loculated ascites, adherent bowel loops, bowel lumen narrowing, thickening of the peritoneum and peritoneal calcifications can be useful [160, 161]. However, in a retrospective study these typical alterations did not correlate very well with the clinical and macroscopic findings [162].

Peritoneal sclerosis is a severe, sometimes life-threatening complication which has been referred to as 'a sword of Damocles for peritoneal dialysis' [163]. Peritoneal sclerosis usually occurs in long-term peritoneal dialysis [162], but has also been diagnosed 1.5 years after only 10 days of intermittent peritoneal dialysis [164]. Depending upon the diagnostic criteria used, the incidence varies between 1.5 and 4.6 per 1000 patient-years [158, 162]. Mortality rates due to sclerosing peritonitis are high, varying from 37% to 93% [162]. Peritoneal sclerosis is always accompanied by loss of mesothelial cells, which is reflected in low dialysate CA 125 concentrations [158]. Although the aetiology of sclerosing peritonitis is not entirely clarified, continuous exposure to unphysiologically high glucose concentrations is likely to be a causative factor [162].

Treatment of ultrafiltration failure

When a patient presents with ultrafiltration failure, first the cause of the problem should be established. Malfunction of the catheter, fluid leaks and extensive adhesion formation should be excluded. Patients with loss of ultrafiltration due to an increased solute transport can usually be managed by shortening their dwell times. Most of these patients will benefit from automated peritoneal dialysis. Replacement of

glucose for the long dwell by 7.5% icodextrin is indicated [70]. As peritoneal lymphatic absorption increases with increasing intra-abdominal pressure, large dialysate volumes should be avoided in patients with a high effective lymphatic absorption rate. When the diagnosis of sclerosing peritonitis is suspected, discontinuation of CAPD or the use of glucose-free dialysate (amino acid solutions, glycerol, icodextrin) should be considered.

Nutritional and metabolic complications

Malnutrition

The possibility of malnutrition has long been recognized in patients undergoing maintenance peritoneal dialysis and has been described as the 'depletion syndrome' [165]. Therefore, the prevention of malnourishment has been a concern from the beginning of the CAPD era. A 'full' abdomen, loss of proteins and other nutrients such as amino acids and vitamins, by the peritoneal route, inadequate dialysis and inflammatory stimuli may contribute to the development of malnutrition in patients treated with peritoneal dialysis.

Nutritional assessment is important to detect protein energy malnutrition. For measurement of nutritional status many methods are available [166]. In most studies on the nutritional status of CAPD patients the number of patients was limited and a variety of variables was measured, making the results of the studies not really comparable. The most extensive study included 224 patients in six centres in Europe and North America [167]. In that study a 'subjective nutritional assessment' was made, using 21 variables derived from history and clinical examination, or anthropometry and biochemistry. Eighteen patients (8%) were severely malnourished, 32.6% were mildly to moderately malnourished and 59.4% did not show any evidence of malnutrition. There was a striking difference among centres. Fifteen of the 18 severely malnourished patients came from two centres. This difference was related to patient age, nutritional status at the commencement of CAPD, the length of time on CAPD and residual renal function. The absence of renal function contributed significantly to anorexia and symptoms of severe malnutrition. In a cross-sectional study in 147 clinically stable patients in one centre the 'composite nutritional index' was used [168], consisting of anthropometric variables, albumin and subjective global assessment (SGA)

[169]. According to this composite nutritional index 17% of patients were severely malnourished. The SGA *per se* was used in a modified version (seven scales instead of three) in the CANUSA study [170]. In this longitudial study, performed in 680 new CAPD patients, a higher SGA was associated with a lower risk of death. The SGA is easy to perform and is recommended by the Dialysis Outcome Quality Initiative (DOQI) [171].

Malnutrition is above all determined by dietary intake. Usually a daily protein intake of 1.0 g/kg or even 1.2 g/kg [172, 173] has been recommended. Despite this, in most patients the actual daily protein intake is about 0.9 g/kg [174, 175], and in the majority of these patients this seems to be adequate. Malnourished patients with a low oral protein intake may benefit from treatment with one or two amino acid-based solutions [176].

Bergström *et al.* [174] found a dietary energy intake consisting of 43% carbohydrate, 39% fat and 19% protein. In CAPD patients the oral intake of carbohydrates is usually relatively low. It appears that in CAPD patients the oral intake of carbohydrates is suppressed to compensate for the peritoneal glucose absorption [177]. It is of importance, however, that in spite of taking into consideration the energy intake provided by the glucose in the dialysate, the recommended daily energy intake (30 kcal/kg) was achieved in only 37% of the patients studied by Jacob *et al.* [175]. Similar results were found by others [174]. These results indicate that, despite the peritoneal energy supply, a low total energy intake is not uncommon in CAPD patients. As utilization of dietary protein depends largely upon energy supply, this may add significantly to the occurrence of protein malnutrition in CAPD patients.

Consequences of glucose absorption

The continuous absorption of glucose from the dialysate has several disadvantages. As about two-thirds of the glucose instilled in the peritoneal cavity is absorbed, the total daily amount of glucose delivered by the peritoneal route can amount to about 300 g in patients using only 4.25% glucose solutions. This large amount of glucose can result in loss of appetite, but also in obesitas. In many patients weight is below the ideal weight when CAPD is started, but increases during CAPD [174, 178, 179]. Overweight can be an especial problem in patients being already obese at the start of CAPD.

Although CAPD with 1.5% glucose exchanges has only marginal effects on glucose and insulin concentrations [180, 181], especially after a hypertonic exchange with 4.25% glucose, changes similar to an oral glucose load have been observed [182]. As a consequence, some CAPD patients may develop 'de-novo' diabetes mellitus.

Hyperlipidaemia

It is well known that in CAPD patients triglyceride and cholesterol concentrations increase during the first months of renal replacement therapy but stabilize thereafter [178, 179, 183]. Regarding the continuous absorption of glucose from the dialysate this stabilization is remarkable. This may indicate a metabolic or dietary adaptation to the glucose load.

More recently it has been shown, however, that CAPD patients have a highly atherogenic serum profile with triglyceride-rich lipoprotein abnormalities [184, 185]. O'Neal *et al.* [185] found a preponderance of small, dense LDL particles in 48% of CAPD patients, compared to 23% of subjects on haemodialysis and 7% of healthy volunteers. Small, dense LDL particles have been associated with an increased risk of myocardial infarction in patients without end-stage renal disease [186].

Several mechanisms can contribute to these abnormalities. Besides hyperinsulinaemia, the continuous absorption of glucose may increase triglyceride synthesis, which can result in a further increase in the concentration of triglyceride-rich lipoproteins. Loss of apolipoprotein AI and AII in the dialysate [187] can result in low concentrations of HDL. Finally, reduced activities of lipolytic enzymes can be responsible for lipoprotein abnormalities. In CAPD patients significantly lower than normal values for hepatic lipase activity have been found [188].

In view of the high prevalence of cardiovascular disease in CAPD patients, treatment of hyperlipidaemia with diet and lipid-lowering agents is recommended when LDL cholesterol levels are 130 mg/dl or greater [189]. However, as long-term trials with lipid-lowering treatment in CAPD patients do not exist, the value of drug therapy reducing cardiovascular risk in CAPD patients is still uncertain.

Losses of nutrients with the dialysate

In CAPD patients the continuous loss of nutrients in the dialysate may result in deficiencies. Weekly losses of free amino acids are in the same magnitude or smaller than with haemodialysis [166]. These losses are small compared with the substantial loss of proteins in the dialysate, varying between 5 and

15 g per day [166, 190, 191]. These losses can increase significantly during peritonitis.

Considerable losses of water-soluble vitamins have been found in CAPD patients. When compared to the excretion of vitamins in the urine of healthy subjects, loss in the dialysate was high for vitamin C and folic acid [192]. Excretion in the dialysate was moderate for vitamin B2 and B6 and relatively low for vitamin B1. When compared to the recommended daily dietary intake, intake was especially low for vitamin B1 and B6. As a result of excretion in the dialysate and insufficient oral intake, deficient blood concentrations for vitamin B1, B6, C and folic acid were seen in a considerable number of patients. Daily oral supplementation comparable with an ample recommended dietary allowance of 2 mg vitamin B, 2 mg vitamin B6, 100 mg vitamin C and 400 µg folic acid is indicated.

Gastrointestinal complications

Nausea, vomiting, upper abdominal discomfort and pain are common features in patients with chronic renal failure. In CAPD patients these symptoms may be aggravated by increased intra-abdominal pressure due to the presence of dialysate in the peritoneal cavity. Two studies showed abnormally delayed gastric emptying in about half of the patients treated with CAPD [193, 194]. It is suggested that the addition of 2 L of dialysate to the abdomen may retard gastric emptying, possibly by mechanical or neurogenic (reflex) mechanisms [193].

In diabetic CAPD patients the administration of intraperitoneal erythromycin (100 mg/2 L of dialysate, making exchanges approximately $\frac{1}{2}$ h before meals) has been successful in the treatment of gastroparesis [195].

Intestinal perforations in CAPD patients result in faecal peritonitis; they usually require surgical intervention. The most common cause of intestinal perforation is diverticulitis. Perforations of the small bowel are usually related to pressure necrosis from the peritoneal dialysis catheter [196]. Appendicitis is as common in CAPD patients as in the general population. Early diagnosis is important as a delay in treatment can result in perforation with subsequent faecal peritonitis. The same applies to gastric or duodenal ulcer. As CAPD patients usually have some air beneath the diaphragm, this symptom is not very helpful in establishing the diagnosis of perforated ulcer.

The prevalence of gallstone disease in CAPD patients is similar to that in the general population. In a prospective study 25% of patients with gall-

stones required cholecystectomy after 1–14 months on CAPD [197]. It was suggested that peritoneal dialysis may promote the development of cholecystitis in patients with asymptomatic gallstones. As in appendicitis, acute cholecystitis bears an additional risk of peritonitis. After laparotomic or laparoscopic cholecystectomy patients may be transferred temporarily to haemodialysis, or have to use intermittent peritoneal dialysis with small volume exchanges for a period of 2 weeks.

In CAPD patients the liver is subject to high concentrations of glucose, both via direct contact of dialysate to the surface of the liver and via the portal vein draining the peritoneal cavity. In diabetic CAPD patients, treated with intraperitoneal insulin, a unique form of hepatic steatosis has been described, with triglyceride depositions in the subcapsular region of the liver [198]. The clinical consequences of this abnormality are not well established. As a complication of peritonitis, abscess formation in the liver can occur. As ultrasound of the liver may be normal, sometimes an exploratory laparotomy is indicated [199].

Hepatic dysfunction in CAPD patients is mostly due to hepatotoxic drugs. In contrast to haemodialysis, the CAPD procedure itself does not increase the risk for hepatitis B or hepatitis C. Despite this, as HBsAg has been demonstrated in the dialysis fluid [200], special precautions are important also in CAPD. Both patients and staff are recommended to be vaccinated against hepatitis B.

Acute pancreatitis in patients on CAPD is an uncommon but serious complication. The prevalence of this complication in CAPD patients is similar to the prevalence in patients on haemodialysis [201]. The clinical diagnosis can be easily confused with dialysis-associated peritonitis. Presenting symptoms are abdominal pain and vomiting, with normal temperature and normal peristalsis. The dialysate can be clear, haemorrhagic or cloudy. Serum amylase concentrations exceeding three times the upper limit of normal, and dialysate amylase concentrations exceeding 100 U/L, may be helpful in diagnosing acute pancreatitis [202]. The 34–58% mortality of acute pancreatitis in patients on CAPD is high when compared to 10% mortality in the normal population [202]. This high mortality rate can be explained by the rapid spread of pancreatic enzymes through the dialysate-filled peritoneal cavity.

Acute pancreatitis in CAPD patients cannot be attributed to one single aetiological factor. It has been postulated that the CAPD procedure itself may be a causative factor. The non-physiological character of the dialysate may irritate the peritoneum overlying the pancreas. Peritonitis and subsequent instillation of possible irritants (antibiotics, anticoagulants) may render the pancreas susceptible to autodigestion [203]. Other possible causes of acute pancreatitis such as hyperlipidaemia, hypercalcaemia and hyperparathyroidism are frequently present in CAPD patients [202]. Continuation of CAPD did not have an apparent effect on the outcome when compared to transfer to haemodialysis.

Anaemia

In most CAPD patients haemoglobin concentrations increase during the first 3–6 months on CAPD, with a stabilization thereafter. After 4 years of treatment the difference in haemoglobin concentration in patients on CAPD when compared to patients on haemodialysis is no longer significant [204, 205]. There is no clear explanation for this phenomenon The improvement of anaemia during CAPD has been shown to be associated with changes in plasma volume [206], while others reported an increase in red cell mass and an improvement of red cell survival [207–209]. The reason for these changes in red cell mass during CAPD is not defined. It may be related, at least in part, to less extracorporeal blood loss, and better preservation of the remaining renal function on CAPD when compared to haemodialysis. Another possibility is better removal of one or more factors inhibiting erythropoiesis [210–212].

The anaemia of chronic renal failure has been shown to be completely reversible in haemodialysis patients treated with exogenous recombinant human erythropoietin (r-HuEPO) [213]. An intravenous route of r-HuEPO is not practical in CAPD patients and the intraperitoneal route not economical because of higher maintenance doses required [214]. Subcutaneous administration of r-HuEPO is effective in relieving anaemia in patients on CAPD and seems to be the optimal route for these patients [215]. A stepwise correction of anaemia, by subcutaneous administration of r-HuEPO twice or thrice weekly in a dose of 25–50 IU/kg, appeared to be safe, without a high risk of adverse effects (such as hypertension) during treatment [216]. Routine iron supplementation may not be necessary in CAPD patients, but a reduced response to r-HuEPO can be observed in patients who become iron deficient. In CAPD patients serum ferritin concentrations should be maintained at $> 100\ \mu g/L$, transferrin saturation at $> 20\%$ and the proportion of hypochromic red blood cells at $< 10\%$. In patients starting r-HuEPO iron status should initially be evaluated monthly, then every 2–3 months [217]. In the majority of CAPD patients oral iron supplementation with ferrous sulphate 200 mg b.d. or t.d.s. is appropriate. In patients with an inadequate response to iron therapy the intravenous administration of iron gluconate or saccharate, 100 mg every 2 weeks, should be considered [217].

Cardiovascular complications

Cardiovascular complications are common in dialysis patients and are the major cause of death [218, 219]. CAPD has some haemodynamic advantages over haemodialysis: no hypercirculation due to an arteriovenous fistula, constant acid–base balance, constant concentrations of sodium, potassium, calcium and other solutes and a continuous removal of waste products that are possible aetiological factors in uraemic cardiomyopathy [220]. Also, in CAPD intra- or interdialytic changes in cardiac filling and major fluctuations in blood pressure are absent. Early echocardiographic studies have shown a decrease in left ventricular mass in the majority of CAPD patients in whom it was increased at the start of dialysis [221]. However, these results could not be confirmed by others [222], who found an increase in the prevalence of left ventricular hypertrophy from 52% to 70% in 21 CAPD patients followed for 18 months. Mortality was significantly higher in patients with severe left ventricular hypertrophy. The higher risk for mortality in CAPD patients with left ventricular hypertrophy was confirmed in an echocardiographic analysis between survivors and non-survivors on CAPD, showing that non-survivors on CAPD had a lower mean left ventricular (LV) ejection function, higher LV end-systolic volume indices and a shorter mean LV ejection time than survivors [223]. The high prevalence of LV hypertrophy may contribute to cardiovascular mortality rates being comparable in haemodialysis and CAPD patients [224], irrespective the possible advantages of CAPD.

One of the explanations for the high cardiovascular mortality in CAPD patients can be a non-symptomatic fluid overload. After initiation of CAPD an early reduction of blood pressure is seen, probably because of normalization of the body fluid volume [218, 225]. However, long-term follow-up has shown that the reduction in blood pressure is not sustained for longer than 4 or 5 years and that patients have to be treated with increasing doses of antihypertensive drugs in the course of time [178].

This has been ascribed to gradual losses in residual renal function and ultrafiltration capacity of the peritoneal membrane. Increased peritoneal permeability with high transport rates of solutes and decreased fluid removal have been associated with increased mortality rates in CAPD [226, 227]. Although a direct relationship with cardiovascular mortality and hypertension is not yet established, these data point clearly to the importance of appropriate fluid control. Besides restriction of water and salt intake, preservation of residual renal function by the long-term use of loop diuretics, the use of alternative osmotic agents to glucose, biocompatible dialysate, and low-sodium dialysate have been proposed [228].

Another possible explanation for the increased cardiovascular morbidity in CAPD patients was recently proposed by Bergström and Lindholm. They hypothesized a pivotal role of proinflammatory cytokines in the development of reduced cardiac contractility, vascular disease, malnutrition and hypoalbuminaemia [229].

Besides the factors discussed above, many other factors such as smoking, hyperlipidaemia, hyperhomocystinaemia, hyperparathyroidism, endothelial dysfunction and anaemia can contribute to the increased cardiovascular risk of CAPD patients. The elevated intra-abdominal pressure due to dialysis fluid does not seem to affect cardiac function [230].

Not only hypertension, but also a reduction in blood pressure can have deleterious effects. Hypotension can provoke cardiac ischaemia in patients with cardiovascular disease. Is has been suggested that lowered blood pressures in CAPD were responsible for exacerbations of peripheral vascular disease [231].

Skeletoarticular complications

Long-term CAPD patients frequently develop skeletoarticular complications such as renal osteodystrophy and amyloidosis-related disorders.

Many symptoms of renal osteodystrophy are insidious in their onset and may vary in intensity [232]. As well as bone pain, renal osteodystrophy can cause arthritis and periarthritis, myopathy, spontaneous ruptures, pruritus, skeletal deformities, vascular and visceral calcifications, central nervous system disturbances, cardiomyopathy, anaemia and retardation of growth in children. In most patients on long-term CAPD, bone biopsies show high turnover bone disease (hyperparathyroid bone disease; osteitis fibrosa) or low turnover bone disease (osteomalacia and adynamic uraemic bone disease) or a mixture of these two

conditions [233]. Pei *et al.* [234] found a significantly lower prevalence in high turnover bone disease among CAPD than haemodialysis patients (13% versus 44%). Aluminium-related bone disease was found in 22% of peritoneal dialysis patients. Adynamic bone disease was found in almost one-half of the patients on peritoneal dialysis, while in haemodialysis its prevalence was only 18%.

Tetracycline labelling of the bone prior to biopsy provides an accurate method to differentiate between high and low turnover bone diseases. Aluminium deposition in the bone has been thought to be associated with low turnover bone disease, but low turnover bone disease can also be present without aluminium deposits [233]. Suppression of parathyroid hormone by increased concentrations of ionized calcium secondary to the increased use of calcium salts as phosphate binder, and administration of calcitriol have been thought to be responsible for low turnover bone disease [235].

On theoretical grounds it was calculated that a dialysate calcium concentration of 1.25 mmol/L would allow the use of larger doses of calcium carbonate, thus decreasing the risk of hypercalcaemia [236]. Consequently, a low calcium-containing dialysate was developed with a calcium concentration of 1.25 mmol/L, magnesium concentration of 0.25 mmol/L and a slightly higher lactate concentration (40 mmol/L) to improve the mild acidosis found in most CAPD patients [237]. Indeed, short-term studies in a small number of patients using this low-calcium dialysate demonstrated that larger doses of calcium salts can be prescribed, resulting in better phosphorus control. The serum concentration of ionized calcium in most patients remained within normal values [238, 239]. In a randomized controlled trial, a significantly better tolerance of calcium-containing phosphate binders with fewer hypercalcaemic episodes have been observed when low-calcium dialysate was used [240]. However, reduction of calcium levels in the dialysate may also lead to a persistent negative calcium balance, resulting in increasing PTH concentrations [241].

Dialysis-related amyloidosis, a well-recognized complication of standard long-term haemodialysis, is related to prolonged exposure to β_2-microglobulin ($\beta_2 M$) serum levels [242]. It is characterized by deposits of $\beta_2 M$ in bone and connecting tissues. The three main syndromes are carpal tunnel syndrome, arthropathy and skeletal manifestations. In several studies it was found that serum $\beta_2 M$ is lower on CAPD than on standard haemodialysis [220]. However, even on CAPD it was 20 times the normal value. Other studies found no difference in serum $\beta_2 M$ levels in haemodialysis and CAPD [243, 244]. Residual renal function is found to have an important influence on serum $\beta_2 M$ concentration, which is reflected in the significant increase in serum values when residual function decreases below 1 ml/min. There is evidence that residual renal function is better preserved in patients on CAPD than in those on haemodialysis [212]. This factor is probably more important in preventing dialysis-related amyloidosis than the better clearance of $\beta_2 M$ by the peritoneal membrane [245]. However, with longer duration of therapy, CAPD patients will not escape this complication [246, 247].

Adequacy in CAPD

During recent years there has been an ongoing debate about whether removal of small solutes is a good predictor of adequacy in peritoneal dialysis. One of the problems of quality assessment in CAPD is the definition of adequacy of dialysis. When compared to the function of two normal kidneys any type of dialysis treatment is insufficient. The only starting point is to compare peritoneal dialysis to the 'Golden Standard' haemodialysis.

Many solutes have been mentioned as possible toxins in severe renal failure. Unfortunately no specific toxin responsible for signs and symptoms of uraemia has been defined. Therefore, marker solutes are used that correlate with uraemic toxicity but are not very toxic themselves: creatinine and urea. Creatinine generation is relatively constant within each patient and is highly correlated with muscle mass. There is no simple way to correct for muscle mass and there is little or no correlation between creatinine generation and protein intake. Urea is correlated to protein intake and seems to be a better marker of toxicity in renal failure than creatinine, though it is not toxic itself [248].

Data supporting the usefulness of urea as a marker of toxicity were obtained in the National Cooperative Dialyses Study [249]. To this study, however, several objections can be made. The study period was only 24–52 weeks and included only 151 patients. Patients over 70 years of age and patients with significant comorbidity were excluded. Furthermore, a bias was introduced as the high BUN group patients were withdrawn from the study when they developed medical problems. Finally it remains doubtful whether these results, obtained in haemodialysis patients, are true for peritoneal dialysis.

Table 1. Most commonly used formulae for calculating PCR

Randerson	PCR = 0.28 (G_{un} + 40)
Teehan	PCR = 6.25 (UN loss + 1.8 + 0.031 body weight)
Bergström	PNA = 19 + 0.272 UA

Where:

G_{un} (μmol/min) = urea nitrogen generation rate
$$= (V_d \times D_{un} + V_u \times U_{un})/t,$$
where V_d and V_u are dialysate and urine volumes in L, D_{un} and U_{un} are dialysate and urine urea concentrations in μmol/L and t is collection time in minutes.

UN loss (g/day) = urea nitrogen loss
UA (mmol/day) = urea appearance
PNA (g/day) = protein equivalent of nitrogen appearance = PCR

CAPD patients constantly have higher time-averaged urea concentrations than patients on chronic intermittent haemodialysis. Despite this, there is no evidence of differences in uraemic morbidity between haemodialysis and CAPD. For the outcome of treatment it is probably more important to avoid peak concentrations [19, 250].

As with haemodialysis, in peritoneal dialysis there is a significant relationship between PCR (reflecting the daily protein intake) and Kt/V [21, 251]. However, the slope of the regression line for patients treated with peritoneal dialysis is significantly steeper than the slope of the line calculated for haemodialysis [251]. This would mean that at the same value for Kt/V, CAPD patients eat more protein than do haemodialysis patients. However, interpretation of this finding is hampered by differences in the formulae used for calculating Kt/V and PCR in haemodialysis and peritoneal dialysis. Furthermore, we have to realize that mathematical coupling between Kt/V PCR is present [252]. Finally, for the interpretation of the results of studies on adequacy of CAPD treatment, it is important to know which formula for calculating PCR is used. The most commonly used formulae are those of Randerson [253], Teehan [254] and Bergström [174], which are summarized in Table 1.

Values for PCR (= PNA) calculated by using these three formulae are not identical. For example: a 60 kg patient with a daily urea-removal of 200 mmol; this patient would have a normalized PCR (nPCR = PCR/body weight) of 0.83 g/kg/day calculated by the Randerson equation, 0.96 g/kg/day by the Teehan equation and 1.22 g/kg/day when the Bergström formula was used.

Similar differences in nPCR were found by Harty et al. [168], comparing the Randerson, Teehan and Borah equations. In the same study they found a significantly greater nPCR in a severely malnourished group compared to a well-nourished group when they used the patients' actual weight in the calculations. However, when they used ideal body weight, nPCR was significantly greater in the well-nourished population. Especially in underweight patients it seems important to use ideal weight instead of actual weight for calculating nPCR or Kt/V [255].

From nitrogen balance studies it has been estimated that CAPD patients have to eat at least 1.2 g/kg body weight/day to maintain a positive nitrogen balance [256]. It has, however, been reported that patients can maintain a positive nitrogen balance with protein intakes of 0.9 g/kg/day or less [174, 254, 257]. Although in multivariate analyses nPCR was not associated with outcome in CAPD patients [258, 259], the NKF-DOQI committee recommended an nPCR of at least 0.9 g/kg/day in adult patients [260].

The significance of urea and creatinine kinetic modelling for clinical outcome of CAPD has been analysed in several studies. Blake *et al.* [261] analysed retrospectively the predictive value of urea kinetics in 76 patients followed over a period of 3 years with a mean follow-up of 20 months. They concluded that urea kinetic modelling is predictive of some biochemical outcomes but not of clinical outcomes in CAPD patients. Teehan *et al.* [262] followed 51 stable CAPD patients for a median of 24 months with quarterly assessment of Kt/V, dialysis index and PCR. Multivariate analyses showed that lower serum albumin, increased age, longer time on CAPD and lower Kt/V independently predicted decreased patient survival. When survival on CAPD was plotted as a function of Kt/V the probability of surviving for 5 years was greater than 90% for patients with a $Kt/V \geqslant 1.89$/week compared with less than 50% for patients with a lower value. This difference, however, was seen only after 2–3 years. In this study Kt/V was also predictive of serum albumin concentrations but not of days hospitalized. Faller and Lameire [179] performed a longitudinal 7-year survey in 23 CAPD patients. They found a negative correlation between Kt/V urea and the number of hospitalization days, and a positive correlation with peripheral nerve conductivity. Brandes *et al.* [263] showed that Kt/V urea and creatinine clearance could differentiate between clinical outcomes classified as good or poor. Good clinical outcomes were associated with Kt/V values of 2.3 compared to 1.5 for poor. The corresponding values for creatinine clearance were 71 and 35 L/week. In the 3-year prospective study in 68 CAPD patients of Maiorca *et al.* [258] Kt/V and creatinine clearance were predictors of mortality and morbidity. A weekly $Kt/V \geqslant 1.96$ and a weekly creatinine clearance

of $\geqslant 58$ L were associated with a significantly better outcome and regarded as the minimum target for adequate dialysis.

The most valuable study until now, the CANUSA study, included 680 CAPD patients from 14 centres in Canada and the USA [259]. The patients were enrolled between September 1990 and 31 December 1992, with a follow-up until 31 December 1993. A decrease of 0.1 unit Kt/V per week was associated with a 5% increase in the relative risk (RR) of death; a decrease of 5 L/1.73 m^2 creatinine clearance per week was associated with a 7% increase in the RR of death. The RR of technique failure was increased with decreased albumin concentration and decreased creatinine clearance. Hospitalization was increased with decreased serum albumin concentration, worsened nutrition according to subjective global assessment (SGA) and decreased creatinine clearance. Extrapolating from their data the authors suggested a weekly Kt/V of 2.1 and a weekly creatinine clearance of 70 L/1.73 m^2 as acceptable. These targets were associated with an expected 2-year survival of 78%. The clinical outcome goals as given by the NKF-DOQI committee are mainly based on this study. This committee recommend a minimum delivered dialysis dose target Kt/V 2.0 per week and a minimum weekly target creatinine clearance of 60 L/1.73 m^2 [264].

It should be considered, however, that in the CANUSA study the association of small solute removal with outcome is confounded by residual renal function. Total Kt/V and creatinine clearance were strongly predictive of mortality, as was residual renal function. In contrast, peritoneal Kt/V and peritoneal creatinine clearance were not predictive at all. This raises the question as to whether solute removal by residual renal function is equal to solute removal by the peritoneal membrane. We have to be aware of benefits of residual renal function that dialysis alone cannot replace, such as superior control of hydration, greater large-molecule clearance, and better preservation of endocrine and metabolic function. It also raises the question of whether small-solute removal is the only important aspect of adequacy. Data from the CANUSA study [265] and other studies [226, 227] suggest that fluid overload contributes significantly to mortality in CAPD patients.

With a declining renal function it is not always possible to reach the targets set by NKF-DOQI [266]; therefore, preservation of renal function by daily administration of 250–500 mg frusemide should be considered [179]. With declining renal function increasing the peritoneal dialytic dose is the only alternative. However, we do not know if intensifying peritoneal dialysis will have a detrimental effect on the peritoneal membrane. As targets given by CANUSA and NKF-DOQI are not validated in long-term studies they should not be misinterpreted as isolated goals; they are merely tools in the individualized prescription of dialysis treatment.

Peritoneal dialysis versus haemodialysis

Shortly after the introduction of CAPD this dialysis modality was called 'the poor stepchild in therapy for end-stage renal disease' [267], and was seen as a 'second-class treatment by third-class physicians' [268]. From the beginning CAPD had to compete with the 'Golden Standard' haemodialysis. Early studies on patient- and technique-survival on CAPD were discouraging [269–271], and similar to early experiences with haemodialysis. Later studies, however, showed no consistent difference in mortality between the two modalities [109, 272–277]. These survival studies were usually retrospective and in most of them no attempt was made to correct for pretreatment differences. More recently, data from large data systems in the USA [278, 279] and Canada [280] were analysed, but even in these large samples results were conflicting. In an historical prospective sample of 1725 diabetic and 2411 non-diabetic ESRD patients, followed from 30 days after onset of ESRD until 2–4 years post-onset, no difference in outcome was found between non-diabetic ERSD patients treated with CAPD or haemodialysis [278]. In this USRDS case mix study, a higher adjusted mortality for CAPD compared to haemodialysis was found among diabetic patients (RR = 1.26, p = 0.03). This increased mortality was especially associated with elderly diabetic patients on CAPD, and became apparent after the first year of treatment. In another study on data obtained from the USRDS, prevalent patients on haemodialysis and CAPD were included [279]; the follow-up was 1 year. At total of 42 372 deaths occurring in 170 700 patient-years at risk were analysed. A significantly higher mortality rate in peritoneal dialysis than in haemodialysis patients was found except in non-diabetics treated for less than 1 year. Fenton et al. [280] analysed data from the Canadian Organ Replacement Register. The study population consisted of 11 970 ESRD patients initiating treatment in

Canada between 1990 and 1994 with a follow-up for a maximum of 5 years. Estimated by Poisson regression the mortality rate ratio (RR) for peritoneal dialysis relative to haemodialysis was 0.73 (95% confidence interval 0.68–0.78); a significant lower mortality for peritoneal dialysis. No such relationship was found when an intention-to-treat Cox regression model was fitted.

The discrepancy with the USRDS studies can be related to different statistical models, to differences in the populations being studied or to differences in health care between the countries. That differences between countries can influence outcome has been shown in the CANUSA study [170], in which the risks for mortality and for hospitalization were significantly greater in the USA compared to Canada.

The conflicting results, even in large studies, make clear that real differences between haemodialysis and CAPD can only be assessed in prospective studies in unselected, randomly allocated patients, and it seems questionable if such a study will ever be possible.

In contrast to outcome studies related to mortality, most studies on technique-survival are consistent in showing a shorter technique-survival in CAPD than in haemodialysis patients [109, 277, 281]. The difference in technique failure is mainly due to peritonitis, but other factors are also of influence. Maiorca et al. [281] found a statistically significant difference in the six dialysis centres participating in a multicentre study. These differences could not be explained by a higher peritonitis rate. Other factors, such as differences in patient selection, treatment and training, are also important, as is the centre's propensity to change methods.

Psychological aspects of CAPD

Although dialysis is a life-saving procedure, we have to realize the heavy burden of disease in patients with end-stage renal disease (ESRD). They have received a lifelong sentence, they will never be carefree healthy persons. Most patients will have an 'ESRD career', alternating dialysis treatments – haemodialysis and peritoneal dialysis – with renal transplantation. Regarding this permanent physical and psychological burden it is not surprising that depression is the most prevalent psychological problem in patients on dialysis [282]. Despite this, most patients adapt to their disruption of lifestyle and reduction in independence. It is likely that the social environment of the patient, especially support from the family, is essential for coping with the disease [283, 284].

Compliance has been shown to influence morbidity and mortality [284]. Patient distress, decreasing satisfaction, poor attendance, severe untreatable illness, medically unexplained symptoms and coexisting social problems have been reported as crucial factors for compliance [285]. Compliance in chronic dialysis patients has been studied in haemodialysis patients [286, 287], where the percentage of time dialysed, compared with the total dialysis time prescribed, seems one of the best parameters of outcome. Less is known about compliance in CAPD. However, it has been suggested that differences in compliance might have been responsible for the differences in treatment outcome between the USA and Canada in the CANUSA study [288]. To optimize compliance in chronically ill patients, patient education is essential. CAPD is a self-care treatment and we have to teach patients to feel responsible for themselves. As CAPD will often continue for years, it is also important to adapt the treatment as much as possible to the patient's lifestyle.

For the assessment of physical and psychosocial factors influencing disease a variety of methods measuring quality of life can be used. An overview of the most often used quality-of-life instruments used among patients on chronic dialysis was given by Ahlmén [289]. Quality-of-life assessment is difficult because of its complexity. Different instruments can be used for measuring functional, mental, psychological, emotional, disease-specific or global aspects of quality of life [289]. For the measurement of the burden of disease several indexes have been proposed [290]. The most widely used instrument for this purpose is the QALY (quality-adjusted life years), measuring survival years adjusted for quality gained through health interventions [291]. Establishing quality of life and burden of disease always raises questions about differences in demography, epidemiology comorbidity, health measures, socioeconomic development, and philosophical conceptions. These differences can make it impossible to compare results from studies in different countries and different groups of patients. Nevertheless, because there are several different dialysis modalities, it is important to know the relative impact of each on the patients' quality of life [292].

It is not surprising that most studies on quality of life in ESRD patients agree upon patients with a renal transplant having a better quality of life than patients on dialysis [293–296]. Inconsistent results, however, have been obtained in studies comparing quality of life in patients on haemodialysis and on CAPD.

Some studies showed no significant difference [297–300]. Other studies have reported a higher qual-

ity of life in CAPD patients when compared to in-centre haemodialysis patients [296, 301]. Another study found better psychological adjustment along several dimensions in haemodialysis when compared to peritoneal dialysis patients, despite the fact that the haemodialysis patients were more severely ill and appeared to suffer from physical symptomatology to a greater degree than peritoneal dialysis patients [302]. Until now all studies on quality of life in dialysis patients were cross-sectional and hampered by differences in the composition of the patient groups studied. Furthermore, among factors influencing quality of life, the use of recombinant erythropoietin has been shown to be important [303, 304]. Therefore, the results of studies conducted before the availability of erythropoietin are questionable as they did not adjust for haemoglobin concentrations. Merkus *et al.* described the results of a study on quality of life conducted by the NECOSAD Study Group [305]. In this study the SF–36, a 36-item Short Form Health Survey Questionnaire, was used encompassing eight dimensions of physical and psychological well-being [306]. In this study in 120 haemodialysis and 106 peritoneal dialysis patients 3 months after the start of chronic dialysis only a marginal superiority of peritoneal dialysis on the mental health dimension was found when compared to haemodialysis. This study also shows that patients with a lower residual glomerular filtration rate reported a worse quality of life, while no effect of dialysis Kt/V urea could be demonstrated. However, longitudinal data are needed to obtain insight into long-term effects of dialysis treatment.

Quality of life is not only important from the patients' perspective. As dialysis treatment is expensive, cost-effectiveness related to quality of life is also important as regards health-care expenses. In a study in the Netherlands, comparing quality-of-life adjusted costs of home haemodialysis, low-care haemodialysis, centre haemodialysis, CCPD and CAPD, the latter appeared to be the most cost-effective treatment modality [307]. It has yet to be shown, however, whether cost-effectiveness of CAPD is the same in other countries with different health-care systems.

Starting and stopping CAPD

Patients with ESRD have to choose a treatment modality. Only a minority of patients will receive a renal transplant as first modality. The vast majority of ESRD patients have to make a choice between haemodialysis or peritoneal dialysis. It appears that in about 80% of patients no strong medical or social contraindications exist for one or the other modality. Peritoneal dialysis has only two absolute contraindications: peritoneal fibrosis or severe adhesion formation and inflammatory bowel disease. Relative contraindications to CAPD may have a major or minor impact on modality selection. The importance of this impact depends largely upon the psychosocial situation in which the patient is living. Several relative contraindications for CAPD are listed in Table 2.

For optimal decision-making adequate patient education is essential [308–310]. Sometimes, mostly in elderly, severely impaired patients, the question is not only 'what modality?' but also 'do I want to be dialysed?' Decisions to initiate treatment are sometimes difficult to make. They are influenced by the expected medical benefit, but also by the willingness of patients [311]. The freedom of choice is also important for termination of dialysis. Withdrawal from dialysis is the third most common cause of death in dialysis patients over 65 years [296, 312].

The major reasons for CAPD patients to change their type of dialysis are peritonitis and catheter-related problems [275, 281, 313]. A peritoneal dialysis initiatives meeting in 1989 showed that 36% of patient drop-out from a haemodialysis was primarily related to peritonitis, 14% to catheter-related problems, 21% to 'other medical' reasons, 19% to psychosocial factors and 10% to inadequate dialysis [313]. Regarding the high targets for adequacy set by the DOQI guidelines it is likely that the percentage drop-out due to 'inadequate dialysis' will have increased during recent years. In some cases this drop-out may be questionable, as the DOQI guidelines have not been validated in long-term prospective studies. Drop-out due to 'inadequate dialysis' should not only be a matter of Kt/V, creatinine or nPNA but also of clinical judgement by an experienced physician.

Indications for catheter removal are given in Table 3. The most common causes of temporary catheter removal are infectious complications. When a catheter should be removed because of peritonitis

Table 2. Relative contraindications to CAPD

Pleuroperitoneal leak	Blindness
Hernia	Quadriplegia
Low-back problems	Crippling arthritis
Polycystic kidneys	Amputations
Diverticulosis	Poor motivation
Colostomy	Overt psychosis
Nephrostomy	Severe pulmonary impairment
Obesity	Hyperlipidaemia

Table 3. Indications for catheter removal

Intractable peritonitis
Relapsing peritonitis
Severe exit-site and tunnel infections
Permanently dislocated catheter
Renal transplantation
Withdrawal from peritoneal dialysis

shortly before the operation a few short dwells can be performed in an attempt to prevent adhesion-formation by removal of fibrin present in the dialysate. The optimal time period between catheter removal for infection and reinsertion of a new catheter is not known [98]. A period of at least 2 weeks between removal and reinsertion is recommended, but also simultaneous removal and insertion of the catheter without interruption of peritoneal dialysis has been reported to be successful [314].

A special issue is catheter removal after renal transplantation. Graft and patient survival after peritoneal dialysis are not different from haemodialysis [315]. However, after transplantation the risk for peritonitis is increased [315, 316]. Therefore early catheter removal is recommended [316].

Management of a CAPD programme

Development of the programme

CAPD is an extremely simple technique when compared to haemodialysis. Management of a CAPD programme, however, is less simple. When introducing a new treatment modality it is important to motivate nephrologists, surgeons, nurses, social workers and other health-care workers involved in the treatment of patients. An enthusiastic, dedicated team is the cornerstone for a successful programme. Furthermore, a well-equipped clinical chemical and microbiological laboratory is necessary. Hospital back-up, and back-up facilities for haemodialysis, should be ascertained. A reliable distribution of dialysis fluid and materials to patients' homes should be arranged. A schedule for 24 h a day coverage is required; therefore the availability of a well-trained medical and nursing staff is necessary. Depending upon the experience of the centre one nurse to each 10–15 patients and one doctor to each 40–50 patients should be available.

Training

Training can be practised in the hospital or on an outpatient basis. It is also possible to train patients at home. Usually training starts about 2 weeks after implantation of the catheter, thus allowing wound healing and avoiding early leakage. Training sessions are usually carried out on a daily basis and they last 4–8 h per day, depending upon patients' physical, mental and emotional status. Usually 7–14 days are needed to complete training. During the training the patients must learn the bag-exchange procedure, the principles of fluid and solute removal, interpreting their own fluid status by blood pressure and weight, and adjusting the choice of dialysate concentrations to their fluid status. Sometimes discomfort occurs when 2 L exchanges are used immediately. In this situation the amount of dialysate used should be adjusted to the patient and increased slowly. During training the patient should also be made familiar with management of common complications such as hypotension, muscle cramps, peritonitis and exit-site infections. Great attention should be paid to exit site and catheter care, and instructions should be given on how to cope with unexpected problems such as accidental disconnections or defective equipment. Before the training is completed a checklist should ensure that all theoretical and practical aspects are mastered. This checklist also includes instructions on the 24 h a day availability of the department.

After training the patient is seen in the outpatient-department. Between visits regular telephone contact ensures patients are self-reliant. If necessary, home visits by nurses are made to evaluate the patient's home environment. After about 1–2 months the intervals between visits to the department can be decreased to once in 1–3 months.

Hospital and haemodialysis back-up

For the management of a CAPD programme, back-up facilities for hospital admissions due to treatment-related or -unrelated complications are essential. The mean stay in hospital per year varies from 10.5 to 26.9 days per patient, depending on the patient population studied [109, 271, 317, 318]. A high percentage of patients with diabetes mellitus especially increases mean stay in the hospital.

For temporary discontinuation of CAPD because of peritonitis, catheter failure or surgical complications, haemodialysis back-up is essential. A mean temporary haemodialysis support of 8.5 days per patient per year CAPD treatment has been calculated [319]. This means that in a programme of 50 CAPD patients managed over 1 year, an average of one to two dialysis places will be occupied by patients temporarily withdrawn from CAPD.

Development of protocols

It is not advisable to manage a CAPD programme without the use of protocols. When starting a CAPD programme it may be useful to use a protocol developed by other centres, or protocols and guidelines given in the literature. Afterwards protocols can be adjusted to local needs. Protocols for the training programme and treatment of peritonitis are essential; protocols for laboratory tests and medication, such as the administration of intraperitoneal insulin, are convenient. Protocols should be evaluated critically on a regular basis. Records on results of treatments, such as data on mortality, hospitalization and incidence of peritonitis should be kept. These records are the basis of continuous quality management.

Future developments

Twenty years ago, shortly after the introduction of CAPD, the success of CAPD was not foreseen. Meanwhile worldwide far more than 100 000 patients are now treated with this dialysis modality, and CAPD is regarded as an equivalent alternative to haemodialysis. However, until now only a small number of patients have remained on CAPD for more than 10 years, and it is still not known whether, on a large scale, long-term treatment for more than 10 years is attainable. In this respect evidence-based definitions of adequate and optimal dialysis are essential. The DOQI guidelines can be regarded as a great step forward, but we have to realize that most of the recommendations are opinion-based.

Validation of the DOQI guidelines

In the DOQI guidelines an early start of dialysis is recommended [320]. This recommendation is based on the assumption that renal and peritoneal clearances are equivalent. However, this is still a hypothesis which should be tested [321]. Renal function is determined not only by glomerular filtration but also by tubular functions and production of hormones. Therefore, renal clearance may be more important than peritoneal clearance.

Evidence that an early start of dialysis will improve outcome is based on studies showing that late referral to the nephrologist has detrimental effects in patients with ESRD [322–327]. However, early referral not only means starting dialysis with a better renal function; early referral also means appropriate treatment of hypertension and renal osteodystrophy, attention to malnutrition, patient education and avoidance of temporary vascular access. Furthermore, regarding the early start of dialysis, we should always be aware of the complications of the dialysis procedure itself. Long-term prospective, preferably randomized, follow-up studies are needed to confirm possible benefits of a 'healthy start' [328].

Although it is obvious that inadequate dialysis has detrimental effects on outcome, we have to realize that the DOQI recommendation to achieve a minimum weekly Kt/V of 2.0 in CAPD patients is not validated in long-term studies. In these studies attention has also to be paid to other aspects of outcome, such as overhydration and cardiovascular morbidity.

Preservation of the peritoneal membrane

For long-term peritoneal dialysis preservation of the peritoneal membrane is essential. None of the currently available dialysis solutions can be considered as 'ideal'. Struijk and Douma [329] reviewed this issue and their recommendations for further research are summarized in Table 4. For testing new solutions the development of reliable animal models is essential. An interesting strategy for preserving the peritoneal membrane is genetic modification of the

Table 4. Recommendations for future research on biocompatible peritoneal dialysis fluids

Further development of existing solutions reducing glucose breakdown products with peptides (mol weight 1–2 kDa), glycerol, amino acids and polyglucose
Development of a replacement for glucose
Analysis of optimal molecular weight for high molecular weight solutes
Pharmacological interventions to improve ultrafiltration and solute transport
Solutes capable of binding uraemic toxins
Solutes with protective agents for long-term viability
Peritonitis-specific solutions
Additives
Systems to safely add substances to the dialysate
On-line dialysate production

Modified from ref. 329.

Table 5. Issues of clinical practice that need valuation in clinical trials

Prevention of cardiovascular disease by the administration of lipid-lowering drugs
Effect of intermittent versus continuous dosing of antibiotics in the treatment of peritonitis
Long-term effects of treatment of *S. aureus* carriers by the intranasal application of mupirocin
Establishing an optimal interval between catheter removal and reimplantation in peritonitis
Long-term use of furosemide for maintenance of residual renal function

peritoneal membrane by gene therapy [330]. This seems a promising strategy for the future.

Clinical research

Many guidelines and recommendations for clinical practice of CAPD are not well validated; there are more questions than answers. Several examples of issues waiting for validating studies are given in Table 5. One of the problems in clinical research is the number of patients needed for appropriate statistical analysis. To achieve these large numbers, multicentre trials are inevitable. For the accurate collection of reliable data trial centres with an adequate staff are needed, able to monitor trials and to motivate participants. A promising development is the initiation of the multicentre Infection Study Project [331]. More projects on other clinical fields are necessary.

References

1. Popovich RP, Moncrief JW, Decherd JF *et al.* The definition of a novel portable–wearable equilibrium peritoneal technique. Am Soc Artif Intern Organs 1976; 5: 64 (abstract).
2. Moncrief JW, Popovich RP, Dombros NV *et al.* Continuous ambulatory peritoneal dialysis. In: Gokal R, Nolph KD, eds. Peritoneal Dialysis. Dordrecht: Kluwer, 1994, pp. 357–97.
3. Boen ST. Overview and history of peritoneal dialysis. Dial Transplant 1977; 6: 12–18.
4. Wineman RJ. End-stage renal decease. Dial Transplant 1978; 7: 1034.
5. Popovich RP, Moncrief JW, Nolph KD *et al.* Continuous ambulatory peritoneal dialysis. Ann Intern Med 1978; 88: 449–56.
6. Moncrief JW. Continuous ambulatory peritoneal dialysis. Dial Transplant 1978; 8: 809–10.
7. Moncrief JW, Nolph KD, Rubin J. Additional experience with continuous ambulatory peritoneal dialysis (CAPD). Trans Am Soc Artif Intern Organs 1978; 24: 476–83.
8. Nolph KD, Popovich RP, Moncrief JW. Theoretical and practical implications of continuous ambulatory peritoneal dialysis. Nephron 1978; 21: 117–22.
9. Oreopoulos DG, Robson N, Izatt S. A simple and safe technique for continuous ambulatory peritoneal dialysis (CAPD). Trans Am Soc Artif Intern Organs 1978; 24: 484–7.

10. Oreopoulos DG. Continuous ambulatory peritoneal dialysis in Canada. Can Med Assoc J 1979; 120: 16.

11. Moncrief JW, Popovich RP, Nolph KD et al. Clinical experience with continuous ambulatory peritoneal dialysis. ASAIO J 1979; 2: 114–19.

12. Nolph KD. Peritoneal clearances. J Lab Clin Med 1979; 94: 519–25.

13. Rubin J, Nolph K, Arfania D et al. Follow-up of peritoneal clearances in patients undergoing continuous ambulatory peritoneal dialysis. Kidney Int 1979; 16: 619–23.

14. Oreopoulos DG Robson M, Faller B et al. Continuous ambulatory peritoneal dialysis: a new era in the treatment of chronic renal failure. Clin Nephrol 1979; 11: 125–8.

15. Oreopoulos DG. The coming of age of continuous ambulatory peritoneal dialysis (CAPD). Dial Transplant 1979; 8: 460.

16. Popovich RP, Hlavinka DJ, Bomar JB et al. Consequences of physiological resistances on metabolite removal from the patient–artificial kidney system. Trans Am Soc Artif Intern Organs 1975; 21: 108–15.

17. Gotch FA, Sargent JA. A mechanistic analysis of the National Cooperative Dialysis Study (NCDS). Kidney Int 1985; 28: 526–34.

18. Watson PE, Watson ID, Batt RD. Total body water volumes for adult males and females estimated from simple anthropometric measurements. Am J Clin Nutr 1980; 33: 27–39.

19. Keshaviah PR, Nolph KD, van Stone JC. The peak concentration hypothesis: a urea kinetic approach to comparing the adequacy of continuous ambulatory peritoneal dialysis (CAPD) and hemodialysis. Perit Dial Int 1989; 9: 257–60.

20. Lysaght MJ, Pollock CA, Hallet MD et al. The relevance of urea kinetic modelling to CAPD. Trans Am Soc Artif Intern Organs 1989; 35: 784–90.

21. Keshaviah PR, Nolph KD, Prowant B et al. Defining adequacy of CAPD with urea kinetics. Adv Perit Dial 1990; 6: 173 7.

22. Gotch FA. Application of urea kinetic modeling to adequacy of CAPD therapy. Adv Perit Dial 1990; 6: 178–80.

23. Keshaviah P. Urea kinetic and middle molecule approaches to assessing the adequacy of hemodialysis and CAPD. Kidney Int 1990; 43: S28–38.

24. Gotch FA. The application of urea kinetic modeling to CAPD. In: La Greca G, Ronco C, Feriani M et al., eds. Peritoneal Dialysis. Milan: Wichtig, 1991, pp. 47–51.

25. Tzamaloukas AH, Murata GH, Malhotra D et al. The minimal dose of dialysis required for a target KT/V in continuous peritoneal dialysis. Clin Nephrol 1995; 44: 316–21.

26. NKF-DOQI Committee. Adequate dose of peritoneal dialysis. Am J Kidney Dis 1997; 30 (suppl. 2): S86–92.

27. Twardowski ZJ, Nolph KD, Khanna R et al. Peritoneal equilibrium test. Perit Dial Bull 1987; 7: 138–47.

28. Twardowski ZJ. Clinical value of standardized equilibrium tests in CAPD patients. Blood Purif 1989; 7: 95–108.

29. Krediet RT, Boeschoten EW, Zuijderhoudt FMJ et al. Simple assessment of the efficacy of peritoneal transport in continuous ambulatory peritoneal dialysis patients. Blood Purif 1986; 4: 194–203.

30. Waniewski J, Werynski A, Heimbürger O et al. Simple models for description of small-solute transport in peritoneal dialysis. Blood Purif 1991; 9: 129–41.

31. Pannekeet MM, Imholz ALT, Struijk DG et al. The standard peritoneal permeability analysis: a tool for the assessment of peritoneal permeability characteristics in CAPD patients. Kidney Int 1995; 48: 866–75.

32. Struijk DG, Krediet RT, Koomen GCM et al. Measurement of peritoneal transport for low molecular weight solutes; which test should be used? Nephrol Dial Transplant 1990; 5: 721.

33. Heimbürger O, Waniewski J, Werynski A et al. Dialysate to plasma solute concentration (D/P) versus peritoneal transport parameters in CAPD. Nephrol Dial Transplant 1994; 9: 47–59.

34. Bergström J. Serum middle molecules and continuous ambulatory peritoneal dialysis. Perit Dial Bull 1982; 2: 59–61.

35. Lamperi S, Carozzi S, Icardi A. Improvement of erythropoiesis in uremic patients on CAPD. Int J Artif Organs 1983; 6: 191–4.

36. Arends JP, Krediet RT, Boeschoten EW et al. Improvement of bleeding time, platelet aggregation and platelet count during CAPD treatment. Proc EDTA 1981; 18: 280–5.

37. Twardowski ZJ, Khanna R, Nolph KD. Osmotic agents and ultrafiltration in peritoneal dialysis. Nephron 1986; 42: 93–101.

38. Krediet RT, Boeschoten EW, Zuijderhoudt FMJ et al. The relationship between peritoneal glucose absorption and body fluid loss by ultrafiltration during continuous ambulatory peritoneal dialysis. Clin Nephrol 1987; 27: 51–5.

39. Imholz ALT, Koomen GCM, Struijk DG et al. Effect of dialysate osmolarity on the transport of low molecular weight solutes and proteins during CAPD. Kidney Int 1993; 43: 1339–46.

40. Leypoldt JK, Mistry CD. Ultrafiltration in peritoneal dialysis. In: Gokal R, Nolph KD, eds. Peritoneal Dialysis. Dordrecht: Kluwer, 1994, pp. 135–61.

41. Nolph KD, Mactier RA, Khanna R et al. The kinetics of ultrafiltration during peritoneal dialysis: the role of lymphatics. Kidney Int 1987; 32: 219–26.

42. Struijk DG, Koomen GCM, Krediet RT et al. Indirect measurement of lymphatic absorption in CAPD patients by the disappearance of dextran 70 is not influenced by trapping. Kidney Int 1992; 41: 1668–75.

43. Mactier RA, Khanna R, Twardowski ZJ et al. Contribution of lymphatic absorption to loss of ultrafiltration and solute clearance in continuous ambulatory peritoneal dialysis. J Clin Invest 1987; 80: 1311–16.

44. Imholz ALT, Koomen GCM, Struijk DG et al. The effect of an increased intraperitoneal pressure of fluid and solute transport during CAPD. Kidney Int 1993; 44: 1078–85.

45. Imholz ALT, Koomen GCM, Vorn WJ et al. Day-to-day variability of fluid and solute transport in upright and recumbent positions during CAPD. Nephrol Dial Transplant 1998; 13: 146–53.

46. Hirszel P, Lameire N, Bogaert M. Pharmacologic alterations of peritoneal transport rates and pharmacokinetics of the peritoneum. In: Gokal R, Nolph KD, eds. Peritoneal Dialysis. Dordrecht: Kluwer, 1994, pp. 161–234.

47. Zemel D, Koomen GCM, Hart AAM et al. Relationship of TNFα, interleukin-6 and prostaglandins to peritoneal permeability for macromolecules during longitudinal follow-up of peritonitis in continuous ambulatory peritoneal dialysis. J Lab Clin Med 1993; 122: 686–96.

48. Tenckhoff H, Schechter H. A bacteriological safe peritoneal access device. Trans Am Soc Artif Intern Organs 1968; 14: 181–6.

49. Twardowski ZJ, Nolph KD, Khanna R et al. The need for 'swan-neck' permanently bent arcuate peritoneal catheter. Perit Dial Bull 1985; 5: 219–23.

50. Swartz R, Messana J, Rocher L et al. The curled catheter: dependable device for percutaneous peritoneal access. Perit Dial Int 1990; 10: 231–5.

51. Ash SR. Chronic peritoneal dialysis catheters: effects of catheter design, materials and location. Semin Dial 1990; 30: 39–40.

52. Cruz C. Cruz catheter: implantation technique and clinical results. Perit Dial Int 1994; 14: S59–63.

53. Gokal A, Ash SR, Helfrich GB et al. Peritoneal catheters and exit-site practices: toward optimum peritoneal access. Perit Dial Int 1993; 13: 29–39.

54. Ogden DA, Bernavente G, Wheeler D et al. Experience with the right angle GORE-TEX® peritoneal dialysis catheter. In: Khanna R, Nolph KD, Prowant B et al., eds. Advances in Continuous Ambulatory Peritoneal Dialysis. Toronto: Peritoneal Dialysis Bulletin Inc., 1986, pp. 155–9.

55. Pommer W, Brauner M, Westphale HJ *et al.* The effect of a silver device in preventing catheter-related infections in peritoneal dialysis patients: Silver Ring Prophylaxis at the Catheter Exit Study. Am J Kidney Dis 1998; 32: 752–60.

56. Lye WC, Lee EJC, Tan CC. Prophylactic antibiotics in the insertion of Tenckhoff catheters. Scand J Urol Nephrol 1992; 26: 177–80.

57. Port FK, Held PJ, Nolph KD *et al.* Risk of peritonitis and technique failure by CAPD connection technique: a national study. Kidney Int 1992; 42: 967–74.

58. Maiorca R, Cataluppi A, Cancarini GC *et al.* Prospective controlled trial of a Y-connector and disinfectant to prevent peritonitis in continuous ambulatory peritoneal dialysis. Lancet 1983; 2: 642–4.

59. Boen ST. Peritoneal dialysis. MD thesis. Van Gorcum and Comp., Assen, 1959.

60. Boen ST. Kinetics of peritoneal dialysis. Medicine 1961; 4: 243–87.

61. Dobbie JW. Pathogenesis of peritoneal fibrosis syndromes (sclerosing peritonitis) in peritoneal dialysis. Perit Dial Int 1992; 12: 14–27.

62. Yamada K, Miyakassa Y, Hamaguchi K *et al.* Immunohistochemical study of human advanced glycosylation end-products (AGE) in chronic renal failure. Clin Nephrol 1994; 42: 354–61.

63. Hendriks SMEM, Ho-dac-Pannekeet MM, van Gulik TM *et al.* Peritoneal sclerosis in peritoneal dialysis patients: analysis of clinical presentation, risk factors and peritoneal transport kinetics. Perit Dial Int 1997; 17: 136–43.

64. Faller B, Aparicio M, Faict D *et al.* Clinical evaluation of an optimized 1.1% amino-acid solution for peritoneal dialysis. Nephrol Dial Transplant 1995; 10: 1432–7.

65. Kopple JD, Bernard D, Massana J *et al.* Treatment of malnourished CAPD patients with an amino acid based dialysate. Kidney Int 1995; 47: 1148–57.

66. Matthys E, Dolkart R, Lameire N. Extended use of a glycerol-containing dialysate in diabetic CAPD patients. Perit Dial Bull 1987; 7: 10–15.

67. Matthys E, Dolkart R, Lameire N. Potential hazards of glycerol dialysate in diabetic CAPD patients. Perit Dial Bull 1987; 7: 16–19.

68. Mistry CD, Gokal R. Single daily overnight (12-h dwell) use of 7.5% glucose polymer (mw 18700; mn 7300) + 0.35% glucose solution: a 3-month study. Nephrol Dial Transplant 1993; 8: 443–7.

69. Ho-dac-Pannekeet MM, Schouten N, Langedijk MJ *et al.* Peritoneal transport characteristics with glucose polymer based dialysate. Kidney Int 1996; 50: 979–86.

70. Wilkie ME, Plant MJ, Edwards L *et al.* Icodextrin 7.5% dialysate solution (glucose polymer) in patients with ultrafiltration failure: extension of CAPD technique survival. Perit Dial Int 1997; 17: 84–7.

71. Davies DS. Kinetics of icodextrin. Perit Dial Int 1994; 14: (suppl. 2): S45–50.

72. Boeschoten EW, Krediet RT. Biocompatiblity of PD fluids. Nephrol Dial Transplant 1996; 11: 1907–11.

73. Lewis S, Holmes C. Host defense mechanisms in the peritoneal cavity of continuous ambulatory peritoneal dialysis patients. First of two parts. Perit Dial Int 1991; 11: 14–21.

74. Holmes C, Lewis S. Host defense mechanisms in the peritoneal cavity of continuous ambulatory peritoneal dialysis patients. Second of two parts. 2: Humoral defenses. Perit Dial Int 1991; 11: 112–17.

75. Vas SI. Peritonitis. In: Nolph KD, ed. Peritoneal Dialysis. Dordrecht: Kluwer, 1989, pp. 261–88.

76. Tranaeus A, Heimbürger O, Lindholm B. Peritonitis during continuous ambulatory peritoneal dialysis (CAPD): risk factors, clinical severity, and pathogenetic aspects. Perit Dial Int 1988; 8: 253–63.

77. Prowant B, Nolph K, Ryan L *et al.* Peritonitis in continuous ambulatory peritoneal dialysis. Analysis of an 8-years experience. Nephron 1986; 43: 105–9.

78. Bernardini J, Holley JL, Johnston JR *et al.* Analysis of ten-year trends in infections in adults on continuous ambulatory peritoneal dialysis (CAPD). Clin Nephrol 1991; 36: 29–34.

79. Churchill DN, Taylor DW, Vas SI *et al.* Canadian CAPD Clinical Trials Group. Peritonitis in continuous ambulatory peritoneal dialysis (CAPD): a multi-centre randomized clinical trial comparing the Y-connector disinfectant system to standard systems. Perit Dial Int 1989; 9: 159–63.

80. Port FK, Held PJ, Nolph KD *et al.* Risk of peritonitis and technique failure by CAPD connection technique: a national study. Kidney Int 1992; 42: 967–74.

81. Bommardeaux A, Quimet D, Galarnean A *et al.* Peritonitis in continuous ambulatory peritoneal dialysis. Impact of a compulsory switch from a standard to a Y-connector system in a single North American center. Am J Kidney Dis 1992; 19: 364–70.

82. Sweinburg FB, Seligman AM, Fine J. Transmural migration of intestinal bacteria. N Engl J Med 1950; 242: 747–51.

83. Wu G, Khanna R, Vas S *et al.* Is extensive diverticulosis of the colon a contra-indication to CAPD? Perit Dial Bull 1983; 3: 180–3.

84. Tranaeus A, Heimbürger O, Granqvist S. Diverticular disease of the colon: a risk factor for peritonitis in continuous ambulatory peritoneal dialysis. Nephrol Dial Transplant 1990; 5: 141–7.

85. Pepersack F, d'Haene M, Toussaint C *et al. Campylobacter jejuni* peritonitis complicating continuous ambulatory peritonitis. J Clin Microbiol 1988; 16: 739–41.

86. Singh MM, Bhargava AN, Jain KP. Tuberculous peritonitis. An evaluation of pathogenic mechanisms, diagnostic procedures and therapeutic measures. N Engl J Med 1969; 281: 1091–4.

87. Williams P, Khanna R, Oreopoulos DG. Treatment of peritonitis in patients on CAPD: no longer a controversy. Dial Transplant 1981; 10: 272.

88. Millikin SP, Matzke GR, Keane WF. Antimicrobial treatment of peritonitis associated with continuous ambulatory peritoneal dialysis. Perit Dial Int 1991; 11: 252–60.

89. The ad hoc advisory committee on peritonitis management. Peritoneal dialysis-related peritonitis treatment recommendations 1993 update. Perit Dial Int 1993; 13: 14–28.

90. Frieden TR, Munsiff SS, Low DE *et al.* Emergence of vancomycin-resistant enterococci in New York City. Lancet 1993; 342: 76–9.

91. Bonten MJM, Hayden MK, Nathan C *et al.* Epidemiology of colonisation of patients and environment with vancomycin-resistant enterococci. Lancet 1996; 348: 1615–19.

92. Troidle L, Kliger HS, Gorban-Brennan N *et al.* Nine episodes of CPD-associated peritonitis with vancomycin resistant enterococci. Kidney Int 1996; 50: 1368–72.

93. Noble WC, Virani Z, Cree RG. Co-transfer of vancomycin and other resistance genes from *Enterococcus faecalis* NCTC 12201 to *Staphylococcus aureus*. FEMS Microbiol Lett 1992; 72: 195–8.

94. Hiramatsu K, Hanaki H, Ino T *et al.* Methicillin-resistant *Staphylococcus aureus* clinical strain with reduced vancomycin susceptibility. J Antimicrob Chemother 1997; 40: 135–6.

95. Centers for Disease Control and Prevention: *Staphylococcus aureus* with reduced susceptibility to vancomycin. United States, 1997. MMWR 1997; 46: 813.

96. Vandamme P, Vercauteren E, Lammens C *et al.* Survey of enterococcal susceptibility patterns in Belgium. J Clin Microbiol 1996; 34: 2572–6.

97. Lameire N, Vogelaers D, Verschraegen G *et al.* Vancomycin resistant enterococci – a treat to the nephrologist on the horizon? Glycopeptide-resistant enterococci and the ICDC-recommendations for limited use of glycopeptides. Nephrol Dial Transplant 1996; 11: 2402–6.

98. Keane WE, Alexander SR, Bailie GR *et al.* Peritoneal dialysis-related peritonitis treatment recommendations: 1996 update. Perit Dial Int 1996: 16: 557–73.

99. Anding K, Krumme B, Pelz K *et al*. Pharmacokinetics and bactericidal activity of a single daily dose of netilmicin in the treatment of CAPD-associated peritonitis. Int J Clin Pharmacol Ther 1996; 34: 465–9.

100. van der Hulst RJ, Boeschoten EW, Nielsen FW *et al*. Ototoxicity monitoring with ultra-high frequency audiometry in peritoneal dialysis patients treated with vancomycin or gentamicin. Otorhinolaryngology 1991; 53: 19–23.

101. Vas SI. Microbiological aspects of chronic amubulatory peritoneal dialysis. Kidney Int 1983; 23: 83–92.

102. Bunke M, Brier ME, Golper TA. Culture-negative CAPD peritonitis: the Network 9 Study. Adv Perit Dial 1994; 10: 174–8.

103. Lye WC, Wong PL, Leong SO *et al*. Isolation of organisms in CAPD peritonitis: a comparison of two techniques. Adv Perit Dial 1994; 10: 166–8.

104. Nubé MJ, Vet JA, van Geelen JA. Bacterial and clinical sequelae of the twinbag system in continuous ambulatory peritoneal dialysis. A single centre study. Neth J Med 1994; 44: 191–8.

105. Gokal R, Ramos JM, Ward MK *et al*. 'Eosinophilic' peritonitis in continuous ambulatory peritoneal dialysis (CAPD). Clin Nephrol 1981; 15: 328–30.

106. Fenton P. Laboratory diagnosis of peritonitis in patients undergoing continuous ambulatory peritoneal dialysis. J Clin Pathol 1982; 35: 1181–4.

107. Report of a working party of the BSAC: Diagnosis and management of peritonitis in CAPD. Lancet 1987; 1: 845–8.

108. Von Graevenitz A, Amsterdam D. Microbiological aspects of peritonitis associated with CAPD. Clin Microbiol Rev 1992; 5: 26.

109. Gokal R, Jakubowski C, King J *et al*. Outcome in patients on continuous ambulatory peritoneal dialysis and hemodialysis: 4-years analysis of a prospective multicentre study. Lancet 1987; 2: 1105–9.

110. Fenton SSA. Peritonitis-related death among CAPD patients. Perit Dial Bull 1983; 3: 9–11.

111. Digenis GE, Abraham G, Savin E *et al*. Peritonitis-related deaths in continuous ambulatory peritoneal dialysis (CAPD) patients. Perit Dial Int 1990; 10: 45–7.

112. Tzamaloukas AH, Obermiller CE, Gibel LJ *et al*. Peritonitis associated with intra-abdominal pathology in continuous ambulatory peritoneal dialysis patients. Perit Dial Int 1993; 13 (suppl. 2): S335–7.

113. Wakeen MJ, Zimmerman SW, Bidwell D. Viscus perforation in peritoneal dialysis patients: diagnosis and outcome. Perit Dial Int 1994; 14: 371–7.

114. Bazzato G, Candini S, Coli U *et al*. A new technique of continuous ambulatory peritoneal dialysis (CAPD): double-bag system for freedom of patients and significant reduction of peritonitis. Clin Nephrol 1980; 13: 251–4.

115. Buoncristiani U, Cazzari M, Quintaliani G *et al*. Abatement of exogenous peritonitis risk using the Perugia CAPD system. Dial Transplant 1983; 12: 14.

116. Maiorca R, Cancarini GC, Brasa S *et al*. Y system with disinfectant in the prevention of peritonitis in CAPD. Contr Nephrol 1987; 57: 178–84.

117. Scalamogna A, De Vecchi A, Castelnovo C *et al*. Long-term incidence of peritonitis in CAPD patients treated by the Y set technique: experience in a single center. Nephron 1990; 55: 24.

118. Zimmerman SW, O'Brien M, Wiedenhoeft FA, Johnson CA. *Staphylococcus aureus* peritoneal catheter-related infections: a cause of catheter loss and peritonitis. Perit Dail Int 1988; 8: 191–5.

119. Davies SJ, Ogg CS, Cameron JS *et al*. *Staphylococcus aureus* nasal carriage, exit-site infections and catheter loss in patients treated with continuous ambulatory peritoneal dialysis (CAPD). Perit Dial Int 1989; 9: 61–4.

120. Pierratos A. Peritoneal dialysis glossary. Perit Dial Bull 1984; 1: 2–3.

121. Holley JL, Bernardini JB, Piraino B. Risk factors for tunnel infections in continuous ambulatory peritoneal dialysis. Am J Kidney Dis 1991; 18: 344–8.

122. Twardowsky ZJ. Peritoneal catheter exit-site infections: prevention, diagnosis, treatment and future directions. Semin Dial 1992; 5: 305–15.

123. Twardowski ZJ (ed.) Peritoneal Catheter Exit-Site Morphology and Pathology. Perit Dial Int 1996; 16: (suppl.) 3.

124. Holley JL, Foulks CJ, Moss AH *et al*. Ultrasound as a tool in the diagnosis and management of exit-site infections in continuous ambulatory peritoneal dialysis. Am J Kidney Dis 1989; 14: 211–16.

125. Plum J, Atrik S, Busch T *et al*. Oral versus intraperitoneal application of clindamycin in tunnel infections. A prospective, ramdomized study in CAPD patients. Perit Dial Int 1997; 17: 486–92.

126. Piraino B, Bernandini J, Sorkin M. A five-year study of the microbiologic results of exit-site infections and peritonitis in continuous ambulatory peritoneal dialysis. Am J Kidney Dis 1987; 10: 281–6.

127. Luzar MA, Brown C, Balf D *et al*. Exit-site care and exit-site infection in CAPD: results of a randomized multicenter trial. Perit Dial Int 1990; 10: 25–9.

128. Burkhart JM. Significance, epidemiology and prevention of peritoneal dialysis catheter infections. Perit Dial Int 1996; 16 (suppl. 1): S340–6.

129. Luzar MA. Exit-site infection in continuous ambulatory dialysis: a review. Perit Dial Int 1991; 11: 333–40.

130. Khanna R, Twardowski ZJ. Peritoneal catheter exit-site (editorial). Perit Dial Int 1988; 8: 119–23.

131. Copley JP. Prevention of peritoneal dialysis catheter-related complications. Am J Kidney Dis 1987; 10: 401–7.

132. Holley JL, Piriano BM. Complications of peritoneal dialysis: diagnosis and management. Semin Dial 1990; 3: 245–8.

133. Wanten GJA, Koolen MI, van Liebergen FJHM *et al*. Outcome and complications in patients treated with continuous ambulatory peritoneal dialysis (CAPD) at a single centre during 11 years. Neth J Med 1996; 49: 4–12.

134. Robinson RJ, Leapman SB, Wetherington GM *et al*. Survival considerations of continuous ambulatory peritoneal dialysis. Surgery 1984; 96: 723–9.

135. Twardowski ZJ, Khanna R. Peritoneal dialysis access and exit site care. In: Gokal R, Nolph KD, eds. Peritoneal Dialysis. Dordrecht: Kluwer, 1994, pp. 271–314.

136. Diaz-Buxo. Mechanical complications of chronic peritoneal dialysis catheters. Semin Dial 1991; 4: 106–11.

137. Bargman JM. Complications of peritoneal dialysis related to increased intra-abdominal pressure. Kidney Int 1993; 43: S75–80.

138. Litherland J, Cupton EW, Ackrill PA *et al*. Computed tomographic peritoneography: CT manifestations in the investigation of leaks and abnormal collections in patients on CAPD. Nephrol Dial Transplant 1994; 9: 1449–52.

139. Hemmeloff Andersen ICE, Dangaard-Morch P. Catheterography in the diagnosis of catheter failure in peritoneal dialysis. Clin Nephrol 1981; 16: 142–5.

140. Twardowski ZJ, Khanna R, Nolph KD *et al*. Intra-abdominal pressure during natural activities in patients treated with continuous ambulatory peritoneal dialysis. Nephron 1986; 44: 129–34.

141. Rocco MV, Stone WJ. Abdominal hernias in chronic peritoneal dialysis patients: a review. Perit Dial Bull 1985; 5: 171–4.

142. Boeschoten EW, Krediet RT, Roos CM *et al*. Leakage of dialysate across the diaphragm: an important complication of continuous ambulatory peritoneal dialysis. Neth J Med 1986; 26: 242–6.

143. Heimbürger O, Waniewski J, Werynski A *et al*. Peritoneal transport in CAPD patients with permanent loss of ultrafiltration capacity. Kidney Int 1990; 38: 495–506.

144. Twardowski ZJ, Nolph KD, Khanna R *et al*. Peritoneal equilibrium test. Perit Dial Bull 1987; 7: 138–47.

145. Davies SJ, Brown B, Bryan J *et al.* Clinical evaluation of the peritoneal equilibration test: a population based study. Nephrol Dial Transplant 1993; 8: 64–70.

146. Krediet RT, Imholz ALT, Struijk DG *et al.* Ultrafiltration failure in continuous ambulatory peritoneal dialysis. Perit Dial Int 1992; 12 (suppl. 2): S59–66.

147. Krediet RT, Boeschoten EW, Zuijderhoudt FMJ *et al.* Peritoneal transport characteristics of water, low-molecular weight solutes and protein during long-term continuous ambulatory peritoneal dialysis. Perit Dial Bull 1986; 2: 61–5.

148. Virga G, Amici G, da Rin G *et al.* Comparison of fast peritoneal equilibration tests with 1.36% and 3.86% glucose solutions. Blood Purif 1994; 12: 113–20.

149. Ho-dac-Pannekeet MM, Atasever B, Struijk DG *et al.* Analysis of ultrafiltration failure in peritoneal dialysis patients by means of standard peritoneal permeability analysis. Perit Dial Int 1997; 17: 144–50.

150. Struijk DG, Krediet RT, Koomen GCM *et al.* Functional characteristics of the peritoneal membrane in long-term continuous ambulatory peritoneal dialysis. Nephron 1991; 59: 213–20.

151. Selgas R, Fernandez-Reyes M-J, Bosque E *et al.* Functional longevity of the human peritoneum: how long is continuous peritoneal dialysis possible? Results of a prospective median long-term study. Am J Kidney Dis 1994; 23: 64–73.

152. Davies SJ, Bryan J, Philips L *et al.* Longitudinal changes in peritoneal kinetics: the effect of peritoneal dialysis and peritonitis. Nephrol Dial Transplant 1996; 11: 448–506.

153. Monquil MCJ, Imholz ALT, Struijk DG *et al.* Does impaired transcellular water transport contribute to net ultrafiltration failure during CAPD? Perit Dial Int 1995; 15: 42–8.

154. Krediet RT, Zuyderhoudt FMJ, Boeschoten EW *et al.* Alterations in peritoneal transport and water during peritonitis in continuous ambulatory peritoneal dialysis patients. Eur J Clin Invest 1987; 17: 43–52.

155. Panasikk E, Pietrzak B, Klos M *et al.* Characteristics of peritoneum after peritonitis in CAPD patients. Adv Perit Dial 1988; 4: 42.

156. Verger C, Cilicout B. Peritoneal permeability and encapsulating peritonitis. Lancet 1985; 1: 986–7.

157. Krediet RT, Struijk DG, Boeschoten EW *et al.* The time course of peritoneal transport kinetics in continuous ambulatory peritoneal dialysis patients who develop sclerosing peritonitis. Am J Kidney Dis 1989; 13: 299–307.

158. Krediet RT. The peritoneal membrane in chronic peritoneal dialysis. Nephrology forum. Kidney Int 1999; 55: 341–56.

159. Dobbie JW. Pathogenesis of peritoneal fibrosing syndromes (sclerosing peritonitis) in peritoneal dialysis. Perit Dial Int 1992; 12: 14–27.

160. Marichal JF, Faller B, Brignon P. Progressive calcifying peritonitis: a new complication of CAPD? Nephron 1987; 45: 229–32.

161. Korzets A, Korzets Z, Peer G *et al.* Sclerosing peritonitis: possible early diagnosis by computerized tomography of the abdomen. Am J Nephrol 1988; 8: 143–6.

162. Hendriks PMEM, Ho-dac-Pannekeet MM, van Gulik TM *et al.* Peritoneal sclerosis in chronic peritoneal dialysis patients: analysis of clinical presentation, risk factors, and peritoneal transport kinetics. Perit Dial Int 1997; 17: 136–43.

163. Schmidt RW, Blumenkrantz M. Peritoneal sclerosis: a sword of Damocles for peritoneal dialysis? Arch Intern Med 1981; 141: 1265–7.

164. Mutoh S, Machida J, Ueda S *et al.* Sclerosing encapsulating peritonitis occurring after very-short-term intermittent peritoneal dialysis. Nephron 1992; 62: 119–20.

165. Palmer RA, Newell JE, Gray ES *et al.* Treatment of chronic renal failure by prolonged peritoneal dialysis. N Engl J Med 1966; 274: 248–54.

166. Lindholm B, Bergström J. Nutritional reguirements of peritoneal dialysis patients. In: Gokal R, Nolph KD, eds. Textbook of Peritoneal Dialysis. Dordrecht: Kluwer, 1994, pp. 443–72.

167. Young GA, Kopple JD, Lindholm B *et al.* Nutritional assessment of continuous ambulatory dialysis patients: an international study. Am J Kidney Dis 1991; 17: 462–71.

168. Harty JC, Boulton H, Curwell H *et al.* The normalized protein catabolic rate is a flawed marker of nutrition in CAPD patients. Kidney Int 1994; 43: 103–9.

169. Detsky AS, McLaughlin JR, Baker JP *et al.* What is subjective global assessment of nutritional status? J Parent Ent Nutr 1987; 11: 8–13.

170. Churchill DN, Taylor W, Keshaviah PR. Adequacy of dialysis and nutrition in continuous peritoneal dialysis. Association with clinical outcomes. J Am Soc Nephrol 1996; 7: 198–207.

171. NKF-DOQI clinical practice guidelines for peritoneal dialysis adequacy. Am J Kidney Dis 1997; 3 (suppl. 2): S67–133.

172. Blumenkrantz MJ, Kopple JD, Moran JK *et al.* Metabolic balance studies and dietary protein requirement in patients undergoing continuous ambulatory peritoneal dialysis. Kidney Int 1982; 21: 849–61.

173. Blake PG, Sombolos K, Abraham G *et al.* Lack of correlation between urea kinetic indices and clinical outcomes in CAPD patients. Kidney Int 1991; 39: 700–6.

174. Bergström J, Fürst P, Alvestrand A *et al.* Protein and energy intake, nitrogen balance and nitrogen losses in patients treated with continuous ambulatory peritoneal dialysis. Kidney Int 1993; 44: 1048–57.

175. Jacob V, Marchant PR, Wild G *et al.* Nutritional profile of continuous ambulatory peritoneal dialysis patients. Nephron 1995; 71: 16–22.

176. Jones M, Hagen T, Algrim Boyle C *et al.* Treatment of malnutrition with 1.1% amino acid peritoneal dialysis solution: results of a multicenter outpatient study. Am J Kidney Dis 1998; 32: 761–9.

177. Bayer H von, Gahl GM, Riedinger H *et al.* Adaptation of CAPD patients to the continuous peritoneal energy uptake. Kidney Int 1983; 23: 29–34.

178. Boeschoten EW, Zuyderhoudt FMJ, Krediet RT *et al.* Changes in weight and lipid concentrations during CAPD treatment. Perit Dial Int 1988; 8: 19–25.

179. Faller B, Lameire N. Evolution of clinical parameters and peritoneal function in a cohort of CAPD patients followed over 7 years. Nephrol Dial Transplant 1994; 9: 280–6.

180. Heaton A, Johnston DG, Burrin JM *et al.* Carbohydrate and lipid metabolism during continuous ambulatory peritoneal dialysis: the effect of a single dialysis cycle. Clin Sci 1983; 65: 539–45.

181. Amstrong VW, Creutzfeldt W, Ebert R *et al.* Effect of dialysis glucose load on plasma and glucoregulatory hormones in CAPD patients. Nephron 1985; 39: 141–5.

182. Wideroe TE, Smeby LC, Myking OL. Plasma concentrations and transperitoneal transport of native insulin and C-peptide in patients on continuous ambulatory peritoneal dialysis. Kidney Int 1984; 25: 82–7.

183. Lameire N, Matthys E, Boheydt R. Effects of long-term CAPD on carbohydrate and lipid metabolism. Clin Nephrol 1988; 30: S53–8.

184. Llopart R, Doňate T, Oliva JA *et al.* Triglyceride-rich lipoprotein abnormalities in CAPD-treated patients. Nephrol Dial Transplant 1995; 10: 537–40.

185. O'Neal D, Lee P, Murphy B *et al.* Low-density lipoprotein particle size distribution in end-stage renal disease treated with hemodialysis or peritoneal dialysis. Am J Kidney Dis 1996; 27: 84–91.

186. Austin MA, Breslow JL, Hennekens CH *et al.* Low density lipoprotein subclass pattern and the risk of myocardial infarction. JAMA 1988; 260: 1917–21.

187. Saku K, Sasaki J, Naito S *et al.* Lipoprotein and apolipoprotein losses during continuous ambulatory peritoneal dialysis. Nephron 1989; 51: 220–4.

188. Shoji T, Nishizawa Y, Nishitani H *et al.* Roles of hypoalbuminemia and lipoprotein lipase on hyperlipoproteinemia in

continuous ambulatory peritoneal dialysis. Metabolism 1991; 10: 1002–8.

189. Levey AS, Beto JA, Coronado BE *et al.* Controlling the epidemic of cardiovascular disease in chronic renal disease. What do we need now? What do we need to learn? Where do we go from here? Am J Kidney Dis 1998; 32: 853–906.

190. Blumenkrantz MJ, Gahl GM, Kopple JD *et al.* Protein losses during peritoneal dialysis. Kidney Int 1981; 19: 593–602.

191. Krediet RT, Imholz ACT, Zemel D *et al.* Clinical significance and detention of individual differences and changes in transperitoneal transport. Blood Purif 1994; 12: 211–32.

192. Boeschoten EW, Schrijver J, Krediet RT *et al.* Deficiencies of vitamins in CAPD patients. The effect of supplementation. Nephrol Dial Transplant 1988; 2: 187–93.

193. Brown-Cartwright D, Smith HJ, Feldman M. Gastric emptying of an indigestible solid in patients with end-stage renal disease on continuous ambulatory peritoneal dialysis. Gastroenterology 1988; 95: 49–51.

194. Bird NJ, Streather CP, O'Doharty MJ *et al.* Gastric emptying in patients with chronic renal failure on continuous ambulatory peritoneal dialysis. Nephrol Dial Transplant 1993; 9: 287–90.

195. Gallar P, Oliet A, Vigil A *et al.* Gastroparesis: an important cause of hospitalization in continuous ambulatory peritoneal dialysis patients and the role of erythromycin. Perit Dial Int 1993; 13: (suppl. 2): S183–86.

196. Korzets Z, Golan E, Ben-Dahan J *et al.* Decubitus small-bowel perforation in ongoing continuous ambulatory peritoneal dialysis. Nephrol Dial Transplant 1992; 7: 79–81.

197. Nelson W, Khanna R, Mathews R *et al.* Gallbladder stones, cholecystitis and cholecystectomy in patients on continuous ambulatory peritoneal dialysis. Perit Dial Bull 1984; 4: 245–8.

198. Bargman JM. The impact of intraperitoneal glucose and insulin on the liver. Perit Dial Int 1996; 16 (suppl. 1): S211–14.

199. Luciani L, Gentile M, Scarduelli B *et al.* Multiple hepatic abscesses complicating continuous ambulatory peritoneal dialysis. Br Med J 1982; 285: 543.

200. Goodman W, Gallagher N, Sherrard DJ. Peritoneal dialysis fluid as a source of hepatitis antigen. Nephron 1981; 29: 107–9.

201. Gupta A, Yuan ZY, Balaskas EV *et al.* CAPD and pancreatitis: no connection. Perit Dial Int 1992; 12: 309–16.

202. Pannekeet MM, Krediet RT, Boeschoten EW *et al.* Acute pancreatitis during CAPD in the Netherlands. Nephrol Dial Transplant 1993; 8: 1376–81.

203. Donnelly S, Levy M, Prichard S. Acute pancreatitis in continuous ambulatory peritoneal dialysis (CAPD). Perit Dial Int 1988; 8: 187–90.

204. Movilli E, Natale C, Cancarini GC *et al.* Improvement of iron utilization and anemia in uremic patients switched from hemodialysis to continuous ambulatory peritoneal dialysis. Perit Dial Bull 1986; 6: 147–9.

205. Salahudeen AK, Keavey PM, Hawkins T *et al.* Is anemia during CAPD really better than during hemodialysis? Lancet 1983; 2: 1046–9.

206. Kurtz SB, Wong VH, Anderson CF *et al.* Continuous ambulatory peritoneal dialysis. Three years' experience at the Mayo Clinic. Mayo Clin Proc 1983; 58: 633–9.

207. De Paepe MB, Schelstraete KGH, Ringoir SM *et al.* Influence of continuous ambulatory peritoneal dialysis on the anemia of end stage renal disease. Kidney Int 1983; 23: 744–8.

208. Saltissi D, Coles GA, Napier JAF *et al.* The hematological response to continuous ambulatory peritoneal dialysis. Clin Nephrol 1984; 22: 21–7.

209. Lameire N. Matthys E, de Paepe M, *et al.* Red-cell survival in patients on continuous ambulatory peritoneal dialysis. Perit Dial Bull 1986; 6: 65–8.

210. Lamperi S, Carozzi S, Icardi A. *In vitro* and *in vivo* studies of erythropoiesis during continuous ambulatory peritoneal dialysis. Perit Dial Bull 1983; 3: 94–6.

211. Nakagawa S. An introductory approach to recently invested metabolic and endocrinological problems in uremia. Nephrol Dial Transplant 1989; 4 (suppl.): 123–6.

212. Rottembourg J. Residual renal function and recovery of renal functions in patients treated by CAPD. Kidney Int 1993; 43 (suppl. 40): S106–10.

213. Eschbach JW, Egrie JC, Downing MR *et al.* Correction of the anaemia of end-stage renal disease with recombinant human erythropoietin. Results of a combined phase I and II clinical trial. N Engl J Med 1987; 316: 73–8.

214. Boelaert JR, Schurgers MC, Matthys EG *et al.* Comparative pharmacokinetics of recombinant erythropoietin administered by the intravenous, subcutaneous and intraperitoneal routes in continuous ambulatory peritoneal dialysis (CAPD) patients. Perit Dial Int 1989; 9: 95–8.

215. Piraino B, Johnston JR. The use of subcutaneous erythropoietin in CAPD. Clin Nephrol 1990; 33: 200–2.

216. Stevens JM, Auer J, Strong CA *et al.* Stepwise correction of anaemia by subcutaneous administration of human recombinant erythropoietin in patients with chronic renal failure maintained by continuous ambulatory peritoneal dialysis. Nephrol Dial Transplant 1991; 6: 487–94.

217. Hörl WH, Cavill I, Macdougall IC *et al.* How to diagnose and correct iron deficiency during r-hu EPO therapy – a consensus report. Nephrol Dial Transplant 1996; 11: 246–50.

218. Lameire N, Bernaert P, Lambert M-C *et al.* Cardiovascular risk factors and their management in patients on continuous ambulatory peritoneal dialysis. Kidney Int 1994; 46 (suppl. 48): S31–8.

219. Luke RG. Chronic renal failure – a vasculopathic state. N Engl J Med 1998; 339: 841–3.

220. Maiorca R, Cancarini GC, Lamerini C *et al.* Is CAPD competitive with hemodialysis for long-term treatment of uremic patients? Nephrol Dial Transplant 1989; 4: 244–53.

221. Leenen F, Smith D, Khanna R *et al.* Changes in left ventricular anatomy and function on CAPD. Perit Dial Bull 1983; 3 (suppl.): S26–8.

222. Eisenberg M, Prichard S, Barre P *et al.* Left ventricular hypertrophy in end-stage renal disease on peritoneal dialysis. Am J Cardiol 1987; 60: 418–19.

223. Huting J, Schutterle G. Cardiovascular factors influencing survival in end-stage renal disease treated by continuous ambulatory peritoneal dialysis. Am J Cardiol 1992; 69: 123–7.

224. Held PJ, Port FK, Webb RL. Excerpts from United States Renal Data System 1991; Annual Data Report. Am J Kidney Dis 1991; 18 (suppl. 2): 1–127.

225. Stablein DM, Hamburger RJ, Lindblad AS *et al.* The effect of CAPD on hypertension control: a report of the National CAPD Registry. Perit Dial Int 1988; 8: 141–4.

226. Davies SJ, Phillips L, Russell GI. Peritoneal solute transport predicts survival on CAPD independently of residual renal function. Nephrol Dial Transplant 1998; 13: 962–8.

227. Wang T, Heimbürger O, Waniewski J *et al.* Increased peritoneal permeability is associated with decreased fluid and small-solute removal and higher mortality in CAPD patients. Nephrol Dial Transplant 1998; 13: 1242–9.

228. Coles GA. Have we underestimated the importance of fluid balance for the survival of PD patients? Perit Dial Int 1997; 17: 321–7.

229. Bergström J, Lindholm B. Malnutrition, cardial disease and mortality: an integrated point of view. Am J Kidney Dis 1998; 32: 834–41.

230. Besselink RA, Schröder CH, van Oort AM. Influence of dialysate exchange on cardial left ventricular function in children treated with CAPD. Perit Dial Int 1991; 11: 141–3.

231. Brown P, Johnston K, Fenton S *et al.* Symptomatic exacerbation of peripheral vascular disease with chronic

ambulatory peritoneal dialysis. Clin Nephrol 1981; 16: 258–61.

232. Llach F, Bover J. Renal osteodystrophy. In: Brenner BM, ed. The Kidney. Philadelphia, PA: WB Saunders, 1996, pp. 2187–273.

233. Malluche HH, Faugere MC. Renal bone disease 1990: an unmet challenge for the nephrologist. Kidney Int 1990; 38: 193–211.

234. Pei Y, Hercz G, Greenwood C et al. Non-invasive prediction of aluminium bone disease in hemo and peritoneal dialysis patients. Kidney Int 1992; 41: 1374–82.

235. Sherrard DJ, Hercz G, Pei Y et al. The spectrum of bone disease in end-stage renal failure. An evolving disorder. Kidney Int 1993; 43: 436–42.

236. Martis L, Serkes K, Nolph KD. Calcium carbonate as a phosphate binder: is there a need to adjust peritoneal dialysate calcium concentrations for patients using calcium carbonate? Perit Dial Int 1989; 9: 325–8.

237. Digenis G, Khanna R, Pierratos A et al. Renal osteodystrophy in patients managed on CAPD for more than three years. Perit Dial Bull 1983; 3: 81–6.

238. Cunningham J, Beer J, Coldwell RD et al. Dialysate calcium reduction in CAPD patients treated with calcium carbonate and alfacalcidol. Nephrol Dial Transplant 1992; 7: 63–8.

239. Hutchison AJ, Gokal R. Towards tailored dialysis fluids in CAPD/the role of reduced calcium and magnesium in dialysis. Perit Dial Int 1992; 12: 199–203.

240. Weinreich T, Passlick-Deetjen, Ritz E. Low dialysate calcium in continuous ambulatory peritoneal dialysis. A randomized controlled multicenter trial. Am J Kidney Dis 1995; 25: 452–60.

241. Buijsen C, Struijk DG, Huijgen H et al. The PTH-ionized calcium (i Ca) relationship in CAPD patients (pt) during low calcium solution. Perit Dial Int 1994; 14: S33 (abstract).

242. Warren DJ, Otieno LS. Carpal tunnel syndrome in patients on intermittent hemodialysis. Postgrad Med J 1975; 51: 450–2.

243. Gagnon RF, Somerville P, Kaye M. β_2-Microglobulin levels in patients on long-term dialysis. Perit Dial Bull 1987; 7: 29–31.

244. Blumberg A, Bürgi W. Behavior of β_2-microglobulin in patients with chronic renal failure undergoing haemodialysis, haemofiltration and continuous peritoneal dialysis (CAPD). Clin Nephrol 1987; 27: 245–9.

245. Tieleman C. Dratwa M, Bergmann P et al. Continuous ambulatory peritoneal dialysis vs hemodialysis: a lesser risk of amyloidosis. Nephrol Dial Transplant 1988; 3: 291–4.

246. Cornelis F, Bardin T, Faller B et al. Rheumatic syndromes and β_2-M amyloidosis in patients receiving long-term peritoneal dialysis. Arthritis Rheum 1989; 32: 785–8.

247. Benz RL, Siegfried JW, Teehan BP. Carpal tunnel syndrome in dialysis patients; comparison between continuous ambulatory peritoneal dialysis and hemodialysis population. Am Quart J Med 1988; 11: 473–6.

248. Deppner TA. Prescribing Hemodialysis: a guide to urea modelling. Dordrecht: Kluwer, 1991, pp. 25–38.

249. Lowrie EG, Laird NM, Parker TF, Sargent JA. Effect of the hemodialysis prescription on patient morbidity. N Engl J Med 1981; 305: 1176–81.

250. Deppner TA. Quantifying hemodialysis and peritoneal dialysis: examination of the peak concentration hypothesis. Semin Dial 1994; 7: 315–17.

251. Lindsay RM, Spanner E. A hypothesis: the protein catabolic rate is dependent upon the type and amount of treatment in dialyzed uremic patients. Am J Kidney Dis 1989; 13: 382–9.

252. Harty JC, Farragher B, Boulton H et al. Is the correlation between the normalized catabolic rate and Kt/V the result of mathematical coupling? J Am Soc Nephrol 1993; 4: 407.

253. Randerson DH, Chapman GV, Farrell PC. Animo acid and dietary status in long-term CAPD patients. In: Atkins RC, Farrel PC, Thomson N, eds. Peritoneal Dialysis. Edinburgh: Churchill Livingstone, 1981, pp. 179–91.

254. Teehan BP, Schleifer CR, Sigler MH et al. A quantitative approach to the CAPD prescription. Perit Dial Bull 1985; 5: 152–6.

255. NKF-DOQI Committee. Appendix E: a detailed rationale for guideline 9. Am J Kidney Dis 1997; 30 (suppl. 2): S122–5.

256. Blumenkrantz MJ, Kopple JD, Moran JK et al. Nitrogen and urea metabolism during continuous ambulatory peritoneal dialysis. Kidney Int 1981; 20: 78–82.

257. Nolph KD, Moore HL, Prowant B et al. Cross sectional assessment of weekly urea and creatinine clearances and indices of nutrition in continuous ambulatory peritoneal dialysis patients. Perit Dial Int 1993; 13: 178–83.

258. Maiorca R, Brunori G, Zubani R et al. Predictive value of dialysis adequacy and nutritional indices for mortality and morbidity in CAPD and HD patients. A longitudinal study. Nephrol Dial Transplant 1995; 10: 2295–305.

259. Churchill DN, Taylor W, Keshaviah PR. Adequacy of dialysis and nutrition in continuous peritoneal dialysis: association with clinical outcomes. J Am Soc Nephrol 1996; 7: 198–207.

260. NKF-DOQI Committee. Clinical outcomes goals for adequate peritoneal dialysis. Am J Kidney Dis 1997; 30 (suppl. 2): S95–100.

261. Blake PG, Sombolos K, Abraham G et al. Lack of correlation between urea kinetic indices and clinical outcomes in CAPD-patients. Kidney Int 1991; 39: 700–6.

262. Teehan BP, Schleifer CR, Brown J. Urea kinetic modeling in an appropriate assessment of adequacy. Semin Dial 1992; 5: 189.

263. Brandes JC, Piering WF, Beres JA et al. Clinical outcome of continuous ambulatory peritoneal dialysis predicted by urea and creatinine kinetics. J Am Soc Nephrol 1992; 2: 140–3.

264. NKF-DOQI Committee. Adequate dose of peritoneal dialysis. Am J Kidney Dis 1997; 30 (suppl. 2): S86–92.

265. Churchill DN, Thorpe KE, Nolph KD et al. CAPD patient and technique survivals are worse with increased membrane permeability. Perit Dial Int 1996; 16 (suppl. 2): S21.

266. Tattersall JE, Doyle S, Greenwood RN et al. Maintaining adequacy in CAPD by individualizing the dialysis prescription. Nephrol Dial Transplant 1994; 9: 749–52.

267. Manis T, Friedman EA. Dialytic therapy for irreversible uremia. N Engl J Med 1979; 301: 1321–8.

268. Mignon F, Michel C, Viron B et al. Why so much disparity of PD in Europe? Nephrol Dial Transplant 1998; 13: 1114–17.

269. Jacobs C, Broyer M, Brunner FP et al. Combined report on regular dialysis and transplantation in Europe. Proc EDTA 1981; 18: 2–58.

270. Kramer P, Brayer M, Brunner FP et al. Combined report on regular dialysis and transplantation in Europe. Proc EDTA 1982; 19: 4–59.

271. Ramos JM, Gokal R, Siamopolous K et al. Continuous ambulatory peritoneal dialysis: three years' experience. Quart J Med 1983; 206: 165–86.

272. Clarytan C, Spinowitz BS, Galler M. A comparative study of continuous ambulatory peritoneal dialysis and center hemodialysis. Efficacy, complications and outcome in the treatment of end-stage renal disease. Arch Intern Med 1986; 146: 1138–43.

273. Burton PR, Walls J. Selection-adjusted comparison of life-expectancy of patients on continuous ambulatory peritoneal dialysis, hemodialysis and renal transplantation. Lancet 1987; 1: 1115–18.

274. Maiorca R, Vonesh E, Cancarini GC et al. A six-year comparison of patient and technique survivals in CAPD and HD. Kidney Int 1988; 34: 518–24.

275. Serkes KD, Blagg CR, Nolph KD et al. Comparison of patient and technique survival in continuous ambulatory peritoneal dialysis (CAPD) and hemodialysis: a multicenter study. Perit Dial Int 1990; 10: 15–19.

276. Wolfe RA, Port FK, Hawthrone VM et al. A comparison of survival among dialytic therapies of choice: in-center

hemodialysis versus continuous ambulatory peritoneal dialysis at home. Am J Kidney Dis 1990; 15: 433–40.

277. Gentil MA, Carriazo A, Paron MI et al. Comparison of survival in continuous ambulatory peritoneal dialysis and hospital hemodialysis: a multicentric study. Nephrol Dial Transplant 1991; 6: 444–51.

278. Held PJ, Port FK, Turenne MN et al. Continuous ambulatory peritoneal dialysis and hemodialysis: comparison of patient mortality with adjustment for comorbid conditions. Kidney Int 1994; 45: 1163–9.

279. Bloembergen WE, Port FK, Mauger EA et al. A comparison of mortality between patients treated with hemodialysis and peritoneal dialysis. J Am Soc Nephrol 1995; 6: 177–83.

280. Fenton SSA, Schaubel DE, Desmeules M et al. Hemodialysis versus peritoneal dialysis: a comparison of adjusted mortality rates. Am J Kidney Dis 1997; 30: 334–42.

281. Maiorca R, Vonesh EF, Cavalli PL et al. A multicenter selection-adjusted comparison of patient and technique survivals on CAPD and hemodialysis. Perit Dial Int 1991; 11: 118–27.

282. Wilson PG. Psychiatric aspects of the dialysis patient. In: Jacobs C, Kjellstrand CM, Koch KM, Winchester JF, eds. Replacement of Renal Function by Dialysis. Dordrecht: Kluwer, 1996, pp. 1455–65.

283. Reiss D. Patient, family, and staff responses to end-stage renal disease. Am J Kidney Dis 1990; 15: 194–200.

284. O'Brien ME. Compliance behaviour and long-term maintenance dialysis. Am J Kidney Dis 1990; 15: 209–14.

285. Sharpe M, Mayou R, Seagroatt V et al. Why do doctors find some patients difficult to help? Q J Med 1994; 87: 187–93.

286. Morduchowicz G, Sylkes J, Aizic S et al. Compliance in hemodialysis patients: a multivariate regression analysis. Nephron 1993; 64: 365–8.

287. Kobrin SM, Kimmel PL, Simmens SJ et al. Behavioral and biochemical indices of compliance in hemodialysis patients. ASAIO Trans 1991; 37: M378–80.

288. Blake PG. Do mortality rates differ between hemodialysis and CAPD? A look at the Canadian vs U.S. data. Dial Transplant 1996; 25: 75.

289. Ahlmén J. Quality of life in the dialysis patient. In: Jacobs C, Kjellstrand CM, Koch KM, Winchester JF, eds. Replacement of Renal Function by Dialysis. Dordrecht: Kluwer, 1996, pp. 1466–79.

290. Robine J-M. Measuring the burden of disease. Lancet 1998; 352: 757–8.

291. Weinstein MC, Stason WB. Foundations of cost effective analysis for health and medical practices. N Engl J Med 1977; 296: 716–21.

292. Simmons RG, Abress L. Quality of life issues for end-stage renal disease patients. Am J Kidney Dis 1990; 15: 201–8.

293. Evans RW, Manninen DL, Garrison LP et al. The quality of life of patients with end-stage renal failure. N Engl J Med 1985; 312: 553–9.

294. Morris P, Jones B. Transplantation versus dialysis: a study of quality of life. Transplant Proc 1988; 20: 23–6.

295. Petrie K. Psychological well-being and psychiatric disturbance in dialysis and renal transplant patients. Br J Med Psychol 1989; 62: 91–6.

296. Simmons RG, Anderson BA, Kamstra L. Comparison of quality of life of patients on continuous ambulatory peritoneal dialysis, hemodialysis, and after transplantation. Am J Kidney Dis 1984; 4: 253–5.

297. Churchill DN, Torrance GW, Taylor W et al. Measurement of quality of life in end-stage renal disease: the time trade-off approach. Clin Invest Med 1987; 10: 14–20.

298. Wolcott DL, Nistenson AR. Quality of life in chronic dialysis patients: a clinical comparison of continuous ambulatory peritoneal dialysis (CAPD) and hemodialysis. Am J Kidney Dis 1988; 11: 402–12.

299. Bremer BA, McCauley CR, Wrona RM et al. Quality of life in end-stage renal disease: a reexamination. Am J Kidney Dis 1989; 13: 200–9.

300. Tucker CM, Ziller RL, Smith WR et al. Quality of life of patients on in-centre hemodialysis versus continuous ambulatory peritoneal dialysis. Perit Dial Int 1991; 11: 341–6.

301. Gokal R. Quality of life in patients undergoing renal replacement therapy. Kidney Int 1993; 40 (suppl.): S23–7.

302. Griffin KW, Wadhwa NK, Friend R et al. Comparison of quality of life in hemodialysis and peritoneal dialysis. Adv Perit Dial 1994; 10: 104–8.

303. Canadian Erythropoietin Study Group. Association between recombinant human erythropoietin and quality of life and exercise capacity of patients receiving hemodialysis. Br Med J 1990; 300: 573–8.

304. Auer J, Simon G, Oliver DO et al. Improvements in quality of life of CAPD patients treated with subcutaneously administered erythropoietin for anemia. Perit Dial Int 1992; 12: 40–2.

305. Merkus MP, Jager KJ, Dekker FW et al. Quality of life in patients on chronic dialysis: self-assessment 3 months after the start of treatment. Am J Kidney Dis 1997; 29: 584–92.

306. Garrat AM, Ruta DA, Abdalla MI et al. The SF-36 health survey questionnaire: an outcome measure suitable for routine use within the NHS? Br Med J 1993; 306: 1437–40.

307. de Wit A, Ramsteijn PG, de Charro FTh. Economic evaluation of end-stage renal disease treatment. Health Policy 1998; 44: 215–32.

308. Campbell J, Ewigman B, Hosokawa M et al. The timing of referral of patients with end stage renal disease. Dial Transplant 1989; 18: 660.

309. Stephenson K, Villano R. Results of a predialysis education program. Dial Transplant 1993; 22: 566.

310. Hood SA, Sandheimer JH. Impact of pre-ESRD management on dialysis outcomes: a review. Semin Dial 1998; 11: 175–80.

311. Kilner JF. Ethical issues in the initiation and termination of treatment. Am J Kidney Dis 1990; 15: 218–27.

312. Port FK. Mortality and causes of death in patients with end-stage renal failure. Am J Kidney Dis 1990; 15: 215–17.

313. Finkelstein FO, Sorkin M, Cramton CW et al. Initiatives on peritoneal dialysis: where do we go from here? Perit Dial Int 1991; 11: 274–8.

314. Posthuma N, Borgstein PJ, Eijsbouts Q et al. Simultaneous peritoneal dialysis catheter insertion and removal in catheter-related infections without interruption of peritoneal dialysis. Nephrol Dial Transplant 1998; 13: 700–3.

315. O'Donoghe D, Manos J, Pearson R et al. Continuous ambulatory peritoneal dialysis and renal transplantation: a ten-year experience in a single center. Perit Dial Int 1992; 12: 242–9.

316. Bakir N, Surachno S, Sluiter WJ et al. Peritonitis in peritoneal dialysis patients after renal transplantation. Nephrol Dial Transplant 1998; 13: 3178–83.

317. Kurtz SB, Wong VH, Andersson CF et al. Continuous ambulatory peritoneal dialysis. Three years' experience at the Mayo Clinic. Mayo Clin Proc 1983; 58: 633–9.

318. Nolph KD, Cutler SJ, Steinberg SM et al. Continuous ambulatory peritoneal dialysis in the United States: a three year study. Kidney Int 1985; 28: 198–205.

319. Gokal R, Baillod R, Boyle S et al. Multi-centre study on outcome of treatment in patients on continuous ambulatory peritoneal dialysis and hemodialysis. Nephrol Dial Transplant 1987; 2: 172–8.

320. NKF-DOQI Committee. Initiation of dialysis. Am J Kidney Dis 1997; 30 (suppl. 2): S70–3.

321. Churchill DN. Adequacy of peritoneal dialysis: research needs. Semin Dial 1998; 11: 205–6.

322. Bonomini V. Early dialysis. Nephron 1979; 24: 157–60.

323. Ratcliffe PJ, Phillips RE, Oliver DO. Late referral for maintenance dialysis. Br Med J 1984; 288: 441–3.

324. Jungers P, Zingraff J, Page B et al. Detrimental effects of late referral in patients with chronic renal failure: a case-control study. Kidney Int 1993 (suppl. 41): S170–3.

325. Hakim RM, Lazarus JM. Initiation of dialysis. J Am Soc Nephrol 1995; 6: 1319–28.

326. Sesso R, Belasco AG. Late diagnosis of chronic renal failure and mortality on maintenance dialysis. Nephrol Dial Transplant 1996; 11: 2417–20.

327. Infudu O, Dawood M, Homel P *et al*. Excess morbidity in patients starting uremia therapy without prior care by a nephrologist. Am J Kidney Dis 1996; 28: 841–5.

328. Methrotra R, Nolph KD. 'Healthy' initiation of chronic dialysis. Current research needs. Semin Dial 1998; 11: 213–15.

329. Struijk DG, Douma CE. Future research in peritoneal dialysis fluids. Semin Dial 1998; 11: 207–12.

330. Hoff CM, Shockley TR. Genetic modification of the peritoneal membrane: potential for improving peritoneal dialysis through gene therapy. Semin Dial 1998; 11: 218–27.

331. Golper TA. Research directions in peritonitis. Semin Dial 1998; 11: 216–17.

12 | Continuous ambulatory peritoneal dialysis in the elderly

E. GRAPSA AND D. G. OREOPOULOS

Introduction

Commonly an individual is designated as elderly at 65 years. During this century the number of people living beyond age 65 has increased. In 1900 only 4% of the Western world's population was over 65 years of age, but now this fraction is 12% and rising [1]. By the year 2040, 21% of the population in the United States will be over 65, and by the year 2050 one in 20 people in the USA will be older than 85 [2, 3]. This progressive increase in the elderly and the success of dialysis have produced a dramatic increase in the numbers of elderly dialysis patients worldwide. Thus, in the USA 47% of those on dialysis are over 65; this fraction is expected to increase to over 60% by the end of this century [4–6]. In Canada, in 1989, 35% of end-stage renal disease (ESRD) patients were over the age of 65 compared to 25% in 1981 [7]. In 1990, in a UK dialysis centre that provides the sole nephrological service for a population of 1.2 million people, those over 65 constituted more than 25% of all new patients accepted for dialysis [8]. The European Renal Association Registry has reported a similar trend. In 1977 only 9% of those patients starting renal replacement therapy were older than 65 years; in 1980, 11%; in 1983, 30%; whereas by 1992 this population had increased to nearly 37% [9, 10]. Thus, elderly patients, who previously were excluded from dialysis, now are the fastest-growing segment of the dialysis population [10, 11].

In most countries haemodialysis is the principal form of therapy in the elderly with ESRD [12, 13]. Chronic peritoneal dialysis, while used extensively in Canada, the UK and some other countries, has been systematically neglected in others such as the USA. Only 16% of the elderly with ESRD in the USA are on peritoneal dialysis [5]. As a mode of treatment in the elderly with ESRD [12–15], renal transplantation and home haemodialysis remain limited and controversial.

Criteria for selection

A dialysis modality for elderly patients can be selected only after a comprehensive evaluation. The choice will be influenced by what is available and by the biases – therapeutic and financial – of the individual nephrologist. When both dialytic modalities are equally available the decision between home versus centre dialysis is influenced by many factors, including patients' preference, as well as medical and social considerations [16, 17]. In addition, a number of physiological changes associated with ageing may influence the choice in these patients [18]. Common in this population [19] are such comorbid conditions as diminished cardiovascular reserve, clinical or subclinical, and atherosclerosis and impaired baroreceptor function, all of which may contribute to poor compensatory response to fluid removal with dialysis [20]. The incidence of dangerous arrhythmias is higher in dialysis patients more than 50 years of age [21]. Bleeding diathesis, which is common in the elderly, partly explains the increased transfusion rate in these patients. Thus elderly patients received a mean of 6.9 ± 0.2 units of blood per year compared with 3.4 ± 0.6 units per year for younger controls ($p < 0.02$) [22].

Vascular disease is also common in the elderly but the literature contains conflicting reports concerning the success and morbidity of the arteriovenous fistula [23, 24] in these patients. The incidence of comorbid chronic illness increases with advancing age. Thus 70% of individuals older than 65 have chronic illness and 30% of these have three or more comorbid conditions [25]. Of the systemic diseases that lead to ESRD in the elderly, hypertension and diabetes taken together account for 40–65% [26, 27]. Constipation and chronic diverticulosis, which may complicate the clinical course of older ESRD patients, may be accelerated by the constipating effects of aluminium-based phosphate binders [28, 29].

R. Gokal, R. Khanna, R.Th. Krediet and K.D. Nolph (eds.), Textbook of Peritoneal Dialysis, 2nd Edition, 419–433.

Underlying pulmonary disease, which compromises oxygenation, may also influence the choice of ESRD treatment.

The selection of dialysis may also be influenced by metabolic characteristics such as chronic bone loss from osteoporosis, altered protein metabolism, a high rate of malnutrition, a tendency to carbohydrate intolerance [11] and alterations in metabolism produced by a variety of drugs. Also, poor tissue turgor and impaired wound healing in the elderly may lead one to select haemodialysis. It must be emphasized that peritoneal dialysis is the only method that permits the home treatment that many elderly people desire. When patients have difficulty in learning dialysis techniques (because of dementia or depression), the help of members of their family, or paramedical staff, may be crucial. Similarly peritoneal dialysis is also suitable for elderly living in nursing homes [16, 30–35].

Advantages of peritoneal dialysis in the elderly

Continuous ambulatory peritoneal dialysis (CAPD) is now used worldwide as treatment for ESRD patients and has a particular place in the management of ESRD elderly patients. Various authors have recognized the medical and/or social advantages for the elderly on CAPD [16, 30–35]. Comorbid diseases such as hypertension, ischaemic heart disease and diabetes are more common in these patients [34]. CAPD achieves better control of hypertension with fewer antihypertensive medications [36, 37], better fluid balance with minimal haemodynamics stress and better blood glucose control through intraperitoneal insulin therapy [38]. The anaemia of chronic renal failure is often less severe in patients on CAPD due to lower blood losses, removal of inhibitors of erythropoiesis and reduced haemolysis [40, 41]. These considerations are important for the elderly with ischaemic heart failure [39–41].

ESRD patients may develop cardiac arrhythmias due to such factors as coronary atherosclerosis and advancing age. CAPD does not seem to provoke or aggravate arrhythmias even in elderly or cardiac patients [42, 43]. Furthermore this modality does not require vascular access [44].

Some additional medical advantages of CAPD for the elderly are better maintenance of residual renal function and a more efficient removal of β_2-microglobulin and middle molecules such as parathyroid hormone [43–48].

Table 1. Advantages of peritoneal dialysis in the elderly

1. Good control of hypertension
2. Requires few antihypertensive medications
3. Good fluid balance
4. Minimal haemodynamic stress
5. Efficacy of intraperitoneal insulin therapy in diabetics
6. Good control of anaemia; requires less erythropoietin
7. Good control of cardiac arrhythmias
8. No need for vascular access
9. Maintenance of residual renal function for longer periods than haemodialysis
10. Removal of β_2-microglobulin and other middle molecules such as parathyroid hormone
11. Home dialysis in a familial environment
12. Low hospitalization rates

Although most older people living in the community are cognitively intact and fully independent in their daily activities, a substantial number report major limitations in activity due to chronic disease. Peritoneal dialysis allows the elderly person to be dialysed at home. Those who live a long distance from a dialysis centre, or those who live in a nursing home, also will do better on peritoneal dialysis [31]. Performed by trained home nurses, CAPD provides the elderly patient with a convenient, comfortable and safe means of home dialysis in a familiar environment without reliance on family members. Thus because of all these advantages, and its low reported rate of hospitalizations and peritoneal dialysis-related complications, we consider CAPD/APD to be a successful alternative to centre dialysis. Table 1 summarizes the advnatages of peritoneal dialysis in the elderly.

Disadvantages of CAPD for the elderly

ESRD is a severe illness; its treatment requires a change in the lifestyles of both the patient and his/ her family, especially in the elderly. Inability to perform self-dialysis, due to dementia, mental impairment, blindness, hemiplegia and other physical handicaps, is an important relative contraindication of CAPD when family social support is inadequate [30, 49]. Some relative contraindications in the elderly are similar to those in young ESRD patients, such as hernia, peripheral vascular disease, extensive diverticulosis, polycystic kidney disease, low-back pain and obesity; any of these might force discontinuation of CAPD, once started. Any of these relative contraindications may be minimized by continuous cyclic peritoneal dialysis (CCPD) performed mainly at night [50, 51].

Reduced peritoneal surface area due to adhesions from previous extensive abdominal operations is an absolute contraindication of CAPD while chronic ostomies, recurrent pancreatitis and recent aortic prosthesis are major contraindications [52]. CAPD may exacerbate rather than improve the condition of malnourished patients [53, 54].

Due to poor salt and fluid intake and increased ultrafiltration, patients on CAPD who have chronic hypotension may develop vascular ischaemic syndromes, particularly of the lower extremities [55].

Nutrition and adequacy of dialysis in the elderly on CAPD

The impact of malnutrition increases significantly with age. Nutritional deficiencies are due to a combination of social, economic, psychological and biochemical factors that keep older people from acquiring and assimilating an adequate and balanced diet [56]. Because renal failure impairs the mechanisms that conserve lean body mass, malnutrition is also a common complication of uraemia. Potential reasons for this association are an inadequate diet due to anorexia and the excessive catabolism stimulated by uraemia [57]. Protein calorie malnutrition is frequent among the general population treated with haemodialysis or CAPD [58, 59]. Finally, during CAPD the loss of proteins and amino acids into dialysis fluid, which is accelerated during peritonitis, may increase the likelihood of malnutrition, especially in the presence of an inadequate protein intake [60].

After an international study Young *et al.* reported that the incidence of malnutrition was related to the patient's age, nutritional status at the start of CAPD, the length of time on CAPD and the residual renal function [61]. Ross and Rutsky found malnutrition in 20% of the elderly and 2% of young CAPD patients [18]. Cianciaruso *et al.* also reported that calorie malnutrition is common among regular dialysis patients and that it is more prevalent in the elderly (51% vs. 35% in the young); however they found no difference in incidence of malnutrition between the two dialysis modalities, viz. haemodialysis and CAPD [54]. Shimomura *et al.* reported that the key factor for the poor outcome of dialysis in elderly patients is low dietary protein intake; they found that a large proportion of elderly CAPD patients were assigned to the 'poor' group. Com-

pared with the 'fairly well-to-do' and 'intermediate' groups, the latter group did not show definitive differences in the urea kinetic parameters but they had the lowest values of blood urea nitrogen (BUN) and protein catabolic rate (PCR) (g/kg/day) [62]. These authors also suggest that protein and nutrient supplement can improve the abnormal biochemical and physical nutritional parameters of the elderly. After the administration of nutrients they found that the values of Kt/V urea increased simultaneously with increases in PCR; they also observe a significant possible correlation between Kt/V urea and NPCR in elderly patients [63]. Nolph *et al.*, who reported similar results, found that the relationship between normalized protein catabolic rate (NPCR) and weekly urea clearance, normalized to total body water, and serum albumin levels, are similar for older and younger CAPD patients. These authors concluded that poor protein intake in the elderly should not be attributed to advanced age if weekly urea clearances are low. Increases in protein intake in response to increases in urea clearances are similar in older and younger CAPD patients [64]. Mooraki *et al.* [65] reported similar weekly Kt/V, weekly creatinine clearance (WCC), PCR, serum albumin levels and weekly (EPO) requirements in elderly and in young CAPD patients.

Cancarini *et al.* found that PCR decreased significantly as the patient's age increased ($p = 0.007$) but this decrease was not correlated with time on CAPD, gender, or serum albumin. Serum albumin did not change as age increased. These authors concluded that long-term CAPD does not necessarily impair nutritional status, and suggested that the oldest patients can maintain adequate serum albumin concentration with lower protein intake than can younger ones [66]. Abdo *et al.*, [67], who studied adequacy of dialysis and nutritional status of continuous cyclic peritoneal dialysis (CCPD) and CAPD patients, also found a statistically significant inverse correlation between age and PCR. Kt/V was also lower as age advanced, although this did not reach statistical significance [67]. Russell *et al.* reported a high incidence of malnutrition among CAPD patients (59%), as evidenced by anthropometric data. Using subjective global assessment, 49% of peritoneal dialysis patients had scores that indicated some degree of malnutrition; of the malnourished patients 86% were mild to moderately malnourished, and 14% were severely malnourished (all of the latter were more than 70 years of age). These authors suggest that the first stage of dietetic intervention is determination of the degree of malnutrition; then one will establish dietary requirements accordingly [68].

Quality of life

Quality of life is the result of many influences on the individual's personal and social environment. More than 10% of elderly persons living in the community show significant symptoms of depression [69]. In most instances such syndromes are related to physical disability such as ESRD or other life stresses [18].

More than 29% of a consecutive sample of ESRD patients awaiting cadaveric transplantation showed depressive symptoms of at least moderate severity [70]. The quality of life of the older dialysis patients depends on the group to which they are compared. When they are compared with older people without ESRD, elderly dialysis patients report not only significantly greater functional impairment but also significantly more emotional distress, more negative psychological effects and lower life satisfaction levels [71]. When they were compared with younger people on dialysis (CAPD-haemodialysis), Stout et al. [72] found (on several scales of assessment) that those less than 60 years of age appeared less satisfied with life. In contrast, the elderly group, with and without risk factors, perceived life to be less stressful than did younger patients. These investigators concluded that the elderly had a good perceived quality of life even when risk factors had been added. Using the Karnofsky and Campbell Happiness Scale, Moody et al. found that patients on dialysis, more than 75 years of age, were less active and less outgoing; however, these older patients perceived their health to be quite good and they took life more positively than did younger dialysis patients. These very old subjects were neither particularly happy nor unhappy [73].

In another study, 30% of the haemodialysis patients (age 14–85 years old) were not satisfied with their life in general compared to 17% in the CAPD group (age 22–77 years) and 5% in the transplanted sample (age 17–72 years). On average, elderly patients reported more marked complaints, less general life satisfaction and higher satisfaction with partnership and family life [74]. McDonald et al. reported that the elderly tolerated self-care home dialysis well and were able to maintain their independence with a good quality of life [75]. However, Diax-Buxo et al. [76] found lower scores among elderly patients in all modalities compared to young

patients but those on CCPD and home haemodialysis had a higher score than those on centre haemodialysis.

As indicated by Karnofsky score, McKevitt et al. reported a high degree of disability among those over 60 years of age on dialysis. Only 32% of patients scored 70 or over and 33% of patients had mild to severe intellectual impairment on the Pfeiffer Short Portable Mental Status Questionnaire, while 62% demonstrated depressive symptoms on the Beck Depression Inventory [77].

The study of Carey et al. [78] shows the important role of family support among CAPD elderly patients. These authors found that among CAPD elderly patients with mild- and high-functioning families, only 9% and 5%, respectively, had been transferred to haemodialysis for psychosocial reasons at 1 year and 21% and 16% at 2 years. On the contrary, in low-functioning families, 67% of elderly CAPD patients had transferred to haemodialysis by 1 year [76]. Older patients who lost their spouses, and had no adequate family support, grieve for prolonged periods – an experience that predisposes them to a major depression. However, despite the presence of such patients, Ross and Rutsky reported low frequency of depression in elderly dialysis (CAPD) patients [18].

Recently De Vecchi reported that 29 of 39 elderly patients on CAPD (74%) and 30 of 53 younger patients (57%) considered their lifestyle 'acceptable' after 1 year of dialysis. Thirty-four of 39 elderly patients (87%) and 32 of 53 (60%) of the younger patients ($p < 0.02$) rated their physical and social state as better than or comparable to that which they had enjoyed before the onset of terminal uraemia [79].

Complications in elderly patients on CAPD

Catheter-related complications

Among CAPD patients many complications are related to the catheter, such as early or late pericatheter leak, exit-site infections, cuff extrusion or herniation at the peritoneal tunnel [80]. Holley et al. found no differences in age and rate of catheter complications among 411 CAPD patients, with and without tunnel infections [81]. Others have reported similar tunnel infection rates in young and elderly CAPD patients [18, 79]. Gentile et al. reported a lower incidence of complications among the elderly

(17.4%) than among younger patients (21%) [12]. Lupo *et al.* found that catheter failure was more frequent in younger patients < 40 years old (24%) mainly due to exit-site tunnel infections, while in patients older than 60 years this incidence did not exceed 16% [82]. In another study that compared 103 elderly CAPD patients with those 18–40 years old, Holley *et al.* [83] found a lower tunnel-infection rate in the elderly (0.15 vs. 0.25 episode per patient-year) compared to the younger group. Similarly, Nissenson *et al.* [84] found that only 9% of the elderly CAPD patients required catheter replacement compared to 20% of younger patients; 7% of the elderly had tunnel infection vs. 13% of the younger. Contrary to these findings, Tzamaloukas *et al.* [85] analysed 120 episodes of peritonitis and found that the variables associated with catheter removal were: advanced age, prolonged duration of peritonitis and coexisting exit-site and tunnel infection.

Hernias

Frequently CAPD patients develop one or more of several types of hernias such as umbilical, inguinal, at the site of a previous laparotomy, at catheter insertion, and in the epigastric area [12, 18, 82, 86]. Poor tissue turgor is a frequent accompaniment of ageing and conceivably could contribute to an increased incidence of hernia in elderly CAPD patients. Despite this, several authors have reported a similar frequency of hernia development between younger and elderly CAPD patients (7.8% vs. 9.9%) [12, 18, 82].

Constipation

Constipation is common in any age group but may be even more frequent in the elderly. Chronic constipation is associated with an increased risk of bowel perforation in patients with ESRD. Sometimes, bowel perforation is associated with the presence of multiple diverticuli. Lower gastrointestinal bleeding due to diverticulitis leads to faecal peritonitis and may necessitate partial colectomy and cessation of peritoneal dialysis. However, the rate of lower gastrointestinal bleeding seems to be similar in young and elderly CAPD patients [18].

Hyperlipidaemia

This is common among patients on CAPD [87–89]. Maiorca *et al.* reported that, in both women and men, blood cholesterol was significantly higher in elderly patients on CAPD compared to those on haemodialysis. However, they found no significant differences in triglyceride levels between the patients on these two modalities [90]. Panarello *et al.* [89] reached similar conclusions.

Peritonitis

The incidence of peritonitis in elderly patients on CAPD varies among centres from 0.42 to 2.8 episodes per patient-year, depending on the connection system used [33, 79, 82, 84, 91–97] and whether the patients themselves are able to do the exchanges [90]. In a recent survey of CAPD in Japan, Kawaguchi found a lower incidence of peritonitis in that country compared to other countries [98]. The average age at which chronic dialysis is begun is 61.5 ± 14 years and elderly patients there tend to shun CAPD. A multicentre analysis conducted by Imada *et al.* in Japan demonstrated a peritonitis rate of one episode per 53.4 patient-month (0.22 year). The data were derived from 1428 patients who were treated in 25 dialysis units; each unit managed over 40 CAPD cases between November 1994 and September 1996 [99]. Peritonitis is the main reason for hospitalization of patients on CAPD [12, 33, 82, 84, 86, 92, 93, 100–109].

Several authors [12, 40, 80, 83, 84, 90, 106] have reported no difference in the incidence of peritonitis between young and elderly patients. Among 3188 patients followed under the United States Renal Data System (USRDS) on various connection systems, Port *et al.* [97] found a significantly higher relative risk (RR) for peritonitis among younger and black patients. Similarly Nebel and Finke [104] reported better results in the elderly, but others [18, 79, 96, 97] have found worse results. The distribution of organisms responsible for peritonitis was similar between elderly and young patients [84]. With respect to the bacteria responsible for these infections in all CAPD patients in Japan, Imada *et al.* [99] found that the distribution was similar to those from series reported elsewhere in the world [91]; these included *Staphylococcus anureus* (25.5%), *Staphylococcus* sp. (17.8%) and *Staphylococcus epidermidis* (12.5%). In 10 CAPD patients aged 68 years or older, Joglar and Saade [108] found a high incidence of fungal peritonitis (33.3%). As a cause of drop-out among 231 young and elderly CAPD patients, Piccoli *et al.* [109] found the contribution of peritonitis was similar (21% vs. 20%). As a cause of death, peritonitis was more common among patients older than 65 years (2.3%) and among those older than 75 (3.2%), than among those younger than 65 years (1.4%).

Morbidity of elderly patients on CAPD

An important element in the morbidity of dialysis patients is hospitalization; such confinement impairs the patient's quality of life and increases the costs of dialysis therapy. Cardiovascular disease, infections – pneumonia and peritonitis, diabetic complications, fluid overload and gastrointestinal disease – are some of the causes for hospitalization [90, 110, 111]. The elderly, who have a variety of comorbid conditions, may require additional hospitalization. Many investigators have reported a greater number of hospitalization days per year for the elderly patients (~22 vs. 17 day/patient-year) [79, 80, 112–114]. Among the elderly who cannot do their own dialysis exchanges the differences become greater (44 days/patient-year). However, Wadhwa *et al.* [115] found lower hospitalization rates and shorter durations of stay (one admission/6 patient-months) among elderly disabled CAPD patients with home nurses, than among those without such assistance (one admission/4 patient-months).

Anderson [91] reported a hospitalization rate of 22.4 days/patient-year among CAPD patients (age 31–88 ($x \pm SD = 62.7 \pm 12.8$)) living in a nursing home. Gangrenous stump infections and peritonitis accounted for 14% and 10% of admissions respectively. These complications, along with delirium, hyperglycaemia, acute cardiovascular accident events, volume depletion, volume overload and pneumonia, accounted for 62% of admissions.

After a multicentre study Malberti *et al.* [114] reported that the average number of hospital admissions in 1983 was 236 for a total of 31 433 hospital days (9.21 days/patient-year); this number increased to 4295 in 1992 for a total of 49 793 hospital days (9.92 days/patient-year). For each patient the mean hospitalization days/year is directly proportional to age at entry, namely 4.6 days/year in those aged 15–24 years, 10.2 in those aged 25–44, 19.8 in those aged 45–65, 31.7 in those aged 65–74 and 34.3 in those over 75 years old. There was no significant difference in the hospitalization rate between males and females. The hospitalization rate of elderly patients on peritoneal dialysis did not differ from that of patients on haemodialysis [114]. According to the USRD's 1998 annual data, the mean numbers of admissions in the older and younger age group

are 1.4 and 1.5 respectively. Members of both age groups spent 30 or more days in hospital. In both dialysis modalities, admission rates increased with age [113].

Generally, hospitalization rates among CAPD/CCPD patients are slightly higher than for haemodialysis patients in each age group until the age of 65; after this age, CAPD/CCPD patients have a lower hospitalization rate. This finding is consistent with trends reported in 1996 and 1997 USRDS reports. In 1996 it was reported that hospitalization rates for CAPD/CCPD patients had been falling steadily while those for haemodialysis patients were relatively stable [113].

Mortality of elderly patients on CAPD

The risk of death in ESRD patients increases with age and with coexisting diseases [115–119]. Several studies have reported that age, the presence of diabetes and cardiovascular disease are associated with a shorter survival rate [10, 16, 79, 82, 91, 120–123]. Early (within 90 days) mortality among elderly patients on dialysis increased significantly from 15% for those aged 65–75, to 20% for those aged 79–84, and 30% for those more than 84 years old [124]. Most of these deaths were related to comorbid conditions.

The 5-year survival was 15% lower for patients older than 65 years old than it was for younger ones in Europe (European Dialysis Transplantation Association Registry, 1995) [10].

Mignon *et al.* [16] found 2- and 4-year survival rates of 47% and 25% respectively in the elderly. These authors excluded from this analysis those who died before the 90th day of treatment. Salomone *et al.* [125] report an increase in 2-year survival for the elderly between the years 1981–85 and 1986–92 (54.6% vs. 59%, $p < 0.05$). In a review of their experiences over a 10-year period, Lupo *et al.* [82] found that the elderly over 70 years old on CAPD has a 12-month survival rate of 80%, 24-month survival rate of 60% and 48-month survival rate of 40%. Age was an independent relative risk of death, independent of cardiovascular disease, diabetes and neoplasm.

Malberti *et al.* [114] reported that elderly patients undergoing dialysis (haemodialysis and CAPD) during the period 1983–92 had a 64% 2-year survival rate, 39% at 4 years and 13% at 8 years.

In elderly patients the absence of systemic diseases leads to a better Kaplan–Meier cumulative 2-year survival: 75.8% vs. 62.5% among those with systemic disease [114]. At the start of Renal Replacement Therapy the presence of one or more comorbid risk factors is associated with a lower cumulative survival rate [122]. Survival decreases as age increases. Thus the 5-year survival of patients over the age of 65 is 20%, compared to 85% for those aged 15–44 years [122]. Survival of diabetic patients is also influenced by age; those over 65 years have a 5-year survival rate of only 10%, compared with 58% for those with diabetes aged 15–44 years. Compared to those on haemodialysis, the comorbidity experience shows that patients on CAPD/CCPD had a 12% lower hazard ratio (0.80) or a 12% increase in survival compared to those on haemodialysis (hazard ratio 1.0) while those in the intermittent peritoneal dialysis group had a 97% increase in hazard ratio (1.97) [122].

Churchill *et al.* report a higher 18-month survival for those ⩾65 years of age in Canada (82%) compared to those in the USA (61.1%) [126]. According to DeVecchi [79], patient survival was significantly worse in the elderly on CAPD compared to young patients – 12-month 80% vs. 90%, 24-month 70% vs. 80%, 36-month 46% vs. 75%, 60-month 20% vs. 60%.

The USRDS 1998 annual data reported an overall improvement in survival of dialysis patients. Thus between 1985 and 1995 [127], first-year death rates for the 65–74-year age group decreased from 40.4 to 30.3 per 100 patient-years of risk.

Death rates for dialysis patients 65 years and over are almost twice as high as for those 44–64 years old [127]. Non-diabetic haemodialysis and peritoneal dialysis patients have similar death rates for all cardiac causes. Cardiac arrest accounts for the deaths of 20% of non-diabetic patients on haemodialysis vs. 19% of those non-diabetic peritoneal dialysis patients. A larger proportion of diabetic haemodialysis patients (24%) die of cardiac arrest than diabetic peritoneal dialysis patients (20%). A higher percentage of peritoneal dialysis patients, both non-diabetics and diabetics, die of infections (20%) than do haemodialysis patients (16%). A larger proportion of non-diabetic patients on haemodialysis (7%) die of malignancy than do those on peritoneal dialysis (4%) [127].

Cardiac causes – cardiac arrest, acute myocardial infarction and other cardiac diseases – account for almost one-half of the reported deaths of dialysis patients in all age groups.

Infection accounts for almost one-quarter of all deaths in the 20–44 age group, but only 17% and 14% of deaths in the 45–64 age group and >65-year-old age groups, respectively. Of the infection category, more than 75% have septicaemia, about 6% have cerebrovascular disease in each age group of all patients while 1% to 4% of deaths in dialysis patients is attributed to malignancy [128].

One out of every five dialysis patients withdraws from dialysis before death; the overall withdrawal rate was 39 per 1000 dialysis patients/year. Patients aged 65 years and older have a much higher rate of withdrawal than do younger patients. Almost one-quarter of all dialysis patients aged 65 years and older withdrew from dialysis before death [128].

Comparison of haemodialysis and peritoneal dialysis in elderly patients

Haemodialysis and peritoneal dialysis have been regarded as equivalent replacement therapies for elderly ESRD patients. The outcomes of these two modalities have been compared using mortality rates, hospitalization days, technique survival, complications, biochemical status, clinical status and life satisfaction [86, 90, 92, 129, 130]. While most of these studies showed no difference in mortality between CAPD and HD [8, 103, 109, 121, 131], some have described better results for CAPD than for HD in elderly patients [90, 107, 131, 132]. Age and comorbid conditions seem to have a statistically significant impact on patient survival but the type of dialysis does not [107].

Elderly diabetic patients on CAPD appear to have a higher relative risk of death than diabetic HD patients in the USA, although the comparisons of more recent cohorts show no difference [132]. On the contrary, in Canada the survival – at least for the first 2 years – is better in PD than HD for all age groups [122].

In their 10-year study (1983–93), Marcelli *et al.* [133] reported that survival of 895 diabetic patients was similar between the two modalities. In a multivariate analysis that took into account all possible confounding factors – sex, age, pretreatment risk factors such as severe heart disease, severe vascular disease, cirrhosis of the liver, cachexia and other risk factors such as the presence of malignancy – these authors showed that age, type of diabetes, pretreatment presence of severe vascular disease and cachexia were independent factors significantly related to survival [133]. However, the modality of dialysis was not an independent significant variable. Among those patients without any baseline risk factor(s), the mean life expectancy was about 4 years for those 45–64 years of age, 2.2 years for those 65–74 years of age, and 1.8 years for patients older than 75 years [133].

Gentil *et al.* have reported that the elderly diabetics on centre haemodialysis have a higher probability of changing to CAPD, whereas those on CAPD showed a trend to remain on this treatment [121].

Analysis of the USRDS 1997 report shows that, among younger (<55 years) diabetic patients, mortality rates tended to be higher on haemodialysis than on CAPD, while the opposite was true among older patients [134].

According to the 1998 USRDS report, even though the average age and proportion of diabetics among new patients has increased steadily each year, death rates during the 5 years on the two dialysis modalities not only did not increase, but instead declined by 12% during 1988–98 [127].

After reviewing data from the Canadian Organs Replacement Register Fenton *et al.* reported that the combined CAPD/CCPD group has a 12% decrease in hazard ratio (0.88) or a 12% increase in survival, compared to haemodialysis – a group hazard ratio 1.0; the intermittent peritoneal dialysis group had a 97% increase in hazard ratio (1.97), but in this group survival decreases as age increases [122].

In a 10-year follow-up Maiorca *et al.* [135, 136] found no difference between the survival of CAPD and haemodialysis patients; the survival curves were very close for the adults and the differences were non-significant for the elderly. Those over 75 years of age had a better survival on CAPD in the first year of treatment. 'Drop-outs' from dialysis, which were higher on CAPD, decreased with age; patient retention on CAPD was worse than on haemodialysis for all patients except for the elderly, for whom it was similar. Technique failure was significantly higher on CAPD and was inversely related to age [136].

Comparison of access methods between HD and peritoneal dialysis

In 122 patients Kim *et al.* [137] found that the cumulative survival rate of all peritoneal catheters was significantly longer than the arteriovenous fistula (AVF) survival rate in 172 HD patients: 84% vs 74% at 1 year, 73% vs 61% at 2 years, and 63% vs 48% at 3 years ($p = 0.029$). They saw no differ-

ences in peritoneal catheter survival according to gender, age or diabetes. Compared with AVF, peritoneal catheters survived for a significantly longer period in the male elderly population ($p = 0.0092$) and in diabetic patients ($p = 0.0022$) [137].

Geriatric HD patients required more access procedures than did those on CAPD [40], but more elderly CAPD patients were transferred to HD [8, 112, 131].

Comparison of hospitalization rates between elderly on HD and peritoneal dialysis

The hospitalization rate (days per year) was similar in elderly patients on HD and on CAPD (31 HD and 30 CAPD) [40]. Benevent *et al.* [92] reported that elderly CAPD patients had fewer days in hospital per month of treatment (4.74 ± 0.53 days) but more admissions (2.29 per year) than those on HD (6 ± 2.72 days per month, 1.48 admissions per year).

Malberti found that hospitalization rate was related to age, sex, presence of systemic nephropathies or malignancy, but not to treatment modality [114].

The USRDS 1998 annual report also recorded a lower hospitalization rate for the CAPD elderly patients [113]. Peritonitis was the primary cause of hospitalization (31%) in this group; other causes were cardiovascular diseases (22%), neurological symptoms (11%) and technique-related complications other than peritonitis (9%). In the HD group the main cause of hospitalization was cardiovascular diseases (26%), while other causes were thrombosis of vascular access (15%), technique-related difficulties other than vascular access (12%) and neurological complications (8%) [113].

Habach *et al.* [112] found the admission rate per patient-year at risk for peritoneal dialysis patients was 14% higher than the rate for HD patients (RR 1.4, $p < 0.001$), after adjusting for race, gender, age and cause of ESRD. Admission rate per patient-year was 1.8 HD vs 2.03 PD and hospital days 13.79 HD vs 25.35 PD for patients up to 65 years of age. Similarly Brunori *et al.* [129] reported fewer hospital days per patient year for 51 patients on HD >65 years (17.6 days/patient-year), and 24.0 days/ patient-year for 109 patients on CAPD >65 years old. The number of admissions per patient-year was 1.8 for HD and 1.7 for CAPD patients >65 years old [129].

Among 2319 older dialysis patients in Georgia and South Carolina between 1982 and 1986 [117] cardiovascular complications (23%) and access-related complications (18.5%) were the most common causes of hospitalization.

Clinical and biochemical status

The incidence of hypertension in the Japan series was similar in the two groups (HD–CAPD) [98] but was higher in the HD elderly [40]; arrhythmias were more frequent in the elderly on HD than among those on CAPD [88]. The incidence of malnutrition was similar in the two groups [88, 100]. There were no significant differences in levels of blood urea nitrogen, serum creatinine, calcium or phosphorus [40]. Cholesterol levels were lower and serum albumin levels higher in elderly HD patients [40, 88, 89].

Elderly patients on CAPD are said to have a better quality of life (QOL) than those on HD [90], but others reported that this feature is similar in the two groups [138]. Diaz-Buxo reported higher QOL scores in elderly patients on CAPD and home HD, than those on centre HD [76].

Access of the elderly to dialysis

Many elderly patients, who are suitable for renal replacement treatment, are not referred for a nephrological opinion and so are denied dialysis [139]. This policy may be responsible in large part for the great difference in the numbers of new patients who present for dialysis in various countries.

Thus in the UK [140] of 16 hypothetical patients (most of them elderly), who were described in brief vignettes, non-nephrologist consultants and general practitioners on average considered 6.9 and 7.4 patients respectively as unsuitable for dialysis. This figure was significantly higher than the 4.7 patients considered unsuitable by nephrologists.

In the US, Sekkarie and Moss [141] did a prospective study of 76 primary-care physicians and 22 nephrologists and found that the former withheld dialysis from 22% of ESRD patients, compared with only 7% withheld by nephrologists. In deciding not to refer a patient for dialysis, 25% of these primary-care physicians did not consult a nephrologist and 60% cited age as a reason not to refer. (It should be noted that the Institute of Medicine Committee for the study of the Medicare ESRD programme explicitly rejected age as a criterion for patient acceptance.)

Non-referral for dialysis also occurs in Ontario, Canada. Among the physicians who responded to the questionnaire circulated by Mendelssohn *et al.* [142], 14% of family physicians and 45% of internists indicated that in the previous 3 years they recalled not referring patients for dialysis, who died subsequently with ESRD. These physicians based their decisions on the wishes of a competent patient (94%), short life-expectancy (88%), poor quality of life (87%) and age (64%).

Among physicians, both increasing age and co-morbidity were associated with a greater stated choice of non-referral. Other factors affecting the referral pattern were distance from the dialysis centre and overcrowding of the nearest dialysis centre. Age increased the non-referral pattern in all these categories.

Low referral by primary-care physicians may be based on inadequate knowledge of the indications for and prognosis of modern dialysis, which then may be imparted unchallenged to the potential patient [142].

In the USA the expanding role of the primary-care physician and the diminishing role of the specialist, a pattern promoted by managed care, will undoubtedly change the practice of medicine in general, and dialysis in particular [141].

In the Canadian study mentioned above, 67% of the physicians believed that health care is rationed in Ontario. We want to stress that the government of Ontario has no explicit policy to ration dialysis among its citizens who require this treatment. Thus physicians seem to be responding to the government's indirect measures by conducting a form of rationing, something the government, or in the USA, the managed-care organizations, will avoid doing overtly.

In the USA the health-care providers, who compete to obtain the 'business' of the various managed-care agencies (business here, represented by the illness of patients), have to make a profit by minimizing expenditures in various aspects of their operations; this they achieve mainly by keeping hospitalization rates low and by keeping to a minimum referrals to specialists. This approach falls most heavily on those patients, like the elderly, who require frequent hospitalization and often have multisystem disease, which requires the care of specialists. Nevertheless, the managed-care industry will not acknowledge this approach as policy (hidden rationing) – hence managed-care organizations and their physicians join in a kind of conspiracy against the elderly and all those who may require expensive care.

The existence of this conspiracy is reflected in the vocabulary used. Thus we talk about managed 'care' when in essence we mean managed expenditures. The patients are consumers and the money spent on them represents lost income, and those who are ravaged by disease or old age are considered as financial burdens. Furthermore, we believe that, as has been set out in a recent article in *Lancet* [143], with the legalization of assisted suicide and subsequent euthanasia, the elderly with ESRD will be coerced covertly into believing that it is 'the right thing to do' and be encouraged to choose 'death with dignity' rather than submit to the 'indignities of this wretched treatment'. Eventually primary-care physicians will fall in with this 'conspiracy' and will do their part: they will stop referring these patients to the nephrologist, as they have started doing already [141].

Another more sinister way of encouraging/enticing primary-care physicians to maintain the earnings of the managed-care corporation is the policy of incentives. The more the physician saves the agency the greater his/her bonus at the end of the year. This policy is sinister because it takes advantage of the greed latent in all of us, and eventually it will undermine the patient/doctor relationship.

What should we do?

We will repeat here some of the recommendations Hall and Berenson made to those physicians who want to preserve their patients' trust and be their advocates in a managed-care environment [144]:

(a) Maintain high scientific standards by practising evidence-based medicine.
(b) Be impartial, i.e. use the same clinical criteria for all patients even when they have different degrees of insurance protection.
(c) Do not enter into any incentive arrangement that is not common use elsewhere, especially one that you would be embarrassed to describe to your patients.

At the same time insurance companies should be encouraged and, if necessary, required by legislation, to describe to prospective clients their incentive policies. Governments should ban and make illegal 'gag' clauses that prevent physicians from protesting or revealing what they believe is unethical in these managed-care plans.

Finally when, because of forces beyond our control, we cannot offer a treatment to a new patient, we should tell such patients the unpleasant truth that they are deprived of care because of economic policies of the government or the managed-care organization.

In conclusion non-referral of elderly for dialysis does occur in North America and we expect that, in the near future, the elderly will have even greater difficulty in gaining access to life-supporting chronic treatment.

We believe that in their professional goals nephrologists should include education of primary-care physicians and geriatricians about what dialysis (HD and PD) does and what the dialysis team can offer in terms of life prolongation and quality of life on dialysis.

With a few exceptions, such as the demented patients or the patient who has a life-expectancy of less than 2 or 3 months and the patient who requires restraint before he/she can be dialysed, all other ESRD patients, after they have been fully informed, should be allowed to decide for themselves whether they want to be dialysed.

Finally, we believe that physicians (all of us, nephrologists, geriatricians and primary-care physicians) should focus and refocus continuously on our primary goal, that is, on being our patient's advocate. Whenever there is a conflict between our patients' interests and our own, or those of the organization that employs us, the interests of the patients always take precedence.

Dialysis withdrawal

The USA has seen a recent increase in deaths due to withdrawal from dialysis; the percentage of such deaths increased from 9.7% in 1988 to 17.6% in 1996 [145]. Almost all reports confirm that deaths due to dialysis withdrawal are much more frequent among the elderly than among younger patients [146, 147]. With the anticipated increase in the number of elderly patients on dialysis (approximately 60% of dialysis patients by the year 2000), nephrologists are encountering the issue of withdrawal with increasing frequency [148].

Patients who die following withdrawal from dialysis may be divided into two main categories:

(a) those with decision-making capacity; and
(b) those without decision-making capacity.

Sekkarie's prospective study [141] showed that 37% of those who died after withdrawal from dialysis lacked decision-making capacity.

When he/she is capable of making the decisions to withdraw, the patient decides that the quality of life on dialysis is not acceptable and eventually the nephrologist has to comply with the patient's wishes. Here the patient's right to autonomy overrides all other ethical principles.

On the other hand, the patient who has lost his/her decision-making capacities poses more difficult ethical and legal problems. An important factor in the management of this group is the presence (or not) of an advance directive and/or the designation of a surrogate decision maker.

Despite all efforts to encourage them to sign advance directives, only 20% of patients in the USA have completed an advance directive [149]. A survey in Pittsburgh showed that many patients were unwilling to sign an advance directive; 50% of these said they feared that, by signing a living will, they might influence the subsequent conduct of their physicians [149]. This lack of trust is particularly prominent among black patients who receive their care from a predominantly white medical profession [144]. Why this lack of trust? What aspects of our practice or behaviour convince our patients that we will not act in their best interests when they are no longer able to decide for themselves [150]?

What should we do for the 20% of patients who, in their advance directives, indicate that they want dialysis to be continued if they lose their decision-making capacity, or for the patients without advance directive whose families request the continuation of dialysis? We believe that, when we encourage a patient to give an advance directive, we enter into a contract that commits us to respect and follow their wishes, whatever is decided. However, it seems that, although we are prepared to follow such wishes if patients ask for discontinuation of treatment, we do not know what to do, and become uncomfortable when they ask for continuation of treatment. If patient autonomy is the primary ethical principle behind such decisions, one should continue dialysing these patients even if the health-care team believes such treatment is futile. However, in increasing numbers nephrologists are acknowledging that they find it difficult to follow through when an advance directive clashes with their own beliefs [151], for example, they believe that continuing to offer medical care to a patient in a persistent vegetative state (PVS) is futile and offends their moral integrity [152].

We believe that resolving such ethical dilemmas requires patience, understanding and compassion. In North America, societal attitudes and principles seem to be changing from a model that gives primacy to the principle of patient autonomy, to a com-munity-based model that values societal objectives and the common good above the wishes of the individual, as eloquently described by Callahan in his book *Setting Limits* [152–155]. Arnold Eiser believes that, under these new circumstances, the community shall (should) have the capacity to set, develop and administer guidelines concerning such problem areas of decision making [152]. The communitarian perspective holds that the community has an interest in assisting the profession of medicine to maintain its integrity and will not compel it to provide non-beneficial futile medical care [152]. An additional benefit of such a policy is that it saves money; for example, the cost of care for those who have completed an advance directive to discontinue treatment is less than one-third the cost of those without such a directive [156].

We disagree with this approach and believe that under these circumstances advance directives would lose their force and meaning.

The main risk in adopting the communitarian approach is that some individuals, who believe that they should continue being dialysed for religious reasons (such as orthodox Jews and some Catholics) may conclude that they are being discriminated against; but worse [157, 158], this approach may be used predominantly for economic reasons. In conclusion, we believe that the expected dramatic increase in the numbers of elderly who suffer from ESRD in the next decade will bring into play economic pressures that will make death due to withdrawal from dialysis an increasingly common event [159, 160].

References

1. Gambert SR. Who are the 'elderly'? Geriat Nephrol Urol 1994; 4: 3–4.
2. Mignon F, Michel C, Mentre F, Viron B. Worldwide demographics and future trends of the management of renal failure in the elderly. Kidney Int 1993; 43 (suppl. 41): S19–26.
3. Calkins ME. Ethical issues in the elderly ESRD patients. ANN J 1993; 20: 569–71.
4. Nissenson AR. Peritoneal dialysis in geriatric patients: an overview and introduction. Adv Perit Dial 1990; 6 (suppl.): 1.
5. USRDS 1997. Annual Data Report. International Comparison of ESRD Therapy. Am J Kidney Dis 1997; 30 (suppl. 1): S187–94.
6. USRDS 1998. Annual Data Report. Treatment Modalities for ESRD Patients. Am J Kidney Dis 1998; 32 (suppl. 1): S50–9.
7. Ismail N, Hakim RM, Oreopoulos DG, Patrikarea A. Renal replacement therapies in the elderly. Part I: Hemodialysis and chronic peritoneal dialysis. Am J Kidney Dis 1993; 27: 759–82.
8. Walls J. Dialysis in the elderly: some UK experience. Adv Perit Dial 1990; 6 (suppl.): 82–5.
9. Geerlings W, Tufveson G, Brunner FP *et al.* Combined report on regular dialysis and transplantation in Europe, XXI, 1990. Nephrol Dial Transplant 1991; 6 (suppl. 4): 5–29.

10. Valderrabano F, Jones EH, Mallick NP. Report on management of renal failure in Europe, XXIV, 1993. Nephrol Dial Transplant 1995; 10 (suppl. 5): 1–25.

11. Nissenson AR. Dialysis therapy in the elderly patient. Kidney Int 1993; 43 (suppl. 40): S51–7.

12. Gentile DE, and Geriatric Committee. Peritoneal dialysis in geriatric patients: a survey of clinical practices. Adv Perit Dial 1990; 6 (suppl.): 29–32.

13. Nissensson AR. Chronic peritoneal dialysis in the elderly. Geriat Nephrol Urol 1991; 1: 3–12.

14. Mattern WD, McGaghie WC, Rigby RJ, Nissenson AR, Dunham CB, Khayrallah MA. Selection of ESRD treatment: an international study. Am J Kidney Dis 1989; 13: 457–64.

15. Nyberg G, Nilsson B, Norben G, Karlberg I. Outcome of renal transplantation in patients over the age of 60: a case–control study. Nephrol Dial Transplant 1995; 10: 91–4.

16. Mignon F, Siohan P, Legallicier B, Khayat R, Viron B, Michel C. The management of uraemia in the elderly: treatment choices. Nephrol Dial Transplant 1995; 10 (suppl. 6): 55–9.

17. Latos DL. Chronic dialysis in patients over age 65. J Am Soc Nephrol 1996; 7: 637–46.

18. Ross CJ, Rutsky EA. Dialysis modality selection in the elderly patient with end-stage renal disease. Advantages and disadvantages of peritoneal dialysis. In: Nissenson AR, ed. Peritoneal Dialysis in the Geriatric Patient. Adv Perit Dial 1990; 6 (suppl.); 11–18.

19. Vlachojannis J, Kurz P, Hoppe D. CAPD in elderly patients with cardiovascular risk factors. Clin Nephrol 1988; 30 (suppl. 1): S13–17.

20. Wizeman U, Timio M, Alpert MA, Kramer W. Options in dialysis therapy: significance of cariovascular findings. Kidney Int 1993; 43 (suppl. 40): S85–91.

21. Niwa A, Taniguchi K, Ito H et al. Echocardiographic and Holter findings in 321 uremic patients on maintenance hemodialysis. Jpn Heart J 1985; 26: 403–11.

22. Chester AC, Rakowski TH, Argy WP Jr, Giacaolone A, Schreiner GE. Hemodialysis in the eighth and ninth decades of life. Arch Intern Med 1979; 139: 1001–5.

23. Feldman HI, Held PJ, Hutchinson JT, Stoiber E, Hartigan MF, Berlin JA. Hemodialysis vascular access morbidity in the United States. Kidney Int 1993; 43: 1091–6.

24. Grapsa EJ, Parakevopoulos AP, Moutafis SP et al. Complications of vascular access in hemodialysis: aged vs. adult patients. Geriat Nephrol Urol 1998; 8: 21–4.

25. Williams P, Rush DR. Geriatric polypharmacy. Hosp Pract 1986; 21: 112, 115–20.

26. Blagg CR. Chronic renal failure in the elderly. In: Oreopoulos DG, ed. Geriatric Nephrology. Boston, MA: Martinus Nijhoff, 1986, pp. 285–313.

27. Porush JG, Faubert PF. Chronic renal failure. In: Porush JG, Faubert PF, eds. Renal Diseases in the Aged. Boston, MA: Little Brown, 1991, pp. 285–313.

28. Lipschutz DE, Easterling RE. Spontaneous perforation of the colon in chronic renal failure. Arch Intern Med 1973; 132: 758–9.

29. Stacy W, Sica D. Dialysis of the elderly patient. In: Zawada ET, Sica DA, eds. Geriatric Nephrology and Urology. Littleton, MA: PSG, 1985, pp. 229–51.

30. Michel C, Bindi P, Viron B. CAPD with private home nurses: an alternative treatment for elderly and disabled patients. Adv Perit Dial 1990; 6 (suppl.): 92–4.

31. Oreopoulos D. Dialyzing the elderly: benefits or burden? Perit Dial Int 1997; 17 (suppl. 2): S7–12.

32. Gorban-Brennan N, Kliger AS, Finkelstein FO. CAPD therapy for patients over 80 years of age. Perit Dial Int 1993; 13: 140–1.

33. Soreide R, Svarstad E, Iversen BM. CAPD in patients above 70 years of age. Adv Perit Dial 1991, 7: 73–6.

34. Nissenson AR. Peritoneal dialysis in elderly patients. In: Gokal R, Nolph KD, eds. Textbook of Peritoneal Dialysis. Dordrecht: Kluwer, 1994: pp. 661–78.

35. Jagose JT, Afthentopoulos JE, Shetty A, Oreopoulos DG. Successful use of continuous ambulatory peritoneal dialysis in octogenarians. Adv Perit Dial 1996; 12: 126–31.

36. Young MA, Nolph KD, Dutton S, Prowant P. Antihypertensive drug requirements in CAPD. Perit Dial Bull 1984; 4: 85–8.

37. Cheigh JS, Serur D, Paguirigan M, Stenzel KH, Rubin A. How well is hypertension controlled in CAPD patients? Adv Perit Dial 1994; 10: 55–8.

38. Copley JB, Lindberg JS. Insulin: its use in patients on peritoneal dialysis. Semin Dial 1988; 1: 143–50.

39. Saltissi D, Coles GA, Napier JA, Bentley P. The hematological response to continuous ambulatory peritoneal dialysis. Clin Nephrol 1984; 22: 21–7.

40. O'Brien M, Zimmerman S. Comparison of peritoneal dialysis and hemodialysis in the elderly. Adv Perit Dial 1990; 6 (suppl.): 65–7.

41. Movilli E, Natale C, Cancarini GC, Maiorca R. Improvement of iron utilization and anemia in uremic patients switched from hemodialysis to continuous ambulatory peritoneal dialysis. Perit Dial Bull 1986; 6: 147–9.

42. Peer G, Korzets A, Hochhauzer E, Eschchar Y, Blum M, Avram A. Cardiac arrhythmia during chronic ambulatory peritoneal dialysis. Nephron 1987; 45: 192–5.

43. Timio M. Ruolo terapeutico della dialisi peritoneale. In: Timio M, ed. Clinica Cardiologi Nell Uremia. Milan: Wichtig, 1990, p. 8.

44. Joffe P, Skov R, Olsen F. Do patients on continuous ambulatory peritoneal dialysis need arteriovenous fistula? In: Khanna R, Nolph KD, Prowant B, Twardowski Z, Oreopoulos DG, eds. Advances in Continuous Ambulatory Peritoneal Dialysis. Proceedings of the Sixth Annual CAPD Conference. Kansas City, MO, 1986, pp. 84–6.

45. Rottembourg J. Residual renal function and recovery of renal function in patients treated by CAPD. Kidney Int 1993; 43 (suppl. 40): S106–10.

46. Gagnon RF, Somerville P, Kaye M. Beta-2 microglobulin serum levels in patients on long term dialysis. Perit Dial Bull 1987; 7: 29–31.

47. Lysaght M, Pollock CA, Moran JE, Ibels LS, Farrell PC. Beta-2 microglobulin removal during continuous ambulatory peritoneal dialysis. Perit Dial Int 1989; 9: 29–35.

48. Delmez JA, Slatopolsky E, Martin K, Gearing B, Harter H. The effects of continuous ambulatory peritoneal dialysis (CAPD) on parathyroid hormone (PTH) and mineral metabolism. Kidney Int 1981; 19: 145 (abstract).

49. Rowe JW. Health care of the elderly. N Engl J Med 1985; 312: 827–35.

50. Diaz-Buxo JA. Clinical use of peritoneal dialysis. In: Nissenson AR, Fine RN, Gentile DE, eds. Clinical Dialysis. Norwalk, CT: Appleton & Lange, 1990, pp. 256–300.

51. Bargman JM. Complications of peritoneal dialysis related to increased intraabdominal pressure. Kidney Int 1993; 43 (suppl. 40): S75–80.

52. Nolph KD. Peritoneal dialysis. In: Brenner BM, Rector FC, eds. The Kidney, vol. II. Philadelphia, PA: WB Saunders, 1991, pp. 2299–335.

53. Sombolos K, Berkelhammer C, Baker J, Wu G, McNamee P, Oreopoulos DG. Nutritional assessment and skeletal muscle function in patients on continuous ambulatory peritoneal dialysis. Perit Dial Bull 1986; 6: 53–8.

54. Dombos NV, Oreopoulos DG. Nutritional aspects of patients on CAPD. In: La Greca G, Chiramonte S, Fabris A, Feriani M, Ronco C, eds. Peritoneal Dialysis. Proceedings of Third International Course on Peritoneal Dialysis, Vicenza, Italy, 1988. Milan: Wichtig, 1988, pp. 113–18.

55. Brown PN, Johnston KW, Fenton SSA, Cattran DC. Symptomatic exacerbation of peripheral vascular disease with chronic ambulatory peritoneal dialysis. Clin Nephrol 1981; 16: 258–61.

56. Cianciaruso B, Brunori G, Traverso G *et al.* Nutritional status in the elderly patients with uraemia. Nephrol Dial Transplant 1995; 10 (suppl. 6): 65–8.

57. Mitch WE. Uremia and the control of protein metabolism. Nephron 1988; 49: 89–93.

58. Hakim RM, Levin NL. Malnutrition in hemodialysis patients. Am J Kidney Dis 1993; 21: 125–37.

59. Piccoli G, Bonello F, Massara C *et al.* Death in conditions of cachexia: the price for the dialysis treatment of the elderly? Kidney Int 1993; 43 (suppl. 41): S282–6.

60. Kagan A, Bar-Khayim Y. Role of peritoneal loss of albumin in the hypoalbuminemia continuous ambulatory peritoneal dialysis patients: relationship to peritoneal transport of solutes. Nephron 1995; 71: 314–20.

61. Young GA, Kopple JD, Lindholm B, Vonesh EF, de Vecchi A, Scalamogna A. Nutritional assessment of continuous ambulatory peritoneal dialysis patients: an international study. Am J Kidney Dis 1991; 17: 462–71.

62. Shimomura A, Tahara D, Azekura H, Matsuo H, Kamo M. Key factors to improve survival of elderly patients on CAPD. Adv Perit Dial 1992; 8: 166–72.

63. Shimomura A, Tahara D, Azekura H. Nutritional improvement in elderly CAPD patients with additional high protein foods. Adv Perit Dial 1993; 9: 80–6.

64. Nolph KD, Moore HL, Prowant B *et al.* Age and indices of adequacy and nutrition in CAPD patients. Adv Perit Dial 1993; 9: 87–91.

65. Mooraki A, Kliger AS, Juergensen P, Gorban-Brennan N, Finkelstein FO. Selected outcome criteria and adequacy of dialysis in diabetic and elderly patients on CAPD therapy. Adv Perit Dial 1994; 10: 89–93.

66. Cancarini G, Constantino E, Brunori G *et al.* Nutritional status of long term CAPD patients. Adv Perit Dial 1992; 8: 84–7.

67. Abdo F, Clemente L, Davy J, Grant J, Ladouceur D, Morton AR. Nutritional status and efficiency of dialysis in CAPD and CCPD patients. Adv Perit Dial 1993; 9: 76–9.

68. Russell L, Davies S, Russell G. Current nutritional recommendations in peritoneal dialysis. Perit Dial Int 1996; 16 (suppl. 1): S459–60.

69. Blazer D. Depression in the elderly. N Engl J Med 1989; 320: 164–6.

70. Rodin G, Voshart K. Depressive symptoms and functional impairment in the medically ill. Gen Hosp Psychiatry 1987; 9: 251–8.

71. Kutner NG, Brogan DJ. Assisted survival, aging, and rehabilitation needs: comparison of older dialysis patients and age-matched peers. Arch Phys Med Rehabil 1992; 73: 309–15.

72. Stout JP, Gokal R, Hillier VF *et al.* Quality of life of high risk and elderly dialysis patients in the UK. Dial Transplant 1987; 16: 674–7.

73. Moody H, Moody C, Szabo E, Kejllstrand C. Are old dialysis patients happy and can they fend for themselves or not? XII International Congress on Nephrology, Jerusalem, Israel, 1993, p. 518 (abstract).

74. Muthny FA, Koch U. Quality of life of patients with end stage renal failure: a comparison of hemodialysis CAPD and transplantation. Contrib Nephrol 1991; 89: 265–73.

75. McDonald M, McPhee PD, Walker R. Successful self-care home dialysis in the elderly: a single center's experience. Perit Dial Int 1995; 15: 33–6.

76. Diaz-Buxo JA, Adcock A, Nelms M. Experience with continuous cyclic peritoneal dialysis in the geriatric patient. Adv Perit Dial 1990; 6 (suppl.): 61–4.

77. McKevitt PM, Jones JF, Marion RR. The elderly on dialysis. Physical psychosocial functioning. Dial Transplant 1986; 15: 130–7.

78. Carey H. Finkelstein S, Santacroce S *et al.* The impact of psychosocial factors and age on CAPD dropout. Adv Perit Dial 1990; 6 (suppl.): 26–8.

79. de Vecchi AF, Maccario M, Braga M, Scalamogna A, Castelnovo C, Ponticelli C. Peritoneal dialysis in non-diabetic patients older than 70 years. Comparison with patients aged 40 to 60 years. Am J Kidney Dis 1998; 31: 479–90.

80. Shah GM, Sabo A, Nguyen T, Juler GL. Peritoneal catheter: a comparative study of column disk and Tenckhoff catheters. Int J Artif Organs 1990; 13: 267–72.

81. Holley JL, Bernardini J, Piraino B. Risk factors for tunnel infections in continuous ambulatory peritoneal dialysis. Am J Kidney Dis 1991; 18: 344–8.

82. Lupo A, Tarchini R, Cancarini G *et al.* Long-term outcome in continuous ambulatory peritoneal dialysis: a 10-year survey by the Italian Cooperative Peritoneal Dialysis Study Group. Am J Kidney Dis 1994; 24: 826–37.

83. Holley JL, Bernardini J, Perlmutter JA, Piraino B. A comparison of infection rates among older and younger patients on continuous peritoneal dialysis. Perit Dial Int 1994; 14: 66–9.

84. Nissenson AR, Gentile DE, Soderblom R. Continuous peritoneal dialysis in the elderly – Southern California/Southern Nevada experience. Adv Perit Dial 1990; 6 (suppl.): 51–5.

85. Tzamaloukas AH, Murata GH, Fox L. Peritoneal catheter loss and death in continuous ambulatory peritoneal dialysis peritonitis: correlation with clinical and biochemical parameters. Perit Dial Int 1993; 13 (suppl. 2): S338–40.

86. Williams AJ, Nicholl JP, el-Nahas AM, Moorhead PJ, Brown CB. Continuous ambulatory peritoneal dialysis and haemodialysis in the elderly. Q J Med 1990; 74: 215–23.

87. Atkins RC, Wood C. Hyperlipemia in CAPD. Perit Dial Int 1993; 13 (suppl. 2): S415–17.

88. Nakagawa S, Ozawa K. Protective aspects for atherogenesis and lipid abnormalities in continuous ambulatory peritoneal dialysis patients. Perit Dial Int 1993; 13 (suppl. 2): S418–20.

89. Panarello G, Calianno G, De Baz H, Signori D, Cappelletti P, Tesio F. Does continuous ambulatory peritoneal dialysis induce hypercholesterolemia? Perit Dial Int 1993; 13 (suppl. 2): S421–3.

90. Maiorca R, Cancarini G, Brunori G *et al.* Continuous ambulatory peritoneal dialysis in the elderly. Perit Dial Int 1993; 13 (suppl. 2): S165–71.

91. Anderson JE. Ten years' experience with CAPD in a nursing home setting. Perit Dial Int 1997; 17: 255–61.

92. Benevent D, Benzakour M, Peyronnet P, Legarde C, Leroux-Robert C, Charmes JP. Comparison of continuous ambulatory peritoneal dialysis and hemodialysis in the elderly. Adv Perit Dial 1990; 6 (suppl.): 68–71.

93. Gorban-Brennan N, Kliger AS, Finkelstein FO. CAPD therapy for patients over 80 years of age. Perit Dial Int 1993; 13: 140–1.

94. De Fijter CWH, Oe PL, Nauta JJP *et al.* A prospective, randomized study comparing the peritonitis incidence of CAPD and Y-connector (CAPD-Y) with continuous cyclic peritoneal dialysis (CCPD). Adv Perit Dial 1991; 7: 186–9.

95. Strauss FG, Holmes DL, Dennis RL, Nortman DF. Prespiking dialysate bags: improved peritonitis prevention in patients on CAPD. Adv Perit Dial 1991; 7: 193–5.

96. Grutzmachere P, Tsobanelis T, Bruns N, Kurz P, Hoppe D, Vlachojannis J. Decrease in peritonitis rate by integrated disconnect system in patients on continuous ambulatory peritoneal dialysis. Perit Dial Int 1993; 13 (suppl. 2): S326–8.

97. Port FK, Held PH, Nolph KD, Turenne MN, Wolfe RA. Risk of peritonitis and technique failure by CAPD connection technique: a national study. Kidney Int 1992; 42: 967–74.

98. Kawaguchi Y. Present status of CAPD in Japan. Am J Kidney Dis 1998; 32: xlix–lii.

99. Imada A, Kawaguchi Y, Kumano K, Nomoto YU, Chiku T, Yamabe K. The peritonitis study group in Japan and Baxter Health Care. A multicenter study of CAPD related peritonitis in Japan. J Am Soc Nephrol 1997; 8: 264A (abstract).

100. Segoloni GP, Salomone M, Piccoli GB. CAPD in the elderly: Italian multicenter study experience. Adv Perit Dial 1990; 6 (suppl.): 41–6.

101. Posen GA, Fenton SA, Arbus GS, Churchill DN, Jeffery JR. The Canadian experience with peritoneal dialysis in the elderly. Adv Perit Dial 1990; 6 (suppl.): 47–50.

102. Nolph KD, Lindblad AS, Novak JW, Steinberg SM. Experiences with the elderly in the National CAPD Registry. Adv Perit Dial 1990; 6 (suppl.): 33–7.

103. Gokal AR. CAPD in the elderly – European and UK experience. Adv Perit Dial 1990; 6 (suppl.): 38–40.

104. Nebel M, Finke K. CAPD in patients over 60 years of age. Review from 1984–1989. Adv Perit Dial 1990; 6 (suppl.): 56–60.

105. Ramos JM, Gokal R, Siamopoulos K, Ward MK, Wilkinson R, Kerr DN. Continuous ambulatory peritoneal dialysis: three years experience. Q J Med 1983; 52: 165–86.

106. Maiorca R, Cancarini GC, Camerini C et al. Is CAPD competitive with haemodialysis for long-term treatment of uraemic patients? Nephrol Dial Transplant 1989; 4: 244–53.

107. Lupo A, Cancarini G, Catizone L et al. Comparison of survival in CAPD and hemodialysis: a multicenter study. Adv Perit Dial 1992; 8: 136–40.

108. Joglar F, Saade M. Improved overall survival of elderly patients on peritoneal dialysis. Adv Perit Dial 1991; 7: 63–7.

109. Piccoli G, Quarello F, Salomone M et al. Dialysis in the elderly: comparison of different dialytic modalities. Adv Perit Dial 1990; 6 (suppl.): 72–81.

110. Tsai TJ, Tsai HF, Chen YM, Hsieh BS, Chen WY, Yen TS. CAPD in patients unable to do their own bag change. Perit Dial Int 1991; 11: 356–8.

111. USDRS Annual Data Report. Renal Data System, 1991. Hospitalization for dialysis patients. Am J Kidney Dis 1991; 18 (suppl. 2): 74–8.

112. Habach G, Bloembergen WE, Mauger EA, Wolfe RA, Port FK. Hospitalization among United States dialysis patients: hemodialysis versus peritoneal dialysis. J Am Soc Nephrol 1995; 5: 1940–8.

113. USRDS Annual Data Report. Hospitalization. Am J Kidney Dis 1998; 32 (suppl. 1): S109–17.

114. Malberti F, Conte F, Limido A et al. Ten years experience of renal replacement treatment in the elderly. Geriat Nephrol Urol 1997; 7: 1–10.

115. Wadhwa NK, Suh H, Cabralda T, Sokol E, Sokumbi D, Solomon M. Peritoneal dialysis with trained home nurses in elderly and disabled end-stage renal disease patients. Adv Perit Dial 1993; 9: 130–3.

116. URSDS 1995. Annual Data Report. ESRD Treatment Modalities. Am J Kidney Dis 1995; 26 (suppl. 2): 551–68.

117. Brogan D, Kutner NG, Flagg E. Survival differences among older dialysis patients in the southeast. Am J Kidney Dis 1992; 20: 376–86.

118. Verbeeten D, De Neve W, Van der Viepeen P, Sennesael J. Dialysis in patients over 65 years of age. Kidney Int 1993; 43 (suppl. 41): S27–30.

119. Khan IH, Catto GR, Edward N, Fleming LW, Henderson LS, McLeod AM. Influence of coexisting disease on survival on renal replacement therapy. Lancet 1993; 341: 415–18.

120. Neves PL. Chronic haemodialysis in elderly patients. Nephrol Dial Transplant 1995; 10 (suppl. 6): 69–71.

121. Gentil MA, Carriazo A, Pavon MI et al. Comparison of survival in continuous ambulatory peritoneal dialysis and hospital haemodialysis: a multicentre study. Nephrol Dial Transplant 1991; 6: 444–51.

122. Fenton SS, Schaubel DE, Desmeules M et al. Hemodialysis versus peritoneal dialysis: a comparison of adjusted mortality rates. Am J Kidney Dis 1997; 30: 334–42.

123. Byrne C, Vernon P, Cohen JJ. Effect of age and diagnosis on survival of older patients beginning chronic dialysis. JAMA 1994; 271: 34–6.

124. Michel C, Khayat R, Virion B, Siohan P, Mignon F. Early mortality during renal replacement therapy (RRT) in ESRD patients 65 years and over. J Am Soc Nephrol 1993; 4: 369.

125. Salomone M, Piccoli GB, Quarello F et al. Dialysis in the elderly: improvement of survival results in the eighties. Nephrol Dial Transplant 1995; 10 (suppl. 6): 60–4.

126. Churchill DN, Thorpe KE, Vonesh EF, Keshaviah PR. Lower probability of patient survival with continuous peritoneal dialysis in the United States compared with Canada. CANADA–USA (CANUSA) peritoneal dialysis study group. J Am Soc Nephrol 1997; 8: 965–71.

127. USRDS 1998 Annual Data Report Patient Mortality and Survival. Am J Kidney Dis 1998; 32 (suppl. 1): S69–80.

128. USRDS 1998 Annual Data Report. Causes of Death. Am J Kidney Dis 1998; 32 (suppl. 1): S81–8.

129. Brunori G, Camerini C, Canacrini G et al. Hospitalization: CAPD versus hemodialysis and transplant. Adv Perit Dial 1992; 8: 71–4.

130. Gokal R, Jakubowski C, King J et al. Outcome in patients on continuous ambulatory peritoneal dialysis and haemodialysis: 4-year analysis of a prospective multicentre study. Lancet 1987; 2: 1105–9.

131. Maiorca R, Vonesh E, Cancarini GC et al. A six-year comparison of patient and technique survivals in CAPD and HD. Kidney Int 1988; 34: 518–24.

132. Lunde NM, Port FK, Wolfe RA, Guire KE. Comparison of mortality risk by choice of CAPD versus hemodialysis among elderly patients. Adv Perit Dial 1991; 7: 68–72.

133. Marcelli D, Spotti D, Conte F et al. Survival of diabetic patients on peritoneal dialysis or hemodialysis. Perit Dial Int 1996; 16 (suppl. 1): S283–7.

134. USRDS Annual Data Report 1991. Incidence and causes of treated ESRD. Methods of ESRD treatment. Survival probabilities and causes of death. Am J Kidney Dis 1991; 18 (suppl. 2): 30–60.

135. Maiorca R, Cancarini GC, Brunori G et al. Comparison of long-term survival between hemodialysis and peritoneal dialysis. Adv Perit Dial 1996; 12: 79–88.

136. Maiorca R, Cancarini GC, Zubani R et al. CAPD viability: a long-term comparison with hemodialysis. Perit Dial Int 1996; 16: 276–87.

137. Kim YS, Yang CW, Jin DC et al. Comparison of peritoneal catheter survival with fistula survival in hemodialysis. Perit Dial Int 1995; 15: 147–51.

138. Westlie L, Umen A, Nestrud S, Kjellstrand C. Mortality, morbidity, and life satisfaction in the very old dialysis patient. Trans Am Soc Artif Intern Organs 1984; 30: 21–30.

139. Feest TG, Mistry CD, Grimes DS, Mallick NP. Incidence of advanced chronic renal failure and the need for end stage renal replacement treatment. Br Med J 1990; 301: 897–900.

140. Challah S, Wing AJ, Bauer R, Morris RW, Schroeder SA. Negative selection for dialysis and transplantation in the United Kingdom. Br Med J 1984; 288: 1119–22.

140. Sekkarie A, Moss AH. Withholding and withdrawing dialysis: the role of physician speciality and education and functional status. Am J Kidney Dis 1998; 31: 464–72.

142. Mendelssohn DC, Kua BT, Singer PA. Referral for dialysis in Ontario. Arch Intern Med 1995; 155: 2473–8.

143. Radcliffe-Richards J, Daar AS, Guttmann RD et al. The case for allowing kidney sales. International Forum for Transplant Ethics. Lancet 1998; 351: 1950–2.

144. Hall MA, Berenson RA. Ethical practice in managed care: a dose of realism. Ann Intern Med 1998; 128: 395–402.

145. United States Renal Data System. 1996 Annual Report. Am J Kidney Dis 1996; 28 (suppl. 2): S1–165.

146. Office Technology Assessment. Dialysis for chronic renal failure. In Life-sustaining Technologies and the Elderly. OTA-BA-306. Washington, DC: US Government Printing Office, 1987, pp. 2–7.

147. Port FK, Wolfe RA, Hawthorne VM, Ferguson CW. Discontinuation of dialysis therapy as a cause of death. Am J Nephrol 1989; 9: 145–9.

148. Bhatnagar V, Maruenda J, Lowenthal DT. Ethical issues involved in dialysis for the elderly. Geriat Nephrol Urol 1998; 8: 111–14.

149. Holley JL, Nespor S, Rault R. Chronic in-center hemodialysis patients' attitudes, knowledge and behavior towards advance directives. J Am Soc Nephrol 1993; 3: 1405–8.

150. Maiorca R. Ethical issues in dialysis: prospects for the year 2000. Nephrol Dial Transplant 1998; 13 (suppl. 1): 1–9.

151. Rutecki GW, Cugino A, Jarjoura D, Kilner JF, Whittier FC. Nephrologists' subjective attitudes towards end-of-life issues and the conduct of terminal care. Clin Nephrol 1997; 48: 173–80.

152. Eiser AR. Withdrawal from dialysis: the role of autonomy and community-based values. Am J Kidney Dis 1996; 27: 451–7.

153. Beauchamp TL. Reversing the protections. Hastings Center Report 1994; 24: 18–19.

154. Murray TH. Communities need more than autonomy. Hasting Center Report 1994; 24: 32–3.

155. Callahan D. Setting Limits: medical goals in an aging society. New York: Simon & Schuster; 1987.

156. Chambers CV, Diamond JJ, Perkel RL *et al.* Relationship of advanced directives to hospital charges in a Medicare population. Arch Intern Med 1994; 154: 541–7.

157. Anonymous. Bishop warns against withdrawing life supports. Hosp Ethics 1992; 8: 9–10.

158. Jacobovits I. Ethical problems regarding termination of life. In: Meier L, ed. Jewish Values in Bioethics. New York: Human Sciences, 1986, pp. 84–95.

159. Moss AH, Stocking CB, Sachs GA, Siegler M. Variation in attitudes of dialysis unit medical directors towards decisions to withhold and withdraw dialysis. J Am Soc Nephrol 1993; 4: 229–34.

160. Bleyer AJ, Tell GS, Evans GW, Ettinger WH, Burkart JM. Survival of patients undergoing renal replacement therapy in one center with special emphasis on racial differences. Am J Kidney Dis 1996; 28: 72–81.

13 | Automated peritoneal dialysis

P. Kathuria and Z. J. Twardowski

Introduction

Automated peritoneal dialysis (APD) is a term used to refer to all forms of peritoneal dialysis that employ a mechanized device to assist in the delivery and drainage of dialysate. Automated cyclers are used in intermittent peritoneal dialysis (IPD), nocturnal intermittent peritoneal dialysis (NIPD), continuous cyclic peritoneal dialysis (CCPD), and tidal peritoneal dialysis (TPD) [1, 2]. In addition, some patients on continuous ambulatory peritoneal dialysis (CAPD) may receive one or more nocturnal exchanges with a night exchange device [3].

Automated PD has become the fastest-growing modality for renal replacement therapy. Limitations with CAPD, including a higher incidence of peritonitis, ultrafiltration failure, complications of increased intra-abdominal pressure, treatment fatigue, and failure to achieve clearance goals, have heralded this change. More so, increasing physician knowledge and acceptance and improved design of cyclers have contributed to the growth of this modality.

According to industry sources, approximately 26% of the peritoneal dialysis patients across the world are managed on APD. The United States Renal Data System [4] report states that while the percentage of patients with ESRD on peritoneal dialysis has remained constant over the past decade, the percentage of patients on APD has increased significantly. In 1991 CCPD was the treatment modality for 1.9% of end-stage renal disease (ESRD) patients and 17% of total peritoneal dialysis patients. The percentage of patients treated with CCPD had grown to 4.2% of the ESRD population (31.5% of total peritoneal dialysis patients) in 1996 (Fig. 1). Industry sources quote a much higher utili-

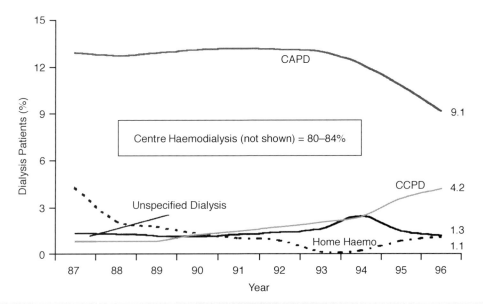

Figure 1. Percentage distribution of prevalent dialysis patients, by treatment modality and year, 1987–96. Centre haemodialysis is not shown. Unspecified dialysis includes other PD and uncertain dialysis. Percentages include Puerto Rico and US territories (USRDS Data 1996) [4].

R. Gokal, R. Khanna, R.Th. Krediet and K.D. Nolph (eds.), Textbook of Peritoneal Dialysis, 2nd Edition, 435–463.
© 2000 *Kluwer Academic Publishers. Printed in Great Britain.*

zation of APD in the United States. Among patients who initiated ESRD therapy in 1996 and opted for peritoneal dialysis, almost one-third were started on APD. Of these, 21.6% were on CCPD, 6.9% on NIPD, and 3.4% on a combination of CAPD and APD (Fig. 2) [5]. In Europe between 30% and 35% of peritoneal dialysis patients are on APD, while in Japan the figure is approximately 20%. Among children and adolescents, the North American Pediatric Renal Transplant Cooperative Study 1995 [6] reported that peritoneal dialysis was used by 63% of patients with ESRD. Of these, almost 70% were treated with APD.

History of APD

The first peritoneal cycler was described by Fred Boen *et al.* [7, 8] in the early 1960s. This device used a sterile dialysate prepared in the hospital and delivered to the bedside in 40-L carboys. Therapy consisted of multiple 2-L exchanges delivered over a 10-h period. An automatic solenoid device controlled delivery of the dialysate into the peritoneal cavity. In 1966 Norman Lasker and co-workers [9] described an automated cycler that became the forerunner of modern cyclers. This gravity-based machine utilized 2-L bottles of dialysate and disposable tubing. A preset volume of dialysate was delivered to the patient and was drained after a prescribed dwell time. At the same time as Lasker, Tenckhoff *et al.* [10] designed an automated system that mixed dialysate concentrate with distilled water processed by a 'miniature still'. This system proved to be expensive, bulky, and time-consuming to use, and was soon abandoned. After the development of reverse-osmosis water, Tenckhoff *et al.* [11] adapted the

technology to develop a new cycler. This cycler used reverse-osmosis water and a proportioning system to mix treated water with dialysate concentrate. Large amounts of dialysate could be easily prepared at a relatively lower cost. Higher glucose concentrations were achieved by adding hypertonic glucose to the mixture.

Cyclers were initially used for intermittent peritoneal dialysis (IPD). IPD was popular between 1970 and 1976 because the simplicity of the procedure permitted patients to perform home dialysis with or without the help of a partner [12]. Patients on IPD also enjoyed relative freedom between treatments, to carry out other activities. However, IPD fell out of favour by the late 1970s because of poor outcomes due to inadequate dialysis and malnutrition [13–15]. In 1976 Popovich and co-workers [16, 17] described the concept of equilibrium peritoneal dialysis, moving the focus away from cycler-dependent treatments. They proposed that fluid left in the abdominal cavity over 4 h would equilibrate with blood urea. Five exchanges of 2 L each and 2 L of ultrafiltration would be required for controlling uraemia. This method came to be called continuous ambulatory peritoneal dialysis (CAPD) [17]. The real revolution for CAPD came with the development of collapsible plastic bags for dialysate [18].

Interest in APD was revived by Diaz-Buzo *et al.* [19] and by Price and Suki [20]. They described the procedure called continuous cyclic peritoneal dialysis (CCPD) which is a form of automated equilibrium peritoneal dialysis. Patients receive three or four exchanges automatically at night and an additional exchange that remains in the abdomen through the day. The catheter is capped during the day and the patient starts the nocturnal exchange by emptying the peritoneal cavity. Connections and disconnections are minimized, reducing the incidence of peritonitis.

A dialysis procedure that combined intermittent and continuous-flow technology was introduced in the late 1960s and early 1970s to increase the efficiency of IPD. This technique was initially introduced as reciprocating peritoneal dialysis [21] and was later revived by Twardowski in 1989 and renamed tidal peritoneal dialysis (TPD) [22]. During this procedure, after an initial fill volume is instilled into the abdominal cavity, only part of the dialysate is drained and replaced by fresh peritoneal dialysis fluid with each cycle. The hypothesis behind this procedure is that leaving a 'sump volume' in the cavity would improve clearances, as there would be constant contact between the peritoneal membrane and dialysate.

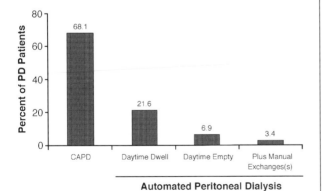

Figure 2. Method of peritoneal dialysis used by patients (USRDS: Dialysis Morbidity and Mortality Study (Wave 2) 1996) [5].

Peritoneal dialysis solutions

Peritoneal dialysis solutions are discussed in Chapter 8. The peritoneal dialysis solutions used for APD are similar in composition to those used in CAPD. The solutions are available in three different dextrose concentrations (1.5%, 2.5% and 4.25% dextrose). The dextrose concentrations used for shorter dwells are generally 1.5% or 2.5%; while for the long dwell the preferable concentration is 2.5% or 4.25% to prevent excessive fluid absorption. The composition of the standard peritoneal dialysis solution is provided in Table 1. A problem occasionally seen in APD modalities using short dwells (NIPD, TPD) is the development of hypernatraemia due to sodium sieving [23–26]. Dialysis solutions with lower sodium concentration should offset this problem.

There has been some concern that the more frequent exchanges during APD would cause a more rapid deterioration of the peritoneal membrane when compared with CAPD. The low pH and hyperosmolality of current dialysis solutions is toxic to mesothelial cells and peritoneal macrophages [27–29]. Glucose, *per se*, also affects the function and viability of peritoneal cells [28, 29]. Furthermore, glucose diffuses freely through the mesothelial layer and exposes the submesothelium to high dextrose concentrations [30]. This leads to the reduplication of the vascular basement membrane and the formation of advanced glycosylation end-products (AGEs) [31, 32]. In addition, it has been seen that degradation products of glucose that are produced during heat sterilization of dialysis solutions promote more rapid generation of AGEs [33]. These problems, plus the fact that glucose is rapidly absorbed from the peritoneal cavity causing a loss of ultrafiltration ability, metabolic complications and obesity, have prompted a search for newer osmotic agents.

Among all alternative osmotic agents, glucose polymers such as icodextrin appear most promising for APD [34]. Icodextrin can sustain ultrafiltration in long dwells with minimal absorption or damage

to the peritoneum. Furthermore, it produces less glycation of protein and appears more biocompatible [33]. The use of icodextrin in APD has been studied formally in two trials so far. In the first trial [35], which was of crossover design, patients received 7.5% icodextrin or were dry for the duration of the daytime dwell for 6 weeks; when on icodextrin, patients had improved Kt/V urea and creatinine clearances. In the second trial [36], patients were randomly selected to receive icodextrin or glucose based peritoneal dialysis solutions for 2 years. The study is ongoing, but published results available so far have shown that the use of icodextrin instead of glucose improved ultrafiltration and required less restriction of fluid intake. The icodextrin group also experienced a significant increase in their 24-h dialysate creatinine clearance; the gain in clearance could be explained by the improvement in ultrafiltration. Amino-acid-based peritoneal dialysis solutions may be an option for the malnourished patient on APD. A multicentre study has demonstrated a slight nutritional benefit with the use of a 1.1% amino acid solution in CAPD patients [37]. Further studies are required to see if the improvement in nutrition will equate to better outcomes. For adequate absorption on APD, the amino acid solutions would have to be used for the long dwell. A 1% amino acid solution provides ultrafiltration roughly equivalent to a 1.36% dextrose solution [38]. To achieve adequate ultrafiltration the amino acid solution may need to be combined with a glucose polymer [39].

Another new innovation, from the standpoint of APD, is the development of bicarbonate solutions. Automated cyclers, much like haemodialysis machines, can easily mix bicarbonate into the dialysate without requiring dual-chamber bags. Such bicarbonate-based solutions are more physiological, especially so for patients requiring dialysis for acute renal failure or those with hepatic dysfunction.

Peritoneal dialysis cyclers

The use of sophisticated software and hardware has made the present generation of cyclers safe, reliable, and easy to use. Current cyclers offer built-in programmes with options for all the varied modalities of automated peritoneal dialysis, including CCPD, classical IPD, NIPD, and TPD. These machines are programmable for dialysis modality, inflow volume, fill, dwell and drain times per cycle, and last bag fill options. The cyclers are equipped with a variety of

Table 1. Composition of standard solutions for automated peritoneal dialysis

Dextrose (%)	1.5–4.25
Sodium (mEq/L)	132
Potassium (mEq/L)	0
Calcium (mEq/L)	2.5–3.5
Magnesium (mEq/L)	0.5–1.5
Lactate (mEq/L)	35–40

alarms for the safety of the patient. These alarms monitor fill and drain volumes and rates, and the temperature of the fluid. Pump-based systems also monitor the pressure and resistance in the system.

Cyclers are now equipped with easy-to-install disposable tubing. The tubing manifold has several prongs for spiking dialysate bags and a single prong leading to the patient. The use of large-volume dialysate bags has reduced the costs of treatment, as well as the number of required connections. The dialysate is moved from the dialysate bags to a reservoir bag and then instilled into the patient. After the designated dwell time is complete, the dialysate is either emptied into a bag or drained directly. The movement of dialysate through the cycler and in and out of the patient is mediated by gravity, pump-driven systems, or a combination of the two. Fluid is preheated in the reservoir bag which is placed on a heater cradle. The preheating of the fluid is done more for the patients' comfort rather than to prevent hypothermia. Integrated scales allow accurate delivery of the fill volume and measurement of drainage and ultrafiltration volumes. Cyclers with paediatric treatment options can deliver volumes as small as 50 ml in 10 ml increments.

Some cyclers automatically monitor infusion and drainage rates and increase treatment efficacy by eliminating lag-time between exchanges. The machines also record and display details of various parameters of the treatment. Treatment data may be stored for up to 30 days on certain machines and transmitted by telephone line to the dialysis centre, allowing an assessment of compliance, as well as documentation of delivered dialysis. Cyclers have become increasingly compact, providing easy portability and convenience for patients.

Physiology

Physiological principles of solute and water transport are discussed extensively in Chapter 5. APD modalities differ from CAPD by the use of short dwell exchanges during the night. The shorter dwells during APD make membrane transport characteristics an important determinant of solute clearances.

Membrane transport characteristics

A major determinant of solute transport by diffusion is the diffusive mass transfer coefficient (MTC). The MTC is a term that represents the clearance rate that would be achieved in the absence of ultrafiltration and solute accumulation in the dialysate. Mathematically, MTC may be expressed as the product of membrane permeability and surface area [40–42]. The MTC values may be calculated from data acquired routinely during peritoneal equilibration tests [40, 43]. These calculations are complicated and the MTC is rarely ever estimated but for research purposes.

Today, the most commonly used technique to evaluate the peritoneal transport characteristic is to measure the dialysate to plasma solute concentration (D/P) for particular solutes during an exchange with conventional peritoneal fluid. This procedure has been standardized by Twardowski *et al.* and named the peritoneal equilibration test (PET) [44]. Patients are classified into four membrane categories: high, high average, low average, and low [44, 45].

High or rapid transporters tend to equilibrate small solute concentrations between dialysate and blood early in a dwell. These patients also absorb glucose early in the dwell. Once the osmotic gradient has dissipated, ultrafiltration ceases, and the dialysate returns are reduced because of reabsorption of fluid. These patients are best served by short dwell treatments. On the other hand, patients with low transport rates achieve peak ultrafiltration late during the dwell, and D/P ratios increase almost linearly over a long dwell. These patients benefit from continuous regimens, as the total dialysis time is crucial for adequate clearances [46]. These principles are illustrated in Table 2 and Fig. 3.

Table 2. Prognostic value of the baseline peritoneal equilibration test results

Solute transport	Ultrafiltration	Clearance	Preferred modality
High	Poor	Adequate	NIPD, CCPD, TPD
High-average	Adequate	Adequate	CAPD, CCPD, NIPD + CAPD, TPD + CAPD
Low-average	Good	Adequate or inadequate	CAPD, CCPD, CCPD + CAPD
Low	Excellent	Inadequate	CAPD, HD

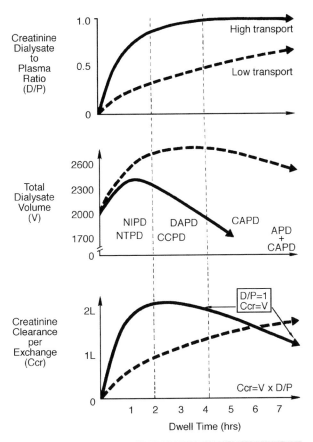

Figure 3. Idealized curves of creatinine and water transport during exchange with 2 L of 2.5% glucose dialysis solution in patients with extremely low and high peritoneal transport characteristics. Upper panel shows dialysate to plasma ratio (D/P); middle panel shows total dialysate volume (V), which is the sum of infusion volume and ultrafiltration; lower panel shows creatinine clearance per exchange (C_{cr}). The curves in the lower panel are derived from those of the upper and middle panels. ———, high peritoneal transport; – – – –, low peritoneal transport. (From ref. 46 with permission.)

Diffusive transport of solutes

The diffusive transport of solutes is a function of the MTC, dialysate flow rate, peritoneal capillary blood flow rate, concentration gradient, and time allowed for transport [47]. In a graph of urea clearance versus dialysate flow (Fig. 4), there is an initial portion of the curve that corresponds with the dialysate flow rates typical of CAPD (three to five exchanges per day). In this region of the curve there is a steep correlation between urea clearance and dialysate flow rates. CAPD is, therefore, dialysate flow limited, and improved clearances may be achieved by increasing the number and/or the volume of exchanges. The second region of this curve is typical

for APD. This region is affected both by the dialysate flow rate and MTC. As dialysate flow is increased in automated regimens, the dwell times become shorter, and an increasing proportion of exchange time is occupied by the inflow and drainage times [48]. Although clearances may be improved by increasing dialysate flow, a point of diminished return will eventually be reached.

Several factors impact the MTC; important from the APD standpoint are the position during dialysis and the dialysate exchange volume (V_{ip}). Using the same V_{ip}, the MTC for urea and creatinine were increased 24% and 19% in one study [49], and 15% and 9%, respectively in another study [50] in the supine position when compared with the upright position. In the supine position the dialysate layers throughout the entire abdominal cavity, while in the upright position dialysate pools in the subumbilical region of the abdomen. The increase in the MTC is caused by increased contact of dialysate with the peritoneal membrane. Additionally, in the supine position, dialysate is more accessible to the peritoneal membrane around the liver [50]. The peritoneal membrane around the liver accounts for up to 45% of the total MTC for the entire peritoneal cavity [51]. Portal blood flow also increases in the supine position [52].

Schoenfeld *et al.* [53] observed a strong linear relationship between the peritoneal transport constant and V_{ip}. These correlations occurred over a range of 1 to 3.8 L of V_{ip}. Keshaviah *et al.* [54] found that the V_{ip} associated with peak MTC increased with increasing body surface area, being approximately 2.5 L for an average-sized patient, and increasing to between 3 and 3.5 L for patients with surface areas larger than 2 m². Once the maximal MTC is achieved, further increases in the V_{ip} provide no additional benefit and may actually cause a decline in the MTC. In summary, increasing the V_{ip} is a more effective means of increasing solute clearances than more frequent exchanges with lower V_{ip}. This practice also reduces dialysate transit time, or the non-dialytic period, and improves clearances.

Solute transport by convection

The magnitude of convective transport is determined by the ultrafiltration rate for the peritoneal membrane, the average solute concentrations within the membrane [55] and the sieving coefficient (S, describing the fraction of solute which passes through the membrane with a water flow: $0 \leqslant S \leqslant 1$) [25, 26].

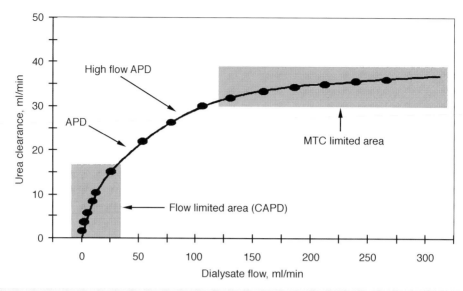

Figure 4. Relationship between urea clearance in peritoneal dialysis and dialysate flow rate. (From ref. 48 with permission.)

Although the sieving effect influences each solute, the important clinical consequence of sieving is related to sodium. The ultrafiltrate is usually low in sodium. Thus, dialysate sodium concentration is initially reduced in the dialysate and tends to increase late in the dwell due to diffusion of sodium into the dialysate and diminished ultrafiltration in longer dwells [23–26]. During APD with shorter dwells, the net electrolyte removal per litre of ultrafiltrate remains far below the extracellular fluid concentration and severe hypernatraemia and hyperosmolality may develop [56]. For such purposes the use of lower sodium dialysate may be necessary [24].

Ultrafiltration

The net ultrafiltration is determined by the difference between the transcapillary ultrafiltration and absorption of fluid from the peritoneal cavity. The transcapillary ultrafiltration gradient is dependent on the hydraulic permeability of the peritoneum, its effective surface area, the hydrostatic pressure gradient, and the colloid and crystalloid osmotic pressure gradients [55, 57–60]. We have already discussed issues regarding the membrane permeability characteristics and their influence on ultrafiltration. The hydrostatic pressure in the peritoneal capillaries may be assumed to be 17 mmHg [61]. The opposing hydraulic pressure in the peritoneal cavity (intra-abdominal pressure) varies depending on posture and activities, and the V_{ip} [62, 63]. Durand *et al.* [64] evaluated the effects of intra-abdominal pressure (IAP) on net ultrafiltration volume. Twenty-

three patients were studied; all received a 2-L exchange (4.25% dextrose) and had a dwell time of 2 h. The net ultrafiltration varied inversely with mean IAP. An increase in the mean IAP by 1 cmH$_2$O caused a decrease of 74 ml in net ultrafiltration at the end of the 2-h dwell. Elevated IAP, however, increases lymphatic absorption significantly more than it decreases transcapillary ultrafiltration [65].

The colloid osmotic gradient in the peritoneal capillaries averages 26 mmHg [61]. The dialysate contains little protein and thus does not generate a colloid osmotic pressure. Therefore, the capillary osmotic pressure supports back-filtration [66]. The transperitoneal crystalloid osmotic gradient is established by dextrose. The gradient is maximal at the beginning of the dwell and gets dissipated during the dwell following glucose absorption from the dialysate and the dilutional effect contributed by ultrafiltration. Shorter dwells capitalize on the maximal rate of net ultrafiltration, especially in rapid transporters. Most of the net ultrafiltration takes place during the short dwells in APD [44, 45]. Patients with prolonged day dwells may absorb a significant percentage of their diurnal dwell even with the use of 4.25% dextrose solutions.

Lymphatic absorption

Along with ultrafiltration, there is a constant absorption of fluid from the peritoneal cavity. Fluid and solutes are reabsorbed directly by the lymphatics and also by a process of back-filtration into the peritoneal interstitium [58–60]. Fluid and solutes entering the peritoneal interstitium are taken up by the local lymphatics and capillaries. The IAP is a major determinant of ergress of fluid from the abdominal cavity into the tissues lining the peritoneal membrane [59, 60, 67, 68] and consequently the IAP influences the lymphatic absorption rate [65].

The subdiaphragmatic lymphatics account for the major portion of the fluid reabsorbed by lymphatics [58]. Lymphatic absorption is dependent on diaphragmatic movements and contact of fluid with the diaphragm. There is an increased contact of fluid with the subdiaphragm in the supine position and enhanced fluid absorption [69]. Thus, in supine APD, two conflicting variables affect lymphatic fluid reabsorption: one, the lower IAP and two, the increased contact of fluid with the subdiaphragm.

Relationship between intraperitoneal volume and IAP

The empty peritoneal cavity has an IAP of 0.5–2.2 cmH$_2$O. The IAP rises in direct proportion to the amount of fluid infused into the abdominal cavity. This relationship is maintained regardless of the patient's position, but the slope of the curve does shift with changes in position. For any intraperitoneal volume, IAP is minimized by assuming the supine position; sitting leads to the highest pressures, and standing results in intraperitoneal pressures between those seen with sitting and lying down [62, 63, 70, 71]. Therefore, the same or larger volumes of dialysate are better tolerated while the patient is supine than during times of activity (Fig. 5).

Measurement of IAP may be an optimal method for determining the appropriate fill volume for dialysis. The maximal acceptable IAP in APD is probably 18 cmH$_2$O. IAP above 20 cmH$_2$O are associated with symptoms and a decrease in the vital capacity [72].

Dialysate fill and drain profiles

It is generally known that dialysate fill rate is a function of fill height and patient position. Fill rate in the supine position is greater, in part, due to the lower intraperitoneal pressure in the supine position than in the upright position. The characteristic drain profile shows a bimodal pattern with high drain volumes for the initial 5–7 min, during which time over 80% of the dialysate is drained; followed by a very abrupt transition to a very slow drain rate (Fig. 6) [49, 73]. The reason for this abrupt transition between outflow rates may be due to the

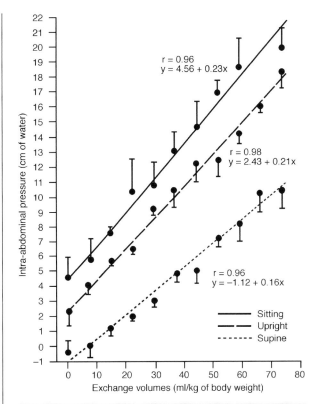

Figure 5. Comparative effect of dialysate volume and patient position on intra-abdominal pressure. Mean $\pm$ SEM. Symbols are: ———, sitting position; ––––––, upright position; ......, supine position during dialysis. (From ref. 71 with permission.)

bowels collapsing on the catheter as the transition volume is approached, causing a significant reduction in outflow.

From the above discussion it is clear that a majority of the drain time during each cycle in APD is spent removing a small percentage of the total dialysate. Shortening the total drain time to include only the initial high outflow period will increase urea clearance up to 10% during an 8-h APD treatment assuming six cycles with a total dialysate flow of 12 L in a patient with average membrane permeability (urea MTC approximately 15 ml/min). The increase in urea clearance is the result of increased dwell time with maximal dialysate volume [49]. Tidal peritoneal dialysis, wherein a tidal volume is exchanged in each cycle, utilizes only the rapid drain segment and obtains maximal benefit of this mechanism. Increasing drain height can also shorten the drain rates. Larger-bore catheters do not provide better fill rates, but may decrease the drain time [49].

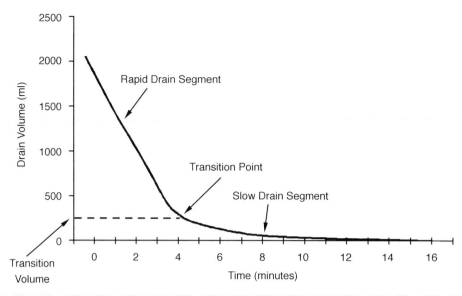

Figure 6. Representative dialysate drain profile. (From ref. 49 with permission.)

Factors influencing selection of APD

APD is the fastest-growing modality of peritoneal dialysis worldwide. However, there is a high variance in the use of APD in different areas of the world. Medical limitations, physician education and biases, availability and cost of equipment and supplies, patient preferences, social reasons, and reimbursement concerns impact the selection of dialysis modality [74].

The choice of APD over CAPD should initially be based on the patient's preference [75]. The increased convenience of these treatments makes them more suitable for patients who have work commitments during the day or are dependent on assistance from others. APD is the modality of choice in children and adolescents. The main reasons for these are the following: peritoneal diffusion is higher in children [76], freedom from bag exchanges in the daytime, no need for venipunctures, and no major effect on the work schedule of their parents [77, 78]. Elderly patients and those with manual or visual impairments, desirous of home peritoneal dialysis are best treated by APD to prevent overwhelming their partners or helpers [78, 79]. Patients, especially children who develop psychosocial problems due to distortion of body image by a protruding abdomen, should also be treated by APD [77].

From a physiological standpoint the choice of peritoneal dialysis modality is best guided by the nature of the peritoneal membrane transport charac-teristics. Optimum therapy is achieved by matching dwell times to the transport type of the patient. These principles have been discussed earlier and are well illustrated in Table 2 and Fig. 3 [44–46]. NIPD may be an option for patients with ultrafiltration failure due to rapid glucose absorption [75].

APD is a viable option for patients with complications due to increased intra-abdominal pressure (hernias, dialysate leaks, haemorrhoids, uterine prolapse, and back pain). From our earlier discussion, IAP is much lower in the supine position for the same dialysate exchange volume. Patients with frequent peritonitis episodes may benefit by switching to APD with its lower incidence of peritonitis [75].

However, APD is not an option for all patients. Higher costs due to the need of a cycler, disposable tubing, and generally larger dialysis volumes serve as a deterrent. Some patients may not accept the prolonged restriction to bed for the duration of overnight cycles or the dependence on a machine. There is a potential for sleep disturbances by machine alarms [79]. Sodium sieving may lead to hypernatraemia, increased thirst, and poor blood pressure control [56].

Different regimens of APD

Continuous cyclic peritoneal dialysis

Continuous cyclic peritoneal dialysis (CCPD) is the only continuous automated peritoneal dialysis regimen (Fig. 7). The technique is essentially a reversal

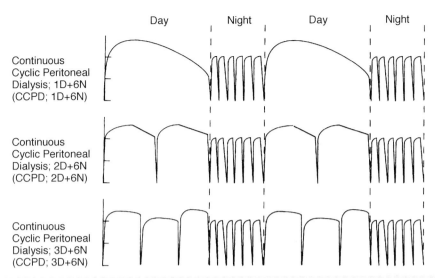

Figure 7. Continuous cyclic peritoneal dialysis (CCPD). Upper panel shows standard CCPD with last bag fill; middle and lower panels show CCPD combined with additional daytime exchanges. (From ref. 2 with permission.)

of CAPD where the shorter exchanges are automatically provided at night while the longer exchanges are performed during the day. An automated cycler is used to deliver three to five nocturnal cycles, each lasting 2.5–3 h. After the last nocturnal cycle the cycler is programmed to deliver a final exchange (last bag fill) of hypertonic dialysate [2].

Small solute clearances are slightly lower in CCPD than in CAPD for the same dialysate flow [80, 81]. The total weekly clearances of middle molecules are the same as CAPD. The solute clearances may be improved by increasing the V_{ip}, increasing the number of nightly exchanges and occasionally combining one or more daytime exchanges [81, 82]. These daytime exchanges may be performed manually or by hooking back to the cycler.

This regimen is best suited for schoolchildren and employed patients who are frequently unable or unwilling to perform daytime exchanges. Patients requiring assistance in performance of dialysis are better served by CCPD than CAPD. Connections and disconnections may be minimized to two, reducing burden on the provider. This is obviously an ideal choice for institutionalized patients. CCPD may be combined with CAPD for patients with below-average peritoneal membrane permeability who are under-dialysed on CAPD.

Classical intermittent peritoneal dialysis

Intermittent peritoneal dialysis (IPD) is a term used for dialysis regimens wherein periods on dialysis alternate with those when the peritoneal cavity is dry [2]. During classical IPD the patient receives several short dwell exchanges over 12–24 h with a dialysis dose between 40 and 60 L, several times a week but usually not every day. Though the procedure can be performed manually, automated cyclers or systems with on-line generation of dialysate are more practical. Treatments may take place in-centre or at home.

Classical IPD has fallen into disfavour as a modality of chronic renal replacement therapy because of poor clearances and high morbidity and mortality [13–15]. However, the procedure continues to be used in countries where there are few alternatives for dialysis [83]. A recent report recommended the use of IPD for patients with ESRD and significant residual renal function [84]. IPD may serve as an alternative to haemodialysis for short-term therapy in patients needing immediate dialysis after peritoneal catheter placement. Small-volume supine dialysis is recommended during this period of catheter break-in. Cheng *et al.* [85] reported a higher incidence of pericatheter leaks, especially amongst diabetics started on IPD during the break-in period. IPD may be used as a transient therapy for patients who have hernias or leaks or those who have recently undergone abdominal surgery. Some leaks may spontaneously seal off with lower intra-abdominal pressures on supine IPD.

Another area of application of IPD is refractory heart failure on maximal medical therapy. Several studies have documented the reduction in morbidity days, and improvement in functional status [86–88].

Nocturnal intermittent peritoneal dialysis

Nocturnal intermittent peritoneal dialysis (NIPD) is an intermittent dialysis regimen performed every night, and may be considered to be similar to CCPD with a dry day (Fig. 8) [2]. NIPD treatments are performed overnight on a cycler. The dialysis usually lasts between 8 and 12 h. Dialysate volumes of 8–12 L per night are used for therapy, and even larger volumes of dialysate are required for anuric patients.

The dry days eliminate about 20% of small solute clearances achieved in a patient who is an average transporter on nightly cycles plus a wet day. Treatment of patients with NIPD has a greater impact on the clearance of middle molecules. The clearance of middle molecules is a time-dependent process, and dry days reduce clearances by 50% [89].

NIPD has been recommended as an optimal modality for those with complications due to elevated intraperitoneal pressure who are unwilling or are not candidates for haemodialysis. Patients with high transport characteristics and those with type I ultrafiltration failure may also be treated with NIPD [46, 75]. Those patients with high levels of residual renal function may initially be treated with NIPD. This modality is not an option for large body surface area subjects and those with average or below-average transport characteristics without significant residual renal function as adequacy parameters cannot be met [89]. NIPD does offer the psychosocial advantage of a better body image and lower glucose absorption leading to a better appetite. The costs of treatment run higher than with CAPD, and patients often do not accept the prolonged confinement to bed. Additionally, sodium sieving and the consequent low sodium in the ultrafiltrate may lead to hypernatraemia, increased thirst, and worsening hypertension [56]. Most NIPD patients use dialysis solutions with a standard sodium concentration of 132 mEq/L. A 5% glucose solution (D5W) may be mixed with peritoneal dialysis solutions in appropriate proportions to achieve lower dialysate sodium concentrations [46]. The marketing of dialysis solutions with lower sodium should eventually overcome this problem.

Tidal peritoneal dialysis

Tidal peritoneal dialysis (TPD) is a regimen combining intermittent and continuous-flow technology. The procedure increases efficiency by maintaining a reserve volume in the peritoneal cavity at all times, providing for uninterrupted solute clearance [22, 90]. A tidal volume is introduced and drained during each cycle (Fig. 8). Prediction of ultrafiltration is important to assure the reserve volume remains unchanged. If ultrafiltration volumes are overestimated, the reserve volume would gradually be depleted. If ultrafiltration volumes are underestimated, the reserve volume will

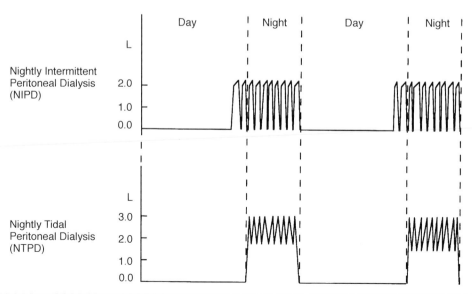

Figure 8. Nightly peritoneal dialysis. Upper panel shows nightly intermittent peritoneal dialysis; lower panel shows nightly tidal peritoneal dialysis. (From ref. 2 with permission.)

gradually increase leading to abdominal discomfort. The most efficient dialysis may be achieved by maintaining a reserve volume of at least 15 ml/kg body weight. With such reserve volume the major determinants of TPD efficiency are the MTC and the dialysate flow rates [91].

Initial studies by Twardowski *et al.* [22] demonstrated that TPD was approximately 20% more effective than NIPD at dialysis flow rates of 3.25–3.5 L per hour. Flanigan and co-workers [90] have shown that TPD can provide equivalent clearances to CCPD in 8 h as compared to 10 h, however, utilizing 16.0 L of dialysate versus 9.5 L for CCPD. Protein losses were not increased on TPD.

A study comparing solute clearances and ultrafiltration on TPD and NIPD found with dialysate flow rates of 18.5 ml/min, solute clearances and ultrafiltration volumes were higher on IPD than on TPD. With flow rates of 25.9 ml/min the ultrafiltration volume was higher on IPD, but no difference was found for solute clearance. At flow rates of 44.4 ml/min there was no difference in ultrafiltration or solute clearances between the two modalities [92]. Another study utilizing very high dialysate flow rates (158.7 ml/min for TPD and 103.0 ml/min for IPD) found higher clearances on TPD [93]. These studies show that at low flow rates the clearances on IPD are better than TPD. Exchanges are few and little time is lost performing exchanges. The advantage of TPD with a continuous contact between the peritoneal surface and dialysis fluid may be offset by the negative influence of a smaller concentration gradient between dialysate and blood. It has been suggested that this result may be caused by inadequate mixing of the tidal volume with the reserve volume. At higher flow rates, clearances for intermittent techniques reach a plateau and fall as more time is required to fill and drain the peritoneal cavity. In this setting TPD allows for higher clearances than IPD.

The indications for TPD are the same as NIPD. Patients experiencing pain at the beginning of inflow and/or the end of drain may obtain relief by switching to TPD (see Chapter 9). Combining CAPD and TPD may extend the option to larger anuric patients or those with low transport characteristics [94]. The major disadvantage is the use of large volumes of dialysate, making the costs of treatment prohibitive. On-line production of dialysate at lower costs may be the future for this method.

Night exchange device and the peritoneal dialysis plus concept

The night exchange device (NXD) allows CAPD patients one or more night-time exchanges while reducing patient burden and improving clearances (Fig. 9). Though several patients on four or less exchanges may opt for this device as a lifestyle choice, the NXD is extremely helpful for patients prescribed five or more exchanges [3].

There is a physiological and kinetic advantage to using this system. Equilibrium of urea between peritoneal dialysis solutions and plasma occurs within 3–6 h of dwell. Dwell times longer than 6 h do not contribute any further to the removal of small solutes and require higher concentrations of dextrose to maintain ultrafiltration. In terms of efficiency, four exchanges every 6 h are more effective than two short and two long dwells [95]. The supine position for the night-time exchange(s) offers an opportunity to use higher V_{ip} maximizing the MTC without an increase in the IAP [54, 63, 71]. Furthermore, patients retaining fluid due to the longer dwell at night on CAPD may also benefit from using the NXD. Patients switching to NXD only for lifestyle reasons, with no change in the number of exchanges, experience only a slight improvement in their solute clearances over baseline. In patients advised an additional exchange, the clearances increase significantly [96]. However, higher clearances would have been achieved by increasing the V_{ip} using a similar total dialysate volume without changing the number of exchanges [54].

The major advantage of NXD is to help achieve adequacy in CAPD, as well as positive fluid balance in patients retaining fluid overnight. Further aspects of this concept are discussed in depth elsewhere in this book.

Adequacy of peritoneal dialysis

Solute clearances and adequacy

Adequate dialysis is defined as the dose of dialysis below which one observes a significant worsening of morbidity and mortality. The National Cooperative Dialysis Study (NCDS) [97] on haemodialysis gave rise to the concept that small solute clearances influence patient morbidity and mortality significantly, and these data were extrapolated to the peritoneal dialysis population. Several studies have confirmed the importance of small solute clearances in defining adequacy among peritoneal dialysis patients [98–104]. At the present time, either urea clearance [Kt, (L/week)] normalized to total body water [V, (L)] and/or total creatinine clearance (C_{cr}) normalized to standardized body surface area (BSA) are used to monitor solute clearances. The con-

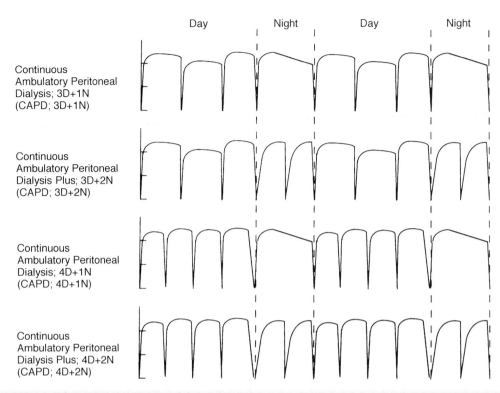

Figure 9. Continuous ambulatory peritoneal dialysis (CAPD) and the use of the night exchange device (NXD). Panel 1 shows CAPD – three daytime exchanges and one bedtime exchange; panel 2 shows CAPD Plus – three daytime exchanges, one bedtime exchange, and an additional exchange delivered by the NXD; panel 3 shows CAPD – four daytime exchanges and one bedtime exchange; panel 4 shows CAPD Plus – four daytime exchanges, one bedtime exchange and an additional night-time exchange delivered by the NXD.

tribution of middle molecules (500–30 000 Da) to uraemic toxicity is controversial. Large solutes such as β_2-microglobulin (MW $\sim$ 12 000), parathormone (MW $\sim$ 9000), and granulocyte inhibition protein (MW $\sim$ 28 000) have been shown to have a pathogenetic role in causing some of the manifestations of uraemia [105–107]. Thus, removal of these solutes could have a bearing on dialysis-related morbidity and mortality [108]. Middle molecules are cleared via diffusive transport, as well as ultrafiltration. The removal of middle molecules is a function of the membrane area, membrane permeability, and time. Since time is the only variable, the total duration of dialysis is critical for the removal of middle molecule waste. During automated peritoneal dialysis the shorter night-time exchanges provide a higher urea clearance than creatinine clearance. Long dwells during the day contribute significantly to the clearance of middle molecules. The clearance of middle molecules in CCPD appears to be similar to CAPD. However, in NIPD with dry days, the time available for dialysis is reduced by 50%, and this dramatically reduces the clearance of middle molecules [89].

Besides the biochemical markers for adequacy, adequate dialysis should provide a feeling of well-being, absence of uraemic symptoms, and a reasonable control of acid–base and electrolyte disturbances. Adequate nutrition, prevention of atherosclerosis and bone disease are equally important considerations.

The adequacy data

The CANUSA Study [98] was a prospective cohort study of nutrition and adequacy in peritoneal dialysis involving 680 patients from 14 centres in Canada and the United States (see Chapter 27). A total of 97.9% of the patients were treated with CAPD and 2.1% with CCPD. During the study, peritoneal clearances were not increased to offset declines in renal function. Since the residual renal function (RRF) decreased over time and the dialysis dose did not change, one of the important predictors of outcome was not peritoneal solute clearance, but RRF. Furthermore, the CANUSA, as well as other studies, have not been able to show a predictive effect on outcome for peritoneal clearances of small molecules independent of RRF. Nevertheless, there is a general consensus that such a relationship exists. A total creatinine clearance at the start of therapy of 70 L/week and a total of Kt/V of 2.1 (i.e. peritoneal plus RRF) was associated with a patient survival of 78% at 2 years. Teehan et al. [99] found the 5-year survival for patients with a Kt/V urea >1.89 exceeded 90%. A prospective study by Maiorca and colleagues [100], describing a group of patients who had been on peritoneal dialysis for a mean duration of 35 months and had relatively lower levels of RRF, showed that patients with a $Kt/V > 1.96$ had improved survival compared to those with a $Kt/V < 1.96$. Again, the difference between survivals was attributed to the level of RRF. Genestier and associates [101] reported that patients with an initial weekly $Kt/V < 1.7$ had a relative risk of death of 1.69; and the relative risk of death with $C_{cr} < 50$ L/1.73 m² was 4.88. There is very little data available on the relationship of solute clearances with outcomes on automated peritoneal dialysis.

The adequacy recommendations

For CAPD, the CANUSA authors [98] suggested a target Kt/V of 2.1 and a total creatinine clearance of 70 L/1.73 m² BSA. A more realistic goal for CAPD would be a total weekly Kt/V of >2.0 and a total weekly creatinine clearance of >60 L/1.73 m². These are in accord with the guidelines by the Dialysis Outcomes Quality Initiative (DOQI) Committee of the National Kidney Foundation [109]. As previously mentioned, there is a paucity of studies on the relationship of solute clearances to outcomes for patients on automated peritoneal dialysis. Data from studies on CAPD patients have been extrapolated for arriving at recommendations for adequacy for APD modalities. The rationale for these recommendations is discussed below.

NIPD is an intermittent therapy. It is reasonable to aim for higher target clearances for intermittent therapies than for continuous therapies. This reasoning finds its basis in the peak concentration hypothesis of Keshaviah et al. [110] which states the peak concentration of uraemic wastes corresponds to the development of uraemic symptoms. They indicated that for a weekly haemodialysis Kt/V of 4.0, the corresponding CAPD weekly Kt/V would be 2.0 [111]. This consideration has further been supported by the finding that survival of CAPD and haemodialysis patients is similar after adjusting for

comorbid conditions provided the dialysis dose is comparable [112].

Using calculations based on the 200% increase in the intermittent haemodialysis clearance required to achieve the same solute clearance as in CAPD while holding protein intake constant, the theoretical difference between CAPD and NIPD clearance would be 8%. Based on this assumption, the Working Group of DOQI [109] recommended that the delivered dose of NIPD would need to be 8% higher than CAPD (108% of 2.0 = 2.16, rounded up to 2.2). The Working Group also assumed that the requisite delivered dose of CCPD would be intermediate between those for CAPD and NIPD. Some variations of CCPD with diurnal exchanges of less duration than the nocturnal exchange of CAPD may be considered equal to CAPD. However, to simplify recommendations, the target Kt/V for CCPD is 2.1. The recommendations for creatinine clearance are percentage adjustments corresponding to the changes in Kt/V urea targets for these groups (Table 3).

The variables in achieving adequacy

To optimize a patient's peritoneal dialysis prescription, one must be cognizant of the patient's body surface area (BSA), peritoneal membrane permeability properties and amount of residual renal function [80, 113]. The presence of RRF makes it easier to achieve clearance guidelines. Each 1 ml/min of corrected residual renal creatinine clearance (C_{cr}) adds approximately 10 L/week/1.73 m² of creatinine clearance to the total C_{cr}. Similarly, for each 1 ml/min of urea clearance, 0.25 is added to the total weekly Kt/V for a 70 kg male. The RRF declines with time, and peritoneal dialysis prescriptions should be adjusted to maintain adequacy criteria. Though renal function is better preserved in peritoneal dialysis patients than in haemodialysis patients [114–116], there has been a report suggesting a

Table 3. Target doses of dialysis for peritoneal dialysis [109]

Modality	Weekly Kt/V urea	Weekly creatinine clearance (corrected to 1.73 m² BSA)
CAPD	>2.0	>60 L
CCPD	>2.1	>63 L
NIPD	>2.2	>60 L

These recommendations are based on total clearance (renal and peritoneal). The renal creatinine clearance is calculated as the sum average of the renal urea and creatinine clearance.

more rapid rate of decline of RRF in APD than CAPD [117].

The peritoneal transport characteristics are determined by the PET [45], by mass transfer of urea coefficients [40–42], or by the standard permeability analysis [118]. The effect of peritoneal transport in influencing dialysis prescription is both direct via solute clearance, and indirect via influencing ultrafiltration. A study assessing peritoneal transport characteristics of 806 patients found the group consisted of 5.6% low transporters, 30.9% low average transporters, 53.1% high average transporters, and 10.6% high transporters [119]. Low transporters are difficult to treat with APD for reasons mentioned earlier. Body surface area and body weight affect the requirements for dialysis. Among the US dialysis population, 75% of patients have a BSA >1.71 m^2 and a median BSA of 1.85 m^2 [119].

The variables that may be manipulated in achieving adequacy are the dialysis modality, fill volume, number of exchanges and spacing, and duration of exchanges [80]. Several computer-assisted kinetic modelling programs are available that help in modelling prescriptions [120–122]. These prescriptions have reasonably close correlation with the actual measurement of 24-h urine and dialysate clearances. Kinetic modelling is not meant to replace the actual measurement of clearance.

Achieving the adequacy guidelines

For some patients, achieving the recommended clearance guidelines may require a substantial increase in dialysis prescription. This raises the concern that targets may be achieved by an unacceptable increase in the cost of dialysis and/or a deterioration in the patients' quality of life. The benefits of increasing clearance must be balanced with the risks for some patients associated with larger fill volumes. The increase in intra-abdominal pressure associated with large V_{ip} may lead to hernias in predisposed individuals and may also lead to increased fluid absorption and less net ultrafiltration. Increased glucose absorption associated with larger fill volumes is also another important consideration [81].

Computer prescription programs have been used to model 12 standardized patients on different dialysis regimens and to predict clearances. These standardized patients were based on one of three ranges of BSA (those with BSA <1.71 m^2, those between 1.71 and 20 m^2, and those >2.0 m^2) and four PET categories. NIPD prescriptions of 15 L of 2.5%

dextrose over 9 h failed in all patients to achieve the recommended NIPD target creatinine clearance of 66 L/week/1.73 m^2 BSA (Fig. 10); increasing the dialysate volume to 20 L and delivering this over 10 h also failed (Fig. 11) [89]. These observations are consistent with earlier reports [123, 124]. Jensen *et al.* [123] found that anephric low transporters above 33 kg standard body weight cannot achieve adequate clearances, while high transporters weighing up to 66 kg may achieve clearance targets. Thus, the use of NIPD (dry days) should be restricted to patients with very small BSA, generally high transporters, or those with significant residual renal function [89, 124, 125]. Increasing the overnight total solution may not always provide additional clearance, especially in low and low-average transporters. Adding a 'wet day' may be more beneficial than increasing the number of overnight exchanges. Total clearance may also be improved by increasing the fill volume and/or lengthening the dwell time and the total treatment time (Fig. 12) [81].

Concerning CCPD in anuric patients, Blake and colleagues [81] observed that, even for small patients with a BSA of <1.71 m^2, a prescription of 4×2 L at night and 2 L during the day, would achieve the target clearance only in high transporters. With a fill volume of 2.5 L, adequacy still would not be achieved in the low and low-average transporters. In patients with a BSA of 1.71–2.0 m^2 on 2.5 L $\times$ 4 at night, 2.5 L during the day prescription, adequacy would only be achieved in the high transporters; increasing the fill volume to 3 L would yield adequacy for all except low transporters. For patients with a BSA >2.0 m^2, a 3 L $\times$ 4 nightly and a 3 L daytime exchange regimen achieves adequacy only in the high and high-average transport category. Adding one or more daytime exchanges may help in achieving adequacy (Fig. 12). In patients who have lost residual renal function, it may not be possible to achieve the DOQI guidelines for both creatinine and Kt/V urea. This is particularly notable in patients with less than high solute transport rates [126].

Tidal peritoneal dialysis utilizes the principle of restricting outflow time to increase efficiency. In large, muscular anuric patients, Twardowski and Nolph [94] have theoretically calculated the possibility of increasing dialysis efficiency by using nightly TPD (NTPD) combined with high-volume exchanges during the day. Using 40 L of dialysis solution in 6 h with a 30-min exchange time for NTPD, the authors were hypothetically able to achieve weekly clearances at levels that can only

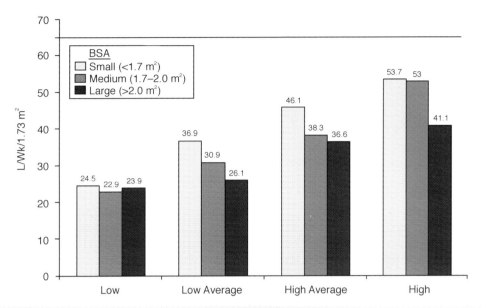

Figure 10. Creatinine clearance, NIPD 2.5 L exchange over 9 h, total volume 15 L, 2.5% dextrose, functionally anephric. (From ref. 89 with permission.)

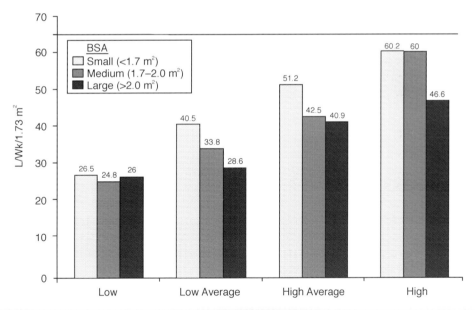

Figure 11. Creatinine clearance, NIPD 2.5 L exchange over 10 h, total volume 21 L, 2.5% dextrose, functionally anephric. (From ref. 89 with permission.)

be achieved in patients on NIPD who have residual renal function. They hypothesized that this modality may be acceptable to some patients and preferable to a switch to haemodialysis. These are, however, entirely hypothetical calculations which need to be validated by clinical studies. At present no cyclers are capable of delivering this amount of therapy.

For patients initiating therapy and desirous of APD, NIPD should probably not be used until a PET has been performed, unless they have substantial residual renal function. Initial guidelines for APD treatment based on BSA and residual renal function have been provided by the Working Group of the DOQI (Table 4) [109]. Further, general guidelines for APD therapy are provided in Table 5.

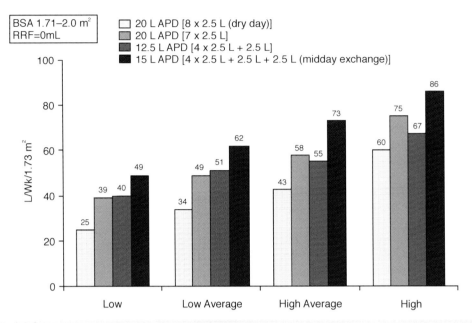

Figure 12. The effect on creatinine clearance of wet days, increasing the number of exchanges, and adding a midday exchange to APD therapy prescriptions. The difference compared with a dry day is illustrated clearly in the first two bars of each membrane transport type. The effect of a midday exchange is shown in the last bar. (From ref. 81 with permission.)

Table 4. Possible initial empirical dialysis prescriptions for CCPD [109]

For patients with an estimated underlying GFR >2 ml/min
  BSA <1.7 m²   4 × 2.0 L (9 h/night) + 2.0 L/day
  BSA 1.7–2.0 m²   4 × 2.5 L (9 h/night) + 2.0 L/day
  BSA >2.0 m²   4 × 3.0 L (9 h/night) + 3.0 L/day

For patients with an estimated underlying GFR ⩽2 ml/min
  BSA <1.7 m²   4 × 2.5 L (9 h/night) + 2.0 L/day
  BSA 1.7–2.0 m²   4 × 3.0 L (9 h/night) + 2.5 L/day
  BSA >2.0 m²   4 × 3.0 L (10 h/night) + 2 × 3.0 L/day[a]

GFR = glomerular filtration rate; BSA = body surface area.
[a] Consider combined haemodialysis/peritoneal dialysis or transfer to haemodialysis if the clinical situation suggests the need. These empirical prescriptions are based on modelling for patients with dialysate-to-plasma creatinine concentration ratio on PET of 0.71 at 4 h, BSA in the range above, and corrected residual renal function of 2 ml/min or 0 ml/min.

Incremental peritoneal dialysis

The decision to initiate dialysis was until recently based on the development of uraemic symptoms or complications. Current recommendations adopted by the Working Group of the DOQI [127] suggest that dialysis should be initiated once the renal Kt/V urea falls below 2.0 or the normalized protein nitrogen appearance spontaneously declines below 0.8 g/kg/day. A renal Kt/V urea of 2.0 corresponds to a urea clearance of 7.0 ml/min and a creatinine clearance between 9 and 14 ml/min/1.73 m² BSA.

Table 5. General guidelines for APD therapy

1. APD prescriptions should be individualized based on membrane permeability, RRF, and BSA.
2. Dialysis modality should be based on the ability of the regimen to provide adequate dialysis, the patients' preference, and their ability to perform the procedure.
3. Computer prescription programs may be useful in designing prescriptions. Kinetic modelling, however, cannot replace actual clinical measurements of clearance.
4. Nightly intermittent peritoneal dialysis regimens should be avoided in all patients except high transporters with small body surface area or substantial RRF.
5. Anuric patients with low or low-average membrane transport characteristics should not be offered APD.
6. Delivered dose of dialysis and RRF should be periodically monitored. Prescriptions should be modified for a decline of RRF.
7. Clearances may be maximized by increasing the V_{ip}, minimizing drain time, and adding daytime exchanges.
8. Icodextrin may be used for the long dwell to improve clearances and ultrafiltration.
9. The V_{ip} should be optimized by using IAP measurements. The maximal tolerated IAP is 18 cmH₂O of water measured from the mid-axillary line.
10. Compliance with prescriptions should be verified periodically.

RRF = residual renal function; BSA = body surface area; V_{ip} = intra-peritoneal exchange volume; IAP = intra-abdominal pressure.

The rationale behind early or 'healthy start' is to avoid malnutrition and uraemic complications. The data of Ikizler *et al.* [128], McCusker *et al.* [129], and Pollock *et al.* [130] strongly demonstrate a linkage between declining renal function and worsening nutritional status. Malnutrition in dialysis patients has been shown to be associated with poor outcomes [99, 131, 132]. While the cause-and-effect relationship of nutritional status and patient mortality is unclear, malnutrition is clearly a good indicator of increased risk of adverse events in ESRD patients. Further, the effect of delaying dialysis may be analogous to the experience in the National Cooperative Dialysis Study (NCDS) [97]. In this study, patients who had been randomized to 24 weeks of low-dose dialysis protocols had twice the mortality in the subsequent year in spite of returning to standard-dose dialysis.

There are no controlled studies yet available documenting the benefits of early dialysis. However, several studies have shown improved survival for patients starting dialysis with higher levels of RRF. Bonomini *et al.* [133], in 1978, had published data showing a poorer prognosis for patients starting dialysis with a residual renal creatinine clearance of <5 ml/min than patients starting incremental haemodialysis with a mean residual renal creatinine clearance of 11 ml/min. Tattersall and colleagues [134] reported an increased rate of hospitalization among patients commencing CAPD with a residual renal Kt/V urea <1.05 per week. Patients who failed to survive had a lower initial Kt/V urea of 0.63 than those who survived (Kt/V urea = 1.05). Schulman and Hakim [135] have reported that patients starting dialysis with a creatinine clearance of >10 ml/min had an 88% 10-year survival compared to 55% in those who initiated dialysis with a creatinine clearance of <10 ml/min (mean 4 ml/min).

APD offers an option for incremental peritoneal dialysis. Patients with significant RRF may initially be started on NIPD. With decline in RRF, clearances may be augmented by switching to high-dose NIPD or to CCPD. Later, clearances may be improved by combining APD with CAPD (Fig. 13) [136]. Early start of peritoneal dialysis is associated with some risks. These risks include infection and the possibility that increasing the length on peritoneal dialysis may contribute to eventual patient 'burn out' [127]. The reduced interference with daily routine, lower work burden, and fewer complications with APD make this a preferable procedure for early start.

Complications of APD

Qualitatively, the complications of APD are similar to those encountered with CAPD. However, quanti-

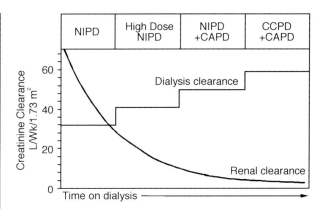

Figure 13. Schematic drawing of the adaptation of APD to change in residual renal function. (From ref. 136 with permission.)

tative differences may exist in the incidence of these complications in the two modalities. Here, we will discuss selective complication of APD.

Peritonitis

Although the incidence of peritonitis in patients treated with peritoneal dialysis has decreased during recent years, it remains a major complication and frequent cause of hospitalization and discontinuation of peritoneal dialysis. The first study discussing the incidence of peritonitis on CCPD was authored by Price and Suki [20] in 1981. They found the incidence of peritonitis was one episode every 18.2 patient-month on CCPD as compared to one episode every 7.2 patient-month on CAPD. Subsequently, Walls *et al.* [137], Diaz-Buxo *et al.* [138], Levy *et al.* [139] and several other authors reported similar results.

With the introduction of disconnect systems, the incidence of peritonitis on CAPD fell significantly. In a randomized prospective study, de Fijter and associates [140] observed that peritonitis occurred significantly less often in those patients receiving CCPD than in those on CAPD with Y-connectors (0.51 compared with 0.94 episode per patient-year; $p = 0.03$). The median time to the first episode of peritonitis was 11 months for patients receiving CAPD with Y-connectors compared with 18 months for CCPD patients ($p = 0.06$). Patients on CAPD with Y-connectors developed their second episode of peritonitis in 6 months compared to 25 months for CCPD patients ($p = 0.18$). In contrast, Burkart *et al.* [141], in another prospective study, found no difference in the incidence of peritonitis between patients on APD (0.58 episode per patient-year) and patients on the Y-set (0.61 episode per patient-year). Their patients using the standard spike system developed peritonitis at a significantly higher rate of 1.62 episodes per patient-year. Viglino *et al.* [142] found the incidence of peritonitis once in 37.5 months for APD and once in 40 months for CAPD with a Y-set (*p* = n.s.). Williams and co-workers [143] reported the incidence of peritonitis on APD to be similar to CAPD with disconnect systems with one episode occurring every 31 months and 29 months, respectively. The incidence of peritonitis for CAPD without disconnect systems was one in 13 months. Troidle *et al.* [144], in a retrospective analysis of 239 patients on ultrabags and 106 patients on CCPD, found the incidence of peritonitis to be similar in the two groups. The incidence for Gram-negative peritonitis was higher for CCPD, but the difference was not statistically significant. A cross-sectional industry-sponsored study collected data from 94 centres and 2965 patients [145]. The data were reported on 6703 patient-months on CAPD and 6791 patient-months on APD. The annual incidence of peritonitis was 0.60 per patient-year for CAPD and a lower incidence of 0.46 per patient-year for APD.

The data on the incidence of peritonitis on APD and CAPD, though somewhat conflicting, suggest that APD patients have a lower incidence of peritonitis. The bases for these findings are many. The reduced number of connections to, and disconnections from, the abdominal catheter may be of significance. Furthermore, most of these connections in APD occur between two sterile surfaces (a new connection line and a new bag), while in CAPD most connections are between the new set and a reusable transfer line and peritoneal catheter. Improved patient technique due to performance of all connections in the same environment, less patient fatigue due to performance of fewer connections and assistance of a helper may help reduce peritonitis rate. Most APD systems now employ flush-before-fill technology, further reducing infection by touch contamination.

Peritoneal dialysis has been shown to have adverse effects on the local immune system. The low pH, high osmolality, and the lactate buffer of the dialysate inhibit phagocytosis and killing by peritoneal macrophages and granulocytes [146–152]. The frequent exchanges also cause a washout of opsonins and peritoneal macrophages [153, 154]. These macrophages are replaced by immature monocytes from the blood. During the prolonged daytime interval without peritoneal exchanges in CCPD and NIPD, the cytotoxic effect of the dialysate solution disappears. There is an increase in the number of mature macrophages in the peritoneal cavity that provide the first line of defence against infection. It is to be noted that mature macrophages have increased chemotactic and phagocytic activity compared to immature cells. Furthermore, the potential for cytokine release, which is inhibited (possibly by dialysate effects) after APD is often restored during the 12–14-h interval without peritoneal dialysis exchanges [154]. IgG levels, C_3, and opsonic activity of dialysis effluent have been shown to increase with increasing dwell time [155]. The dry days in NIPD provide no additional beneficial effect on recovery of host defences compared with CCPD which has a wet day [154]. Thus, the absence of dialysate during the day in NIPD and the prolonged dwell of CCPD allow a period for the recovery of host defences. These improved first-line host defences may well be able to eradicate a small bacterial inoculum introduced at the time of connecting to the cycler.

During TPD, the presence of a reserve volume prevents extreme changes in intraperitoneal pH and the phagocytic function of peritoneal macrophages is better preserved. Early during treatment with TPD there is a lesser washout and dilution of cells and opsonins compared to CCPD. However, overall loss of cells and IgG do not differ if the total amount of peritoneal dialysis fluid used and total treatment time are made equal for both procedures [156].

The diagnostic criteria for peritonitis were established based on clinical experience with CAPD patients whose dwell times are 4–6 h long. The use of shorter dwell times by APD patients with suspected peritonitis could potentially result in misleading low dialysate cell counts and falsely negative cultures. However, data from paediatric patients on APD suggest the criteria for CAPD peritonitis can be accurately applied to adult APD. Cloudy fluid and/or fever and/or abdominal pain suggest the diagnosis of peritonitis. A dialysate white blood cell count > $100/\text{mm}^3$, with more than 50% polymorphonuclear neutrophils, is supportive of the diagnosis, as is a positive Gram stain [157]. In equivocal cases, or in patients with systemic and abdominal symptoms in whom dialysate appears to be clear, a second exchange is performed with a dwell of at least 1 h but preferably 3–4 h. A count of > $100/\text{mm}^3$ mostly polymorphonuclear cells, or a positive Gram stain, dictates treatment; otherwise simple observation is recommended. On occasions the initial drain of stagnant fluid present in the abdomen all day in patients with only partial daytime exchanges or dry days will appear cloudy in the absence of peritonitis. The white blood cell count may exceed 100/mm^3, but mononuclear cells will predominate. More important, dialysate rapidly clears with the initiation of peritoneal dialysis.

The diagnosis of peritonitis in APD may often be delayed in patients using cyclers that dispose of dialysate directly without a drain bag [158]. To avoid those problems, patients should be trained to collect a small amount of the dialysate from the initial drain at the start of the night therapy and inspect it for cloudiness. If abdominal pain is experienced, a manual exchange for inspection and possible cell count with culture is recommended.

The organisms causing peritonitis in APD are similar to CAPD [140, 143]. *Pasteurella multocida* has been identified as the cause of peritonitis in a few patients. This infection is caused by cats biting into the cycler tubing [159]. The antibiotic treatment of peritonitis is no different from CAPD. Continuous antibiotics may be administered after switching the patient to every 3 or 4-h exchanges until the fluid clears. Alternately, a single, daily dose of antibiotic may be administered in the long dwell [157]. Patients may require adjustment of the APD prescription to account for the increased permeability of the peritoneal membrane during peritonitis.

Catheter infections (exit site and tunnel)

Catheter-related infections are becoming the most common infection associated with peritoneal dialysis. These infections are an important cause of morbidity, peritonitis, and catheter failure. The Final Report of the National CAPD Registry [160] reported an equal incidence of exit-site and tunnel infections of 0.6 episode per patient-year of observation in CAPD and CCPD. The incidence of catheter replacement was 0.2 per patient-year for CAPD and 0.3 episode per patient-year for CCPD. In data reported by Burkart *et al.* [141], the incidence of exit-site infections was 0.41 episode per patient-year for APD, 0.32 per patient-year for patients on Y-sets, and 0.62 per patient-year for patients on a standard spike. Statistical significance was only seen for the comparison between Y-set and standard spike ($p = 0.01$). de Fijter *et al.* [140] found exit-site infections occur with a mean incidence of 0.38 per patient-year in both CAPD patients on a Y-connector and CCPD. Holley and co-workers [161], on the other hand, reported a significant decrease of exit-site infections for cycler patients (0.5 episode per patient-

year) in contrast to CAPD patients using disconnect systems (0.86 episode per patient-year). Patients on non-disconnect systems developed exit-site infections at an incidence of 1.2 episodes per patient-year. The duration on dialysis may be a factor impacting on the incidence of exit-site infections in different studies. A decrease in exit-site infections is noted with increasing time on dialysis [161, 162]. Other factors may be surgical technique, catheter type, and exit-site care. Overall, disconnect systems, including APD, have fewer catheter infections than non-disconnect systems. It may be postulated that, by disconnecting, the exits are subject to lesser trauma, tension, torque, or pulling [141].

Complications of increased IAP

Hernias and dialysate leaks

The complications of increased IAP are seen predominantly among CAPD and CCPD patients. As discussed earlier, the IAP is maximal while sitting, intermediate while standing, and least in a supine position [63, 71]. The increased pressure in the abdomen causes an increase in the abdominal wall tension and may cause hernias or dialysate leaks. Interestingly, a few recent studies [163, 164] have not been able to find a correlation between V_{ip} and the incidence of hernias. Furthermore, Durand *et al.* [165] found no relationship between IAP and mechanical complications. It may be possible that the IAP required to cause hernias are much higher than achieved under usual clinical conditions, and patients who develop hernias have structural weakness of the abdominal wall. Susceptible patients include older multiparous females, patients with autosomal dominant polycystic kidney disease, those with prior hernias or dialysate leaks, and prolonged corticosteroid treatment [166, 167]. The incidence of hernias on CAPD ranges between 10% and 25%, while on IPD the incidence is 2% to 5%; for CCPD the incidence is approximately 9%. The usual sites for hernias are inguinal, umbilical, pericatheter, and incisional [168, 169]. Susceptible patients on CCPD should receive smaller diurnal dwells. Surgery is recommended for most hernias because of the risk of bowel or omental incarceration and strangulation. Post-surgery, once patients return to peritoneal dialysis, low volume and/or supine dialysis should be used.

Dialysate leaks are another complication of elevated IAP. These may present as abdominal or genital oedema, pericatheter pseudohernias, and rarely as a vaginal leak of dialysate. Leaks are characterized by dissection of fluid through tissue planes and may or may not be associated with hernias. Fluid leaks may be detected by radionucleotide imaging [170] or by computerized tomography scans with contrast in the dialysate [171]. Sometimes, leaks without associated hernias resolve by utilizing low-volume supine dialysis or a temporary transfer to haemodialysis. Surgical repair may eventually be required. Additional information on hernias and leaks is detailed in Chapter 9.

Respiratory function

The presence of fluid in the abdomen and elevated IAP impact on pulmonary indices. There is a greater decline in pulmonary indices in the supine position compared to the upright or sitting positions. CAPD patients generally have better pulmonary indices than patients on APD. A good measure of the tolerance of intraperitoneal volumes is the forced vital capacity (FVC) in the supine position [63]. Thieler *et al.* [172] described that the FVC in the supine position declined by a mean of 3.4% after the infusion of 2 L of dialysate into the peritoneal cavity. Pulmonary indices were not significantly affected by the presence of 2 L of fluid in the sitting or upright positions. Gotloib and co-workers [70] reported a 62% reduction in FVC with a V_{ip} of 2.5 L in four patients treated with NIPD. In a study by Durand *et al.* [72] vital capacity decreased linearly by 4.42% per litre of V_{ip}. During sleep, the drop in vital capacity is reflected by a reduction in the pulmonary reserve volume and decreases in vital capacity by 20% or more may affect blood oxygenation. Clinical symptoms and discomfort are generally not seen with an IAP of less than 20 cmH$_2$O. Based on this observation, and the fact that vital capacity may be significantly compromised by an IAP of 20 cmH$_2$O or more, Durand has recommended a maximal acceptable IAP of 18 cmH$_2$O measured from the mid-axillary line. The measurement of IAP is simple and may serve as an easy guide for optimizing dialysate-fill volumes. It has to be stressed that some patients may feel discomfort and shortness of breath at lower IAP, possibly due to the reduced strength of the diaphragm [63]. The ultimate guide of the appropriate intraperitoneal volume is the subjective assessment of the patient.

Hydrothorax is another pulmonary complication. Hydrothorax usually develops on the right side. Patients may range from being asymptomatic to having severe respiratory compromise. Most patients developing hydrothorax are females; multiparity confers an additional risk. Fluid transverses the diaphragm through lymphatics or through defects in the diaphragm [173, 174]. This complication occurs very rarely in NIPD and may be treated by low-volume supine dialysis, pleurodesis, or surgical repair [175].

Back pain

Back pain is another complication related to increased IAP. The increased IAP can pull lumbar vertebrae into a more lordotic position and increase the stress on the spine. Poor muscle tone, osteoporosis and degenerative joint disease can worsen the process. The treatment is aimed at reducing IAP by switching to APD, preferably with dry days [169].

Residual renal function

The residual renal function contributes significantly to the adequacy of dialysis and the excretion of middle and large molecules. The kidneys are also the principal sites for formation of erythropoietin and activation of vitamin D. Anuric patients have very low erythropoietin levels [176] and are unable to synthesize activated vitamin D [177]. Various studies have shown a more rapid decline of RRF in haemodialysis patients than CAPD patients [114–116]. The generation of inflammatory mediators by the extracorporeal circuit and possible ischaemia due to rapid fluid shifts and episodes of hypotension may be responsible [178–180].

A disconcerting study published by Hiroshige *et al.* [117] found that RRF declined more rapidly with APD compared to CAPD over a 6-month period. For the eight patients on NIPD the rate of decline in creatinine clearance was -0.29 ml/min/month and for the four CCPD patients -0.34 ml/min/month. These rates were significantly higher compared to the authors' own CAPD data, as well as the data of others. Nephrotoxic insults were ruled out, and the more rapid decline of renal function was attributed to the intermittent nature of APD.

Peritoneal dialysis in high transporters

High transporters are patients with a D/P creatinine of 0.82–1.03 on the peritoneal equilibration test [44]. Between 10% and 15% of the peritoneal dialysis population are high transporters [44, 119]. These patients equilibrate small solutes early in a dwell and also have the most rapid absorption of glucose causing a quick loss of the osmotic gradient for ultrafiltration [45, 46]. For this reason, drain volumes may decrease leading to a lower Kt/V urea on CAPD in high transporters compared to high-average transporters as was shown in the CANUSA study. Furthermore, high transporters on CAPD may develop oedema, especially with loss of RRF.

High transporters have an excessive risk of developing hypoalbuminaemia and having adverse outcomes including death [181–187]. Several different mechanisms have been proposed to explain the hypoalbuminaemia: high transporters have excessive protein losses in dialysate [181–183], problems with ultrafiltration may lead to haemodilution [187], and lastly, the greater proportion of dialysate glucose absorbed may lead to satiety and poor food intake [181, 182]. On the other hand, the high absorption of dialysate glucose could benefit by promoting nitrogen balance [188].

Nolph et al found high transporters to have a lower daily creatinine production indicating a smaller muscle mass compared to patients with lower D/P values on the PET [181]. In contrast, Harty and associates [187] found no difference in anthropometrics, lean body mass, fat mass, and protein intake between low and high transporters on CAPD. The CANUSA study [183] found lower serum albumin amongst the high transporters, but no difference in nutritional assessment by subjective global assessment, percentage lean body mass, and normalized protein catabolic rate across the board. The failure of the D/P creatinine ratio to correlate with direct measurements of body composition supports the absence of a relationship between membrane permeability and malnutrition.

An association of increased morbidity and mortality has been found with high membrane transport for patients on CAPD. The CANUSA study [183] has shown a gradation of the adverse effects based on transport category. For low, low-average, high and high-average transporters, the 2-year survival was 91%, 80%, 72% and 71%, and the technique survival was 80%, 61%, 52% and 48%, respectively. This was despite the fact that high transporters had superior creatinine clearances. Davies et al. [185] reported a 70.5% 3-year survival for high transporters, compared with >85% for low, low-average and high transporters. The mechanisms of the poor outcome are unclear. High transporters have a low serum albumin which is a variable associated with increased risk of death. However, there is strong statistical correlation and multicollinearity in re-gression models between low serum albumin and high transport characteristics, making it difficult to interpret the influence of each as an independent variable on outcome [189]. Fried [186] in his study established a poorer survival of high transporters independent of serum albumin. Lindholm and co-workers [190] have shown that more permeable membranes have less effective sodium and water removal. This may be related to a reduced number of water pores in the peritoneal membrane of these patients. Thus, high transporters are likely to be volume overloaded, which is likely to affect their clinical outcomes.

Automated peritoneal dialysis with short dwell may be the answer for these patients. Patients requiring daytime dwell may be managed by early drainage of the day dwell, introduction of an evening dwell or use of one or two daytime exchanges. With these techniques, ultrafiltration can be maximized with less glucose absorption and less suppression of appetite. Kathuria et al. have reported that dialysate protein losses, however, remain the same on NIPD as compared to CAPD [191]. Newer osmotic agents such as icodextrin may prove useful for the day dwell. Some patients need to switch to haemodialysis if refractory fluid overload and hypoalbuminaemia develops. Further research needs to be done to compare survival of high transporters on APD versus CAPD and whether improving fluid balance has a positive impact on outcome.

Treatment of diabetics with APD

Diabetes mellitus is the most common cause of new patients requiring renal replacement therapy and accounts for 42% of new patients in the United States [5]. Renal transplantation offers the best outcome for diabetics with ESRD [192]. The choice of dialysis modality (haemodialysis or peritoneal dialysis) is influenced among other things by comorbid conditions, social circumstances, the ability to tolerate volume shifts, and the status of the vasculature. The reasons for choosing APD for diabetics are no different than for non-diabetics. No studies have compared survival for diabetics on APD versus CAPD. As mentioned earlier, diabetics with visual or manual impairment may be better treated by APD because of the lesser number of connections and reduced workload on assistants. Nightly peritoneal dialysis offers an advantage to high transporters who can receive enormous glucose loads from rapid glucose absorption during continuous peritoneal dialysis. In addition to raising the blood glucose, the rapid glucose absorption lowers the osmotic gradient between dialysate and blood, resulting in reduced ultrafiltration, diminished solute removal, and fluid retention [193, 194]. With APD, adequate ultrafiltration may be achieved with lower absorption of glucose [194]. Further details of management of diabetics on peritoneal dialysis are discussed in Chapter 21.

Peritoneal dialysis in the treatment of acute renal failure

Peritoneal dialysis offers a safe, effective, low-cost, and biocompatible intracorporeal dialysis system for the treatment of acute renal failure (ARF). The peritoneal membrane has excellent permeability for uraemic toxins up to 50 kDA and a limited permeability to molecules above 300 kDa. There is almost perfect impermeability to bacteria and the rare instance of peritonitis is easily diagnosed by the development of cloudy bags. The procedure avoids anticoagulation making it safe for those with bleeding problems, recent surgery, and intracranial haemorrhage [195]. Peritoneal dialysis offers gentle fluid removal, which is of added benefit for patients with a compromised cardiovascular status [196]. The gradual removal of solutes with peritoneal dialysis minimizes the risk for disequilibrium syndrome. Neurosurgical patients have a lesser tendency to develop brain oedema on peritoneal dialysis than when treated with haemodialysis. Peritoneal dialysis allows easy correction of electrolyte and acid–base problems in most circumstances [197]. The potential for early recovery of renal function is better for patients treated with peritoneal dialysis than haemodialysis [195, 198]. During haemodialysis, patients are subjected to episodes of hypotension which lead to recurrent ischaemic injury to the tubules [198, 199]. Interaction of blood and dialysis membrane can release harmful inflammatory mediators and cause neutrophilic infiltration of the kidneys, prolonging the duration of ARF [200, 201].

In spite of the multiple advantages of peritoneal dialysis, ARF is increasingly being treated by haemodialysis or continuous extracorporeal replacement techniques. The changing spectrum of patients with acute renal failure and increasing sophistication of extracorporeal replacement techniques has heralded this change. Patients developing ARF have more serious underlying diseases than in the past. They are often septic and hypercatabolic and may have multi-organ failure. Extracorporeal techniques offer significantly higher clearances and fluid removal than peritoneal dialysis. Furthermore, aggressive nutrition in catabolic patients increases the need for solute and water clearances, which may not be met on peritoneal dialysis [197]. Although peritoneal blood flow in patients with hypotension is usually maintained by autoregulation [202], the use of catecholamine pressors, especially norepinephrine, may cause a decline in the peritoneal blood flow and solute clearances [203, 204]. A postoperative or traumatized abdomen is a contraindication for peritoneal dialysis. Even though earlier reports have discussed the successful use of peritoneal dialysis in such situations [205], the risks of peritoneal dialysis are unacceptable with the availability of present-day alternatives. Caution should be used for patients with hernias, pleuroperitoneal connections, bowel ileus and abdominal adhesions. Elevation of IAP may further compromise lung function in patients with respiratory distress [206]. Peritoneal dialysis is also not suited for severely hyperkalaemic patients as the maximal rate of potassium removal is restricted to 12 mEq/h [207]. Other contraindications include faecal and fungal peritonitis and abdominal wall cellulitis [206].

Peritoneal dialysis remains a viable option for facilities lacking expertise and personnel for performing extracorporeal dialysis. It remains the procedure of choice for young children [208] and infants [209]. It may be the only option for patients with access failure due to excessive burns or advanced vascular disease. Severe hypothermia is another indication for peritoneal dialysis [206]. Patients with pancreatitis were often treated with peritoneal dialysis based on the belief that removal of pancreatic enzymes and inflammatory mediators may help control the inflammation and necrotic process. A large randomized multicentric trial has shown no benefit of peritoneal lavage over maximal supportive care [210].

Technique

Peritoneal dialysis access may be obtained by the insertion of a rigid catheter or a soft-cuffed catheter. The rigid catheters may be inserted easily at the bedside. These catheters are designed for single use and should not be used for more than 3 days because of the high risk for peritonitis and bowel perforation [211]. Because of these complications, and the unpredictable course of ARF and need for subsequent dialysis, most centres now place chronic catheters. These catheters are generally inserted under direct visualization during a mini-laparotomy or by using a peritoneoscope. The reader is referred to Chapter 9 for technical details of obtaining peritoneal access.

The dialysis regimens that may be used for acute renal failure are intermittent peritoneal dialysis and continuous equilibrium peritoneal dialysis [197]. The intermittent peritoneal dialysis session usually lasts 48–72 h. Dialysis is delivered by manual exchanges or automated delivery systems. The use of an automated device eliminates the need for constant nursing supervision, provides timed exchanges, and can monitor ultrafiltration. The usual exchange volume for adults is 2 L. Patients with smaller body size, recent abdominal surgery, pulmonary disease and hernias should receive smaller volumes. In larger patients, in the absence of contraindications, 2.5- or 3-L fill volumes should be used to augment clearances. The usual exchange lasts for 60 min with approximately 5–10 min devoted to inflow and 10–20 min for outflow. Hypercatabolic patients may require dialysate flow rates of 4 L or more per hour. With the use of shorter dwells, infusion and drainage take up an increasing proportion of time; the contact time for dialysate and the peritoneal membrane is reduced and the drained dialysate is only partially saturated with urea. This increases the costs of treatment significantly and provides only a modest improvement in clearances. A maximal clearance of 25 ml/min may be achieved with rapid cycling [206]. Ultrafiltration may be adjusted by altering the dextrose concentration in the dialysate. Heparin should be added to most exchanges performed immediately after catheter insertion.

Continuous equilibrium peritoneal dialysis is a continuous regimen that utilizes relatively long dwells of 2–6 h and thereby differs from intermittent, short-dwell acute peritoneal dialysis which has been traditionally used for ARF [212, 213]. The procedure is similar to CAPD except the patients are not ambulatory. Exchanges are delivered manually or by automated means. Clearances of 5–7 ml/min may be achieved with 9–10 L of drainage per day [206].

Complications and outcome

Infective complications such as peritonitis and catheter infections are more common with the rigid catheter. Peritonitis is often caused by endogenous organisms. Patients may develop catheter-related problems including haemorrhage, hollow viscus perforation, catheter obstruction and inflow pain [206]. A host of metabolic complications are also seen: hypokalaemia, hypernatraemia, hyperglycaemia,

respiratory alkalosis and metabolic alkalosis. The absorption of large amounts of glucose from the dialysate can lead to hepatic steatosis, hyperglycaemia, increase in carbon dioxide production, and worsening respiratory failure [214]. An occasional patient may have worsening of lactic acidosis due to the lactate in the peritoneal dialysis solution [215]. Significant amounts of protein may be lost into the dialysate, which should be taken into consideration while assessing nutritional needs [195]. Other complications include hypotension due to excessive ultrafiltration; hypothermia; leaks, hernias, and respiratory compromise due to elevated IAP; and rare cases of chyloperitoneum.

Although a random survey of American nephrologists has reported that 25% practise acute peritoneal dialysis, there is a paucity of data on outcomes of ARF treated by peritoneal dialysis, suggesting marked under-reporting [216]. Firmat and Zucchini [217] in 1979 compiled data on 1101 cases of ARF treated by peritoneal dialysis from their own experience and published literature. They found no difference in outcomes between those treated by either peritoneal dialysis or haemodialysis. Sepsis was the major cause of mortality. Rodgers and associates [218] reported their clinical experience acquired over 27 years on 246 geriatric patients with ARF. The survival of patients, whether treated by peritoneal dialysis or haemodialysis, was no different. Survival improved over the years from 31% to 42% in patients treated with haemodialysis, and from 15% to 32% in patients treated with peritoneal dialysis. Ash and colleagues [219], in their report of 100 patients treated by either peritoneal dialysis or haemodialysis, found 48% of their peritoneal dialysis patients recovered renal function versus 38% of their haemodialysis patients. The mortality was similar in the two groups. A subsequent review of an additional 145 patients with ARF by the same authors found similar outcomes as the initial study [195].

Clinical results with APD

Despite the recent increases in the number of patients being treated with APD, there is, as yet, little data on long-term morbidity and mortality in comparison with other means of renal replacement therapy. Most registry reports combine the results for CAPD and APD. Data that do exist consist of experience from single centres. Some of these data are discussed here.

Most studies reveal that the choice of APD is generally guided by social issues or the development of complications on CAPD, including ultrafiltration failure, hernias, and dialysate leaks [140, 142, 143, 220, 221]. Recently some centres have started using NIPD as a modality in early or 'healthy' start as the first step in incremental peritoneal dialysis [136]. Adequate dialysis can be achieved for most patients with APD, although some patients require a combination of APD with additional daytime exchanges [142, 143, 220]. Haemoglobin and haematocrit were similar in studies comparing APD with CAPD, as were the erythropoietin requirements [140, 220, 221]. Metabolic parameters were well controlled [140, 220], though a study by Woodrow *et al.* [221] found higher levels of potassium, phosphorus and creatinine in NIPD patients. Hypertension is generally well controlled on APD with one-third to one-half the patients being able to either discontinue or decrease medications [140, 220].

The incidence of ultrafiltration failure increases from 2.6% after 1 year of CAPD to 30.9% after 6 years of CAPD [222]. The risk of ultrafiltration failure is extremely low on APD [220] and is possibly related to the long diurnal rest in most APD modalities. Overall, the incidence of peritonitis and exit-site infections is markedly lower on APD when compared to CAPD. However, the use of disconnect systems, especially ultrabags, has decreased the incidence of infective complications on CAPD and made it comparable to APD. de Fijter *et al.* [140] have reported that the average number of hospitalizations per patient-year was 1.0 using CAPD with a disconnect system, and 0.60 per patient-year for CCPD ($p = 0.02$). The mean duration of hospitalization per admission for CAPD was 10.8 days, and for CCPD 9.6 days ($p =$ n.s.) [140]. Brunkhorst *et al.* [220] also reported that patients on APD averaged 10 hospital days per year.

Diaz-Buxo *et al.* [13] in 1984 had reported the technique survival for CCPD to be 80%, 62%, and 56% at 1, 2 and 3 years, respectively. The 3-year patient survival was 83%. In a more recent study by Viglino *et al.* [142] the 5-year technique survival was 82% on APD, 87% on haemodialysis, and 62% on CAPD. The transfer rate to haemodialysis for APD is between 8% and 12% in the first year [140, 143, 220], which is significantly lower than the 10–30% transfer rate in the first year for CAPD [5]. Most patients accept APD well and report convenience over CAPD. In Brunkhorst *et al.*'s study, 74% of the patients less than 60 years were employed [220]. In summary, APD is comparable if not superior to CAPD.

The future of APD

In the future we should expect to see an increasing automation of peritoneal dialysis. Improving technology and an increase in the number of elderly patients requiring dialysis will cause a significant increase in the use of APD. Future machines will be more advanced and highly automatic, and yet simpler to operate. 'On-line' production of contemporary compound solutions individualized for each patient will provide not only toxin and fluid removal, but also appropriate nutrition [223]. The cyclers would incorporate on-line monitoring of urea, creatinine, and middle molecules in the effluent, allowing close monitoring of peritoneal clearances. Connection systems and catheter technology will need to be further improved, leading to further improvement in quality of life, a decrease in both the incidence of peritonitis and total drop-out rate on peritoneal dialysis. The adequacy targets on APD will be better defined with the completion of prospective outcome studies. The day is not far away when we will be able to revolutionize the practice of peritoneal dialysis through the remodelling of the peritoneum using gene therapy.

Acknowledgements

The authors thank Mariann Duca for her excellent secretarial assistance.

References

1. Twardowski ZJ. Peritoneal dialysis glossary II. Perit Dial Int 1988; 8: 15–77.
2. Twardowski ZJ. Peritoneal dialysis glossary III. Perit Dial Int 1990; 10: 173–5.
3. Cruz C, Dumler F, Schmidt R, Gotch F. Enhanced peritoneal dialysis delivery with PD Plus™. Adv Perit Dial 1992; 8: 288–90.
4. United States Renal Data System. USRDS 1998 Annual Report. National Institutes of Health, National Institute of Diabetes and Kidney Diseases, Bethesda, MD, 1998.
5. United States Renal Data System: USRDS 1997 Annual Data Report. The USRDS Dialysis Morbidity and Mortality Study (Wave 2). National Institutes of Health, National Institute of Diabetes and Digestive and Kidney Disease, Bethesda, MD, 1997.
6. Warady BA, Hebert D, Sullivan EK, Alexander SR, Tejani A. Renal transplantation, chronic dialysis, and chronic renal insufficiency in children and adolescents. The 1995 Annual Report of the North American Pediatric Renal Transplant Cooperative Study. Pediatr Nephrol 1997; 11: 49–64.
7. Boen ST, Mulinari AS, Dillard DH, Schribner BH. Periodic peritoneal dialysis in the management of chronic uremia. Trans Am Soc Artif Intern Organs 1962; 8: 256–65.
8. Boen ST, Mion CM, Curtis FK, Schilipetar G. Periodic peritoneal dialysis using the repeated puncture technique and an

automatic cycling machine. Trans Am Soc Artif Intern Organs 1964; 10: 409–14.

9. Lasker N, McCauley EP, Passarotti CT. Chronic peritoneal dialysis. Trans Am Soc Artif Intern Organs 1966; 12: 94–7.

10. Tenckhoff H, Shilipetar G, van Paasschen WH, Swanson E. A home peritoneal dialysate delivery system. Trans Am Soc Artif Intern Organs 1969; 15: 103–7.

11. Tenckhoff H, Weston B, Shilipetar G. A simplified automatic peritoneal dialysis system. Trans Am Soc Artif Intern Organs 1972; 18: 436–40.

12. Boen ST. Overview and history of peritoneal dialysis. Dial Transplant 1977; 6: 12–13.

13. Diaz-Buxo JA, Walker PJ, Chandler JT, Burgess WP, Farmer CD. Experience with intermittent peritoneal dialysis and continuous cyclic peritoneal dialysis. Am J Kidney Dis 1984; 4: 242–8.

14. Ahmad S, Gallagher N, Shen F. Intermittent peritoneal dialysis: status reassessed. Trans Am Soc Artif Intern Organs 1979; 25: 86–9.

15. Schmidt RW, Blumenkrantz MJ. IPD, CAPD, CCPD, CRPD – peritoneal dialysis: past, present and future. Int J Artif Organs 1981; 4: 124–9.

16. Popovich RP, Moncrief JW, Decherd JF et al. The definition of a portable–wearable equilibrium peritoneal technique. ASAIO Abstracts 1976; 5: 64 (abstract).

17. Popovich RP, Moncrief JW, Nolph KD, Ghods AJ, Twardowski ZJ, Pyle WK. Continuous ambulatory peritoneal dialysis. Ann Intern Med 1978; 88: 449–56.

18. Oreopoulos DG, Robson M, Izatt S, Clayton S, deVerber GA. A simple and safe technique for continuous ambulatory peritoneal dialysis (CAPD). Trans Am Soc Artif Intern Organs 1978; 24: 484–9.

19. Diaz-Buxo JA, Farmer CD, Walker PJ, Chandler JT, Holt KL. Continuous cyclic peritoneal dialysis: a preliminary report. Artif Organs 1981; 5: 157–61.

20. Price CG, Suki WN. Newer modifications of peritoneal dialysis: options in the treatment of patients with renal failure. Am J Nephrol 1981; 1: 97–104.

21. Stephen RL, Atkin-Thore E, Kolff WJ. Reciprocating peritoneal dialysis with a subcutaneous peritoneal catheter. Trans Am Soc Artif Intern Organs 1976; 22: 575–84.

22. Twardowski ZJ, Prowant BF, Nolph KD, Khanna R, Schmidt LM, Satalowich RJ. Chronic nightly tidal peritoneal dialysis. ASAIO Trans 1990; 36: M584–8.

23. Nolph KD, Hano JE, Teschan PE. Peritoneal sodium transport during hypertonic peritoneal dialysis. Physiologic mechanisms and clinical implications. Ann Intern Med 1969; 70: 931–41.

24. Ahearn DJ, Nolph KD. Controlled sodium removal with peritoneal dialysis. Trans Am Soc Artif Intern Organs 1972; 18: 423–8.

25. Nolph KD, Twardowski ZJ, Popovich RP, Rubin J. Equilibration of peritoneal dialysis solutions during long-dwell exchanges. J Lab Clin Med 1979; 93: 246–56.

26. Nolph KD, Sorkin MI, Moore H. Autoregulation of sodium and potassium removal during continuous ambulatory peritoneal dialysis. Trans Am Soc Artif Intern Organs 1980; 26: 334–8.

27. Jorres A, Topley N, Witowski J, Liberek T, Gahl GM. Impact of peritoneal dialysis solutions on peritoneal immune defense. Perit Dial Int 1993; 13 (suppl. 2): S291–4.

28. Topley N, Coles GA, Williams JD. Biocompatibility studies on peritoneal cells. Perit Dial Int 1994; 14 (suppl. 3): S21–8.

29. Coles GA. Biocompatibility of various osmotic solutes. Perit Dial Int 1995; 15 (suppl. 7): S71–5.

30. Flessner MF. Osmotic barrier of the parietal peritoneum. Am J Physiol 1994; 267 (5 Pt 2): F861–70.

31. Yamada K, Miyahara Y, Hamaguchi K et al. Immunohistochemical study of human advanced glycosylation end-products (AGE) in chronic renal failure. Clin Nephrol 1994; 42: 354–61.

32. Nakayama M, Kawaguchi Y, Yamada K et al. Immunohistochemical detection of advanced glycosylation end-products in the peritoneum and its possible pathophysiological role in CAPD. Kidney Int 1997; 51: 182–6.

33. Dawnay AB, Millar DJ. Glycation and advanced glycation end-product formation with icodextrin and dextrose. Perit Dial Int 1997; 17: 52–8.

34. Peers E, Gokal R. Icodextrin: overview of clinical experience. Perit Dial Int 1997; 17: 22–6.

35. Cooper A, Henderson IS, Jones MC. Daytime dwell with 7.5% icodextrin in automated peritoneal dialysis (APD). J EDTNA-ERA 1995; 21 (suppl. 1): 21.

36. Posthuma N, ter Wee PM, Verbrugh MA et al. Icodextrin instead of glucose during the daytime dwell in CCPD increases ultrafiltration and 24-hour dialysate creatinine clearance. Nephrol Dial Transplant 1997; 12: 550–3.

37. Kopple JD, Bernard D, Messana J et al. Treatment of malnourished CAPD patients with an amino acid based dialysate. Kidney Int 1995; 47: 1148–57.

38. Goodship TH, Lloyd S, McKenzie PW et al. Short-term studies on use of amino acids as an osmotic agent in continuous peritoneal dialysis. Clin Sci 1987; 73: 471–8.

39. Faller B, Shockley T, Genestier S, Martis L. Polyglucose and amino acids: preliminary results. Perit Dial Int 1997; 17 (suppl. 2): S63–7.

40. Randerson DH. Continuous ambulatory peritoneal dialysis – a critical appraisal. Thesis, University of New South Wales, Sydney, Australia, 1980.

41. Pyle WK, Popovich RP, Moncrief JW. Mass transfer in peritoneal dialysis. In: Gahl GM, Kessel M, Nolph KD, eds. Advances in Peritoneal Dialysis. Amsterdam: Excerpta Medica, 1981, pp. 41–6.

42. Garred LJ, Canaud B, Farrell PC. A simple kinetic model for assessing peritoneal mass transfer in chronic ambulatory peritoneal dialysis. ASAIO J 1983; 6: 131–7.

43. Kush RD, Hallett MD, Ota K et al. Long-term continuous ambulatory peritoneal dialysis. Mass transfer and nutritional and metabolic stability. Blood Purif 1990; 8: 1–13.

44. Twardowski ZJ, Nolph KD, Khanna R et al. Peritoneal equilibration test. Perit Dial Bull 1987; 7: 138–47.

45. Twardowski ZJ. Clinical value of standardized equilibration tests in CAPD patients. Blood Purif 1989; 7: 95–108.

46. Twardowski ZJ. Nightly peritoneal dialysis. Why, who, how, and when? ASAIO Trans 1990; 36: 8–16.

47. Popovich RP, Moncrief JW. Kinetic modeling of peritoneal transport. Contrib Nephrol 1979; 17: 59–72.

48. Ronco C. Limitations of peritoneal dialysis. Kidney Int 1996; 50 (suppl. 56): S69–74.

49. Brandes JC, Packard WJ, Watters SK, Fritsche C. Optimization of dialysate flow and mass transfer during automated peritoneal dialysis. Am J Kidney Dis 1995; 25: 603–10.

50. Curatola G, Zoccali C, Crucitti S. Effect of posture on peritoneal clearance in CAPD patients. Perit Dial Int 1988; 8: 58–9.

51. Flessner MF, Dedrick RL. Importance of the liver in peritoneal dialysis. J Am Soc Nephrol 1993; 4: 404 (abstract).

52. Fukudome Y, Ozawa K, Shoji T et al. How is the portal vein flow in CAPD? Evaluation of postural change by colour flow-doppler ultrasound (CFDU). Perit Dial Int 1992; 12 (suppl. 2): S4 (abstract).

53. Schoenfeld P, Diaz-Buzo JA, Keen M, Gotch FA. The effect of body position, surface area, and intraperitoneal exchange volume on the peritoneal transport constant (KoA). J Am Soc Nephrol 1993; 4: 416 (abstract).

54. Keshaviah P, Emerson PF, Vonesh EF, Brandes JC. Relationship between body size, fill volume, and mass transfer area coefficient in peritoneal dialysis. J Am Soc Nephrol 1994; 4: 1820–6.

55. Heimbürger O, Waniewski J, Werynski A, Lindholm B. A quantitative description of solute and fluid transport during peritoneal dialysis. Kidney Int 1992; 41: 1320–32.

56. Shen FH, Sherrard DJ, Scollard D, Merritt A, Curtis FK. Thirst, relative hypernatremia, and excessive weight gain in

maintenance peritoneal dialysis. Trans Am Soc Artif Intern Organs 1978; 24: 142–5.

57. Renkin EM. Relation of capillary morphology to transport of fluid and large molecules: a review. Acta Physiol Scand Suppl 1979; 463: 81–91.

58. Flessner MF. Peritoneal transport physiology: insights from basic research. J Am Soc Nephrol 1991; 2: 122–35.

59. Flessner MF. Net ultrafiltration in peritoneal dialysis: role of direct fluid absorption into peritoneal tissue. Blood Purif 1992; 10: 136–47.

60. Zakaria ER, Simonsen O, Rippe A, Rippe B. Transport of tracer albumin from peritoneum to plasma: role of diaphragmatic, visceral, and parietal lymphatics. Am J Physiol 1996; 270 (5 Pt 2): H1549–56.

61. Rose BD. Clinical Physiology of Acid–Base and Electrolyte Disorders, 2nd edn. New York: McGraw-Hill, 1984, p. 33.

62. Twardowski ZJ, Khanna R, Nolph KD et al. Intraabdominal pressures during natural activities in patients treated with continuous ambulatory peritoneal dialysis. Nephron 1986; 44: 129–35.

63. Twardowski ZJ, Prowant BF, Nolph KD, Martinez AJ, Lampton LM. High volume, low frequency continuous ambulatory peritoneal dialysis. Kidney Int 1983; 23: 64–70.

64. Durand PY, Chanliau J, Gamberoni J, Hestin D, Kessler M. Intraperitoneal pressure, peritoneal permeability and volume of ultrafiltration in CAPD. Adv Perit Dial 1992; 8: 22–5.

65. Imholz AL, Koomen GC, Struijk DG, Arisz L, Krediet RT. Effect of an increased intraperitoneal pressure on fluid and solute transport during CAPD. Kidney Int 1993; 44: 1078–85.

66. Struijk DG, Krediet RT, Imholz AL, Koomen GC, Arisz L. Fluid kinetics in CAPD patients during dialysis with a bicarbonate-based hypo-osmolar solution. Blood Purif 1996; 14: 217–26.

67. Flessner MF, Schwab A. Pressure threshold for fluid loss from peritoneal cavity. Am J Physiol 1996; 270 (2 Pt 2): F377–90.

68. Zakaria ER, Rippe B. Peritoneal fluid and tracer albumin kinetics in the rat. Effects of increases in intraperitoneal hydrostatic pressure. Perit Dial Int 1995; 15: 118–28.

69. Courtice FC, Steinbeck AW. The effect of lymphatic obstruction and of posture on the absorption of protein from the peritoneal cavity. Austral J Exp Biol Med Sci 1951; 29: 451–8.

70. Gotloib L, Mines M, Garmizo L, Varka I. Hemodynamic effects of increased intra-abdominal pressure in peritoneal dialysis. Perit Dial Bull 1981; 1: 41–3.

71. Diaz-Buxo JA. CCPD is even better than CAPD. Kidney Int 1985; 28 (suppl. 17): S26–8.

72. Durand PY, Chanliau J, Gamberoni J, Hestin D, Kessler M. APD: clinical measurement of the maximal acceptable intraperitoneal volume. Adv Perit Dial 1994; 10: 63–7.

73. Kumano K, Yokota S, Sakai T, Kazama H, Sofue K. Minimizing the drainage period for continuous ambulatory peritoneal dialysis. Perit Dial Int 1994; 14: 52–5.

74. Nissenson AR, Prichard SS, Cheng IK et al. Non-medical factors that impact on ESRD modality selection. Kidney Int 1993; 43 (suppl. 40): S120–7.

75. Diaz-Buxo JA. Peritoneal dialysis modality selection for the adult, the diabetic, and the geriatric patient. Perit Dial Int 1997; 17 (suppl. 3): S28–31.

76. Ellis EN, Watts K, Wells TG, Arnold WC. Use of the peritoneal equilibrium test in pediatrics dialysis patients. Adv Perit Dial 1991; 7: 259–61.

77. Salusky IB, Holloway M. Selection of peritoneal dialysis for pediatric patients. Perit Dial Int 1997; 17 (suppl. 3): S35–7.

78. Cancarini GC. The future of peritoneal dialysis: problems and hopes. Nephrol Dial Transplant 1997; 12 (suppl. 1): 84–8.

79. Hiroshige K, Iwamoto M, Ohtani A. Clinical benefits and problems in recent automated peritoneal dialysis treatment. Int J Artif Organs 1998; 21: 367–70.

80. Keshaviah P. Establishing kinetic guidelines for peritoneal dialysis modality selection. Perit Dial Int 1997; 17 (suppl. 3): S53–7.

81. Blake P, Burkart JM, Churchill DN et al. Recommended clinical practices for maximizing peritoneal dialysis clearances. Perit Dial Int 1996; 16: 448–56.

82. Diaz-Buxo JA, Farmer CD, Chandler JD et al. Continuous cyclic peritoneal dialysis (CCPD) – 'wet' is better than dry. Perit Dial Bull 1987; 7: S22.

83. Nissenson AR. Dialysis modality selection: harsh realities. Perit Dial Int 1996; 16: 343–4.

84. Okada K, Takahashi S. Modification of peritoneal dialysis: intermittent automated peritoneal dialysis. Nephron 1997; 77: 109–10.

85. Cheng YL, Chau KF, Choi KS, Wong FK, Cheng HM, Li CS. Peritoneal catheter-related complications: a comparison between hemodialysis and intermittent peritoneal dialysis in the break-in period. Adv Perit Dial 1996; 12: 231–4.

86. Mailloux LU, Swartz CD, Onesti G, Heider C, Ramirez O, Brest AN. Peritoneal dialysis for refractory congestive heart failure. JAMA 1967; 199: 873–8.

87. Ryckelynck JP, Lobbedez T, Valette B et al. Peritoneal ultrafiltration and refractory congestive heart failure. Adv Perit Dial 1997; 13: 93–7.

88. Freida Ph, Ryckelynck JPh, Potier J et al. Place de l'ultra-filtration peritoneale dans le traitement medical de l'insuffisance cardiaque au stade IV de la NYHA. Bull Dial Perit 1995; 5: 7–18.

89. Goel S, Saran R, Nolph KD, Moran J, Vonesh EF, Dunham T. Dry days in chronic peritoneal dialysis: whether whither or wither? Semin Dial 1997; 10: 134–6.

90. Flanigan MJ, Doyle C, Lim VS, Ullrich G. Tidal peritoneal dialysis: preliminary experience. Perit Dial Int 1992; 12: 304–8.

91. Flanigan MJ, Lim VS, Pflederer TA. Tidal peritoneal dialysis: kinetics and protein balance. Am J Kidney Dis 1993; 22: 700–7.

92. Aasarod K, Wideroe TE, Flakne SC. A comparison of solute clearances and ultrafiltration volume in peritoneal dialysis with total or fractional (50%) intraperitoneal volume exchange with the same dialysate flow rate. Nephrol Dial Transplant 1997; 12: 2128–32.

93. Cocchi R, Catizone L, Boggs R et al. High flow tidal peritoneal dialysis versus IPD: a short-term comparison study. In: Ota K, Winchester JF, Maher JF, Hirzel P, eds. Current Concepts in Peritoneal Dialysis. Amsterdam: Elsevier, 1992, pp. 802–5.

94. Twardowski ZJ, Nolph KD. Is peritoneal dialysis feasible once a large muscular patient becomes anuric? Perit Dial Int 1996; 16: 20–3.

95. Diaz-Buxo JA. Enhancement of peritoneal dialysis: the PD Plus concept. Am J Kidney Dis 1996; 27: 92–8.

96. Page DE. CAPD with a night-exchange device in the only true CAPD? Adv Perit Dial 1998; 14: 60–3.

97. Gotch FA, Sargent JA. A mechanistic analysis of the National Cooperative Dialysis Study (NCDS). Kidney Int 1985; 28: 526–34.

98. Canada-USA (CANUSA) Peritoneal Dialysis Study Group. Adequacy of dialysis and nutrition in continuous peritoneal dialysis: association with clinical outcomes. J Am Soc Nephrol 1996; 7: 198–207.

99. Teehan BP, Schleifer CR, Brown JM, Sigler MH, Raimondo J. Urea kinetic analysis and clinical outcomes on CAPD: a five-year longitudinal study. Adv Perit Dial 1990; 6: 181–5.

100. Maiorca R, Brunori G, Zubani R et al. Predictive value of dialysis and nutritional indices for mortality and morbidity in CAPD and HD patients. A longitudinal study. Nephrol Dial Transplant 1995; 10: 2295–305.

101. Genestier S, Hedelin G, Schaffer P, Faller B. Prognostic factors in CAPD patients: a retrospective study of a 10-year period. Nephrol Dial Transplant 1995; 10: 1905–11.

102. Lameire NH, Vanholder R, Veyt D, Lambert MC, Ringoir S. A longitudinal five-year survey of urea kinetic modeling parameters in CAPD patients. Kidney Int 1992; 42: 426–32.

103. De Alvaro F, Bajo MA, Alvarez-Ude F *et al.* Adequacy of peritoneal dialysis: Does *Kt/V* have the same predictive value as in HD? A multicenter study. Adv Perit Dial 1992; 8: 93–7.

104. Brandes JC, Piering WF, Beres JA, Blumenthal SS, Fritsche C. Clinical outcome of continuous ambulatory peritoneal dialysis predicted by urea and creatinine kinetics. J Am Soc Nephrol 1992; 2: 1430–5.

105. Gejyo F, Odani S, Yamada T *et al.* β-2 microglobulin: a new form of amyloid protein associated with chronic hemodialysis. Kidney Int 1986; 30: 385–90.

106. Massry SG, Goldstein DA. The search for uremic toxin(s) '*x*': '*x*' – PTH. Clin Nephrol 1979; 11: 181–9.

107. Horl WH, Haag-Weber M, Georgopoulos A, Block LH. Physicochemical characteristics of a polypeptide present in uremic serum that inhibits the biological activity of polymorphonuclear cells. Proc Natl Acad Sci USA 1990; 87: 6353–7.

108. Cheung AK. Quantification of dialysis. The importance of membrane and middle molecules. Blood Purif 1994; 12: 42–53.

109. Practice Guidelines of the National Kidney Foundation's Dialysis Outcomes Quality Initiative (DOQI). Adequate dose of peritoneal dialysis. Am J Kidney Dis 1997; 30 (suppl. 2): S86–92.

110. Keshaviah PR, Nolph KD, Van Stone JC. The peak urea concentration hypothesis: a urea kinetic modeling approach to comparing adequacy of continuous ambulatory peritoneal dialysis (CAPD) and hemodialysis. Perit Dial Int 1989; 9: 257–60.

111. Keshaviah P. Adequacy of CAPD: a quantitative approach. Kidney Int 1992; 42 (suppl. 38): S160–4.

112. Keshaviah PK, Ma J, Thorpe K *et al.* Comparison of 2-year survival on hemodialysis (HD) and peritoneal dialysis with dose of dialysis matched using the peak concentration hypothesis. J Am Soc Nephrol 1995; 6: 540 (abstract).

113. Burkart JM, Schreiber M, Korbet SM *et al.* Solute clearance approach to adequacy of peritoneal dialysis. Perit Dial Int 1996; 16: 457–70.

114. Rottembourg J, Issad B, Gallego JL *et al.* Evolution of residual renal function in patients undergoing maintenance hemodialysis or continuous ambulatory peritoneal dialysis. Proc Eur Dial Transplant Assoc 1993; 19: 397–403.

115. Cancarini GC, Brunori G, Camerini C *et al.* Renal function recovery and maintenance of residual diuresis in CAPD and hemodialysis. Perit Dial Bull 1986; 6: 77–9.

116. Lysaght MJ, Vonesh EF, Gotch F *et al.* The influence of dialysis treatment modality on the decline of remaining renal function. ASAIO Trans 1991; 37: 598–604.

117. Hiroshige K, Yuu K, Soejima M, Takasugi M, Kuroiwa A. Rapid decline of residual renal function in patients on automated peritoneal dialysis. Perit Dial Int 1996; 16: 307–15.

118. Pannekeet MM, Imholz AL, Struijk DG *et al.* The standard permeability analysis: a tool for the assessment of peritoneal permeability characteristics in CAPD patients. Kidney Int 1995; 48: 866–75.

119. Baxter Healthcare Corporation. Internal Baxter Evaluation of 806 Patients at 60 U.S. Centers. McGraw Park, Illinois, January 1990.

120. Vonesh EF, Burkart J, McMurray SD, Williams PF. Peritoneal dialysis kinetic modeling: validation in a multicenter clinical study. Perit Dial Int 1996; 16: 471–81.

121. Vonesh EF, Keshaviah PR. Applications in kinetic modeling using PD Adequest®. Perit Dial Int 1997; 17 (suppl. 2): S119–25.

122. Gotch FA, Lipps BJ, Keen ML, Panlilio F. Computerized urea kinetic modeling to prescribe and monitor delivered *Kt/V* (*pKt/V*, d*Kt/V*) in peritoneal dialysis. Fresenius Randomized Dialysis Prescriptions and Clinical Outcome Study (RDP/CO). Adv Perit Dial 1996; 12: 43–5.

123. Jensen RA, Nolph KD, Moore HL. Weight limitations for adequate therapy using commonly performed CAPD and NIPD regimens. Semin Dial 1994; 7: 61–4.

124. Rocco MV. Body surface area limitations in achieving adequate therapy in peritoneal dialysis patients. Perit Dial Int 1996; 16: 617–22.

125. Misra M, Nolph KD, Khanna R. Will automated peritoneal dialysis be the answer? Perit Dial Int 1997; 17: 435–9.

126. Twardowski ZJ. Relationship between creatinine clearances and *Kt/V* in peritoneal dialysis patients: a critique of the DOQI document. Perit Dial Int 1998; 18: 252–5.

127. Practice Guidelines of the National Kidney Foundation's Dialysis Outcomes Quality Initiative (DOQI). Initiation of peritoneal dialysis. Am J Kidney Dis 1997; 30 (suppl. 2): S70–3.

128. Ikizler TA, Greene JH, Wingard RL, Parker RA, Hakim RM. Spontaneous dietary protein intake during progression of chronic renal failure. J Am Soc Nephrol 1995; 6: 1386–91.

129. McCusker FX, Teehan BP, Thorpe KE, Keshaviah PR, Churchill DN. How much peritoneal dialysis is required for the maintenance of a good nutritional state? Kidney Int 1996; 50 (suppl. 56): S56–61.

130. Pollock CA, Ibels LS, Zhu FY *et al.* Protein intake in renal disease. J Am Soc Nephrol 1997; 8: 777–83.

131. Harter HR. Review of significant findings from the National Cooperative Dialysis Study and recommendations. Kidney Int 1983; 23 (suppl. 13): S107–12.

132. Lowrie EG, Lew NL. Death risk in hemodialysis patients: the predictive value of commonly measured variables and an evaluation of death rate differences between facilities. Am J Kidney Dis 1990; 15: 458–82.

133. Bonomini V, Vangelista A, Stefoni S. Early dialysis in renal substitutive programs. Kidney Int 1978; 13 (suppl. 8): S112–16.

134. Tattersall J, Greenwood R, Farrington K. Urea kinetics and when to commence dialysis. Am J Nephrol 1995; 15: 283–9.

135. Schulman G, Hakim RM. Improving outcomes in chronic hemodialysis patients: should dialysis be initiated earlier? Semin Dial 1996; 9: 225–9.

136. Wrenger E, Krautzig S, Brunkhorst R. Adequacy and quality of life with automated peritoneal dialysis. Perit Dial Int 1996; 16 (suppl. 1): S153–7.

137. Walls J, Smith BA, Feehally J, Travernel D, Turgan C. CCPD – an improvement on CAPD. In: Grahl GM, Keisel M, Nolph KD, eds. Advances in Peritoneal Dialysis. Amsterdam: Excerpta Medica, 1981, pp. 141–3.

138. Diaz-Buxo JA, Walker PJ, Burgess WP, Chandler JR, Farmer CD, Holt KL. Current status of CCPD in prevention of peritonitis. Adv Perit Dial 1985, 2: 145–8.

139. Levy M, Balfe JW, Geary D, Fryer-Keene SP. Factors predisposing and contributing to peritonitis during chronic peritoneal dialysis in children: a ten-year experience. Perit Dial Int 1990; 10: 263–9.

140. de Fijter CW, Oe LP, Nauta JJ *et al.* Clinical efficacy and morbidity associated with continuous cyclic compared with continuous ambulatory peritoneal dialysis. Ann Intern Med 1994; 120: 264–71.

141. Burkart JM, Jordan JR, Durnell TA, Case LD. Comparison of exit-site infections in disconnect versus disconnect systems for peritoneal dialysis. Perit Dial Int 1992; 12: 317–20.

142. Viglino G, Gandolfo C, Virga G, Cavalli PL. Role of automated peritoneal dialysis within a peritoneal dialysis program. Adv Perit Dial 1995; 11: 134–8.

143. Williams P, Cartmel L, Hollis J. The role of automated peritoneal dialysis (APD) in an integrated dialysis programme. Br Med Bull 1997; 53: 697–705.

144. Troidle LK, Gorban-Brennan N, Kliger AS, Finkelstein FO. Continuous cycle therapy, manual peritoneal dialysis therapy, and peritonitis. Adv Perit Dial 1998; 14: 137–41.

145. Diaz-Buzo JA. Management of peritonitis in automated peritoneal dialysis patients. Adv Perit Dial 1998; 14: 131–6.

146. Lewis S, Holmes C. Host defence mechanisms in the peritoneal cavity of continuous ambulatory peritoneal dialysis patients. Perit Dial Int 1991; 11: 14–21.

147. de Fijter CW, Verbrugh HA, Peters ED et al. *In vivo* exposure to the currently available peritoneal dialysis fluids decreases the function of peritoneal macrophages in CAPD. Clin Nephrol 1993; 39: 75–80.

148. de Fijter CW, Verbrugh HA, Oe LP et al. Biocompatibility of a glucose-polymer-containing peritoneal dialysis fluid. Am J Kidney Dis 1993; 21: 411–18.

149. Topley N, Alobaidi HM, Davies M, Coles GA, Williams JD, Lloyd D. The effect of dialysate on peritoneal phagocyte oxidative metabolism. Kidney Int 1988; 34: 404–11.

150. Bos HJ, Vlaanderen K, Van der Meulen J, De Veld J, Oe LP, Beelen RHJ. Peritoneal macrophages in short dwell time effluent show diminished phagocytosis. Perit Dial Int 1988; 8: 199–202.

151. Alobaidi HM, Coles GA, Davies M, Lloyd D. Host defence in continuous ambulatory peritoneal dialysis: the effect of the dialysate on phagocyte function. Nephrol Dial Transplant 1986; 1: 16–21.

152. Duwe AK, Vas SI, Weatherhead JW. Effects of the composition of peritoneal dialysis fluid on chemiluminescence, phagocytosis, and bactericidal activity in vitro. Infect Immun 1981; 33: 130–5.

153. Bennett-Jones DN, Yewdall VM, Gillespie CM, Ogg CS, Cameron JS. Strain differences in the opsonization of *Staphylococcus epidermidis*. Perit Dial Int 1989; 9: 333–9.

154. Wrenger E, Baumann C, Behrend M, Zamore E, Schindler R, Brunkhorst R. Peritoneal mononuclear cell differentiation and cytokine production in intermittent and continuous automated peritoneal dialysis. Am J Kidney Dis 1998; 31: 234–41.

155. Vlaanderen K, de Fijter CW, Bos HJ et al. The effect of dwell time on peritoneal phagocytic defense of chronic peritoneal dialysis patients. Adv Perit Dial 1989; 5: 151–3.

156. de Fijter CW, Verbrugh HA, Oe PL, Heezius EC, Verhoef J, Donker AJ. Antibacterial peritoneal defence in automated peritoneal dialysis: advantages of tidal over continuous cyclic peritoneal dialysis. Nephrol Dial Transplant 1994; 9: 156–62.

157. Keane WF, Alexander SR, Bailie GR et al. Peritoneal dialysis-related peritonitis treatment recommendations: 1996 Update. Perit Dial Int 1996; 16: 557–73.

158. Steele M, Kwan JT. Potential problem: delayed detection of peritonitis by patients receiving home automated peritoneal dialysis. Perit Dial Int 1997; 17: 617.

159. Uribarri J, Bottone EJ, London RD. *Pasteurella multocida* peritonitis: are peritoneal dialysis patients on cyclers at increased risk? Perit Dial Int 1996; 16: 648–9.

160. Lindblad AS, Novak JW, Nolph KD et al. Complications of treatment. In Final Report of the National CAPD Registry of the National Institutes of Health. 1988: 4-1–4-13.

161. Holley JL, Bernardini J, Piraino B. Continuous cycling peritoneal dialysis is associated with lower rates of catheter infections than continuous ambulatory peritoneal dialysis. Am J Kidney Dis 1990; 16: 133–6.

162. Fellin G, Gentile MG, Manna GM et al. Peritonitis prevention: a Y-connector and sodium hypochlorite. Three years experience. Report of the Italian CAPD study group. Adv Perit Dial 1987; 3: 114–18.

163. Hussain SI, Bernardini J, Piraino B. The risk of hernia with large exchange volumes. Adv Perit Dial 1998; 14: 105–7.

164. Bleyer AJ, Casey MJ, Russell GB, Kandt M, Burkart JM. Peritoneal dialysate fill-volumes and hernia development in a cohort of peritoneal dialysis patients. Adv Perit Dial 1998; 14: 102–4.

165. Durand PY, Chanliau J, Gamberoni J, Hestin D, Kessler M. Routine measurements of hydrostatic intraperitoneal pressures. Adv Perit Dial 1992; 8: 108–12.

166. Digenis G, Khanna R, Mathews R et al. Abdominal hernias in patients undergoing continuous ambulatory peritoneal dialysis. Perit Dial Bull 1982; 2: 115–17.

167. O'Connor JP, Rigby RJ, Hardie IR et al. Abdominal hernias complicating continuous ambulatory peritoneal dialysis. Am J Nephrol 1986; 6: 271–4.

168. Rocco MV, Stone JW. Abdominal hernias in chronic peritoneal dialysis patients: a review. Perit Dial Bull 1985; 5: 171.

169. Bargman JM. Complications of peritoneal dialysis related to increased intra-abdominal pressure. Kidney Int 1993; 43 (suppl. 40): S75–80.

170. Mandel P, Faegenburg D, Imbriano LJ. The use of technetium-99m sulfur colloid in the detection of patent processus vaginalis in patients on continuous ambulatory peritoneal dialysis. Clin Nucl Med 1985; 10: 553–5.

171. Osborne TM. CT peritoneography in peritoneal dialysis patients. Australas Radiol 1990; 34: 204–6.

172. Thieler H, Riedel E, Pielesch W et al. Continuous ambulatory peritoneal dialysis and pulmonary function. Proc Eur Dial Transplant Assoc 1980; 17: 333–6.

173. Boeschoten EW, Krediet RT, Roos CM, Kloek JJ, Schipper ME, Arisz L. Leakage of dialysate across the diaphragm: an important complication of continuous ambulatory peritoneal dialysis. Neth J Med 1986; 29: 242–6.

174. Lieberman FL, Hidemura R, Peters RL, Reynolds TB. Pathogenesis and treatment of hydrothorax complicating cirrhosis with ascites. Ann Intern Med 1966; 64: 341–51.

175. Green A, Logan M, Medawar W et al. The management of hydrothorax in continuous ambulatory peritoneal dialysis (CAPD). Perit Dial Int 1990; 10: 271–4.

176. Caro J, Brown S, Miller O, Murray T, Erslev AJ. Erythropoietin levels in uremic nephric and anephric patients. J Lab Clin Med 1979; 93: 449–58.

177. Jongen MJ, van der Vijgh WJ, Lips P, Netelenbos JC. Measurements of vitamin D metabolites in anephric subjects. Nephron 1984; 36: 230–4.

178. Hallett M, Owen J, Becker G et al. Maintenance of residual renal function: CAPD versus HD. Perit Dial Int 1992; 12 (suppl. 2): S42 (abstract).

179. Schulman G. A review of the concept of biocompatibility. Kidney Int 1993; 43 (suppl. 41): S209–12.

180. Iest CG, Vanholder RC, Ringoir SM. Loss of residual renal function in patients on regular hemodialysis. Int J Artif Organs 1989; 12: 159–64.

181. Nolph KD, Moore HL, Prowant B et al. Continuous peritoneal dialysis with a high flux membrane. ASAIO J 1993; 39: 904–9.

182. Heaf J. CAPD adequacy and dialysis morbidity: detrimental effect of a high peritoneal equilibration rate. Ren Fail 1995; 17: 575–87.

183. Churchill DN, Thorpe KE, Nolph KD, Keshaviah PR, Oreopoulos DG, Page D. Increased peritoneal membrane transport is associated with decreased patient and technique survival for continuous peritoneal dialysis patients. J Am Soc Nephrol 1998; 7: 1285–92.

184. Wu CH, Huang CC, Huang JY, Wu MS, Leu ML. High flux peritoneal membrane is a risk factor in survival of CAPD treatment. Adv Perit Dial 1996; 12: 105–9.

185. Davies SJ, Phillips L, Russell GI. Peritoneal solute transport predicts survival on CAPD independently of residual renal function. Nephrol Dial Transplant 1998; 13: 962–8.

186. Fried L. Higher membrane permeability predicts poorer patient survival. Perit Dial Int 1997; 17: 387–9.

187. Harty JC, Boulton H, Venning MC, Gokal R. Is peritoneal permeability an adverse risk factor for malnutrition in CAPD patients? Miner Electrol Metab 1996; 22: 97–101.

188. Bergstrom J, Furst P, Alvestrand A, Lindholm B. Protein and energy intake, nitrogen balance, and nitrogen losses in patients treated with continuous ambulatory peritoneal dialysis. Kidney Int 1993; 44: 1048–57.

189. Blake PG. What is the problem with high transporters? Perit Dial Int 1997; 17: 317–20.

190. Wang T, Waniewski J, Heimbürger O, Werynski A, Lindholm B. A quantitative analysis of sodium transport and

removal during peritoneal dialysis. Kidney Int 1997; 52: 1609–16.

191. Kathuria P, Moore HL, Khanna R, Twardowski ZJ, Goel S, Nolph KD. Effect of dialysis modality and membrane transport characteristics on dialysate protein losses of patients on peritoneal dialysis. Perit Dial Int 1997; 17: 449–54.

192. Najarian JS, Kaufman DB, Fryd DS *et al.* Long-term survival following kidney transplantation in 100 type I diabetic patients. Transplantation 1989; 47: 106–13.

193. Diaz-Buxo JA. Blood glucose control in diabetes: I. Semin Dial 1993; 6: 392.

194. Twardowski ZJ, Nolph KD, Khanna R, Gluck Z, Prowant BF, Ryan LP. Daily clearances with continuous ambulatory peritoneal dialysis and nightly peritoneal dialysis. Trans Am Soc Artif Intern Organs 1986; 32: 575–80.

195. Ash SR, Bever SL. Peritoneal dialysis for acute renal failure: the safe, effective, and low cost modality. Adv Ren Replace Ther 1995; 2: 160–3.

196. Sugino N, Kubo K, Nakazoto S *et al.* Therapeutic modalities and outcome in acute renal failure. In: Solez K, Ruzen LC, eds. Acute Renal Failure. New York: Marcel Dekker, 1991, pp. 443–54.

197. Lameire N. Principles of peritoneal dialysis and its application in acute renal failure. In: Ronco C, Bellomo R, eds. Critical Care Nephrology. Dordrecht: Kluwer, 1998, pp. 1357–71.

198. Brady HR, Singer GG. Acute renal failure. Lancet 1995; 346: 1533–40.

199. Conger JD. Does hemodialysis delay recovery from acute renal failure? Semin Dial 1990; 3: 146–8.

200. Schulman G, Hakim R. Hemodialysis membrane biocompatibility in acute renal failure. Adv Ren Replace Ther 1994; 1: 75–82.

201. Lang S, Kuchle C, Fricke H, Schiffl H. Biocompatible intermittent hemodialysis. New Horiz 1995; 3: 680–7.

202. Erbe RW, Greene JA Jr, Weller JM. Peritoneal dialysis during hemorrhagic shock. J Appl Physiol 1967; 22: 131–5.

203. Nolph KD, Miller L, Husted FC, Hirszel P. Peritoneal clearance in scleroderma and diabetes mellitus: effects of intraperitoneal isoproterenol. Int Urol Nephrol 1976; 8: 161–9.

204. Hirszel P, Lasrich M, Maher JF. Divergent effects of catecholamines on peritoneal mass transport. Trans Am Soc Artif Intern Organs 1979; 25: 110–13.

205. Tzamaloukas AH, Garella S, Chazan JA. Peritoneal dialysis for acute renal failure after major abdominal surgery. Arch Surg 1973; 106: 639–43.

206. Nolph KD. Peritoneal dialysis for acute renal failure. Trans Am Soc Artif Intern Organs 1988; 34: 54–5.

207. Brown ST, Ahearn DJ, Nolph KD. Potassium removal with peritoneal dialysis. Kidney Int 1973; 4: 67–9.

208. Latta K, Offner G, Brodehl J. Continuous peritoneal dialysis in children. Adv Perit Dial 1992; 8: 406–9.

209. Zaramella P, Andreeta B, Zanon GF *et al.* Continuous peritoneal dialysis in newborns. Perit Dial Int 1994; 14: 22–5.

210. Mayer AP, McMohan MJ, Corfield AP *et al.* Controlled clinical trial of peritoneal lavage for the treatment of acute pancreatitis. N Engl J Med 1985; 312: 399–404.

211. Barton IK, Inada-Kim M. Acute peritoneal dialysis: how to do it. Br J Hosp Med 1997; 57: 134–6.

212. Posen GA, Luisello J. Continuous equilibration peritoneal dialysis in the treatment of acute renal failure. Perit Dial Bull 1980; 1: 6–7.

213. Steiner RW. Continuous equilibration peritoneal dialysis in acute renal failure. Perit Dial Int 1989; 9: 5–7.

214. Manji S, Shikora S, McMahon M, Blackburn GL, Bistrian BR. Peritoneal dialysis for acute renal failure: overfeeding resulting from dextrose absorbed during dialysis. Crit Care Med 1990; 18: 29–31.

215. Vande Walle J, Raes A, Castillo D, Lutz-Dettinger N, Dejaegher A. Advantages of HCO3 solution with low sodium concentration over standard lactate solutions for acute peritoneal dialysis. Adv Perit Dial 1997; 13: 179–82.

216. Tape TG, Wigton RS, Blank LL, Nicolas JA. Procedural skills of practicing nephrologists. A national survey of 700 members of the American College of Physicians. Ann Intern Med 1990; 113: 392–7.

217. Firmat J, Zucchini A. Peritoneal dialysis in acute renal failure. Contrib Nephrol 1979; 17: 33–8.

218. Rodgers H, Staniland JR, Lipkin GW, Turney JH. Acute renal failure: a study of elderly patients. Age Aging 1990; 19: 36–42.

219. Ash SR, Wimberly AL, Mertz SL. Peritoneal dialysis for acute and chronic renal failure: An update. Hosp Pract 1983; 2: 179–210.

220. Brunkhorst R, Wrenger E, Krautzig S, Ehlerding G, Mahiout A, Koch KM. Clinical experience with home automated peritoneal dialysis. Kidney Int 1994; 46 (suppl. 48): S25–30.

221. Woodrow G, Turney JH, Cook JA *et al.* Nocturnal intermittent peritoneal dialysis. Nephrol Dial Trans 1994; 9: 399–403.

222. Heimbürger O, Waniewski J, Werynski A, Tranaeus A, Lindholm B. Peritoneal transport in CAPD patients with permanent loss of ultrafiltration capacity. Kidney Int 1990; 38: 495–506.

223. Henderson LW. Dialysis in the 21st century. Am J Kidney Dis 1996; 28: 951–7.

14 | Adequacy of peritoneal dialysis

J. M. Burkart

Introduction

As a renal replacement therapy, dialysis, at best, only approximates normal renal function (Table 1). Despite these deficiencies, however, dialysis has extended the lives of end-stage renal disease (ESRD) patients, some for over 20 years [1]. Although many patients do very well on dialysis, data compiled by the Health Care Financing Administration (HCFA) and analysed by the United States Renal Disease System (USRDS) have shown that the gross mortality rate for the United States ESRD population (predominantly haemodialysis (HD) patients) in 1990 was 24% [2]. The extent to which uraemia in the form of underdialysis contributed to this overall mortality rate in ESRD patients is unknown. Some have suggested that inadequacies in the prescribed dose of dialysis were contributing to these high mortality rates [3, 4]. As a result, more attention has been paid to patient outcome and to optimizing total solute clearance. The mean Kt/V for subpopulations of HD patients has increased from 1.0/Rx in patients starting dialysis during 1986–87 to 1.22/Rx in a random sample of prevalent HD patients in December 1993 [5]. Associated with this change there has been a gradual increase in the adjusted 1-, 2- and 5-year patient survival percentages for patients starting dialysis over the years 1979–73.

Although 'adequate' dialysis is crucial for the well-being of any ESRD patient, adequacy of peritoneal dialysis or any renal replacement therapy is difficult to define. The word 'adequacy' comes from the Latin word '*adequare*' [6], which means 'to equalize'. Idealistically, this would mean that adequate dialysis would return the patients' lifestyle and life-expectancy to what it would have been if the patient never had renal disease. 'Optimal' dialysis prescriptions are said to be those in which there is no further incremental improvement in patient outcome as the dose is increased further while also imparting minimal negative effects on the patient's quality of life.

One indisputable reason for the lower life-expectancy in ESRD patients is that they have at least one chronic medical condition and therefore are 'patients', and not healthy individuals. In addition, ESRD patients tend to have multiple comorbid diseases at initiation of dialysis that can also adversely influence outcome [7], the prevalence of which is increasing. We can influence the patient's total solute clearance. Nephrologists must do their best to provide enough renal replacement therapy so we are sure that the amount of dialysis delivered is not the rate-limiting step that determines whether the patient lives or dies. One example of this concept is the data by Charra *et al.* [8], who reported on long-term [20 years) follow-up for 445 unselected HD patients, all of whom received 24 hours/week of conventional HD using Kiil plate dialysers. The mean Kt/V for these 445 patients was 1.67, much higher than the estimated average prescribed Kt/V in the USA at that time ($Kt/V = 1.02$) [9]. Each gender subgroup was then split into two equal-numbered subgroups as a function of Kt/V and mean arterial pressure (MAP). For these subgroups outcome was not a function of Kt/V, but was correlated with blood pressure, and age. The overall 20-year patient survival was 43%, approaching that for healthy individuals of the same age! This is an example of an optimal dialysis prescription – i.e. one in which patient outcome is dependent not on the amount of dialysis delivered, but on the other comorbid dis-

Table 1. Solute removal by dialysis and the natural kidney

	Natural solute kidney	HD–standard flux	HD–Hi flux	CAPD
Urea (L/week)	750	130	130	70
Vitamin B$_{12}$ (L/week)	1200	30	60	40
Inulin (L/week)	1200	10	40	20
β$_2$-microglobulin (mg/wk)	1000	0	300	250

(Keshaviah P. Adequacy of CAPD: a quantitative approach. Kidney Int 1992; 42 (suppl. 28): S160–4.)

R. Gokal, R. Khanna, R.Th. Krediet and K.D. Nolph (eds.), Textbook of Peritoneal Dialysis, 2nd Edition, 465–497.
© 2000 *Kluwer Academic Publishers. Printed in Great Britain.*

eases that are present. Our goal as nephrologists is to provide this optimal dose of dialysis.

This chapter discusses adequacy issues for peritoneal dialysis (PD) in terms of total solute clearance and other issues related to the PD prescription. It acknowledges that adequacy of dialysis addresses more than just total solute clearance issues. Optimal treatment of a patient with ESRD must additionally address multiple issues such as blood pressure, volume control, treatment of acidosis, anaemia and prevention of metabolic bone disease, most of which are beyond the scope of this chapter.

What yardstick for adequacy of dialysis should we use?

Many of the known clinical manifestations of uraemia, such as decreased appetite, metallic taste, nausea, vomiting, pericarditis, pleuritis and encephalopathy, are obvious [10]. There is evidence to suggest that underdialysis may be associated with hypertension [11] and lipid abnormalities [12], both of which may increase the risk of atherogenesis, cardiovascular disease and mortality. Uraemic neuropathy may not be diagnosed until it is far advanced, at which time it may be irreversible [13]. Because of the insidious onset and potentially fatal or irreversible nature of some manifestations of uraemia, nephrologists needed a laboratory parameter that measures the delivered amount of solute clearance, while predicting patient outcome. There is no documented single substance that has been shown to be the 'uraemic toxin'. Undoubtedly, the clinical manifestations of the uraemic syndrome are the result of the synergistic effect of an entire family of uraemic toxins of both small and moderate molecular weights. Therefore, because there is no single uraemic toxin, we will have to rely on surrogate markers for uraemia. Currently, solutes such as urea nitrogen, creatinine and β_2-microglobulin are commonly used.

There are data to suggest that the outcome for both HD and PD patients [14, 15] is related to total solute clearance. However, it would be appropriate to ask, whether protein intake, nutritional status or middle molecule clearance should be used as the yardstick for dialysis dose.

It has been suggested that dietary protein intake (estimated by obtaining the protein equivalent of nitrogen balance or PNA) tends to correlate with total solute clearance [16]. A higher Kt/V is generally associated with a higher protein energy intake,

both in HD and in PD. Would it suffice to only monitor normalized PNA, and if it is stable and in an adequate range, assume that the dose of dialysis is 'adequate?' Anecdotal clinical data would suggest the answer is no. Furthermore, their relationship may be more mathematical than physiological. Our current practical ways to measure protein intake are estimations of protein intake [17] and can be very misleading when the patient is not in a steady state. The protein equivalent of nitrogen appearance or PNA will often overestimate dietary protein intake (DPI) in a catabolic state and may underestimate DPI when anabolic. The relationship between protein intake, solute clearance, and the manifestations of uraemia is likely to be different in each patient. Certainly, small molecular weight clearance is not the only factor that determines dietary protein intake. Comorbid diseases have a significant impact. Therefore, although PNA should be an adequacy target, it cannot be the only target used.

It is a common clinical experience that when PD patients manifest uraemic symptoms they improve after increasing the volume or number of exchanges/ day. Figure 1 demonstrates the theoretical influence of the number of PD exchanges on the weekly solute clearance for a wide range of molecular weights. It is clear that increasing the number of exchanges per day results in only a minimal increase in large or middle molecule clearance, but a marked increase in small solute clearance (MW <500 Da). Therefore, based on Keshaviah's theoretical projections [18] and the available clinical experience, it seems that overall small solute clearance, not middle or large molecular weight clearance, is most closely related to uraemic toxicity, and that small solute clearance

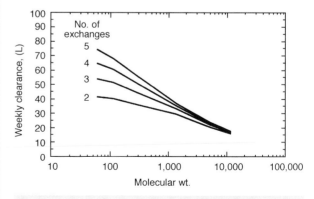

Figure 1. The influence of the number of CAPD exchanges on the weekly solute clearance for a range of solute molecular weights derived from a computerized model of peritoneal transport. (Keshaviah P. Adequacy of CAPD: A quantitative approach. Kidney Int 1992; 42 (suppl. 38): S160–4.)

in terms of urea or creatinine kinetics should be used for monitoring dialysis dose.

Total solute clearance ($K_{renal} + K_{peritoneal} = K_{rp}$) for PD is commonly estimated in terms of urea clearance as weekly Kt/V_{urea} or if using creatinine as weekly creatinine clearance (CCr) normalized to 1.73m^2. These calculations assume that residual renal and peritoneal clearances are equal, although there are no data to prove this. Residual renal CCr is typically determined as the sum of urea and creatinine clearances/2 (corrected creatinine clearance), and is felt to be an estimate of glomerular filtration [19]. The equations for calculating total solute clearance can be found in the Appendix.

Minimal target dose for PD – outcome studies

Many studies have looked at patient outcomes in terms of relative risk of death or morbidity and its relationship to total solute clearance. Their significance and relevance to predicting patient outcome have been reviewed elsewhere [20–22]. The multiple-outcome studies published to date differ in methodology and number of patients enrolled. All tend to conclude that outcome (relative risk of death) is in some way related to total solute clearance. However, the recommended minimal total solute clearance goal one should attempt to achieve is slightly different in each study. These studies are briefly reviewed below.

Kt/V data

Theoretical constructs

In the original description of CAPD, Popovich and Moncrief predicted that an anephric 70 kg patient (total body water or $V = 42$ L) would remain in positive nitrogen balance when prescribed five 2 L exchanges/day [23]. Based on theoretical data, others felt a patient would need the equivalent of a weekly Kt/V of 2.0–2.25 [18, 24].

Based on theoretical constructs, if maintenance of positive nitrogen balance was the desired outcome, a target weekly Kt/V of 2.0–2.25 would be appropriate.

Univariate analysis

A series of cohort studies attempted to provide clinical validation of the above theoretical data. Blake *et al.* [25], using urea kinetics and an anthropomet-

ric method to calculate V, found limited value in predicting patient outcome by total Kt/V (patients with a total Kt/V of <1.5 had a higher relative risk of death). Lameire *et al.* [26] reported that the mean weekly total Kt/V in a group of 16 patients who had been on PD at least 5 years was >1.89 (most of whom were anuric), while DeAlvaro *et al.* [27] found that patients with a weekly Kt/V of >2.0 were more likely to survive. In summary, these studies using univariate analysis, which did not examine the role of other important variables (such as diabetes, cardiovascular disease, age), suggested that a total Kt/V of <1.9 was associated with an increased risk of death.

Multivariate analysis

Using multivariate analysis of data, Teehan *et al.* [28] suggested that increased patient age, time on dialysis, lower serum albumin levels and lower weekly total Kt/V were predictive of decreased patient survival. The 5-year survival for patients with a total Kt/V of >1.89 was $>90\%$. Maiorca *et al.* [29] evaluated a group of *prevalent* PD patients who had been on dialysis for a mean of 35 ± 26 months and followed them for up to 3 years. Patients with a mean weekly total Kt/V during the study period of at least 1.96 had a better overall survival. They did not find an increased survival rate for patients with a mean weekly total Kt/V of >2.03 versus those with a total Kt/V of 1.96–2.03. It is important to note that these prevalent patients had a mean residual renal glomerular filtration rate (GFR) of 1.73 ml/min at enrolment into the study. Genestier *et al.* [30] retrospectively evaluated 201 CAPD patients followed for 23.95 ± 21.37 months using baseline values only. They found that baseline weekly total Kt/V must be higher than 1.7 for optimal survival, and their data did not support a decrease in the relative risk with any further increase in Kt/V. None of these studies evaluated the effect of the decline in overall solute clearance over time, and it was uncertain as to what benefit, if any, patients would achieve if the weekly Kt/V was higher than the recommended cutoffs.

A prospective multicentre cohort study of *incident* patients in North America (Canadian and USA Study – CANUSA) evaluated the association of total solute clearance (Kt/V, creatinine clearance) and nutrition as time-dependent covariates with patient mortality, technique failure and hospitalization [14]. Baseline residual renal GFR in this cohort was approximately 3.8 ml/min at enrolment into the study [39 L/week]. These data suggested that total solute clearance (K_{pr}) predicted outcome. Every 0.1 unit increase in total weekly Kt/V was associated with a 6% decrease in the relative risk of death; similarly, every 5 L/1.73m^2/week increase in total creatinine clearance (CCr) was associated with a 7% decrease in the relative risk of death. Over the range of the clearances studied there was no evidence of a plateau effect. The predicted 2-year survival associated with a constant Kt/V of 2.1 was 78%. The weekly total CCr that was associated with a 78% 2-year survival was 70 L/1.73m^2.

Although the CANUSA study gives us the best evidence that survival on PD is related to total solute clearance, it is important to note that the results are based on theoretical constructs and two very important assumptions: (1) total solute clearance remained stable over time, and (2) one unit or ml/min of clearance due to residual renal function is equal to one unit or ml/min of clearance due to PD. In fact, total solute clearance decreased over time as residual renal function decreased with no corresponding increase in the peritoneal component (Figure 2). Therefore, because the peritoneal component of total solute clearance tended not to change over the course of the study, one interpretation of CANUSA would be to say that the more residual renal function the better. The CANUSA conclusions must be interpreted with some caution. These survival curves are statistical models that require clinical validation, and to date there are no data to prove that these assumptions are true. The clinical conclusion of CANUSA and their controversies have been recently reviewed [31]. Interventional studies with a constant total solute clearance are needed for more definitive proof of these results.

More recently published data in abstract form look only at relative risk of death in relationship to solute clearance in a group of anuric patients [32]. These patients had been on PD a mean of 16.5 (range 0–110) months on enrolment into the study (development of anuria). Their total solute clearance was thus due to peritoneal clearance only. Using multiple regression analysis, outcome was related to total solute clearance in terms of Kt/V and creatinine clearance. In these patients the best survival was associated with a Kt/V of >1.8/week and creatinine clearance >50 L/1.73 m^2/week, which was associated with a 58% reduction in risk of mortality. There was no demonstrated incremental improvement for higher values.

In summary, data from studies using multivariate analysis would suggest that for continuous therapies

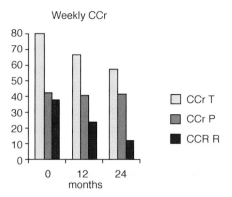

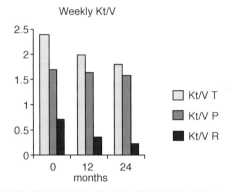

Figure 2. Total solute clearance over time for residual renal function (RRF) and peritoneal clearance (K_p) for both *Kt/V* and creatinine clearance (CCr). (Churchill DN, Taylor DW, Keshaviah PR. Adequacy of dialysis and nutrition in continuous PD: Association with clinical outcomes. J Am Soc Nephrol 1996; 7: 198–207.)

such as CAPD a weekly total Kt/V_{urea} of at least 2.0–2.1 would be a reasonable minimal total solute clearance target.

Creatinine clearance data

Studies measuring total solute clearance in terms of creatinine clearance (CCr) have also suggested that clearance predicted outcome [24, 25, 33]. In the CANUSA study total CCr predicted not only death, but also technique survival and hospitalization [14]. Analysis of those data suggested that a total weekly CCr of >70 L/1.73 m^2 would predict a 78% 2-year patient survival. In the report by Maiorca *et al.* [29] in which a total weekly Kt/V of 1.98 corresponded to a total weekly CCr of 58 L/1.73 m^2, patients with a mean weekly total CCr of <50 L/1.73 m^2 did significantly worse than those with higher clearances. Genestier *et al.* [30] reported that total CCr was a sensitive predictor of death. Patients with a weekly total CCr of <50 L/1.73 m^2 had a five times higher risk of death than those with higher levels; while in anuric patients [32] the best survival was associated with a weekly creatinine clearance of > 50 L/1.73 m².

These data would suggest that for continuous therapies the minimal weekly CCr should be at least 60 L/1.73 m².

Recommended acceptable total solute clearance targets for PD

An ad hoc committee on adequacy of peritoneal dialysis [21] has reviewed the literature published as of mid-1997 and has recommended the following minimal total weekly solute clearances (Table 2). For continuous therapies such as CAPD, available evidence would support a target total weekly Kt/V of > 2.0 or a minimal weekly total CCr of > 60 L/1.73 m².

For continuous cycling peritoneal dialysis (CCPD) the recommended targets are a weekly $Kt/V \geqslant 2.1$ and a weekly creatinine clearance of $\geqslant 63$ L/1.73 m². This slight increase in weekly total solute clearance goals when compared to CAPD is based on the fact that the daytime dwell for CCPD (14–15 h) tends to be longer than the night-time dwell (9–10 h) for CAPD. During the long daytime dwell for CCPD, diffusive transport tends to stop because equilibrium between dialysis and plasma has been reached in most patients and, hence, the therapy is less 'continuous' than CAPD.

For intermittent therapies such as nightly intermittent peritoneal dialysis (NIPD) or daily intermittent peritoneal dialysis (DAPD), the weekly Kt/V should be at least 2.2, and the weekly total CCr should be at least 66 L/1.73 m². These higher targets were calculated by Gotch and Keen [34].

There are no clinical outcome data to prove that higher total solute clearance goals are needed for CCPD and NIPD. Reasons for the higher recom-

mended solute clearances for intermittent therapies are based on the following theoretical arguments.

1. The possibility that the peak concentration of retained solutes [35], not the time-averaged concentration of retained solutes, relates to uraemic symptoms and perhaps inhibits appetite.
2. Data which suggest that when one adjusts for differences in comorbid diseases and scales for differences in the dose of dialysis for PD and HD, expected 2-year survival is the same [36].

Are the NKF-DOQI total solute guidelines on target?

Bhaskaran *et al.* [32] have reported that only 57% of CAPD and 81% of APD patients had a weekly Kt/V of $\geqslant 2.0$ and 2.2 respectively. Additionally, only 35% of CAPD and 35% of APD patients reached the creatinine clearance of 60 and 66 L/1.73 m²/week respectively. Others have found that 38.7% of patients met both Kt/V and CCr targets, while in 6.3% only Kt/V was at target, and in another 16.4% CCr, but not Kt/V was at target. Thirty-eight per cent did not reach either target [37].

Using kinetic modelling, one would predict that in anuric patients the average patient with a Kt/V of 2.0 is unlikely to have a creatinine clearance greater than 60 L/week [34, 38]. Clinical experience in anuric patients would confirm these findings. The NKF-DOQI Guidelines [21] are based on outcome data published as of June 1997. There were no outcome data in anuric patients published at that time.

The NKF-DOQI Committee felt that these minimal total solute clearance values (i.e. for CAPD, $Kt/V = 2.0$; CCr = 60 L/1.73 m²) would be constant no matter the relative contribution of residual renal function, stating that *both* yardsticks should be above target and that if any one is at target, that one yardstick should be Kt/V. If one were to review minimal total solute clearance recommendations in anuric patients, one notes that the minimal total solute clearance values are less than the NKF-DOQI Guidelines, and they are relatively lower for CCr than for Kt/V (Fig. 3). Once more data are available the guidelines may need to be modified, as noted in editorials regarding the adequacy of PD [39, 40]. However, as of 1 November 1998 these are the recommended guidelines to follow.

Table 2. Minimal recommendations for dialysis dose

Continuous ambulatory peritoneal dialysis (CAPD)
  $Kt/V \geqslant 2.0$ per week
  Creatinine clearance $\geqslant 60$ L/week/1.73 m²

Continuous cycling peritoneal dialysis (CCPD)
  $Kt/V > 2.1$ per week
  Creatinine clearance > 63 L/week/1.73 m²

Intermittent peritoneal dialysis (NIPD, DAPD)
  $Kt/V \geqslant 2.2$ per week
  Creatinine clearance > 66 L/week/1.73 m²

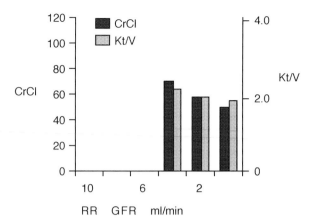

Figure 3. Recommended weekly targets for *Kt/V* and creatinine clearance from published studies plotted in relationship to residual renal (RR) GFR in mls/min at baseline. (Churchill DN, Taylor DW, Keshaviah PR. Adequacy of dialysis and nutrition in continuous PD: association with clinical outcomes. J Am Soc Nephrol 1996; 7: 198–207; Maiorca R, Brunori G, Zubani R *et al.* Predictive value of dialysis adequacy and nutritional indices for morbidity and mortality in CAPD and HD patients. A longitudinal study. Nephrol Dial Transplant 1995; 10: 2295–305; Bhaskaran S, Schaubel DE, Jassal V *et al.* The effect of small solute clearance on survival of anuric PD patients (abstract). Perit Dial Int 1999 (in press).)

Impact of nutritional status on patient outcome

Nutritional issues in PD patients are extensively reviewed in Chapter 16 of this book. Their relevance to 'adequacy' of dialysis is briefly reviewed below. A patient's underlying nutritional status is dependent on many non-ESRD-related factors (comorbid diseases, depression, gastroparesis, etc.). Additionally, chronic renal failure is associated with a variety of metabolic and nutritional abnormalities. It is well known that nausea, vomiting and appetite suppression are symptoms of uraemia, and that uraemic patients tend to have decreased dietary protein intake (DPI) [41]. Furthermore, spontaneous DPI decreases as residual renal GFR decreases to less than 50 to 25 ml/min [42]. These tendencies may be exacerbated during the period prior to the initiation of dialysis when many patients are not only anorexic but are acidotic and are treated with low-protein 'renal protective' diets. As a result, patients may exhibit signs of protein malnutrition when they present for dialysis. Earlier initiation of dialysis (see later) may prevent this.

Dialysis itself is associated with unique metabolic and nutritional problems. Peritoneal dialysis patients are known to have a decreased appetite and early satiety [43,44]. PD patients typically lose 5–15 g of protein and 2–4 g of amino acids in their dialysate/day [45]. These losses amount to a net loss equivalent to 0.2 g protein/kg/day. Rapid transporters lose more protein than low transporters. These losses are increased during episodes of peritonitis [46] and can double even after a mild episode.

In the most extensive evaluation of a cross-section of CAPD patients published to date, 49.6% (111/224) were found to have signs of malnutrition [47]. Eight per cent were severely malnourished, and these patients tended to have minimal to no residual renal function. Malnutrition was present in 18.1% of patients on CAPD treated for less than 3 months, compared to 41.6% of patients on CAPD for longer than 3 months. In this study there was no attempt to increase total solute clearance as residual renal function decreased. Hence, total solute clearance tended to be less in long-term PD patients with minimal residual renal function. Marckmann evaluated 16 CAPD patients using mid-arm circumference/skin thickness measurements and found that only 44% had normal nutritional status [48], while Pollock *et al.* [49] found that 23% of CAPD patients had <80% of normal total body nitrogen with a mean of 88% of normal for the group.

Repeated studies in both ESRD (50–53) and non-ESRD [54] patients have shown that one of the most important predictors of outcome is the patient's underlying nutritional status. Data by Lowrie *et al.* best exemplify this point [50]. In HD patients, as the serum albumin decreases from the reference value of 4.5 to 4.0 g/dl to an albumin of less than 2.5 g/dl, the risk of death increased to 18 times that of the reference group. This is corroborated by data from the USRDS [55]. The link between malnutrition and poor clinical outcome does not rely solely on serum albumin as a marker. Loss of muscle mass as indicated by lower serum creatinine or total body-nitrogen levels, low prealbumin levels and subjective global assessment score are all good predictors of morbidity and mortality. Hence for optimal PD therapy the effect of total solute clearance on nutrition must be known and minimized.

Measurements of nutritional status

Of the readily available measures of nutritional status, serum albumin levels, protein equivalent of nitrogen balance (PNA) and subjective global assessment scores (SGA), have traditionally been used.

Serum albumin levels

Serum albumin levels are a measure of visceral protein storage and are a predictor of patient outcome in ESRD populations. Teehan et al. [28] have reported that serum albumin was a more immediate and more sensitive predictor of death than dialysis dose. Others have shown that in PD patients a low serum albumin concentration was a marker for increased morbidity and mortality, no matter if obtained at the initiation of therapy [56], over the duration of dialysis, [28, 57], or measured at a stable period while on dialysis [58, 59]. In the CANUSA study, serum albumin and subjective global assessment scores were powerful predictors of patient outcome [14] even at initiation of dialysis.

It is important to recognize that different assays for serum albumin give markedly different results [60]. The Bromocresol green assay is preferred. Using this, the mean albumin level in 1202 PD patients in late 1994/early 1995 was 3.5 g/dl [61].

PD patients tend to have a lower serum albumin than HD patients, for reasons that are unclear. Although serum albumin appears to be a very good marker of overall nutritional status in PD patients, its overall significance in an individual patient must be viewed with caution. The causes of hypoalbuminaemia are multifactorial (Table 3), and when evaluating an individual patient all causes must considered, including the possibility that a chronic inflammatory state exists in both HD [62, 63] and PD [64, 65].

During PD the peritoneal cavity is repeatedly exposed to unphysiological fluids [66, 67]. Morphological studies reveal that the morphology of the peritoneum changes over time on PD [68]. These changes may be related to cytotoxicity due to hyperosmolality, low pH, lactate buffers, and glycosylation of protein. Additionally, it has been debated that current PD solutions may [69] or may not [70] induce a chronic inflammatory state. This chronic inflammatory state may eventually lead to changes in peritoneal transport and the development of a sclerosing syndrome of the peritoneal cavity [71, 72]. Serum C-reactive protein (sCRP) levels, an acute-phase protein thought to be a marker of a chronic/acute inflammatory state, were a predictor of survival at 2 years at initiation of PD [73] and while on HD [62]. Of note is that it has also been reported that sCRP levels in PD patients were lower than those in HD patients and comparable to those with chronic renal insufficiency [74]. It is possible that our current 'standard' solutions need to be modified to maintain vaiability of membrane clearance capacity and membrane durability. However, it is difficult to prove that the abnormalities noted in vitro are the sole reason for the long-term detrimental effects on the peritoneum [75]. Once more is known the future discussions of adequacy may also involve discussions about controlling/modifying the chronic inflammatory state.

Protein equivalent of nitrogen balance

PNA is a useful tool for monitoring estimated protein intake. Estimated DPI is calculated from urea nitrogen appearance (UNA) in dialysate and urine. Multiple equations have been suggested, some of which have been validated in CAPD (not NIPD) patients (i.e. PNA = PCR + protein losses) (Table 4). Most [95%] of nitrogen intake in humans is in the form of protein. Therefore, when the patient is in a steady state (not catabolic or anabolic), total nitrogen excretion multiplied by 6.25 (there are about 6.25 g protein/g of nitrogen) is a good estimation of DPI [76]. This calculation was initially called the protein catabolic rate (PCR). PCR actually represents the amount of protein catabolism exceeding synthesis required to generate an amount of nitrogen that is excreted. PCR is actually a net catabolic equivalent. Thus, because these calculations are based on nitrogen appearance, the term is more

Table 3. Causes of hypoalbuminaemia

Dilutional (volume overload)
Decreased synthesis
Increased body losses
    Urine
    Dialysate
Chronic inflammatory states

Table 4. Commonly used formulas of dietary protein intake (DPI)

Formula for calculating PNA

Randerson I	PNA = 10.76 (UNA/1.44 + 1.46], where UNA is in g/day
Randerson II	PNA = 10.76 (UNA + 1.46], where UNA is in mg/min
Modified Borah	PNA = $9.35 G_{un}$ + $.294 V$ + protein losses
Teehan	PNA = 6.25 (UN_{loss} + 1.81 + 0.031 body weight)
Kjelldahl	PNA = 6.25 × N. loss
Bergstrom	PNA = 19 + 7.62 × UNA

(Modified from Kopple JD, Jones MR, Keshaviah PK et al. A proposed glossary for dialysis kinetics. Am J Kidney Dis 1995; 26: 963–81 and Keshaviah P, Nolph K. Protein catabolic rate calculations in CAPD patients. ASAIO Trans 1991; 37: M400–2.)

appropriately called the protein equivalent of nitrogen appearance, or PNA.

Keshaviah and Nolph [77] have compared these formulae and recommended the Randerson equation [78], where PNA = 10.76 (UNA + 1.46), and UNA is in mg/min, or PNA = 10.76 (UNA/1.44 + 1.46), and UNA is in g/day. These equations assume that the patient is in a steady state where UNA = urea nitrogen output which equals urea generation. The Randerson equation also assumes that the average protein loss in the dialysate is 7.3 g/day. In dialysis patients with substantial urinary or dialysate protein losses these direct protein losses must be added to the equation to yield a true PNA.

The PNA must be normalized for patient size (nPNA). What weight to use for normalization is controversial. Depending on what weight is used in calculating nPNA, there may or may not be a statistical relationship between malnutrition and nPNA values below target. PNA normalized by standard weight or actual weight tends to be high in malnourished individuals. For instance, a malnourished patient's nPNA may not be low, or may seem to be increasing over time if a malnourished, lesser 'weight' is used for normalization compared to the patient's baseline weight [79]. In this case, over time, the absolute PNA may decrease, causing malnutrition, while the normalized values remain the same. This fact is important not only for patient-to-patient comparisons, but more importantly when comparing serial measurements in an individual patient. The DOQI working group recommends using standard weight or $V/0.58$ for normalization [80]. The weight used in this case for normalization does not change, and nPNA is more likely to reflect these changes. However, it has been shown that protein intake, not nPNA, correlates best with outcome and signs of malnutrition [79].

A nPNA should be obtained at baseline during training. Decreasing values would then suggest a decreasing protein intake. One cause for this may be a suboptimal total solute clearance.

Subjective global assessment score

The subjective global assessment (SGA) score [81] modified for PD, is a valid estimate of nutritional status in PD patients [82]. In the CANUSA study a modified SGA using a seven-point scale addressing four items (weight change, anorexia, subcutaneous tissue and muscle mass) predicted outcome [14]. On multivariate analysis, poorer SGA scores were associated with a higher relative risk of death. It is

recommended that this simple test be obtained sequentially (twice a year) in PD patients to evaluate nutritional status. If a decline is noted, evaluate for comorbid diseases and consider a suboptimal total solute clearance as the cause.

Dietary protein requirements in peritoneal dialysis

There is some controversy as to what amount of dietary protein intake (DPI), in terms of grams of protein per kilogram of body weight, is needed to maintain positive nitrogen balance in peritoneal dialysis patients. Early studies suggested that a dietary protein intake of at least 1.2 g/kg/day was needed to maintain nitrogen balance [83, 84], a value considerably higher than that recommended for normal individuals. Total energy intake (including PD glucose absorption) is recommdended to be at least 35 kcal/kg body weight – similar to that for healthy individuals [85]. However, cross-sectional studies by Bergstrom *et al.* [86] and Nolph [87] suggest that their patients who show no signs of malnutrition seem to eat less (0.99, 0.88 g protein/kg/day respectively). If a DPI, estimated by nPNA, of at least 1.0 g/kg/day is considered adequate to maintain normal nutrition in these patients, then a 'minimal' dose of PD needed to achieve this can be estimated from published data (Fig. 4). These data would suggest that for PD patients to achieve a nPNA of approximately 1.0 g/kg/day, a total Kt/V of 1.9–2.1/week is needed, similar to the minimal targets suggested by outcome data. Note from the

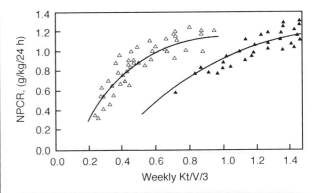

Figure 4. Correlation between *Kt/V* (weekly *Kt/V*/3) and protein catabolic rate (NPCR) for HD patients (solid triangles) and CAPD patients (open triangles). In contrast to previous reports, the nonlinear correlation appears to be the stronger relationship. (From ref. 207, Ronco C, Bosch JP, Lew SQ, *et al.* Adequacy of continuous ambulatory peritoneal dialysis: comparison with other dialysis techniques. Kidney Int 1994; 46 (suppl. 48): S18–24.)

figures that a HD dose of 1.2–1.3 /Rx would also be needed for a similar target nPNA.

Relationship between solute clearance and estimations of dietary protein intake

Strategies aimed at preventing malnutrition in PD patients have been reviewed elsewhere [88, 89]. Although nephrologists may not be able to modify pre-existing comorbid diseases, by preventing malnutrition one may be able to prevent the development of cardiac disease while on dialysis [90]. Hence, if it is possible to minimize malnutrition by providing 'adequate' clearance of solute, this should be attempted.

Lindsay *et al.* [16] have shown that attempts to increase DPI by dietary counselling or protein supplementation alone were unsuccessful without first increasing the dialysis dose in HD patients. This observation suggests that patients must be adequately dialysed to assure a satisfactory DPI. In cross-sectional analyses of data, a linear relationship between PNA and Kt/V was found, suggesting that DPI was partly dependent on Kt/V [86, 87, 91]. However, it is argued that this may be due to mathematical coupling of data [92]. Definitive data which show that, for an individual patient, as total solute clearance (dialysis dose) is increased, protein intake, nutritional status and predicted outcome all similarly increase, are lacking.

Data correlating PNA to serum albumin in PD patients is scarce [93]. Although it is clear that there are other factors that determine the serum albumin concentration, the relationship between DPI and serum albumin concentration or nutritional status is a significant one. Thus, in PD patients who do not normalize their serum albumin concentrations, inadequate DPI and/or inadequate total solute clearance must be considered as the possible cause. In fact, some have recommended that protein intake, estimated from nPNA, be monitored as a yardstick for adequacy of dialysis [94]. Preliminary data have shown that a change in total solute clearance is associated with a corresponding change in serum albumin [18, 95, 96]. Similarly, it was noted in the CANUSA Study that nutritional parameters increased as dialysis was initiated [56]. These data suggest that for adequate dialysis the solute clearance must be sufficient to allow for adequate protein intake in order to optimize patient outcome. At our centre, if the patient has a low albumin (<4.0 g/dl),

underdialysis is always part of the differential diagnosis.

Interestingly, when comparing the slope of the line for Kt/V verses PNA in HD and CAPD patients, there tends to be a much steeper slope for CAPD patients than for HD patients (Fig. 4). Perhaps the stimulus for dietary protein and energy intake is related to the peak concentration of retained uraemic toxins. HD is an intermittent therapy, associated with peaks and valleys for serum concentrations of urea and other solutes, while CAPD maintains a stable concentration of uraemic toxins during the week. Therefore, HD may require a relatively higher overall dose/week to assure that the peak concentrations of solutes achieved are not higher than those maintained with standard CAPD (Fig. 5). This theory, termed the 'peak concentration hypothesis' [35], may explain why the average weekly solute clearance measured in Kt/V is less for CAPD than it is for HD (2.0 versus 3.4/week). The observation that CAPD patients tend to have a greater dietary protein intake than HD patients for a given Kt/V would support this hypothesis. Again, note that in these data for both HD and PD patients the relationship between Kt/V and PNA tended to level off at a PNA of about 0.9–1.2 g/kg/day. This point on the curve for PD patients corresponds to a weekly Kt/V of 2.0, similar to the recommended minimal weekly target determined from review of clinical outcome data. This is one reason the NKF-DOQI Guidelines recommended higher clearances for intermittent PD therapies such as CCPD and NIPD.

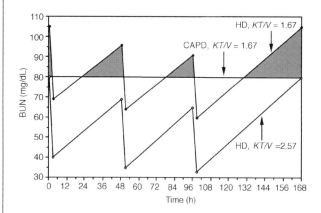

Figure 5. Theoretical weekly BUN profiles for haemodialysis patients with a weekly *Kt/V* of 1.67 and 2.57 compared to the steady state BUN of CAPD with a weekly *Kt/V* of 1.67. (Keshaviah PR, Nolph KD, Van Stone JC. The peak concentration hypothesis: a urea kinetic approach to comparing the adequacy of continuous ambulatory PD (CAPD) and HD. Perit Dial Int 1989; 9: 257–60.)

Summary of dialysis dosing

To summarize the available information regarding dialysis dosing in CAPD patients, several key points should be emphasized: (1) total solute clearance predicts outcome; (2) nutritional status predicts outcome; (3) total solute clearance is correlated with PNA in patients in whom there are no other significant diseases that interfere with dietary protein intake; (4) inadequate clearance may result in subtle irreversible or slowly reversible uraemic changes; (5) solute clearance should be monitored; (6) minimal target weekly total solute clearances have been established (Table 2); (7) monitoring and dose adjustments should be proactive, not reactive.

Major determinants of total solute clearance

Residual renal function

Each 1 ml/min of corrected residual renal creatinine clearance adds approximately 10 L/week/1.73 m² for the average patient with a BSA of 1.73 m². Similarly, for each 1 ml/min of residual renal urea clearance, approximately 0.25 Kt/V is added to the total weekly Kt/V urea for a 70 kg male. For instance, if a patient starts PD with a residual renal creatinine clearance of 5 ml/min (not an unusual scenario), the corrected renal creatinine clearance (GFR) would be about 4 ml/min, adding approximately 40 L/week of creatinine clearance to overall solute clearance (see Appendix), while the residual renal urea clearance might be about 3 ml/min. Considering that a total of 60 L/1.73 m²/week of creatinine clearance is recommended for 'adequate therapy', one can readily see how residual renal function could represent a significant portion of the patient's overall clearance. In one report it represented 39% of total clearance [97] while in another residual renal clearance represented 25% of the total [98].

As residual renal function decreases, overall clearance expressed as Kt/V or CCr decreases. (Fig. 2). Unless the dialysis dose is adjusted as the residual renal function declines, the patient may receive inadequate therapy. In one study of 147 CAPD patients receiving four 2 L exchanges per day once anuric only one patient had a weekly CCr >60 L/1.73 m² and only 17% had a Kt/V >1.9 [99]. Some have suggested that residual renal function is better preserved with PD than HD [100–103]. The creatinine clearance was stable [10 ml/min) in the majority of patients at 2 years after

starting PD [100, 103]. This may not have been well appreciated in the past because of the previously high drop-out rate from peritoneal dialysis to HD because of peritonitis. Now that peritonitis rates have decreased [104], technique survival may increase [105], and more cases of inadequate dialysis may become apparent if nephrologists do not adjust the PD prescription to compensate for decreases in residual renal function. These data highlight the need to regularly monitor residual renal function and total solute clearance and proactively adjust the peritoneal portion of total clearance as indicated to compensate for any loss of residual renal function. Tattersall *et al.* found that as the residual renal component of Kt/V fell it was possible to compensate for declining residual renal function in some patients by increasing dialysis dose [106].

When calculating the CCr due to underlying residual renal function, it is important to remember that at very low glomerular filtration rates (GFR) or creatinine clearances, much of the creatinine in the urine is due to proximal tubular secretion rather than actual glomerular filtration. As a result, traditional measurements of creatinine clearance (24-h collection) can significantly overestimate the true GFR. The clearance of most other small molecular weight substances by the kidney, such as urea, involve only glomerular filtration and little or no tubular secretion. Creatinine and urea are used as surrogate markers for small molecular weight clearance. Therefore, when attempting to determine the actual clearance of small molecular weight substances due to residual renal function, only the clearance due to GFR is needed. If using creatinine kinetics as the surrogate, it is recommended that the sum of the measured urea clearance and creatinine clearance divided by 2 be used to approximate underlying residual renal GFR [18]. This amount in litres/day is then added to the daily peritoneal creatinine clearance to determine total daily CCr. If one is measuring dialysis dose using urea kinetics, no adjustment for tubular secretion is needed (see Appendix).

Peritoneal membrane transport characteristics

The first step in tailoring an individual patient's peritoneal dialysis prescription is to know that patient's peritoneal membrane transport characteristics. Unlike HD, where the physician has a wide menu of dialysers to choose from for each individual patient, peritoneal dialysis patients are 'born' with their membrane. A change in peritoneal dialysis dose can usually be accomplished only by changing dwell time, dwell volume, or the number of exchanges per day. At present there is no clinically proven way to favourably change membrane transport.

The peritoneal equilibration test (PET), popularized by Twardowski [107], is now the standard way to characterize the peritoneal membrane transport properties of an individual patient. The PET is a standardized test in which, after an overnight dwell, 2 L of 2.5% dextrose dialysate is instilled (time 0) and allowed to dwell for 4 h. Dialysate urea, glucose, sodium, and creatinine are measured at time 0, and after 2 and 4 h of dwell time, and serum values are drawn after 2 h. Four-hour drain volume is also measured. For each of these dwell times, dialysate to plasma ratios (D/P) of creatinine and urea are determined, as is the ratio of glucose at the drain time to the initial dialysate glucose concentration (D/D_0) (Figs 6 and 7). Based on published data the patient's peritoneal membrane type can be characterized as high, high-average, low-average and low. In a review of 806 patients, 10.4% were found to be high transporters, 53.1% high-average, 30.9% low-average, and 5.6% low transporters [108]. The PD prescription that would best match the patient's

transport characteristics can be then chosen (Table 5). One should also be aware of differences in transport for urea and creatinine. As shown in Fig. 6, urea (MW 60 Da) is transported faster than creatinine (MW 112 Da), so that most patients are greater than 90% equilibrated for urea after a 4-h dwell; whereas for creatinine the average patient is only 65% equilibrated at 4 h.

Solute clearance by PD is related to the D/P ratio of creatinine or urea times the drain volume (DV). Patients with small drain volumes tend to have lower clearances. It is important to point out that rapid transporters of creatinine/urea also tend to be rapid absorbers of dialysate glucose. Therefore, in these patients, although the D/P ratios of urea and creatinine at 4 h or longer dwells tend to be close to unity, their drain volumes tend to be small due to reabsorption of fluid once the glucose gradient is mitigated [109] (Fig. 8). As noted in Fig. 7, as ultrafiltration occurs, there is seiving of solute in the ultrafiltration so that the sodium concentration in the ultrafiltrate is less than that in plasma. As a result, when using standard glucose-containing solutions, dialysate

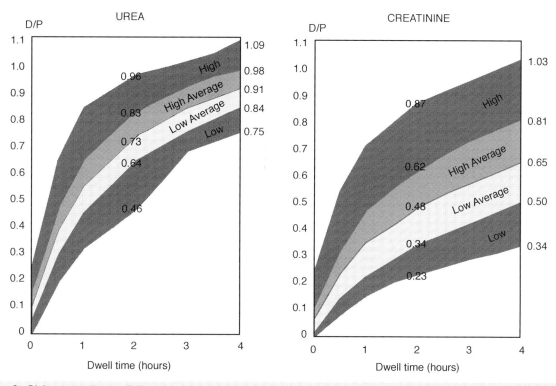

Figure 6. Dialysate to plasma (D/P) ratios for urea and creatinine during the standard peritoneal equilibration test (PET). Exact values at 2 and 4 h are shown. (Modified from: Twardowski ZJ, Nolph KD, Khanna R *et al.* Peritoneal equilibration test. Perit Dial Bull 1987; 7: 138–47 and Twardowski ZJ, Khanna R, Nolph KD. Peritoneal dialysis modifications to avoid CAPD dropouts. In: Khanna R, Nolph KD, Prowant BF, Twardowski ZJ, Oreopoulos DG, eds. Advances in Continuous Ambulatory Peritoneal Dialysis. Proceedings of the Seventh Annual CAPD Conference, Kansas City, Missouri, February 1987. Peritoneal Dialysis Bulletin, Inc., Toronto, 1987, pp. 171–8.)

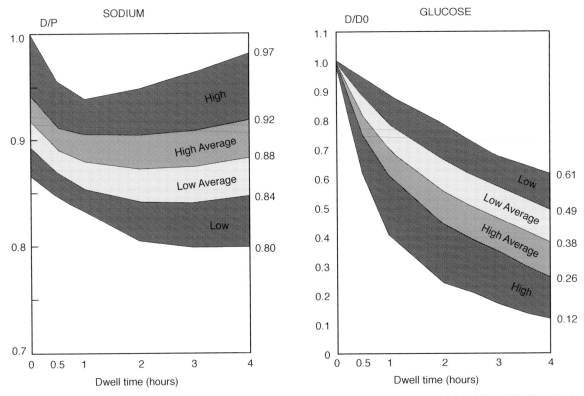

Figure 7. Dialysate to plasma (D/P) ratio of sodium and glucose dialysate to dialysate at time zero (D/D$_0$) ratio versus dwell time. Sodium concentration decreases rapidly at the beginning of dwell time due to sieving. The decrease is more pronounced in low transporters. (Twardowski ZJ. Influence of different automated PD schedules on solute and water removal. Nephrol Dial Transplant 1998; 13 (suppl. 6): 103–11.)

Table 5. Baseline PET prognostic value

Solute transport	UF	Predicted response to CAPD dialysis	Preferred peritoneal dialysis modality
High	Poor	Adequate	NIPD, DAPD
High-average	Adequate	Adequate	Standard volume PD
Low-average	Good	Adequate	Standard volume PD
Low	Excellent	Inadequate	High volume PD

NIPD = nightly intermittent PD; DAPD = daytime ambulatory PD; CAPD = continuous ambulatory PD; CCPD = continuous cycling PD. (Twardowski ZJ. Clinical value of standardized equilibration tests in CAPD patients. Blood Purif 1989; 7: 95–108.)

sodium concentration falls during ultrafiltration, and once the glucose concentration gradient is mitigated and ultrafiltration ceases, the sodium in the dialysate approaches that of plasma due to diffusion. This change in dialysate sodium can be used when evaluating a patient with true ultrafiltration failure. In fact, as is shown in Fig. 9, with dwell times associated with standard CAPD, rapid transporters may have drain volumes that are actually less than the instilled

volume. For these patients short dwell times are needed to reduce or minimize fluid reabsorption and optimize clearances. In patients who are low transporters, peak ultrafiltration occurs later during the dwell and net ultrafiltration can be obtained even after prolonged dwells. In these patients the D/P ratio increases almost linearly during the dwell. It is not until 8–10 h that the D/P ratio reaches unity. For these patients dwell time is the crucial determinant of overall clearance, and they will do best with continuous therapies such as standard CAPD or CCPD, which utilize 24 h/day for dialysis and maximize dwell time/exchange. If a patient has a large body surface area he/she may need high doses (i.e. large volumes of these therapies) which in practice may be difficult to achieve.

To put these differences in perspective one can appreciate that after only a 2-h dwell time, a rapid transporter will probably have achieved 2 L of creatinine clearance, whereas the creatinine clearance in a low-transport individual may be only 1 L or less, despite a larger drain volume (Fig. 8). It may take the low transporter up to 7–8 h of dwell time to

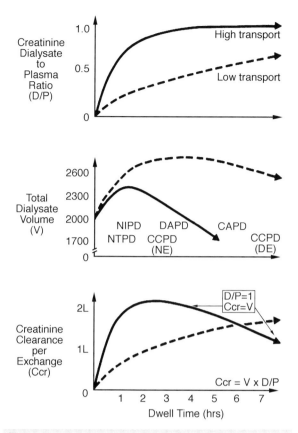

Figure 8. Idealized curves of creatinine and water transport during an exchange with 2 L of 2.5% glucose dialysis solutions in patients with extremely low and high transport characteristics. (Twardowski ZJ.   Nightly peritoneal dialysis (Why? who? how? and when?). ASAIO Trans 1990; 36: 8–16.)

achieve the same clearance that a rapid transporter achieves after only a 2 h dwell. These differences must be taken into account when attempting to tailor an individual patient's peritoneal dialysis prescription.

There are other ways to classify a patient's peritoneal membrane transport, but in the usual clinical setting the PET is the most practical. Mass transfer area coefficients (MTAC) [110, 111] are more precise and more succinctly define transport. These define transport independent of ultrafiltration (convection-related solute removal), and hence are not influenced by dwell volume or glucose concentration. The practical use of MTAC for modelling a PD prescription requires additional laboratory measurements and computer models but once these are obtained MTAC can be easily used in the clinical setting [112.] The standard peritoneal permeability analysis is another less-often-used test to follow transport and ultrafiltration characteristics [113].

The major difference in this test is that it is better able to determine sodium sieving and can better differentiate the causes of ultrafiltration failure. Nine cross-sectional and 16 longitudinal studies of peritoneal transport were reviewed by Rippe and Krediet [114]. In 14/25 there was no change in peritoneal transport over time on PD; in the other 11/25 there was a slight increase in low/medium molecular weight substances over time. Others found no change in peritoneal transport in 23 patients followed for at least 7 years [115], while Selgas et al. found no significant change in transport over time (some up to 7 years) in patients with a low incidence of peritonitis [116]. However, in subsequent follow-up these authors noted that there was a tendency towards increase in small solute transport for creatinine and loss of ultrafiltration, especially in patients with greater episodes of peritonitis [117, 118], similar to the findings by Heimburger et al. who found that 30.9% developed ultrafiltration failure (change in transport) after 6 years on PD [119]. These data emphasize the importance of monitoring membrane transport and adjusting the PD prescription if needed. To optimize solute clearance, drain volumes, blood volume and ultrafiltration, while minimizing hypertonic glucose use, rapid transporters on CAPD may need to change to a form of CCPD or NIPD.

Influence of body size on solute clearance

It is intuitive that removing the same amount of solute from a 55 kg elderly female would represent relatively more clearance than the same amount of solute removed from an 80 kg muscular male. These patients probably have different metabolic rates. Therefore, the absolute daily clearance must be normalized for differences in body size (by V or volume of distribution for Kt/V and by BSA or body surface area for CCr). Based on the patient's body size, one can predict whether or not an individual patient would be adequately dialysed using four 2.0 L exchanges once that patient was anuric [120–122]. This modelling also predicts that, if one were to increase the instilled volume/exchange from 2.0 L to 2.5 L or greater, under similar conditions total solute clearance should increase, and the instilled volumes needed to achieve your target solute clearances can be predicted [121–123] (Fig. 10).

In a review of 806 PD patients the median BSA was 1.85 m² (not 1.73 m²), whereas the 25th percentile was 1.71 m² and the 75th percentile was 2.0 [108]. Despite this finding that most PD patients

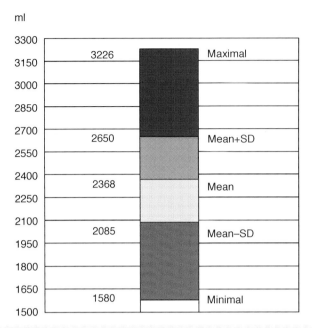

Figure 9. Drain volumes after 4 h dwell time in the study population. Because patients with high solute transport rates have usually low drain volumes and vice-versa the stack bar areas are shaded in the patterns per category. (Based on data from: Twardowski ZJ, Khanna R, Nolph KD. Peritoneal dialysis modifications to avoid CAPD dropouts. In: Khanna R *et al.* eds. Advances in Continuous Ambulatory Peritoneal Dialysis. Proceedings of the Seventh Annual CAPD Conference, Kansas City, Missouri, February 1987. Perit Dial Bull, Inc., Toronto, 1987: 171–8; Twardowski ZJ, Nolph KD, Khanna R *et al.* Peritoneal equilibration test. Perit Dial Bull 1987; 7: 138–47.)

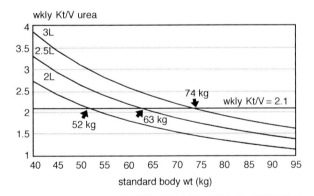

Figure 10. Weekly renal urea clearance normalized to total body water (*Kt/V*) urea (vertical axis) as a function of standard body weight (horizontal axis) in anephric patients using four 2-, 2.5-, or 3-L exchanges daily (curves). The weight above which weekly *Kt/V* urea falls below the target of 2.1 is indicated for each curve. Four exchanges daily CAPD in anephric patients, dialysate/plasma urea = 0.95, drain volume = inflow + 1.5 L. (Modified from Jensen RA, Nolph KD, Moore HL, Khanna R, Twardowski ZJ. Weight limitations for adequate therapy using commonly performed CAPD and NIPD regimens. Semin Dial 1994; 7: 61–4.)

are larger than the 'standard' BSA of 1.73 m², based on clearances predicted by kinetic modelling, if one were able to individualize therapy (increased instilled volumes, daytime exchange for CCPD, nightly exchange device), one should be able to achieve the recommended acceptable target total solute clearances for most patients on PD. Those patients who are low transporters and those who have large body surface areas (> 1.8 m²) would not be likely to obtain these targets once anuric.

Special considerations

Rapid transporters

As mentioned above, individual patient peritoneal membrane transport characteristics are important in determining total solute clearance and ultrafiltration rates in PD patients. Rapid transporters tend to optimize both solute clearance and ultrafiltration after a short dwell time (approximately 2 h) and therefore are likely to do well on short dwell therapies such as NIPD, with or without one or two 2–4-h daytime dwells. One would predict that they would easily reach total solute clearance goals for Kt/V and creatinine clearance [108]. Despite this relative ease in the ability to achieve recommended total solute clearance goals, these patients have recently been shown to have an increased relative risk of death and a decreased technique survival

[124]. In the CANUSA Study, patients with a 4-h D/P creatinine of >0.65 (high) were compared to those with a 4-h D/P creatinine of <0.65 (low). The 2-year probability for technique survival was 79% among low transporters compared to 71% for high transporters. The probability of 2-year patient survival was 82% among low transporters versus 72% for high transporters with a relative risk of death of 2.18 for high versus low transporters using this definition for high transporters (D/P creatinine >0.65).

Other investigators have made similar observations [125]. Nolph, *et al.* [126] noted that high transporters (D/P >0.81) had increased incidence of malnutrition. Heaf [127] noted increased morbidity in rapid transporters. These findings were not confirmed by other investigators [128].

The reason(s) for this increased relative risk while on CAPD are unclear [129]. One thought is that there is a tendency towards malnutrition because of the increased protein losses in rapid transporters. Many have shown that as the D/P ratio at 4 h increases, there tends to be increased protein loss. As dialysate protein losses increase, serum albumin levels decrease, and serum albumin correlates inversely with peritoneal membrane transport [130–132]. Another way to explain the low levels may be overt or subtle volume overload. The typical dwells associated with CAPD would tend to be associated with problems with ultrafiltration in these patients. This volume overload may lead to increased blood pressure and/or increased left ventricular hypertrophy with its associated increased risks of death. Furthermore, to optimize ultrafiltration, these patients will probably increase the percentage glucose in their fluids, leading to better ultrafiltration, but increased glucose absorption. This increased glucose absorption may [133–136] or may not [137] inhibit appetite.

It has been recommended that these patients change to NIPD with or without a short daytime dwell. This change maintains total solute clearance, while decreasing the need for hypertonic glucose exchanges, therefore decreasing the relative amount of glucose absorption [138]. There are no data, however, to evaluate outcome for these patients who change to NIPD, although there may be an increase in nutritional parameters. If one does change to NIPD, it is important to remember that it is recommended that one must now increase total solute clearance goals to $Kt/V > 2.2$ and creatinine clearance $> 661/1.73$ m^2/week because of the intermittent nature of the therapy. There may be a small but insignificant decrease in protein losses when changing from CAPD to NIPD [130, 138].

Acid–base metabolism

An essential component of providing 'optimal' dialysis is correction of acidosis. Chronic acidosis has a detrimental effect on protein, carbohydrate and bone metabolism. In CAPD patients, body base balance is self-regulated by feedback between plasma bicarbonate levels and bicarbonate gain/loss [139]. Dialysis must provide sufficient replenishment of buffers to compensate for the daily acid load. Lactate (concentration 35–40 mmol/L) is the standard buffer in currently available PD solutions. Lactate is converted to pyruvate and oxygenated or used in gluconeogenesis with the consumption of H^+ and the generation of bicarbonate [140]. Some CAPD patients remain acidotic. With lactate-containing buffer solutions, buffer balance is governed by the relative amounts of H^+ generation, bicarbonate loss, lactate absorption, and lactate metabolism [141–143].

Ultrafiltration volume can affect bicarbonate loss [139, 141]. Acid–base status is also related to peritoneal membrane transport type [144]. These authors showed that D/P creatinine ratio from PET was positively correlated with lactate gain, dialysate base gain, and arterial bicarbonate concentration. Rapid transporters gain more lactate during the typical dwell and tended to have higher arterial bicarbonate levels. In 44 patients with metabolic alkalosis the mean D/P creatinine was 0.66 ± 0.12, whereas in those with metabolic acidosis the mean D/P creatinine was 0.59 ± 0.09 ($p < 0.005$) (Table 6). Most CAPD patients have stable mean plasma bicarbonate levels of about 25.6 mmol/L using a dialysate lactate of 35 mmol/L. Increasing dialysate lactate results in a higher serum bicarbonate level [145]. Lowrie and Lew [146] noted no correlation between serum albumin levels and bicarbonate concentration, and this was confirmed by Bergstrom [147]. Control of acidosis is important to prevent protein catabolism [148, 149]. More data are needed to evaluate the effect of PD fluid lactate levels on outcome.

Which is the preferred target – *Kt/V* or CCr?

Currently, either total Kt/V or total CCr can be used to monitor solute clearance. There are no data to suggest that one index is better than the other. Although these two yardsticks do not fall on the same linear scale, the two values usually correlate [150]. However, in up to 20% of patients there is a significant discrepancy between the two [37, 151,

Table 6. Comparison of acid–base parameters and buffer transport according to membrane transport type

	High (n = 10)	High-average (n = 54)	Low-average (n = 66)	Low (n = 13)
pH	7.44 ± 0.03	7.42 ± 0.05	7.41 ± 0.03	7.38 ± 0.03[a]
HCO$_3$ (mmol/L)	26.7 ± 3.2	24.8 ± 2.9	24.3 ± 3.8	23.4 ± 2.8[a]
LG (mmol/day)	284.5 ± 52.3	259.3 ± 44.4[a]	238.4 ± 48.9[b]	205.7 ± 40.8[c]
DBL (mmol/day)	229.7 ± 32.8	242.9 ± 40.0	225.3 ± 39.9	211.1 ± 31.2
DBG (mmol/day)	40.8 ± 18.2	22.1 ± 47.4[a]	13.83 ± 50.3[b]	5.9 ± 12.3[c]
D/D$_0$ lactate	0.08 ± 0.02	0.09 ± 0.03	0.12 ± 0.04	0.13 ± 0.08[b]
D/P$_{bicarbonate}$	1.02 ± 0.15	1.06 ± 0.12	1.00 ± 0.12	1.07 ± 0.12

LG = lactate gain; DBL = dialytic bicarbonate loss; DBG = dialytic base gain.

[a] $p < 0.05$ versus high.

[b] $p < 0.05$ versus high and high-average.

[c] $p < 0.05$ versus high, high-average, and low-average.

(Kang DH, Yoon K, Lee HY, Han DS. Impact of peritoneal membrane transport characteristics on acid–base status in CAPD patients. Perit Dial Int 1998; 18: 294–302.)

152]. In these situations, one is often presented with a clinical dilemma. For instance, one may find a Kt/V that appears adequate while CCr is not, and yet the patient seems to be doing well. Similarly, one may have seen a patient who is gaining weight and eating well, yet the parameters are below target. How can one explain these findings? What does one do?

The reasons for these discrepancies are multifactorial and include: the amount of residual renal function present and its relative contribution to total Kt/V or CCr, the difference in peritoneal transport of urea and creatinine, and the influence of patient size on normalization.

Residual renal clearance is the result of glomerular filtration and tubular manipulation of that filtrate. For creatinine, in addition to the glomerular filtration, there is also proximal tubular secretion of creatinine which adds to the total solute clearance of creatinine. This is especially true in the advanced stages of renal insufficiency where the absolute amount of creatinine secretion can increase by as much as 30%, accounting for up to 35% of urinary creatinine [153]; whereas for urea there is filtration, but also tubular reabsorption. Therefore, in advanced stages of renal disease, even when estimations of GFR (mean of creatinine and urea clearances) are used for creatinine clearance, the residual renal clearance of creatinine will be relatively greater than that for urea. In contrast, peritoneal clearance is predominantly diffusion-driven. (There is also a component of convective clearance due to ultrafiltration, but this contribution is relatively smaller than that due to diffusion.) Therefore, because urea is of a smaller molecular weight than creatinine, the numerical value for peritoneal clearance of urea

tends to be relatively greater than that for creatinine clearance. This is most pronounced in patients who are low transporters. In summary, the ratio of CCr : Kt/V (reference is $60 : 2.0 = 30$) tends to be higher at the initiation of dialysis when patients tend to have a significant amount of residual renal function; whereas, once anuric, the ratio of CCr : Kt/V tends to be lower (Fig. 2).

Peritoneal membrane transport characteristics may also explain this discrepancy. The diffusive clearance for urea is relatively greater than that for creatinine. Therefore, the urea clearance/dwell tends to be greater than that for creatinine. This is most pronounced in low transporters where the ratio of CCr : Kt/V tends to be lower than in high transporters (Fig. 11). During the typical dwells associated with CAPD the dialysate to plasma ratio (D/P) for urea tends to reach unity (equilibration between blood and dialysate) in all patients, whereas the D/P for creatinine tends to reach unity only in high transporters. The NKF-DOQI Guidelines for adequacy of PD made the assumption that the ratio of dialysis creatinine clearance to dialysis urea clearance in CAPD was 0.8. However, the basis for this assumption is not noted in the document.

The guidelines do not differentiate between genders. As shown in Table 7, the patient's weight has a different effect on normalization (V or BSA) for male or female and for CCr versus Kt/V. These differences are noted in Fig. 12. In patients with similar BSA, instilled volume transport type and gender has a significant effect on Kt/V calculations but not CCr calculations. The mathematical relationship between BSA and V is not fixed; it is disturbed by both gender and obesity. Furthermore, the actual V is different if 'obesity' is due to a change

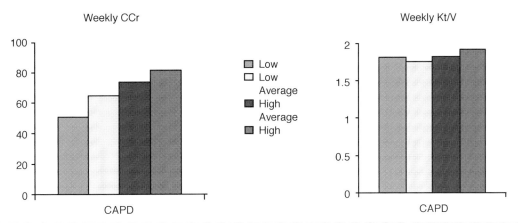

Figure 11. *Kt/V* and creatinine clearance values for low, low-average, high-average and high transport with a BSA between 1.71 and 2.0 m², no residual renal function and 2.5L fill volumes. (Modified from: Blake P, Burkart JM, Churchill DN *et al.* Recommended clinical practices for maximizing PD clearances. Perit Dial Int 1996; 16: 448–56.)

Table 7. Equations for normalization (calculating *V* for *Kt/V* or BSA for creatinine clearance)

V male (L)	$= 2.447 + 0.3362 \times$ weight (kg) $+ 0.1074$ $\times$ height (cm) $- 0.09516 \times$ Age (years)
V female (L)	$= -2.097 + 0.2466 \times$ weight (kg) $+ 0.1069$ $\times$ height (cm)
BSA	$= 0.007184 \times$ body weight (kg)$^{0.425} \times$ height (cm)$^{0.725}$

(Watson PE, Watson ID, Batt RD. Total body water volumes for adult males and females estimated from simple anthropometric measurements. Am J Clin Nutr 1980; 33: 27–39 and Dubois D, Dubois EF. A formula to estimate the approximate surface area if height and weight be known. Arch Intern Med 1916; 17: 863–71.)

in body fat versus a change in body water (overhydration) [154] and if the patient has had an amputation [155]. The problems with current 'normalization' practices were reviewed by Tzamaloukas *et al.* [156] and these authors propose using *V* for normalization of both *Kt/V* and CCr despite the above descriptions. Further outcome studies with various means of normalization are needed.

Therefore, in the average anuric patient on five 2 L exchanges/day with average peritoneal transport characteristics, peritoneal creatinine clearance will be 73% of urea clearance [157]. Thus in an anuric average transporter with a weekly peritoneal *Kt/V* of 2.0, the expected creatinine clearance is about 55 L/1.73 m²/week in males and 47 L/1.73 m²/week in females. Similarly, for NIPD patients with average transport, the peritoneal creatinine clearance will be 64% of urea. Thus, for an anuric average transporter on NIPD, with a weekly *Kt/V* of 2.2, the expected weekly creatinine clearance will be 53 L/1.73 m² in males and 45 L/1.73 m² in females. As shown in

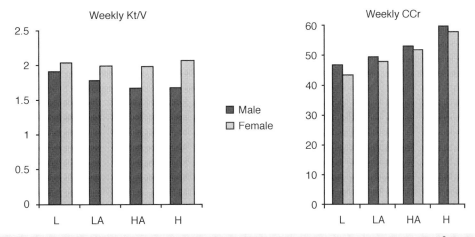

Figure 12. Actual mean clearances corresponding to 8.0 L prescriptions in 90 PD patients with BSA < 1.7 m² based on peritoneal transport types. (Ref. 208; modified from Vonesh EF, Moran J. Discrepancies between urea *Kt/V* versus normalized creatinine clearance. Perit Dial Int 1997; 17: 13–16.)

Table 8, in anuric patients at Kt/V target creatinine clearance is more often than not going to be below NKF-DOQI recommendations.

There are no clinical outcome data to support the use of one solute clearance yardstick (CCr or Kt/V) over the other. Most of the published outcome data are related to Kt/V. These solute clearance goals are based on reported outcomes predicted by certain amounts of solute clearance. Based on this discussion, it is apparent that in most cases the two values correlate, and that either could be used as an index of adequacy. There are no data which show that one is better than the other. However, as outlined above, at times it is not practical to achieve both targets. My recommendation is that one should use both, and strive to have both measurements above target. If neither is above target, one should consider increasing the dose of dialysis. If only one is above target, one needs to follow that patient, particularly his/her nutritional status, closely. If malnourished, or if the albumin is decreasing, consider increasing dialysis dose so that both are above target based on patient lifestyle constraints. DOQI Guidelines suggest having at least Kt/V at target [21]. Based on the above discussions, others [158] and myself feel that a Kt/V target of 2.0/week for CAPD [2.1 for CCPD and 2.2 for NIPD) is likely to be adequate, and that one should always strive to at least have Kt/V above target.

Table 8. Creatinine clearance (L) at Kt/V of 2.2 in NIPD and 2.0 in CAPD

	NIPD		CAPD	
Transport category	Females	Males	Females	Males
Minimal value	32.90	38.80	30.70	36.30
Low transporters	33.70	39.80	35.70	41.60
Mean − SD	34.30	40.50	39.40	46.50
Low-average transporters	40.00	47.20	43.20	51.00
Mean	44.70	52.70	46.70	55.10
High-average transporters	48.00	56.60	50.10	59.10
Mean + SD	50.80	59.90	53.20	62.80[a]
High transporters	55.60	65.60	58.10	68.50[a]
Maximal value	59.40	70.00[a]	62.70[a]	73.90[a]

Assumptions: Total body water in males = 41.7 L; total body water in females = 32.1 L; body surface area in males = 1.92 m²; body surface area in females = 1.74 m²; NIPD (nocturnal intermittent PD): hourly 2-L exchanges: CAPD (continuous ambulatory PD): five 2-L exchanges.
[a] Values are above the DOQI guidelines for creatinine clearance at recommended Kt/V.
(Twardowski ZJ. Relationships between creatinine clearances and Kt/V in PD patients: a critique of the DOQI document. Perit Dial Int 1998; 18: 252–5.)

Normalization

Severely malnourished patients would tend to have a low ratio of total CCr to total Kt/V_{urea}. This is because malnutrition causes a relatively greater decrease in V than in BSA (Table 9). Therefore, when normalizing Kt or CCr, the Kt/V is increased proportionally more than CCr. Total body water (V) can be estimated as a fixed percentage of body weight, or more accurately, by using anthropometric formulas based on sex, age, height and weight such as the Watson [159] or Hume [160] formulas in adults. These equations provide unrealistic estimates for V in patients whose weights are markedly different from normal body weight (NBW). BSA is usually calculated using the formula by Dubois and Dubois [161]. Jones [162] noted that when ABW was used for normalization there was no difference in total solute clearance (Kt/V or CCr) between well-nourished and malnourished patients. However, when calculated V and BSA were determined using desired body weight (DBW), there was a statistically significant difference between the groups for both weekly Kt/V (1.68 ± 0.46 vs. 1.40 ± 0.41, $p < 0.05$) and for creatinine clearance in L/1.73 m²/week (52.5 ± 10.3 vs. 41.6 ± 19.0, $p < 0.01$). These data suggest that in malnourished, underweight individuals, if ABW is used to calculate V, the resultant V will be much smaller than that found if the larger DBW is used. In these instances, when Kt is divided by V, the resultant Kt/V may be acceptable despite progressive anorexia and weight loss in the patient.

For well-nourished patients with a stable weight who are not markedly different from desired or ideal weight, the patient's actual body weight can be used in these equations for determinations of V and BSA. However, when markedly different from ideal, the choice of which weight to use in clearance calculations becomes important. At our unit we determine the patient's 'desired body weight' 'during PD train-

Table 9. Adequacy calculations: what weight should you use?

BW ratio	⩽0.9	0.9–1.1	>1.1
Percentage	19	33	48
BWa/BWd	0.82	1.01	1.37
Kt/V_a	1.95	2.08	1.94
Kt/V_d	1.74	2.08	2.25
CCra (L/week)	68.1	71.5	64.1
CCrd (L/week)	62.6	71.7	72.4

(Satko SG, Burkart JM. Frequency and causes of discrepancy between Kt/V and creatinine. Perit Dial Int 1997; 17: S23.)

ing' and always use that weight in adequacy calculations, to avoid this problem if the weight changes significantly. DBW is expressed in kilograms, and is the midpoint of the range of body weights associated with the greatest longevity for normal individuals of the same age range, sex, and skeletal frame size as the individual in question. These body weights are published in the Metropolitan Life Insurance Company actuarial tables. The NKF-DOQI Guidelines suggest that in malnourished patients one must adjust the total solute clearance goals for that patient. In an attempt to promote anabolism the following adjustment was recommended. Using the patient's actual weight, the minimal weekly total solute clearance goals should be adjusted by the ratio of desired/actual body weight. In this case, for a malnourished patient on CAPD the weekly Kt/V target would be higher than 2.0 (i.e. $2.0 \times$ desired/actual body weight). Further studies are needed to confirm the appropriateness of this recommended adjustment of weekly total solute clearance goals.

How to monitor dialysis dose

The most accurate way to measure dialysis dose is to measure the total amount of the solute in question cleared from the body during a specific time interval. In practice, for CAPD, this means that 24-h collections of dialysate and urine should be obtained. Total solute clearance is calculated as described in the Appendix. An alternative would be to estimate the daily clearance either mathematically or with the use of computer-assisted kinetic modelling programs. It is important to remember that these estimations are truly approximations and, therefore, this is not recommended. Although they do tend to correlate with the actual clearance measured from 24-h collections, there is a high degree of discordance [163, 164]. Therefore, the gold standard for measurement of dialysis dose is to obtain 24-h collections of both urine and dialysate to document the delivered dose of dialysis. These studies should be obtained quarterly and within 1 month of any prescription change. Despite these recommendations, data from the United States suggest that adequacy studies are not done in many PD patients [165] (Fig. 13).

PET data are obtained in order to characterize the patient's peritoneal membrane transport characteristics (see above), not to determine clearance. The two tests are complementary to each other and are routinely used together for developing a patient's dialysis prescription and for problem solving.

Several studies have documented that an individual patient's peritoneal membrane tends to be stable over time [166–168]. However, in some patients it may change. Therefore, peritoneal transport should be monitored to optimize clearance and ultrafiltration. PET is the most practical way to do this, and it is recommended that it be obtained twice a year. It has been shown that over time, if there tends to be any change in transport characteristics, the D/P ratios were likely to increase slightly, associated with a small decrease in ultrafiltration. Alternatively, one can estimate D/P values for PET from D/P values on 24° dialysate collections (Dialysis Adequacy and Transport Test, or DATT) when followed sequentially in an individual patient [169]. These values tend to be slightly higher than the D/P for creatinine on the standard PET. The DATT is not recommended for work-up of ultrafiltration failure, but if the patient's dialysis prescription has not changed (i.e. instilled volume and percentage glucose), sequential DATT measurements do predict peritoneal membrane transport as long as instilled volume/exchange has not changed. Twenty-four-hour collections can also be used to calculate lean body mass (LBM), creatinine generation rates and estimate protein intake (Table 10).

Non-compliance

Non-compliance with a medical regimen is not uncommon, and can adversely affect patient outcome. The degree of non-compliance with the dialysis prescription itself is easily documented in in-centre HD populations [170, 171], although its impact on outcome has been difficult to define. Certainly there is an element of non-compliance with a home therapy such as PD. Until recently there have been no simple ways to evaluate non-compliance in these populations. Recent publications have suggested that a value above unity for the ratio of measured to predicted creatinine production may be an indication of recent periods of non-compliance [172–174]. From these studies it has been estimated that only 78% of the prescribed therapy is actually delivered [172]. These authors speculated that, if the patient had been non-compliant prior to collecting 24 h of dialysate and urine for adequacy studies, but was compliant on the day of collection, then a 'washout' effect would occur. In such a case the creatinine production would be higher than would be predicted from standard equations, resulting in an elevated ratio of measured to predicted creatinine production. Others have shown that the index is *not*

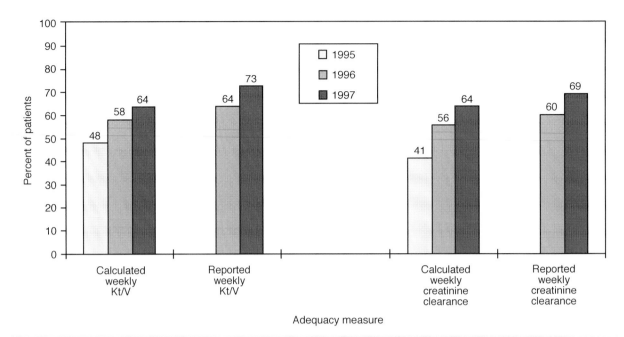

Figure 13. Significant differences 1995–97 for calculated measures and 1996–97 for reported measures; $p < 0.0001$. (Frankenfield DL, Prowant BF, Flanigan MJ *et al.* for the ESRD Core Indicators Workgroup. Trends in clinical indicators of care for adult PD patients in the U.S., 1995–97. Kidney Int 1999 (in press).)

Table 10. Usefulness of 24-h collections of dialysis and urine collection

Creatinine kinetics	Urea kinetics
Creatinine clearance[D]	Urea clearance[D]
Creatinine clearance[U]	Urea clearance[U]
Total creatinine clearance[D + U]	Total urea clearance[D + U]
Creatinine production[D + U]	PNA[D + U]
Lean body mass[D + U]	Urea generation[D + U]
D/P creatinine[D]	
Ratio of measured to predicted creatinine generation	

Creatinine and urea kinetics	24 h urine

Estimated GFR (modified creatinine clearance)	Drain volume – UF rates

D = dialysis only; U = urine only.
(Burkart JM, Schreiber M, Korbet S *et al.* Solute clearance approach to adequacy of peritoneal dialysis. Perit Dial Int 1996; 16: 457–70.)

a good indicator of compliance [175, 176]. More data are needed. Perhaps sequential rather than individual ratios will be helpful. Nevertheless, non-compliance with the prescription is a real issue, as documented by patient questionnaires [177] and by looking at patient home inventories [178]. Interestingly, non-compliance may be more of an issue in the USA than in other countries such as Canada.

At present there is no definitive test, short of asking patients and looking at home inventories, to determine patient compliance. More importantly, one should discuss compliance with the patient and have a heightened awareness of the problem. Be sure to design PD prescriptions with patients' lifestyle needs and abilities in mind. Five manual exchanges a day is not realistic for most patients. Automated therapies may help. Education and importance of compliance with prescription should be emphasized.

Prescription dialysis

Timing for initiation of dialysis – 'healthy start'

The NKF-DOQI Guidelines [21] and others [179, 180] have highlighted the need to treat patients throughout the stages of chronic renal failure (CRI) as a continuum. Data are emerging which suggest that the patient's clinical status, especially nutritional status and left ventricular functional status, at the onset of dialysis is a major predictor of eventual morbidity and mortality.

The traditional absolute indications for initiation of dialysis, such as pericarditis, encephalopathy, refractory hyperkalaemia, nausea, vomiting and volume overload, raise little controversy. Weight loss and signs of malnutrition are other more subtle, 'relative' indications for initiation. Interestingly, as opposed to ESRD when minimal target values for weekly total solute clearance have been established (i.e. $Kt/V > 2.0$, CCr > 60 L/1.73 m^2, for CAPD), minimal values for total solute clearance by residual renal function alone prior to initiation of dialysis have not been established. This seems paradoxical. In fact, in the CANUSA Study the mean RR GFR at initiation was approximately 3.38 ml/min (CANUSA), while a recent evaluation of the HCFA 2728 data by the USRDS suggested that the median creatinine clearance level in 90 987 patients who started dialysis was 8.9 ml/min. The proportion of patients with a GFR >10, 5–10 and <5 ml/min was 14%, 63% and 23%, respectively [181]. If there are very compelling data for both PD and HD which suggest that weekly solute clearance is a predictor of long-term outcomes, would this not be true for patients with advanced renal insufficiency? There are indirect data to suggest that, in general, patients who start dialysis with relatively more residual renal function have better outcomes and tend to be less malnourished.

The DOQI working group for PD adequacy has developed the following guideline 'Unless certain conditions are met, patients should be advised to initiate some form of renal replacement therapy when residual renal Kt/V_{urea} falls below 2.0/week. The conditions that indicate dialysis may not yet be needed are: (1) stable too increasing oedema free body weight *and* (2) a nPNA >0.8 gm/kg/d *and* (3) complete absence of clinical signs and symptoms attributable to uraemia' [21].

This guideline does not preclude the importance of quality-of-life issues, blood pressure control, treatment of anaemia and consideration of protein restriction and use of acetylcholinesterase inhibitors to prevent progression of disease. It still suggests individualization of therapy initiation. The recommendations are based on the following indirect evidence.

Baseline nutritional status is a strong predictor of outcome

Data suggest that baseline nutritional parameters such as serum albumin, lean body mass, nPNA or subjective global assessment score are strong predictors of outcome. For instance the predicted 2-year survivals for patients in the CANUSA study with baseline serum albumins of >35, 30–35 and <30 g/L were 85%, 75% and 64%, respectively [14].

Although not well studied, it is a clinical impression that patients begin to eat better once dialysis is initiated. Data from CANUSA would support this concept. Statistically significant increases in the absolute values of SGA and %LBM but not albumin which correlated with the increase in Kt/V or creatinine clearance were demonstrated over the first 6 months of dialysis [56].

As residual renal GFR declines, so does spontaneous DPI

In a study of 90 patients with CRI, Ikizler *et al.* [182] have shown that as GFR decreased to below 25–50 ml/min, spontaneous DPI also decreased. In that report, patients with a CCr of >50 ml/min had a mean DPI of 1.01 g/kg/day, vs. A DPI of 0.54 g/kg/day (less than currently recommended minimal requirements) in patients with a CCr <10 ml/min. A similar statistically significant trend was also observed for serum cholesterol, transferrin and total creatinine excretion. Cross-sectional data from the Modification of Diet in Renal Disease study (MDRD) (both the pilot and full-scale study) have suggested that there was a significant positive correlation between residual renal function and DPI [183]. These observations were supported by reports from others [184, 185]. Because of the significant effect of malnutrition on subsequent patient survival once on dialysis, once DPI is less than 0.8 g/kg/day, initiation of dialysis should be considered.

Relationship between *Kt/V* and DPI may be the same for CRI and for continuous PD

Mehrotra *et al.* [184] have reported that the relationship between DPI and small solute clearance measured in terms of Kt/V is similar for CRI and CAPD patients. This is supported by data from our unit which suggest that the relationship between DPI and total Kt/V is similar to that observed for these two parameters in the MDRD patients with advanced chronic renal insufficiency who reached end-stage. In these databases, for both CAPD and CRI, DPI of <0.8 g/kg/day are typically seen when Kt/V is <2.0/week, suggesting that to prevent malnutrition in these patients initiation of dialysis should be considered.

Outcome data

Some databases suggest that outcomes are better for patients who start dialysis 'early' than in those who start 'late'. Bonomini *et al.* [186] showed that the 5-year survival in 34 patients who started dialysis when their residual renal CCr was >10 ml/min was

100% compared to an 85% survival in 158 patients starting dialysis with a CCr <5 ml/min. Tattersall *et al.* [187] have shown that the level of renal function at the initiation of dialysis was an independent predictor of patient outcomes, while others [188] reported that survival and hospitalization during the first 6 months after initiation of HD was related to baseline residual renal Kt/V. Jungers *et al.* [189] have shown that those referred late (<1 month prior to initiation of dialysis) had a higher hospitalization rate and cost, while Radcliffe *et al.* [190] similarly reported that late referral (< 1 month before ESRD) had higher complications and mortality.

Taken in aggregate these studies suggest, at least in part, that outcome on dialysis is related to the level of residual renal function at the initiation of dialysis. One explanation for these observations may be the influence of residual renal solute clearance on the patient's nutritional status.

Approach to the near-ESRD patient

How should one approach the near-ESRD patient? While protein-restricted diets and the use of erythropoietin may ameliorate some symptoms of uraemia, delaying the 'clinical' need to start dialysis, other uraemic problems (acidosis, osteodystrophy, neuropathy, etc.) continue to progress. One could initiate dialysis once patients have obvious symptoms or begin to lose weight.

The alternative approach recommended by the DOQI working group is to avoid malnutrition and irreversible changes from uraemia by keeping the target total weekly solute clearance (in terms of Kt/V) above the minimal recommended Kt/V targets for maintenance ESRD patients. Based on the published data for ESRD patients, dialysis should be recommended when the weekly residual renal Kt/V is <2.0. The overall goal would be to keep total weekly Kt/V >2.0 at all times. This can be achieved by the incremental use of either PD or HD with consideration of patient quality-of-life issues and minimal interruption of lifestyle.

Initial prescription

When a patient presents with near-ESRD or ESRD, and PD is elected, two alternatives for writing the initial prescription exist. These are based on the patient's residual renal function and symptoms. For those patients with minimal residual renal function the initial prescription should consist of a 'full dose' of PD in order to meet minimal total solute clear-ance goals. If the patient has a significant amount of residual renal function (but residual renal Kt/V <2.0), 'incremental' dosage of PD can be inititated.

In both instances the initial prescription is based on the patient's body size (BSA) and amount of residual renal function (both potentially known variables at initiation of dialysis). At initiation, peritoneal transport is not known. Initial prescriptions are based on the assumption that the patient's peritoneal transport is average. Once an individual patient's transport type is known, his/her prescription can be more appropriately tailored. During training, transport type can be predicted from drain volume during a timed (4-h) dwell with 2.5% glucose and compared to those predicted by PET [107].

Because peritoneal transport can change over first 1–4 weeks of therapy, it is recommended that baseline PET be delayed until after 2–3 weeks on PD.

'Full dose' implementation

Examples of empirical initial PD prescription based on BSA and residual renal clearance using the 'full dose' approach are found in Table 11 [191]. These prescriptions are based on kinetic modelling and require 24-h collections of dialysate and urine to confirm that targets are met.

'Incremental' dialysis

Similarly, one can use empirical prescriptions based on kinetic modelling for implementing PD using an 'incremental' approach. These are also based on BSA and residual renal clearance (Table 12 and Fig. 14). Incremental dialysis requires close monitoring and proactive adjustment of dialysis prescriptions and 24-h collection of dialysate and urine to document clearances. Residual renal clearance should be obtained every 1–2 months so that the peritoneal component can be modified if indicated to make sure total weekly Kt/V is 2.0 or higher. The argument for incremental dialysis and the suggestions that this approach could be better/more practical for PD are reviewed elsewhere [192].

Pitfalls in prescribing PD

There are some common pitfalls in prescribing the peritoneal component of total solute clearance. The following is a brief summary of some of these, and should be considered whenever a patient appears underdialysed. Because PD is a home therapy, non-compliance with the prescription must always be considered as a reason for underdialysis [177]. Cer-

Table 11. Empirical 'full dose' PD prescriptions

BSA	Residual renal GFR	
	$\leqslant 2$ mL/min	> 2 mL/min
BSA < 1.71 m^2	4×2.5 L CAPD 5×2.0 L NXD* 4×2.5 L APD 3×2.5 L $+ 2.0$ L $+ 2.0$ L APD	4×2.0 L CAPD 4×2.0 L $+ 2.0$ L APD
BSA 1.71–2.0 m^2	4×2.5 L CAPD 3×2.5 L $+ 3.0$ L CAPD 3×2.0 L $+ 2 \times 2.5$ L NXD 4×3.0 L $+ 2.5$ L APD	4×2.0 L CAPD 4×2.5 L APD
BSA > 2.0 m^2	4×3.0 L CAPD 4×3.0 L CAPD 3×2.5 L $+ 2 \times 3.0$ L NXD 3×3.0 L $+ 3.0$ L $+ 3.0$ L APD	4×2.5 L CAPD 4×2.5 L $+ 2.5$ L APD

* NXD uses nightly exchange device to do a mid night exchange.
(Blake PG, Burkart JM, Dunham TK. *et al.* Peritoneal Dialysis Prescription Management Tree: A Need for Change. Baxter Healthcare Corporation, 1997.)

Table 12. Empirical 'incremental' PD prescription

	Case 1	Case 2	Case 3
BSA	1.71 m^2	1.86 m^2	2.0 m^2
Fill volume of bags	2.0	2.5	3.0
At indicated GFR, ml/min			
Start with one exchange	10	11	12
Switch to two	7	8	9
Full therapy	5	6	7

(Lysaght, M. Personal communication, 1998.)

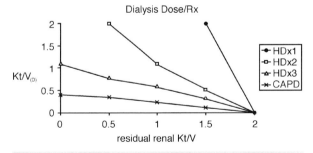

Dialysis Dose/Rx

Figure 14. Equivalent total dialysis doses for incremental replacement of $K_r t/V_{urea}$ calculated with the assumptions that [1] K_r, K_p, and K_d are clinically equivalent clearance terms and [2] the intermittent dialysis dose schedule is equivalent to continuous dialysis when average pre-dialysis BUN equals steady-state BUN with continuous therapy at equal nPCR. Note that $eK_d t/V_{urea}$ equals the equilibrated (double-pool), delivered, and normalized haemodialysis dose. (Peritoneal Dialysis Adequacy Work Group of the National Kidney Foundation. Dialysis Outcomes Quality Initiative (DOQI): Clinical Practice Guidelines. Am J Kidney Dis 1997; 30 (suppl. 2): S67–136.)

tainly, patients may be compliant with their prescription when bringing in their 24-h collections; however, if the patient is non-compliant at home, he/she may be underdialysed on a daily basis. Home visits to monitor the amount of supplies on hand, and keeping track of monthly orders, may help sort this out [193].

Some issues to consider in patients on standard CAPD would be: (1) inappropriate dwell times (a rapid transporter would do better with short dwells); (2) failure to increase dialysis dose to compensate for loss of residual renal function; (3) inappropriate instilled volume (patient may only infuse 2 L of a 2.5 L bag) [194]; (4) multiple rapid exchanges and one very long dwell (patient may do three exchanges between 9 a.m. and 5 p.m., and a long dwell from 5 p.m. to 9 a.m., limiting overall clearances) [195]; finally, (5) inappropriate selection of dialysate glucose for long dwells which may not maximize ultrafiltration and consequently clearance.

In general, when the goal is to increase total solute clearance, it is best to increase dwell volume, not number of exchanges. Increasing the number of exchanges decreases dwell time/exchange, making the therapy less effective for the average patient (Fig. 15).

Other problems are specific for those patients on cycler therapy. The drain time may be inappropriately long (> 20 min), thus increasing the time the patient must be connected to the cycler, perhaps limiting the number of exchanges a patient would tolerate. Inappropriately short dwell times may also be prescribed, making the therapy less effective for the average patient in whom length of dwell is cru-

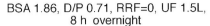

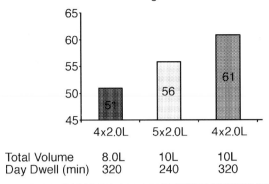

	4×2.0L	5×2.0L	4×2.0L
Total Volume	8.0L	10L	10L
Day Dwell (min)	320	240	320

Figure 15. Increasing the prescription from 4 × 2.0 L to 5 × 2.0 L increased the clearance only 10%. Increasing the prescription from 4 × 2.0 L to 4 × 2.5 L increased clearance by 21%. This demonstrates the need, in CAPD, for 2.5 L fill volume. (Blake PG, Burkart JM, Dunham TK *et al.* Peritoneal Dialysis Prescription Management Tree: A Need for Change. Baxter Healthcare Corporation, 1997.)

cial. Failure to augment total dialysis dose with a daytime dwell ('wet' day versus 'dry' day) could also result in underdialysis. Cycler patients typically 'cycle' for 9–10 h per night. Therefore, the daytime dwell is long (15–14 h). During this long dwell (longer than the 'long' night-time dwell for typical CAPD patients), diffusion stops and reabsorption often begins, minimizing clearance. Use of a midday exchange is an effective way to optimize both clearance and ultrafiltration in these patients (Fig. 16). Also, use of alternative osmotic agents such as icodextrin, which maintains ultrafiltration during long

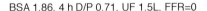

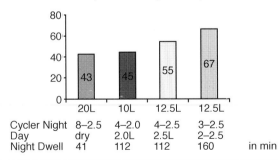

	20L	10L	12.5L	12.5L
Cycler Night	8–2.5	4–2.0	4–2.5	3–2.5
Day	dry	2.0L	2.5L	2–2.5
Night Dwell	41	112	112	160	in min

Figure 16. A 10 L wet day (CCPD) delivers 8% more clearance than a 20 L dry day (NIPD). A 12.5 L prescription with a wet day and a daytime exchange improved clearance 57% over the 20 L dry day prescription. This demonstrates the need, in APD, for 2.5 L fill volume, wet day, and a daytime exchange. (Blake PG, Burkart JM, Dunham TK *et al.* Peritoneal Dialysis Prescription Management Tree: A Need for Change. Baxter Healthcare Corporation, 1997.)

dwells, will be helpful [196]. These optimze both clearance and ultrafiltration without hypertonic glucose. Finally, poor selection of dialysate glucose may not allow maximization of ultrafiltration, resulting in less total clearance.

When changing from standard CAPD (long dwells) to cycler therapy (short dwells), it is important to remember the difference in transport rates of urea and creatinine and the effect that this change will have on the patient's overall clearance. These differences and their relevances for CAPD, CCPD, NIPD and other modifications are reviewed by Twardowski [197]. Typical instilled volumes, dwell times and number of exchanges per day/night for CAPD, CCPD, DAPD, etc. are outlined in Table 13. Transport of urea into the dialysate tends to occur faster than for creatinine. Therefore, if total solute clearance targets are measured using urea kinetics, keeping Kt/V constant going from long to short dwells may decrease creatinine clearance. In contrast, if creatinine clearance is the total solute clearance target, keeping creatinine clearance constant when changing from long to short dwells will keep Kt/V constant, or even increase it. This concept has been termed 'Horizontal modelling' [198] (Fig. 17).

Knowledge of the individual patient's peritoneal transport characteristics and familiarity with the differences in dialysis needs for rapid versus slow transporters is imperative to avoid problems or confusion.

Adjusting dialysis dose

Minimal established dialysis doses are outlined in Table 2. When determining an individual patient's prescription, one should aim for a total solute clearance that is above this minimum, but also allow for other indexes of adequate dialysis such as quality-of-life issues, blood pressure control, and dietary protein intake. If during routine monitoring or clinical evaluation of the patient the delivered dose of dialysis needs to be altered, this can easily be done in a scientific manner if you know the patient's present transport characteristics (PET), the present total clearance of urea or creatinine, and you understand the relationship between dialysis clearance, drain volume, and dwell time based on the measured D/P ratios. It is important that these relationships are understood because increasing the instilled volume does not always result in an increase in clearance. For instance, in a patient who is a low transporter and in whom clearance is critically dependent on dwell time, changing from standard CAPD (infused

Table 13. Characteristics of CAPD, CCPD, DAPD, NIPD and NTPD in adults

	CAPD	CCPD	DAPD	NIPD	NTPD
Regimen	Continuous	Continuous	Intermittent	Intermittent	Intermittent
Flow technique	Intermittent	Intermittent	Intermittent	Intermittent	Tidal
Method	Manual	Automated	Manual	Automated	Automated
Interrupted day	Yes	No or yes	Yes	No	No
Interrupted night with possible alarms	No	Yes	No	Yes	Yes
Helper convenience	No	Yes or no	No	Yes	Yes
Travel convenience	Yes	No	Yes	No	No
Intra-abdominal pressure with fluid	High	High	High	Low	Low
Leaks/hernias	Common	Common	Common	Rare	Rare
Night (h/24 h)	8–10	8–10	0	8–12	8–11
Night (no. of exchanges)	1	4–10	0	4–10	15–40
Night (exchange volume L)	1.5–3.0	1.0–3.0	0	1.0–3.0	1.0–2.5
Night (reserve volume L)	0	0	0	0	0.5–1.5
Daytime (h/24 h)	14–16	14–16	14–16	0	0
Daytime (exchange volume L)	1.5–3.0	1.5–3.0	1.5–3.0	0	0
Daytime (no. of exchanges)	4–5	1–3	4–5	0	0
Total volume (1/24 h)	8.0–15.0	10.0–20.0	8.0–12.0	10.0–20.0	15.0–40.0
Preferred transport category	Average/low	Average/low	High	High/average	High/average
Glucose absorption/UF (g/L)	60–160	50–150	80–120	30–70	50–90
Na removal/UF (mEq/L)[a]	120–140	80–130	120–140	20–90	30–100
Blood pressure control	Easy	Easy	Easy	Less easy	Less easy
Preferred solution Na (mEq/L)	132	132	132	126–132	120–132

[a] With dialysis solution sodium concentration of 132 mEq/L.
(Modified and updated from Twardowski ZJ. Practical issues in prescribing PD. In: Andreucci VE, Fine LG, eds. International Yearboook of Nephrology, London: Springer, 1993, pp. 287–310.)

volume – 8 L) to a form of cycler therapy using 2-h dwells, where the infused volume may be as high as 10–14 L may not always result in an overall increase in that patient's clearance (Fig. 16).

Once familiar with these relationships, to adjust the dialysate prescription you would need to know the D/P ratios at the anticipated dwell time and the patient's drain volume for that dwell time. By altering dwell time you change the D/P ratio and the drain volume. By altering instilled volume you will also affect total drain volume and therefore clearance. In general, increasing the instilled volume without changing dwell time will result in an increase in solute clearance.

Another means to tailor a dialysis prescription would be with the use of computer-assisted kinetic modelling programs [199, 200] which allow for ease in adjusting a patient's dialysis prescription. Baseline PET data, drain volumes, and patient weights are needed for input data. Use of these programs usually allows one to set targets for solute clearance, glucose absorption, and anticipated dietary protein intake. These computer simulations then give you a menu of prescriptions that should achieve these targets, and you can choose the one that would best suit the patient's lifestyle.

Tidal peritoneal dialysis is a form of automated dialysis in which, after an initial dialysate fill, only a portion of the dialysate is drained from the peritoneum, and this is replaced with fresh dialysate after each cycle. This leaves the majority of the dialysate in constant contact with the peritoneal membrane. A typical tidal dialysis prescription would usually require 23–28 L of instilled volume, but preliminary studies suggest that tidal dialysis may be approximately 20% more efficient than nightly PD at dialysate flow rates of about 3.5 L/h [201].

Risk of complications from increased intra-abdominal pressure

Intraperitoneal pressure increases almost linearly with increases in installed volumes [202]. For any instilled volume, pressure is greatest sitting, with the lowest pressures observed when supine. This increased pressure leads to increased tension of the abdominal wall and the potential for hernia formation in areas of weakness. Studies in individual units have reported an incidence of hernia formation between 10% and 20% [203, 204]. Patients should be instructed to avoid activities that lead to increases in intra-abdominal pressure, such as lifting. Theo-

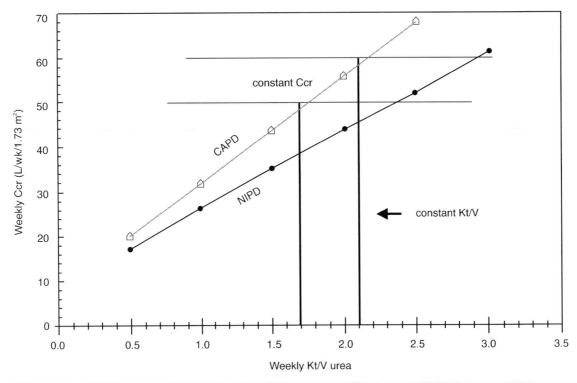

Figure 17. Weekly creatinine clearance (Ccr) is related to weekly *Kt/V* on 1 h cycles (NIPD) and 6 h cycles (CAPD) in patients with average transport characteristics. Grey horizontal lines and black lines indicate constant weekly creatinine clearances and constant *Kt/V*, respectively. Horizontal modelling maintains creatinine clearance and increases *Kt/V* while switching from CAPD to NIPD; vertical modelling maintains *Kt/V* and decreases creatinine clearance. (Modified from Nolph KD, Twardowski ZJ, Keshaviah PK. Weekly clearances of urea and creatinine on CAPD and NIPD. Perit Dial Int 1992; 12: 298–303.)

retically, as one increases instilled volume to compensate for loss of residual renal function (RRF), the incidence of hernias should increase. Our data suggest this is not true [205]. At this time there are no definitive studies which state that, as dialysis dose is increased by increasing instilled volume, the risk of hernias increases.

Clinical assessment of adequacy

As mentioned at the beginning of this chapter, the clinical assessment of adequate dialysis does not just consist of any one laboratory measurement. It includes lack of signs or symptoms of uraemia, as well as a patient's feeling of 'well-being', control of blood pressure and anaemia and other biochemical parameters [206]. The minimal target dialysis dose should be delivered and an adequate PNA achieved. If the clinical judgement is that the patient is manifesting signs of uraemia despite what appears to be adequate laboratory measurements of 'dialysis dose', it would be prudent to increase the patient's dialysis

dose if no other cause for this symptomatology is found. Certainly, a patient could be very compliant with the prescription during the period of dose monitoring but, because this is a home therapy, there may not be compliance during the rest of the therapy interval. Another explanation would be the effect a decreasing weight has on calculation of *V* and the effect normalization of *Kt* in a malnourished patient has on *Kt/V* calculation (described in the section on discrepancy, above). Furthermore, if the dose of dialysis appears inadequate despite an adequate clinical assessment, these patients should be monitored very closely. I would anticipate that, if the dose of dialysis is truly inadequate, subtle signs and symptoms of uraemia will begin to develop that may not be readily reversible.

Summary

The dose of dialysis delivered does influence outcome, and does correlate with dietary protein intake. When considering adequacy of dialysis one must monitor both of these parameters in addition to clinical assessment, blood pressure control, treatment of anaemia, osteodystrophy, and other comorbid diseases. Periods of inadequate dialysis can result in subtle symptoms of uraemia that are insidious in onset and may not be reversible. These can influence outcome in a negative way. To prevent this symptomatology, and provide as close to optimal dialysis as possible it is important to monitor dialysis dose so that changes in dialysis prescription can be made proactively rather than reactively. The minimal dose of dialysis needed to maximize outcome has been established, and when tailoring PD prescriptions it is important that the prescribed dialysis dose be targeted to at least achieve these minimal doses.

Acknowledgement

The author thanks Amanda Burnette for all her secretarial assistance in the preparation of this chapter.

Appendix: Calculation of dialysis dose

The gold standard for determining the daily clearance of any solute is to measure the actual amount of that solute removed from the body during a day. For solute lost in the urine this is classically done by measuring the concentration of that solute (mg/dl or g/L) in a volume (V) of urine and dividing the product by the concentration of the solute in body fluids (mg/dl or g/L).

$$\text{Creat}_u \times V_u \div \text{Creat}_p$$
$$= \text{daily renal creatinine clearance (L/day)} \quad (1)$$

where Creat_u is urinary creatinine concentration in mg/dl, V_u is volume of urine in L/day and Creat_p is plasma creatinine concentration in mg/dl. To calculate the weekly renal creatinine clearance one would multiply the daily creatinine clearance (eq. 1) by 7 days (eq. 2).

$$(\text{Creat}_u \times V_u \div \text{Creat}_p \times 7$$
$$= \text{weekly creatinine clearance (L/week)} \quad (2)$$

To calculate daily renal urea clearance one would substitute urea for creatinine in eq. (1) (eq. 3) and use a similar substitution in eq. (2) for weekly urea clearance, where Urea_u is the concentration of urea

in urine in mg/dl and Urea_p is the concentration of urea in plasma in mg/dl.

$$\text{Urea}_u \times V_u \div \text{Urea}_p$$
$$= \text{daily renal urea clearance (L/day)} \quad (3)$$

Calculation of residual renal creatinine clearance (RRCCr) for use in determination of total solute clearance is the sum of the daily renal urea and creatinine clearances divided by 2 (eq. 4) (see above for rationale).

$$\text{RRCCr} = (\text{eq. 1} + \text{eq. 3}) \div 2 \quad (4)$$

Urea kinetic modelling, as developed for HD, can also be applied to PD. This modelling uses the dimensionless term Kt/V, or total urea clearance divided by the volume of urea distribution (V). As with creatinine kinetics, the daily clearance of urea due to residual renal function is supplemental to that achieved from dialysis. The calculation of the residual renal function (RRF) contribution to total daily Kt/V is as follows. KT is the daily renal urea clearance in L/day (eq. 3). Urea volume of distribution (V) is either estimated (60% of the patient's weight in kilograms if male, and 55% of patients weight if female) or preferably obtained from standardized nomograms or equation such as the Watson equation (eq. 5A or 5B).

$$V \text{ male (L)} = 2.447 + 0.3362 \times \text{weight (kg)}$$
$$+ 0.1074 \times \text{height (cm)}$$
$$- 0.09516 \times \text{age (year)} \quad (5A)$$
$$V \text{ female (L)} = -2.097 + 0.2466 \times \text{weight (kg)}$$
$$+ 0.1069 \times \text{height (cm)} \quad (5B)$$
$$Kt/V \text{ (RRF)} = \text{eq. 3} \div \text{eq. 5A or 5B}$$
$$Kt/V \text{ (RRF)} = [(\text{Urea}_U \times V_V \div \text{Urea}_P] \div V \quad (6)$$

To calculate total (urinary and dialysate) creatinine clearance or Kt/V, the contributions from residual renal function are added to the clearance from dialysis. Daily dialysate creatinine clearance (DialCCr) is calculated by modifying eq. (1) to represent measurements obtained from 24-h dialysate collections. Dialysate creatinine concentration (Creat_D) is substituted for urinary creatinine and total daily dialysate drain volume (DV_D) is substituted for urine volume (eq. 7).

$$\text{DialCCr (L/day)} = \text{Creat}_D \times DV_D \div \text{Creat}_P \quad (7)$$

Total weekly creatinine clearance is the sum of daily

dialysate (DialCCr) and residual renal (RRCCr) creatinine clearances times 7 days/week (eq. 8).

$$\text{Weekly Creat Cl} = (\text{eq. 7} + \text{eq. 4}) \times 7$$
$$\text{Weekly Creat Cl} = (\text{DialCCr} + \text{RRCCr}) \times 7 \tag{8}$$

This value must then be adjusted for patient size, using a nomogram for body surface area (eq. 8A). The recommended minimal dose for continuous therapy is $\geqslant 60$ L/week/1.73 m^2.

$$\text{Weekly Creat Cl} = (\text{eq. 8} \times 1.73 \text{ m}^2/\text{patient's BSA})$$
$$\text{or} \tag{8A}$$
$$\text{Weekly Creat Cl} = (\text{eq. 8} \times 1.73 \text{ m}^2/\text{eq. 9})$$

Where patient's BSA is calculated:

$$\text{BSA} = 0.007184 \times \text{body weight (kg)}^{0.425}$$
$$\times \text{height (cm)}^{0.725} \tag{9}$$

Daily dialysate Kt/V is calculated in the following way. KT is simply the daily clearance of urea from dialysate. This is calculated by substituting Urea$_D$ for Urea$_u$ and the drain volume of dialysate (DV$_D$) for urine volume in eq. 3 (see eq. 10), and dividing this by the volume of distribution for urea, estimated using eq. (5A or 5B) or from a nomogram to get Kt/V (eq. 11).

$$\text{Dialysate urea clearance/day} = \text{urea}_D \times V_D \div \text{urea}_P \tag{10}$$

$$\text{Daily dialysate } Kt/V = \text{eq. 10} \div \text{eq. 5 (A or B)}$$

$$\text{Daily dialysate } Kt/V$$
$$= \text{Dialysate urea clearance/day} \div V \tag{11}$$

The daily dialysate Kt/V (eq. 11) is then added to the daily residual renal Kt/V (eq. 6) and multiplied by 7 to determine the total daily Kt/V (eq. 12).

$$\text{Total daily } Kt/V = (\text{eq. 11} + \text{eq. 6})$$

$$\text{Total daily } Kt/V = Kt/V \text{ dialysate} + Kt/V \text{ (RRF)} \tag{12}$$

Total weekly Kt/V is simply the total daily $Kt/V \times$ (eq. 13).

$$\text{Total weekly } Kt/V = \text{eq. 12} \times 7$$
$$\text{Total weekly } Kt/V = \text{Total daily } Kt/V \times 7 \tag{13}$$

As mentioned in the text, the minimal target weekly Kt/V for continuous therapy should be $\geqslant 2.0$.

References

1. Lundin PA III. Prolonged survival on hemodialysis. In: Maher JF, ed. Replacement of Renal Function, 3rd edn. Dordrecht: Kluwer, 1989, pp. 1133–40.
2. USRDS Annual Data Report 1992. Bethesda: National Institutes of Health, NIDDKD, 1992.
3. Sargent JA. Shortfalls in the delivery of dialysis. Am J Kidney Dis 1990; 15: 500–510.
4. Parker TF, Husni L. Delivering the prescribed dialysis. Semin Dial 1993; 6: 13–15.
5. USRDS Annual Data Report 1996. Bethesda: National Institutes of Health, NIDDKD, 1996.
6. Webster's II New Riverside Dictionary. New York: Berkley, 1984.
7. Collins AJ, Hanson G, Umen A, Kjellstrand C, Keshaviah P. Changing risk factor demographics in end-stage renal disease patients entering hemodialysis and the impact on long-term mortality. Am J Kidney Dis 1990; 15: 422–32.
8. Charra B, Calemard E, Ruffet M *et al.* Survival as an index of adequacy of dialysis. Kidney Int 1992; 41: 1286–91.
9. Delmez J, Windus D. Hemodialysis prescription and delivery in a metropolitan community. Kidney Int 1991; 41: 1023–8.
10. May RC, Kelly RA, Mitch WE. Pathophysiology of uremia. In: Brenner BM, Rector FC, eds. The Kidney. Philadelphia: WB Saunders, 1991, pp. 1997–2018.
11. Luik AJ, Kooman JP, Leunissen KML. Hypertension in haemodialysis patients: is it only hypervolaemia? Nephrol Dial Transplant 1997; 12: 1557–60.
12. Bagdade JD, Porte D, Bierman EL. Hypertriglyceridemia: a metabolic consequence of chronic renal failure. N Engl J Med 1968; 279: 181–5.
13. Neilsen VK. The peripheral nerve function in chronic renal failure. VII. Longitudinal course during terminal renal failure and regular hemodialysis. Acta Med Scand 1974; 195: 155.
14. Churchill DN, Taylor DW, Keshaviah PR. Adequacy of dialysis and nutrition in continuous peritoneal dialysis: association with clinical outcomes. J Am Soc Nephrol 1996; 7: 198–207.
15. Lowrie EG, Laird NM, Parker TF, Sargent JA. Effect of the hemodialysis prescription on patient morbidity. N Engl J Med 1981; 305: 1176–81.
16. Lindsay RM, Spanner E. A hypothesis: the protein catabolic rate is dependent upon the type and amount of treatment in dialyzed uremic patients. Am J Kidney Dis 1989; 13: 382–9.
17. Kopple J, Jones M, Keshaviah P *et al.* A proposed glossary for dialysis kinetics. Am J Kidney Dis 1995; 26: 963–81.
18. Keshaviah P. Adequacy of CAPD: a quantitative approach. Kidney Int 1992; 42 (suppl. 38): S160–4.
19. Van Olden RW, Krediet RT, Struijk DG, Arisz L. Measurement of residual renal function in patients treated with continuous ambulatory peritoneal dialysis. J Am Soc Nephrol 1996; 7: 745–50.
20. Churchill DN. Adequacy of peritoneal dialysis: how much do we need? Kidney Int 1994; 46 (suppl. 48): S2–6.
21. Peritoneal Dialysis Adequacy Work Group of the National Kidney Foundation. Dialysis Outcomes Quality Initiative (DOQI): Clinical Practice Guidelines. Am J Kidney Dis 1997; 30 (suppl. 2): S67–136.
22. Burkart JM, Schreiber M, Korbet S *et al.* Solute clearance approach to adequacy of peritoneal dialysis. Perit Dial Int 1996; 16: 457–70.
23. Popovich RP, Moncrief JW. Kinetic modeling of peritoneal transport. Contrib Nephrol 1979; 17: 59–72.
24. Teehan BP, Schliefler CR, Sigler MH, Gilgore GS. A quantitative approach to CAPD prescription. Perit Dial Bull 1985; 5: 152–6.
25. Blake PG, Balaskas E, Blake R, Oreopoulos DG. Urea kinetic modeling has limited relevance in assessing adequacy of dialysis in CAPD: In: Khanna R, Nolph KD, Prowant BF, Twardowski ZJ, Oreopoulous DG, eds. Advances in Peritoneal

Dialysis. Toronto: Peritoneal Dialysis Bulletin, 1992, pp. 65–70.

26. Lameire NH, Vanholder R, Veyt D, Lambert M, Ringoir S. A longitudinal, five year survey of urea kinetic parameters in CAPD patients. Kidney Int 1992; 42: 426–32.

27. De Alvaro F, Bajo MA, Alvarez-Ude F, Vigil A, Molina A, Selgas CR. Adequacy of peritoneal dialysis: does Kt/V have the same predictive value as for HD? A multicenter study. In: Khanna R, Nolph KD, Prowant BF, Twardowski ZJ, Oreopoulos DG, eds. Advances in Peritoneal Dialysis. Toronto: Peritoneal Dialysis Bulletin, 1992, pp. 93–7.

28. Teehan BP, Schleifer CR, Brown JM, Sigler MH, Raimondo J. Urea kinetic analysis and clinical outcome on CAPD. A five year longitudinal study. In: Khanna R, Nolph KD, Prowant BF, Twardowski ZJ, Oreopoulos DG, eds. Advances in Peritoneal Dialysis. Toronto: Peritoneal Dialysis Bulletin, 1990, pp. 181–5.

29. Maiorca R, Brunori G, Zubani R et al. Predictive value of dialysis adequacy and nutritional indices for morbidity and mortality in CAPD and HD patients. A longitudinal study. Nephrol Dial Transplant 1995; 10: 2295–305.

30. Genestier S, Hedelin G Schaffer P, Faller B. Prognostic factors in CAPD patients. A retrospective study of a 10-year period. Nephrol Dial Transplant 1995; 10: 1905–11.

31. Churchill DN. Implications of the Canada–USA (CANUSA) study of the adequacy of dialysis on peritoneal dialysis schedule. Nephrol Dial Transplant 1998; 13 (suppl. 6): 158–63.

32. Bhaskaran S, Schaubel DE, Jassal V et al. The effect of small solute clearance on survival of anuric peritoneal dialysis patients. Perit Dial Int 1999 (in press) (abstract).

33. Brandes JC, Piering WF, Beres JA, Blumenthal SS, Fritsche C. Clinical outcome of continuous ambulatory peritoneal dialysis predicted by urea and creatinine kinetics. J Am Soc Nephrol 1992; 2: 1430–5.

34. Gotch FA, Keen ML. Kinetic modeling in peritoneal dialysis. In: Nissenson AR, Fine RN, Genile DE, eds. Clinical dialysis, 3rd edn. Norwalk, CT: Appleton & Lange, 1997, pp. 343–75.

35. Keshaviah PR, Nolph KD, Van Stone JC. The peak concentration hypothesis: a urea kinetic approach to comparing the adequacy of continuous ambulatory peritoneal dialysis (CAPD) and hemodialysis. Perit Dial Int 1989; 9: 257–60.

36. Keshaviah PK, Ma J, Thorpe K, Churchill D, Collins A. Comparison of 2 year survival on hemodialysis (HD) and peritoneal dialysis with dose of dialysis matched using the peak concentration hypothesis. J Am Soc Nephrol 1995; 6: 540 (abstract).

37. Satko SG, Burkart JM. Frequency and causes of discrepancy between Kt/V and creatinine. Perit Dial Int 1997; 17: S23.

38. Meyer KV, Venkataraman V, Twardowski ZJ. Creatinine kinetics in peritoneal dialysis. Semin Dial 1998; 11: 88–94.

39. Gokal R, Harty J. Are there limits for CAPD? Adequacy and nutritional considerations. Perit Dial Int 1996; 16: 437–41.

40. Blake PG. A review of the DOQI recommendations for peritoneal dialysis. Perit Dial Int 1998; 18: 247–51.

41. Gilbert R, Goyal RK. The gastrointestinal system. In: Eknoyan G, Knochel JP, eds. The Systemic Consequences of Renal Failure. New York: Grune & Stratton, 1984, p. 133.

42. Ikizler TA, Wingard RL, Hakim RM. Malnutrition in peritoneal dialysis patients: etiologic factors and treatment options. Perit Dial Int 1995; 15: S63–6.

43. Hylander B, Barkeling B, Rossner S. What contributes to poor appetite in CAPD patients? Perit Dial Int 1991; 11 (suppl. 1): 117.

44. Hylander B, Barkeling B, Rossner S. Appetite and eating behavior – a comparison between CAPD patients, HD patients, and healthy controls. Perit Dial Int 1992; 12 (suppl. 1): 137A.

45. Lindholm B, Bergstrom J. Nutritional management of patients undergoing peritoneal dialysis. In: Nolph KD, ed. Peritoneal Dialysis, 3rd edn. Boston: Kluwer, 1989, pp. 230–60.

46. Bannister DK, Archiardo SR, Moore LW. Nutritional effects of peritonitis in continuous ambulatory peritoneal dialysis (CAPD) patients. J Am Diet Assoc 1987; 87: 53–6.

47. Young GA, Kopple JD, Lindholm B et al. Nutritional assessment of CAPD patients: an international study. Am J Kidney Dis 1991; 17: 462–71.

48. Marckmann P. Nutritional status of patients on hemodialysis and peritoneal dialysis. Clin Nephrol 1988; 29: 75–8.

49. Pollock CA, Allen BJ, Warden RA et al. Total body nitrogen by neutron activation in maintenance dialysis. Am J Kidney Dis 1990; 16: 38–45.

50. Lowrie EG, Lew NL. Death risk in hemodialysis patients: the predictive value of commonly measured variables and an evaluation of death rate differences between facilities. Am J Kidney Dis 1990; 15: 458–82.

51. Degoulet P, Legrain M, Reach I et al. Mortality risk factors in patients treated by chronic hemodialysis. Nephron 1982; 31: 103–10.

52. Kupin W, Zasuwa G, Kilates MC, Smith J, Johnson M, Levin NW. Protein catabolic rate (PCR) as predictor of survival in chronic hemodialysis patients. Council Renal Nutr QJ 1986; 10: 15–17.

53. Acchiardo SR, Moore LW, Latour PA. Malnutrition as main factor in morbidity and mortality of hemodialysis patients. Kidney Int 1983; 24 (suppl. 15): S199–203.

54. Harris T, Cook EF, Garrison R, Higgins M, Kannel W, Goldman L. Body mass index and mortality among nonsmoking older persons. The Framingham Heart Study. JAMA 1988; 259: 1520–4.

55. Held PJ, Port FK, Agadoa LYC. Survival probabilities and causes of death. In: Agadoa LYC, Held PJ, Port FK, eds. USRDS Annual Data Report 1991, 2nd edn. Bethesda: National Institutes of Health, NIDDKD, 1991, pp. 31–40.

56. McCusker FM, Teehan BP, Thorpe K, Keshaviah P, Churchill D. How much peritoneal dialysis is requried for the maintenance of a good nutritional state? Kidney Int 1996; 50: S56–61.

57. Blake PG, Flowerdew G, Blake RM, Oreopoulos DG. Serum albumin in patients on continuous ambulatory peritoneal dialysis – predictors and correlations with outcomes. J Am Soc Nephrol 1993; 3: 1501–7.

58. Spiegel DM, Anderson M, Campbell U et al. Serum albumin: a marker for morbidity in peritoneal dialysis patients. Am J Kidney Dis 1993; 21: 26–30.

59. Rocco MV, Burkart JM. Lack of correlation between efficacy number and traditional measures of peritoneal dialysis adequacy. J Am Soc Nephrol 1992; 3: 417.

60. Koomen GCM, van Straalen JP, Boeschoten EW, Gorgels JPMC, Hoek FJ. Comparison between dye binding methods and nephelometry for the measurement of albumin in plasma of dialysis patients. Perit Dial Int 1992; 12 (suppl. 1): S133.

61. Rocco MV, Flanigan MJ, Beaver S et al. Report from the 1995 core indicators for peritoneal dialysis study group. Am J Kidney Dis 1997; 30: 165–73.

62. Bergstrom J, Heimburger O, Lindholm B, Qureshi AR. Elevated serum C-reactive protein is a strong predictor of increased mortality and low serum albumin in hemodialysis (HD) patients. J Am Soc Nephrol 1995; 6: 573.

63. Qureshi AR, Anderstam B, Danielsson A, Gutierrez A, Lindholm B, Bergstrom J. Predictors of malnutrition in maintenance hemodialysis (HD) patients. J Am Soc Nephrol 1995; 6: 586 (abstract).

64. Han DS, Lee SW, Kang SW et al. Factors affecting low values of serum albumin in CAPD patients. In: Khanna R, ed. Advances in Peritoneal Dialysis. Toronto: Peritoneal Dialysis Publications, 1996, 12, pp. 288–92.

65. Yeun JY, Kaysen GA. Active phase proteins and peritoneal dialysate albumin loss are the main determinants of serum albumin in peritoneal dialysis patients. Am J Kidney Dis 1997; 30: 923–7.

66. Liberek T, Topley N, Jörres A, Coles GA, Gahl GM, Williams JD. Peritoneal dialysis fluid inhibition of phagocyte function:

Effects of osmolality and glucose concentration. J Am Soc Nephrol 1993; 3: 1508–15

67. Dawnay A. Advanced glycation end products in peritoneal dialysis. Perit Dial Int 1996; 16: S50–3.

68. Dobbie JW. Morphology of the peritoneum in CAPD. Blood Purif 1989; 7: 74–85.

69. Beelen RHJ, van der Meulen J, Verbrugh HA et al. CAPD, a permanent state of peritonitis: a study on peroxidase activity. In: Maher JF, Winchester JF, eds. Frontiers in Peritoneal Dialysis. New York: Field & Rich, 1986, pp. 524–30.

70. Dobbie JW. Durability of the peritoneal membrane. Perit Dial Int 1995; 15: S87–92.

71. Slingeneyer A, Canaud B, Mion C. Permanent loss of ultrafiltration capacity of the peritoneum in long-term peritoneal dialysis: an epidemiological study. Nephron 1983; 33: 133–8.

72. Afthentopoulos IE, Passadakis P, Oreopoulos DG. Sclerosing peritonitis in continuous ambulatory peritoneal dialysis patients: one center's experience and review of the literature. Adv Ren Replacement Ther 1998; 5: 157–67.

73. Noh H, Lee SW, Kang SW et al. Serum C-reactive protein: a predictor of mortality in continuous ambulatory peritoneal dialysis patients. Perit Dial Int 1998; 18: 387–94.

74. Haubitz M, Brunkhorst R, Wrenger E, Forese P, Schulze M, Koch KM. Chronic induction of C-reactive protein by hemodialysis, but not by peritoneal dialysis therapy. Perit Dial Int 1996; 16: 158–62.

75. Coles GA. Towards a more physiologic solution for peritoneal dialysis. Semin Dial 1995; 8: 333–5.

76. Kopple JD, Jones MR, Keshaviah PK et al. A proposed glossary for dialysis kinetics. Am J Kidney Dis 1995; 26: 963–81.

77. Keshaviah P, Nolph K. Protein catabolic rate calculations in CAPD patients. ASAIO Trans 1991; 37: M400–2.

78. Randerson DH, Chapman GV, Farrell PC. Amino acid and dietary status in CAPD patients. In: Atkins RC, Farrell PC, Thompson N, eds. Peritoneal Dialysis. Edinburgh, UK: Churchill Livingstone, 1981, pp. 171–91.

79. Harty JC, Boulton H, Curwell J et al. The normalized protein catabolic rate is a flawed marker of nutrition in CAPD patients. Kidney Int 1994; 45: 103–9.

80. Nolph KD, Moore HL, Prowant B et al. Cross sectional assessment of weekly urea and creatinine clearances and indices of nutrition in continuous ambulatory peritoneal dialysis patients. Perit Dial Int 1993; 13: 178–83.

81. Detsky AS, McLaughlin JR, Baker JP et al. What is subjective global assessment of nutritional status. J Parent Ent Nutr 1987; 11: 8–13.

82. Enia G, Sicuso C, Alati G, Zoccali C. Subjective global assessment of nutrition in dialysis patients. Nephrol Dial Transplant 1993; 8: 1094–8.

83. Blumenkrantz MJ, Kopple JD, Moran JK, Coburn JW. Metabolic balance studies and dietary protein requirements in patients undergoing continuous ambulatory peritoneal dialysis. Kidney Int 1982; 21: 849–61.

84. Diamond SM, Henrich WL. Nutrition and peritoneal dialysis. In: Mitch WE, Klahr S, eds. Nutrition and the Kidney. Boston: Little, Brown, 1988, pp. 198–223.

85. Lindholm B, Bergstrom J. Nutritional requirements of peritoneal dialysis. In: Gokal R, Nolph KD, eds. Textbook of Peritoneal Dialysis. Dordrecht: Kluwer, 1994, pp. 443–72.

86. Bergstrom J, Lindholm B. Nutrition and adequacy of dialysis. How do hemodialysis and CAPD compare? Kidney Int 1993; 43 (suppl. 40): S39–50.

87. Nolph KD. What's new in peritoneal dialysis – an overview. Kidney Int 1992; 42 (suppl. 38): S148–52.

88. Jones MR. Preventing malnutrition in the long-term peritoneal dialysis patient. Semin Dial 1995; 8: 347–54.

89. Lindholm B, Wang T, Heimburger O, Bergstrom J. Influence of different treatments and schedules on the factors conditioning the nutritional status in dialysis patients. Nephrol Dial Transplant 1998; 13: 66–73.

90. Foley R, Parfrey P, Harnett J, Kent G, Murray D, Barre P. Hypoalbuminemia, cardiac morbidity, and mortality in end-stage renal disease. J Am Soc Nephrol 1996; 7: 728–36.

91. Gotch FA. Dependence of normalized protein catabolic rate on Kt/V in continuous ambulatory peritoneal dialysis: not a mathematical artifact. Perit Dial Int 1993; 13: 173–5.

92. Harty J, Farragher B, Boulton H et al. Is the correlation between normalized protein catabolic rate and Kt/V due to mathematic coupling? Am J Soc Nephrol 1993; 4: 407.

93. Kaysen GA, Schoenfeld P. Albumin homeostasis in patients undergoing continuous ambulatory peritoneal dialysis. Kidney Int 1984; 25: 107–14.

94. Nolph KD, Keshaviah P, Emerson P et al. A new approach to optimizing urea clearances in hemodialysis and continuous ambulatory peritoneal dialysis. ASAIO J 1995; 41: M446–51.

95. Burkart JM, Jordan J, Garchow S, Jones M. Using a computer kinetic modeling program to prescribe peritoneal dialysis. Perit Dial Int 1993; 13 (suppl. 1): S77.

96. Lindsay RM, Spanner E, Heidenheim RP et al. Which comes first, Kt/V or PCR – chicken or egg? Kidney Int 1992; 42 (suppl. 38): S32–6.

97. Lutes R, Perlmutter J, Holley JL, Bernadini J, Piraino B. Loss of residual renal function in patients on peritoneal dialysis. In: Khanna R, Nolph KD, Prowant BF, Twardowski ZJ, Oreopoulos DG, eds. Advances in Peritoneal Dialysis. Toronto: Peritoneal Dialysis Publications, 1993; 9: 165–8.

98. Gotch FA, Gentile DE, Schoenfeld P. CAPD prescription in current clinical practice. In: Khanna R, Nolph KD, Prowant BF, Twardowski ZJ, Oreopoulos DG, eds. Advances in Peritoneal Dialysis. Toronto: Peritoneal Dialysis Publications, 1993; 9: 69–72.

99. Harty JC, Boulton H, Uttley L, Heelis N, Venning M, Gokal R. Limitations of urea kinetic modeling as predictors of nutritional and dialysis adequacy in CAPD. Am J Nephrol 1993; 13: 454–63.

100. Rottembourg J, Issad B, Gallego JL et al. Evolution of residual renal functions in patients undergoing maintenance hemodialysis or continuous ambulatory peritoneal dialysis. Proc EDTA 1993; 19: 397–403.

101. Cancarini GC, Brunori G, Camerini C, Brasa S, Manili L, Maiorca R. Renal function recovery and maintenance of residual diuresis in CAPD and hemodialysis. Perit Dial Bull 1986; 5: 77–9.

102. Lysaght MJ, Vonesh EF, Gotch F et al. The influence of dialysis treatment modality on the decline of remaining renal function. Trans ASAIO 1991; 37: 598–604.

103. Hallet M, Owen J, Becker G, Stewart J, Farrell P. Maintenance of residual renal function: CAPD versus HD. Perit Dial Int 1992; 12 (suppl. 1): 124 (abstract).

104. Port FK, Held PJ, Nolph KD, Turenne MN, Wolfe RA. Risk of peritonitis and technique failure by CAPD connection technique: a national study. Kidney Int 1992; 42: 967–74.

105. Jindal KK, Hirsch DJ. Long-term peritoneal dialysis in the absence of residual renal function. Perit Dial Int 1996; 16: 77–89.

106. Tattersall JE, Doyle S, Greenwood RN, Farrington K. Maintaining adequacy in CAPD by individualizing the dialysis prescription. Nephrol Dial Transplant 1994; 9: 749–52.

107. Twardowski ZJ. Clinical value of standardized equilibration tests in CAPD patients. Blood Purif 1989; 7: 95–108.

108. Blake P, Burkart JM, Churchill DN et al. Recommended clinical practices for maximizing peritoneal dialysis clearances. Perit Dial Int 1996; 16: 448–56.

109. Twardowski ZJ. Nightly peritoneal dialysis (why? who? how? and when?). ASAIO Trans 1990; 36: 8–16.

110. Garred LJ, Canaud B, Farrell PC. A simple kinetic model for assessing peritoneal mass transfer in chronic ambulatory peritoneal dialysis. ASAIO J 1983; 3: 131–7.

111. Popovich RP, Moncrief SW. Transport kinetics. In: Nolph KD, ed. Peritoneal dialysis, 2nd edn. Boston: Martinus Nijhoff, 1985, pp. 115–58.

112. Vonesh EF, Lysaght MJ, Moran J. Kinetic modeling as a prescription aid in peritoneal dialysis. Blood Purif 1991; 9: 246–70.

113. Krediet RT, Struijk DG, Koomen GCM, Arisz L. Peritoneal fluid kinetics during CAPD measured with intraperitoneal dextran 70. ASAIO Trans 1991; 37: 662–7.

114. Rippe B, Krediet R. Peritoneal physiology – transport of solutes. In: Gokal R, Nolph KD, eds. The Textbook of Peritoneal Dialysis. Dordrecht: Kluwer, 1994, pp. 69–113.

115. Faller B, Lameire N. Evolution of clinical parameters and peritoneal function in a cohort of CAPD patients followed over 7 years. Nephrol Dial Transplant 1994; 9: 280–6.

116. Selgas R, Fernandez-Reyes MJ, Bosque E *et al.* Functional longevity of the human peritoneum: how long is continuous peritoneal dialysis possible? Results of a prospective medium long-term study. Am J Kidney Dis 1994; 23: 64–73.

117. Selgas R, Bajo MA, del Peso G, Jimenez C. Preserving the peritoneal dialysis membrane in long-term peritoneal dialysis patients. Semin Dial 1995; 8: 326–32.

118. Selgas R, Bajo MA, Paiva A, del Peso G, Diaz C, Aguilera A, Hevia C. Stability of the peritoneal membrane in long-term peritoneal dialysis patients. Adv Ren Replace Ther 1998; 5: 168–78.

119. Heimburger O, Waniewski J, Werynski A, Tranaeus A, Lindholm B. Peritoneal transport characteristics in CAPD patients with permanent loss of ultrafiltration. Kidney Int 1990; 38: 495–506.

120. Jensen RA, Nolph KD, Moore HL, Khanna R, Twardowski ZJ. Weight limitations for adequate therapy using commonly performed CAPD and NIPD regimens. Semin Dial 1994; 7: 61–4.

121. Nolph KD. Has peritoneal dialysis peaked? The impact of the CANUSA study. ASAIO Trans 1996; 42: 136–8.

122. Rocco MV. Body surface area limitations in achieving adequate therapy in peritoneal dialysis patients. Perit Dial Dial 1996; 16: 617–22.

123. Blake PG. Targets in CAPD and APD prescription. Perit Dial Int 1996; 16: S143–6.

124. Churchill DN, Thorpe KE, Nolph KD, Keshaviah PR, Page D, Oreopoulos DG. Increased peritoneal transport is associated with decreased CAPD technique and patient survival. J Am Soc Nephrol 1997; 8: 189A.

125. Davies SJ, Phillips L, Russell GI. Peritoneal solute transfer is an independent predictor of survival on CAPD. J Am Soc Nephrol 1996; 7: 1443.

126. Nolph KD, Moore HL, Prowant B *et al.* Continuous ambulatory peritoneal dialysis with a high flux membrane: a preliminary report. ASAIO J 1993; 39: M566–8.

127. Heaf J. CAPD adequacy and dialysis morbidity: detrimental effect of a high peritoneal equilibrium rate. Renal Failure 1995; 17: 575–87.

128. Harty JC, Boulton H, Venning M, Gokal R. Is peritoneal permeability an adverse risk factor for malnutrition in CAPD patients? Miner Electrolyte Metab 1996; 22: 97–101.

129. Blake P. What is the problem with high transporters? Perit Dial Int 1997; 17: 317–20.

130. Burkart JM. Effect of peritoneal dialysis prescription and peritoneal membrane transport characteristics on nutritional status. Perit Dial Int 1995; 15: S20–35.

131. Kagan A, Bar-Khayim Y, Schafe Z, Fainaru M. Heterogeneity in peritoneal transport during continuous ambulatory peritoneal dialysis and its impact on ultrafiltration, loss of macromolecules and plasma level of proteins, lipids and lipoproteins. Nephron 1993; 63: 32–42.

132. Struijk DG, Krediet RT, Koomen GC *et al.* Functional characteristics of the peritoneal membrane in long term continuous ambulatory peritoneal dialysis. Nephron 1991; 59: 213–20.

133. Mamoun H, Anderstam B, Lindholm B, Södersten P, Bergström J. Peritoneal dialysis solutions with glucose and amino acids suppress appetite in the rat. J Am Soc Nephrol 1994; 5: 498.

134. Lindholm B, Bergstrom J. Nutritional requirements of peritoneal dialysis. In: Gokal R, Nolph KD, eds. Textbook of Peritoneal Dialysis. Dordrecht: Kluwer, 1994, pp. 443–72.

135. Balaskas EV, Rodela H, Oreopoulos DG. Effect of intraperitoneal infusion of dextrose and amino acids on the appetite of rabbits. Perit Dial Int 1993; 13: S490–8.

136. Mamoun AH, Anderstam B, Sodersten P, Lindholm B, Bergstrom J. Influence of peritoneal dialysis solutions with glucose and amino acids on ingestive behavior in rats. Kidney Int 1996; 49: 1276–82.

137. Davies S, Russell L, Bryan J, Phillips L, Russell G. Impact of peritoneal absorption of glucose on appetite, protein catabolism and survival in CAPD patients. Clin Nephrol 1996; 45: 194–8.

138. Twardowski ZJ, Nolph KD, Khanna R, Gluck Z, Prowant BF, Ryan LP. Daily clearances with CAPD and NIPD. ASAIO Trans 1986; 32: 575–80.

139. Feriani M. Adequacy of acid base correction in continuous ambulatory peritoneal dialysis patients. Perit Dial Int 1994; 14: S133–8.

140. Feriani M, Ronco C, La Greca G. Acid–base balance with different CAPD solutions. Perit Dial Int 1996; 16: S126–9.

141. La Greca G, Biasioli S, Chiaramonte S *et al.* Acid–base balance on peritoneal dialysis. Clin Nephrol 1981; 16: 1–7.

142. Uribarri J, Buquing J, Oh MS. Acid–base balance in chronic peritoneal dialysis patients. Kidney Int 1995; 47: 269–73.

143. Graham KA, Reaich D, Goodship THJ. Acid–base regulation in peritoneal dialysis. Kidney Int 1994; 46 (suppl. 48): S47–50.

144. Kang DH, Yoon K, Lee HY, Han DS. Impact of peritoneal membrane transport characteristics on acid–base status in CAPD patients. Perit Dial Int 1997; 18: 294–302.

145. Walls J, Pickering W. Does metabolic acidosis have clinically important consequences in dialysis patients? Semin Dial 1998; 11: 18–19.

146. Lowrie EG, Lew NL. Commonly measured laboratory variables in hemodialysis patients: relationships among them and to death risk. Semin Nephrol 1992; 12: 276–83.

147. Bergstrom J. Why are dialysis patients malnourished? Am J Kidney Dis 1995; 26: 229–41.

148. Bailey JL, Mitch WE. Does metabolic acidosis have clinically important consequences in dialysis patients? Semin Dial 1998; 11: 23–4.

149. Graham KA, Reaich D, Channon SM *et al.* Correction of acidosis in CAPD decreases whole body protein degradation. Kidney Int 1996; 49: 1396–400.

150. Acchiardo SR, Kraus AP, Kaufman PA, LaHatte G, Adkins D, Moore LW. Evaluation of CAPD prescription. In: Khanna R, Nolph KD, Prowant BF, Twardowski ZJ, Oreopoulos DG, eds. Advances in Peritoneal Dialysis. Toronto: Perit Dial Bull 1991; 7: 47–50.

151. Chen HH, Shetty A, Afthentopoulos IE, Oreopoulos DG. Discrepancy between weekly Kt/V and weekly creatinine clearance in patients on CAPD. In: Khanna R, ed. Advances in Peritoneal Dialysis. Toronto: Peritoneal Dialysis Publications, 1995, pp. 83–7.

152. Vonesh EF, Burkart JM, McMurray S, Williams PF. Peritoneal dialysis kinetic modeling: validation in a multicenter clinical study. Perit Dial Int 1996; 16: 471–81.

153. Doolan PD, Alpen EL, Theil GB. A clinical appraisal of the plasma concentration and endogenous clearance of creatinine. Am J Med 1962; 32: 65–79.

154. Tzamaloukas AH. Effect of edema on urea kinetic studies in peritoneal dialysis. Perit Dial Int 1994; 14: 398–400.

155. Tzamaloukas AH, Saddler MC, Murphy G *et al.* Volume of distribution and fractional clearance of urea in amputees on continuous ambulatory peritoneal dialysis. Perit Dial Int 1994; 14: 356–61.

156. Tzamaloukas AH, Malhotra D, Murata GH. Indicators of body size in peritoneal dialysis: their relation to urea and creatinine clearances. Perit Dial Int 1998; 18: 366–70.

157. Twardowski ZJ. Relationships between creatinine clearances and *Kt/V* in peritoneal dialysis patients: a critique of the DOQI document. Perit Dial Int 1998; 18: 252–5.

158. Nolph KD. Is total creatinine clearance a poor index of adequacy in CAPD patients with residual renal function? Perit Dial Int 1997; 17: 232–3.

159. Watson PE, Watson ID, Batt RD. Total body water volumes for adult males and females estimated from simple anthropometric measurements. Am J Clin Nutr 1980; 33: 27–39.

160. Hume R, Weyers E. Relationship between total body water and surface area in normal and obese subjects. J Clin Pathol 1971; 24: 234–8.

161. Dubois D, Dubois EF. A formula to estimate the approximate surface area if height and weight be known. Arch Intern Med 1916; 17: 863–71.

162. Jones MR. Etiology of severe malnutrition: results of an international cross-sectional study in continuous ambulatory peritoneal dialysis patients. Am J Kidney Dis 1994; 23; 412–20.

163. Burkart JM, Jordan JR, Rocco MV. Assessment of dialysis dose by measured clearance versus extrapolated data. Perit Dial Int 1993; 13: 184–8.

164. Misra M, Reaveley DA, Ashworth J, Muller B, Seed M, Brown EA. Six-month prospective cross-over study to determine the effects of 1.1% amino acid dialysate on lipid metabolism in patients on continuous ambulatory peritoneal dialysis. Perit Dial Int 1997; 17: 279–86.

165. Frankenfield DL, Prowant BF, Flanigan MJ et al. for the ESRD Core Indicators Workgroup. Trends in clinical indicators of care for adult peritoneal dialysis patients in the U.S., 1995–1997. Kidney Int 1999 (in press).

166. Blake PG, Abraham G, Sombolos K et al. Changes in peritoneal membrane transport rates in patients on long term CAPD. In: Khanna R et al., eds. Advances in Peritoneal Dialysis, vol. 15. Toronto: Peritoneal Dialysis Publication, 1989, pp. 3–7.

167. Burkart JM, Freedman BI, Rocco MV. Effect of hematocrit on peritoneal clearance in CAPD patients. Perit Dial Int 1992; 12 (suppl. 1): 103.

168. Korbet SM, Vonesh EF, Firanek CA. The effect of hematocrit on peritoneal transport. Am J Kidney Dis 1991; 18: 573–8.

169. Rocco MV, Jordan JR, Burkart JM. 24-hour dialysate collection for determination of peritoneal membrane transport characteristics: longitudinal follow-up data for the dialysis adequacy and transport test. Perit Dial Int 1996; 16: 590–3.

170. Rocco MV, Burkart JB. Prevalence of missed treatments and early signoffs in hemodialysis patients. J Am Soc Nephrol 1993; 4: 1178–83.

171. Parker TF, Husni L. Delivering the prescribed dialysis. Semin Dial 1993; 6: 13–15.

172. Keen ML, Lipps BJ, Gotch FA. The measured creatinine generation rate in CAPD suggests that only 78% of prescribed dialysis is delivered. In: Khanna R, Nolph KD, Prowant BF, Twardowski ZJ, Oreopoulos DG, eds. Advances in Peritoneal Dialysis. Toronto: Peritoneal Publications, 1993, pp. 73–5.

173. Warren PJ, Brandes JC. Compliance with the peritoneal dialysis prescription is poor. J Am Soc Nephrol 1994; 4: 1627–9.

174. Nolph KD, Twardowski ZJ, Khanna R, Moore HL, Prowant BF. Predicted and measured daily creatinine production in CAPD: identifying noncompliance. Perit Dial Int 1995; 15: 22–5.

175. Burkart JM, Bleyer AJ, Jordan JR, Zeigler NC. An elevated ratio of measured to predicted creatinine production in CAPD patients is not a sensitive predictor of noncompliance with the dialysis prescription. Perit Dial Int 1996; 16: 142–6.

176. Blake PG, Spanner E, McMurray S, Lindsay RM, Ferguson E. Comparison of measured and predicted creatinine excretion is an unreliable index of compliance in PD patients. Perit Dial Int 1996; 16: 147–53.

177. Blake PG, Korbet S, Blake R et al. for the North American PD Compliance Study Group. Admitted noncompliance with CAPD exchanges is more common in US than Canadian patients. J Am Soc Nephrol 1998 (in press).

178. Bernardini J, Piraino B. Measuring compliance with prescribed exchanges in CAPD and CCPD patients. Perit Dial Int 1997; 17: 338–42.

179. Obrador GT, Arora P, Kausz AT, Pereira BJG. Pre-end stage renal disease care in the United States: a state of disrepair. J Am Soc Nephrol 1998; 9: S44–54.

180. Nolph KD. Rationale for early incremental dialysis with continuous ambulatory peritoneal dialysis. Nephrol Dial Transplantation 1998; 13 (suppl. 6): 117–19.

181. Obrador GT, Ruthazer R, Arora P, Pereira BJG, Levey AS. What is the level of GFR at the start of dialysis in the U.S. ESRD population? J Am Soc Nephrol 1998; 9: 156A.

182. Ikizler TA, Greene JH, Wingard RL, Parker RA, Hakim RM. Spontaneous dietary protein intake during progression of chronic renal failure. J Am Soc Nephrol 1995; 6: 1386–91.

183. Kopple JD, Berg R, Houser H, Steinman TI, Teschan P (Modification of Diet in Renal Disease Study Group). Nutritional status of patients with different levels of chronic renal insufficiency. Kidney Int 1989; 26: S184–94.

184. Mehrotra R, Saran R, Moore H, Nolph KD. Towards targets for imitation of dialysis: the relationship of protein catabolic rate to *Kt/V*~urea~ in chronic renal failure patients. J Am Soc Nephrol 1996; 7: 1521.

185. Pollock CA, Ibels LS, Zhu FY et al. Protein intake in renal disease. J Am Soc Nephrol 1997; 8: 777–83.

186. Bonomini V, Feletti C, Scolari MP, Stefoni S. Benefits of early initiation of dialysis. Kidney Int 1985; 28: S57–9.

187. Tattersall J, Greenwood R, Farrington K. Urea kinetics and when to commence dialysis. Am J Nephrol 1995; 15: 283–9.

188. Schulman G, Hakim R. Improving outcomes in chronic hemodialysis patients: should dialysis be initiated earlier? Semin Dial 1996; 9: 225–9.

189. Jungers P, Zingraff J, Page B, Albouze G, Hannedouche T, Man N. Detrimental effects of late referral in patients with chronic renal failure: a case control study. Kidney Int 1993; 43: S170–3.

190. Ratcliffe PJ, Phillips RE, Oliver DE. Late referral for maintenance dialysis. Br Med J 1984; 288: 441–3.

191. Blake PG, Burkart JM, Dunham TK et al. Peritoneal Dialysis Prescription Management Decision Tree: A Need for Change. Baxter Healthcare Corporation, 1997.

192. Nolph KD. Rationale for early incremental dialysis with continuous ambulatory peritoneal dialysis. Nephrol Dial Transplant 1998; 13: 117–19.

193. Bernardini J, Piraino B. Measuring compliance with prescribed exchanges in CAPD and CCPD patients. Perit Dial Int 1997; 17: 338–42.

194. Caruana RJ, Smith KL, Hess CP, Perez JC, Cheek PL. Dialysate dumping: a novel cause of inadequate dialysis in continuous ambulatory peritoneal dialysis patients. Perit Dial Int 1989; 9: 319–20.

195. Sevick MA, Levine DW, Burkart JW, Rocco MV, Keith J, Cohen SJ. Measurement of CAPD adherence using a novel approach. Perit Dial Int 1999 (in press).

196. Mistry CD, Mallick NP, Gokal R. Ultrafiltration with an isosmotic solution during long peritoneal dialysis exchanges. Lancet 1987; 2: 178–82.

197. Twardowski ZJ. Influence of different automated peritoneal dialysis schedules on solute and water removal. Nephrol Dial Transplant 1998; 13 (suppl. 6): 103–11.

198. Nolph KD, Twardowski ZJ, Keshaviah PR. Weekly clearances of urea and creatinine on CAPD and NIPD. Perit Dial Int 1992; 12: 298–303.

199. Vonesh EF, Keshaviah PR. Applications in kinetic modeling using PD Adequest. Perit Dial Int 1997; 17: S119–25.

200. Gotch FA, Lipps BJ. Pack PD. A urea kinetic modeling computer program for peritoneal dialysis. Perit Dial Int 1997; 17: S126–30.

201. Twardowski ZJ. New approaches to intermittent peritoneal dialysis therapies. In: Nolph KD, ed. Peritoneal Dialysis, 3rd edn. Boston: Kluwer, 1990, pp. 133–51.

202. Twardowski Z, Khanna R, Nolph K *et al.* Intra-abdominal pressures during natural activities in patients treated with continuous ambulatory peritoneal dialysis. Nephron 1986; 44: 129–35.

203. Digenis G, Khanna R, Mathews R, Oreopoulos DG. Abdominal hernias in patients undergoing continuous ambulatory peritoneal dialysis. Perit Dial Bull 1982; 2: 115–17.

204. Rocco M, Stone W. Abdominal hernias in chronic peritoneal dialysis patients: a review. Perit Dial Bull 1985; 5: 171–4.

205. Bleyer AJ, Russell G. The relationship between intermittent hemodialysis and sudden and cardiac death events. J Am Soc Nephrol 1998; 9: 200A.

206. Coles GA. Have we underestimated the importance of fluid balance for the survival of PD patients. Perit Dial Int 1997; 17: 321–6.

207. Ronco C, Bosch JP, Lew SQ *et al.* Adequacy of continuous ambulatory peritoneal dialysis: comparison with other dialysis techniques. Kidney Int 1994; 46 (suppl. 48): S18–24.

208. Vonesh EF, Moran J. Discrepancies between urea Kt/V versus normalized creatinine clearance. Perit Dial Int 1997; 17: 13–16.

15 | Ultrafiltration failure

S. MUJAIS

Definitions

Ultrafiltration failure can be defined as failure of peritoneal fluid removal to match the volume balance needs of the patient being treated by peritoneal dialysis. It represents a failure to maintain volume homeostasis. The complex implications of this definition are readily apparent: the maintenance of volume homeostasis is dependent on the balance of input and output; hence failure to maintain volume homeostasis may reside in disturbances in either, or in a mismatch of the two operations. Further, volume removal is usually dependent on both renal and peritoneal components. As renal fluid removal declines over time, the peritoneal component needs to be adjusted to compensate for the loss. Failure of such adjustment will disrupt volume homeostasis without necessarily implying a failure of peritoneal fluid removal capacity. Hence, when faced with a disruption of volume homeostasis, the clinician needs to determine where the fault lies: is it failure of the peritoneum to respond to an adequate osmotic stimulus, or the failure of the prescription to provide such an osmotic stimulus, or the failure of the patient to comply with dietary restrictions and guidelines? Taken a step further, it can be argued that failure at the peritoneal level is also complex, as the response to the osmotic stimulus may be adequate, but overshadowed by other operative processes (such as lymphatic/tissue reabsorption) whereby the net observed ultrafiltration response is inadequate.

The implications of the above discourse are clinically relevant as they affect the interventions required to alleviate the consequences of failure of volume homeostasis. They can be restated thus: failure of volume homeostasis is not necessarily the result of inadequate peritoneal fluid removal. It can result from excessive salt/water intake. Failure of peritoneal fluid removal does not necessarily imply a pathological alteration of the peritoneal membrane. It may be due to an erroneous prescription that does not offer optimal conditions for peritoneal ultrafiltration, or the operation of contrary mechanisms that thwart the effects of proper peritoneal membrane response.

The proper incidence of ultrafiltration failure (UFF) is difficult to determine because of the variability in case definition [1–8]. If one considers failure of peritoneal response to adequate osmotic stimulus as an operational definition, then the incidence is rather low. However, if failure to achieve volume homeostasis is the criterion used, then a larger number of patients may be at risk of being labelled as having UFF. This is further affected by the availability of alternative therapeutic options. Patients who have fluid management problems on standard continuous ambulatory peritoneal dialysis (CAPD), may do well with the use of alternative osmotic agents such as icodextrin [9–15], or by transfer to automated peritoneal dialysis (APD) [16]. Should, then, the definition be failure to maintain fluid balance on current therapy, or failure after more appropriate alternative therapies have been attempted? With the increasing tendency to tailor peritoneal dialysis (PD) modality selection (CAPD vs. APD) to individual patient characteristics, and wide utilization of icodextrin, it is likely that older prevalence data will become irrelevant to guide current clinical practice.

Classification

Table 1 offers a classification of causes of failure of volume homeostasis divided into the operative mechanisms. This is an aetiological classification that is useful as a framework for discussion of the various conditions. It divides the possible causes into groups based on a pathophysiological approach, and will be used in the discussion of the various entities. The linear approach to causation classification, however, does not always capture the complexity of clin-

R. Gokal, R. Khanna, R.Th. Kromiet and K.D. Nolph (eds.), Textbook of Peritoneal Dialysis, 2nd Edition, 499–513.
© 2000 Kluwer Academic Publishers. Printed in Great Britain.

Table 1. Causes of volume homeostasis failure

Input-dependent cause
Excessive salt/water intake

Output-dependent causes
Uncompensated loss of residual renal function
Inadequate provision of ultrafiltration conditions
   Long dwells
   Inappropriate tonicity
   Mismatch of prescription and peritoneal equilibration test
   (PET) status
Exaggerated contrary mechanisms
   Lymphatic/tissue reabsorption
Failure of peritoneal response
   High transport status
   Aquaporin deficiency
   Loss of functional peritoneum
Mechanical failure of dialysis procedure
   Obstruction and other catheter malfunctions
   Leaks

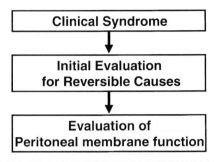

Figure 1. Step-wise diagnostic scheme.

ical situations. It is not uncommon for causative mechanisms to coexist in the same patient. The most intuitively obvious example of mixed causality is the mismatch between fluid intake and dialysis prescription when the former is excessive and the latter is inadequate. More complex examples would be situations of ultrafiltration capacity failure due to high transport coupled with enhanced lymphatic/tissue reabsorption. Such occurrences of mixed causality are not rare in nephrology. They can be likened to mixed acid–base disorders and, like the latter, require a sharp diagnostic acumen coupled to a systematic approach to unravel their intricacies.

Diagnosis

Aetiological classifications, however, do not always offer the most clinically usable diagnostic approach as the exigencies of the latter are based more on frequency of occurrence and logistical simplification. Indeed, input-dependent causes, inadequate provision of optimal ultrafiltration conditions, and mechanical failures of the dialysis procedure are more common than the other conditions [7, 8]. Hence, the diagnostic approach needs to account for the frequency hierarchy of causes to be most efficient and practical. The more frequently occurring aetiologies need to be addressed first in a stepwise diagnostic scheme. Such a diagnostic approach is illustrated in Fig. 1.

In the work-up of volume homeostasis failure it is important to consider the multitude of factors that can alter fluid balance (Fig. 2). The clinical history

may readily disclose the probable causation that can then be pursued with definitive diagnostic testing. A history of non-compliance with either dietary advice or PD prescription may direct the evaluation to more interventional pathways and preclude the need for expensive and tedious diagnostic work-up. Understandably, the detection and resolution of patient non-compliance are not easy tasks. Parallel evidence for non-compliance in other aspects of the therapy, or generalized evidence for non-adequacy of the therapy, may be helpful. Concomitant small solute inadequacy and inadequate fluid removal are rarely due to true peritoneal membrane pathology. The clinical profile of the syndrome is also helpful when it is associated with a persistent reduction in drain volume. Reductions in drain volume due to mechanical problems have a more acute presentation. A positional dialysate flow suggests a malpositioned catheter, whereas sluggish outflow (and/or inflow) may result from a partially obstructed or entrapped catheter. Findings of oedema localized to the abdomen or inguinal area on clinical examination can be important clues to the presence of a peritoneal leak.

At the time of the initial office evaluation a quick 'fill and drain' with 2 L of dialysate is beneficial in order to directly observe the nature and rate of in-flow and out-flow. The presence of fibrin clots may explain abnormalities with flow, which reduce the efficiency of drainage and volume removal and can often be resolved with intraperitoneal heparin. If incomplete drainage or positional drainage is observed, a flat-plate radiograph of the abdomen will assess the possibility of a malpositioned catheter. When an entrapped catheter or peritoneal leak is suspected, peritoneography or peritoneal computerized tomography are valuable in their diagnosis [17–20]. Diagnostic and therapeutic approaches to these conditions should be sought in the appropriate chapters in this volume.

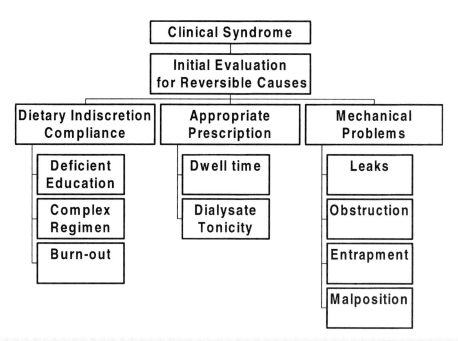

Figure 2. Work-up of volume homeostasis failure.

The exclusion of rapidly resolvable causes of impaired fluid removal has diagnostic and therapeutic advantages. The causes discussed above can frequently be resolved with standard therapeutic approaches and the clinical syndrome hence resolved. Streamlining of the diagnostic approach is also aided by the exclusion of the mechanical causes. The next diagnostic step is to evaluate the ultrafiltration and transport functions of the peritoneal membrane (Fig. 3).

Traditionally, peritoneal membrane function has been assessed by the peritoneal equilibration test (PET). The PET has been standardized both procedurally and interpretably to classify membrane function [21]. It is, however, directed primarily at small solute clearance and although ultrafiltration capacity is closely linked to the latter, the current PET test does not address the issue of quantifying pathological variations in ultrafiltration. For the purposes of diagnosing presence and causation of impaired fluid removal, the required test is one which will: (1) measure ultrafiltration under optimal conditions (to avoid false-positive results); (2) evaluate small solute transport to aid in defining causation; and (3) have validated criteria that correlate with clinical behaviour (to avoid both false-negative and false-positive results). The current PET test does provide a thorough evaluation of small solute transport, but because of the modest osmotic challenge of a 2.5%/2.27% dextrose concentration utilized in the test the osmotic drive for ultrafiltration is not optimal. Further, the normal ranges for ultrafiltration volume expected for each transport category have not been fully defined, nor have they been validated against clinical behaviour.

A modification of the standard PET test introduced by Krediet and his colleagues [22, 23] offers a reasonable alternative and is recommended as the main test for determining the appropriateness of peritoneal ultrafiltration response (Fig. 4). The modification consists of replacing the 2.5%/2.27% dextrose solution of the standard PET with a 4.25%/3.86% dextrose solution, thereby satisfying the criterion of maximal osmotic drive defined above as required for proper evaluation of ultrafiltration capacity. A value of less than 400 ml of net ultrafiltration in a 4 h dwell correlates well with clinical behaviour and avoids any false-positive results. An additional advantage of this approach is that it allows for determination of sodium sieving by profiling the changes in dialysate sodium concentration induced by osmotically driven water flow. As water influx into the peritoneal cavity is mediated in part by aquaporins, the enhanced osmotic drive

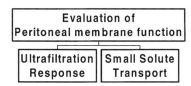

Figure 3.

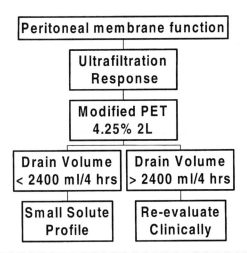

Figure 4.

will draw water into the peritoneal cavity, thereby diluting the sodium concentration. The greater the influx of water via aquaporins the greater the decline in dialysate sodium. Impaired aquaporin-mediated water transport will lead to obliteration of the decline in dialysate sodium. Hence, measurement of sodium sieving will allow better diagnostic discrimination of the causes of impaired ultrafiltration [24–27]. The characterization of small solute transport with this approach correlates well with the results of the standard PET test with 2.5%/2.27%.

After initial exclusion of mechanical, compliance, dietary and other relevant clinical causes of impaired fluid removal, the patient needs to undergo an evaluation of ultrafiltration response. A modified PET test is performed and dialysate and plasma sampling obtained as usual. The modified test allows for both fluid removal and small solute profiles to be evaluated. The former is the primary discriminating measurement, and determination of small solute profile becomes relevant only if fluid removal is deemed abnormal. If the ultrafiltration response is normal, then there is no need to assay the dialysate for small solute profile. If the ultrafiltration response is abnormal, then the relevant dialysate sample would be at hand for further evaluation. This approach limits the testing to a single session without need to inconvenience the patient.

The primary intent of the test is to quantify the net ultrafiltration in response to a 4.25%/3.86% dextrose dialysis solution challenge. If net ultrafiltration is greater than 400 ml/4 h (drain volume greater than 2400 ml/4 h), the subsequent diagnostic sequence needs to focus on the following possible aetiologies: (1) dietary indiscretion or dialysis non-

compliance; (2) inappropriate prescription; and (3) recent loss of residual renal function for which no adjustments were made in prescription. In effect, a net ultrafiltration greater than 400 ml/4 h (a drain volume greater than 2400 ml/4 h) effectively rules out any alterations in peritoneal functional parameters as being responsible for the inadequate fluid removal and the ensuing clinical syndrome. If net ultrafiltration is less than 400 ml/4 h (drain volume lower than 2400 ml/4 h), the subsequent diagnostic sequence is dependent on an examination of the results of small solute profile measurement (Fig. 5). Once it has been determined that the net ultrafiltration is lower than the discriminatory value, then the samples obtained during the test can be assayed for small solute concentrations. When using the values for net ultrafiltration or drain volume indicated above, the physician should keep in mind the possibility of overfill of dialysis bags, which may be in the order of 50 ml, and account for this volume in their evaluation of the observed response.

Causes of volume homeostasis failure

Input-dependent causes

Excessive salt and water intake in end-stage renal disease (ESRD) is so frequent that it invites neglect, either because of familiarity or resigned frustration. Below the apparent simplicity of the clinical imperative to limit intake lies a complex web of factors that make the task very difficult. Patient-related factors such as established habits, difficulties in altering behaviour, resentment and contrariness, and simple and pure gluttony, are familiar to the practising physician and so are the barriers to their modification. Resigned frustration with the latter, however, should not be allowed to become a pattern of clinical approach. The attention to intake issues has to focus additionally on three other aspects. First, is avoidance of being lulled by the impression that because PD is a continuous daily therapy the dangers of fluid overload are attenuated [28]. The potential advantages of PD are real only if they are used properly. The ability to control fluid removal on a daily basis is a significant advantage, but only if it is used appropriately. The tolerance of PD patients for greater food and fluid intake than haemodialysis patients should not be abused by neglect of proper dietary guidelines. Second, attempts at limiting salt and water intake should be balanced against provi-

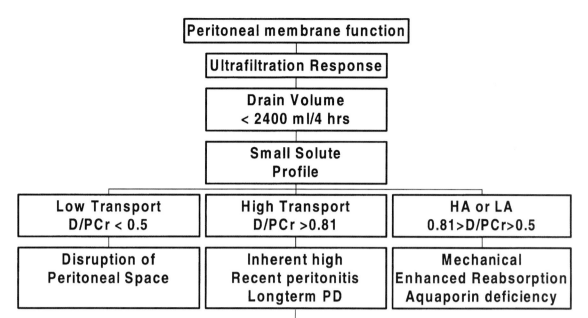

Figure 5.

sion of adequate nutrition. Salt and water are obligatory components of food, and the zeal to control the former should not lead to restrictions imposed on the latter that may hinder proper nutrition. Third, some physicians have used excessive fluid intake coupled with large ultrafiltration volume achieved with high glucose dialysate as a method of enhancing solute clearance. The contribution of ultrafiltration to clearance in PD is quite significant and the success of the above approach in the hands of expert users is testimony to this fact. Caution is necessary, however, when such an approach is used in both the selection and education of the patient in whom this approach is contemplated. Failure of the ultrafiltration to occur because of non-compliance with prescribed regimen, and excessive licence in increasing intake by the unwary patient, are risks to consider.

Output-dependent causes

Uncompensated loss of residual renal function

The contribution of residual renal function to fluid balance is major at the time of usual initiation of dialysis. Patients started on dialysis at a glomerular filtration rate of 5–10 ml/min per 1.73 m^2 usually have over a litre of urine output per day. They are able to maintain such an output for over a year unless an intercurrent illness (peritonitis) or event (contrast dye study) causes a sudden loss of renal function. It is usually in such settings that a discrepancy between fluid balance needs and suitability of

ongoing prescription arises most acutely. As renal function will inevitably undergo further declines in all patients, failure to adjust the dialytic prescription to the fluid balance requirements will lead to incipient fluid overload. The rate loss of renal function varies among patients, and the impact of declining glomerular filtration rate (GFR) on urine output is also variable. GFR may decline without a perceptible change in urine output until advanced failure sets in. It is therefore useful to evaluate urine output on a quarterly basis and adjust prescription as needed.

Inadequate provision of optimal ultrafiltration conditions

From a clinical standpoint, inadequate provision of optimal ultrafiltration conditions can be reduced to two situations: a mismatch between prescription and PET status best exemplified by use of long dwells in high transporters, and mismatch between dwell time and tonicity exemplified by use of low tonicity solutions in both high transport states and long dwells.

Long dwells. Glucose is an unsuitable osmotic agent for long dwells because of its rapid absorption. By 4 h, in patients with high transport, less than 25% of the original glucose concentration persists in the dialysate. Glucose concentration continues to fall, albeit less dramatically, with further prolongation of the dwell. The two critical periods for ultrafiltration failure in a diurnal cycle of treatment are then the overnight dwell in CAPD and the day-time dwell in APD [16]. The former can be short-ened by the use of an automated night-time exchange device and the latter by earlier drainage, either man-ually or by re-attachment to the cycler for that function exclusively. Alternatively, and probably preferable from a quality-of-life standpoint, the use of alternative osmotic agents such as icodextrin would provide enhanced ultrafiltration with less disruption of lifestyle. When problems with fluid removal arise, examination of the long dwell first is worthwhile, as this is the most vulnerable compo-nent of the therapy.

Inappropriate tonicity. While improvements in fluid removal can be achieved by modifications in dwell time and, as discussed in another section, prescrip-tions with lower glucose content can be modelled and used, provision of appropriate tonicity for the chosen dwell duration and the peritoneal transport type is nevertheless necessary [16]. It is not uncom-mon to find patients labelled as having UFF when the cause of fluid excess is the reluctance of the physician to prescribe even 2.5%/2.36% dialysate. Indeed, the areas of the world where 'ultrafiltration failure' is most frequently cited as a cause of tech-nique failure are those that have the lowest utiliza-tion of solutions with tonicity higher than 1.5% glucose [29]. In contrast, experts have suggested that UFF be defined as failure to obtain adequate fluid removal despite use of two or more exchanges with 4.25%/3.86% glucose! In the United States, where 'ultrafiltration failure' is seldom listed as a cause of technique failure, over 50% of dialysate used is in the 2.5%/2.36% formulation. With the advent of icodextrin as an alternative osmotic agent, enhanced ultrafiltration without an increase in glu-cose exposure may be obtained.

Exaggerated contrary mechanisms

The peritoneal absorptive flow consists of two different pathways: (1) *direct lymphatic absorption* and (2) *fluid absorption into tissues.* The peritoneal absorptive flow is independent of the intraperitoneal *osmotic* pressure and thus not influenced by ultrafiltration induced by the osmotic agent in the dialysate (i.e. osmotic pressure-driven convective flow). On the other hand, the peritoneal fluid and protein absorption rates in animal experiments have been shown to be directly proportional to the intra-eritoneal *hydrostatic* pressure. Hydrostatic pressure-driven convection is the most likely mechanism

driving the fluid and protein transport into adja-cent tissues.

Increased lymphatic/tissue absorption (or overall peritoneal tissue reabsorption) can lead to a low drain volume despite an adequate response to an osmotic challenge [30, 31]. Since enhanced lym-phatic/tissue reabsorption is ongoing, the response to the osmotic challenge is obscured if one relies solely on final drain volume or even on peritoneal volume. Lymphatic/tissue absorption of peritoneal fluid negatively influences the overall removal of water (decreases net ultrafiltration) and solute (par-tially negating the effect of diffusive and convective solute transport). Since the lymphatic/tissue absorp-tion of peritoneal fluid does not alter the concen-tration of solutes in the dialysate, the D/P creatinine ratio remains unchanged even though net ultra-filtration can be significantly decreased. Lymphatic/ tissue absorption rates average 0.95–1.0 ml/min in the upright position and increase to 1.5 ml/min in the supine position, possibly due to an increase in intraperitoneal pressure in the subdiaphragmatic area where a large proportion of the lymphatic sto-mata exist. This postural change in lymphatic/tissue absorption has not been uniformly observed. An overall increase in intraperitoneal pressure causes a decline in net ultrafiltration, primarily by the increase in lymphatic/tissue absorption rate.

The relative contribution of increased lymphatic/ tissue reabsorption to fluid removal problems is not definitively established. Proper assessment of fre-quency of the condition, however, will require fur-ther work. Impaired net ultrafiltration associated with the disappearance of intraperitoneally adminis-tered macromolecules was found in two out of the nine patients with UFF described by Heimbürger *et al.* [4]. Krediet and his group [23] found a dextran disappearance rate exceeding 2 ml/min in seven out of 19 patients with inadequate ultrafiltra-tion (net UF < 400 ml/4 h on 4.25%/3.86% glu-cose), often in combination with the presence of a large peritoneal surface area. Up to now no evidence is present suggesting that the prevalence of this cause of impaired peritoneal fluid removal would increase with the duration of PD.

Definitive proof of the condition requires identifi-cation of high macromolecule clearance from the peritoneal cavity to plasma as a surrogate marker for fluid removal by the lymphatic pathway [32, 33]. The point bears emphasis: clearance of macro-molecules is used as an indicator of fluid clearance, but the two are not necessarily identical. In the absence of such a test the diagnosis is made by exclusion of mechanical catheter problems, and aquaporin deficiency in patients with low average or high average solute transport on the modified PET. The rate of lymphatic absorption is estimated by measuring the disappearance of macromolecules such as albumin or dextran 70 from the peritoneal cavity (molecules too large for transcapillary transfer by either diffusion or convection). As described by Pannekeet et al. [23], this can be done by adding 1 g of dextran 70 per litre to a 2 L 4 h 4.25%/3.86% dextrose dwell. The dialysate would be sampled at 0, 10, 20, 30, 60, 120, 180 and 240 min and the lymphatic or tissue resorption rate of dialysate would be calculated from the dextran clearance from the peritoneal cavity. Measurement of lymphatic flow is uncommon in clinical practice due to the complexity of the procedure. Since transcapillary ultrafiltration is essentially normal in this situation, osmotically mediated water transport into the intraperitoneal cavity results in the normal dilution of the sodium concentration of the dialysate (because the sieving coefficient for sodium is less than 1.0, the sodium concentration in ultrafiltrate is less than that of serum, leading to an increase in intraperitoneal sodium free water which dilutes the initial dialysis solution sodium concentration). A 2–4 mEq/L decrease in the dialysate sodium concentration will normally be observed within 2 h of a 2 L 2.5%/2.27% dextrose dialysate dwell (this decrease in sodium concentration can be augmented by the use of 4.25%/3.86% dialysate), and has been used as indirect evidence of normal transcapillary ultrafiltration. In patients with reduced net ultrafiltration secondary to increased lymphatic absorption the normal decline in sodium concentration is maintained.

Failure of peritoneal response

High transport status. Patients with a low drain volume (<2400 ml/4 h with a 4.25%/3.86% modified PET) and D/P creatinine >0.81, and D/D_0 glucose < 0.30 probably represent the largest group of patients with inadequate filtration due to peritoneal membrane characteristics. These patients fall into three groups: (1) patients with an inherent high small solute transport profile at initiation of dialysis; (2) patients with peritonitis; and (3) patients who develop a high transport profile in the course of long-term PD. These patients tend to have good small molecular weight solute transport, but have poor ultrafiltration during standard CAPD using glucose-containing dialysate due to rapid absorption

of glucose and dissipation of the osmotic gradient. If their dwell times are mismatched for their membrane transport characteristics they often appear to have inadequate ultrafiltration as they lose residual renal function and no longer have urine flow to supplement net daily peritoneal fluid removal.

Inherent high transport. Ten per cent of patients starting PD display this transport profile. This proportion appears to be constant in various population groups and stable over medium periods of observation [34]. Patients in this group have very efficient membranes for small solute clearance, but may have difficulty in ultrafiltration, particularly in long dwell cycles. These patients are at risk of high protein losses in the peritoneum. A high level of technique failure has been described on CAPD therapy, probably related to fluid management. Retrospective analysis also suggests higher mortality in this group [35–37]. These patients typically do well on CAPD until residual renal volume decreases, at which time it may become difficult to maintain euvolaemia and blood pressure control on standard CAPD with glucose-containing solutions. APD and icodextrin for long dwell are recommended therapeutic approaches in this group (see below).

Recent peritonitis. It is a common clinical observation for PD patients to experience fluid retention during episodes of peritonitis [38–41]. These patients often need a temporary change in their standard dialysis prescription (shorter dwell times or increased tonicity of fluids) to achieve net ultrafiltration. When compared to baseline, PET data during peritonitis reveal an increase in the D/P ratio for creatinine and a decrease in the D/D_0 ratio for glucose. There is also an increase in protein losses and a significant decrease in net ultrafiltration. These clinical and physiological changes associated with peritonitis are usually reversible and, after recovery from the episode, membrane transport usually returns to baseline. Several studies have indicated that ultrafiltration during an episode of peritonitis can be satisfactorily achieved with the use of icodextrin [42].

High transport during long-term PD. An increase in small solute transport during the course of long-term therapy on PD is thought to be due to an increase in peritoneal membrane functional surface area [43–48]. Peritoneal equilibration testing shows an increase in D/P ratio for creatinine, a decrease in the D/D_0 ratio for glucose and a smaller than usual decrease in dialysate sodium during the dwell. In contrast to the situation seen with peritonitis, in which transport changes are usually transient and protein losses are increased, the small solute transport changes in this group tend to be permanent, and protein mass transport does not change. It is often easy to maintain total solute clearance goals in these patients despite a tendency towards clinical volume overload.

These changes in peritoneal membrane function were originally described with acetate-containing dialysis solutions [1, 49], but have also been seen in patients who have used only lactate-containing dialysis. A history of recurrent peritonitis and extensive use of hypertonic exchanges has been observed in some, but not all, studies. The incidence seems to increase with time on PD, implicating repeated exposure of the peritoneum to dialysis solution as a cause.

The natural history of peritoneal membrane transport over time has been debated [34, 48, 50–54]. This is mainly due to non-comparability of the methods used. A small number of studies have used standardized 4 h dwell evaluations with examination of both ultrafiltration and solute transport, while a larger number utilized clearance monitoring. The latter may mask opposing directional changes in solute and fluid transport. The potential increase in solute clearance due to an increase in D/P creatinine may be masked by the potential decline due to lower ultrafiltration. The emerging picture, however, is that during long-term observations (>2 years) some degree of increase in D/P creatinine does occur in patients on PD.

Aquaporin deficiency. This is a relatively rare condition and only a small number of cases with suspected diagnosis have been reported [55]. Nevertheless, greater awareness and more systematic evaluation may allow a more precise determination of its true prevalence. Further, this condition offers a very interesting model to understand peritoneal transport and its alteration by pathological states. The peritoneal capillary membrane is not freely permeable to solutes but is a highly selective barrier, with the ability to impede diffusion and convection of relatively small molecules while restricting large macromolecules, but to a lesser degree than standard haemodialysis membranes. This suggests that the peritoneal capillaries contain populations of varying 'pores', which alter solute transport. This has led, through computer simulations [56–61] and animal work [62–65], to the 'three-pore theory' of water

and solute transport across the peritoneal membrane (mainly transcapillary movement of solute and fluid). This theory proposed three populations of pores: a large number of transcellular pores (4–5 Å radius), a large number of small pores (40–50 Å) and a small number of large pores (200–300 Å). This theory predicted that 40–50% of the total ultrafiltrate is obtained through the transcellular path and therefore will be solute free, when driven by an osmotic pressure differential. Animal work and indirect human research has pointed strongly to the aquaporins being the water channel transcellular pores (ultra-small pore). Aquaporins have been demonstrated by *in-situ* techniques to be present in the human peritoneal capillary endothelium and mesothelium [66, 67]. The small pores are also involved in water transport through colloid osmosis and hydrostatic pressures which are in balance; these are also the pores through which most of the small solute transport occurs. Aquaporin deficiency is that situation in which there is damage to, or a diminished number of, water channel ultra-small pores, which can lead to deficient crystalloid-induced ultrafiltration [55, 68].

Various indirect methods can be applied in clinical practice to estimate the magnitude of aquaporin-mediated water transport. The so-called sieving of sodium is the simplest one [24–27]. The dialysate concentration of Na^+ decreases during the initial phase of a dialysis dwell using a hypertonic glucose solution (4.25%/3.86% glucose). The minimum value is usually reached after 30–60 min. It is likely that the dissociation between the transport of Na^+ and that of water is caused by aquaporin-mediated water transport. Consequently the magnitude of the dip in D/P Na^+ provides information on channel-mediated water transport. However, in situations of a large vascular surface area the diffusion and/or convection of Na^+ from the circulation to the dialysate through small pores will also increase, thereby blunting the decrease of D/P Na^+. Therefore, a blunting of Na sieving is not an absolute proof of aquaporin deficiency.

Another way to assess aquaporin-mediated transport is to calculate the difference in net ultrafiltration obtained after a 4 h dwell with 1.5%/1.36% glucose and with 4.25%/3.86% glucose dialysate; 1.5%/1.36% glucose induces only a small crystalloid osmotic pressure gradient, and therefore limited transport through water channels. On the other hand, 4.25%/3.86% glucose induces a very high crystalloid osmotic pressure gradient and the net ultrafiltration obtained with it is therefore much more dependent on the number and function of water channels. Consequently Δ ultrafiltration 4.25%/3.86%–1.5%/1.36% will decrease in situations with impaired aquaporin-mediated water transport. D/P Na^+ or ΔNa^+ are probably the simplest ways for rough assessment of channel-mediated water transport, but a correction for diffusion should probably be applied when the difference between the plasma and the initial dialysate concentration of Na^+ exceeds e.g. 5 mmol/L.

Loss of functional peritoneum. The combination of low drain volume in the face of adequate osmotic challenge and low small solute transport is very rare, and reflects a major disruption of the peritoneal membrane and/or intraperitoneal fluid distribution. It is usually due to adhesions and the functional consequences may be related to fluid trapping in small spaces. Peritoneography may be helpful in making the diagnosis by identifying sequestered spaces. Poor ultrafiltration in association with low transport is reported to occur in the advanced stages of sclerosing peritonitis [69–72]. It is important, however, to realize that a high transport rate has also been described prior to a diagnosis of sclerosing peritonitis [69–72]. Unfortunately no large prospective study of fluid problems in PD patients has been performed, so it is not possible to state how often UFF together with low transport occurs. Because this condition results in both inadequate volume and inadequate solute removal, transfer to haemodialysis is required for adequate management in anuric patients [6]. In patients with residual renal function, management by PD and oral loop diuretics may be successful.

A caveat on the diagnostic criteria is in order: patients with underlying low transport rate and leaks or mechanical problems or high lymphatic/tissue reabsorption may also present with the composite picture of low drain volume and low small solute transport. It is therefore important to exclude these latter causes before accepting low transport as the reason for the difficulty with peritoneal fluid removal.

Mechanical failure of dialysis procedure

Catheter malfunctions. Catheter-related problems contributing to poor drain volumes include obstruction, entrapment, or malposition [7, 8]. Catheter obstruction, either partial or complete, often results from fibrin plugs or build-up within the catheter lumen, but can be due to omentum obstructing the

catheter ports or even a kinked catheter. These lead to sluggish or intermittent inflow/outflow of dialysate and thus alter the efficiency of fluid removal. Fibrin strands seen in the dialysate should raise suspicion of the problem but the diagnosis is otherwise one of exclusion, as radiographic evaluation is generally not helpful except in identifying kinked catheters. Treatment consists of aggressive 'flushing' of the catheter with a dialysate-filled syringe, and if this is unsuccessful the use of fibrinolytic agents when fibrin-related occlusion is suspected.

The intra-abdominal portion of the catheter may become 'entrapped' in a compartment formed by adhesions. This can lead to a reduction in intraperitoneal capacity resulting in pain on inflow once the compartment volume has been surpassed. With the use of peritoneography the compartment can be demonstrated. Treatment may be attained with surgical lysis of the adhesions if they are not too extensive.

Catheter malposition may occur because of improper placement, but this often results from the migration of catheters originally in a good position [73]. A malpositioned catheter has positional outflow and does not drain the peritoneal cavity effectively, leading to an increase in residual volume. A normal residual volume (R) is approximately 200–250 ml [21] and can be measured from information obtained during the PET using the following equation:

$$R = V_{in}(S_3 - S_2)/(S_1 - S_3)$$

where V_{in} = instillation volume, S_1 = solute concentration (urea or creatinine) in the pre-test drain, S_2 = solute concentration of the instilled fluid (0 for urea or creatinine) and S_3 = solute concentration immediately following instillation [21]. An increase in residual volume dilutes the glucose concentration in the freshly instilled dialysate. The effect is usually less than 10%. This decreases the osmotic gradient and thus reduces the rate of transcapillary ultrafiltration without any significant effect on solute transport. Net ultrafiltration is decreased while the D/P creatinine ratio remains essentially unchanged. An increase in the calculated residual volume should raise the suspicion of a malpositioned catheter. However, the presence of this problem is often clinically apparent and the diagnosis is easily made with the aid of simple radiographic techniques (flat-plate of the abdomen) as peritoneal dialysis catheters have radiopaque material imbedded within.

Leaks. Dialysate leaks from the abdominal cavity result in a decrease in drain volume and net fluid removal. In the case of external leaks the impact is greater on drain volume. In leaks into the abdominal wall or pleural space the net fluid removal is diminished either because of reabsorption from the interstitial spaces or sequestration in the pleural space. Leaks into the interstitial space are commonly accompanied by abdominal wall oedema with or without genital oedema. Leaks can occur at any time but are often seen after being on PD for several months (>4–6 months) and usually occur at the catheter insertion site but can also be associated with an abdominal wall hernia or a history of multiple abdominal surgeries [17, 18, 74, 75]. Localized abdominal wall oedema or subcutaneous fluid collections are often evident. Diagnosis is confirmed by utilizing radiographic techniques that include intraperitoneal infusion of a dialysis solution in which radiographic contrast has been added with computed tomography, or through the intraperitoneal infusion of radioisotope with peritoneal scintigraphy [17–20, 74–78].

Peritoneal membrane function is not compromised; therefore peritoneal transport as evaluated by the PET is not changed compared to baseline, but the secondary increase in lymphatic absorption leads to reduced fluid removal. Leaks associated with hernias usually require surgical repair and a temporary transfer to haemodialysis until adequate healing has occurred. Leaks occurring in the absence of a hernia usually represent a tear in the parietal peritoneum. In this situation there is frequently a history of multiple abdominal surgeries, pregnancies, recent corticosteroid usage, or abdominal straining (coughing, Valsalva manoeuvre). Small leaks may respond to peritoneal rest with haemodialysis support, or the use of intermittent PD without the need for surgical repair. Recurrence may require surgical repair.

Therapy

General guidelines

A summary of guidelines for the prevention of fluid overload is presented in Table 2.

Routine standardized monitoring

Routine standardized monitoring of desired weight, course of residual renal function, and achieved ultrafiltration with current dialysis prescription should be emphasized in the care protocols of all patients on PD. This approach will allow for early detection of developing problems and early interven-

Table 2. Guidelines for prevention of volume overload in patients on peritoneal dialysis

General guidelines
Routine standardized monitoring, including awareness of PET status
Dietary counselling concerning appropriate salt and water intake
Protection of residual renal function (RRF)
Loop diuretics if RRF present
Enhanced compliance – education
Appropriate prescription
Hyperglycaemia control
Preservation of peritoneal membrane function

CAPD
Avoidance of long dwells with low glucose concentrations
Use of night-time exchange device
Tailoring prescription to transport profile determined by PET

APD
Avoidance of long dwells with low glucose concentrations
Use of short day dwells even when no additional exchange is needed for clearance

tion with corrective measures. The volume status of patients on PD should be used as a core indicator of dialysis adequacy. Constant re-evaluation by physicians and nurses of the patient's target weight in the light of blood pressure and other features suggestive of fluid overload is required. Particular emphasis should be placed on the desirability of normalizing blood pressure by using fluid removal alone, without antihypertensive drugs, until it is proven that this strategy is not adequate. Routine performance of PET with a view to identifying high and high average transporters in whom monitoring of fluid status is particularly critical is greatly encouraged. Use of icodextrin for the long dwell and utilization of APD may be preferred approaches in these patients.

Dietary counselling

Avoidance of dietary indiscretion can be enhanced by detailed counselling and regular re-enforcement of taught guidelines. The tendency to be more liberal in dietary restrictions with PD patients compared to patients on haemodialysis should be tempered by the need to maintain desired weight and reduction of cardiovascular risk. The general assumption that patients on PD tolerate greater dietary salt and fluid indiscretion should not be construed as an endorsement for such indiscretion [79]. Tepid indifference that allows patients to hover close to mild oedema may have pernicious long-term consequences. It is recognized that dietary interventions are the hardest to implement as they involve an elaborate process of education and lifestyle modification.

Protection of residual renal function

Residual renal function (RRF) plays an important role in both small solute adequacy and volume control. The protective zeal that has become a cornerstone of nephrological management in the pre-ESRD phase needs to be sustained after initiation of dialysis. This is particularly important in the context of the new directions in dialysis initiation where patients are started on dialytic therapy at higher levels of residual renal function than previously. Attention to the nephrotoxic potential of over-the-counter medications should become a component of regular patient interviews. Further, the use of aminoglycosides in the management of peritonitis should be limited to cases in which no safer effective alternative is available. Protection from the nephrotoxic potential of contrast agents is limited by the obvious inability of using hydration methods. The promise of adenosine antagonists (e.g. aminophylline) has not been explored in this population, and may be considered by inference until tested. Avoidance of nephrotoxic agents should be practised rigorously.

Diuretic use

Routine use of high-dose loop diuretics to maintain urine output in patients with residual renal function is a viable consideration. Usually large oral doses are needed (furosemide range 250–1000 mg) with or without addition of a thiazide-like diuretic (metolazone 5–10 mg given 30 min prior to the loop diuretic). Urine volume can be successfully increased even in advanced renal failure by the use of large doses of loop diuretics alone or in combination with thiazides. While these agents do not help preserve RRF, they do increase urine output [80]. The concern over the potential ototoxicity finds its origin in the experience with large intravenous doses. Oral administration seems not to carry the same risk.

Education and enhanced compliance

Emphasis should be placed in the initial training period on the education of the patient in the diagnosis and significance of fluid overload (e.g. awareness of importance of hypertension, peripheral oedema, shortness of breath, etc.). Additionally, patients should be provided appropriate education in what the indications are to use more hypertonic PD solutions. Routine monitoring of patient compliance with PD exchanges and education of the patient in the importance of this issue are highly desirable. Better techniques to determine and detect non-compliance need to be developed.

Appropriate prescription

Choosing the correct prescription for the peritoneal transport type of the patient is crucial. While historically patients with high transport and high average transport have been managed with CAPD, their ultrafiltration requirements have been met with the utilization of higher glucose concentrations. It is possible in such patients to achieve adequate ultrafiltration using APD (four to five night cycles and short day dwell) and lower total glucose exposure than with CAPD [16]. In patients with low transport or low average transport greater ultrafiltration for the same glucose load can be achieved with the use of an automated night-time exchange device.

Hyperglycaemia control

In diabetic patients hyperglycaemia can adversely affect the maintenance of an osmotic gradient across the peritoneal membrane. Control of the hyperglycaemia may allow improved ultrafiltration without the need to use hypertonic glucose solutions unnecessarily. As glucose control is, under current practice conditions, mostly monitored and modified by the patients independently, education of the patient on the relevance of this activity to the adequacy of dialysis is important.

Preservation of peritoneal membrane function

The impact of peritonitis on membrane function acutely, and possibly chronically, has been discussed above. Minimization of damage to the peritoneal membrane by implementation of strategies to decrease the peritonitis rate should be universally applied. The use of more biocompatible solutions may also influence membrane preservation, partly via reduction in peritonitis rate. Temporary cessation of PD has been used in a few patients with high small solute transport characteristics with some success, and may be a reasonable option to consider if other approaches are unsuccessful [81–83]. Alternatively, reduction of peritoneal membrane glucose exposure may lead to some improvement in transport parameters [84].

Therapeutic guidelines for specific diagnostic categories

Failure of peritoneal response

High transport status. In addition to the universal guidelines discussed above, therapeutic interventions in patients with high small solute transport need to address the basic pathophysiological mechanism of rapid dissipation of the osmotic gradient. The latter phenomenon is particularly prominent during the long overnight dwell in CAPD and the daytime dwell in APD. The most appropriate intervention is the use of large molecular weight substitutes for glucose such as icodextrin [10–15]. Dialysate solutions containing this polyglucose have been shown to be superior to glucose-based solutions in achieving net ultrafiltration during long dwells in the majority of patients, and particularly in high transporters. In areas where icodextrin dialysis solutions are not available, shortening dwell time is the preferred approach. In CAPD patients this can be achieved with the use of an automated night-time exchange device. This approach will shorten dwell time, and has the additional benefit of improving small solute clearance with little impact on patient lifestyle. Alternatively, patients can be switched to APD where the use of short dwell times in the night phase enhances ultrafiltration. In patients on APD, forgoing the daytime exchange and optimizing the night-time regimen may be sufficient [16]. If small solute clearance suffers, then a short daytime exchange with mid-day drainage will supplement night-time clearance without compromising ultrafiltration. If the preceding options are insufficient, then high glucose concentrations may be required. In a few patients adjunctive, temporary, or permanent haemodialysis may be required.

Preventive measures remain limited and speculative because of a lack of thorough understanding of the factors underlying high transport [85–87]. In patients with inherent high transport there are no clear associations with reversible conditions that can be therapeutically addressed. The possible association with higher indices of chronic systemic inflammatory response remains unproven. The clearest category for intervention is that of the transient small solute high transport rate associated with peritonitis. Approaches to reduce and prevent infections with improved connectology, patient training, and local prophylaxis have been successful, but more remains to be achieved. In patients who develop a high transport profile in the course of chronic PD the approach is more a question of considered opinion rather than evidence-based. Reinforcing universal measures before relying on the chronic intensive use of 4.25%/3.86% glucose dialysate is generally preferable. Further, where available, use of icodextrin in lieu of any high glucose dialysate for the long dwell is recommended.

Loss of functional peritoneum. The combination of reduced solute clearance and diminished ultrafiltration represents a state of significant shortcomings in delivery of appropriate renal replacement by peritoneal dialysis. If therapeutic targets for both azotaemia and volume homeostasis cannot be met, then adjunctive haemodialysis or permanent transfer to haemodialysis may be required in anuric patients. In patients with residual renal function the use of loop diuretics may allow achievement of adequate fluid balance while continuing on PD.

Aquaporin deficiency. Adherence to the universal measures detailed above is necessary in all conditions whatever the underlying aetiology of the impaired ultrafiltration. Patients with aquaporin deficiency continue to have significant ultrafiltration via non-aquaporin pathways. This can be enhanced by the use of icodextrin in long dwells allowing for sustained fluid removal [12, 15, 87, 88]. For the glucose-based exchanges, short dwells are preferable as in patients with high transport profile with the same provisions of maintained solute clearance optimization.

Exaggerated contrary mechanisms

When enhanced tissue reabsorption results in reduced net ultrafiltration, interventions to maximize overall ultrafiltration are required to reach a state favourable to fluid removal. Ultrafiltration needs to exceed reabsorption to allow proper volume homeostasis. All interventions that maximize ultrafiltration (short dwell time, high tonicity of dialysate) need to be combined. As tissue resorption is a continuous process, and as ultrafiltration tends to decline with time, short cycle therapy is required to keep the balance of operation earlier than the convergence of the two processes. Adjusting cycle number and overall cycler time in APD, or cycle number in CAPD, to the requirements of both ultrafiltration and solute clearance needs to be done meticulously [16]. Although there is much promising investigative evidence to show that tissue resorption can be reduced [89–93], no pharmacological intervention can be recommended at this time for the lack of definitive clinical studies.

References

1. Faller B, Marichal JF. Loss of ultrafiltration in continuous ambulatory peritoneal dialysis. A role for acetate. Perit Dial Bull 1984; 4: 10.

2. Bazzato G, Coli U, Landini S *et al.* Restoration of ultrafiltration capacity of peritoneal membrane in patients on CAPD. Int J Artif Organs 1984; 7: 93.

3. Verger C, Larpent L, Celicout B. Clinical significance of ultrafiltration failure on CAPD. In: La Graeca G, Chiaramonte S, Fabris A, Feriani M, Ronco C, eds. Peritoneal Dialysis. Milan: Wichtig Editore, 1986, pp. 91–4.

4. Heimbürger O, Wanieski J, Werynski A, *et al.* Peritoneal transport in CAPD patients with permanent loss of ultrafiltration capacity. Kidney Int 1990; 38: 495–506.

5. Ronco C, Ferianai M, Chiaramonte S *et al.* Pathophysiology of ultrafiltration in peritoneal dialysis. Perit Dialysis Int 1990; 10: 119.

6. Mactier RA. Investigation and management of ultrafiltration failure in CAPD. In: Khanna R, Nolph KD, Prowant BF *et al.*, eds. Advances in Peritoneal Dialysis, vol. 7, Nashville: Perit Dial Bull, Inc., 1991, p. 57.

7. Korbet SM, Rodby RA. Causes, diagnosis, and treatment of peritoneal membrane failure. In: Henrich WL, ed. Principles and Practice of Dialysis, 2nd edn. Baltimore: Williams & Wilkins, 1998, pp. 185–206.

8. Korbet SM. Work-up of ultrafiltration failure. Adv Renal Repl Ther 1998; 5: 194–204.

9. Imholz ALT, Brown CB, Koomen GCM, Arisz L, Krediet RT. The effect of glucose polymers on water removal and protein clearances during CAPD. Adv Perit Dial 1993; 9: 25–30.

10. Ho-dac-Pannekeet MM, Schouten N, Langendijk MJ *et al.* Peritoneal transport characteristics with glucose polymer based dialysate. Kindey Int 1996; 50: 979–86.

11. Peers E, Gokal R. Icodextrin: overview of clinical experience. Perit Dial Int 1997; 17: 22–6.

12. Peers E, Gokal R. Icodextrin provides long dwell peritoneal dialysis and maintenance of intraperitoneal volume. Artif Organs 1998; 22: 8–12.

13. Posthuma N, ter Wee PM, Verbruh HA *et al.* Icodextrin instead of glucose during the daytime dwell in CCPD increases ultrafiltration and 24-h dialysis creatinine clearance. Nephrol Dial Transplant 1997; 12 (suppl. 1): 550–3.

14. Woodrow G, Stables G, Oldroyd R, Gibson J, Turney JH, Brownjohn AM. Comparison of icodextrin and glucose solutions for the daytime dwell in automated peritoneal dialysis. Nephrol Dial Transplant 1999; 14: 1530–5.

15. Wilkie ME, Plant MJ, Edwards L, Brown CB. Icodextrin 7.5% dialysate solution (glucose polymer) in patients with ultrafiltration failure: extension of technique survival. Perit Dial Int 1997; 17: 84–7.

16. Mujais S. Ultrafiltration management in automated peritoneal dialysis. In: Ronco C, Amici G, Feriani M, Virga G, eds. Automated Peritoneal Dialysis. Contrib Nephrol. Basel: Karger, 1999, vol. 129, pp. 255–66.

17. Litherland J, Gibson M, Sambrook P, Lupton E, Beaman M, Ackrill P. Investigation and treatment of poor drains of dialysate fluid associated with anterior abdominal wall leaks in patients on chronic ambulatory peritoneal dialysis. Nephrol Dial Transplant 1992; 7: 1030–4.

18. Litherland J, Lupton EW, Ackrill PA, Venning M, Sambrook P. Computed tomographic peritoneography: CT manifestations in the investigation of leaks and abnormal collections in patients on CAPD. Nephrol Dial Transplant 1994; 9: 1449–52.

19. Scanziani R, Dozio B, Caimi F, De Rossi N, Magfri F, Surian M. Peritoneography and peritoneal computerized tomography: a new approach to non-infectious complications of CAPD. Nephrol Dial Transplant 1992; 7: 1035–8.

20. Cochran ST, Do HM, Ronaghi A, Nissenson AR, Kadell BM. Complications of peritoneal dialysis: evaluation with CT peritoneography. Radiographics 1997: 17: 869–78.

21. Ho-dac Pannekeet MM, Atasever B, Struijk DG, Krediet RT. Analysis of ultrafiltration failure in peritoneal dialysis patients by means of standard peritoneal permeability analysis. Perit Dial Int 1997; 17: 144–50.

22. Twardowski ZJ, Nolph K, Khanna R *et al.* Peritoneal equilibration test. Perit Dial Bull 1987; 7: 138–47.

23. Pannekeet MM, Imholz AL, Struijk DG *et al.* The standard peritoneal permeability analysis: a tool for the assessment of peritoneal permeability characteristics in CAPD patients. Kidney Int 1995; 48: 866–75.

24. Nolph KD, Twardowski ZJ, Popovich RP, Rubin J. Equilibration of peritoneal dialysis solutions during long-dwell exchanges. J Lab Clin Med 1979; 93: 246–56.

25. Chen TW, Khanna R, Moore H, Twardowski ZJ, Nolph KD. Sieving and reflection coefficients for sodium salts and glucose during peritoneal dialysis. J Am Soc Nephrol 1991; 2: 1092–100.

26. Waniewski J, Heimburger O, Werynski A, Lindholm B. Aqueous solute concentrations and evaluation of mass transport coefficients in peritoneal dialysis. Nephrol Dial Transplant 1992; 7: 50–6.

27. Zweers MM, Struijk DG, Krediet RT. Correcting sodium sieving for diffusion from circulation. Perit Dial Int 1999 (In press) (abstract).

28. Coles GA. Have we underestimated the importance of fluid balance for the survival of PD patients? Perit Dial Int 1997; 17: 321–6.

29. Kawaguchi Y, Hasegawa T, Nakayama M, Kubo H, Shigematu T. Issues affecting the longevity of the continuous peritoneal dialysis therapy. Kidney Int 1997; 52 (suppl. 62): S105–7.

30. Mactier R, Khanna R, Twardowski Z, Nolph K. Contribution of lymphatic absorption to loss of ultrafiltration and solute clearances in continuous ambulatory peritoneal dialysis. J Clin Invest 1987; 80: 1311–16.

31. Heimbürger O, Waniewski J, Werynski A, Sun Park M, Lindholm B. Lymphatic absorption in CAPD patients with loss of ultrafiltration capacity. Blood Purif 1995; 13: 327–39.

32. Abensur H, Romao J, Prado E, Kakehashi E, Sabbaga E, Marcondes M. Use of dextran 70 to estimate peritoneal lymphatic absorption rate in CAPD. Adv Perit Dial 1992; 8: 3–6.

33. Krediet RT, Struijk DG, Koomen GCM, Arisz L. Peritoneal fluid kinetics during CAPD measured with intraperitoneal dextran 70. ASAIO Trans 1991; 37: 662–7.

34. Selgas R, Bajo MA, Paiva A *et al.* Stability of the peritoneal membrane in long-term peritoneal dialysis patients. Adv Renal Repl Ther 1998; 5: 168–78.

35. Davies SJ, Phillips L, Russel GI. Peritoneal solute transport predicts survival on CAPD independently of residual renal function. Nephrol Dial Transplant 1998; 13: 962–8.

36. Churchill DN, Thorpe KE, Nolph KD, Keshaviah PR, Page D, Oreopoulos DG. Increased peritoneal transport is associated with decreased CAPD technique and patient survival. J Am Soc Nephrol 1997; 8: 189A.

37. Wang T, Heimbürger O, Waniewski J, Bergström J, Lindholm B. Increased peritoneal permeability is associated with decreased fluid and small-solute removal and higher mortality in CAPD patients. Nephrol Dial Transplant 1998; 13: 1242–9.

38. Panasiuk E, Pietrzak B, Klos M *et al.* Characteristics of peritoneum after peritonitis in peritonitis in CAPD patients. Adv Perit Dial 1988; 4: 42.

39. Krediet RT, Zuyderhoudt FMJ, Boeschoten EW, Arisz L. Alterations in the peritoneal transport of water and solutes during peritonitis in continuous ambulatory peritoneal dialysis patients. Eur J Clin Invest 1987; 17: 43–52.

40. Gotloib L, Shostak A, Bar-Shella P, Cohen R. Continuous mesothelial injury and regeneration during long-term peritoneal dialysis. Perit Dial Int 1987; 7: 148–55.

41. Hagmolen of ten Have W, Ho-dac-Pannekeet MM, Struijk DG, Krediet RT. Mesothelial regeneration after peritonitis in dialysis patients. J Am Soc Nephrol 1997; 180A.

42. Posthuma N, ter Weel PM, Donnker AJM, Peers EM, Oe PL, Vergrugh HA. Icodextrin use is CCPD patients during peritonitis: ultrafiltration and serum disaccharide concentrations. Nephrol Dial Transplant 1998; 13: 2341–4.

43. Krediet RT, Boeschoten EW, Zuyderhoudt FMJ, Arisz L. Peritoneal transport characteristics of water, low molecular weight solutes and proteins during long-term continuous ambulatory peritoneal dialysis. Perit Dial Bull 1986; 6: 61–5.
44. Krediet RT, Zemel D, Imholz ALT, Koomen GCM, Struijk DG, Arisz L. Indices of peritoneal permeability and surface area. Perit Dial Int 1993; 13 (suppl. 2): S31–4.
45. Krediet RT, Zemel D, Imholz ALT, Struijk DG. Impact of surface area and permeability on solute clearances. Perit Dial Int 1994; 14 (suppl. 3): S70–7.
46. Krediet RT. Prevention and treatment of peritoneal dialysis membrane failure. Adv Renal Repl Ther 1998; 5: 212.
47. Ho-dac-Pannekeet MM, Hiralall JK, Struijk DG, Krediet RT. Longitudinal follow-up of CA 125 in peritoneal effluent. Kidney Int 1997; 51: 888–93.
48. Wideroë FE, Smeby LC, Mjåland S, Dahl K, Berg KJ, Aas TW. Long-term changes in transperitoneal water transport during continuous ambulatory peritoneal dialysis. Nephron 1984; 38: 238–47.
49. Rottembourg J, Brouard R, Issad B et al. Role of acetate in loss of ultrafiltration during CAPD. Contrib Nephrol 1987; 57: 197.
50. Selgas R, Fernandez-Reyes MJ, Bosque E et al. Functional longevity of the human peritoneum: how long is continuous peritoneal dialysis possible? Results of a prospective medium long-term study. Am J Kidney Dis 1994; 23: 64–73.
51. Davies SJ, Bryan J, Phillips L Russel GI. Longitudinal changes in peritoneal kinetics: the effects of peritoneal dialysis and peritonitis. Nephrol Dial Transplant 1996; 11: 448–56.
52. Lamiere N, Vanholder R, Veys D et al. A longitudinal five year survey of urea kinetic parameters in CAPD patients. Kidney Int 1992; 42: 426–33.
53. Struijk DG, Krediet RT, Koomen GCM, Boeschoten EW, Hoek FJ, Arisz L. A prospective study of peritoneal transport in CAPD patients. Kidney Int 1994; 45: 1739–44.
54. Faller B, Lameire N. Evolution of clinical parameters and peritoneal function in a cohort of CAPD patients followed over 7 years. Nephrol Dial Transplant 1994; 9: 280–6
55. Monquil MC, Imholz AL, Struijk DJ, Krediet R. Does impaired transcellular water transport contribute to net ultrafiltration failure during CAPD? Perit Dial Int 1995; 15: 42–8.
56. Rippe B, Stelin G. Simulations of peritoneal solute transport during CAPD. Application of two pore formalism. Kidney Int 1989; 35: 1234–44.
57. Rippe B, Stelin G, Haraldsson B. Computer simulations of peritoneal transport in CAPD. Kidney Int 1991; 40: 315–25.
58. Rippe B, Simonsen O, Stelin G. Clinical implication of a three pore model of peritoneal transport. Adv Perit Dial 1991; 7: 3–9.
59. Rippe B, Krediet R. Peritoneal physiology – transport of solutes. In: Gokal R, Nolph KD, eds. The Textbook of Peritoneal Dialysis. Dordrecht: Kluwer, 1994, pp. 69–113.
60. Stelin G, Rippe B. A phenomenological interpretation of the variation in dialysate volume with dwell time in CAPD. Kidney Int 1990; 38: 465–72.
61. Vonesh EF, Rippe B. Net fluid absorption under membrane transport models of peritoneal dialysis. Blood Purif 1992; 10: 209–26.
62. Flessner MF. Peritoneal transport physiology: insights from basic research. J Am Soc Nephrol 1991; 2: 122–35.
63. Hasegawa H, Kamijo T, Takahashi H et al. Regulation and localisation of peritoneal aquaporins expression during long-term peritoneal dialysis in rats. J Am Soc Nephrol 1998; 9: 19A.
64. Yang B, Folfesson HG, Yang J, Ma T, Matthay MA, Verkman SA. Reduced osmotic water permeability of the peritoneal barrier in AQP1 knockout mice; AQP1 provides a 'water-only' pathway in peritoneal dialysis. J Am Soc Nephrol 1998; 9: 29A.

65. Carlsson O, Nielsen S, Zakaria ER, Rippe B. *In vivo* inhibition of transcellular water channels (Aquaporin-1) during acute peritoneal dialysis in rats. Am J Physiol 1996; 271: H2254–62.
66. Pannekeet MM, Mulder JB, Weening JJ, Struijk DG, Zweers MM, Krediet RT. Demonstrations of aquaporin-CHIP in peritoneal tissue of uremic and CAPD patients. Perit Dial Int 1995; 15 (suppl. 1): S54–7.
67. Ho-dac-Pannekeet MM, Krediet R. Water channels in the peritoneum. Perit Dial Int 1996; 16: 255–9.
68. Goffin E, Combet S, Jamar F, Cosyns J-P, Devuyst O. Expression of aquaporin-1 (AQP1) in a long-term peritoneal dialysis patient with impaired transcellular water transport. Am J Kidney Dis 1999 (In press).
69. Verger C, Celicout B. Peritoneal permeability and encapsulating peritonitis. Lancet 1985; 1: 986.
70. Krediet RT, Struijk DG, Boescheten EW et al. The time course of peritoneal transport kinetics in continuous ambulatory peritoneal dialysis patients who develop sclerosing peritonitis. Am J Kidney Dis 1989; 13: 299–307.
71. Hendriks PMEM, Ho-dac-Pannekeet MM, van Gulik TM et al. Peritoneal sclerosis in chronic peritoneal dialysis patients: analysis of clinical presentation, risk factors and peritoneal transport kinetics. Perit Dial Int 1997; 17: 136–43.
72. Campbell S, Clarke P, Hawley C, Wigan M, Kerlin P, Butler J, Wall D. Sclerosing peritonitis: identification of diagnostic, clinical and radiological features. Am J Kidney Dis 1994; 24: 819–25.
73. Schleifer C, Ziemek H, Teehan B, Benz R, Sigler M, Gilgore G. Migration of peritoneal catheters: personal experience and survey of 72 other units. Perit Dial Bull 1987; 7: 189–93.
74. Tzamaloukas A, Gibel L, Eisenberg B et al. Early and late peritoneal leaks in patients on CAPD. Adv Perit Dial 1990; 6: 64–71.
75. Twardowski ZJ, Tully R, Nichols W. Computerized tomography CT in the diagnosis of subcutaneous leak sites during continuous ambulatory peritoneal dialysis (CAPD). Perit Dial Bull 1984; 4: 163–6.
76. Schultz S, Harmon T, Nachtnebel K. Computerized tomographic scanning with intraperitoneal contrast enhancement in a CAPD patient with localized edema. Perit Dial Bull 1984; 4: 253–4.
77. Wankowicz Z, Pietrzak B, Przedlacki J. Colloid peritoneoscintigraphy in complications of CAPD. Adv Perit Dial 1988; 4: 138–43.
78. Kopecky R, Frymoyer P, Witanowski L, Thomas F, Wojtaszek J, Reinitz E. Prospective peritoneal scintigraphy in patients beginning continuous ambulatory peritoneal dialysis. Am J Kidney Dis 1990; 15: 228–36.
79. Fine A, Fontaine B, Ma M. Commonly prescribed salt intake in continuous ambulatory peritoneal dialysis is too restrictive: results of a double-blind crossover study. J Am Soc Nephrol 1997; 8: 1311–14.
80. Medcalfe JF, Harris KPG, Walls J. Frusemide increases urine volume but does not preserve residual renal function in patients on CAPD – results of a six months randomized controlled study. Perit Dial Int 1998; 18 (suppl. 2): S1.
81. Miranda B, Selgas R, Celadilla O et al. Peritoneal resting and heparinization as an effective treatment for ultrafiltration failure in patients on CAPD. Contrib Nephrol 1991; 89: 199.
82. De Alvaro F, Castro MJ, Dapena F et al. Peritoneal resting is beneficial in peritoneal hyperpermeability and ultrafiltration failure. Adv Perit Dial 1993; 9: 56–61.
83. Burkhart J, Stallard R. Result of peritoneal membrane (PM) resting (R) on dialysate (d) CA125 levels and PET results. Perit Dial Int 1997; 17 (suppl. 1): S5.
84. Ho-dac-Pannekeet MM, Struijk DG, Krediet R. Improvement of transcellular water transport by treatment with glucose free dialysate in patients with ultrafiltration failure. Nephrol Dial Transplant 1996; 11: 255.
85. Selgas R, Bajo MA, Del Peso G, Jiménez C. Preserving the peritoneal dialysis membrane in long-term peritoneal dialysis patients. Semin Dial 1995; 8: 326–32.

86. Krediet RT. Preserving the integrity of the peritoneal membrane in chronic peritoneal dialysis. Nephrology Forum. Kidney Int (In press).

87. Krediet R, Ho-dac-Pannekeet MM, Imholz AL, Struijk DG. Icodextrin's effects on peritoneal transport. Perit Dial Int 1997; 17: 35–41.

88. Rippe B, Zakaria ER, Carlsson O. Theoretical analysis of osmotic agents in peritoneal dialysis: what size is an ideal osmotic agent? Perit Dial Int 1996; 16 (suppl. 1): S97–103.

89. Mactier RA, Khanna R, Moore H, Twardowski ZJ, Nolph KD. Pharmacological reduction of lymphatic absorption from the peritoneal cavity increases net ultrafiltration and solute clearances in peritoneal dialysis. Nephron 1988; 50: 229–32.

90. Chan PCK, Tam SCF, Robinson JD *et al.* Effect of phosphatidylcholine on ultrafiltration in patients on continuous ambulatory peritoneal dialysis. Nephron 1991; 59: 100–3.

91. Mactier RA, Khanna R, Twardowski ZJ, Moore H, Nolph KD. Influence of phosphatidylcholine on lymphatic absorption during peritoneal dialysis in the rat. Perit Dial Int 1988; 8: 179–86.

92. Struijk DG, van der Reijden HJ, Krediet RT, Koomen GCM, Arisz L. Effect of phosphatidylcholine on peritoneal transport and lymphatic absorption in a CAPD patient with sclerosing peritonitis. Nephron 1989; 51: 577–8.

93. Baranowska-Daca E, Torneli J, Popovich RP, Moncrief JW. Use of bethanechol chloride to increase available ultrafiltration in CAPD. Adv Perit Dial 1995; 11: 69–72.

16 | Nutritional aspects of peritoneal dialysis

C. A. POLLOCK, B. A. COOPER, L. S. IBELS AND E. DE KANTZOW

Abstract

Maintaining the nutritional status of the patient is recognized as an important aspect of peritoneal dialysis therapy. Patients commencing dialytic therapy are at risk of malnutrition due to factors inherent in progressive renal failure including the metabolic and hormonal effects of uraemia, comorbid disease, the effects of drugs prescribed, and psychosocial factors associated with chronic disease. It has been estimated that up to two-thirds of patients on peritoneal dialysis may be malnourished, and this group has a higher risk of both morbidity and mortality. Several groups of patients appear to be a higher risk of complications of malnutrition, in particular the elderly and patients with renovascular disease, where the risk of vascular disease may be magnified. Once dialysis is commenced additional mechanisms which promote progressive malnutrition occur. In peritoneal dialysis these include inadequate dialysis, loss of protein and amino acids during dialysis, which may be more marked in patients with increased peritoneal permeability, and the catabolic efects of peritonitis. Glucose-based dialysate may displace other food sources and amplify abnormalities in carbohydrate metabolism. Bioincompatible dialysate and peritonitis may stimulate cytokine production and promote malnutrition. Nutritional adequacy is not easy to assess in peritoneal dialysis, largely due to dependence of traditional markers of nutrition on body water content, which varies in end-stage renal failure. Total body nitrogen (TBN) provides the most accurate means of measuring protein stores and has significant and predictable prognostic value. In the absence of access to measurement of TBN, several parameters should be considered in parallel to achieve an overall assessment of nutrition, as all other methods may be variably affected by the presence of renal failure, the mode and adequacy of dialysis delivery and fluid status at the time of assessment. Serum albumin is the visceral protein marker most well established as having important prognostic value and should be regularly assessed, but both its sensitivity and specificity in detecting nutritional impairment prior to severe malnutrition are poor. However, no single alternative serum protein measure confers improved sensitivity in detecting malnutrition in dialysis patients. Alternative measures of lean body mass, such as bioelectrical impedance and dual-energy X-ray absorptiometry when measured with an accurate determination of total body water may well prove to be useful, but as yet their prognostic usefulness is unclear. The subjective global assessment is a useful prognostic tool, but is not specific for nutritional adequacy and is likely to be significantly affected by comorbid illness. Nutritional supplementation in small studies with either oral, intravenous intradialytic parenteral nutrition or intraperitoneal amino acids has been shown to improve several nutritional markers, provided the profile of the supplemental solution is appropriate to the deficiencies observed in renal failure and adequate energy is concurrently supplied. However, the impact of improving nutrition in benefiting prognosis awaits confirmation.

Introduction

It is increasingly recognized that chronic renal failure is associated with a high incidence of malnutrition, which is due to factors inherent to a progressive loss of renal function, the underlying disease process and the treatment strategies employed in chronic renal failure (Table 1).

Many of these factors persist into end-stage renal failure, and additional challenges to nutritional adequacy are faced once dialysis is commenced. In peritoneal dialysis, malnutrition may manifest as protein malnutrition with low muscle mass and hypoproteinaemia; as energy malnutrition with a decrease in body weight, low fat mass and low carbohydrate

R. Gokal, R. Khanna, R.Th. Krediet and K.D. Nolph (eds.), Textbook of Peritoneal Dialysis, 2nd Edition, 515–543.

Table 1. Causes of malnutrition in chronic renal failure

Inadequate intake
Uraemic toxicity
Unpalatable or inadequate diet
Gastrointestinal illness
Comorbid disease
Polypharmacy
Psychosocial and socioeconomic factors

Excessive losses
Proteinuria

Increased catabolism
Primary disease
Endocrine disorders of uraemia
Drugs
Acidosis

---

stores; or most commonly, as combined protein–energy malnutrition. It is increasingly recognized that protein–energy malnutrition underlies many of the manifestations of the uraemic syndrome such as increased susceptibility to infection, impaired wound healing, poor rehabilitation, vascular disease and anaemia and, indeed, has a significant impact on prognosis once end-stage renal failure is reached. Continued emphasis on prevention of malnutrition in uraemia and in patients on dialysis is necessary, with the aims of both improving the quality of life and reducing the complications associated with end-stage renal failure.

The nutritional requirements which relate specifically to peritoneal dialysis form the focus of this chapter. As factors in the predialysis period also have significant effects on the dialytic phase of renal failure, these aspects will be explored, as will appropriate comparative studies with patients treated with haemodialysis. However, it should be borne in mind that comparisons between patients on peritoneal dialysis and haemodialysis may not always be valid, even using the same methods of assessment, due to differences in the patients selected for each treatment modality, and differences in biochemical parameters and steady-state fluid balance. To date no prospective study has compared nutritional status in patients randomized to receive either haemodialysis or peritoneal dialysis. The majority of studies concerning nutrition in peritoneal dialysis have related to patients on continuous ambulatory peritoneal dialysis, and few have been performed in adult patients using automated peritoneal dialysis. Hence, unless otherwise specified, the studies discussed here concern patients on continuous ambulatory peritoneal dialysis (CAPD).

Malnutrition in chronic renal failure

As renal dysfunction progresses, and endogenous renal clearances fall, protein intake is reduced and the patient's nutrient intake needs to be closely monitored [1–3]. This reduction is independent of dietary advice [1] and has been shown to be in the order of 0.06 g of protein/kg body weight/day for each reduction of 10 ml/min in glomerular filtration [3]. Indeed, at the time of enrolment into end-stage renal failure programmes, in the absence of prescribed guidelines as to the stage at which dialysis should be commenced, patients are uniformly ingesting a diet which predictably results in a negative nitrogen balance, and this fails to increase within 3 months of the commencement of CAPD [1]. The observation that malnutrition is more common in the early stages of dialysis [1, 4, 5], and the correlation observed with nutrition at the commencement of dialysis and the nutritional state 2 years later [6], suggests that an increased effort to improve the patient's nutritional state prior to commencement of dialysis will decrease the malnutrition observed once end-stage renal failure is reached, and ultimately result in an improved outcome.

Well-defined abnormalities occur in protein and energy utilization in chronic renal failure. There is no evidence that patients with chronic renal failure have a reduced protein requirement compared with that of the normal population, and indeed, the additional catabolic stresses that are present in renal failure (discussed below) would suggest that protein requirements may be higher. The recommended daily protein intake for the normal population was revised upwards from 0.6 to 0.76 g/kg per day in 1984 [7], as it was recognized that healthy subjects may be in a negative nitrogen balance when protein intake is less than this amount. In chronic renal failure the adaptive mechanisms which maintain nitrogen balance are similar to those which exist in the normal population [8]. However, in the presence of additional 'metabolic challenges' such as acidosis, or coexistent catabolic processes, or indeed if the protein intake falls below 0.6 g/kg body weight per day, then a negative nitrogen balance ensues.

Because of the undoubted high morbidity and mortality associated with commencing dialysis in a malnourished state, the benefits of a low protein diet in ameliorating uraemic symptoms and retarding the progression of renal failure need to outweigh the risks of malnutrition. Although low protein diets are commonly prescribed to prolong endogenous renal function [9] and to reduce the uraemic symptoms which develop with progressive renal failure, these studies have not been extended to examine the prognosis of these patients who have commenced dialysis later by virtue of dietary restrictions. Our own studies [1], in which 52 patients were assessed prior to the commencement of dialysis, demonstrated a protein intake that was spontaneously lower than the recommended dietary protein intake in the normal Australian population. This failed to increase within 3 months of the commencement of dialysis, despite concerted efforts by trained dietitians. Increased blood sugar, cholesterol and triglyceride levels were observed in patients consuming a low protein diet, which were likely to be secondary to a proportionate increase in carbohydrate and fat intake. Hence the adverse metabolic effects in this population, already at risk of cardiovascular complications, in addition to the inability to adjust dietary habits to accommodate the catabolic effects of dialysis, may be an unrecognized detrimental effect of a long-term low protein diet. Careful monitoring of the nutritional state is therefore mandatory in patients as they progress to renal failure. Because of the controversy regarding the benefits of protein restriction in renal impairment, a recent workshop convened to develop management recommendations for the prevention of chronic renal disease [10] concluded that 'the evidence that prescription of a low protein diet slows the progression of renal disease is inconclusive'. Present recommendations are that a standard protein intake should be advised, but if progressive renal impairment or uraemic symptoms occur, a reduction to 0.8 g/kg per day should be instituted.

Several groups of patients appear to be at higher risk of complications of malnutrition, in particular the elderly and patients with renovascular disease. Increasing age has been demonstrated to have an adverse effect on many nutritional markers, which is reflected in the decrease in muscle mass with ageing. Many factors may contribute to this, including comorbid illnesses and the effects of drugs needed to treat these illnesses – depression, lack of access to food due to difficulties in shopping, or food prices, and inanition or inability to cook [11]. Piccoli *et al.* [12] have demonstrated an association between advancing age and poor nutrition, and both this study and our own investigations [13] have demonstrated the striking association between vascular disease and poor nutrition. Ritz *et al.* [14] have hypothesized that the increased vascular risk in malnourished patients is due to a deficiency of

L-arginine, with a resultant decrease in nitric oxide synthase causing local vasoconstriction and hypertension.

Patients with diabetes mellitus entering end-stage renal failure programmes in increasing numbers, may be at particular risk due to concomitant dietary limitations and the presence of coexistent pathology, such as gastroparesis, which limits nutrient intake. Patients commencing dialysis after prolonged therapy with corticosteroids, such as failed allograft recipients, would be predicted to begin treatment with diminished protein stores and hence to tolerate the catabolic stresses of dialysis poorly. However, no study to date has addressed this issue.

Magnitude of the problem

Both cross-sectional and longitudinal studies suggest that up to two-thirds of patients on haemodialysis and continuous ambulatory peritoneal dialysis [4, 13, 15–26] are malnourished. In many patients, particularly on CAPD, malnutrition may occur in spite of the frequent presence of marked obesity. Recent large-scale prevalence data from the CANUSA study [27] showed 55% of the 680 patients as having some degree of malnutrition, while 4.2% were considered severely malnourished as determined by serum albumin and subjective global assessment. Similarly, the 1996 Peritoneal Dialysis Core Indicators study [28] showed that 47% of peritoneal dialysis patients had an albumin below 35 g/L and 70% had an estimated protein intake of less than 1 g/kg body weight per day. This occurred despite a tendency to obesity in the population as a whole.

In a large Italian multicentre study of 487 patients [24] malnutrition, as determined by blood protein estimation, anthropometry and a modified subjective global assessment, was present to some extent in 42% of CAPD patients and 31% of haemodialysis patients. Within the CAPD group, serum proteins, including albumin, were low, although anthropometric measurements did not confirm a loss of somatic protein. In this study the subjective global assessment was felt to correlate with visceral and somatic protein measures, body fat stores and energy intake.

Marckmann [22] assessed 16 CAPD patients, again using multiple parameters to arrive at a single assessment of nutrition, including the objective markers of body weight, mid-arm muscle circumference, triceps skinfold thickness and serum transferrin. This study classified 19% of patients as having protein–calorie malnutrition and 37% severe malnutrition. Nelson *et al.* [23] demonstrated that the mid-arm muscle circumference was below the 25th centile for sex-, age- and race-matched individuals in 59% of 138 CAPD patients.

Prognostic implications of malnutrition

Malnutrition is clearly associated with a substantial increase in morbidity and mortality in patients with end-stage renal failure [13, 15, 16, 29–31]. The gold standard measure of body protein stores, total body nitrogen, strongly predicts mortality in end-stage renal failure. In a longitudinal study of 154 patients on maintenance dialysis (76 on CAPD), we observed that the patients who died had a lower total body nitrogen than those who survived [13]. The probability of death within 12 months in the patients with a nitrogen index (ratio of the measured nitrogen to the predicted nitrogen for a sex-, age-, and height-matched control) less than 80% of the predicted normal value was 48%. The relative risk of death in this population was 4.1.

Other studies have documented an association between a decrease in serum albumin and a poor prognosis in patients on CAPD [13, 31–33]. Teehan *et al.* [32], in a longitudinal 5-year study of CAPD patients, reported that a low serum albumin level was a better predictor of mortality than kinetic studies. Avram *et al.* [31] reported that CAPD patients with a serum albumin concentration <3.2 g/dl had only a 30% 2-year survival. In a subsequent study of 169 patients followed up to 60 months, the nutritional markers of serum albumin and creatinine were predictive of mortality for up to 5 years [34]. Spiegel and Breyer [33] have also demonstrated that serum albumin in CAPD patients is a powerful predictor of short-term morbidity and long-term mortality. However, the mean serum albumin in the patients who died was extremely low at 27 ± 0.7 g/dl and it is therefore unlikely that they would not have been recognized as being malnourished or at risk from comorbid conditions on clinical grounds. The serum albumin may nevertheless be normal despite significant reductions in total body nitrogen stores, and is thus a late marker of malnutrition [13]. The relative value of serum albumin as the sole marker of nutrition is discussed below.

Malnutrition also has a substantial impact on morbidity. In our own studies we [35] observed significant associations between more numerous hospital admissions and lower normalized protein catabolic rates, serum albumin and total protein levels, between the duration of periods in hospital and lower serum albumin and total protein levels, and between more frequent episodes of infection and reduced total body nitrogen levels.

Factors contributing to malnutrition in peritoneal dialysis

Once dialysis is commenced a number of additional mechanisms promote progressive malnutrition in both peritoneal dialysis and haemodialysis [36]. Collectively, these mechanisms include anorexia, inadequate dialysis, loss of amino acids, protein and other nutrients during the dialysis procedure, acidosis, progressive endocrine abnormalities and the activation of cellular catabolic pathways, frequent blood-letting, the catabolic effects of the dialysis membrane in haemodialysis, and the displacement of other energy sources by glucose in peritoneal dialysis. Although severe malnutrition is easily recognized, it is of more importance to identify milder forms of poor nutrition in order to prevent the progression to a more severe nutritional disorder.

Carbohydrate metabolism

Uraemia is associated with universal abnormalities in carbohydrate metabolism as a result of hyperinsulinaemia caused by decreased degradation of insulin by functional renal tissue, and insulin resistance due to both post-receptor defects [37] and hormonal factors which impair glucose disposal. Intolerance to a glucose load may be further exacerbated by an inability to regulate insulin secretion from pancreatic beta cells induced by hyperparathyroidism and decreased action of 1,25-hydroxyvitamin D [38].

In CAPD, due to the continuous glucose load associated with glucose-based dialysate, the abnormalities in carbohydrate metabolism are amplified. Up to 20% of the carbohydrate intake comes from the peritoneal absorption of glucose [39], resulting in persistent hyperinsulinaemia, which is reflected by increased C-peptide levels. This constant energy source leads to obesity, but paradoxically may exacerbate malnutrition in some patients, due to a reduction in appetite, and specifically in protein intake. Further abnormalities in nutrient utilization occur as a consequence of derangements in carbohydrate metabolism, including reduced gluconeogenesis and ketogenesis and inhibition of lipolysis, whereas elevations in glucagon, alanine and lactate concentrations persist [40]. Improved insulin sensitivity has been observed in patients on cycled peritoneal dialysis compared to haemodialysis, but this has not translated into a beneficial effect on nutritional status as assessed by serum albumin and anthropometric measurements after 3 months [41]. In patients with high peritoneal transport rates the worsening malnutrition observed may be at least partly induced by excessive peritoneal glucose absorption.

Protein and amino acid metabolism

The substantial losses of protein (5–15 g/24 h) from the peritoneal cavity contribute to the negative nitrogen balance often observed in peritoneal dialysis [39]. These losses increase substantially in peritonitis, resulting in a vicious cycle of worsening malnutrition and an attendant increase in susceptibility to infection. Nutrient intake is often concurrently reduced, further exacerbating the negative nitrogen balance.

Serum amino acid profiles are similar in patients on CAPD and haemodialysis [42–44]. In general, plasma essential amino acid levels are low and nonessential amino acid concentrations are normal or increased, in a pattern similar to that seen in protein–calorie malnutrition, except that in this instance intake is normal. Plasma amino acid levels reflect more recent nutritional intake rather than the nutritional steady state, and in chronic renal failure do not reflect intracellular amino acid levels [44]. Decreases in the serum of essential amino acids with decreased ratios of valine to glycine, and tyrosine to phenylalanine are observed. Up to 3.4 g of amino acid are lost in the dialysate in patients on CAPD [45]. Substantial increases in plasma levels of N- and O-carbamoylated amino acids which may inhibit protein synthesis have also been reported in CAPD [46].

The specific combinations of *intracellular amino acids* have been shown in biostatistical analyses to predict the levels of cell biosynthesis, such as protein synthesis and energy, in health and disease [47]. The abnormalities observed in chronic renal failure lead to functional defects in protein and energy metabolism that constitute cellular malnutrition. Specific intracellular deficiencies occur in the essential branched-chain amino acids valine, isoleucine and leucine, as well as in methionine [48]. In CAPD the muscle amino acid profiles reflect the abnormal serum amino acid profile, with reduced tyrosine and taurine and increased lysine, asparagine, aspartic acid, glutamine and citrulline [49].

Acidosis

It has become increasingly evident that metabolic acidosis accelerates the malnutrition associated with a reduced dietary intake in chronic renal failure. Both *in vitro* and *in vivo* animal studies have shown that acidosis promotes malnutrition via the dual mechanisms of increased muscle degradation, by up-regulating enzymes involved in these catabolic pathways and a reduction in the ability to limit oxidation of essential amino acids [50–52]. Cellular mechanisms promoting protein catabolism include activation of lysosomal and calcium-activated proteases and energy-requiring pathways, specifically the ATP-ubiquitin-proteasome proteolytic and branched-chain ketoacid dehydrogenase pathways. In patients with chronic renal failure and a mean serum bicarbonate of 15 mmol/L, correction of acidosis has been shown to result in a reduction of protein catabolism by 28–30% [53]. Furthermore, as acidosis decreases albumin synthesis [54], it may be directly or indirectly related to the increased mortality in chronic renal failure that is associated with a low serum albumin.

Recently, Graham *et al.* [55] have shown that correction of acidosis in CAPD decreases protein degradation and synthesis, but has no effect on leucine oxidation, which is regarded as a measure of whole-body protein metabolism. Indeed, correction of acidosis in these CAPD patients does not alter the plasma amino acid profile, except for a fall in methylhistidine levels, which has been shown to be a valid marker for skeletal breakdown in humans [56]. It is possible that the dialysis procedure alters muscle branched-chain amino acid metabolism by blunting branched-chain ketoacid dehydrogenase activity, resulting in normal leucine oxidation in both CAPD and haemodialysis patients when compared to normal controls [55, 57]. Following correction of acidosis there is a fall in plasma urea consistent with a reduction in protein degradation [55]. Stein *et al.* [58] found in a randomized controlled trial that CAPD patients using a high alkali dialysate (40 mmol/L lactate) had a greater increase in anthropometric measurements in comparison to patients treated with a low alkali dialysate (35 mmol/L). Similar improvements in anthropometric measurements occur in haemodialysis patients when dialysate bicarbonate is increased from 30 to 40 mmol/L, which revert when a low dialysate bicarbonate is reinstituted [59].

Although normalization of systemic acidosis is likely to be associated with improved protein utilization, a higher protein intake is associated with a higher acid load, and increased dialysis is likely to be necessary to maintain a normal serum bicarbonate [60].

Recent recommendations suggest that in the predialysis stage the optimal serum bicarbonate level is > 21 mmol/L, and after commencement of CAPD this should be increased to 24 mmol/L.

Adequacy of dialysis

It has been well demonstrated that an adequate nutrient intake is dependent on adequate dialysis and both these factors affect prognosis [27, 32, 35, 61–64], although their net effect is not uniform [65]. The CANUSA study demonstrated that an increase in the clearance of creatinine in the CAPD population from 40 to 95 litres per week is associated with an increase in 2-year patient survival from 65% to 86% [27]. Similarly, Blake *et al.* [66] showed that the death rate increased if the creatinine clearance measured less than 48 L/week. More controversial issues relate to whether the adequacy of dialysis, determined by Kt/V, and the protein intake, determined from total nitrogen appearance, are mathematically or physiologically related [67–70], and whether continued residual renal function confers a benefit on nutritional status independent of total clearance achieved.

It is clear from studies which use measures of dialytic and renal clearance and/or nutritional state independent of urea kinetic modelling, that a relationship between total clearance and protein intake exists [1]. Although these studies are not confounded by the interdependence of measured urea output in each parameter, they remain co-dependent on the urine and dialysate volume. In the CANUSA study [27], creatinine clearance correlated positively with protein intake; however, these effects could not be dissociated from the effects of a higher residual renal function. An increase in protein intake, determined by the normalized protein catabolic rate, or an increase in dialysis delivery, measured as Kt/V, does not uniformly result in an increase in serum albumin [25, 70, 71]. It has been found that in the Asian population a Kt/V lower than that currently recommended in Caucasians has no negative impact on prognosis [72], although data are unavailable on the nutritional status of this group. In particular, no measure of protein intake in these patients relative to the control population, who would be expected to have a protein intake lower than their Caucasian counterparts, is available.

The interdependence of protein intake and Kt/V when both are derived from measured urea losses is less conclusive. Certainly cross-sectional studies demonstrate a close correlation between the two indices [70], but this does not confirm a biological relationship. Longitudinal studies in which Kt/V is increased and a higher steady-state PNA is reached confirm that a measured change in nitrogen balance is achieved [73–75]. Additional observations, such as the non-linear correlation between Kt/V and protein catabolic rate and the differing values for protein catabolic rate with the same measured Kt/V when different membranes are used, support the use of kinetically derived markers of dialytic adequacy and protein intake as independent prognostic variables. A recent study in which solute clearances were increased by means of increasing dialysate drainage volumes did not result in any increase in protein intake or serum albumin [76]. Two other studies, attempting to increase dialysis dose, showed no impact on DNA or serum albumin [77, 78]. Indeed, it is has not yet been shown in appropriate clinical trials that increasing the dialysis dose can in itself improve nutritional state and positively influence outcome.

Residual renal function

The importance of maintaining residual renal function is increasingly appreciated as much in the dialysis population as in patients with chronic renal dysfunction. Data from several sources [1, 2, 27, 35, 79] suggest that a lesser degree of residual renal function at the initiation of dialysis is associated with a poorer nutritional state, and results in poorer patient survival. In the multicentre study of Young *et al.* [21], there was a marked difference in residual renal function between patients regarded as well-nourished versus those who were malnourished. In 43 stable patients on CAPD [80] the protein intake, estimated as the normalized protein catabolic rate (nPCR), correlated with total weekly clearances of creatinine and residual renal function. All patients with residual renal function contributing more than 40 L/week had a nPCR of greater than 1.0 g/kg per day. Residual renal function therefore contributes significantly to the maintenance of adequate nutrition in CAPD. Confounding issues exist in these retrospective analyses, and a prospective assessment of nutritional state and prognosis in patients commencing dialysis at an earlier stage in evolution of renal failure is necessary. It is interesting to note that, in the prospective study by Harty *et al.* [76], the dietary protein intake declined in keeping the declining residual function. There is evidence that residual renal function is maintained in patients on CAPD to a greater extent than in haemodialysis [81, 82], and this has been considered to confer a nutritional advantage. It has been suggested that increased dialysate volumes, which are now more frequently prescribed to maintain dialytic clearances, may result in accelerated loss of residual renal function and impair the nutritional state of the patient. These observations, however, are not yet supported by clinical data.

Peritoneal permeability and nutrition

An increase in peritoneal permeability, which is estimated to be present in up to 15% of patients at the start of dialysis, has been associated with an increase in peritoneal protein loss and a low serum albumin [64, 83], and therefore has been implicated in the development of malnutrition in CAPD [84, 85]. It is not known whether patients who commence dialysis with a highly permeable membrane have a different prognosis in comparison to those who develop an increase in peritoneal permeability during dialysis. It has been suggested that the poor ultrafiltration typically observed in patients with high transport rates is associated with more frequent use of hypertonic dialysate, with a resultant increase in glucose absorption and suppression of appetite, all of which factors would amplify a nutritional deficit. Diabetics tend to have increased peritoneal permeability, and this may contribute to the lower albumin observed in this population. However, concurrent comorbid states, including diabetes mellitus, have a more significant impact on serum albumin and outcome than does the presence of an increase in peritoneal membrane permeability [86, 87]. Consistent with this is the observation that, although patients with rapid transport have a lower serum albumin, other markers of nutrition in this group are not necessarily indicative of a malnourished state [88]. This suggests a dissociation between the prognostic value of a low albumin concentration due to excessive dialysate losses and a low albumin due to malnutrition. This is not surprising given that the kinetics of albumin synthesis and catabolism are markedly different in the two circumstances (reviewed in ref. 89).

Hormones and cytokines

In the haemodialysis population, high predialysis serum cortisol has been associated with both an increased rate of hospitalization, and the presence of markers suggestive of a catabolic state [90]. A low T3 has been reported in malnutrition in dialysis, but this may well represent a compensatory response and have protective effects in limiting protein catabolism in chronic renal failure [91]. Similar hormonal disturbances are likely to be inherent in end-stage renal failure and to extend to the CAPD population, rather than being specific to the haemodialysis population.

More recently, interest has increased in the insulin-like growth factor-1 (IGF-1) and growth hormone axis. It is well known that IGF-1 is the major mediator of the anabolic effects of growth hormone [92]. IGF-1 levels are generally normal in renal failure, but there are marked abnormalities in the growth hormone-IGF-1 axis, with associated abnormalities in IGF–1 pharmacokinetics [93, 94]. However, some studies have reported an association between low serum IGF-1 and malnutrition [19, 95]. The lack of a tight relationship between IGF-1 and malnutrition is due to two factors: first a resistance to the action of both growth hormone and IGF-1, and second, the close dependence of the action of IGF-1 on IGF binding proteins (IGFBP), which is likely to be altered in uraemia [96]. Studies in children on peritoneal dialysis suggest that the most important IGF-binding protein in modulating IGF actions in uraemia is the 29 kDa fragment of IGFBP-3 [97].

The interrelationship between acidosis, malnutrition and IGF-1 is of interest as the presence of acidosis is likely further to reduce the anabolic effects of IGF-1 in chronic renal impairment. In uraemia, reductions in hepatic growth hormone receptor and IGF-1 mRNA expression occur, which are reproduced by metabolic acidosis [98–100].

The relationship of elevated cytokines to the development of malnutrition in renal failure is an area of active study. Peritoneal dialysate which is bioincompatible is more likely to stimulate cytokine production from peritoneal mesothelial cells, as well as through the activation of monocytes and neutrophils, which contributes to increased catabolism in CAPD [101]. Peritonitis is likely to cause a further increase in peritoneal cytokine production, with production of prostaglandins, proteoglycans, growth factors, monocyte chemoattractant protein-1 (MCP-1), interleukin-1, -4, -5, -6 and -8, and tumour necrosis factor (TNF) [102, 103]. Interleukins-1 and -6 and tumour necrosis factor are known to suppress caloric intake and are elevated in chronic renal failure. The additional contribution of comorbid disease and renal failure to cytokine elevation is as yet undetermined. Recently Bergstrom and Lindholm [104] have hypothesized that cardiac failure may cause malnutrition, and that infection/inflammation may predispose to atherosclerosis as well as catabolism and hypoalbuminaemia. Proinflammatory cytokines (IL-1, IL-6, TNF) appear to play a pivotal role by causing muscle wasting, hypoalbuminaemia and anorexia, as well as reduced cardiac contractility and atherosclerotic vascular disease. Malnutrition rarely may be the direct cause of death, but may contribute to a poor prognosis by aggravating pre-existing heart failure and increasing the susceptibility to infections. In support of this is a recent report by Stenvinkel *et al.* [105] in advanced chronic renal failure. They assessed the cross-sectional carotid intima-media area and carotid plaques in 109 predialysis patients. They found that rapidly developing atherosclerosis is caused by a synergism of different mechanisms such as malnutrition, inflammation, oxidative stress and genetic components. Apart from the classical risk factors, low vitamin E levels and elevated C-reactive protein (CRP) levels were associated with increased carotid intima-media area.

Comorbid illness

The association between malnutrition and a poor prognosis is not necessarily causative, as many comorbid conditions present in the dialysis population are likely to cause malnutrition independent of renal failure [106]. Thus the presence of malnutrition may be a marker of illness rather than the direct cause of subsequent morbidity. The presence of comorbid disease has been found to be an independent risk factor for both poor nutrition and poor outcome in CAPD, and for mortality in haemodialysis and CAPD patients [27, 87, 107, 108]. In particular, vascular disease and left ventricular dysfunction profoundly affect prognosis and have been associated with a poor nutritional state [35, 109]. Comorbidity is strongly associated with an older age, and with poorer nutrition as indicated by a lower dietary protein and caloric intake and a lower plasma creatinine level independent of the dialytic dose.

Bergstrom *et al.* [110] have demonstrated, using a Cox proportional hazard model, that an increase in CRP is an independent predictor of survival, whereas serum albumin lost its significance as a survival factor when corrected for CRP. Serum albumin was inversely correlated with CRP, suggesting that comorbid illnesses (inflammation, infection,

tissue injury) which increase CRP may lower serum albumin. The relationships between an elevation in CRP, infection or inflammation and a low serum albumin have more recently been confirmed by several groups [111–113].

The CANUSA study [27], which is discussed in detail elsewhere, similarly demonstrated that the presence of comorbidity has a stronger impact on prognosis than do the nutritional markers.

CAPD compared to haemodialysis: nutritional considerations

As has already been stated, the tools used to identify patients who are malnourished are different in each dialysis population. There are inherent differences in the selection of patients for each mode of therapy, the adequacy of dialysis delivery and the degree of residual renal function, and most studies have been neither prospective nor adequately controlled. As a result of these factors a nutritional advantage of one form of dialysis over another remains to be properly assessed. Although peritoneal dialysis has been reported to have a lower adjusted mortality rate relative to haemodialysis (relative risk 0.73), similar problems exist with comparative studies on treatment modality and mortality [114]. With these caveats in mind it has been reported that CAPD confers a nutritional advantage over haemodialysis. It has been speculated that this advantage of CAPD may be due to a number of factors including control of acidosis, reduced protein turnover, maintenance of residual renal function, the absence of the catabolic effects of a bioincompatible membrane and a stable blood urea concentration [13]. The peak concentration hypothesis [115] suggests that appetite suppression in haemodialysis patients is due to the peak toxin level just prior to dialysis therapy. Thus, although the time-averaged urea concentration (TAC_{urea}) may be similar in haemodialysis and CAPD, appetite is better maintained in CAPD.

Despite the factors which may positively influence nutrition in the CAPD population, there are additional catabolic stresses specific to the treatment modality. Peritoneal protein losses range between 8 and 10 g/day and amino acid losses between 3 and 4 g/day. Although serum albumin may be lower in the patients with higher peritoneal protein loss, this is not uniformly the case; hence these losses may not necessarily be implicated in the development of malnutrition [116]. Constant glucose absorption, which has been estimated to be as much as 16–22% of the total caloric intake [13, 117, 118], has been reported to displace other caloric sources and to limit protein intake, while still maintaining energy intake. However, peritoneal glucose absorption has been also shown to be an important energy source which contributes to nutritional well-being [119]. Importantly, we have shown it to be as important as protein intake in determining nutritional state [13]. Goodship *et al.* [120], using whole-body leucine turnover, showed that the balance between protein synthesis and breakdown was significantly higher in CAPD patients compared to uraemic subjects. Berkelhammer *et al.* [121] have performed similar studies in HD patients and reported that, although protein breakdown was similar to that in controls, rates of protein synthesis were lower and protein oxidation rates in the post-absorptive state were higher. Hence these differences in protein synthetic/ catabolic rates may further explain the differences observed in CAPD versus haemodialysis patients.

The balance of the competing influences on nutrition in end-stage renal failure appears to favour CAPD over haemodialysis. We have demonstrated that nutrition is relatively better maintained, and that anabolism is possible in CAPD compared to haemodialysis [13]. Fenton *et al.* [4] assessed 118 CAPD patients on three occasions. In the 24 patients on CAPD for less than 3 months, 42% were malnourished; conversely, 18% of patients on CAPD for greater than 3 months were regarded as being malnourished, suggesting that overall CAPD improves nutrition in malnourished patients commencing dialysis. The Toronto group found, in contrast, a decline in total-body nitrogen during the first year on CAPD [122], the difference perhaps being attributed to the improvement in CAPD techniques during the time interval between the individual studies.

Lipid metabolism in CAPD

Cardiovascular disease is the leading cause of death in patients with end-stage renal disease on both HD and CAPD [117, 118, 123]. Although the atherogenic lipid disturbances that accompany uraemia are likely to be primarily involved, the cause of the high incidence of vascular disease is clearly multifactorial. These factors include elevated total cholesterol and triglyceride concentrations, low levels of high-density lipoprotein cholesterol (HDLC), raised cholesterol to HDLC ratios as well as increased levels of

intermediate particles (due, in part to impaired lipoprotein lipase activity). In addition, impairment of 'reverse' cholesterol transport from cell is due in part to low levels of HDL and of lecithin cholesterol acyl transferase activity, low apolipoprotein (apo) A-1 to apo B ratios, and raised lipoprotein (a) concentrations [39, 124–130].

Increased serum cholesterol and triglyceride concentrations are seen within 6 months of commencement of CAPD [39, 125, 128, 131] and it has been postulated that at least part of the observed initial increase in serum lipids could occur as a consequence of correction of the malnutrition which accompanies end-stage renal failure.

Compared to patients on maintenance haemodialysis, CAPD patients have more atherogenic serum lipid profiles with higher serum cholesterol, LDLC and apo B concentrations, higher cholesterol to HDLC ratios, and lower apo A-1 to apo B ratios, in most [124, 126, 129, 130], but not all studies [132]. HDLC concentrations, however, may be higher in CAPD patients [130, 133].

Correlations have been observed between lipid disturbances in dialysis patients and manifest vascular disease [1]. On the other hand, overall mortality has been reported by Avram *et al.* [8] to be greater in patients with lower cholesterol and apo B concentrations and higher apo A–1 to apo B ratios, which is likely to represent the increased mortality associated with malnutrition. In this study, positive correlations were found between serum albumin concentrations and both total cholesterol and apo B, which may reflect the adverse effects of malnutrition on the synthesis of visceral proteins such as albumin and lipoproteins [126]. Patients on CAPD with elevations in lipoprotein (a) and fibrinogen have been shown to have an increased prevalence of coronary artery disease, increased lipoprotein (a) levels being more likely to occur in patients with low molecular weight apo (a) isoforms [134].

Some [125], but not all [127], studies have reported correlations between glucose absorption from the peritoneum and the levels of total cholesterol, LDLC, triglycerides and very low-density lipoprotein (VLDL) cholesterol and triglycerides in CAPD patients. Low HDLC levels may be partly due to peritoneal losses of HDL [84, 127]. The ratio of peritoneal clearance of apolipoprotein A-1/clearance of apolipoprotein B, a measure of relative loss of protective factors into the peritoneal effluent, may be a novel atherogenic risk measure in patients maintained on CAPD [131]. A more atherogenic plasma lipid profile has been seen in patients with high peritoneal transport characteristics [84], which may reflect either increased glucose absorption or increased peritoneal protein loss [127].

Mineral and trace elements: considerations in peritoneal dialysis and supplemental recommendations

Due to the continuous nature of peritoneal dialysis, dietary restriction of fluids, electrolytes and minerals is less stringent in CAPD compared to intermittent therapies (Table 2).

Minerals

A diet with 'no added salt' is recommended due to the frequent coexistence of hypertension and vascular disease. Potassium restriction is rarely required, but serum potassium should be measured and if necessary dietary modifications made. Potassium intake correlates with protein intake, and if it is necessary to increase the protein intake beyond 1.2 g/kg per day, a positive potassium balance will occur [45].

Table 2. Mineral, vitamin and trace element recommended intakes in peritoneal dialysis

Nutrient	Recommended intake
Protein	1.2–1.5 g/kg ideal body weight/day
Energy	>35 kcal/ideal body weight/day
Fat	Low fat diet (up to 30% of calories): mono- and polyunsaturated fats encouraged
Sodium	80–100 mmol/day
Potassium	Usually no restriction of a moderate intake
Phosphorus	1000–2000 mmol/day (+phosphate binders)
Calcium	Individualized (usually no less than 1000 mg/day)
Magnesium	200–300 mg/day (may be individualized if used as a phosphate binder)
Iron	Individualized (depending on EPO use)
Zinc	15 mg/day
Fluid	0.8–1.5 L (depending on fluid balance)
Vitamins*	
B$_1$	1.5 mg/day
B$_2$	1.7 mg/day
B$_6$	10 mg/day
B$_{12}$	6 µg/day
C	60 mg/day
Niacin	20 mg/day
Pantoethenate	10 mg/day
Biotin	300 µg/day
Folic acid	1 mg/day
D	Individualized dose (see text)

*Other fat-soluble vitamins not routinely recommended.

Magnesium levels are generally normal in CAPD, but again correlate with protein intake. The use of magnesium-containing phosphate binders may increase serum magnesium levels, which should then be routinely monitored in such patients.

Calcium and phosphate metabolism and their interrelationship between vitamin D and parathyroid hormone are discussed elsewhere in this book. However, the extent of the effects on nutritional parameters of hyperparathyroidism, and deficiency of and resistance to vitamin D, deserves emphasis. Hyperparathyroidism, like dysregulation of vitamin D, is associated with abnormalities in skeletal turnover, anaemia and immune deficiencies, as well as disturbances in insulin secretion [135, 136]. In addition, it impairs both skeletal muscle fatty acid oxidation [137] and protein catabolism [136], while vitamin D deficiency is associated with muscle atrophy [135]. Clearly, the development of hyperparathyroidism and altered vitamin D metabolism in chronic renal failure both contributes to and exacerbates the nutritional abnormalities observed. CAPD has been reported to ameliorate some aspects of disordered calcium and phosphate homeostasis; hence it has been postulated that an improvement in nutrition observed in CAPD is due to its beneficial effects on these parameters, and secondarily on hyperparathyroidism and vitamin D metabolism. The more liberal use of vitamin D and its analogues in CAPD has clearly had additional nutritional benefits in CAPD.

The recommended intake of calcium varies, depending on the prevailing calcium and phosphate homeostasis and the calcium concentration in the dialysate. A minimum daily requirement of 1000 mg is advocated, but clearly this is modified by concurrent necessity for phosphate-binding therapy, the presence of hyperparathyroidism and requirement for vitamin D therapy. A lower dialysate calcium may allow greater use of calcium-containing oral phosphate binders, which can be advantageous in some patients.

Iron deficiency is increasingly encountered in patients on CAPD due to the high prevalence of patients on erythropoietin and the associated increased iron requirement which is common to all dialysis patients. The preferred method of iron delivery varies between dialysis units, the recent recommendation of the Dialysis Outcome and Quality Initiative (DOQI) being for intravenous iron administration as the optimal means of maintaining sufficient iron stores to achieve a target haemoglobin level.

Elevations in serum aluminium remain the most widely recognized perturbation in trace element balance associated with disease in dialysis patients. Although the morbidity reported has principally occurred in haemodialysis patients in the presence of unrecognized high concentrations of aluminium in the dialysate, significant complications have also arisen from the use of aluminium-containing phosphate binders. Although highly effective, their use has fallen dramatically due to the anaemia, bone disease and cognitive dysfunction now known to be associated with the accumulation of aluminium. This is discussed in greater detail elsewhere in the book.

Zinc deficiency has been reported in CAPD [138, 139]. However, the clinical significance of such observations is not clear. Many of the symptoms of zinc deficiency, such as altered taste, anorexia, hyperprolactinaemia, weakness and impotence, are part of the uraemic syndrome, and the causative role of zinc is not established. Deviations from normal levels of the trace elements chromium, cobalt and bromine have also been reported [139, 140].

Low selenium concentrations have been recorded in patients with chronic renal failure on both HD and CAPD [141], with associated low levels of platelet glutathione activity. Although not proven, it is postulated that this may be associated with accelerated vascular disease. Low selenium levels in malnutrition and CAPD have also been associated with increased myopathy and deranged immune function [142].

Vitamins and carnitine

Depletion of water-soluble vitamins has been reported in patients on CAPD, thought to be related to dialytic losses rather than reflecting a generalized poor nutrient intake, as similar deficiencies of fat-soluble vitamins (with the exception of biologically active vitamin D) have not been described. Specifically, no increased requirement for cobalamin, biotin, niacin, pantothenic acid, and vitamins A, E and K is reported [143]. Deficiencies of vitamin C, B6, B1 and B2 and folate similar to those occurring in the haemodialysis population have been reported in CAPD patients. Replacement doses in the form of multivitamin tablets containing only water-soluble vitamins are generally recommended, particularly if there are additional concerns regarding nutritional status. Patients should be advised that these multivitamin tablets should not contain additional elements or fat-soluble vitamins, due to the risk of accumulation and toxicity. Folate supplemen-

tation may have the additional benefit of reducing elevated homocysteine levels in CAPD patients [144], which has been aetiologically associated with accelerated vascular disease in patients with end-stage renal failure [145, 146].

Carnitine is a quaternary amine essential for transport of fatty acids to the oxidative site in the mitochondria. Carnitine deficiency has been reported in CAPD and correlates positively with plasma levels of the precursors lysine and methionine, with the estimated protein intake, and correlates inversely with losses of protein in the dialysate [147]. In uraemia it is also associated aetiologically with the development of hypertriglyceridaemia, but the benefits of carnitine supplementation in ameliorating the triglyceride abnormalities seen in CAPD patients have not been proven.

Methods of assessment of nutritional status: overview

Nutritional status is difficult to assess in end-stage renal failure, particularly in the early stages of malnutrition when intervention to improve nutritional adequacy is theoretically more likely to be successful. Many markers of nutrition and assessment techniques are available (Table 3).

However, the majority of these nutritional markers have not been validated in the dialysis population. The most appropriate methods of estimating nutrition in end-stage renal disease determine

Table 3. Assessment of nutritional status

Recorded/recalled dietary intake
Serum creatinine
Creatinine appearance
Urea kinetic modelling
Serum albumin
Other serum markers (lymphocyte count, haemoglobin, prealbumin, immunoglobulins, complement, transferrin, retinal-binding protein, insulin-like growth factor-1)
Anthropometric measurements (body weight, body mass index, skinfold thickness, mid-arm muscle circumference)
Subjective global assessment
Bioelectrical impedance
Dual-energy X-ray absorptiometry
Total-body nitrogen
Total-body potassium
Delayed-type hypersensitivity
Research tools to determine nutrition
   Metabolic balance studies
   Radiolabelled amino acid turnover
   Amino acid profiles
   Muscle protein analyses

current nutritional intake, nutrient intake in the immediate or recent past, and the longer-term overall state of nutrition. Because the assessment of the energy intake is more difficult than assessment of protein intake, an estimate of protein intake is generally made and a sufficient energy intake is assumed on the basis of effective protein utilization. In practice the current dietary adequacy is determined by a combination of dietary history and a measure of urea nitrogen appearance; the nutrient intake in the recent past by biochemical markers; and the longer-term state of nutrition by a measure of body composition in addition to some biochemical markers. Measures used in each of these settings have some advantages, but also some disadvantages, which will be discussed. In the absence of the ability to measure total-body nitrogen, several parameters should be considered in parallel to achieve an overall assessment of nutrition, as all other methods may be affected to some degree by the presence of renal failure, the mode and adequacy of dialysis delivery and fluid status at the time of assessment. These considerations are incorporated into the Dialysis Outcome Quality Initiative (DOQI) guidelines for nutritional surveillence, (summarized in ref. 148), in which recommendations include measuring a variety of indices including the protein equivalent of nitrogen appearance (PNA) as determined by urea kinetics, subjective global assessment, fat-free oedema free body mass and serum albumin.

Methods of determining nutritional state which are largely investigational research tools will not be discussed, as they are less applicable to clinical practice. These include metabolic balance studies, whole-body leucine turnover and the use of plasma and intracellular amino acid profiles as indices of nitrogen balance. Although they yield important information in a research setting, these methods are time-consuming and expensive, and their use has been largely limited to validation of alternative forms of measuring nutrient intake rather than in clinical practice.

Dietary review

A dietary history is a simple, easily available technique for determining nutrient intake. The nutrient intake needs to be carefully evaluated by a dietitian skilled in assessing patients with end-stage renal failure, the most useful method being a prospective record of food intake over 3 days. However, even this method presupposes that this is the 'usual' diet ingested by the patient. Dietary histories based on the patient's recollection of food intake, whilst of some value [149, 150], show a high individual variance [151] and in general cannot be relied upon for quantitative assessment of food intake [152, 153]. They are of more value for determining qualitative food intake where a redirection in the overall diet may be required. More accurate recording of dietary intake requires a more intensive approach, including the use of duplicate proportion techniques and weighing of both food servings and residual portions.

Serum creatinine and creatinine appearance

Serum creatinine is variably affected by age, dietary intake and muscle mass in the dialysis patient as well as the patient who is not on dialysis. A low serum creatinine on dialysis reflects a poor nutritional state, and is associated with an increased risk of death [16, 34, 154]. In patients on peritoneal dialysis, creatinine clearance (derived from both dialytic and renal clearances) is a useful marker of the adequacy of therapy, and has been shown to correlate with the protein intake, as measured by protein catabolic rate and serum albumin [64].

Serum albumin

Serum albumin is perhaps the most widely used and easily measured marker of nutrition. It is the best-established visceral protein marker in terms of its prognostic value, and should be regularly assessed, although the sensitivity and specificity of this marker in detecting nutritional impairment prior to the development of severe malnutrition are poor. However, given that no single alternative serum protein measure has been shown to confer improved sensitivity in detecting malnutrition in dialysis patients, serum albumin remains an important index of nutritional status and does have prognostic significance in patients both with and without renal failure [13, 16, 21, 25, 32, 33, 39, 107, 153–157]. The method of albumin measurement is important in comparative studies as the bromocresol green method overestimates albumin in comparison with immunonephelometry [107, 158]. The reason for this overestimation is that the dye is not completely specific for albumin and is taken up by other proteins, and this difference is exaggerated in CAPD patients. Bromocresol purple yields serum albumin levels that are closer to the immunonephelometric method, although it does slightly underestimate the level in CAPD patients by 1–2 g/L.

It should be kept in mind that although nutritional state is an important regulator of albumin synthesis, and hence of serum albumin, it may be affected by factors other than nutrition, especially in dialysis. Bianchi *et al.* [159] in 1970 determined that there were discrepancies in the total-body distribution of albumin in dialysis patients as compared with the normal population, particularly with regard to the fraction of albumin in the extravascular space. Plasma albumin is decreased in dialysis and particularly in CAPD due to fluid retention, alterations in vascular permeability with loss of albumin from the intravascular to extravascular space, reduction in lymphatic return and increased catabolism and decreased synthesis [160]. Kayser and Schoenfeld [161] had earlier shown that in CAPD patients the total albumin pool is normal, thus indicating fluid overload as a major component of the hypoalbuminaemia. In addition, peritoneal protein loss and the effects of an excessive peritoneal glucose load in the presence of a low protein intake also act to depress serum albumin levels [162]. Comorbidity also serves to depress serum albumin, the severity of intercurrent illness modifying both serum albumin and prognosis independent of nutritional reserves [106].

More recently, Foley *et al.* [109] followed a cohort of 432 patients with end-stage renal failure, including 171 peritoneal dialysis patients, for 41 months, assessing factors associated with the development of cardiac disease. They showed that a 10 g/L fall in serum albumin was independently associated with the development of left ventricular dilation, *de novo* cardiac failure with a relative risk of 4.2 and overall mortality with a relative risk of 2.06. These results remained valid even after adjustment for baseline comorbidity. However, these associations were not as strong as those observed between serum albumin and cardiac disease in the haemodialysis population.

Despite these observations, albumin and transferrin levels can remain unchanged at low levels in longitudinal studies with no increase in mortality [163], suggesting that the low albumin need not reflect a generalized nutritional deficit. Goodship *et al.* [120] compared patients on CAPD and normal subjects, showing that somatic muscle protein reserves were similar, but serum albumin and plasma amino acid levels were lower after 3 months of CAPD. In Young *et al.*'s study [21], 24% of patients classified as being well-nourished had serum albumin levels less than 35 g/dl, with no other marker suggestive of poor nutrition. De Fijter *et al.*

[164] found that, although serum albumin was lower in CAPD patients compared to HD patients, their lean body mass determined by bioelectrical impedance analysis (BIA) was higher. There was no correlation between the BIA assessment and albumin levels in the CAPD group. Furthermore, the protein intake, measured as the protein catabolic rate, is often high, and the albumin low, in CAPD [64, 165], which suggests that factors other than nutrition may affect serum albumin [166]. These results, taken collectively, also suggest that a low serum albumin may well be a marker of systemic disease, rather than primarily a reflection of the nutritional state.

Held *et al.*, in the 1992 report of the US Renal Data System [167], found that the relative risk for mortality was higher for haemodialysis patients whose serum albumin was 30–35 g/dl than for those with a serum albumin level of 35–40 g/dl. In contrast, for CAPD patients no increase in risk for mortality was observed until the serum albumin was less than 30 g/dl. Struijk *et al.* [107] similarly found that patients commencing CAPD with a serum albumin less than 30.9 g/dl had a significantly poorer survival than patients whose serum albumin was greater than this value. However, a Cox's proportional hazards analysis failed to demonstrate an independent effect of serum albumin on survival, which was much more closely linked with the presence of comorbid illness, age and haemoglobin concentration. Comorbidity was in turn associated with a low serum albumin. Similarly, the CANUSA study demonstrated an increased risk of mortality in patients with a lower serum albumin [27], but due to the presence of comorbid illness and its inherent effect on albumin, a direct relationship between serum albumin and mortality cannot be drawn.

Several studies have demonstrated a higher hospital admission rate in patients with a low serum albumin [25, 156, 157, 168], in addition to poorer nerve conduction studies and technique failure [25]. Germain *et al.* [169] have shown that a low albumin level and low protein catabolic rates correlate with increased mortality and intra-abdominal complications. In CAPD, however, serum albumin levels correlate poorly with Kt/V and PCR [65] due to increasing peritoneal transport resulting in increasing albumin loss, although this finding has not been universal [32, 157].

Overall it appears that a serum albumin of less than 40 g/dl is of concern in the haemodialysis population, but because of different mechanisms of synthesis and loss in CAPD, an albumin of 35 g/dl in the CAPD population should raise the same measure of concern. As a decrease in serum albumin is not an early indicator of malnutrition, by the time the albumin falls, nutrition may be grossly impaired [170–172].

Other serum markers of nutrition

In addition to albumin, other serum protein markers of malnutrition have been assessed in renal failure, but are difficult to interpret due to the influence of factors other than nutritional considerations. They include serum levels of total proteins, transferrin, prealbumin, the third component of complement, immunoglobulins and retinol-binding protein. In general, the prognostic value in finding an abnormal value in serum proteins has been to date poorly assessed in longitudinal studies.

Prealbumin and transferrin have been suggested as better markers of short-term nutritional state, as they have a shorter half-life than serum albumin. Prealbumin, in addition to albumin, has been shown in a prospective study to predict mortality in CAPD patients [34]. In this study of single baseline measurements of serum biochemical markers of nutrition in 250 haemodialysis and 140 CAPD patients, low levels of serum albumin, prealbumin, and creatinine predicted a poor prognosis, in addition to older age and the presence of diabetes [34]. In the haemodialysis patients, low cholesterol and an increased time of dialysis were further associated with a poor prognosis [173]. In contrast, Kaufmann *et al.* [174] have demonstrated a high rate of cutaneous anergy, low lymphocyte count, low serum albumin and total protein levels in predialysis patients. These levels reverted towards normal after the initiation of chronic dialysis therapy, while serum prealbumin, the third component of complement, and anthropometric measures remained normal in both predialysis and maintenance dialysis patients.

Transferrin is markedly affected by factors, other than the nutritional state, which often coexist in chronic renal failure. Low levels are seen in the presence of tumour, infection or chronic inflammatory disease, whereas high levels are seen in iron deficiency, which is frequent with widespread erythropoietin use. This therefore limits the value of transferrin as a nutritional marker in end-stage renal failure.

Leptin

Leptin is a recently discovered hormone [175] which is synthesized and secreted by adipose tissue, and postulated to have a direct influence on appetite and body weight [176, 177]. In human obesity, leptin levels are positively correlated with BMI [178–180].

The association between plasma leptin and malnutrition has recently been assessed in renal disease. In a cross-sectional study by Young *et al.* [181], leptin was highly correlated with total fat in all patient groups, and leptin levels relative to total fat mass were higher in renal patients compared to controls. Other studies performed by Howard *et al.* [182] confirmed the fact that leptin levels are significantly higher than normal in patients with renal disease, when normalized for gender and BMI. In a study of CAPD patients leptin levels were significantly higher in both males and females than in normal controls, and female gender and BMI were the strongest predictors of hyperleptinaemia [183]. The leptin/fat ratios were inversely correlated with dietary protein intake, while leptin levels correlated negatively with lean tissue mass in patients with chronic renal failure [182].

The possible mechanisms for increased leptin levels in end-stage renal disease are reduced leptin clearance [184], increased leptin synthesis or altered protein binding of leptin. It is postulated that elevated leptin levels may induce anorexia and contribute to the malnutrition found in renal failure. However, the predictive value of plasma leptin as a marker of malnutrition in patients on peritoneal dialysis needs to be assessed further in prospective studies.

Anthropometric measurements

A body weight in the lower centiles of the ideal body weight range, low BMI or a history of recent weight loss clearly raise concern regarding nutritional adequacy or comorbid illness. However, poor nutrition, particularly in CAPD, often does not present with these signs or symptoms, and hence more specific anthropometric measures of fat and lean body mass are required. Variations in total body water in end-stage renal failure limit the usefulness of anthropometric measurements as markers of nutrition. Expected values for age and sex have been derived from the normal population, but these values are unlikely to reflect nutritional state in end-stage renal disease. We have found no correlation between nutritional state as measured by total body nitrogen and anthropometric measurements in haemodialysis or CAPD [13, 185], which clearly indicates that these measurements underestimate the degree of protein malnutrition and hence the mortality risk [185, 186].

Urea kinetic modelling

Urea kinetic modelling is increasingly utilized for assessment of the adequacy of dialysis in both peritoneal dialysis and haemodialysis. In many respects the validity of using this method is stronger in peritoneal dialysis, as the concentrations of urea and volumes are directly measured rather than calculated, as is the case in haemodialysis. The use of urea kinetic modelling to determine the adequacy of dialysis is discussed elsewhere in this book, and will be addressed here only as it relates to nutrition.

Many investigators have established the urea nitrogen appearance (UNA) as an index of protein metabolism, and therefore of protein intake [187, 188]. The UNA is the net production of urea and its appearance in body fluids and in measurable losses. It has been shown in stable patients that there is a predictable correlation between UNA and total urea nitrogen appearance (TNA). The production of urea nitrogen is directly related to protein intake, but the production of nitrogen from sources other than urea is minimally affected by diet [189] and is constant over a wide variety of renal function [186]. Given that daily changes in body nitrogen are usually negligible in stable patients on peritoneal dialysis, the UNA is usually represented as the sum of dialysate and urinary losses. The protein equivalent of total nitrogen appearance (PNA) expresses the nitrogen appearance in terms of protein. In the steady state it is assumed that the PNA is equal to the dietary intake of protein. Based on the assumption that nitrogen constantly accounts for 16% of protein, the following equation applies.

PNA (grams of protein/24 h) = TNA
(grams of nitrogen/24 h) × 6.25.

Because of the constant relationship between the measured UNA and the total nitrogen appearance, the PNA is determined from the UNA, or from the urea appearance (UA) by the following formulae [190]:

PNA (g/day) = 20.1 + 7.5 × UNA (g/24 h)

or

PNA (g/day) = 20.1 + 0.209 × UA (mmol/24 h)

Several alternative equations have been derived to calculate the PNA in CAPD patients. Comparisons

performed by Keshaviah and Nolph [191] have shown that all equations correlate closely with each other and do not show any significant difference from measured protein intake. However, if dialysate protein loss is excessive (greater than 10–15 g protein per day), this needs to be additionally accounted for in making an estimate of protein intake [192]. In this case it is recommended that the protein intake be determined from the UNA by determining the protein equivalent of non-protein nitrogen appearance (PNPNA), which in the individual patient is equal to the PNA minus protein losses. This should reflect the net protein intake under steady-state conditions, i.e. the total intake of protein minus dialysate and urinary protein losses [190]. Thus by determining the PNPNA (see below) and adding dialysate and urinary protein loss, a more accurate estimate of the PNA may be made.

PNPNA (g/day) = 15.1 + 6.95 × UNA (g/24 h)

or

PNPNA (g/day) = 15.1 + 0.195 × UA (mmol/24 h)

The terminology is often loosely applied, so that the terms used in applying urea kinetic modelling to nutrition in CAPD have recently been redefined [193]. For practical purposes the PNA can be substituted for the older terminology referring to it as the 'protein catabolic rate' or PCR. It should be reiterated that the assumptions on which the equations are based hold true only if the patient is in steady state. As the half-life of urea varies in renal failure from about 7 h to in excess of 1 month [189], a steady state cannot be assumed if a dietary or treatment intervention has occurred within the previous month. In addition, because small differences in rates of protein synthesis and degradation can result in large alterations in lean body mass, small errors are important and therefore careful repeated measurements should be undertaken. Indeed, Panzetta et al. [194] have found significant variability in the estimated daily intake of protein in 25% of clinically stable patients. Studies assessing the benefits of the kinetically derived protein intake suggest that relaying the information back to the patient results in an improved compliance with dietary recommendations [195].

Conventionally, the calculated protein intake has been expressed as g of protein ingested per kg of body weight. Although this standardization allows for uniformity of expression between patients, recommendations for protein and caloric intake calculated on the basis of amounts per kilogram of body weight perpetuate overeating in overweight patients and undereating in malnourished patients [26, 196].

Clearly, both the dialysis dose and the protein intake may potentially be misinterpreted when results are normalized to actual rather than the ideal body weight for an individual patient. Malnourished patients are more likely to be below the ideal body weight, and therefore urea clearances and protein intake, normalized to 58% actual body weight, may be similar in both malnourished and well-nourished patients. However, as both estimates are normalized to ideal body weight, their values may be significantly lower in the malnourished population [116]. Current recommendations are to express both protein and caloric intake based on ideal, rather than actual, body weight, and to promote dietary guidelines based on this normalization [116, 196, 197]. Ideal body weight is generally determined by a BMI of 22–25, with some allowance for differences in racial subgroups. Alternatively, protein intake can be normalized to lean body mass, determined by generation of creatinine [198]. This creates potential problems since if dietary prescription is based on lean body mass, patients with low lean body mass are likely to need an individualized recommendation for a higher protein and caloric intake to normalize lean body mass. Hence, uniform dietary advice based on ideal body weight is likely to be more 'user-friendly' in a clinical setting.

Bioelectrical impedance

Lean body mass, containing protein, water and bone compartments, is widely utilized as a measure of nutritional status. In the normal population protein and water should be positively correlated, although this relationship does not necessarily hold true in renal failure. The measurement of body water has been shown to be possible by measurement of the body's impedance to a small alternating electric current. Several regression equations, established in normal volunteers, then allow the prediction of total body water. A relatively new approach which has not yet been validated in renal failure applies this principle using a swept frequency bioimpedance monitor which allows measurement of the extracellular component of body water as well as total body water [199]. The importance of this development is that the intracellular water may be a better predictor of body cell mass and hence of body protein than is total body water. It should be emphasized that the impedance of human tissue depends on its fluid and electrolyte content. A fixed ratio exists between total body water and lean body mass in normal individuals, and the latter can therefore be calculated from impedance values [200]. However, reliable bioelectrical impedance-based lean body mass measurements can only be obtained when patients are euvolaemic, which may be difficult to assess [201]. This discrepancy in measurement of lean body mass with varying degrees of renal dysfunction has been demonstrated by Nielsen *et al.* [202], the differences being explained in both predialysis and dialysis populations by the presence of excessive amounts of fluid. In a further study comparing deuterium dilution, as the gold standard of total body water, and bioelectrical impedance assessments of total body water, bioelectrical impedance estimates were less accurate in patients with chronic renal failure compared to normal controls [203]. In a prospective study of CAPD patients followed from the commencement of dialysis with serial anthropometric and bioelectrical impedence measurements, a rise in total body water accounted for the initial observed gain in weight [204]. Subsequently, an increase in total body fat occurred. In this study bioelectrical impedance measurements, compared with anthropometric measurements, consistently underestimated nutritional stores.

Conversely, other studies have [205] found a good relationship between total body water derived from bioelectrical impedence measurement and that determined by antipyrine dilutional volume.

Despite the limitations, bioelectrical impedance has been used to determine the nutritional state successfully in patients on peritoneal dialysis [206, 207]. Although there is good correlation between estimates of total body water by electrical impedance and by measurement against a 'gold standard' technique, the limits of agreement are wide [208, 209]. In a group of 18 CAPD patients where fat free mass was assessed by bioelectrical impedence and compared to total body nitrogen and dual-energy X-ray absorptiometry (DEXA), the limits of agreement were similarly large: −5.9 kg to 18.1 kg [210].

Thus, although the available data suggest that bioelectrical impedance measurement in dialysis patients appear to correlate well with other assessments of body composition, the accuracy and sensitivity of the method has not yet been confirmed in this group. Abnormal composition of body water in patients on dialysis, with its subsequent alteration in the measured resistance, may explain the inaccuracies. Although the validity of bioelectrical impedance measurements in predicting outcome has not been assessed, the technique warrants further study as it is relatively easy to perform and can be undertaken easily on a large scale, and easily repeated.

Computerised tomography

Saxenhofer *et al.* [211] studied two groups of dialysis patients at least 6 months after commencement of dialysis, using computerized tomography of mid-thigh muscle mass and peripheral and central fat stores. The coefficient of variation of each method was less than 2%. In CAPD patients there was a significant correlation between central fat stores and serum cholesterol, and between mid-thigh muscle mass and serum albumin. No such correlations were found in the haemodialysis patients, although the reasons for this are not clear. No significant difference in body composition was found between the two dialysis groups, but when compared to a normal population, both groups exhibited increased central fat deposits and a reduction in muscle stores.

Dual-energy X-ray absorptiometry (DEXA)

Dual-energy X-ray absorptiometry (DEXA) utilizes the same principles as dual photon absorptiometry, which has been been shown to be clinically useful in the measurement of body composition [212, 213], but overcomes the problems associated with a decaying radionuclide source by utilizing a small X-ray tube [214]. DEXA measures three body components separately: bone mineral, fat mass and lean mass. Lean body mass is defined by DEXA as fat free mass [214]. Horber *et al.* [215] have advocated the use of DEXA in haemodialysis patients. However, *in-vitro* studies have shown that the addition of saline to a phantom results in significant reductions in the DEXA fat measurements [216], thus limiting the usefulness of this technique in end-stage renal failure, given the variability in hydration and the resultant variability in the assessment of lean body mass. Similarly, clinical studies [217] indicate that errors are introduced by variations in body thickness induced by changes in hydration.

Total body nitrogen (TBN)

The established gold standard for measurement of body protein is the direct measurement of protein stores by prompt *in-vivo* neutron capture analysis. The technique was initially introduced in 1973 and

has been shown to correlate directly with muscle mass [218, 219].

TBN provides important information regarding the prognosis of patients [13, 185], the probability of death within 12 months in patients having a TBN of less than 80% of the predicted value being 48% [13]. This technique is clearly able to detect patients likely to do poorly on dialysis over a period of 12 months follow-up, which is not predictable from anthropometry in either haemodialysis or CAPD, nor from serum albumin measurements in the haemodialysis population. Other groups have also utilized TBN measurements to assess nutrition in dialysis patients, and have found a similar degree of malnutrition in both the haemodialysis and CAPD population. Some variability is evident, in part due to a 'centre effect' or 'laboratory effect', but also because of variability in dialysis techniques and prescription of dialysis over the periods of study [122, 186, 220–222]. TBN measurements in both CAPD and haemodialysis have further been shown to correlate with a higher protein catabolic rate and a reduction in episodes of infection [35].

Total body potassium

Total body potassium is a direct measure of fat free mass in the normal population. The technique assesses the amount of naturally occurring ^{40}K and then applies the Forbes constant to determine body cell mass [223]. However, the Forbes constant was developed in the normal population and is unlikely to apply in renal failure, in which alterations in total body potassium, independent of nutrition, are known to occur [122]. Importantly, changes in total body potassium may result from changes in intracellular water and are not independent of total body water. Hence, in addition to its limited availability, total body potassium is unlikely to be of significant use in determining the nutritional state in patients on peritoneal dialysis.

Subjective global assessment

It is clear that in the dialysis population, with the exception of TBN, a single marker is insufficient to detect even significant degrees of nutritional impairment [224] and a combination of markers should be considered as a global nutritional assessment. This has led to development of the 'subjective global assessment' (SGA) [225] which involves the judgement of malnutrition by several markers, but is principally dependent on body weight and gastrointestinal symptoms and not on serum albumin. However, in a study comparing SGA with anthropometry, bioelectrical impedance and biochemical measures in 59 dialysis patients, the investigators found that SGA could significantly predict patients with low serum albumin in both haemodialysis and CAPD patients [226]. Conversely, in a cross-sectional study by Jones [227] in 76 CAPD patients, SGA identified patients who had abnormal body mass (determined by weight and body mass index), muscle mass and muscle strength, but these factors did not correlate with serum albumin levels, which was considered to indicate the lack of validity of serum albumin, rather than the SGA, as a marker of nutrition.

The subjective global assessment is a useful prognostic tool, but is not specific for nutritional adequacy and is likely to be significantly affected by comorbid illness. The subjective measures include the patient's history of weight loss, anorexia and vomiting, and the physician's estimate of muscle wasting, oedema and loss of subcutaneous fat. The SGA overall 'score' is based on clinical judgement, which is both a strength and a weakness, and makes interpretion of the score in different centres less reliable. Its validity has been established using objective measures in CAPD patients [4, 21]. Cianciaruso et al. [24] used the SGA to assess 224 CAPD and 263 haemodialysis patients in a multicentre study, and demonstrated that 42% of CAPD and 31% of haemodialysis patients were malnourished. The study by Young et al. [21] using the SGA, and also including measurement of serum albumin, similarly found that 41% of patients on CAPD had variable degrees of malnutrition, which correlated with residual renal function and less prescribed dialysis. Compared to haemodialysis patients the CAPD patients tended to have a lower albumin and total protein, higher body weight, skinfold thicknesses and percentage body fat, but similar serum transferrin and mid-arm muscle circumference. Fenton et al. have shown, using the SGA, that CAPD patients judged as having mild/moderate malnutrition have a significantly reduced survival [4].

In the CANUSA study SGA, as modified by Baker et al. [228], was the best nutritional estimate to predict clinical outcome. The patients were classified as having normal nutrition or mild to moderate or severe malnutrition [229]. The 2-year survival probabilities were 80.5%, 77.3% and 47.2% respectively. However, it is difficult to assess comorbid factors independently from nutritional factors that may contribute to a poor SGA. Twenty-five per cent of

patients commencing haemodialysis in Canada have a serum albumin less than 30 g/dl [230], whereas 16% in the CANUSA study had a serum albumin less than 30 g/dl [27]. Because of the inherent differences between populations selected for different forms of dialysis, prognostic data derived from the CAPD patients cannot be extrapolated to the haemodialysis population Indeed, extrapolations drawn from particular dialysis centres may well not be applicable to other centres, as again borne out in the CANUSA study, which reported that dialysis in the USA relative to Canada was associated with a higher mortality.

The use of multiple markers to increase the validity of the nutritional assessment has been advocated by the recent National Institutes of Health Consensus Development Conference on Morbidity and Mortality of Dialysis [230]. They consider that a minimum assessment, in the absence of access to measurement of TBN, should include weight, height, a record of recent weight loss, anthropometric measurements, serum protein, albumin, transferrin, prealbumin and the use of urea nitrogen appearance to calculate the protein catabolic rate. However, no relative value is placed on individual parameters. This report acknowledges that, while newer techniques such as bioelectrical impedance measurements and dual energy X-ray absorptiometry are being explored, they are as yet not routinely recommended as their prognostic value is unclear.

Total body water

The estimation of TBW remains one of the major factors affecting the reliability of the various methods of determination of nutrition. TBW varies significantly in end-stage renal failure, and a reliable measure is necessary to determine nutritional state as well as the estimated delivery of dialysis. The majority of commonly used estimates of body water have been shown to be inaccurate when compared to the gold standard of deuterium dilution [231, 232]. The Watson formula [233] has been applied to the determination of body water in normal subjects, but it has not been adequately validated in renal disease. In CAPD patients the Watson formula and bioelectrical impedance measures underestimate TBW [208], whereas TBW estimated as 58% body weight results in overestimation, particularly in obese patients as fat contains no water. Indeed, in obese patients the error in estimated TBW using all methods is magnified, and deuterium oxide dilution has been recommended as a more accurate direct measure [208] although clearly this technique is more labour-intensive and less likely to be used on a routine basis. In CAPD patients with a more normal body mass index the Watson equation has been shown to correlate best with directly measured body water [234].

Panzetta *et al.* [235] have shown that in CAPD patients the mean value of TBW is normal, but abnormally distributed, with a reduction in extracellular and an increase in intracellular water. This is in contrast to patients with chronic renal failure and the haemodialysis population, in whom extracellular water is consistently normal or increased when compared to normal subjects.

Automated peritoneal dialysis (APD)

Limited studies are available assessing the nutritional adequacy in continuous cycled peritoneal dialysis (CCPD). Many are uncontrolled, and biased in that patients who are rapid transporters are usually recommended for short-dwell automated peritoneal dialysis in which net glucose absorption and protein losses can be minimized and ultrafiltration maximized. In a small cross-sectional study comparing 19 CAPD and 13 CCPD patients no significant differences were observed in serum albumin, Kt/V or nPCR. However, there was a trend for each value to be higher in the CCPD-treated group [236]. In the 1996 Peritoneal Dialysis Core Indicators Study, a random audit of 1317 patients on peritoneal dialysis in the United States, no differences in nutritional markers were observed between the 785 patients using CAPD and the 423 patients using APD [28]. These results have been confirmed by studies demonstrating that dialysis delivered in equal amounts to patients on CAPD and CCPD results in similar biochemical nutritional parameters over a period of up to 24 months [237–239]. In an additional small study [89], switching patients from CAPD to APD resulted in an increase in dialysate clearances and PNA and a reduction in peritoneal protein loss, with only a marginal increase in serum albumin. The reasons for this are no doubt manifold. However, on the basis of the peak urea hypothesis alluded to above, clearance targets should be higher in APD compared to CAPD. Whether increased dialysis delivery improves the nutritional state and ultimately the prognosis in patients treated with APD remains to be studied.

Therapy of malnutrition in peritoneal dialysis

It will be evident from the above discussion that malnutrition in peritoneal dialysis patients is best addressed by attention to both predialysis factors and dialytic factors independent of nutrient intake. In addition to regular assessment and maintenance of nutrient intake, specific attention towards correction of acidosis, avoidance of drugs which exacerbate anorexia, prevention and control of hyperparathyroidism and maintenance of vitamin D homeostasis needs to be addressed in the predialytic phase. Clearly, catabolic comorbid conditions should be optimally treated. The timing of initiation of dialysis and its effect on nutrition has not been well studied. However, intuitive reasoning suggests that clearances prior to initiation of dialysis should not have fallen below the target clearances aimed for on dialysis.

Once dialysis is commenced, dietary protein and energy intake should be increased, the dialytic prescription should be tailored to maximize dialytic clearances and to minimize the use of hypertonic glucose-based dialysate, and the most biocompatible dialysate solutions available should be preferentially used. Connection systems should be used to limit infectious complications, particularly peritonitis, in view of the inherent increase in peritoneal protein losses. Ongoing interventions directed to normalizing metabolic derangements in chronic renal failure and maintenance of renal function should persist into the dialytic phase of renal disease. Regular review by both the renal physician and dietitian, with detailed nutritional assessment, should be regularly undertaken, and specific nutritional therapy advocated if malnutrition is present or, indeed, if nutritional reserves are being depleted even in the absence of overt malnutrition. Nutritional support will be of value only in patients in whom an inadequate nutrient intake is the cause of malnutrition, and where additional factors are promoting malnutrition these need to be concurrently addressed.

Protein and energy

Metabolic studies determining the protein intake required to maintain a positive nitrogen balance have recommended a protein intake of 1.0–1.4 g/kg per day and a caloric intake of 35–45 kcal/kg in CAPD [240]. Although the recommendations are conventionally made on a per-kg basis, it should be reiterated that it is preferable to recommend nutrient intake adjusted to ideal rather than actual body weight. Current recommendations are that dietary protein should be of high biological value, i.e. have a high content of essential amino acids such as occurs in beef and fish. However, it appears that if patients are encouraged to ingest protein from a variety of sources a sufficient supply of essential amino acids will be ensured. Older patients should not be expected to have a reduced protein intake, as occurs in healthy subjects, and may indeed have a higher minimum protein requirement than younger patients on CAPD [241]. Clearly, as the CAPD population is ageing and the elderly population has additional risk factors for malnutrition, these patients need close nutritional surveillence.

An insufficient caloric intake even in the face of adequate dietary protein intake is in itself likely to result in a negative nitrogen balance [242]. Indeed, body protein as measured by neutron activation analysis in both haemodialysis and CAPD is more likely to correlate with estimated energy intake than with protein intake [13, 185]. As CAPD is associated with an obligatory energy intake by virtue of peritoneal glucose absorption, this has been postulated as one of the means whereby nutrition is better maintained in CAPD. Because of the glucose load and its attendant adverse effect on the lipid profile, the dietary intake of simple carbohydrates, cholesterol and saturated fats should be modified. It is currently recommended that 35% of energy intake be in the form of fat, and use of mono- and polyunsaturated fats be encouraged. Carbohydrates should be predominantly in the form of starches. Individualized dietary advice for obese and undernourished patients is required. Obese patients usually require limitation of their use of hypertonic glucose-based solutions, and a reduction in caloric intake. Malnourished patients require a stepwise approach to therapy, ranging from optimization of dialysis and comorbid conditions to oral and parenteral supplementation and, in rare circumstances, promotion of anabolism through pharmacological means (see below).

In patients unable to ingest the minimum protein requirement of 1.2 g/kg per day and caloric intake of 35 kcal/kg per day (and more if a low BMI is present), nutritional support should begin with counselling from a trained dietitian. Specific issues such as cost and limited access to food may be identified and rectified. If palatability is a concern, alternative food sources may be suggested. As a consequence of the increased nutrient load, dialysis and/or medication prescriptions may need to be modified. However, this should not be regarded as a deterrent to improving nutrient intake.

Supplements are available in the form of high protein ± calorie formulations, which may be an acceptable alternative source of some nutrients. The efficacy of oral nutritional supplementation has not been subjected to a randomized controlled trial in CAPD patients. However, small non-randomized studies have demonstrated that in the elderly patient with a low albumin, biochemical markers of nutrition may improve after oral supplementation [243].

Appetite stimulants such as megesterol acetate, a semisynthetic derivative of progesterone, have been used in malnourished patients outside the setting of renal failure with some success. As yet there are no data on their efficacy in renal failure. The anabolic steroid nandrolone decanoate has been trialled in small numbers of cachectic CAPD patients and found to exert an anabolic effect. However, in this non-randomized study no improvement was observed if intraperitoneal amino acids were concurrently used [244].

Lipids

Correction of hyperlipidaemia should be part of the management of all patients on peritoneal dialysis, and indeed in renal disease in general. The cornerstone of any therapeutic regimen should be dietary modification, restricting cholesterol, saturated fats, and excess carbohydrates. Other non-pharmacological measures to be undertaken include cessation of smoking, daily regular exercise, weight reduction in obese patients, and avoidance of drugs likely to elevate plasma lipids [245]. Unfortunately these measures often prove inadequate, and drug therapy has to be considered. The HMG-CoA reductase inhibitors reduce total cholesterol and LDLC while maintaining or increasing HDLC. The bile acid sequestrants reduce total cholesterol and LDLC, without affecting HDLC, but there is a high incidence of gastrointestinal side-effects and the potential to interfere with the absorption of other medications. Fibric acid derivatives reduce total triglycerides, as well as total cholesterol and LDLC, while maintaining or increasing HDLC. Nicotinic acid is effective in lowering lipoprotein (a), triglycerides, total cholesterol and LDLC, and raising HDLC, but compliance is poor because of side-effects. Probucol lowers total cholesterol and LDLC, but can also lower HDLC and thus cannot be recommended. L-Carnitine lowers triglyceride levels and increases HDLC concentrations in some dialysis patients, but appears to be more efficacious in haemodialysis than in CAPD patients. Fish oil supplementation (omega-3-fatty acids) decreases serum triglycerides by inhibiting VLDL synthesis, but may increase LDL-apolipoprotein B [240]. In a meta-analysis comparing and contrasting the relative efficacy of various antilipaemic therapies Massy et al. [246] found that the HMG-CoA reductase inhibitors and fibric acid analogues consistently reduced cholesterol in patients on CAPD, while only HMG-CoA reductase inhibitors decreased LDL and increased HDL. Triglycerides were reduced by fibric acid analogues. Erythropoietin treatment has also been shown to provide beneficial effects on serum lipids in both haemodialysis and CAPD patients, reducing total cholesterol, apoprotein B, and serum triglycerides [247].

Acidosis

An essential component of therapy aimed at improving nutrition in end-stage renal failure is to correct systemic acidosis. Mild acidosis may be best corrected by calcium carbonate as it both provides the necessary calcium to offset the negative calcium balance and in addition reduces intestinal phosphate absorption. However, as the ionization of calcium carbonate is inhibited by the physicochemical conditions of the gastric fluid (such as occurs if a patient is concurrently taking a H_2 receptor blocker or hydrogen pump inhibitor) the alkalinizing action of calcium carbonate may be strongly reduced.

In CAPD plasma bicarbonate is generally held constant when a lactate concentration of 37.5 mmol/L is used. A considerable proportion of patients develop serum bicarbonate levels above 28 mmol/L when the dialysate lactate is increased to 40 mmol/L. An increased lactate concentration should be advocated if the serum bicarbonate level is consistently below normal on standard dialysate. An alternative is to prescribe a low calcium dialysate (which has a higher lactate concentration) and oral calcium carbonate, which adds a significant alkali source as well as an effective phosphate binder. However, the effect on acid–base homeostasis is very difficult to predict. Indeed, with progressive reduction in renal clearances, an increase in dialysis delivery has been complicated by alkalosis with attendant soft tissue calcification, hypoxaemia, kidney stones, etc., all of which may be significant problems.

The increasing use of intraperitoneal amino acids to supplement nutrition has been associated with the development of acidosis, impairing utilization of the amino acids. With refinements in the delivery of these supplements acidosis is now more effectively controlled (see below).

Growth factors

An improvement in nitrogen balance has been observed in many catabolic states with the use of recombinant human growth hormone. Its effect is thought to be due to induction of insulin-like growth factor-1, which promotes anabolism and reduces protein degradation. Although serum IGF-1 levels are low in uraemia, and animal studies suggest both receptor and post-receptor defects in IGF-1 action in uraemia, limited studies in CAPD patients have shown a short-term improvement in nitrogen balance following growth hormone treatment [248]. This benefit has been translated to a significant improvement in lean body mass [249].

Specific use of IGF-1 as nutritional support in malnourished patients on CAPD has additionally confirmed a positive benefit on nitrogen balance [250], which is not seen in healthy subjects [251].

However, as yet, no improvement in outcome has been observed as a consequence of growth factor use. To advocate such expensive therapy a clear benefit needs to be documented in ongoing prospective trials.

Intraperitoneal amino acids

Gjessing [252] first demonstrated absorption of amino acids from the peritoneal cavity in 1968. However, initial studies using amino acid-based dialysate were not shown to improve the abnormal plasma amino acid profile, which may have been due to a suboptimal dialysate amino acid profile or the lack of effective utilization of infused amino acids [253]. Modification of the amino acid-based dialysate to a solution containing an increased proportion of essential amino acids, arginine and branched-chain amino acids, in association with a lower alanine and glycine content, has resulted in improved utilization of amino acids, which again has translated into an improvement in nutritional parameters [254, 255]. Using this dialysate, the negative nitrogen balance is reversed, with improvement in the plasma lipoprotein levels and normalization of the plasma amino acid profile. In general, improvement in the nutritional state is best observed in patients whose malnutrition is due to inadequate nutrient intake, rather than in those with increased catabolism.

Although initial studies did not uniformly show an improvement in nutritional status as a consequence of intraperitoneal amino acid, more recent studies, utilizing an amino acid solution designed to have a decreased propensity to cause acidosis, have shown an improvement in nutritional state as measured by the serum albumin [256], blood urea and TBN concentrations, an increase in plasma proteins after amino acid-based dialysate [256–259], normalization of the amino acid profile [254, 259, 260] an improvement in nitrogen balance [254] and weight gain [254, 256]. If systemic acidosis develops as a consequence of intraperitoneal amino acid administration, this should be treated to prevent the negative impact on protein utilization [257, 259, 260]. This potential problem has decreased since the introduction of a 1.1% amino acid solution with an increased buffer from the standard of 35 mmol to 40 mmol lactate [255].

Kopple *et al.* prospectively studied nitrogen balance in 19 malnourished CAPD patients [260] treated with intraperitoneal amino acids. Following administration of amino acids a positive nitrogen balance in association with protein anabolism occurred. The fasting amino acid profile returned to normal, the greatest increase being observed in the essential amino acids. Total serum protein and transferrin concentrations significantly increased and serum albumin levels also tended to increase.

It has been reported that only severely malnourished patients benefit from the use of intraperitoneal amino acid [253] and in patients with lesser degrees of malnutrition, supplemental amino acids are less likely to confer benefit [261]. This finding has not been universal [255], but indeed cost considerations usually preclude their use in patients with lesser degrees of nutritional depletion which is usually responsive to oral supplementation. Any changes in the amino acid profile induced by intraperitoneal supplementation are manifest by day 10 of treatment [260], which is not suprising given that oral intake is reflected in the plasma profile within days [262].

Intraperitoneal amino acids appear to be most effectively utilized when administered after meals, as this provides concurrent energy, thereby maximizing protein synthesis, with no adverse effect on the plasma amino acid profile [257]. Nightly administration of amino acid-based dialysate has the disadvantage of no concurrent energy supply and hence poor utilization of the amino acids, in addition to a limited ultrafiltration capacity because of the rapid dissipation of the osmotic gradient in an overnight dwell. This was confirmed by Dombros *et al.* [253],

who demonstrated that no nutritional advantage was conferred after 12 weeks' nightly intraperitoneal administration of 1% amino acid. In this study TBN showed a tendency to fall, although not significantly, over the 12-week study period. This is consistent with the initially net negative nitrogen balance observed in haemodialysis patients supplemented with intradialytic parenteral nutrition [263], probably as a consequence of inadequate calories being concurrently administered. In contrast, afternoon administration of intraperitoneal amino acids appears to confer a benefit [256], although this is difficult to correlate in the absence of randomized studies assessing the relative benefits of different installation times.

The increased buffering capacity, and hence the biocompatibility of amino acid-based dialysate involves a theoretical risk of an increased number of episodes of peritonitis [264], but this has not been a clinically significant complication. The efficacy in ultrafiltration and small molecule clearance of a 1% amino acid solution has been estimated to be equivalent to that of a 1.36% dextrose solution [265]. Ultrafiltration capacity is limited in amino acid-based dialysate by the development of nitrogenous wastes, and therefore amino acids cannot be substituted for hypertonic glucose dialysate. Nausea, vomiting and associated appetite suppression have been reported as complications of the increased nitrogen load [253]. However, such symptoms generally develop in the setting of multiple exchanges of amino acid-based dialysate, or the use of dialysate containing more than 1.1% amino acids. Peritoneal membrane permeability has not been shown to be affected by the use of 1.1% amino acid-based dialysate. However, higher concentrations of amino acid may affect peritoneal permeability [266].

References

1. Pollock CA, Ibels LS, Zhu F-Y *et al.* Protein intake in renal disease. J Am Soc Nephrol 1997; 8: 777–83.
2. Mehrotra R, Saran R, Moore HL *et al.* Towards targets for initiation of chronic dialysis. Perit Dial Int 1997; 17: 497–508.
3. Ikizler TA, Greene JH, Wingard RL, Parker RA, Hakim RM. Spontaneous dietary protein intake during progression of chronic renal failure. J Am Soc Nephrol 1995; 6: 1386–91.
4. Fenton SSA, Johnston N, Delmore T *et al.* Nutritional assessment of continuous ambulatory peritoneal dialysis patients. Trans Am Soc Artif Intern Organs 1987; 33: 650–3.
5. Marckmann P. Nutritional status and mortality of patients in regular dialysis therapy. J Intern Med 1989; 226: 429–32.
6. Salusky IB, Fine RN, Nelson P. Factors affecting growth and nutritional status in children undergoing CAPD. Kidney Int 1984; 25: 260.
7. Rand WM, Uany R, Scrimshaw S, eds. Protein Energy Requirement in Developing Countries: Results of interna-

tional research. FAO/WHO/UNU. United Nations Bulletin, 1984 (suppl. 10): 327.

8. Tom K, Young VR, Chapman T, Masud T, Dixon A, Maroni BJ. Long-term adaptive responses to dietary protein restriction in chronic renal failure. Am J Physiol 1995; 268: E668–77.

9. Klahr S, Levey AS, Beck GJ et al. For the Modification of Diet in Renal Disease Study Group: The effects of dietary protein restriction and blood pressure control on the progression of renal disease. N Engl J Med 1994; 330: 877–84.

10. Jacobson HR, Striker GE. Report on a workshop to develop management recommendations for the prevention of progression in chronic renal disease. Am J Kidney Dis 1995; 25: 103–6.

11. Nissenson AR. Dialysis therapy in the elderly patient. Kidney Int 1993 (suppl. 40): S51–7.

12. Piccoli G, Bonello F, Massara C et al. Death in conditions of cachexia: the price for the dialysis treatment of the elderly? Kidney Int 1993 (suppl. 41): S282–6.

13. Pollock CA, Ibels LS, Allen BJ et al. Total body nitrogen as a prognostic marker in maintenance dialysis. J Am Soc Nephrol 1995; 6: 82–8.

14. Ritz E, Vallance P, Nowicki M. The effect of malnutrition on cardiovascular mortality in dialysis patients: is L-arginine the answer? Nephrol Dial Transplant 1994; 9: 129–30.

15. Maiorca R, Cancarini GC, Brunori G, Camerini C, Manili L. Morbidity and mortality of CAPD and hemodialysis. Kidney Int 1993 (suppl. 40): S4–15.

16. Lowrie EG, Lew NL. Death risk in hemodialysis patients: the predictive value of commonly measured variables and an evaluation of death rate differences between facilities. Am J Kidney Dis 1990; 15: 458–82.

17. Bilbrey G, Cohen T. Identification and treatment of protein calorie malnutrition in chronic haemodialysis patients. Dial Transplant 1989; 18: 669–700.

18. Guarnieri G, Toigo G, Situlin R et al. Muscle biopsy studies in chronically uremic patients: evidence for malnutrition. Kidney Int 1983 (suppl. 16): S187–93.

19. Jacob V, LeCarpentier JE, Salzano S et al. IGF-1, a marker of undernutrition in hemodialysis patients. Am J Clin Nutr 1990; 52: 39–44.

20. Hakim RM, Levin N. Malnutrition in hemodialysis patients. Am J Kidney Dis 1993; 21: 125–37.

21. Young GA, Kopple JD, Lindholm B et al. Nutritional assessment of continuous ambulatory peritoneal dialysis patients: an international study. Am J Kidney Dis 1991; 17: 462–71.

22. Marckmann P. Nutritional status of patients on hemodialysis and peritoneal dialysis. Clin Nephrol 1988; 29: 75–8.

23. Nelson EE, Hong CD, Pesce AL, Peterson DW, Singh SE, Pollak VE. Anthropometric norms for the dialysis population. Am J Kidney Dis 1990; 16: 32–7.

24. Cianciaruso B, Brunori G, Kopple JD et al. Cross-sectional comparison of malnutrition in continuous ambulatory peritoneal dialysis and hemodialysis patients. Am J Kidney Dis 1995; 26: 475–86.

25. Blake PG, Flowerdew G, Blake RM, Oreopoulos DG. Serum albumin in patients on continuous ambulatory peritoneal dialysis – predictors and correlations with outcomes. J Am Soc Nephrol 1993; 3: 1501–7.

26. Harty J, Boulton H, Heelis N, Uttley L, Venning M, Gokal R. Limitations of kinetic models as predictors of nutritional and dialysis adequacy in continuous ambulatory peritoneal dialysis patients. Am J Nephrol 1993; 13: 454–63.

27. Churchill DN, Taylor DW, Keshaviah PR. Adequacy of dialysis and nutrition in continuous peritoneal dialysis: association with clinical outcomes. J Am Soc Nephrol 1996; 7: 198–207.

28. Flanigan MJ, Bailie GR, Frankenfield DL, Frederick PR, Prowant BF, Rocco MV. 1996 peritoneal dialysis core indicators study: report on nutritional indicators. Perit Dial Int 1998; 18: 489–96.

29. Acchiardo SR, Moore LW, Latour PA. Malnutrition as the main factor in morbidity and mortality of hemodialysis patients. Kidney Int 1983 (suppl. 16): S199–203.

30. Degoulet P. Legrain M, Reach I et al. Mortality risk factors in patients treated by chronic hemodialysis. Report of the Diaphane collaborative study. Nephron 1982; 31: 103–10.

31. Avram MM, Goldwasser P, Erroa M, Fein PA. Predictors of survival in continuous ambulatory peritoneal dialysis patients: the importance of prealbumin and other nutritional and metabolic markers. Am J Kidney Dis 1994; 23: 91–8.

32. Teehan BP, Schleifer CR, Brown JM, Sigler MH, Raimondo J. Urea kinetic analysis and clinical outcome in CAPD. A 5 year longitudinal study. Adv Perit Dial 1990; 6: 181–5.

33. Spiegel DM, Breyer JA. Serum albumin: a predictor of long-term outcome in peritoneal dialysis patients. Am J Kidney Dis 1994; 23: 283–5.

34. Avram MM, Fein PA, Bonomini L et al. Predictors of survival in continuous ambulatory peritoneal dialysis patients: a five year prospective study. Perit Dial Int 1996; 16 (suppl. 1): S190–4.

35. Fung L, Pollock CA, Caterson RJ et al. Dialysis adequacy and nutrition determine prognosis in CAPD patients. J Am Soc Nephrol 1996; 7: 1–8.

36. Pollock CA, Ibels LS, Allen BJ. Nutritional markers and survival in maintenance dialysis patients. Nephron 1996; 74: 625–41.

37. DeFronzo RA, Alverstrand A, Smith D, Hendler R, Hendler E, Wahren J. Insulin resistance in uremia. J Clin Invest 1981; 67: 563–8.

38. Cade C, Norman AW. Vitamin D3 improves impaired glucose tolerance and insulin secretion in the vitamin D deficient rat *in vivo*. Endocrinology 1986; 119: 84–90.

39. Pollock CA, Ibels LS, Caterson RJ, Mahony JF, Waugh DA, Cocksedge B. Continuous ambulatory peritoneal dialysis: eight years of experience at a single center. Medicine 1989; 68: 293–308.

40. Heaton A, Johnston DG, Burrin JM et al. Carbohydrate and lipid metabolism during CAPD: the effect of a single dialysis cycle. Clin Sci 1983; 65: 539–45.

41. Mak RHK. Insulin resistance in uremia: effect of dialysis modality. Pediatr Res 1996; 40: 304–8.

42. Randerson DH, Chapman GV, Farrell PC. Amino acid and dietary status in CAPD patients. In: Atkins RC, Farrell PC, Thompson N, eds. Peritoneal Dialysis. Edinburgh: Churchill Livingstone, 1981, pp. 179–91.

43. Jones MR, Kopple JD. Valine metabolism in normal and chronically uremic man. Am J Clin Nutr 1978; 31: 1660–4.

44. Bergstrom J, Furst P, Noree LO, Vinnars E. Intracellular free amino acids in muscle tissue of patients with chronic uremia: effect of peritoneal dialysis and infusion of essential amino acid. Clin Sci Mol Med 1978; 54: 51–60.

45. Blumenkrantz M, Kopple J, Moran J. Metabolic balance studies and dietary protein requirements in CAPD. Kidney Int 1982; 21: 849–61.

46. Kraus LM, Kraus AP Jr. Tyrosine and N-carbamoyl-tyrosine in end-stage renal disease during continuous ambulatory peritoneal dialysis. J Lab Clin Med 1991; 118: 555–62.

47. Metcoff J, Dutta S, Burns G, Pederson J, Matter B, Rennert O. Effects of amino acid infusions on cell metabolism in hemodialyzed patients with uremia. Kidney Int 1983 (suppl. 16): S87–92.

48. Metcoff J. Malnutrition at the cellular level in uremia: a new frontier for research. J Am Coll Nutr 1986; 5: 229–41.

49. Lindholm B, Alverstrand A, Furst P, Bergstrom J. Plasma and muscle free amino acids during continuous ambulatory peritoneal dialysis. Kidney Int 1989; 35: 1219–26.

50. England BK, Chastain JL, Mitch WE. Abnormalities in protein synthesis and degradation induced by extracellular pH in BC3H1 myocytes. Am J Physiol 1991; 260: C277–82.

51. May RC, Kelly RA, Mitch WE. Metabolic acidosis stimulates protein degradation in rat muscle by a glucocorticoid dependent mechanism. J Clin Invest 1986; 77: 614–21.

52. Mitch WE, Medina R, Grieber S *et al.* Metabolic acidosis stimulates muscle protein degradation by activating the ATP-dependent pathway involving ubiquitin and proteasomes. J Clin Invest 1994; 93: 2127–33.

53. Reaich D, Channon SM, Scrimgeour CM, Daley SE, Wilkinson R, Goodship THJ. Correction of acidosis in humans with CRF decreases protein degradation and amino acid oxidation. Am J Physiol 1993; 265: E230–5.

54. Ballmer PE, McNurlan MA, Hulter HN, Anderson SE, Garlick PJ, Krapf R. Chronic metabolic acidosis decreases albumin synthesis and induces negative nitrogen balance in humans. J Clin Invest 1995; 95: 39–45.

55. Graham KA, Reaich D, Channon SM *et al.* Correction of acidosis in CAPD decreases whole body protein degradation. Kidney Int 1996; 49: 1396–400.

56. Long CL, Dillard DR, Bodzin JH, Geiger JW, Blakemore WS. Validity of 3-methylhistidine as an indicator of skeletal muscle protein breakdown in humans. Metabolism 1988; 37: 844–9.

57. Schreiber M, Kalhan S, McCullough A, Savin . Branched amino acid metabolism in chronic renal failure and hemodialysis. Proc EDTA-ERA 1985; 22: 116–20.

58. Stein A, Moorhouse J, Iles-Smith H *et al.* Role of an improvement in acid–base status and nutrition in CAPD patients. Kidney Int 1997; 52: 1089–95.

59. Williams AJ, Dittmer ID, McArley A, Clarke J. High bicarbonate dialysis in haemodialysis patients: effects on acidosis and nutritional status. Nephrol Dial Transplant 1997; 12: 2633–7.

60. Kang SW, Lee SW, Lee IH *et al.* Impact of metabolic acidosis on serum albumin and other nutritional parameters in long-term CAPD patients. Adv Perit Dial 1997; 13: 249–52.

61. Lysaght MJ, Pollock CA, Hallet MD, Ibels LS, Farrell PC. The relevance of urea kinetic modelling to CAPD. Trans Am Soc Artif Intern Org 1989; 35: 784–90.

62. Keshaviah PR, Nolph KD, Prowant B *et al.* Defining adequacy of CAPD with urea kinetics. Adv Perit Dial 1990; 6: 173–7.

63. Acchiardo SR, Kraus AP, LaHatte G, Kaufman PA, Adkins D, Moore LW. Urea kinetics evaluation of hemodialysis and CAPD patients. Adv Perit Dial 1992; 8: 55–8.

64. Nolph KD, Moore HL, Prowant B, Meyer M *et al.* Cross sectional assessment of weekly urea and creatinine clearances and indices of nutrition in continuous ambulatory peritoneal dialysis patients. Perit Dial Int 1993; 13: 178–83.

65. Blake PG, Sombolos K, Abraham G *et al.* Lack of correlation between urea kinetic indices and clinical outcome in CAPD patients. Kidney Int 1991; 39: 700–6.

66. Blake PG, Balaskas EV, Izatt S, Oreopoulos DG. Is total creatinine clearance a good predictor of clinical outcomes in continuous ambulatory peritoneal dialysis. Perit Dial Int 1992; 12: 353–8.

67. Murata GH, Tzamaloukas AH, Malhotra D *et al.* Protein catabolic rate in patients on continuous peritoneal dialysis. ASAIO J 1996; 42: 46–51.

68. Blake PG. The problem of mathematical coupling: how can statistical artefact and biological causation be separated when relating protein intake to clearance in 'predialysis' and dialysis patients. Perit Dial Int 1997; 17: 431–4.

69. Lowrie EG. Thoughts about judging dialysis treatments: mathematics and measurements, mirrors in the mind. Semin Nephrol 1996; 16: 242–62.

70. Harty J, Faragher B, Venning M, Gokal R. Urea kinetic modeling exaggerates the relationship between nutrition and dialysis in CAPD patients (the hazards of cross-sectional analysis). Perit Dial Int 1995; 15: 105–9.

71. Tzamaloukas AH, Murata GH, Malhotra D, Fox L. Predictors of serum albumin in CAPD. Perit Dial Int 1995; 15 (suppl. 4): S10.

72. Lo WK, Jiang Y, Cheng SW, Cheng IKP. Survival of CAPD patients in a center using three two-litre exchanges as a standard regime. Perit Dial Int 1996; 16 (suppl. 1): S163–6.

73. Lindsay RM, Spanner E. A hypothesis: the protein catabolic rate is dependent upon the type and amount of treatment in dialysed uremic patients. Am J Kidney Dis 1989; 13: 382–9.

74. Lindsay RM, Spanner E, Heidenheim RP *et al.* Which comes first, *Kt/V* or PCR – chicken or egg? Kidney Int 1992 (suppl. 38): S32–6.

75. Gotch F. A positive correlation of PCRN to *Kt/V* in cross sectional studies is not proof of a causal relationship. Perit Dial Int 1995; 15: 274–85.

76. Harty J, Boulton H, Faragher B, Venning M, Gokal R. The influence of small solute clearance on dietary protein intake in continuous ambulatory peritoneal dialysis patients: a methodologic analysis based on cross-sectional and prospective studies. Am J Kidney Dis 1996; 28: 553–60.

77. Williams P, Jones J. Marriot J. Do increases in dialysis dose in CAPD lead to nutritional improvement? Nephrol Dial Transplant 1994; 9: 1841–2.

78. Heimburger O, Traneous A, Bergstrom J *et al.* The effect of increasing peritoneal dialysis on *Kt/V*, protein catabolic rate and serum albumin. Perit Dial Int 1992; 12 (suppl. 1): S19 (abstract).

79. Tattersall J. Greenwood R, Farrington K. Urea kinetics and when to commence dialysis. Am J Nephrol 1995; 15: 283–9.

80. Lutes R, Holley JL, Perlmutter J, Piraino B. Correlation of normalised protein catabolic rate to weekly creatinine clearance and *Kt/V* in patients on peritoneal dialysis. Adv Perit Dial 1993; 9: 97–100.

81. Lysaght MJ, Vonesh E, Gotch F *et al.* CA, Prowant B, Farrell P. The influence of dialysis treatment modality on the decline of remaining renal function. ASAIO J 1991; 37: 598–604.

82. Schmidt RJ. Residual renal function in peritoneal dialysis patients. Semin Dial 1995; 8: 343–6.

83. Kagan A, Bar-Khayim Y. Role of peritoneal loss of albumin in the hypoalbuminemia of continuous ambulatory peritoneal dialysis patients: relationship to peritoneal transport of solutes. Nephron 1995; 71: 314–20.

84. Kagan A, Bar-Khayim Y, Schafer Z, Fainaru M. Heterogeneity in peritoneal transport during continuous ambulatory peritoneal dialysis and its impact on ultrafiltration, loss of macromolecules and plasma levels of proteins, lipids and lipoproteins. Nephron 1993; 63: 32–42.

85. Nolph KD. Clinical implications of membrane transport characteristics on the adequacy of fluid and solute removal. Perit Dial Int 1994; 14: 78–82.

86. Davies SJ, Bryan J, Phillips L, Russell GI. The predictive value of *Kt/V* and peritoneal solute transport in CAPD patients is dependent on the type of comorbidity present. Perit Dial Int 1996; 16 (suppl. 1): S158–62.

87. Davies SJ, Russe L, Bryan J, Phillips L, Russell GI. Co-morbidity, urea kinetics, and appetite in continuous ambulatory peritoneal dialysis patients: their interrelationship and prediction of survival. Am J Kidney Dis 1995; 26: 353–61.

88. Harty JC, Boulton H, Venning MC, Gokal R. Is peritoneal permeability an adverse risk factor for malnutrition in CAPD patients. Miner Electrolyte Metab 1996; 22: 97–101.

89. Burkart JM. Effect of peritoneal dialysis prescription and peritoneal membrane transport characteristics on nutritional status. Perit Dial Int 1995; 15: S20–35.

90. Himmelfarb J, Holbrook D, McMonagle E, Robinson R, Nye L, Spratt D. *Kt/V*, nutritional parameters, serum cortisol and insulin growth factor-1 levels and patient outcome in hemodialysis. Am J Kidney Dis 1994; 24: 473–9.

91. Verger MF, Verger C, Hatt-Magnien D, Perrone F. Relationship between thyroid hormones and nutrition in chronic renal failure. Nephron 1987; 45: 211–15.

92. Krieg J Jr, Santos F, Chan JCM. Growth hormone, insulin-like growth factor and the kidney. Kidney Int 1995; 48: 321–36.

93. Blake PG. Growth hormone and malnutrition in dialysis patients. Perit Dial Int 1995; 15: 210–16.

94. Fouque D, Peng SC, Kopple JD. Pharmacokinetics of recombinant human insulin-like growth factor-1 in dialysis patients. Kidney Int 1995; 47: 869–75.

95. Kagan A, Altman Y, Zadik Z, Bar-Khayim Y. Insulin-like growth factor–1 in patients on CAPD and hemodialysis: relationship to body weight and albumin level. Adv Perit Dial 1995; 11: 234–8.

96. Tonshoff B, Blum WF, Wingen AM, Mehls O. Serum insulin-like growth factors (IGFs) and IGF binding proteins 1, 2, and 3 in children with chronic renal failure: relationship to height and glomerular filtration rate. The European Study Group for Nutritional Treatment of Chronic Renal Failure in Childhood. J Clin Endocrinol Metab 1995; 80: 2684–91.

97. Kale AS, Liu F, Hintz RL et al. Characterisation of insulin-like growth factors and their binding proteins in peritoneal dialysate. Pediatr Nephrol 1996; 10: 467–73.

98. Chan W, Valerie KC, Chan JCM. Expression of insulin-like growth factor-1 in uremic rats: growth hormone resistance and nutritional intake. Kidney Int 1993; 43: 790–5.

99. Tonshoff B, Eden S, Weiser E et al. Reduced hepatic growth hormone (GH) receptor gene expression and increased plasma GH binding protein in experimental uremia. Kidney Int 1994; 45: 1085–92.

100. Challa A, Chan W, Krieg RJ Jr et al. Effect of metabolic acidosis on the expression of insulin-like growth factor and growth hormone receptor. Kidney Int 1993; 44: 1224–7.

101. Coles GA. Towards a more physiologic solution for peritoneal dialysis. Semin Dial 1995; 8: 333–5.

102. Topley N. The cytokine network controlling peritoneal inflammation. Perit Dial Int 1995; 15 (suppl. 7): S35–40.

103. Balaskas EV, Bamihas GI, Tourkantonis A. Cytokines (Cys) and C-reactive protein (CRP) in CAPD patients. Perit Dial Int 1998; 18: 85–6.

104. Bergstrom J, Lindholm B. Malnutrition, cardiac disease and mortality: integrated point of view. Am J Kidney Dis 1998; 32: 834–41.

105. Stenvinkel P, Heimburger O, Paultre F et al. Strong association between malnutrition, inflammation and atherosclerosis in chronic renal failure. Kidney Int 1999; 55 (in press).

106. Dombros NV, Digenis GE, Oreopoulos DG. Is malnutrition a problem for the patient on peritoneal dialysis: nutritional markers as predictors of survival in patients on CAPD. Perit Dial Int 1995; 15: S10–29.

107. Struijk DG, Krediet RT, Koomen GC, Boeschoten EW, Arisz L. The effect of serum albumin at the start of continuous ambulatory peritoneal dialysis treatment on patient survival. Perit Dial Int 1994; 14: 121–6.

108. Keane WF, Collins AJ. Influence of comorbidity on mortality and morbidity in patients treated with hemodialysis. Am J Kidney Dis 1994; 24: 1010–18.

109. Foley RN, Parfrey PS, Harnett JD, Kent GM, Murray DC, Barre PE. Hypoalbuminaemia, cardiac morbidity, and mortality in end stage renal disease. J Am Soc Nephrol 1996; 7: 728–36.

110. Bergstrom J, Heimburger O, Lindholm B, Qureshi AR. Elevated serum C-reactive protein is a strong predictor of increased mortality and low serum albumin in hemodialysis patients. J Am Soc Nephrol 1995; 6: 588.

111. McIntyre C, Harper I, Macdougall IC, Raine AEG, Williams A, Baker LRI. Serum C-reactive protein as a marker for infection and inflammation in regular dialysis patients. Clin Nephrol 1997; 48: 371–4.

112. Han DS, Lee SW, Kang SW et al. Factors affecting low values of serum albumin in CAPD patients. Adv Perit Dial 1996; 12: 288–92.

113. Kaysen GA, Yeun J, Depner T. Albumin synthesis, catabolism and distribution in dialysis patients. Miner Electrolyte Metab 1997; 23: 218–24.

114. Schaubel DE, Morrison HI, Fenton SSA. Comparing mortality rates on CAPD/CCPD and hemodialysis: the Canadian experience. Perit Dial Int 1998; 18: 478–84.

115. Keshaviah PR, Nolph KD, Van Stone JC. The peak concentration hypothesis: a urea kinetic approach to comparing the adequacy of continuous ambulatory peritoneal dialysis and hemodialysis. Perit Dial Int 1989; 9: 257–60.

116. Jones MR. Etiology of severe malnutrition: results of an international cross-sectional study in continuous ambulatory peritoneal dialysis patients. Am J Kidney Dis 1994; 23: 412–20.

117. Haire HM, Sherrard DJ, Scardapane D, Curtis FK, Brunzell JD. Smoking, hypertension, and mortality in a maintenance dialysis population. Cardiovasc Med 1978; 3: 1163–8.

118. Burton PR, Walls J. Selection-adjusted comparison of life-expectancy of patients on continuous ambulatory peritoneal dialysis, haemodialysis and renal transplantation. Lancet 1987; 1: 1115–19.

119. Davies SJ, Russell L, Bryan J, Phillips L, Russell GI. Impact of peritoneal absorption of glucose on appetite, protein catabolism and survival in CAPD patients. Clin Nephrol 1996; 45: 194–8.

120. Goodship TH, Lloyd S, Clague MB, Bartlett K, Ward MK, Wilkinson R. Whole body leucine turnover and nutritional status in continuous ambulatory peritoneal dialysis. Clin Sci 1987; 73: 463–9.

121. Berkelhammer CH, Baker JP, Leiter LA et al. Whole-body protein turnover in adult hemodialysis patients as measured by ^{13}C-leucine. Am J Clin Nutr 1987; 46: 778–83.

122. Williams P, Kay R, Harrison J et al. Nutritional and anthropometric assessment of patients on CAPD over one year: contrasting changes in total body nitrogen and potassium. Perit Dial Bull 1981; 1: 82–7.

123. Lindner A, Charra B, Sherrard DJ, Scribner BH. Accelerated atherosclerosis in prolonged maintenance hemodialysis. N Engl J Med 1974; 290: 697–701.

124. Pollock CA, Ibels LS, Ong CS, Caterson RJ, Waugh DA, Mahony JF. Lipoprotein(a): relationship to vascular disease in dialysis and renal transplantation. Nephrology 1995; 1: 213–20.

125. Lindholm B, Norbeck HE. Serum lipids and lipoproteins during continuous ambulatory peritoneal dialysis. Acta Med Scand 1986; 220: 143–51.

126. Avram MM, Goldwasser P, Burrell DE, Antignani A, Fein PA, Mittman N. The uremic dyslipidemia: a cross-sectional and longitudinal study. Am J Kidney Dis 1992; 20: 324–35.

127. Kagan AK, Bar-Khayim Y, Schafer Z, Fainaru M. Kinetics of peritoneal protein loss during CAPD: 11. Lipoprotein leakage and its impact on plasma lipid levels. Kidney Int 1990; 37: 980–90.

128. Ramos JM, Heaton A, McGurk JG, Ward MK, Kerr DNS. Sequential changes in serum lipids and their subfractions in patients receiving continuous ambulatory peritoneal dialysis. Nephron 1983; 35: 20–3.

129. Sniderman A, Cianflone K, Kwiterovich PO, Hutchinson T, Barre P, Prichard S. Hyperapobetalipoproteinemia: the major dyslipoproteinemia in patients with chronic renal failure treated with chronic ambulatory peritoneal dialysis. Atherosclerosis 1987; 65: 257–64.

130. Fuchs C, Armstrong VW, Cremer P et al. An investigation of the lipoprotein profiles of patients on hemofiltration as compared to those on hemodialysis and intermittent peritoneal dialysis. Contrib Nephrol 1982; 32: 92–6.

131. Cantaluppi A, Scalamogna A, Guerra L, Graziani G, Ponticelli C. Plasma lipid and lipoprotein levels in patients treated with CAPD. Perit Dial Bull 1982; 2: 99.

132. Wessel-Aas T, Blomhoff JP, Wideroe TE, Wirum E, Nilsen T. The effect of systemic heparinization on plasma lipoproteins and toxicity in patients on hemodialysis and continuous ambulatory peritoneal dialysis. Acta Med Scand 1984; 216: 85–92.

133. Roxe DM, del Greco F, Hughes J et al. Hemodialysis vs. peritoneal dialysis: results of a 3-year prospective controlled study. Kidney Int 1981; 19: 341–8.

134. Bartens W, Nauck M, Schollmeyer P, Wanner C. Elevated lipoprotein (a) and fibrogen levels increase the cardiovascular risk in continuous ambulatory peritoneal dialysis patients. Perit Dial Int 1996; 16: 27–33.

135. Brown A, Dusso A, Slatopolsky E. Vitamin D. In: Seldin DE, Giebisch G, eds. The Kidney: physiology and pathophysiology. New York: Raven Press, 1992, pp. 1505–52.

136. Massry SG. Parathyroid hormone: a uremic toxin. In: Ringoir S, Vanholder R, Massry SG, eds. Uremic Toxins. New York: Plenum Press, 1987, pp. 1–17.

137. Perna AF, Smogorzewski M, Massry SG. Verapamil reverses PTH- or CRF-induced abnormal fatty acid oxidation in muscle. Kidney Int 1988; 34: 774–8.

138. Gilmour ER, Hartley GH, Goodship THJ. Trace elements and vitamins in renal disease. In: Mitch E, Klahr S, eds. Nutrition and the Kidney. Boston: Little, Brown, 1993, pp. 114–31.

139. Thomson MM, Stevens BJ, Humphrey TJ, Atkins RC. Comparison of trace elements in peritoneal dialysis, hemodialysis and uremia. Kidney Int 1983; 23: 9–14.

140. Wallaeys B, Cornelis R, Mees L, Lameire N. Trace elements in serum, packed cells and dialysate of CAPD patients. Kidney Int 1986; 30: 599–604.

141. Girelli D, Olivieri O, Stanzial AM et al. Low platelet glutathione peroxidase activity and serum selenium concentration in patients with chronic renal failure: relations to dialysis treatments, diet and cardiovascular complications. Clin Sci 1993; 84: 611–17.

142. Dworkin B, Weseley S, Rosenthal WS, Schwartz EM, Weiss L. Diminished blood selenium levels in renal failure patients on dialysis: Correlations with nutritional status. Am J Med Sci 1987; 293: 6–12.

143. Wolk R. Micronutrition in dialysis. Nutr Clin Pract 1993; 8: 267–76.

144. van Guldener C, Janssen MJFM, Lambert J, ter Wee PM, Donker AJM, Stehouwer CDA. Folic acid treatment of hyperhomocysteinemia in peritoneal dialysis patients: no change in endothelial function after long-term therapy. Perit Dial Int 1998; 18: 282–9.

145. Bostom AG, Shemin D, Verhoef P et al. Elevated fasting total plasma homocysteine levels and cardiovascular disease outcomes in maintenance dialysis patients: a prospective study. Arteriosclerosis Thromb Vasc Biol 1997; 17: 2554–8.

146. Moustapha A, Naso A, Nahlawi M et al. Prospective study of hyperhomocysteinemia as an adverse cardiovascular risk factor in end-stage renal disease. Circulation 1998; 97: 138–41.

147. Moorthy AW, Rosenblum M, Rajaram R, Shug AL. A comparison of plasma and muscle carnitine levels in patients on peritoneal and hemodialysis for chronic renal failure. Am J Nephrol 1983; 3: 205–8.

148. Blake PG. A review of the DOQI recommendations for peritoneal dialysis. Perit Dial Int 1998; 18: 247–51.

149. Krantzler NJ, Mullen BJ, Schutz HG, Grivetti LE, Holden CA, Meiselman HL. Validity of telephoned diet recalls and records for assessment of individual food intake. Am J Clin Nutr 1982; 36: 1234–42.

150. Gersovitz M, Madden JP, Smiciklas-Wright H. Validity of the 24-hour dietary recall and seven day food record for group comparisons. J Am Diet Assoc 1978; 73: 48–55.

151. Karvetti RL, Knuts L-R. Validity of the estimated food diary: comparison of 2-day recorded and observed food and nutrient intakes. J Am Diet Assoc 1992; 92: 580–4.

152. Gahl GM, Baeyer HV, Averdunk R et al. Outpatient evaluation of dietary intake and nitrogen removal in continuous ambulatory peritoneal dialysis. Ann Intern Med 1981; 94: 643–6.

153. Fidanza F. Sources of error in dietary servings. Bibl Nutr Dieta 1974; 20: 105–13.

154. Owen WF, Lew NL, Liu Y, Lowrie EG, Lazarus JM. The urea reduction ratio and serum albumin concentration as predictors of mortality in patients undergoing hemodialysis. N Engl J Med 1993; 329: 1001–6.

155. Herman FR, Safran C, Levkoff SE, Minaker KL. Serum albumin level on admission as a predictor of death, length of stay and readmission. Arch Intern Med 1992; 152: 125–130.

156. Spiegel DM, Anderson M, Campbell U et al. Serum albumin: a marker for morbidity in peritoneal dialysis patients. Am J Kidney Dis 1993; 21: 26–30.

157. Marcus RG, Chaing E, Dimaano F, Uribarri J. Serum albumin associations and significance in peritoneal dialysis. Adv Perit Dial 1994; 10: 94–8.

158. Blagg CR, Liedtke RJ, Batjer JD et al. Serum albumin concentration-related Health Care Financing Administration quality assurance criterion is method-dependent: revision is necessary. Am J Kidney Dis 1993; 21: 138–44.

159. Bianchi R, Mariani G, Pilo A. Albumin synthesis measurements by means of an improved two tracer method in patients with chronic renal failure. J Nucl Biol Med 1970; 14: 136.

160. Fleck A. Computer models for metabolic studies on plasma proteins. Ann Clin Biochem 1985; 22: 33–49.

161. Kaysen OA, Schoenfeld PY. Aluminum homeostasis in patients undergoing continuous ambulatory peritoneal dialysis. Kidney Int 1984; 25: 107–14.

162. Lunn PG. Nutritional aspects of plasma protein metabolic studies: protein-energy malnutrition. In: Mariani G, ed. Pathophysiology of Plasma Protein Metabolism. London: Macmillan, 1984, pp. 299–324.

163. Fine A, Cox D. Modest reduction of serum albumin in continuous ambulatory peritoneal dialysis is common and of no apparent clinical consequence. Am J Kidney Dis 1992; 20: 50–4.

164. de Fijter CWH, Oe LP, de Frijter WM, van den Meulen J, Donker AJM, de Vries PMJM. Is serum albumin a marker for nutritional status in dialysis patients? J Am Soc Nephrol 1993; 4: 402.

165. Schoenfeld PY. Is the lower serum albumin concentration in CAPD a reflection of nutritional status? Albumin is an unreliable marker of nutritional status. Semin Dial 1992; 5: 218–23.

166. Heimburger O, Bergstrom J, Lindholm B. Albumin and amino acid levels as markers of adequacy in continuous ambulatory peritoneal dialysis. Perit Dial Int 1994; 14 (suppl. 3): S123–32.

167. Held PJ. US incidence, prevalence and survival in ESRD and diabetes. Report of the USRDS, 12th Annual Conference on Peritoneal Dialysis, Seattle, 1992.

168. Young GA, Young JB, Young SM et al. Nutrition and delayed hypersensitivity during continuous ambulatory peritoneal dialysis in relation to peritonitis. Nephron 1986; 43: 177–86.

169. Germain M, Harlow P, Mulhern G, Lipkowitz G, Braden G. Low protein catabolic rate and serum albumin correlate with increased mortality and abdominal complications in peritoneal dialysis patients. Adv Perit Dial 1992; 8: 113–15.

170. Steinman TI, Mitch WE. Nutrition in dialysis patients. In: Maher JF, ed. Replacement of Renal Function by Dialysis. Boston: Kluwer, 1989, pp. 1088–106.

171. Diaz-Buxo JA. Is continuous ambulatory peritoneal dialysis adequate long-term therapy for end-stage renal disease? A critical assessment. J Am Soc Nephrol 1992; 3: 1039–48.

172. Hylander B, Barkeling B, Rossner S. Eating behaviour in continuous ambulatory peritoneal dialysis and hemodialysis patients. Am J Kidney Dis 1992; 20: 592–7.

173. Avram MM, Mittman N, Bonomini L, Chattopadhyay J, Fein P. Markers for survival in dialysis. Am J Kidney Dis 1995; 26: 209–19.

174. Kaufmann P, Smolle KH, Horina JH, Zach R, Krejs GJ. Impact of long term hemodialysis on nutritional state in patient with end stage renal failure. Clin Invest 1994; 72: 754–61.

175. Zhang Y, Proenca R, Maffei M, Barone M, Leopold L, Friedman JM. Positional cloning of the mouse obese gene and its human homologue. Nature 1994; 372: 425–32.

176. Halaas JL, Gajiwala KS, Maffei M *et al.* Weight-reducing effects of the plasma protein encoded by the obese gene. Science 1995; 269: 543–6.

177. Pelleymounter MA, Cullen MJ, Baker MB *et al.* Effects of the obese gene product on body weight regulation in ob/ob mice. Science 1995; 269: 540–3.

178. Lonnqvist F, Arner P, Nordfors L, Schalling M. Overexpression of the obese (ob) gene in adipose tissue of human obese subjects. Nature Med 1995; 1: 950–3.

179. Hamilton BS, Paglia D, Kwan AY, Deitel M. Increased obese mRNA expression in omental fat cells from massively obese humans. Nature Med 1995; 1: 953–6.

180. Considine RV, Sinha MK, Heiman ML *et al.* Serum immunoreactive-leptin concentrations in normal-weight and obese humans. N Engl J Med 1996; 334: 292–5.

181. Young GA, Woodrow G, Kendall S *et al.* Increased plasma leptin/fat ratio in patients with chronic renal failure: a cause of malnutrition? Nephrol Dial Transplant 1997; 12: 2318–23.

182. Howard JK, Lord GM, Clutterbuck EJ, Ghatei MA, Pusey CD, Bloom SR. Plasma immunoreactive leptin concentration in end-stage renal disease. Clin Sci 1997; 93: 119–26.

183. Dagogo-Jack S, Ovalle F, Landt M, Gearing B, Coyne DW. Hyperleptinemia in patients with end-stage renal disease undergoing continuous ambulatory peritoneal dialysis. Perit Dial Int 1998; 18: 34–40.

184. Sharma K, Considine RV, Michael B *et al.* Plasma leptin is partly cleared by the kidney and is elevated in hemodialysis patients. Kidney Int 1997: 51: 1980–5.

185. Pollock CA, Allen BJ, Warden RA *et al.* Total-body nitrogen by neutron activation in maintenance dialysis. Am J Kidney Dis 1990; 26: 38–45.

186. Rayner HC, Stroud DB, Salamon KM *et al.* Anthropometry underestimates body protein depletion in hemodialysis patients. Nephron 1991; 59: 33–40.

187. Farrell PC, Hone PW. Dialysis induced catabolism. Am J Clin Nutr 1980; 33: 1417–22.

188. Maroni BJ, Steinman TI, Mitch WE. A method for estimating nitrogen intake of patients with chronic renal failure. Kidney Int 1985; 27: 58–65.

189. Mitch WE, Walser M. Nutritional therapy of the uremic patient. In: Brenner BM, Rector FC, eds. The Kidney, 3rd edn. Philadelphia: Saunders, 1986, pp. 1759–90.

190. Bergstrom J, Heimburger O, Lindholm B. Calculation of the protein equivalent of total nitrogen appearance from urea appearance. Which formulas should be used? Perit Dial Int 1998; 18: 467–73.

191. Keshaviah P, Nolph KD. Protein catabolic rate calculations in CAPD patients. ASAIO Trans 1991; 37: M400–2.

192. Usha K, Moore HL, Nolph KD. Protein catabolic rate in CAPD patients: comparison of different techniques. Adv Perit Dial 1996; 12: 284–7.

193. Kopple JD, Jones MR, Keshaviah PR *et al.* A proposed glossary for dialysis kinetics. Am J Kidney Dis 1995; 26: 963–81.

194. Panzetta G, Tessitore N, Faccini G, Maschio G. The protein catabolic rate as a measure of protein intake in dialysis patients: usefulness and limits. Nephrol Dial Transplant 1990; 5 (suppl. 1): 125–7.

195. Goldstein DJ, Frederico CB. The effect of urea kinetic modeling on the nutrition management of hemodialysis patients. J Am Diet Assoc 1987; 87: 474–9.

196. Harty JC, Boulton H, Curwell J *et al.* The normalised protein catabolic rate is a flawed marker of nutrition in CAPD patients. Kidney Int 1994; 45: 103–9.

197. Virga G, Viglino G, Gandolfo C, Aloi E, Cavalli PL. Normalization of protein equivalent of nitrogen appearance and dialytic adequacy in CAPD. Perit Dial Int 1996; 16 (suppl. 1): S185–9.

198. Canaud B, Leblanc M, Garred LJ, Bosc J-Y, Argiles A, Mion C. Protein catabolic rate over lean body mass ratio: a more rational approach to normalise the protein catabolic rate in dialysis patients. Am J Kidney Dis 1997; 30: 672–9.

199. Cornish BH, Thomas BJ, Ward LC. Improved prediction of extracellular and total body water of rats using impedance loci generated by multiple frequency bioelectrical impedance analysis. Phys Med Biol 1993; 38: 337–46.

200. Lukaski HC, Bolonchuk WW, Hall CA, Siders WA. Estimation of fat free mass in humans using the bioelectrical impedance method: a validation study. J Appl Physiol 1986; 60: 1327–32.

201. de Fijter CWH, de Fitjer MM, Oe LP, Donker AJM, de Vries PMJM. The impact of hydration status on the assessment of lean body mass by body electrical impedance in dialysis patients. Adv Perit Dial 1993; 9: 101–4.

202. Nielsen PK, Ladefoged J, Olgaard K. Lean body mass by dual energy X-ray absorptiometry (DEXA) and by urine and dialysate creatinine recovery in CAPD and pre-dialysis patients compared to normal subjects. Adv Perit Dial 1994; 10: 99–103.

203. Woodrow G, Oldroyd B, Turney JH, Davies PS, Day JM, Smith MA. Measurement of total body water and urea kinetic modelling in peritoneal dialysis. Clin Nephrol 1997; 47: 52–7.

204. Bergia R, Bellini ME, Valenti M *et al.* Dionisio P, Pellerey M, Bajardi P. Longitudinal assessment of body composition in continuous ambulatory peritoneal dilaysis patients using bioelectrical impedence and anthropometric measurement. Perit Dial Int 1993; 13 (suppl. 2): S512–4.

205. de Fijter WM, de Fijter CW, Oe PL, ter Wee PM, Donker AJ. Assessment of total body water and lean body mass from anthropometry, Watson formula, creatinine kinetics, and body electrical impedence compared with antipyrine kinetics in peritoneal dialysis patients. Nephrol Dial Transplant 1997; 12: 151–6.

206. Stall S, Ginsberg NS, Lynn RI, Zabetakis PM. Bioelectrical impedence analysis and dual energy X-ray absorptiometry to monitor nutritional status. Perit Dial Int 1995; 15 (suppl. 5): 59–62.

207. Schmidt R, Dumler F, Cruz C, Lubkowski T, Kilates C. Improved nutritional follow-up of peritoneal dialysis patients with bioelectrical impedence. Perit Dial Bull 1992; 8: 157–9.

208. Wong KC, Xiong DW, Borovnicar DJ, Stroud DB, Atkins RC, Strauss BJG. *Kt/V* in CAPD by different estimations of V. Kidney Int 1995; 48: 563–9.

209. Kong CH, Thompson CM, Lewis CA, Hill PD, Thompson FD. Determination of total body water in uremic patients by bioelectrical impedance. Nephrol Dial Transplant 1993; 8: 716–19.

210. Borovnicar DJ, Wong KC, Kerr PG *et al.* Total body protein status assessed by different estimates of fat free mass in adult peritoneal dialysis patients. Eur J Clin Nutr 1996; 50: 607–16.

211. Saxenhofer H, Scheidegger J, Descoeudres C, Jaeger P, Horber FF. Impact of dialysis modality on body composition in patients with end-stage renal disease. Clin Nephrol 1992; 38: 219–23.

212. Heymsfield SB, Wang J, Heshka S, Kehayians JL, Pierson RN. Dual-photon absorptiometry: comparison of bone mineral and soft tissue mass measurements *in vivo* with established methods. Am J Clin Nutr 1989; 49: 1283–9.

213. Mazess RB, Peppler WW, Gibbons M. Total body composition by dual-photon (153Gd) absorptiometry. Am J Clin Nutr 1984; 40: 834–9.

214. Haarbo J, Gotfredsen A, Hassager C, Christiansen C. Validation of body composition by dual energy X-ray absorptiometry (DEXA). Clin Physiol 1991; 11: 331–41.

215. Horber FF, Thomi F, Casez JP, Fonteille J, Jaeger P. Impact of hydration on body composition as measured by dual

energy X-ray absorptiometry in normal volunteers and patients on haemodialysis. Br J Radiol 1992; 16: 895–900.

216. Humphreys I. Accuracy and precision of the dual-energy X-ray absorptiometry (DEXA) technique in measuring body composition with stimulated fluid changes in beef mince phantoms (personal communication).

217. Roubenoff R. Kehayias JJ, Dawson-Hughes B, Heymsfield SB. Use of dual energy X-ray absorptiometry in body-composition studies: not yet a 'gold' standard. Am J Clin Nutr 1993; 58: 589–91.

218. Harvey TC, Dykes PW, Chen NS et al. Measurement of whole body nitrogen by neutron activation analysis. Lancet 1973; 2: 395–9.

219. Allen BJ, Blagojevic N, McGregor BJ, Morgan WD. *In vivo* determination of protein in malnourished patients. In: Ellis KJ, Yasamura S, eds. *In vivo* Body Composition Studies, vol. 3. London: Institute of Physical Sciences and Medicine, 1987, pp. 77–82.

220. Schilling H, Wu G, Pettit J. Nutritional status of patients on long term CAPD. Perit Dial Bull 1985; 5: 12–18.

221. Williams ED, Henderson IS, Boddy K et al. Whole-body elemental composition in patients with renal failure and after transplantation studied using total-body neutron activation analysis. Eur J Clin Invest 1984; 14: 362–8.

222. Cohn SH, Brennan BL, Yasamura S, Vartsky D, Vaswani AN, Ellis KJ. Evaluation of body composition and nitrogen content of renal patients on chronic dialysis as determined by total body neutron activation. Am J Clin Nutr 1983; 38: 52–8.

223. Heymsfield SB, Matthews D. Body composition: research and clinical advances – 1993 ASPEN Research Workshop. J Parent Enter Nutr 1994; 18: 91–103.

224. Morgenstern A, Winkler J, Narkis R et al. Adequacy of dialysis and nutritional status. Nephron 1994; 66: 438–41.

225. Detsky AJ, McLaughlin JR, Baker JP et al. What is subjective global assessment of nutritional status? J Parent Enter Nutr 1987; 11: 8–13.

226. Enia G, Sicuso C, Alati G, Zoccali C. Subjective global assessment of nutrition in dialysis patients. Nephrol Dial Transplant 1993; 8: 1094–8.

227. Jones CH, Newstead CG, Will EJ, Smye SW, Davison AM. Assessment of nutritional status in CAPD patients: serum albumin is not a useful measure. Nephrol Dial Transplant 1997; 12: 1406–13.

228. Baker JP, Detsky AS, Wesson DE et al. Nutritional assessment: a comparison of clinical judgement and objective measurements. N Engl J Med 1982; 306: 969–72.

229. McCusker FX, Teehan BP, Thorpe KE, Keshaviah PR, Churchill DN. How much peritoneal dialysis is required for the maintenance of a good nutritional state? Canada–USA (CANUSA) Peritoneal Dialysis Study Group. Kidney Int 1996 (suppl. 56): S56–61.

230. National Institutes of Health Consensus Development Conference on Morbidity and Mortality of Dialysis. November 1993; Bethesda, National Institutes of Health, 1994; 11: 1–33.

231. Woodrow G, Oldroyd B, Turney JH, Davies PS, Day JM, Smith MA. Measurement of total body water and urea kinetic modelling in peritoneal dialysis. Clin Nephrol 1997; 47: 52–7.

232. Kushner RF, Schoeller DA. Estimation of total body water by bioelectrical impedance analysis. Am J Clin Nutr 1986; 44: 417–24.

233. Watson PE, Watson ID, Batt RD. Total body water volumes for adult males and females estimated from simple anthropometric measurements. Am J Clin Nutr 1980; 33: 27–39.

234. Arkouche W, Fouque D, Pachiaudi C et al. Total body water and body composition in chronic peritoneal dialysis patients. J Am Soc Nephrol 1997; 8: 1906–14.

235. Panzetta G, Guerra U, D'Angelo A et al. Body composition and nutritional status in patients on continuous ambulatory peritoneal dialysis. Clin Nephrol 1985; 23: 18–25.

236. Abdo F, Clemente L, Davy J et al. Nutritional status and efficency of dialysis in CAPD and CCPD patients. Adv Perit Dial 1993; 9: 76–9.

237. Dumler F, Galan M, Cruz C. Impact of peritoneal dialysis modality on nutritional and biochemical parameters. Adv Perit Dial 1996; 12: 298–301.

238. de Fijter CW, Oe LP, Nauta JJ et al. Clinical efficacy and morbidity associated with continuous cyclic compared with continuous ambulatory peritoneal dialysis. Ann Intern Med 1994; 120: 264–71.

239. Strauss FG, Holmes DL, Dennis RL. Dialysis adequacy indices in high membrane transporters treated with short dwell peritoneal dialysis. Adv Perit Dial 1995; 11: 110–13.

240. Bergstrom J, Furst P, Alvestrand A, Lindholm B. Protein and energy intake, nitrogen balance and nitrogen losses in patients treated with continuous ambulatory peritoneal dialysis. Kidney Int 1993; 44: 1048–57.

241. Campbell WW, Crim MC, Dallal GE, Young VR, Evans WJ. Increased protein requirements in elderly people: new data and retrospective reassessments. Am J Clin Nutr 1994; 60: 501–9.

241. Slomowitz LA, Monteon FJ, Grosvenor M, Laidlaw SA, Kopple JD. Effect of energy intake on nutritional status in maintenance hemodialysis patients. Kidney Int 1989; 35: 704–11.

243. Shimomura A, Tahara D, Azekura H. Nutritional improvement in elderly CAPD patients with additional high protein foods. Adv Perit Dial 1993; 9: 80–6.

244. Dombros NV, Digenis GE, Soliman G, Oreopoulos DG. Anabolic steroids in the treatment of malnourished CAPD patients: a retrospective study. Perit Dial Int 1994; 14: 344–7.

245. Mittman N, Avram MM. Dyslipidemia in renal disease. Semin Nephrol 1996; 16: 202–13.

246. Massy ZA, Ma JZ, Louis TA, Kasiske BL. Lipid-lowering therapy in patients with renal disease. Kidney Int 1995; 48: 188–98.

247. Pollock CA, Wyndham R, Collett PV et al. Effects of erythropoietin therapy on the lipid profile in end-stage renal failure. Kidney Int 1994; 45, 897–902.

248. Ikizler TA, Wingard RL, Breyer JA, Schulman G, Parker RA, Hakim RM. Short-term effects of recombinant human growth hormone in CAPD patients. Kidney Int 1994; 46: 1178–83.

249. Kang DH, Lee SW, Kim HS, Choi KH, Lee HY, Han DS. Recombinant human growth hormone (rhGH) improves nutritional status of undernourished adult CAPD patients. J Am Soc Nephrol 1994; 5: 494 (abstract).

250. Peng S, Fouque D, Kopple J. Insulin-like growth factor-1 causes anabolism in malnourished CAPD patients. J Am Soc Nephrol 1993; 4: 414.

251. Mauras N, Horber F, Haymond M. Low dose recombinant human insulin-like growth factor-1 fails to affect protein anabolism but inhibits islet cell secretion in humans. J Clin Endocrinol Metab 1992; 75: 1192–7.

252. Gjessing J. Addition of amino acids to peritoneal dialysis fluid. Lancet 1968; 2: 812.

253. Dombros NV, Prutis K, Tong M et al. Six month overnight intraperitoneal amino-acid infusion in continuous ambulatory peritoneal dialysis (CAPD) patients – no effect on nutritional status. Perit Dial Int 1990; 10: 79–84.

254. Bruno M, Bagnis C, Marangella M, Rovera L, Cantaluppi A, Linari F. CAPD with an amino acid dialysis solution: a long term cross over study. Kidney Int 1989; 35: 1189–94.

255. Faller B, Aparicio M, Faict D et al. Clinical evaluation of an optimised 1.1% amino acid solution for peritoneal dialysis. Nephrol Dial Transplant 1995; 10: 1432–7.

256. Renzo S, Beatrice D, Giuseppe L. CAPD in diabetics: use of amino acids. Adv Perit Dial 1990; 6: 53–5.

257. Oren A, Wu G, Anderson GH et al. Effective use of amino acid dialysate over four weeks in CAPD patients. Perit Dial Bull 1983; 3: 66–73.

258. Young GA, Dibble JB, Hobson SM *et al.* The use of an amino acid based CAPD fluid over 12 weeks. Nephrol Dial Transplant 1989; 4: 285–92.

259. Arfeen S, Goodship TH, Kirkwood A, Ward MK. The nutritional, metabolic and hormonal effects of eight weeks of continuous ambulatory peritoneal dialysis with a 1% amino acid solution. Clin Nephrol 1990; 33: 192–9.

260. Kopple JD, Bernard D, Messana J *et al.* Treatment of malnourished CAPD patients with an amino acid based dialysate. Kidney Int 1995; 47: 1148–57.

261. Misra M, Ashworth J, Reaveley DA, Muller B, Brown EA. Nutritional effects of amino acid dialysate (Nutrineal) in CAPD patients. Adv Perit Dial 1996; 12: 311–14.

262. Saunders SJ, Truswell AS, Barbezat GO, Wittman W, Hansen JDL. Plasma free amino acid pattern in protein calorie malnutrition. Lancet 1967; 1: 795–7.

263. Cooper BA, Caterson RJ, Elliot P, Pollock CA. Intradialytic parenteral nutrition (IDPN) in malnourished haemodialysis patients. Australian and New Zealand Society of Nephrology, 1996 (abstract).

264. Topley N, Mackenzie R, Petersen MM *et al. In vitro* testing of a potentially biocompatible continuous ambulatory peritoneal dialysis fluid. Nephrol Dial Transplant 1991; 6: 574–81.

265. Goodship TH, Lloyd S, McKenzie PW *et al.* Short term studies on the use of amino acids as an osmotic agent in continuous ambulatory peritoneal dialysis. Clin Sci 1987; 73: 471–8.

266. Faller B. Amino acid based peritoneal dialysis solutions. Kidney Int 1996 (suppl. 56): S81–5.

17 | Peritonitis

L. Fried and B. Piraino

Introduction

Peritonitis remains a major complication of peritoneal dialysis, accounting for much of the morbidity associated with the technique. Peritonitis accounts for 15–35% of hospital admissions and is the major cause of transfer to haemodialysis (technique failure) [1–6]. High peritonitis rates are associated with mortality, either as a primary or contributing factor [2, 7–10].

In the early 1980s peritonitis incidence was high, with rates as high as 6.3 episodes/patient year [11]. With improvements in connection technology the rates declined to around 0.5 episodes/patient year (Fig. 1) [4–6, 12]. However, many patients continue to experience frequent peritonitis. Overall rates mask different outcomes based on patient demographics and the organism involved [6, 13–15]. This chapter will review the pathogenesis, diagnosis, treatment and clinical course of peritoneal dialysis-associated peritonitis. Table 1 shows the definition of terms used in the chapter.

Pathogenesis

Pathogens

The most common organisms producing peritonitis are summarized in Table 2 [2, 12, 16–20]. Most

Table 1. Definitions

Peritonitis	>100 WBC/μl, >50% polymorphonuclear cells
Exit-site infection	Erythema and/or drainage from exit site
Tunnel infection	Erythema, oedema or tenderness over the subcutaneous portion of the catheter (may be occult)
Catheter infection	Exit-site and/or tunnel infection
Recurrent peritonitis	Peritonitis with the same organism within 2–4 weeks of stopping antibiotics
Refractory peritonitis	Unresolving peritonitis despite appropriate antibiotics

Table 2. Organisms producing peritoneal dialysis peritonitis*

	Episodes/patient-year
Gram-positive	
Staphylococcus epidermidis	0.17–1.04
Staphylococcus aureus	0.09–0.15
Streptococcus	0.04–0.14
Enterococcus	0.01–0.04
Other Gram-positive	<0.01–0.02
Gram-negative	0.09–0.24
Fungal	<0.01–0.07
Mycobacterial	<0.01
Sterile	0.10–0.20

*From references 2, 12, 16–21.

episodes are due to a single organism [22, 23]. In contrast to surgical peritonitis and spontaneous bacterial peritonitis, the most common organisms are Gram-positive [22]. Table 2 shows rates (versus percentages) to highlight that the wide variability in reported rates is mainly due to differences in the rate of coagulase-negative staphylococcal peritonitis. With declining Gram-positive infection rates secondary to changes in connection technique, the proportion of infections secondary to Gram-negative organisms is increasing [24]. However, the actual rate per year of Gram-negative peritonitis is relatively constant [8]. Although unusual, fungi are

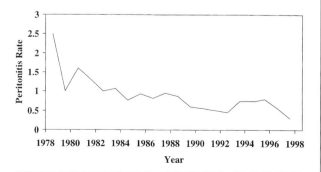

Figure 1. Peritonitis rates over time at the University of Pittsburgh PD Program.

R. Gokal, R. Khanna, R.Th. Krediet and K.D. Nolph (eds.), Textbook of Peritoneal Dialysis, 2nd Edition, 545–564.
© 2000 *Kluwer Academic Publishers. Printed in Great Britain.*

important causes of peritonitis as the sequelae are serious. Fungal peritonitis is predominantly due to *Candida* species, though many species have been reported [25–30]. Anaerobic peritonitis is uncommon and suggests bowel perforation [31–33]. Multi-organism infections that involve more than one Gram-negative organism also suggest bowel perforation. However, polymicrobial peritonitis with Gram-positive organisms can result from touch contamination or a catheter infection [34]. Mycobacterial peritonitis is rare, but may be more common in countries where mycobacterial infections are endemic [35].

Routes of entry

The routes of entry for peritonitis are summarized in Table 3.

Touch contamination

The most common source of peritonitis is contamination at the time of the exchange, leading to infection with predominantly Gram-positive skin flora ('touch contamination') [36]. The organism involved is mainly coagulase-negative *Staphylococcus,* though diphtheroids, *Corynebacterium* and *Bacillus* are also seen [19]. The Y-set with flush-before-fill technique decreased the incidence of peritonitis from touch contamination [19, 24, 37–40]. This has decreased coagulase-negative *Staphylococcus* peritonitis as well as other Gram-positives, but has had no effect on the incidence of *S. aureus* [19, 39]. Some patients' skin is colonized with Gram-negatives, which may be related to prior antibiotic use [16]. In these patients touch contamination can lead to Gram-negative peritonitis. In one study the Y-set decreased the incidence of *Acinetobacter* peritonitis, indicating touch contamination as a route of infection [39].

Catheter-related

Catheter infections account for 10–25% of peritonitis episodes [17, 23, 41, 42]. Exit-site and tunnel infections predispose patients to the development of peritonitis, presumably through contiguous

Table 3. Routes of entry for peritonitis

Touch contamination
Catheter-related
Enteric
Haematogenous
Gynaecological

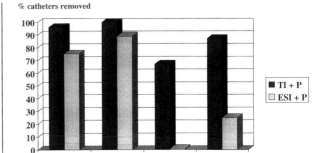

% catheters removed

Figure 2. Catheter removal by organism. From Gupta *et al.*, ref. 42. Reprinted with permission. TI = Tunnel infection, ESI = exit-site infection, P = peritonitis, CNS = coagulase negative *Staphylococcus.*

spread along the catheter surface [43]. In a trial examining the risk factors for peritonitis, the development of an exit-site infection doubled the risk of subsequent peritonitis [24]. Piraino *et al.*, in a study prior to the introduction of the Y-set, found that 64% of those with a history of an exit-site infection developed peritonitis, versus 45% without [44]. The most common organisms causing exit-site infections are *S. aureus*, *Pseudomonas*, and coagulase-negative *Staphylococcus* [45]. Tunnel infections are predominantly caused by *S. aureus*, followed by *Pseudomonas* [42]. In contrast, coagulase-negative Staphylococcus is an unusual cause of tunnel infection, catheter-related peritonitis or catheter loss [42, 45]. In a recent study, none of the coagulase-negative *Staphylococcus* peritonitis episodes associated with an exit-site infection required catheter removal versus 76% with other organisms [42] (Fig. 2). Peritonitis associated with tunnel infections is generally refractory to treatment without removal of the catheter. Except in the case of coagulase-negative *Staphylococcus*, the treatment failure rate was still high even when there was an exit-site infection without clinical evidence of a tunnel infection, suggesting occult tunnel infections. Catheter infections can also produce relapsing peritonitis, recurrent peritonitis with the same organism within 2–4 weeks of stopping antibiotics. This can be due to the presence of a tunnel infection or alternatively to bacterial colonization of a biofilm [46, 47]. Biofilm formation is ubiquitous and does not necessarily result from infection [48]. Recurrent peritonitis in association with a biofilm is most often due to coagulase-negative *Staphylococcus*, while recurrent peritonitis due to a tunnel infection is generally due to *S. aureus* or *Pseudomonas*.

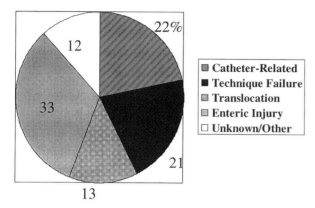

Figure 3. Aetiology of peritonitis involving enteric organisms, including *Streptococcus* sp. and *Torulopsis*. Data derived from ref. 56.

Enteric

Most Gram-negative peritonitis is caused by intestinal flora. This can result from abdominal perforation, instrumentation or other abdominal processes [31, 49–56]. However, in many cases an aetiology of the infection is not found [14]. Enteric organisms may enter the peritoneal cavity by transmural migration across the gastrointestinal tract [57]. Diverticulosis appears to increase the risk of transmural migration, as can acute treatment of constipation [58, 59]. The presence of multiple Gram-negative organisms or an anaerobe suggests perforation [33]. Figure 3 summarizes the aetiology of peritonitis involving enteric organisms.

Haematogenous spread

Bacteraemia can lead to peritonitis, though it is an uncommon cause. Invasive procedures or dental work can produce transient bacteraemia and peritonitis [53, 60, 61]. Routine gastrointestinal endoscopy is associated with bacteraemia in 2–6% of procedures, though oesophageal dilation and variceal sclerotherapy have a significantly higher frequency [62, 63]. Dental procedures can lead to peritonitis from mouth organisms such as *Streptococcus* sp. [60, 61]. These cases are potentially preventable with prophylactic antibiotics.

Gynaecological

In rare cases ascending infections from uterine and vaginal sources can lead to peritonitis. This can lead to infections with vaginal flora, including yeast. Cases have been reported with gynaecological procedures, vaginal leak of dialysate and the use of intrauterine devices [64–66].

Predisposing factors

Risk factors

Studies examining risk factors for the development of peritonitis identified higher rates for children, African Americans, Native Canadians, and those with a history of substance abuse or lower socioeconomic status [23, 67–72]. The higher rate in children is mainly due to Gram-positive organisms [61]. Age (in adults), diabetes and gender do not appear to be significant risks [23, 67, 72, 73]. Recent studies have identified immunosuppression as a risk factor. Prior steroid use is not consistently a predictor, but HIV-positive patients have higher peritonitis rates [23, 74, 75]. In addition, the proportion of Gram-negative and fungal infections is higher in HIV-positive patients [74–76]. Prior antibiotic use is also a risk for fungal peritonitis [25, 26, 77]. Gastric acid inhibitors may increase the risk of Gram-negative peritonitis [58]. Upper respiratory tract infections may predispose children to peritonitis, though the reason for this is not clear [61]. The strongest dialysis-related factors are the type of connection system and staphylococcal nasal carriage.

Connection system

The Y-set was introduced in the late 1970s in Europe but did not gain widespread use until the mid to late 1980s [8, 37]. This system uses a flush-before-fill technique that flushes sterile dialysate into the drain bag after connection to the patient's catheter, but before dialysate is infused into the peritoneum [37]. This decreases the possibility of bacteria from touch contamination reaching the peritoneal cavity. This improvement dramatically decreased the peritonitis rate when compared to the standard spike system [24, 37, 38, 40]. The Canadian CAPD Clinical Trials Group performed a randomized multicentre trial comparing a standard spike to the Y-set [24]. The Y-set reduced the peritonitis rate by 60%. The twin bag system with a pre-attached drain bag, requiring only connection at the catheter, further reduces peritonitis rates [78, 79].

Continuous cycler peritoneal dialysis is currently a popular form of PD. Some studies have found that CCPD patients have a lower peritonitis rate than CAPD [80, 81]. This is presumably secondary to the decreased number of connections between the system and peritoneal catheter. However, the CCPD set-up still requires the patient to 'spike' bags, which is a potential source of contamination. The twin bag system for CAPD has lowered rates to the similar or lower than that reported for CCPD [82, 83]. A modification using an assist device to spike the bags on CCPD may further lower peritonitis rates [84]. No direct comparisons between CAPD with the twin bag system and CCPD with this modification have been performed.

Staphylococcal carriage

Approximately 50% of PD patients are *S. aureus* nasal carriers [85–90]. Nasal carriage increases the risk of *S. aureus* exit-site infections and subsequently peritonitis [86–88, 91, 92]. Phage typing of *S. aureus* from those with peritonitis or exit-site infection found that the isolates were the same as from the nares [85, 87]. Zimmerman *et al.* found that 83% of all *S. aureus* peritonitis episodes were associated with *S. aureus* catheter infection [93]. This is consistent with a failure of the Y-set to reduce *S. aureus* peritonitis.

Compared to non-carriers, carriers have a 2–6-fold higher incidence of *S. aureus* peritonitis [87–91]. Immunosuppressed patients appear to be at particular risk of *S. aureus* peritonitis, regardless of carriage status [94]. Diabetics appear to have an increased rate of nasal carriage [86, 94]. However, it is controversial whether diabetics have an increased risk of *S. aureus* peritonitis after accounting for the higher carriage [86, 89, 90, 94]. Treatment strategies that treat nasal carriage (nasal mupirocin or cyclical rifampin) or treat the exit-site to prevent *S. aureus* exit-site infection (mupirocin), dramatically reduce the incidence of *S. aureus* peritonitis (see below, Prevention) [95–99].

Clinical presentation

The usual symptoms are cloudy fluid and abdominal pain (Table 4) [16, 22, 61]. The presentation can vary from cloudy fluid with no pain to a severe illness [16, 20]. In children, cloudy fluid is almost universal, though the incidence of abdominal pain may be less than in adults [61]. The initial presentation in children may be fever alone [61].

Early studies found that 98–100% of cases presented with cloudy fluid [16, 22, 61]. However, a more recent study found that 6% presented with abdominal pain, in the absence of cloudy fluid or elevated cell count [100]. Usually this represents a delay of leukocytosis, and when re-examined, the dialysate cell count has increased [100, 101]. This delay may be secondary to slower cytokine response to infection [100]; therefore, PD patients with abdominal pain should be considered to have peritonitis, until proven otherwise. Cloudy fluid can, in rare cases, represent malignancy or chylous ascites [102–105]. These cases can be differentiated by cytology and dialysate triglyceride levels. The differential diagnosis of cloudy effluent is outlined in Table 5.

The presentation is somewhat dependent on the organism involved and the aetiology of peritonitis. Episodes due to coagulase-negative *Staphylococcus* and other skin organisms such as *Corynebacterium* are generally milder than episodes with *S. aureus*, *Streptococcus*, fungi or Gram-negative organisms [20, 106, 107]. Peritonitis from bowel perforation or other abdominal processes often produces severe symptoms, but the initial presentation may not differ from typical peritonitis [31–33, 108]. Some investigators have found that the presence of free air associated with peritonitis, or alternatively, increasing free air (as free air results from introduction of air during an exchange) to be a clue to bowel perforation [108, 109]. Tunnel tenderness indicates a tunnel infection, but the sensitivity of the physical examination for tunnel infections is low [110]. Since tunnel infections are generally associated with exit-site infections, the presence of an exit-site infection in a patient with peritonitis should trigger a suspicion of catheter-related peritonitis.

Table 4. Clinical presentation* (percentages)

Cloudy fluid	98–100
Abdominal pain	67–97
Abdominal tenderness	62–79
Rebound tenderness	35–62
Fever	34–36
Chills	18–23
Nausea	30–35
Vomiting	25–30
Diarrhoea	7–15

*From references 16, 22, 61.

Table 5. Differential diagnosis of cloudy effluent

Infectious peritonitis, including culture-negative peritonitis
Eosinophilic peritonitis
Sclerosing peritonitis
Chylous ascites
Malignant ascites
Pancreatitis
Chemical peritonitis

Diagnosis

Cell count

The usual criteria for peritonitis are: (1) cloudy fluid; (2) dialysate white blood cell count $>100/\mu l$; (3) polymorphonuclear cells (PMN) $>50\%$; and (4) positive culture [22, 30]. In the absence of peritonitis the cell count is usually $<30/\mu l$ and is predominantly mononuclear [100, 111, 112]. Some authors have found that PMN $>50\%$ is a better criterion that the total cell count, especially in patients already on antibiotics [113, 114]. Short dwell times can also decrease the number of white cells seen. Antonsen et al. found that if the cell count is not done within 4–6 h of collection the number of leukocytes can decrease by 25–30% [115]. The leukocyte count is more stable if samples are sent in EDTA tubes.

Tuberculous peritonitis may present with a predominance of lymphocytes, but neutrophil predominance is more common [35, 116–118]. Occasionally, eosinophil predominance is seen (eosinophilic peritonitis). Rarely, this is due to fungal peritonitis, but in most cases cultures for bacteria and fungus are negative [119, 120]. In many cases the peritoneal eosinophilia occurs early after the initiation of PD and is felt to represent a reaction to the plasticizers in the PD catheter or plastic dialysate bags [121, 122]. Blood eosinophila may also be seen [123–125]. Antibiotics are not necessary and in most cases the eosinophils resolve without treatment [121, 125, 126]. Persistent cases may respond to steroids or a mast-cell-stabilizing antihistamine [127, 128].

Culture

The handling of the dialysate is important in establishing the aetiological agent. Culturing a large volume improves the diagnosis, as does the use of blood culture techniques [30, 129–134]. In general, at least 10–20 ml of dialysate should be cultured using blood culture media. Lysis-centrifugation may also improve the yield [135]. Blood cultures are rarely positive; therefore routine culturing of the blood is not necessary. Cultures are generally positive within 24–72 h, though coagulase-negative *Staphylococcus* may grow more slowly [136]. Fungal cultures might take longer than the routine time in many laboratories and a high index of suspicion is needed, especially if the patient is not responding to antibiotics. Of course, the growth of

mycobacteria is slow, resulting in a delayed diagnosis.

The use of Gram stain for earlier diagnosis is controversial. Some authors only report a positive Gram stain in 20–30%, while a more recent study was positive in $>90\%$ [30, 137]. The yield of the Gram stain was higher for Gram-negative organisms [137]. The positive predictive value of the Gram stain was 68% for Gram-positive and 95% for Gram-negative organisms. It is important not to base antibiotic therapy solely on the Gram stain. This same study found that in 40% of cases where Gram-positive cocci were seen, another organism was found, or the culture was negative. However, Gram stains can yield an early diagnosis of fungal peritonitis, which can allow prompt initiation of appropriate treatment [27].

Tunnel ultrasound

Ultrasound may be beneficial in diagnosing an occult tunnel infection. The width of a normal tunnel is approximately 6 mm [138]. In the presence of a tunnel infection, ultrasound of the tunnel can show decreased echogenicity around the tunnel, indicating a fluid collection [110, 139]. In one study ultrasound was three times more sensitive in picking up a tunnel infection than were clinical criteria alone [110]. In patients with an exit-site infection a positive ultrasound indicates a high risk of catheter loss [140, 141]. The indications for use of ultrasound in evaluating the patient with peritonitis have not yet been determined.

Differential of culture-negative peritonitis

The incidence of culture-negative peritonitis has decreased with improvement in culture techniques. In a study comparing cultures with Bactec® bottles versus standard culture plates, Luce et al. found a culture-negative rate of 4% for Bactec® versis 22% for standard [130]. In most cases a negative culture represents a problem with culture methods or culturing too small a volume of dialysate [142]. Reculturing sometimes yields an organism [143]. There is debate about the causative organism in these cases, but most studies implicate Gram-positive organisms and the incidence has decreased with the use of the Y-set [18, 19, 144].

Another aetiology of culture-negative peritonitis is the surreptitious use of antibiotics. One study found that in one-third of the culture-negative cases there was antimicrobial activity in the dialysate

[145]. Though antibiotic use is a potential cause of negative cultures that should be explored with patients, it is notable that this study had a particularly high rate of culture-negative peritonitis. Culture-negative peritonitis can also be secondary to unusual or difficult-to-culture organisms, such as mycobacteria or some fungi. These cases do not respond to antibiotics, though there may be an early response of mycobacterial infections to quinolones [146].

Pancreatitis can also present as abdominal pain with an increased cell count. Peritoneal fluid amylase > 100 U/L can help differentiate pancreatitis from usual peritonitis [147]. However, other abdominal processes, such as ischaemic bowel and small bowel perforation, can also produce an elevated amylase in the dialysate [147, 148]. Rare causes of culture-negative peritonitis are chemical peritonitis from medications (Vancoled brand vancomycin, amphotericin, thrombolytics) or presence of endotoxin in the dialysate [149–154].

Treatment

Initial regimen

Once cultures have been sent, antibiotics should be started promptly. Hospitalization is generally based on severity of illness, such as hypotension, need for intravenous fluids and parenteral narcotics. Pain control is important and is often neglected. Intraperitoneal antibiotics are generally preferred as this route may be more effective than the intravenous route, and certainly results in high local levels [155]. There are many published antibiotic regimens for PD peritonitis. In an effort to standardize the treatment of PD peritonitis the Advisory Committee on Peritoneal Management of the International Society for Peritoneal Dialysis reviewed the literature and published guidelines [142]. The guidelines are periodically updated as new information on peritonitis and its treatment becomes available. In 1993 the committee's recommendation for empirical antibiotics was vancomycin plus ceftazidime or an aminoglycoside [156]. However as concern for vancomycin-resistant organisms increased, the committee updated the recommendations in 1996 to decrease the routine use of vancomycin.

Table 6 summarizes the guidelines' initial empirical therapy. The guidelines advocate the use of a first-generation cephalosporin plus an aminoglycoside. Subsequent antibiotic therapy is based on the

Table 6. Initial empirical antibiotic therapy (ISPD Committee Guidelines)*

Intermittent dosing	
Cefazolin or cephalothin	15 mg/kg or 500 mg/L if urine output <500 ml/day; 25% higher if urine output >500 ml
Plus: Aminoglycoside: Gentamicin/tobramycin/netilmicin	0.6 mg/L if urine output <500 ml; 1.5 mg/kg load if urine output greater than 500 ml, then 0.6 mg/kg/day as initial dose, though may need to dose more frequently based on levels
or Amikacin	2 mg/kg if urine output <500 ml; if urine output greater than 500: 5 mg/kg load then 2 mg/kg/day, though may need to dose more frequently based on levels
Continuous dosing	
Cefazolin or cephalothin	500 mg load then 125 mg/L in each exchange
Plus: Aminoglycoside: Gentamicin/tobramycin/netilmicin	8 mg/L load then 4 mg/L in each exchange
or Amikacin	25 mg/L load then 12 mg/L in each exchange

*From reference 142.

culture results (see Table 7 for dosing of other antibiotics [29, 142, 157–163]). Both continuous and intermittent therapy dosing are given, and there are not enough data to recommend one regimen over another. Intermittent dosing is more convenient, and may be associated with less toxicity from the aminoglycoside. Once-daily dosing is also applicable to APD, where the antibiotics can be given in the long day dwell, although few data exist. However, there is concern that intermittent dosing will lead to long periods where the antibiotic level is below the minimal inhibitory concentration (MIC), especially in the presence of significant residual renal function [164]. This theoretically can lead to induction of resistance [165]. There are fewer reported data on dosing of antibiotics in children. For the cephalosporins the dose per litre can still be adjusted for the smaller exchange volume [142]. The aminoglycosides should be dosed on weight and blood levels monitored to avoid toxicity.

The current guidelines are controversial. Some centres have reported high cure rates with the above antibiotic regimen. Weber *et al.* found an overall cure rate of 79% using cefazolin and gentamicin,

Table 7. Dosing of commonly used intraperitoneal antibiotics for peritonitis*

	Intermittent	Continuous dosing
Cephalosporins		
Cefazolin	1–1.5g/day	500 mg load then 125mg/L
Cephalothin	15 mg/kg/day	500 mg load then 125–250 mg/L
Ceftazidime	1 g/day	250 mg load then 125 mg/L
Cefamandole	1 g/day	500 mg load then 250 mg/L
Cefotaxime	2 g/day	500 mg load then 250 mg/L
Ceftriaxone	1 g/day	250 mg load then 125 mg/L
Aminoglycosides		
Amikacin	2 mg/kg	25 mg load then 12 mg/L
Gentamicin	0.6–1 mg/kg[†]	8 mg load then 4 mg/L[‡]
Netilmicin	0.6–1 mg/kg	8 mg load then 4 mg/L[‡]
Tobramycin	0.6–1 mg/kg	8 mg load then 4 mg/L[‡]
Penicillins		
Ampicillin	Data on i.p. not available	125 mg/L
Oxacillin	Data on i.p. not available	125 mg/L
Nafcillin	Data on i.p. not available	125 mg/L
Piperacillin	Data on i.p. not available	3000 mg load then 500 mg/L
Ticarcillin	Data on i.p. not available	125 mg/L
Quinolones		
Ciprofloxacin	Data on i.p. not available (can give p.o. 500 b.i.d.)	25–50 mg/L
Ofloxacin	200 mg/day (i.p. or p.o.)	Data on i.p. not available
Pefloxacin	400 mg/day (i.p. or p.o.)	Data on i.p. not available
Other antibiotics		
Vancomycin	30 mg/kg, up to 2 g/day	1 g load then 25 mg/L
Clindamycin	Data on i.p. not available	300 mg load then 150 mg/L
Imipenem	1 g b.i.d.	500 mg load then 200 mg/L
Teicoplanin	400 mg b.i.d.	400 mg load then 40 mg/L
Aztreonam	1 g	1000 mg load then 250 mg/L

*From references 29, 142, 157, 159–163.
[†]Higher dose for those with residual renal function. Need to dose based on levels.
[‡]Some investigators use 8 mg/L.
i.p., Intraperitonel; p.o., per os.

though the rate was 95% in those without a tunnel infection or intra-abdominal pathology [161]. Lai and Grucek found similarly high cure rates with cefazolin and an aminoglycoside [166, 167]. However, other centres have not found such favourable results [21, 163]. The antibiotics do not adequately cover methicillin-resistant *Staphylococcus aureus* (MRSA) or enterococcus. Methicillin-resistant coagulase-negative *Staphylococcus* may respond as the local antibiotic concentrations are higher than the MIC [142]. However, Vas *et al.* found that treatment with cefazolin cured only 45% of methicillin-resistant coagulase-negative *Staphylococcus* [162]. Centres with a high rate of methicillin resistance should use vancomycin. An alternative approach to the *ad-hoc* committee was recently proposed by van Biesen *et al.* (Fig. 4) [21]. This regimen utilized vancomycin and gentamicin as initial therapy followed by oral ciprofloxacin alone or ciprofloxacin

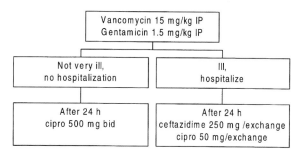

Figure 4. Alternative treatment regimen for empirical antibiotics as proposed by van Biesen. Figure modified with permission from ref. 21.

plus intraperitoneal ceftazidime if the patient was ill and required hospitalization. This produced a coverage rate of 96% versus 78% for the regimen proposed by the *ad-hoc* committee.

The effect of the short courses of aminoglycoside on residual renal function is not known, but theoretically could impact clearances. In an effort to avoid aminoglycosides, centres have tried monotherapy with cefazolin alone, but this appears to be inadequate [168, 169]. Oral quinolones have been tried in order to ease administration and control costs. Quinolones have good peritoneal penetration [170] but as initial monotherapy cover only two-thirds of infections [165, 171]. The regimen misses mainly Gram-positive infections so intermittent vancomycin plus a quinolone may be an effective regimen [172]. Alternatively, the antibiotics can be switched to an oral quinolone once the culture sensitivities have returned. Oral quinolones must be separated in time from any antacid, including phosphate binders, which interfere with absorption of the drug.

Subsequent regimen

Gram-positive organisms

If a Gram-positive organism, especially coagulase-negative *Staphylococcus* or other skin organism, is isolated, the patient should be questioned about a break in technique and a review of connection technique should be made. The course for various Gram-positive organisms differs and is summarized below.

Coagulase-negative staphylococcus *and other Gram-positive skin organisms.*   If the organism isolated is a diphtheroid, *Corynebacterium* or *Bacillus*, a first-generation cephalosporin for 14 days is generally sufficient. In the case of coagulase-negative *Staphylococcus* the course depends on whether the organism is methicillin-resistant. Methicillin-sensitive organisms can be treated with cefazolin and the cure rate is equivalent to vancomycin [162]. The cure rate for methicillin-resistant organisms is much lower with cefazolin (versus vancomycin) [162]. If cephalosporins are the empirical therapy the patient should be changed to clindamycin or vancomycin once methicillin-resistant organisms are identified.

Staphylococcus aureus.   In the majority of cases, *S. aureus* peritonitis is associated with a catheter infection [93, 106, 173]. The peritonitis tends to be severe and patients often require hospitalization [20, 106]. If *S. aureus* catheter infection is present, the catheter should be removed promptly. Once the culture returns the subsequent antibiotic regimen also depends on whether the organism is methicillin sensitive. If the organism is methicillin sensitive the

antibiotics can be switched to an anti-staphylococcal penicillin or the first-generation cephalosporin can be continued [142]. Rifampin can be added if desired, or if the response to treatment is slow [142]. If the organism is methicillin resistant the antibiotics should be changed to vancomycin (or possibly clindamycin). The vancomycin should be dosed every 5–7 days with more frequent dosing for those with residual renal function. Trough vancomycin levels can help guide therapy. Rifampin 600 mg/day should be added to the regimen [142, 174]. Treatment failure for MRSA is higher than for methicillin-sensitive staphylococcal infections [175]. Antibiotics should be continued for 21 days [142].

Streptococcal.   Streptococcal peritonitis accounts for 10–15% of episodes [2, 16, 17, 20]. Most cases are secondary to *S. viridans*, followed by *Enterococcus*. Streptococcal peritonitis also tends to be more severe than coagulase-negative *Staphylococcus* [107]. Beta-haemolytic streptococcal peritonitis can be particularly severe, leading to shock and death [16, 176]. Non-enterococcal streptococcal peritonitis responds well to ampicillin and first-generation cephalosporins [142]. The response to these antibiotics appears to be better than the response to vancomycin [142]. Antibiotics should be continued for 14 days [142]. Pain, often severe, must be adequately treated.

Enterococcal infections are slower to respond to antibiotics. If sensitive, ampicillin 125 mg/L in each exchange is the preferred antibiotic, to avoid selection of vancomycin-resistant *Enterococcus* (VRE) [142]. Once-daily low-dose aminoglycosides may be synergistic. *Enterococcus* is part of the gastrointestinal flora; peritonitis should lead to consideration of work-up for abdominal pathology [56, 177]. The incidence of VRE varies from unit to unit [178–181]. The prevalence is increased by prior use of antibiotics and hospitalization [181]. PD, as a home therapy, may have a lower incidence of VRE carriage. However, VRE peritonitis carries a high mortality [182]. VRE infections may respond to teicoplanin, quinapristin/dalfopristin or chloramphenicol, though experience in PD patients is limited [183–185]. The recommendations for limiting vancomycin are based on concerns of increasing the prevalence of VRE and fear of transmission of resistance to other organisms such as *Staphylococcus aureus*. Indeed, intermediate resistant and heterogeneously resistant MRSA have been described in Japan, the United States and France, and this may represent an ominous preliminary stage to vancomycin resistance [186–188].

Gram-negative peritonitis

General considerations. Once the organisms and the antibiotic sensitivity have been determined, the antibiotics should be narrowed to avoid long-term aminoglycosides, given the risk of ototoxicity and vestibular toxicity [189, 190]. The aminoglycosides may differ in risk of ototoxicity and vestibular toxicity, and the risk of toxicity may increase with repeated courses [191, 192]. A review in patients without renal failure found that the risk of ototoxicity was 14% for amikacin, 8% for gentamicin, 6% for tobramycin and 2.5% for netilmicin [191]. The risk for vestibular toxicity was similar for gentamicin, amikacin and tobramycin at around 3–4%, with netilmicin around 1.5%. However, there are few data for patients on PD. In a study examining the development of ototoxicity using tobramycin, hearing declined in 25% but improved in 17.5% [193].

The most common organisms isolated in Gram-negative peritonitis are *Klebsiella*, *Escherichia coli*, and *Enterobacter* [14, 194]. The presentation is more severe than that seen with coagulase-negative *Staphylococcus*. Gram-negative peritonitis is associated with higher rates of death, hospitalization, catheter loss and transfer to haemodialysis than peritonitis with Gram-positive organisms [6, 14, 15] (see Fig. 6). This is also true for episodes not associated with abdominal perforation.

In uncomplicated episodes the antibiotics should be continued for 2 weeks [142]. Ceftazidime is a highly effective agent for treatment of Gram-negative infections and is an effective empirical antibiotic when Gram-negative infections are suspected (generally given with vancomycin) [195–197]. Quinolones, oral or intraperitoneal, can be effective in sensitive organisms. Infections with *Acinetobacter* and *Xanthomonas* can be difficult to treat. *Acinetobacter* is associated with high prevalence of antibiotic resistance and relapse, and is best treated with two antibiotics for 3 weeks [198, 199]. *Xanthomonas* also produces serious infections and should be treated with two antibiotics for a duration of 21 days [142, 200].

Multiple enteric pathogens or the presence of an anaerobe suggest intra-abdominal pathology and the need for surgical evaluation [33, 201]. If a patient with single-organism peritonitis is not responding to appropriate therapy, this should also prompt an evaluation [202]. Patients may initially respond to antibiotics but then deteriorate [56]. Unlike the case with routine peritonitis, bacteraemia is not uncommon with peritonitis associated with abdominal processes [55, 203].

Pseudomonas. Unlike other Gram-negative organisms, *Pseudomonas* peritonitis is commonly associated with catheter infections [204, 205]. Both current and prior episodes of *Pseudomonas* exit-site infection predispose to peritonitis. One study found that 22% of patients with a history of *Pseudomonas* exit-site infection developed peritonitis after resolution of the exit-site infection [206]. If a patient presents with *Pseudomonas* peritonitis, the exit site and tunnel should be examined for infection, which can be subtle. If present, the likelihood of cure without catheter removal is low, and the catheter should be removed [42, 205]. Peritonitis should be treated with two anti-pseudomonal antibiotics [142]. The duration of antibiotics should be 21 days.

Fungal

The optimal treatment of fungal peritonitis is not known. The mortality rate associated with fungal peritonitis is high in children and adults, 20–45% [25, 26, 28, 207, 208]. There are reports of successful treatment of fungal peritonitis without catheter removal, but most patients will ultimately lose their catheter [26–28]. Larger series have found a cure rate without catheter removal of approximately 10% using fluconazole [209–211]. In the largest reported series Goldie *et al.* examined the outcome of 55 cases of fungal peritonitis. The regimens varied, though approximately 90% received amphotericin and 25% received two antifungal medications. The survival in those whose catheter was removed within 1 week of diagnosis was 85% versus 50% in those whose catheter was not removed, though the series was uncontrolled [25].

Given the poor outcome, we feel that the catheter should be removed in fungal peritonitis. If the decision is made to treat with the catheter in place, the catheter should be removed if there is no sign of improvement within a week of starting treatment. There are no controlled trials of antifungal therapy. Two anti-fungal medications are commonly used. Amphotericin [0.5 mg/kg per day intravenously $\pm$ 1–2 mg/L intraperitoneally) was used in older series, but more recently the azoles have been used [212, 213]. The azoles can be given orally, intravenously or intraperitoneally.

The commonly used agents are ketoconazole [400 mg/day) and fluconazole [100–200 mg/day, 3 mg/kg in children), though micronazole [100–200 mg/day) has also been used [142, 210, 211, 214–216]. Oral fluconazole appears to have better intraperitoneal penetration than ketoconazole [214]. 5-Fluorocytosine [50 mg/L intraperitoneally or 1 g per os q.d.) is often added for synergy [142, 214]. Therapy should generally be continued for 4–6 weeks [142]. Some patients, after catheter removal and treatment, may be able to return to PD but the incidence of adhesions is high and most will need to remain on haemodialysis [27]. The ability to return to PD might be improved by prompt removal of the catheter and anti-fungal therapy, but this is controversial [217].

Mycobacterium

Mycobacteria are rare causes of peritonitis that require a high index of suspicion for diagnosis. Acid-fast bacilli smears are usually negative. Cultures when obtained are positive, but growth is slow, delaying the diagnosis [35, 116]. The number of reported cases is low, but the disease appears to respond to standard anti-tuberculous therapy [35]. CAPD continuation is occasionally possible but ultrafiltration failure may occur [35, 218]. Many patients will have had their catheter removed for unresolving peritonitis before the diagnosis is made. Peritonitis with non-tuberculous mycobacterium, mainly *M. fortuitum*, has been reported and can respond to appropriate antibiotics [219].

Culture-negative

If, after 96 h, the culture is negative but the patient is responding to therapy and the Gram stain did not reveal a Gram-negative organism, the aminoglycoside can be discontinued. The cephalosporin should then be continued for a total of 14 days [142]. If the patient is not responding, the Gram stain and culture should be repeated [143]. If this does not reveal an aetiology for the apparent failure of antibiotics, consideration of catheter removal or culture for unusual organisms should be made.

Follow-up

General. Clinical response is generally seen in 3–5 days, though this is organism-dependent. The dialysate leukocyte count in uncomplicated peritonitis normalizes in 4–5 days [11]. If there has been no improvement by 96 h, re-evaluation is essential. Reculturing might yield an organism not covered by the chosen antibiotics. The patient should be assessed for intra-abdominal pathology or enteric source; the catheter should be evaluated for infection. Unresolving peritonitis predicts a poor outcome and catheter removal is imperative [220].

Catheter removal

The indications for catheter removal during peritonitis are listed in Table 8. Usually a period of 2–4 weeks between catheter removal and insertion of a new catheter is advocated, to avoid reinfection [142, 221]. However, this requires temporary transfer to haemodialysis, which can be inconvenient for the patient and problematic for young children [222]. Experience is growing on simultaneous removal and replacement of catheters for relapsing or recurrent peritonitis [222–228]. In a recent study Postuma *et al.* found that in 38 of 40 procedures the patient could continue PD [228]. Criteria included a peritoneal WBC count less than 100/μl and continued antibiotics for 10 days after the WBC normalized or 7 days after surgery. A dialysate leak developed in two patients and there were two episodes of peritonitis within 30 days. This simultaneous technique appears to be more successful for Gram-positive peritonitis than for *Pseudomonas* or fungal peritonitis [223, 225]. In one small series a dialysate WBC count <200/μl at the time of the procedure predicted success with *Pseudomonas* infections [229]. In many cases haemodialysis was avoided with the simultaneous procedure [223, 227, 228].

Relapsing peritonitis

In relapsing peritonitis, peritonitis with the same organism recurs after completion of antibiotics. Most cases are secondary to the presence of a subcutaneous tunnel infection [47]. Relapse may also be secondary to inadequate treatment of the prior infection. Underdosing of antibiotics increases the risk of relapse. Mulhern *et al.* found that in patients treated

Table 8. Indications for catheter removal during peritonitis

Refractory
Relapsing
Catheter-related
Enteric associated with intra-abdominal process
Fungal

with once-weekly vancomycin a low trough level predicted relapse (9/14 with 4-week mean trough <12 mg/L relapsed versus 0/17 >12 mg/L) [230]. It is important to consider a patient's weight (and hence volume of distribution) and residual renal function when dosing antibiotics. Dosing on a 5-day schedule may be preferred, especially if there is residual renal function.

In some cases relapse is secondary to harbouring of bacteria in a catheter biofilm. Once a tunnel infection has been ruled out, these cases may respond to intraperitoneal streptokinase [750 000 IU) or urokinase [7500–10 000 IU) in addition to antibiotics [231]. This treatment is most successful for coagulase-negative *Staphylococcus* or culture-negative peritonitis [231]. The cure rate is 50–65% in selected patients, though this is lower than with catheter removal [153, 232–234]. If the peritonitis does not respond, the catheter should be removed. In rare cases relapse is secondary to the presence of an abdominal abscess [47].

Outcome and sequelae

Resolution

From 60% to 90% of episodes resolve with antibiotics [20, 235–237]. The rates of resolution are higher in the absence of an exit-site or tunnel infection. Catheter removal rates are higher for *S. aureus* and Gram-negative infections. The higher rate of catheter removal for *S. aureus* is secondary to catheter infections, as the rate of removal in the absence of a catheter infection is similar to coagulase-negative *Staphylococcus* [14].

Abscess formation

Abscess formation occurs in less than 1% of episodes of peritonitis [238]. The patients tend to present with abdominal pain, nausea, vomiting and peripheral leukocytosis [238]. The organisms reported are Gram-negative, fungus and *S. aureus* [47, 238]. CT scan or ultrasound is helpful in making the diagnosis. The disease responds to drainage.

Transfer to haemodialysis (technique failure)

Peritonitis is the major cause of technique failure in PD patients, accounting for 30–80% of permanent transfers [4, 5, 239]. The Y-set reduced peritonitis, but did not significantly impact technique survival in all studies [5, 18]. Peritonitis from coagulase-

negative *Staphylococcus* and other skin organisms tends to be less severe, and as a result reduction in touch contamination has less of an impact on technique survival. Severe episodes of peritonitis are associated with decreasing albumin from increased protein losses, poor intake and inflammatory response [13, 240]. This is associated with a worse long-term outcome. Prompt transfer to haemodialysis is appropriate in severe, poorly responding episodes of peritonitis.

Sclerosing peritonitis

Sclerosing encapsulating peritonitis is an uncommon (1–2% of PD patients) but serious complication of PD. This entity is not infectious, but patients present with abdominal pain, nausea and vomiting, bowel obstruction and malnutrition [241]. A loss of ultrafiltration is seen [241]. The disease can present after transfer to haemodialysis or transplantation. Recurrent peritonitis may be a predisposing factor, but this is not a consistent finding. Nomoto *et al.* found that those with sclerosing peritonitis had a 3.3 times higher peritonitis rate than those without, but Hendriks *et al.* found that the rates were not different [241, 242]. The pathogenesis appears to be injury to the mesothelium that results in a fibrotic reaction. It may not be recurrent peritonitis alone but a severe episode that is important [243, 244]. This is supported by Davies *et al.*, who found that ultrafiltration tends to decline with time on PD and is worsened and accelerated by severe or closely spaced episodes of peritonitis [245].

Death

Peritonitis results in death in 1–6% of episodes [2, 8, 9, 246]. The mortality rate for Gram-negative and fungal peritonitis is significantly higher [4–10% for Gram-negative, 20–45% for fungal) [8, 14, 25, 208] (Fig. 5). Mortality associated with bowel perforation approaches 50% [55, 56]. In contrast, the mortality associated with coagulase-negative *Staphylococcus* peritonitis is less than 1% [8]. There is a high mortality rate in the first year after transfer to haemodialysis, which may be related to poorer nutrition in those with severe peritonitis episodes [5]. Lower albumin rates are associated with increased mortality after peritonitis, but this may be related to the increased protein losses with severe peritonitis and not pre-existing malnutrition. Patients with cardiovascular disease appear to be at increased risk of death after peritonitis [47].

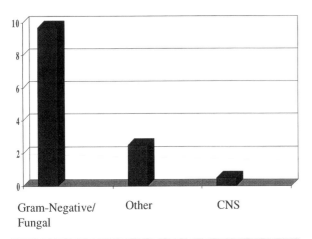

Figure 5. Mortality of peritonitis by organism. Rates expressed as percentage associated with death per episode. CNS = Coagulase-negative *Staphylococcus*. Data derived from ref. 8.

Prevention

General

Careful selection of patients can decrease a programmes peritonitis rate. Transfer to haemodialysis of patients with multiple episodes of peritonitis should be strongly considered. Training by experienced nurses is critical. Dryden *et al.* found that a preventative programme decreased the risk of exit-site infection (10-fold), peritonitis rate (2-fold) and catheter loss (4.5-fold) [247]. The programme was directed at *S. aureus* nasal carriage, intensive training of nurses and aseptic techniques for catheter insertion and care. Tubing changes should be performed by nurses, not patients [248]. Connection technology for CAPD using a twin bag system or APD should be utilized. The spike assist device for APD may also decrease rates [84]. Aggressive nutritional intervention in children may decrease the peritonitis rate [249]. We provide prophylaxis for technique-related contaminations with cefazolin or cephalexin, as well as prophylaxis for invasive procedures.

In terms of training, patients should be instructed to wear masks during exchanges. Careful hand-washing with anti-bacterial soap, and complete drying of the hands, decreases the skin bacterial count by 95–99%, thus reducing the potential transfer of bacteria [250]. The room where exchanges are performed should be isolated from heavy traffic. Pets should be excluded from the room in which exchanges are performed as bacterial transmission from pets has been reported [251, 252].

Prevention of catheter-related peritonitis

The use of prophylactic antibiotics at the time of insertion is controversial. The recent 1998 ISPD guidelines state that it is prudent to use antibiotics, and suggest the use of anti-staphylococcal antibiotics [253]. There have been three randomized prospective trials. Two showed a benefit using cefuroxime (1.5 g intravenously, 250 mg intraperitoneally) or gentamycin [1.5 mg/kg intravenously) [254, 255]. In both cases the incidence of peritonitis was lower in the first month after insertion. In contrast, Lye *et al.* found no benefit using gentamicin (80 mg) and cefazolin (500 mg) [256]. Given the high risk of catheter loss with catheter-related peritonitis, we recommend the use of prophylactic antibiotics. Though the ISPD recommends an anti-staphylococcal antibiotic, it may be more prudent to use an antibiotic that also has Gram-negative coverage (e.g. cefazolin). Staphylococcal infections predominate in those untreated, but Gram-negative infections have also been reported [254, 257]. Double-cuff catheters should be utilized [252], with a downward directed exit site [23, 252]. Swimming should be avoided after catheter insertion, until the catheter is healed, and swimming in lakes and ponds completely avoided. Exit-site infections should be treated promptly. We have found that patients with untreated well water at home are at increased risk for *Pseudomonas* exit-site infections, and we instruct these patients to use bottled water for exit-site care.

Specific organism prophylaxis

Dental procedures

Oral procedures have a high incidence of transient bacteraemia, though the inoculum is generally low [63]. Peritonitis after dental procedures has been reported in children and adults [60, 61]. Though there are no prospective trials, we would recommend prophylaxis prior to dental procedures, using American Heart Association guidelines.

Staphylococcus aureus

S. aureus nasal carriage increases the risk of peritonitis as well as exit-site and tunnel infections [86–88, 91, 92]. There have been a number of studies examining the effect of prophylaxis on peritonitis; these regimens are summarized in Table 9. All the regimens decrease the rate of infection (Fig. 6). In a study directly comparing exit-site mupirocin to cyclical rifampin every 3 months, both were equally

Table 9. *Staphylococcus aureus* prophylactic regimens

	Reference
Rifampin (carriers)	
Adults:	
600 mg/day × 5 days every 3 months	95, 98
Children:	
300 mg/day for children <30 kg, 600 mg/day	
for >30 kg	259*
20 mg/kg/day in two divided doses	97†
Exit-site mupirocin	98, 99
Daily as part of routine exit-site care for all patients	
(not studied in children)	
Nasal mupirocin	
2% b.i.d.–t.i.d. × 5–7 days for carriers with	
retreatment for recolonization based on cultures	
(adults and children)	91, 96
2% b.i.d. for 5 days each month in carriers	258

*Paediatric trial; the rifampin was given with nasal bacitracin.
†Paediatric trial; the mupirocin was given with cloxacillin.

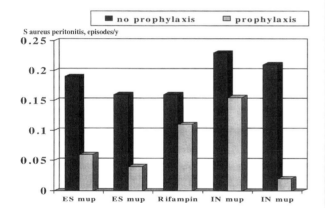

Figure 6. Effect of staphylococcal peritonitis prophylaxis on peritonitis rates. Trials shown are adult trials utilizing only rifampin or mupirocin. Data derived from refs 95, 96, 98, 99, 258. ES mup = Exit-site mupirocin, IN mup = intra-nasal mupirocin.

effective but the incidence of side-effects was greater with the rifampin [98].

In the two studies utilizing mupirocin at the exit site, all patients were treated [98, 99]. The nasal mupirocin trials treated carriers only [91, 96, 258]. Most of the nasal mupirocin trials required subsequent surveillance cultures and retreatment of those who became recolonized [91, 96]. The recolonization rate is high after mupirocin or rifampin treatment, with 40–55% recurrence at 3 months [96, 259]. The Mupirocin Study Group, in contrast, initially screened patients for nasal carriage (two-thirds positive cultures) and then treated identified carriers with nasal mupirocin for 5 days every month [258].

Given the cost of frequent cultures this may be a more economical approach. The definition of carrier varied between the studies, but a conservative definition is one positive of three serial cultures [98]. Persistently positive nasal cultures (two or more out of three), is associated with a greater risk of infection, but the staphylococcal peritonitis rate is still elevated with one positive culture (compared to non-carriers) [88].

There were few side-effects associated with the mupirocin, mainly nasal irritation and discharge for the nasal route [258]. Exit-site mupirocin can degrade polyurethane and should be avoided with these catheters [260]. Increased antibiotic resistance to mupirocin has not been found with use of prophylactic mupirocin, though mupirocin appears to be less effective for MRSA [261, 262]. Given the high morbidity associated with *S. aureus* peritonitis, each dialysis unit should establish a prophylactic regimen to prevent this infection.

Fungal

Prior antibiotic use increases the risk of fungal peritonitis [25, 26, 77]. This introduces a potential target group for prophylaxis. Four trials have studied the effect of prophylaxis, though only one was a prospective, randomized trial (Fig. 7) [263–266]. Three trials utilized oral nystatin: 500 000 U tablet q.i.d., 500 IU t.i.d., or in children 10 000 U/kg/day in three divided doses during the antibiotic course [263, 265, 266]. Lo et al. randomized patients to either nystatin tablets during antibiotic courses or to control [263]. There was a decreased incidence of *Candida* peritonitis (1.9 versus 6.4 per 100 peritonitis episodes and 0.66 versus 1.43 per 100 antibiotic prescription for any indication) with prophylaxis. Two of the trials utilized ketoconazole (10 mg/kg per day in children) or fluconazole (200 mg on day 1, then 100 mg/day) [264, 266]. These studies, which had retrospective controls, also found a decreased incidence of fungal peritonitis.

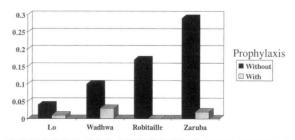

Figure 7. Effect of fungal prophylaxis on fungal peritonitis rates. Data derived from refs 263–266.

No side-effects of the prophylactic regimens were reported. Oral nystatin appears to be a reasonable choice for prophylaxis, especially in high-risk immunosuppressed patients and those on long-term antibiotics.

Gram-negative

Unfortunately, despite the morbidity and mortality associated with Gram-negative peritonitis, there are few effective interventions to reduce the incidence. Trials utilizing neomycin, cotrimoxazole or cephalexin were not effective in decreasing peritonitis [267–269]. Constipation, a possible inciting event, should be avoided with a bowel regimen. Prophylactic antibiotics should be administered for endoscopic and gynaecological procedures. The abdomen should be drained prior to procedures. Further research aimed at preventing Gram-negative peritonitis is necessary.

References

1. Canada–USA (CANUSA) Peritoneal Dialysis Study Group. Adequacy of dialysis and nutrition in continuous peritoneal dialysis: association with clinical outcomes. J Am Soc Nephrol 1996; 7: 198–207.
2. Pollock CA, Ibels LS, Caterson RJ, Mahony JF, Waugh DA, Cocksedge B: Continuous ambulatory peritoneal dialysis: eight years of experience at a single center. Medicine 1989; 68: 293–308.
3. Saade M, Joglar F. Chronic peritoneal dialysis: seven-year experience in a large Hispanic program. Perit Dial Int 1995; 15: 37–41.
4. Viglino G, Cancarini G, Catizone L et al. The impact of peritonitis on CAPD results. Adv Perit Dial 1992; 8: 269–75.
5. Woodrow G, Turney JH, Brownjohn AM. Technique failure in peritoneal dialysis and its impact on patient survival. Perit Dial Int 1997; 17: 360–4.
6. Fried L, Syed Abidi S, Bernardini J, Johnston JR, Piraino B. Hospitalization in peritoneal dialysis patients. Am J Kidney Dis (In press).
7. Bloembergen WE, Port FK. Epidemiological perspective on infections in chronic dialysis patients. Adv Renal Replacement Ther 1996; 3: 201–7.
8. Fried LF, Bernardini J, Johnston JR, Piraino B. Peritonitis influences mortality in peritoneal dialysis patients. J Am Soc Nephrol 1996; 7: 2176–82.
9. Rubin J, Hsu H. Continuous ambulatory peritoneal dialysis: ten years at one facility Am J Kidney Dis 1991; 17: 165–9.
10. Slingeneyer A, Mion C, Beraud JJ, Branger B, Balmes M. Peritonitis, a frequently lethal complication of intermittent and continuous peritoneal dialysis. Proc Eur Dial Transplant Assoc 1981; 18: 212–21.
11. Rubin J, Rogers WA, Taylor HM et al. Peritonitis during continuous ambulatory peritoneal dialysis. Ann Intern Med 1980; 92: 7–13.
12. De Vecchi AF, Maccario M, Braga M, Scalamogna A, Castelnovo C, Ponticelli C. Peritoneal dialysis in nondiabetic patients older than 70 years: comparison with patients age 40 to 60 years. Am J Kidney Dis 1998; 31: 479–90.
13. Tzamaloukas AH, Murata GH, Fox L. Peritoneal catheter loss and death in continuous ambulatory peritoneal dialysis peritonitis: correlation with clinical and biochemical parameters. Perit Dial Int 1992; 13 (suppl. 2): S338–40.
14. Bunke CM, Brier ME, Golper TA, for the Academic Subcommittee of the Network 9 Peritonitis Study. Outcomes of single organism peritonitis in peritoneal dialysis: gram-negatives versus gram positives in the Network 9 Peritonitis Study. Kidney Int 1997; 52: 524–9.
15. Troidle L, Gorban-Brennan N, Kliger A, Finkelstein F. Differing outcomes of gram-positive and gram-negative peritonitis. Am J Kidney Dis 1998; 32: 623–8.
16. Fenton S, Wu G, Cattran D, Wadgymar A, Allen AF. Clinical aspects of peritonitis in patients on CAPD. Perit Dial Bull 1981; 1 (suppl. 6): S4–7.
17. Grefberg N, Danielson BG, Nilsson P. Peritonitis in patients on continuous ambulatory peritoneal dialysis: a changing scene. Scand J Infect Dis 1984; 16: 187–93.
18. Domrongkitchaiporn S, Karim M, Watson L, Moriarty M. The influence of continuous ambulatory peritoneal dialysis connection technique on peritonitis rate and technique survival. Am J Kidney Dis 1994; 24: 50–8.
19. Holley JL, Bernardini J, Piraino B. Infecting organisms in continuous ambulatory peritoneal dialysis patients on the Y-set. Am J Kidney Dis 1994; 23: 569–73.
20. Tranaeus A, Heimburger O, Lindholm B. Peritonitis in continuous ambulatory peritoneal dialysis (CAPD): diagnostic findings, therapeutic outcome and complications. Perit Dial Int 1989; 9: 179–90.
21. Van Biesen W, Vanholder R, Vogelaers D et al. The need for a center-tailored treatment protocol for peritonitis. Perit Dial Int 1998; 18: 274–81.
22. Peterson PK, Matzke G, Keane WF. Current concepts in the management of peritonitis in patients undergoing continuous ambulatory peritoneal dialysis. Rev Infect Dis 1987; 9: 604–12.
23. Golper TA, Brier ME, Bunke M et al. for the Academic Subcommittee of the Steering Committee of the Network 9 Peritonitis and Catheter Survival Studies. Risk factors for peritonitis in long-term peritoneal dialysis: Network 9 Peritonitis and Catheter Survival Studies. Am J Kidney Int 1996; 28: 428–36.
24. Canadian CAPD Clinical Trials Group. Peritonitis in continuous ambulatory peritoneal dialysis (CAPD): a multicenter randomized clinical trial comparing the Y connector disinfectant system to standard systems. Perit Dial Int 1989; 9: 159–63.
25. Goldie SJ, Kiernan-Troidle L, Torres C et al. Fungal peritonitis in a large chronic peritoneal dialysis population: a report of 55 episodes. Am J Kidney Dis 1996; 28: 86–91.
26. Johnson RJ, Ramsey PG, Gallagher N, Ahmad S. Fungal peritonitis in patients on peritoneal dialysis: incidence, clinical features and prognosis. Am J Nephrol 1985; 5: 169–75.
27. Eisenberg ES, Leviton I, Soeiro R. Fungal peritonitis in patients receiving peritoneal dialysis: experience with 11 patients and review of the literature. Rev Infect Dis 1986; 8: 309–20.
28. Michel C, Courdavault L, Al Khayat R, Viron B, Roux P, Mignon F. Fungal peritonitis in patients on peritoneal dialysis. Am J Nephrol 1994; 14: 113–20.
29. Winton MD, Everett ED. Antimicrobial therapy for CAPD-associated peritonitis. Blood Purif 1989; 7: 115–25.
30. Vas SI. The diagnosis and treatment of peritonitis in patients on continuous ambulatory peritoneal dialysis. Semin Dial 1995; 8: 232–7.
31. Rotellar C, Sivarajan S, Mazzoni MJ et al. Bowel perforation in CAPD patients. Perit Dial Int 1992; 12: 396–8.
32. Van Reijden HJ, Struijik DG, van Ketel RJ, Kox C, Krediet RT, Arisz L. Fecal peritonitis in patients on continuous ambulatory peritoneal dialysis, an end-point in CAPD? Adv Perit Dial 1988; 4: 198–203.
33. Bustos E, Rotellar C, Mazzoni MJ, Rakowski TA, Argy WP, Winchester JF. Clinical aspects of bowel perforation in

patients undergoing continuous ambulatory peritoneal dialysis. Semin Dial 1994; 7: 355–9.

34. Holley JL, Bernardini J, Piraino B. Polymicrobial peritonitis in patients on continuous peritoneal dialysis. Am J Kidney Dis 1992; 19: 162–6.

35. Lui SL, Lo CY, Choy BY, Chan TM, Lo WK, Cheng IPK. Optimal treatment and long-term outcome of tuberculous peritonitis complicating continuous ambulatory peritoneal dialysis. Am J Kidney Dis 1996; 28: 747–51.

36. Vas S. Microbiological aspects of peritonitis. Perit Dial Bull 1981; 1: S11–14.

37. Bazzato G, Coli U, Landini S et al. The double bag system for CAPD reduces the peritonitis rate. Trans Am Soc Artif Intern Organs 1984; 30: 690–2.

38. Bonnardeaux A, Ouimet D, Galarneau A et al. Peritonitis in continuous ambulatory peritoneal dialysis: impact of a compulsory switch from a standard to a Y-connector system in single North American center. Am J Kidney Dis 1992; 29: 364–70.

39. Dryden MS, McCann M, Wing AJ, Phillips I. Controlled trial of a Y-set dialysis delivery system to prevent peritonitis in patients receiving continuous ambulatory peritoneal dialysis. J Hosp Infect 1992; 20: 185–92.

40. Grutzmacher P, Tsobanelis T, Bruns M, Kurz P, Hoppe D, Vlachojannis J. Decrease in peritonitis rate by integrated disconnect system in patients on continuous ambulatory peritoneal dialysis. Perit Dial Int 1992; 13 (suppl. 2): S326–8.

41. Vas SI. Etiology and treatment of peritonitis. Trans Am Soc Artif Intern Organs 1984; 30: 682–4.

42. Gupta B, Bernardini J, Piraino B. Peritonitis associated with exit site and tunnel infections. Am J Kidney Dis 1996; 28: 415–19.

43. Read RR, Eberwein P, Dasgupta MK et al. Peritonitis in peritoneal dialysis: bacterial colonization by biofilm spread along the catheter surface. Kidney Int 1989; 35: 614–21.

44. Piraino B, Bernardini J, Sorkin M. The influence of peritoneal catheter exit-site infections on peritonitis, tunnel infections, and catheter loss in patients on continuous ambulatory peritoneal dialysis. Am J Kidney Dis 1986; 8: 436–40.

45. Scalamogna A, Castelnovo C, De Vecchi A, Ponticelli C. Exit-site and tunnel infections in continuous ambulatory peritoneal dialysis. Am J Kidney Dis 1991; 18: 674–7.

46. Dasgupta MK, Costerton JW. Significance of biofilm-adherent bacterial microcolonies on Tenckhoff catheters of CAPD patients. Blood Purif 1989; 7: 144–55.

47. Tzamaloukas AH, Hartshorne MF, Gibel LJ, Murata GH. Persistence of positive dialysate cultures after apparent cure of CAPD peritonitis. Adv Perit Dial 1993; 9: 198–201.

48. Swartz R, Messana J, Holmes C, Williams J. Biofilm formation on peritoneal catheters does not require the presence of infection. Trans Am Soc Artif Intern Organs 1991; 37: 626–33.

49. Verger C, Danne O, Vuillemin F. Colonoscopy and continuous ambulatory peritoneal dialysis. Gastroint Endosc 1987; 33: 334–5.

50. Sprenger R, Neyer U. *Enterococcus* peritonitis after endoscopic polypectomy: need for prophylactic antibiotics. Perit Dial Bull 1987; 7: 263–4.

51. Holley J, Seibert M, Moss A. Peritonitis following colonoscopy: a need for prophylaxis? Perit Dial Bull 1987; 7: 105–6.

52. Maruyama H, Nakamura T, Oya M et al. Posthysteroscopy *Candida glabrata* peritonitis in a patient on CAPD. Perit Dial Int 1997; 17: 404–5.

53. Troidle L, Kliger AS, Goldie SJ et al. Continuous peritoneal dialysis-associated peritonitis of nosocomial origin. Perit Dial Int 1996; 16: 505–10.

54. Ray SM, Piraino B, Holley J. Peritonitis following colonoscopy in a peritoneal dialysis patient. Perit Dial Int 1990; 10: 97–8.

55. Tzamaloukas AH, Obermiller LE, Gibel LJ et al. Peritonitis associated with intra-abdominal pathology in continuous ambulatory peritoneal dialysis. Perit Dial Int 1993; 13: S335–7.

56. Harwell CM, Newman LN, Cacho CP, Mulligan DC, Schulak JA, Friedlander MA. Abdominal catastrophe: visceral injury as a cause of peritonitis in patients treated by peritoneal dialysis. Perit Dial Int 1997; 17: 586–94.

57. Schweinburg FB, Seligman AM, Fine J. Transmural migration of intestinal bacteria: a study based on the use of radioactive *Escherichia coli*. New Engl J Med 1976; 242: 747–51.

58. Caravaca F, Ruiz-Carlo R, Dominguez C. Risk factors for developing peritonitis caused by micro-organisms of enteral origin in peritoneal dialysis patients. Perit Dial Int 1998; 18: 41–5.

59. Singharetnam W, Holley JL. Acute treatment of constipation may lead to transmural migration of bacteria resulting in gram-negative, polymicrobial or fungal peritonitis. Perit Dial Int 1996; 16: 423–5.

60. Kiddy K, Brow PP, Michael J, Adu D. Peritonitis due to *Streptococcus viridans* in patients receiving continuous ambulatory peritoneal dialysis. Br Med J 1985; 290: 969.

61. Levy M, Balfe JW. Optimal approach to the prevention and treatment of peritonitis in children undergoing continuous ambulatory and continuous cycling peritoneal dialysis. Sem Dial 1994; 7: 442–9.

62. Bottoman VA, Surawicz CM. Bacteremia with gastrointestinal endoscopic procedures. Gastroint Endosc 1986; 32: 342–6.

63. Durack DT. Prevention of infective endocarditis. N Engl J Med 1995; 332: 38–44.

64. Coward RA, Gokal R, Wise M, Mallick NP, Warrell D. Peritonitis associated with vaginal leakage of dialysis fluid in continuous ambulatory peritoneal dialysis. Br Med J 1982; 284: 1529.

65. Swartz RD. Recurrent polymicrobial peritonitis from a gynecologic source as a complication of CAPD. Perit Dial Bull 1983; 3: 32–3.

66. Stuck A, Seiler A, Fry FJ. Peritonitis due to an intrauterine device in a patient on CAPD. Perit Dial Bull 1986; 6: 158–9.

67. Oxton LL, Zimmerman SW, Roeker EB, Wakeen M. Risk factors for peritoneal dialysis-related infections. Perit Dial Int 1994; 14: 137–44.

68. Korbet SM, Vonesh EF, Firanek CA. A retrospective assessment of risk factors for peritonitis among an urban CAPD population. Perit Dial Int 1993; 13: 126–31.

69. Fine A, Cox D, Bouw M. Higher incidence of peritonitis in Native Canadians on continuous ambulatory peritoneal dialysis. Perit Dial Int 1994; 14: 227–30.

70. Farias MG, Soucie JM, McClellan W, Mitch WE. Race and the risk of peritonitis: an analysis of factors associated with the initial episode. Kidney Int 1994; 46: 1392–4.

71. Juergensen PH, Juergensen DM, Wuerth DB et al. Psychosocial factors and the incidence of peritonitis. Adv Perit Dial 1996; 12: 196–8.

72. Nolph KD, Cuttler SJ, Steinberg SM, Novak JW. Continuous ambulatory peritoneal dialysis in the United States: a three-year study. Kidney Int 1985; 28: 198–205.

73. Holley JL, Bernardini J, Perlmutter JA, Piraino B. A comparison of infection rates among older and younger patients on continuous peritoneal dialysis. Perit Dial Int 1994; 14: 66–9.

74. Andrews PA, Warr KJ, Hicks JA, Cameron JS. Impaired outcome of continuous ambulatory peritoneal dialysis in immunosuppressed patients. Nephrol Dial Transplant 1996; 11: 1104–8.

75. Tebben JA, Rigsby MO, Selwyn PA, Brennan N, Kliger A, Finkelstein FO. Outcome of HIV infected patients on continuous ambulatory peritoneal dialysis. Kidney Int 1993; 44: 191–8.

76. Lewis M, Gorban-Brennan NL, Kliger A, Cooper K, Finkelstein FO. Incidence and spectrum of organisms causing peritonitis in HIV positive patients on CAPD. Adv Perit Dial 1990; 6: 136–8.

77. Bordes A, Campos-Herrero MI, Fernandez A, Vega N, Rodriguez JC, Palop L. Predisposing and prognostic factors of fungal peritonitis in peritoneal dialysis. Perit Dial Int 1995; 15: 275–6.

78. Kiernan L, Kliger A, Gorban-Brennan N *et al.* Comparison of continuous ambulatory peritoneal dialysis-related infections with different 'Y-tubing' exchange systems. J Am Soc Nephrol 1995; 5: 1835–8.

79. Harris DCH, Yuill EJ, Byth K, Chapman JR, Hunt C. Twin-versus single-bag disconnect systems: infection rates and cost of continuous ambulatory peritoneal dialysis. J Am Soc Nephrol 1996; 7: 2392–8.

80. De Fijter CWH, Oe LP, Nauta JJP *et al.* Clinical efficacy and morbidity associated with continuous cyclic compared with continuous ambulatory peritoneal dialysis. Ann Intern Med 1994; 120: 264–71.

81. Diaz-Buxo JA. Current status of continuous cyclic peritoneal dialysis (CCPD). Perit Dial Int 1989; 9: 9–14.

82. Schmidt R, Bender F, Domico J, Bernardini J, Sorkin M, Piraino B. Peritonitis rates of APD may not better those of CAPD. Perit Dial Int 1998; 18 (suppl. 1): S34.

83. Troidle LK, Gorban-Brennan N, Kliger AS, Finkelstein FO. Continuous cycler therapy, manual peritoneal dialysis therapy, and peritonitis. Adv Perit Dial 1998; 14: 137–41.

84. Bird M, Dacko C, Miller M, Bernardini J, Piraino B. Reducing peritonitis in APD patients. Perit Dial Int (In press).

85. Sewell CM, Clarridge J, Lacke C, Weinman EJ, Young EJ. Staphylococcal nasal carriage and subsequent infection in peritoneal dialysis patients. JAMA 1982; 248: 1493–5.

86. Luzar MA, Coles GA, Faller B *et al. Staphylococcus aureus* nasal carriage and infection in patients on continuous ambulatory peritoneal dialysis. N Engl J Med 1990; 322: 505–9.

87. Davies SJ, Ogg CS, Cameron JS, Poston S, Noble WC. *Staphylococcus aureus* nasal carriage, exit-site infection and catheter loss in patients treated with continuous ambulatory peritoneal dialysis (CAPD). Perit Dial Int 1989; 9: 61–4.

88. Piraino B, Perlmutter JA, Holley JL, Bernardini J. *Staphylococcus aureus* peritonitis is associated with Staphylococcus aureus nasal carriage in peritoneal dialysis patients. Perit Dial Int 1993; 13 (suppl. 2): S332–4.

89. Wanten GJA, van Oost P, Schneeberger PM, Koolen MI. Nasal carriage and peritonitis by *Staphylococcus aureus* in patients on continuous ambulatory peritoneal dialysis: a prospective study. Perit Dial Int 1996; 16: 352–6.

90. Zimakoff J, Pedersen FB, Bergen L *et al.* and additional members of the Danish Study Group of Peritonitis in Dialysis (DASPID). *Staphylococcus aureus* carriage and infections among patients in four haemo- and peritoneal-dialysis centres in Denmark. J Hosp Infect 1996; 33: 289–300.

91. Kingwatanakul P, Warady BA. *Staphylococcus aureus* nasal carriage in children receiving long-term peritoneal dialysis. Adv Perit Dial 1997; 13: 281–4.

92. Lye WC, Leong SO, van der Straten J, Lee EJC. *Staphylococcus aureus* CAPD-related infections are associated with nasal carriage. Adv Perit Dial 1994; 10: 163–5.

93. Zimmerman SW, O'Brien M, Wiedenhoeft FA, Johnson CA. *Staphylococcus aureus* peritoneal catheter-related infections: a cause of catheter loss and peritonitis. Perit Dial Int 1988; 8: 191–4.

94. Vychytil A, Lorenz M, Schneider B, Horl WH, Haag-Weber M. New strategies to prevent *Staphylococcus aureus* infections in peritoneal dialysis patients. J Am Soc Nephrol 1998; 9: 669–76.

95. Zimmerman SW, Ahrens E, Johnson CA *et al.* Randomized controlled trial of prophylactic rifampin for peritoneal dialysis-related infections. Am J Kidney Dis 1991; 18: 225–31.

96. Perez-Fontan M, Rosales M, Rodriguez-Carmona A *et al.* Treatment of *Staphylococcus aureus* nasal carriers in CAPD with mupirocin. Adv Perit Dial 1993; 9: 242–5.

97. Blowley DL, Warady BA, McFarland KS. The treatment of *Staphylococcus aureus* nasal carriage in pediatric peritoneal dialysis patients. Adv Perit Dial 1994; 10: 297–9.

98. Bernardini J, Piraino B, Holley J, Johnston JR, Lutes R. A randomized trial of *Staphylococcus aureus* prophylaxis in peritoneal dialysis patients: mupirocin calcium ointment 2%

applied to the exit site versus cyclic oral rifampin. Am J Kidney Dis 1996; 27: 695–700.

99. Thodis E, Bhaskaran S, Pasadakis P, Bargman JM, Vas SI, Oreopoulos DG. Decrease in *Staphylococcus aureus* exit-site infections and peritonitis in CAPD patients by local application of mupirocin ointment at the catheter exit site. Perit Dial Int 1998; 18: 261–70.

100. Koopmans JG, Boeschoten EW, Pannekeet MM *et al.* Impaired initial cell reaction in CAPD-related peritonitis. Perit Dial Int 1996; 16 (suppl. 1): S362–7.

101. Korzets Z, Korzets A, Golan E, Zevin D, Bernheim J. CAPD peritonitis – initial presentation as an acute abdomen with clear peritoneal effluent. Clin Nephrol 1992; 37: 155–7.

102. Humayan HM, Daugirdas JT, Ing TS, Leehy DJ, Gandhi VC, Popli S. Chylous ascites in a patient treated with intermittent peritoneal dialysis. Artif Organs 1984; 8: 358–60.

103. Bagnis C, Gabella P, Bruno M *et al.* Cloudy dialysate due to adenocarcinoma cells in a CAPD patient. Perit Dial Int 1993; 13: 322–3.

104. Bargman JM, Zent R, Ellis P, Auger M, Wilson S. Diagnosis of lymphoma in a continuous ambulatory peritoneal dialysis patient by peritoneal fluid cytology. Am J Kidney Dis 1994; 23: 747–50.

105. Porter J, Wang WM, Oliveira DBG. Chylous ascites and continuous ambulatory peritoneal dialysis. Nephrol Dial Transplant 1991; 6: 659–61.

106. Kim D, Tapson J, Wu G, Khanna R, Vas SI, Oreopoulos DG. Staph aureus peritonitis in patients on continuous ambulatory peritoneal dialysis. Trans Am Soc Artif Intern Organs 1984; 30: 494–7.

107. De Bustillo EM, Aguilera A, Jimenez C, Bajo MA, Sanchez C, Selegas R. Streptococcal versus *Staphylococcus epidermidis* peritonitis in CAPD. A comparative study. Perit Dial Int 1997; 17: 392–5.

108. Wakeen MJ, Zimmerman SW, Bidwell D. Viscus perforation in peritoneal dialysis patients: diagnosis and outcome. Perit Dial Int 1994; 14: 371–7.

109. Chang JJ, Yeun JY, Harsbargen JA. Pneumoperitoneum in peritoneal dialysis patients. Am J Kidney Dis 1995; 25; 297–301.

110. Plum J, Sudkamp S, Grabensee B. Results of ultrasound-assisted diagnosis of tunnel infections in continuous ambulatory peritoneal dialysis. Am J Kidney Dis 1994; 23: 99–104.

111. Keane WF, Peterson PK. Peritonitis during continuous ambulatory peritoneal dialysis: the role of host defense mechanisms. Trans Am Soc Artif Intern Organs 1984; 30: 684–6.

112. Flanigan MJ, Freeman RM, Lim VS. Cellular response to peritonitis among peritoneal dialysis patients. Am J Kidney Dis 1985; 6: 420–4.

113. Riera G, Bushinsky D, Emmanouel DS. First exchange neutrophilia: an index of peritonitis during chronic intermittent peritoneal dialysis. Clin Nephrol 1985; 24: 5–8.

114. Smoszna J, Raczka A, Fuksiewicz A, Wankowicz Z. Prognostic value of different tests in the early diagnosis of peritonitis during standard peritoneal dialysis (SPD). Adv Perit Dial 1988; 4: 194–7.

115. Antonsen S, Pedersen FB, Wang P, and the Danish Study Group on Peritonitis in Dialysis (DASPID). Leukocytes in peritoneal dialysis effluents. Perit Dial Int 1991; 11: 43–7.

116. Holley HP, Tucker CT, Moffatt TL, Dodds KA, Dodds HM. Tuberculous peritonitis in patients undergoing chronic home peritoneal dialysis. Am J Kidney Dis 1982; 1: 222–6.

117. Mallat SG, Brensilver JM. Tuberculous peritonitis in a CAPD patient cured without catheter removal: case report, review of the literature and guidelines for treatment and diagnosis. Am J Kidney Dis 1989; 13: 154–7.

118. Dunmire RB, Breyer JA. Nontuberculous mycobacterial peritonitis during continuous ambulatory peritoneal dialysis: case report and review of diagnostic and therapeutic strategies. Am J Kidney Dis 1991; 18: 126–30.

119. Sridhar R, Thornely-Brown D, Kant KS. Peritonitis due to *Aspergillus niger*: diagnostic importance of peritoneal eosinophilia. Perit Dial Int 1990; 10: 100–1.

120. Nankivell BJ, Pacey D, Gordon DL. Peritoneal eosinophilia associated with *Paecilomyces variotii* infection in continuous ambulatory peritoneal dialysis. Am J Kidney Dis 1991; 18: 603–5.

121. Gokal R, Ramos JM, Ward MK, Kerr DNS. 'Eosinophilic' peritonitis in continuous ambulatory peritoneal dialysis (CAPD). Clin Nephrol 1981; 15: 328–30.

122. Solary E, Cabanne JF, Tanter Y, Rifle G. Evidence for a role of plasticizers in 'eosinophilic' peritonitis in continuous ambulatory peritoneal dialysis. Nephron 1986; 42: 341–2.

123. Piraino BM, Silver MR, Dominguez JH, Puschett JB. Peritoneal eosinophils during intermittent peritoneal dialysis. Am J Nephrol 1984; 4: 152–7.

124. Chandran PKG, Humayun HM, Daugirdas JT, Nawab ZM, Gandhi VC, Ing TS. Blood eosinophila in patients undergoing maintenance peritoneal dialysis. Arch Intern Med 1985; 145: 114–16.

125. Chan MK, Chow L, Lam SS, Jones B. Peritoneal eosinophilia in patients on continuous ambulatory peritoneal dialysis: a prospective study. Am J Kidney Dis 1988; 11: 180–3.

126. Nassberger L, Arbin A. Eosinophic peritonitis – hypothesis. Nephron 1987; 46: 103–4.

127. Leung ACT, Orange G, Henderson IS. Intraperitoneal hydrocortisone in eosinophilic peritonitis associated with continuous ambulatory peritoneal dialysis. Br Med J 1983; 286: 766.

128. Tang S, Lo CY, Lo WK, Chan TM. Resolution of eosinophilic peritonitis with ketotifen. Am J Kidney Dis 1997; 30: 433–6.

129. Ryan S, Fessia S. Improved method for recovery of peritonitis-causing microorganisms from peritoneal dialysate. J Clin Microbiol 1987; 25: 383–4.

130. Luce E, Nakagawa D, Lovell J, Davis J, Stinebaugh BJ, Suki WN. Improvement in the bacteriologic diagnosis of peritonitis with the use of blood culture media. Trans Am Soc Artif Intern Organs 1982; 28: 259–62.

131. Blondeau JM, Pylypchuk GB, Kappel JE, Pilkey B, Lawler C. Comparison of bedside- and laboratory-inoculated Bactec high- and low-volume resin bottles for the recovery of microorganisms causing peritonitis in CAPD patients. Diagn Microbiol Infect Dis 1998; 31: 281–7.

132. McIntyre M, Trend V, Depoiy C. The microbiological diagnosis of CAPD peritonitis. Perit Dial Bull 1986; 6: 40–1.

133. Lye WC, Wong PL, Leong SO, Lee EJC. Isolation of organisms in CAPD peritonitis: a comparison of two techniques. Adv Perit Dial 1994; 10: 166–8.

134. Sewell DL, Golper TA, Hulman PB et al. Comparison of large volume culture to other methods for isolation of microorganisms from dialysate. Perit Dial Int 1990; 10: 49–52.

135. Forbes BA, Frymoyer PA, Kopecky RT, Wojtaszek JM, Pettit DJ. Evaluation of the lysis-centrifugation system for culturing dialysates from continuous ambulatory peritoneal dialysis patients with peritonitis. Am J Kidney Dis 1988; 11: 176–9.

136. Fenton P. Laboratory diagnosis of peritonitis in patients undergoing continuous ambulatory peritoneal dialysis. J Clin Pathol 1982; 35: 1181–4.

137. Bezerra DA, Silva MB, Caramori JST et al. The diagnostic value of gram stain for initial identification of the etiologic agent of peritonitis in CAPD patients. Perit Dial Int 1997; 17: 269–72.

138. Korzets Z, Erdberg A, Golan E et al. Frequent involvement of the internal cuff segment in CAPD peritonitis and exit-site infection – an ultrasound study. Nephrol Dial Transplant 1996; 11: 336–9.

139. Vychytil A, Lorenz M, Schneider B, Horl WH, Haag-Weber M. New criteria for management of catheter infec-

tions in peritoneal dialysis patients using ultrasonography. J Am Soc Nephrol 1998; 9: 290–6.

140. Holley JL, Foulks CJ, Moss AH, Willard D. Ultrasound as a tool in the diagnosis and management of exit-site infection in patients undergoing continuous ambulatory peritoneal dialysis. Am J Kidney Dis 1989; 14: 211–16.

141. Domico J, Warman M, Jaykamur S, Sorkin MI. Is ultrasonography useful in predicting catheter loss? Adv Perit Dial 1993; 9: 231–2.

142. Keane WF, Alexander SR, Bailie GR et al. Peritoneal dialysis-related peritonitis treatment recommendations: 1996 update. Perit Dial Int 1996; 16: 557–73.

143. Bunke M, Brier M, Golper TA. Culture-negative CAPD peritonitis: the Network 9 Study. Adv Perit Dial 1994; 10: 174–8.

144. Holley JL, Moss AH. A prospective evaluation of blood culture versus standard plate techniques for diagnosing peritonitis in continuous ambulatory peritoneal dialysis. Am J Kidney Dis 1989; 13: 184–8.

145. Eisele G, Adewunni C, Bailie GR, Yocum D, Venezia R. Surreptitious use of antimicrobial agents by CAPD patients. Perit Dial Int 1993; 13: 313–15.

146. Pagniez DC, Vrtovsnik F, Delvallez L, Reade R, Dequiedt P, Tacquet A. Ofloxacin treatment may mask tuberculous peritonitis in CAPD patients. Perit Dial Int 1991; 11: 92–3.

147. Burkhart J, Haigler S, Caruana R, Hylander B. Usefulness of peritoneal fluid amyalse levels in the differential of peritonitis in peritoneal dialysis patients. J Am Soc Nephrol 1991; 1: 1186–90.

148. Caruana RJ, Burkhart J, Segraves D, Smallwood S, Haymore J, Disher B. Serum and peritoneal fluid amylase levels in CAPD. Am J Nephrol 1987; 7: 169–72.

149. Charney DI, Gouge SF. Chemical peritonitis secondary to intraperitoneal vancomycin. Am J Kidney Dis 1991; 17: 76–9.

150. Piraino B, Bernardini J, Johnston J et al. Chemical peritonitis due to intraperitoneal vancomycin (Vancoled). Perit Dial Bull 1987; 7: 156–9.

151. Wong PN, Mak SK, Lee KF, Fung LH, Wong AKM. A prospective study of vancomycin- (Vancoled-)induced chemical peritonitis in CAPD patients. Perit Dial Int 1997; 17: 202–4.

152. Karanicolas S, Oreopoulos DG, Izatt SH et al. Epidemic of aseptic peritonitis caused by endotoxin during chronic peritoneal dialysis. N Engl J Med 1977; 296: 1336–7.

153. Nankivell BJ, Lake N, Gillies A. Intracatheter streptokinase for recurrent peritonitis in CAPD. Clin Nephrol 1991; 35: 20–3.

154. Coronel F, Martin-Rabadan P, Romero J. Chemical peritonitis after intraperitoneal administration of amphotericin B in a fungal infection of the catheter subcutaneous tunnel. Perit Dial Int 1993; 13: 161–2.

155. Bennett-Jones D, Wass V, Mawson P et al. A comparison of intraperitoneal and intravenous/oral antibiotics in CAPD peritonitis. Perit Dial Bull 1987; 7: 31–3.

156. Keane WF, Everett ED, Golper TA et al. Peritoneal dialysis-related peritonitis treatment recommendations: 1993 update. Perit Dial Int 1993; 13: 14–28.

157. Nikolaidis P, Walker SE, Dombros N, Toourkantonis A, Paton TW, Oreopoulos DG. Single-dose pefloxacin pharmacokinetics and metabolism in patients undergoing continuous ambulatory peritoneal dialysis (CAPD). Perit Dial Int 1991; 11: 59–63.

158. Janknegt R. CAPD peritonitis and fluoroquinolones. Perit Dial Int 1991; 11: 48–58.

159. Cheng IKP, Chan CY, Wong WT et al. A randomized prospective comparison of oral versus intraperitoneal ciprofloxacin as the primary treatment of peritonitis complicating continuous ambulatory peritoneal dialysis. Perit Dial Int 1993; 13 (suppl. 2): S351–4.

160. Perez-Fontan M, Rosales M, Fernandez F *et al.* Ciprofloxacin in the treatment of gram-positive bacterial peritonitis in patients undergoing CAPD. Perit Dial Int 1991; 11: 233–6.

161. Weber J, Staerz E, Mettang T, Machleidt C, Kuhlmann U. Treatment of peritonitis continuous ambulatory peritoneal dialysis (CAPD) with intraperitoneal cefazolin and gentamicin. Perit Dial Int 1989; 9: 191–5.

162. Vas S, Bargman J, Oreopoulos DG. Treatment of PD patients of peritonitis caused by gram-positive organisms with single daily dose of antibiotics. Perit Dial Int 1997; 17: 91–4.

163. Lupo A, Rugiu C, Bernich P *et al.* A prospective, randomized trial of two antibiotic regimens in the treatment of peritonitis in CAPD patients: teicoplanin plus tobramycin versus cephalothin plus tobramycin. J Antimicrob Chemother 1997; 40: 729–32.

164. Golper T. Intermittent versus continuous antibiotics for PD-related peritonitis. Perit Dial Int 1997; 17: 11–12.

165. Thomas JK, Forrest A, Bhavnani SM *et al.* Pharmacodynamic evaluation of factors associated with the development of bacterial resistance in acutely ill patients during therapy. Antimicrob Agents Chemother 1998; 42: 521–7.

166. Gucek A, Bren AF, Lindic J, Hergouth V, Mlinsek D. Is monotherapy with cefazolin of ofloxacin an adequate treatment for peritonitis in CAPD patients? Adv Perit Dial 1994; 10: 144–6.

167. Lai MN, Kao MT, Chen CC, Cheung SY, Chung WK. Intraperitoneal once-daily dose of cefazolin and gentamycin for treating CAPD peritonitis. Perit Dial Int 1997; 17: 87–9.

168. Flanigan MJ, Lim VS. Initial treatment of dialysis associated peritonitis: a controlled trial of vancomycin versus cefazolin. Perit Dial Int 1991; 11: 31–7.

169. Gucek A, Bren AF, Hergouth V, Lindic J. Cefazolin and netilmycin versus vancomycin and ceftazidime in the treatment of CAPD peritonitis. Adv Perit Dial 1997; 13: 218–20.

170. Nikolaidis PP. Quinolones: pharmacokinetics and pharmacodynamics. Perit Dial Int 1993; 13 (suppl. 2): S377–9.

171. Cheng IKP, Chan CY, Wong WT. A randomised prospective comparison of oral ofloxacin and intraperitoneal vancomycin plus aztreonam in the treatment of bacterial peritonitis complicating continuous ambulatory peritoneal dialysis (CAPD). Perit Dial Int 1991; 11: 27–30.

172. Nye KJ, Gibson SP, Nwosu AC, Manji MR, Robinson BHB, Hawkins JB. Single-dose intraperitoneal vancomycin and oral ciprofloxacin for the treatment of peritonitis in CAPD patients: preliminary report. Perit Dial Int 1993; 13: 59–60.

173. Piraino B, Bernardini J, Sorkin M. A five year study of the microbiologic results of exit site infections and peritonitis in continuous ambulatory peritoneal dialysis. Am J Kidney Dis 1987; 10: 281–6.

174. Keller E. Pharmacokinetics and pharmacodynamics of antistaphylococcal antibiotics in continuous ambulatory peritoneal dialysis patients. Perit Dial Int 1993; 13 (suppl. 2): S367–70.

175. Lye WC, Leong SO, Lee EJC. Methicillin-resistant *Staphylococcus aureus* nasal carriage and infections in CAPD. Kidney Int 1993; 43: 1357–62.

176. Borra SI, Chandarana J, Kleinfeld M. Fatal peritonitis due to Group B β-hemolytic *Streptococcus* in a patient receiving continuous ambulatory peritoneal dialysis. Am J Kidney Dis 1992; 19: 375–7.

177. Suh H, Wadhwa NK, Cabralda T, Sorrento J. Endogenous peritonitis and related outcome in peritoneal dialysis patients. Adv Perit Dial 1996; 12: 192–5.

178. Low CL, Eisele G, Cerda J *et al.* Low prevalence of vancomycin-resistant *Enterococcus* in dialysis outpatients with a history of vancomycin use. Perit Dial Int 1996; 16: 651–2.

179. Sandoe JAT, Gokal R, Struthers JK. Vancomycin-resistant enterococci and empirical vancomycin for CAPD peritonitis. Perit Dial Int 1997; 17: 617–18.

180. Brady JP, Snyder JW, Harsbargen JA. Vancomycin-resistant *Enterococcus* in end-stage renal disease. Am J Kidney Dis 1998; 32: 415–18.

181. Tokars JI, Miller ER, Alter MJ, Arduino MJ. National surveillance of dialysis associated diseases in the United States, 1995. ASAIO J 1998; 44: 98–107.

182. Troidle LK, Kliger AS, Gorban-Brennan N , Fikrig M, Golden M, Finkelstein FO. Nine episodes of CPD-associated peritonitis with vancomycin resistant enterococci. Kidney Int 1996; 50: 1368–72.

183. Lynn WA, Clutterbuck E, Want S *et al.* Treatment of CAPD-peritonitis due to glycopeptide-resistant *Enterococcus faecium* with quinupristin/dalfopristin. Lancet 1994; 344: 1025–26.

184. Linden PK, Pasculle AW, McDevitt D, Kramer DJ. Effect of quinupristin/dalfopristin on the outcome of vancomycin-resistant *Enterococcus faecium* bacteraemia: comparison with a control cohort. J Antimicrob Chemother 1997; 39 (suppl. A): 1–7.

185. Norris AH, Reilly JP, Edelstein PH, Brennan PJ, Schuster MG. Chloramphenicol for the treatment of vancomycin-resistant enterococcal infections. Clin Infect Dis 1995; 20: 1137–44.

186. Hiramatsu K, Aritaka N, Hanaki H *et al.* Dissemination in Japanese hospitals of strains of *Staphylococcus aureus* heterogeneously resistant to vancomycin. Lancet 1997; 350: 1670–3.

187. Ploy MC, Gelaud C, martin C, de Lumley L, Denis T. First clinical isolate of vancomycin-intermediate *Staphylococcus aureus* in a French hospital. Lancet 1998; 351: 1212.

188. CDC Update – *Staphylococcus aureus* with reduced susceptibility to vancomycin – United States, 1997. MMWR 1997; 46: 813.

189. Chong TK, Piraino B, Bernardini J. Vestibular toxicity due to gentamicin in peritoneal dialysis patients. Perit Dial Trans 1991; 11: 152–5.

190. Lee J, Innes CP, Petyo CM. Vertigo in CAPD patients treated with intraperitoneal gentamicin. Perit Dial Int 1989; 9: no. 97.

191. Kahlmeter G, Dahlager JI. Aminoglycoside toxicity – a review of clinical studies published between 1975 and 1982. J Antimicrob Chemother 1984; 13 (suppl. A): 9–22.

192. Gendeh BS, Said H, Gibb AG, Aziz NS, Kong N, Zahir ZM. Gentamicin ototoxicity in continuous ambulatory peritoneal dialysis. J Laryngol Oto 1993; 107: 681–5.

193. Nikolaidis P, Vas S, Lawson V *et al.* Is intraperitoneal tobramycin ototoxic in CAPD patients? Perit Dial Int 1991; 11: 156–61.

194. Spencer RC. Infections in continuous ambulatory peritoneal dialysis. J Med Microbiol 1988; 27: 1–9.

195. Beaman M, Solaro L, McGonigle RSJ, Michael J, Adu D. Vancomycin and ceftazidime in the treatment of CAPD peritonitis. Nephron 1989; 51: 51–5.

196. Gray HH, Goulding S, Eykyn SJ. Intraperitoneal vancomycin and ceftazidime in the treatment of CAPD peritonitis. Clin Nephrol 1985; 23: 81–4.

197. Shemin D, Maaz D. Gram-negative peritonitis in peritoneal dialysis: improved outcome with intraperitoneal ceftazidime. Perit Dial Int 1996; 16: 638–41.

198. Lye WC, Lee EJC, Leong SO, Kumarasinghe G. Clinical characteristics and outcome of Acinetobacter infections in CAPD patients. Perit Dial Int 1994; 14: 174–7.

199. Ruiz A, Ramos B, Burgos D, Frutos MA, de Novales EL. *Acinetobacter calcoaceticus* peritonitis in continuous ambulatory peritoneal dialysis (CAPD) patients. Perit Dial Int 1988; 8: 285–6.

200. Szeto CC, Li PKT, Leung CB *et al. Xanthomonas maltophilia* peritonitis in uremic patients receiving continuous ambulatory peritoneal dialysis. Am J Kidney Dis 1997; 29: 91–5.

201. Spence PA, Mathews RE, Khanna R, Oreopoulos D. Indications for operation when peritonitis occurs in patients on

continuous ambulatory peritoneal dialysis. Surg Gynecol Obstet 1985; 161: 450–2.

202. Miller GV, Bhandari S, Brownjohn AM, Turney JH, Benson EA. 'Surgical' peritonitis in the CAPD patient. Ann R Coll Surg Engl 1998; 80; 36–9.

203. Morduchowicz G, van Dyk DJ, Wittenberg C, Winkler J, Boner G. Bacteremia complicating peritonitis in peritoneal dialysis patients. Am J Nephrol 1993; 13: 278–80.

204. Bunke M, Brier ME, Golper TA representing the Academic Committee of Network #9. *Pseudomonas* peritonitis in peritoneal dialysis patients: the Network #9 Peritonitis Study. Am J Kidney Dis 1995; 25: 769–74.

205. Krothapalli R, Duffy WB, Lacke C et al. *Pseudomonas* peritonitis and continuous ambulatory peritoneal dialysis. Arch Intern Med 1982; 142: 1862–3.

206. Kazmi HR, Raffone FD, Kliger AS, Finkelstein FO. *Pseudomonas* exit site infections in continuous ambulatory peritoneal dialysis patients. J Am Soc Nephrol 1992; 2: 1498–501.

207. Montane BS, Mazza I, Abitbol C et al. Fungal peritonitis in pediatric patients. Adv Perit Dial 1998; 14: 251–4.

208. Rubin J, Kirchner K, Walsh D, Green M, Bower J. Fungal peritonitis during continuous ambulatory peritoneal dialysis: a report of 17 cases. Am J Kidney Dis 1987; 10: 361–8.

209. Chan TM, Chan CY, Cheng SW, Lo WK, Lo CY, Cheng IPK. Treatment of fungal peritonitis complicating continuous ambulatory peritoneal dialysis with oral fluconazole: a series of 21 patients. Nephrol Dial Transplant 1994; 9: 539–42.

210. Hoch BS, Namboodiri NK, Banayat G et al. The use of fluconazole in the management of *Candida* peritonitis in patients on peritoneal dialysis. Perit Dial Int 1993; 13 (suppl. 2): S357–9.

211. Montengro J, Aguirre R, Gonzalez O, Martinez I, Saracho R. Fluconazole treatment of *Candida* peritonitis with delayed removal of the peritoneal dialysis catheter. Clin Nephrol 1995; 44: 60–3.

212. Oh SH, Conley SB, Rose GM, Rosenblum M, Kohl S, Pickering LK. Fungal peritonitis in children undergoing peritoneal dialysis. Pediatr Infect Dis 1985; 4: 62–6.

213. Vargemezis V, Papadopoulou ZL, Liamos H et al. Management of fungal peritonitis during continuous ambulatory peritoneal dialysis (CAPD). Perit Dial Bull 1986; 6: 17–20.

214. Fabris A, Pellanda MV, Gardin C, Contestabile A, Bolzonella R. Pharmacokinetics of antifungal agents. Perit Dial Int 1993; 13 (suppl. 2): S380–2.

215. Debruyne D, Ryckelynck JP Fluconazole serum, urine, and dialysate levels in CAPD patients. Perit Dial Int 1992; 12: 328–9.

216. Benevent D, Peyronnet P, Lagarde C, Lerouz-Robert C. Fungal peritonitis in patients on continuous ambulatory peritoneal dialysis: three recoveries in five cases without catheter removal. Nephron 1985; 41: 203–6.

217. Nagappan R, Collins JF, Lee WT. Fungal peritonitis in continuous ambulatory peritoneal dialysis – the Auckland experience. Am J Kidney Dis 1992; 20: 492–6.

218. Cheng IKP, Chan PCK, Chan MK. Tuberculous peritonitis complicating long-term peritoneal dialysis. Am J Nephrol 1989; 9: 155–61.

219. White R, Abreo K, Flanagan R et al. Nontuberculous mycobacterial infections in continuous ambulatory peritoneal dialysis patients. Am J Kidney Dis 1993; 22: 581–7.

220. Smith JL, Flanigan MJ. Peritoneal dialysis catheter sepsis: a medical and surgical dilemma. Am J Surg 1987; 154: 602–7.

221. Gokal R, Ash SR, Helfrich GB et al. Peritoneal catheters and exit-site practices: toward optimum peritoneal access. Perit Dial Int 1993; 13: 29–39.

222. Schroder CH, Severijnen RSVM, de Jong MCW, Monnens LAH. Chronic tunnel infections in children: removal and replacement of the continuous ambulatory peritoneal dialysis catheter in a single operation. Perit Dial Int 1993; 13: 198–200.

223. Swartz R, Messana J, Reynolds J, Ranjit U. Simultaneous catheter replacement and removal in refractory peritoneal dialysis infections. Kidney Int 1991; 40: 1160–5.

224. Majkowski NL, Mendley SR. Simultaneous removal and replacement of infected peritoneal dialysis catheters. Am J Kidney Dis 1997; 29: 706–11.

225. Cancarini GC, Manili L, Brunori G et al. Simultaneous catheter replacement–removal during infectious complications in peritoneal dialysis. Adv Perit Dial 1994; 10: 210–13.

226. Fredensborg BB, Meyer HW, Joffe P, Fugleberg S. Reinsertion of PD catheters during PD-related infections performed either simultaneously or after an intervening period. Perit Dial Int 1995; 15: 374–8.

227. Goldraich I, Mariano M, Rosito N, Goldraich N. One-step peritoneal catheter replacement in children. Adv Perit Dial 1993; 9: 325–8.

228. Posthuma N, Borgstein PJ, Eijsbouts Q, ter Wee PM. Simultaneous peritoneal dialysis catheter insertion and removal in catheter-related infections without interruption of peritoneal dialysis. Nephrol Dial Transplant 1998; 13: 700–3.

229. Mayo RR, Messana JM, Boyer CJ, Swartz RD. *Pseudomonas* peritonitis treated with simultaneous catheter replacement and removal. Perit Dial Int 1995; 15: 389–90.

230. Mulhern JG, Braden GL, O'Shea MH, Madden RL, Lipkowitz GS, Germain MJ. Trough serum vancomycin levels predict the relapse of gram-positive peritonitis in peritoneal dialysis patients. Am J Kidney Dis 1995; 25: 611–15.

231. Dasgupta MK. Use of streptokinase or urokinase in recurrent CAPD peritonitis. Adv Perit Dial 1991; 7: 169–72.

232. Murphy G, Tzamaloukas AH, Eisenberg B, Gibel LJ, Avasthi PS. Intraperitoneal thrombolytic agents in relapsing or persistent peritonitis of patients on continuous ambulatory peritoneal dialysis. Int J Artif Organs 1991; 14: 87–91.

233. Williams AJ, Boletis I, Johnson BF et al. Tenckhoff catheter replacement or intraperitoneal urokinase: a randomised trial in the management of recurrent continuous ambulatory peritoneal dialysis (CAPD) peritonitis. Perit Dial Int 1989; 9: 65–7.

234. Innes A, Burden RP, Finch RG, Morgan AG. Treatment of resistant peritonitis in continuous ambulatory peritoneal dialysis with intraperitoneal urokinase: a double-blind clinical trial. Nephrol Dial Transplant 1994; 9: 797–9.

235. Golper TA, Hartstein AI. Analysis of the causative pathogens in uncomplicated CAPD-associated peritonitis: duration of therapy, relapses and prognosis. Am J Kidney Dis 1986; 7: 141–5.

236. Khanna R, Wu G, Vas S, Oreopoulos DG. Mortality and morbidity on continuous ambulatory peritoneal dialysis. ASAIO J 1983; 6: 197–204.

237. Heaton A, Rodger RSC, Sellars L et al. Continuous ambulatory peritoneal dialysis after the honeymoon: review of experience in Newcastle 1979–1984. Br Med J 1986; 293: 938–41.

238. Boroujerdi-Rad H, Juergensen P, Mansourian V, Kliger AS, Finkelstein FO. Abdominal abscesses complicating peritonitis in continuous ambulatory peritoneal dialysis patients. Am J Kidney Dis 1994; 23: 717–21.

239. Maiorca R, Cancarini GC, Zubani R et al. CAPD viability: a long-term comparison with hemodialysis. Perit Dial Int 1996; 16: 276–87.

240. Fox L, Tzamaloukas AH, Murata GH. Metabolic differences between persistent and routine peritonitis in CAPD. Adv Perit Dial 1992; 8: 346–50.

241. Hendriks PMEM, Ho-dac-Pannekeet MM, van Gulik TM et al. Peritoneal sclerosis in continuous peritoneal dialysis patients: analysis of clinical presentation, risk factors, and peritoneal transport kinetics. Perit Dial Int 1997; 17: 136–43.

242. Nomoto Y, Kawaguchi Y, Kubo H, Hirano H, Sakai S, Kurokawa K. Sclerosing encapsulating peritonitis in patients undergoing continuous ambulatory peritoneal dialysis: a report of the Japanese encapsulating peritonitis study group. Am J Kidney Dis 1996; 28: 420–7.

243. Dobbie JW, Henderson I, Wilson LS. New evidence on the pathogenesis of sclerosing encapsulating peritonitis (SEP) obtained from serial biopsies. Adv Perit Dial 1987; 3: 138–49.

244. Dobbie JW. Pathogenesis of peritoneal fibrosing syndromes (sclerosing peritonitis) in peritoneal dialysis. Perit Dial Int 1992; 12: 14–27.

245. Davies SJ, Bryan J, Phillips L, Russell GI. Longitudinal changes in peritoneal kinetics: the effect of dialysis and peritonitis. Nephrol Dial Transplant 1996; 11: 498–506.

246. Tzamaloukas AH. Decreasing morbidity and mortality in long-term peritoneal dialysis patients. Semin Dial 1995; 8: 397–400.

247. Dryden MS, Ludlam HA, Wing AJ, Phillips J. Active intervention dramatically reduces CAPD-associated infection. Adv Perit Dial 1991; 7: 125–8.

248. Oreopoulos DG, Vas SI, Khanna R. Prevention of peritonitis during continuous ambulatory peritoneal dialysis. Perit Dial Bull 1983; 3 (suppl.) S18–22.

249. Dabbagh S, Fassinger N, Clement K, Fleishman LE. The effect of aggressive nutrition on infection rates in patients maintained on peritoneal dialysis. Adv Perit Dial 1991; 7: 161–4.

250. Miller TE, Findon G. Touch contamination of connection devices in peritoneal dialysis – a quantitative microbiologic analysis. Perit Dial Int 1997; 17: 560–7.

251. Joh J, Padmanabhan K, Bastani B. *Pasteurella multocida* peritonitis following cat bite of peritoneal dialysis tubing. With a brief review of the literature. Am J Nephrol 1998; 18: 258–9.

252. Mackay K, Brown L, Hudson K. *Pasteurella multocida* peritonitis in peritoneal dialysis patients: beware of the cat. Perit Dial Int 1997; 17: 608–10.

253. Gokal R, Alexander S, Ash S et al. Peritoneal catheters and exit-site practices toward optimum peritoneal access: 1998 update. Perit Dial Int 1998; 18: 11–33.

254. Wikdahl AM, Engman U, Stemayr BG, Sorensen JG. One-dose cefuroxime IV and IP reduces microbial growth in PD patients after catheter insertion. Nephrol Dial Transplant 1997; 12: 157–60.

255. Bennett-Jones DN, Martin J, Barratt AJ, Duffy TJ, Naish PF, Aber GM. Prophylactic gentamicin in the prevention of early exit-site infections and peritonitis in CAPD. Adv Perit Dial 1988; 4: 147–50.

256. Lye WC, Lee EJC, Tan CC. Prophylactic antibiotics in the insertion of Tenckhoff catheters. Scand J Urol Nephrol 1992; 26: 177–80.

257. Sardegna KM, Beck AM, Strife CF. Evaluation of perioperative antibiotics at the time of dialysis catheter placement. Pediatr Nephrol 1998; 12: 149–52.

258. The Mupirocin Study Group. Nasal mupirocin prevents *Staphylococcus aureus* exit-site infection during peritoneal dialysis. J Am Soc Nephrol 1996; 7: 2403–8.

259. Hanevold CD, Fisher MC, Waltz R, Bartosh S, Baluarte HJ. Effect of rifampin on *Staphylococcus aureus* colonization in children on peritoneal dialysis. Pediatr Nephrol 1995; 9: 609–11.

260. Rao SP, Oreopoulos DG. Unusual complication of polyurethane PD catheter. Perit Dial Int 1997; 17: 410–12.

261. Slocombe B, Perry C. The antimicrobial activity of mupirocin – an update on resistance. J Hosp Infect 1991; 19 (suppl. B): 19–25.

262. Kauffman CA, Terpenning MS, He X et al. Attempts to eradicate methicillin-resistant *Staphylococcus aureus* from a long-term-care facility with the use of mupirocin ointment. Am J Med 1993; 94: 371–8.

263. Lo WK, Chen CY, Cheng SW, Poon JFM, Chan DTM, Cheng IKP. A prospective randomized control study of nystatin prophylaxis for *Candida* complicating continuous ambulatory peritoneal dialysis. Am J Kidney Dis 1996; 28: 549–52.

264. Wadhwa NK, Suh H, Cabralda T. Antifungal prophylaxis for secondary fungal peritonitis in peritoneal dialysis patients. Adv Perit Dial 1996; 12: 189–91.

265. Zaruba K, Peters J, Jungbluth H. Successful prophylaxis for fungal peritonitis in patients on continuous ambulatory peritoneal dialysis: six years' experience Am J Kidney Dis 1991; 17: 43–6.

266. Robitaille P, Merouani A, Clermont MJ, Hebert E. Successful antifungal prophylaxis in chronic peritoneal dialysis: a pediatric experience. Perit Dial Int 1995; 15: 77–9.

267. Churchill DN, Taylor DW, Vas SI et al. Peritonitis in continuous ambulatory peritoneal dialysis (CAPD) patients: a randomized clinical trial of cotrimoxazole prophylaxis. Perit Dial Int 1988; 8: 125–8.

268. Sharma BK, Smith EC, Rodriguez H, Pillay VKG, Gandhi VC, Dunea G. Trial of oral neomycin during peritoneal dialysis. Am J Med Sci 1971; 262: 175–8.

269. Low DE, Vas SI, Oreopoulos DG et al. Prophylactic cephalexin ineffective in chronic ambulatory peritoneal dialysis. Lancet 1980; 2: 753–4.

18 | Peritoneal inflammation and long-term changes in peritoneal structure and function

G.A. COLES, J.D. WILLIAMS AND N. TOPLEY

Introduction

Peritoneal dialysis (PD) is now an established and acceptable mode of treatment for end-stage renal failure. Whilst in short-term studies PD (3–5 years) has been shown to have a comparable outcome in terms of patient survival on haemodialysis [1–3], there are still concerns as to whether this mode of therapy can provide adequate treatment for end-stage renal disease in the longer term. Within the first 3–5 years, however, there is a considerable dropout rate from PD. This is principally due to episodes of peritonitis, loss of ultrafiltration or inadequate solute clearance [2–5].

Over the past decade, hand in hand with improvements in solution delivery systems and better understanding of the physiology of peritoneal transport, has been an increased awareness of the need to understand the basic biology of the peritoneal membrane and how this changes during PD. Investigations in several centres have revealed information about the peritoneum's response to inflammation, as well as some insight into the changes that occur in the structure of this membrane during PD therapy. Peritoneal host defence appears to involve a complex interplay between the resident cells of the peritoneal membrane, infiltrating inflammatory cells and their secreted products in mediating the host's response to PD itself, as well as to episodes of acute inflammation. This increase in our understanding of the cell biology of the peritoneum has enabled us to begin to address two key questions regarding this therapy:

1. Given that clinical data clearly show a deterioration of peritoneal 'function' with time on PD what are the causative factors? Is it related to (a) uraemia, (b) episodes of peritonitis, (c) structural changes in the peritoneal membrane, (d) continuous exposure to dialysis solution components, or (e) any combination of (a)–(d)?

2. If changes in peritoneal structure occur in PD patients, what form do they take and is their development related to the above factors?

The purpose of this review is to provide an overview of our current understanding of peritoneal membrane structure and function, and how this is impacted upon by inflammation and PD solutions over time. Initially we will attempt, based on published literature, to give an overview of the structure of the membrane and subsequently, using recent data from the 'Peritoneal Biopsy Registry', update this to give a more contemporary view of the changes that occur with time on PD. We will then examine the processes by which inflammation is activated and controlled, and investigate the potential link between this and peritoneal dysfunction. Subsequently we will discuss the potential impact of solution biocompatibility on peritoneal membrane structure and function. Finally, we will examine what measures might be taken to preserve the long-term function of the peritoneal membrane and discuss which 'markers' might be of prognostic value in monitoring the status of the peritoneum, as well as predicting adverse changes that might compromise PD therapy.

Peritoneal structure and function: changes over time

The peritoneal cavity

The peritoneum is a continuous, translucent serous membrane that consists of a monolayer of mesothelium resting on a basal lamina. Below this there is a compact zone at the margin of which are discontinuous bands of elastin fibres which give the membrane its normal elasticity. Within this 'compact' zone are interwoven numerous bundles of collagen fibres embedded in a connective tissue stroma. This

R. Gokal, R. Khanna, R.Th. Krediet and K.D. Nolph (eds.), Textbook of Peritoneal Dialysis, 2nd Edition, 565–583.

interstitium appears to be largely composed of glyco-proteins and proteoglycans [6–9], although this precise composition remains to be defined. Within the submesothelial interstitium there are visible occasional fibroblasts and mast cells, and inter-spersed within it are the lymphatics. At the margin of the compact zone reside the majority of small blood vessels. Beneath this layer is largely areolar connective tissue containing some blood vessels.

The peritoneum with its mesothelial monolayer is divided into two parts: the parietal peritoneum which bounds the outer surface of the body cavity and the visceral peritoneum which covers the abdo-minal organs. The space between these layers forms the peritoneal cavity. In addition, the greater omen-tum is a mesenteric apron that is continuous with the peritoneum and hangs freely into the peritoneal cavity, extending from the lower border of the stom-ach and covering the intestines. This consists of a trabecular loose fibrous connective tissue framework covered on its surface by a continuous mesothelial monolayer. It contains fibroblasts, blood and lym-phatic vessels. In the visceral peritoneum the com-pact zone is significantly thinner and contains numerous blood vessels at its margins.

The mesothelium

The mesothelial layer consists of a single layer of squamous epithelial cells of mesodermal origin. In addition to the peritoneal cavity, mesothelial cell monolayers also line the pleural cavity and pericar-dium [10, 11]. The serosal surface of the mesothe-lium contains numerous microvilli. These serve to increase the peritoneal surface area, thereby facilita-ting absorption of materials and reducing friction and facilitating intestinal movement. The mesothe-lial surface is also covered by a microscopic electro-negative 'glycocalyx' composed primarily of proteo-glycans [12, 13]. These highly glycosylated mole-cules are hydrophilic, and this may aid the movement of closely opposed surfaces. This move-ment is also facilitated by the ability of the mesothe-lial cell to secrete specific phospholipid species possibly derived from the large number of lamellar bodies easily identifiable within the cytoplasm of these cells [14–16]. The mesothelial monolayer con-sists of a single layer of cells tightly opposed to each other with desmosomes and tight and gap junctions readily identifiable. In common with endothelium the mesothelial cell has a well-developed system of micropinocytotic vesicles and larger membrane-bound vacuoles.

Following the introduction of PD in the early 1970s interest in understanding the biology of the peritoneal cavity inevitably led to the isolation and culture of the cells lining it. Once it was clear (in common with all other tissue cells) that the mesothe-lium was more than an inert bystander in tissue homeostasis, investigation of the biology of these cells identified their potential role in peritoneal homeostasis and host defence against infection [17–21]. Subsequently, numerous studies, using cul-tured animal or human mesothelium, have identified that these cells have a vast biosynthetic capacity. Through their expression or secretion of various mediators they have the potential to contribute to peritoneal homeostasis as well as to its response to bacterial contamination. In this respect mesothelial secretion of inflammatory mediators (prostaglan-dins, cytokines, chemokines and nitric oxide), media-tors of fibrinolysis (tissue plasminogen activator, its inhibitor and tissue factor), growth factors, phospho-lipids and proteoglycan species has been demon-strated [15, 16, 18–43]. In addition they express on their surface adhesion molecules important in their interaction with migrating leukocyte populations (ICAM-1 and VCAM-1). The list of activities secreted or expressed by mesothelium continues to expand.

The submesothelial interstitium

Ongoing research has clearly identified the contribu-tion of the mesothelium to peritoneal homeostasis. More recently our understanding of the function of the cells that reside within the submesothelial inter-stitium (fibroblasts and capillary endothelium) and changes that occur in the acellular portions of the peritoneal membrane has also increased. The isola-tion and characterization of peritoneal fibroblasts (that reside within the peritoneal tissue) have demon-strated that these cells also have significant biosyn-thetic capacity [44, 45], and probably in common with mesothelium contribute to the peritoneum's response to inflammation. In addition, given the importance of interstitial cells in controlling extra-cellular matrix turnover, these fibroblasts may be important controllers of structural/'fibrotic' changes that have been demonstrated in the dialysed perito-neal cavity. As we will describe later, further investi-gation will expand our understanding of the contribution of these and other 'interstitial' cells to peritoneal homeostasis, and to normal and abnor-mal extracellular matrix turnover in the dialysed peritoneal cavity.

Within the submesothelial interstitium reside the capillaries, and whilst their contribution to solute and water movement is clear, their function (or changes that occur in them) with respect to peritoneal inflammation is yet to be fully elucidated. Evidence, so far based on small numbers of patient samples, suggests that both the structure and number of capillaries changes during PD, particularly in those patients with ultrafiltration problems [46, 47]. These changes – which include increases in capillary number and structure (smooth muscle hyperplasia, subendothelial thickening and collagen deposition) – are suggestive of diabetic microangiopathy [48]. These could clearly modulate endothelial and smooth muscle cell structure and function, as well as altering solute transport. Our recent data, generated from the Peritoneal Biopsy Registry, suggest that these initial observations are indeed accurate, and suggest that the occurrence and severity of the described 'vasculopathy' is dependent on the time on therapy (see later) [49].

Whilst it is clear that structural changes within the peritoneal membrane could contribute to the observed functional alterations, there is to date no direct evidence of what the implication of alterations in capillary function (or 'fibrosis') might have on peritoneal function (both in terms of ultrafiltration and homeostasis/inflammation).

Long-term changes in peritoneal structure

The introduction of PD more than 20 years ago projected the peritoneal membrane into a completely new environment. This has introduced a whole new set of variables to the hitherto protected environment of the peritoneum. Conventional PD solutions by their very nature must be bioincompatible in order to function effectively (see later). The presence of an indwelling catheter within the cavity is a constant irritant, and the need to exchange fluids a minimum of four times a day means that bacterial and/or fungal contamination of the cavity is probably a relatively common occurrence. These features are likely to result in an inflammatory response of varying degree. It is, therefore, not surprising that with time on dialysis both structural and functional changes occur at the level of the peritoneal membrane.

Studies of the development of peritoneal fibrosis in PD patients are relatively limited. Initial observations were made, in small numbers of patients, on samples either taken at catheter replacement or removal or at autopsy. In these biopsies histological and immunocytochemical examination was undertaken [6–9, 48, 50–60]. None of these studies, however, presents a systematic examination of the relationship between therapy (time on PD, solution exposure, peritonitis history, etc.) and the observable changes in peritoneal ultrastructure. The sum of the observations presented suggests that whilst changes certainly occur in both the mesothelium (denudation, loss of microvilli), interstitium (various degrees of undefined 'fibrosis' and leukocyte infiltration) and the vascular bed, they are not systematically described and are thus of limited value in understanding the natural history of the development of peritoneal 'fibrosis' in PD patients.

To date there are two published studies which suggest that repeated episodes of peritonitis may contribute to the loss of membrane function [61, 62]. In contrast, although a number of hypotheses have been put forward suggesting that repeated exposure to high concentrations of glucose may be linked to changes in both membrane structure and function with time on dialysis, there is, as yet, no direct evidence to support this contention.

There are, however, a number of published studies which attempt to address the relationship between morphological changes and clinical events. An autopsy study performed in 1991 examined 16 patients who had been on peritoneal dialysis from times ranging from 1 month to 8 years [50]. Multiple peritoneal sections were taken and examined for fibrosis, serosal thickening, degree of collagen deposition and vascularity. Peritoneal changes – which included thickening, inflammation and adhesion – were unrelated to time on PD; only the number of peritonitis episodes correlated significantly with the chronicity of changes within the membrane (chronicity was defined as the degree of fibroblastic activity, serosal thickness and intensity of chronic inflammation). Neither age nor time on PD correlated with chronic changes. This study supported earlier observations in 51 biopsies that had been taken from 31 patients on continuous ambulatory peritoneal dialysis (CAPD) [8]. Many of these were during episodes of peritonitis. There was loss of mesothelium with time, and disruption of the interstitium. In those patients in whom repeat biopsies were available there was only a partial recovery.

Vascular changes in the peritoneal membrane were also described by the same group in 1989 [52]. A total of 76 specimens were taken from 45 patients, 29 of these before the start of CAPD and 47 after

2–6 months of treatment. Biopsies were taken from patients either when the catheter was being inserted for the first time, or when undergoing surgery for the repositioning of the catheter. The findings described with time on CAPD included replication of the mesothelial and capillary basement membrane. This resulted eventually in considerable thickening of the subendothelial tissue, culminating eventually in occlusion of capillary lumina. Among the patients studied were a group of diabetic patients, and of these latter patients it was noted that 90% showed reduplication of basement membrane before the start of CAPD. The conclusion of the authors in this study was that changes in the peritoneal membrane with time could be likened to changes in diabetic microangiopathy.

Dobbie *et al.* have published extensively on the changes in the peritoneal membranes of patients on peritoneal dialysis [54–59, 63]. They described in detail changes in the mesothelial cells including a loss of microvilli, and an increase in the amount of endoplasmic reticulum and a decrease in the number of micropinocytotic vesicles. Alterations to the submesothelial basement membrane and to the basement membranes of stromal blood vessels were also noted, including thickening and reduplication of the membrane in a manner similar to that seen in diabetics. Dobbie's assertion, however, was that the major changes seen in the stroma and stromal blood vessels were seen mainly in patients who had previously had significant peritonitis. These studies concluded that patients who had few episodes of peritonitis rarely experienced diabetic changes within the peritoneal membrane. The most severe cases of microangiopathy were encountered in the biopsies of diabetic patients with a history of multiple and severe episodes of peritonitis. These changes were attributed to the loss of a barrier preventing the diffusion of glucose into the stroma. The exposure of stroma to high concentrations of glucose would lead to non-enzymatic glycosylation of proteins within the membrane and the induction of pathological changes to both basement membrane serosal blood vessels.

The earliest description of changes to the vasculature of the peritoneal membrane was demonstrated in peritoneal biopsies in which postcapillary venules had several layers of reduplication of basal lamina [53]. These changes to blood vessel structure were described in greater detail by Honda *et al.* when biopsies from three patients with ultrafiltration failure were examined in detail [46]. Light microscopy showed extensive interstitial fibrosis, loss of meso-

thelium and vascular changes. The alterations to the vasculature included severe fibrosis and hyalinization of the media of venules. There was extensive deposition of type IV collagen and laminin in the vascular wall and degeneration of smooth muscle cells in the media.

Interestingly, endothelial cells were relatively well preserved. These pathological alterations were found in patients with ultrafiltration failure, and it was suggested that hyperosmolar dialysis fluids and the exposure to glucose might have been responsible for these changes. More recently the same group have correlated changes in the peritoneal vasculature with the accumulation of the advanced glycosylation endproducts in patients with low ultrafiltration [47]. Biopsies from 14 CAPD patients with varying levels of ultrafiltration were examined immunohistochemically for advanced glycosylation end-products (AGE) deposition (anti-CML antibody) and morphometrically for peritoneal fibrosis and microvascular sclerosis. Despite the relatively small numbers of samples the extent of AGE accumulation correlated with the progression of interstitial fibrosis and vascular sclerosis. In addition, changes in ultrafiltration were inversely correlated to interstitial fibrosis and microvascular sclerosis as well as to microvascular AGE accumulation.

We have recently presented a preliminary morphological quantitative analysis of parietal peritoneal samples from 108 patients worldwide [49]. The median thickness for the submesothelial compact collagenous zone in predialysis patients was 130 μm, for those biopsied during the first year on PD it was 180 μm, for those biopsied from year 2–5 it was 220 μm and for those on PD for more than 5 years it was 460 μm. Vascular changes were seen in 15% of group predialysis patients, 10% of year 1 patients, 33% of patients in years 2–5, and 50% of those on PD more than 5 years. Vascular changes comprised progressive subendothelial hyalinization with luminal narrowing or obliteration. In advanced cases the hyaline material contained calcific deposits. This study clarified and demonstrated a clear temporal relationship between time on dialysis, peritoneal thickening and the development of a hyalinizing vasculopathy. Figure 1 shows a representative biopsy from a predialysis patient compared to one from an individual treated by CAPD for more than 5 years.

Recently, a case-controlled study of biopsies from patients with severe peritoneal fibrosis/sclerosis demonstrated an increase in vessel number in patients with peritoneal fibrosis compared to con-

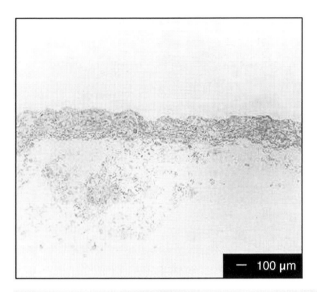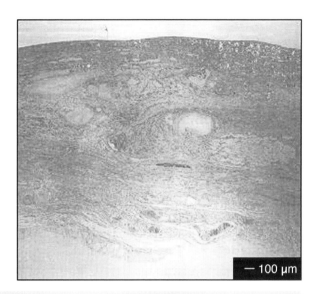

Figure 1. Changes in submesothelial thickness with time on PD. The section on the left is taken from a patient not previously exposed to PD. The section on the right is from a patient with more than 5 years treatment. Note the markedly increased submesothelial thickness in the long-term sample.

trols with thickening of the vessel walls and dilation of capillaries [48]. These changes were thought to be consistent with glucose-induced microangiopathy.

There thus appear to be two significant elements to the structural changes seen in the peritoneum with the time on dialysis. The first is a significant increase in the thickness of the submesothelial compact zone, resulting apparently from the increased deposition of collagen. This is often associated with a loss of surface mesothelial cells, although in many cases the mesothelium is present despite significant degrees of submesothelial thickening. In some studies the changes observed correlated with the incidence and severity of peritonitis. Other studies demonstrate changes in the vascular bed of the peritoneum, which resemble diabetic microangiopathy.

Although it has been suggested that the changes observed are linked to peritonitis, there is little prospective evidence to support this. There is, however, a significant correlation with the degree of AGE deposition within the membrane. Clearly large prospective structure/function studies are required in order to establish the structural/functional relationships within the peritoneal membrane.

A major problem for patients on PD appears to be the progressive thickening of the compact zone, 'fibrosis' within the membrane leading to 'sclerosis'. A distinction has been made between 'fibrosis' and 'sclerosis' by a number of investigators. This distinc-

tion is rarely made by trained hisotpathologists. It is unlikely that fibrosis and sclerosis are two distinct entities; rather that 'sclerosis' is the end-result of a process of interstitial thickening (in this case of the submesothelial compact zone) which finally leads to thickened fibrous tissue encapsulating the bowel. There seems to be a spectrum of changes within the cavity ranging from thickening of the peritoneum, 'tanning of the peritoneum' and sclerosing encapsulating peritonitis resulting in bowel obstruction, obliteration of the peritoneal cavity and adhesion formation. There may also be a mural fibrosis of the bowel with invasion of the outer muscle layers. With increased fibrosis the surface of the peritoneal membrane consists of an acellular band of hyalinized collagen. Mesothelium is absent. This is a rare if increasing complication in PD (0.5–0.9% of the overall PD population) and is manifested mostly in long-term patients (≥ 8 years on therapy) where its incidence rises to 15–20% of patients on PD for more than 8 years [64]. Its incidence does not appear (based on currently available data) to be related to the patient's peritonitis history; however, it is usually precipitated by an infective episode [65–67]. The increasing number of patients on long-term PD (>8 years) has meant that the total number of episodes of SEP has increased, but the overall frequency of its occurrence has not altered, these data strongly suggesting that time on PD is the most important factor in its initiation [64] and that a 'sensitization' process occurs in the long-term dialysed peritoneum.

The progressive thickening of the membrane results in damage to the longitudinal muscle layer of the bowel, obliteration of the capillary plexus and loss of the mesenteric nerve plexus. 'Sclerosing encapsulating peritonitis' results in cocooning of the small bowel by fibrous tissue. Eventually calcification may occur, and the resulting bowel obstruction may cause death. Earliest reports were linked to antiseptics containing chlorhexidine, dialysate fluids containing acetate or severe peritonitis. In an extensive study published in 1998 an analysis of 54 patients diagnosed with sclerosing peritonitis, either by surgical or radiological means, was undertaken [64]. Although the overall prevalence was 0.7% it increased progressively with time on PD; being 2%, 6.4%, 10.8% and 19.4% for patients on dialysis for greater than 2, 5, 6 and 8 years respectively. Peritonitis was associated with 38% of cases, fungal infection with 7%. The overall mortality rate was 56%. A small number of patients were treated with immunosupression [5] and there was a suggestion that this resulted in clinical improvement. Data from Japanese studies would indicate a similar relationship with time on dialysis with the peritonitis [66].

Although our understanding of the changes that occur in the structure of the dialysed peritoneal membrane has increased over the past 20 years, there are still significant gaps in our knowledge. A review of the data suggests that progressive structural changes do occur, the severity of which are linked to the length of time the membrane is exposed to PD. Correlations have been made in small numbers of patients between various parameters, and are suggestive of important causal relationships. One must bear in mind, however, that several changes occur in the PD patients with time on PD. There are progressive changes such as loss of ultrafiltration, changes in solute clearance, increased cumulative exposure to dialysis solution components and to episodes of peritonitis, all of which is against the background of the fact that the patients are uraemic, and in many cases will have a complicated medical history. The implication of those factors as being directly responsible for, or a result of, the structural alterations (submesothelial thickening and vascular changes), although logical and attractive, must be interpreted with caution, as without significant additional structural, functional and clinical data the relationships cannot be considered as abso-

lute. This must be an area of intense investigation over the next 5–10 years.

Mechanisms of peritoneal fibrosis

As mentioned above, there is evidence that the structure of the peritoneal membrane changes during PD therapy. The precise mechanisms by which these alterations, which have been termed 'peritoneal fibrosis and sclerosis', are initiated are poorly understood at the cellular level. Studies on fibrosis development in other organs (lung, liver, kidney and skin) suggest that fibrosis involves a series of overlapping phases, which eventually lead to irreparable damage to the interstitium of the tissue involved [68–73]. The initiation phase is usually related to ongoing inflammation, and to the fact that the presence of macrophages is a key feature in its development. Initial activation is followed by a period of increased extracellular matrix turnover resulting in interstitial collagen deposition and eventually tissue fibrosis. In the early phases of inflammation the infiltration of activated macrophages and their release of cytokines and growth factors [68, 74] is a key process. This activation phase provides the cellular signals for both the attraction and activation of interstitial fibroblasts, and appears to result in increased matrix deposition [68]. Clearly, as mentioned earlier, the processes that govern the development of peritoneal membrane structural changes are complex, and there are many additional variables (acute and chronic inflammation, uraemia, solution exposure, etc.). Understanding how these processes impact on the development of these changes will clearly require *in-vivo* as well as *in-vitro* observations.

Some insight into the cellular mechanisms that contribute to the process of peritoneal fibrosis have come from investigations of the reactions of peritoneal interstitial fibroblasts in *in-vitro* culture systems [44, 45]. These cells, in common with the mesothelium, have significant biosynthetic capacity [44, 45]. Using a three-dimensional cell culture system in which, as *in vivo*, the fibroblasts are maintained within an interstitial type matrix, we observed that repeated activation of peritoneal fibroblasts resulted in sustained cell proliferation and extracellular matrix (collagen and fibronectin) synthesis [75]. These data are of interest when taken in the context of the clinical evidence showing that loss of ultrafiltration appears to occur more rapidly in those patients who suffer repeated or prolonged episodes of peritonitis [62].

Changes in peritoneal function with time on dialysis

Solute transport

Studies on patients treated for up to 10 years, or more, with CAPD show that on average there is a slowly increasing small solute transport rate which can be easily demonstrated by an increasing D/P creatinine and decreasing D/D_0 glucose using the peritoneal equilibration test (PET) [5]. This is confirmed by measurements of mass area transfer coefficient (MTAC) [76]. However, many patients have stable transport rates for 5 years or more [76]. Frequent or severe peritonitis is associated with a permanent increase in small solute transport, but after a period of several years even patients who have experienced little or no peritonitis may have a rising D/P creatinine [5, 61, 62]. It has been suggested that the increase in average small solute transport is due to a minority of patients experiencing a rise whereas the majority have stable function. This stability may be more apparent than real, as individuals with high small solute transport will leave CAPD more quickly [5]. This is because an increased peritoneal clearance of creatinine is associated with a significantly higher technique failure [5, 77, 78]. In addition there is a raised mortality [5, 78]. The cause is not clear, but an association with fluid overload and thus cardiovascular problems is possible, since an increased transport will lead to a more rapid absorption of glucose with abolition of the osmotic gradient. This in turn will lead to reduced ultrafiltration and the chance of overload. The morphological cause for a progressive increase in small solute transport may be the increased number of capillaries demonstrated in biopsies from patients on CAPD for several years [48].

Ultrafiltration

One of the commonest changes in peritoneal function with time on CAPD is a gradual decline in ultrafiltration when using glucose dialysate. It has been suggested that by 3 years some 10% of patients have ultrafiltration problems [79] and by 6 years this has increased to 30% [80]. A study from Japan reported that 50% of those individuals who had survived at least 6 years on CAPD would have technique failure due to fluid overload from ultrafiltration loss [81]. Unfortunately, none of these reports gave details of the exact nature of the ultrafiltration problems. In addition to being one of the commonest causes of

technique failure reduced ultrafiltration is associated with increased mortality [5]. The exact mechanism is not certain, but may involve fluid overload leading to left ventricular failure or hypertension [82]. The commonest cause of loss of ultrafiltration is thought to be an increased effective surface area of peritoneum as judged by increased small solute transport [83]. As a result a more rapid absorption of glucose will occur, leading to dissipation of the osmotic gradient and thus reduced fluid removal. The morphological counterpart of this change in function may well be the increased vascularity being reported in peritoneal biopsies from long-term PD patients, especially those with sclerosing peritonitis [48]. A further mechanism suggested for poor ultrafiltration is the loss of functional water channels [84]. Whether other possible causes of ultrafiltration loss, e.g. a change in fluid reabsorption rate, are time-related remains unknown, as there has been no systematic study of peritoneal fluid removal in a large cohort of patients who have had several years CAPD. All the possible mechanisms and their management are discussed in detail in the chapter on ultrafiltration failure.

Macromolecular clearance

Very few studies have looked at the long-term peritoneal clearances of proteins during PD. The restriction coefficients for macromolecules apparently do not change during the first 2 years of CAPD, but increase after a longer period of treatment [85]. This might be caused by a reduction in the large pore radius or by alterations in the interstitial tissue. The morphological cause might be the increased thickening of the submesothelial layer with collagen deposition (see above). At present this change in restriction coefficient has no obvious clinical significance.

Long-term effects of automated peritoneal dialysis (APD)

At present there are no data available on the effect of long-term APD on peritoneal membrane function. This is in part due to the fact that worldwide only a minority of patients start with APD. Many APD individuals have been switched to this therapy from CAPD because of problems with achieving solute adequacy targets and/or difficulties with fluid removal. As a result long-term experience is so far limited. Whether those who change to APD because of a high small solute transport, and thus poor ultrafiltration, subsequently have further difficulties with fluid removal remains unknown.

Monitoring peritoneal membrane function

In view of the possible changes in peritoneal function that may occur during long-term PD it is important to monitor solute transport and ultrafiltration. At present there is no apparent clinical need to assess macromolecular clearance on a regular basis. How frequently one should measure peritoneal function is unclear, since there are no comparative studies. The dialysis outcomes quality initiative (DOQI) guidelines recommend measurement every 4 months [86]. For a PD unit supporting a large number of patients this is a considerable workload. We would suggest every 6 months, but with a repeat test if any clinical problem arises. A number of different techniques for measuring peritoneal function are available. The most widely used is the PET [87]. This will give an estimate of small solute transport rate as well as current ultrafiltration capacity. As originally described, it uses a 2.27% anhydrous glucose bag. There is some advantage in using a 3.86% anhydrous glucose bag as this will give a better estimate of ultrafiltration. If this is less than 400 ml after a 4-h dwell then ultrafiltration loss is suspected [83]. Furthermore, with a 3.86% bag it is easier to assess sodium sieving and thus aquaporin (water channel) function [84] (see chapter on ultrafiltration loss). It is important to remember that performing the PET alone will not give an assessment of total solute removal, i.e. adequacy. Thus the PET must be combined with measuring 24-h renal and peritoneal clearances of urea and creatinine.

Other tests have also been described including mass transfer area coefficient [88], standard permeability analysis [89], peritoneal dialysis capacity [90] and the apex time [91]. The peritoneal dialysis capacity test in particular does allow calculation of a number of other parameters derived from the three-pore theory, including pore area per unit diffusion distance, but as yet these have not been correlated with clinical outcomes. Computer programs are available commercially to assist in the calculations of the test results using the PET or the peritoneal dialysis capacity.

Peritoneal inflammation

As mentioned previously, inflammation appears to play a central role in modulating the function and possibly structure of the peritoneal membrane. Over the past decade information gleaned from measurements of intraperitoneal inflammatory mediator levels (in PD effluent isolated from patients during stable PD and during peritonitis), as well as a large body of *in-vitro* cell culture data, has identified an outline of the process by which peritoneal inflammation is initiated and amplified, and how it resolves. These data suggest that following bacterial contamination of the peritoneal cavity a coordinated train of events is set in motion to eradicate the invading organisms and resume normal tissue homeostasis. It is also clear that both the resident and infiltrating cells (both tissue cells and resident macrophages and infiltrating leukocytes) participate in these processes.

The normal peritoneal cavity contains a small resident population of leukocytes, predominantly tissue macrophages [92, 93]. In PD patients this number is substantially increased, possibly as a result of the dialysis procedure itself, which results in a constant flux of mononuclear cells into the peritoneal cavity [92, 93], but also possibly resulting from a subclinical activation of cells related to uraemia.

Inflammation in the dialysed peritoneum involves an initiation phase resulting from the activation of resident phagocytes, and probably the mesothelium, by invading microorganisms (or their secreted products) [94, 95]. Next there is an amplification phase in which mesothelial cell activation by peritoneal macrophage-derived proinflammatory cytokines (such as interleukin 1-beta (IL-1β) and tumour necrosis factor alpha (TNF-α)) appears to play a key role. This process results in the generation of chemotactic signals, via the creation of a gradient of chemotactic cytokines (specific for individual leukocyte subpopulations) leading to the recruitment of these inflammatory cells to the site of activation [18, 19, 43, 96]. This infiltration process is facilitated by the up-regulation of leukocyte-specific adhesion molecules of the immunoglobulin superfamily (ICAM-1 and VCAM-1/2) on the mesothelial surface [22, 27, 35, 97].

The process of leukocyte infiltration is tightly controlled such that initially polymorphonuclear leukocytes predominate (6–24 h) and are subsequently replaced by mononuclear cells (mononuclear phagocytes and T and B lymphocytes) [98]. This switch in leukocyte phenotype, which appears to be at least partly controlled by regulation of mesothelial cell-derived chemokines, is presumed to represent the resolution of infection/inflammation, although much less is understood about this process and the return to tissue homeostasis [99].

The link between inflammation and membrane dysfunction

In order to understand how structural changes can occur over time in the dialysed peritoneal membrane, as mentioned earlier it is important to understand which factors could contribute to these processes. Continuous exposure to specific dialysis solution components (glucose and glucose degradation products (GDP)) potentially directly contribute to cell activation and 'pro-fibrotic' events. These factors may also have more indirect effects by modulating (in a negative manner) peritoneal host defence and thus potentially increasing the peritoneum's susceptibility to infection [100]. Whilst there is no direct evidence to support this latter hypothesis, there is clearly a link between peritoneal inflammation and membrane function in PD patients [62]. To develop this thought train we make the assumption (based on reasonable evidence) that the functional changes in the peritoneal membrane (ultrafiltration, solute clearance, etc.) are linked to the changes in its structure that occur in long-term PD patients. Our increasing understanding of peritoneal inflammatory processes and how these events are paralleled in other organ systems also allows us (to some extent) to extrapolate from current understanding of fibrotic processes in these organs to events that might contribute to structural alterations in the peritoneal membrane (see earlier).

As discussed earlier, it is important to define the process of fibrotic development (hypercellularity and changes in extracellular matrix turnover and deposition over months or years that may eventually lead to irreparable deposition of a dense collagenous matrix, occlusion of blood vessels and loss of mesothelium) and to see the process as a continuum, and to avoid confusion with descriptions of end-stage sclerosing membrane syndromes [66, 67]. Data from many centres have clearly identified sclerosing peritonitis, or in its most severe form sclerosing encapsulating peritonitis (SEP), both histologically and functionally.

In defining 'fibrotic' changes within the peritoneum, however, we wish to focus on those events that potentially occur continuously over time (from initiation of the therapy) that impact on peritoneal membrane dysfunction. Although we still understand little about the time-course over which these changes occur, we assume that they have a cumulative effect over years on PD.

Potential markers of peritoneal healing and fibrosis

Having identified that the peritoneal membrane changes both structurally and functionally the goal must be to identify easily achievable and reliable measures of its 'status' that may be predictive of membrane failure or other complications. Whilst the PET (in whatever is the acceptable form) is of value clinically in determining solute transport, etc., it is not accurate enough to be of prognostic value in determining changes in the structure of the membrane that are suggestive of potential problems. There is no accepted way of monitoring the structure of the peritoneal membrane during the course of dialysis treatment; neither, at present, does a body of data exist that can provide us with markers of the natural history of alterations. The markers so far examined, as we will discuss later, are not specific nor do they provide evidence of defined biological processes. The ideal way to monitor membrane changes would be prospective timed biopsies (an impractical option). Radiology is an option, but one which can be applied only at late stages of peritoneal fibrosis (see below). The best current option, as we will discuss, would be to identify a soluble marker present within the PD effluent (to which there is easy and continuous access in nearly all patients) which correlates closely with changes in structure and which can then be compared with changes in function. Thus we would be able to predict (based on changes from normal values) those patients who are likely to develop problems with dialysis adequacy and/or ultrafiltration. In addition, those patients who develop progressive fibrosis might be detectable at an early stage, and measures prescribed to prevent progressive damage.

Imaging techniques

The process of imaging the peritoneal cavity in patients on CAPD was originally applied as a technique to determine the position of the peritoneal catheter. Subsequently it has been used to investigate changes brought about by progressive fibrosis of the peritoneal membrane (sclerosing encapsulating peritonitis). The role of plain abdominal X-rays is confined to the demonstration of dilated bowel loops which accompany obstruction, or the presence of eggshell calcification of the bowel wall and abdominal wall when the fibrotic process is advanced. The role of bowel contrast studies is to define the functional abnormalities which also occur.

Ultrasound examination has a wider application in the investigation of membrane changes with PD. In a study of 14 patients with SEP alterations in peristalsis, bowel tethering to the posterior abdominal wall, intraperitoneal echogenic fibrous strands (adhesions) and thickening of the membrane were described [101]. More recently plain X-rays, ultrasound (US) and computerized tomography (CT) have been used to investigate patients on CAPD with clinical signs of intestinal obstruction [102]. In those patients with mild fibrosis the signs were difficult to distinguish from non-CAPD patients with obstruction. The presence of thickened peritoneal membranes (separation of bowel loops), 'thumb printing', bowel calcification, loculated fluid and the presence of a visible membrane all signified advanced fibrosis. Indeed this latter study indicated that the combination of all three forms of imaging gave the best evaluation of the patient.

Recent studies have also suggested that, in children at least, the thickness of the peritoneum can be estimated by US [103]. In a study of 131 children the thickness of the peritoneal membrane was estimated at a fixed point on the sternal umbilical line. Thickness was correlated to weight, height and age. Children on haemodialysis had normal-thickness membranes. Those on CAPD who had suffered peritonitis showed increased thickness, decreased bowel movement and adhesions.

Ex-vivo markers of peritoneal structural changes

One of the significant advantages of PD is that it provides access to dialysis effluent within which various parameters can be assessed. Indeed measurements (of mediator levels and the cellular components) in drained effluent have provided the basis for our understanding of the process of peritoneal inflammation *in vivo* [98, 104–111]. The ready access to this material has made it an attractive proposition within which to measure levels of markers, which might be indicative of changes in the function of the membrane or its constitutive parts. In this respect, markers of mesothelial cell mass/turnover (CA125) [112–114], markers of endothelial cell function (Factor VIII) and presumed fibrotic or wound healing markers (pro-collagen I/III, hyaluronic acid and transforming growth factor,

Table 1. Potential markers in dialysis effluent

Markers	Possible significance
CA125	Mesothelial cell mass?
Hyaluronic acid	Healing: mesothelial cell integrity: inflammatory status?
Phospholipids	Mesothelial cell integrity?
Factor VIII	Endothelial cell mass: angiogenesis?
Collagen peptides	Collagen turnover: fibrosis?
TGF-β_1	Profibrotic activity?
VEGF	Angiogenesis?

TGF-β1) [115, 116] and angiogenic potential (vascular endothelial growth factor, VEGF) [117] have been measured in PD patients at various points during treatment. Unfortunately, despite the promise and potential importance of this approach, much of the data so far generated has been cross-sectional and based on small patient numbers. This has produced conflicting results in different centres regarding the relationship between markers and time on PD, e.g. CA125 [113, 118]. There is clearly a need for longitudinal studies on CA125 and other markers in individual patients to define the variability and thus usefulness of these tests. Only when such data are available can definitive links between these markers and clinical changes in peritoneal function be established or refuted. Table 1 lists potential effluent markers and their possible significance. Data from the recent clinical trials of 'biocompatible' solutions are certainly indicative in *in-vivo* effects, as indicated by changes in dialysate CA125, hyaluronic acid and procollagen levels. Whilst at present we can only speculate what these changes might represent in terms of the status of the peritoneal membrane, the fact that their levels are impacted upon by therapy modulation does provide evidence that the type of solution infused does affect the status of the peritoneal membrane *in vivo* [119, 120]. Figure 2 shows the changes occurring with various markers during a study of a potentially more biocompatible fluid.

Biocompatibility and the peritoneal membrane: the influence of the dialysate

More than a decade of largely in-vitro data has resulted in an understanding of the potential role that peritoneal dialysis fluid (PDF) components might play in modulating peritoneal membrane structure and function. These data derived initially

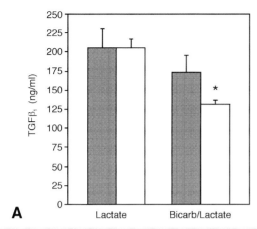
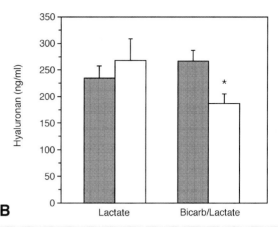

Figure 2. The changes occurring in dialysate effluent markers (**A**), TGF-β_1 and (**B**) hyaluronic acid in a short-term clinical study comparing lactate- and bicarbonate/lactate-buffered peritoneal dialysis solutions [164]. Grey bars represent the run-in phase (both patient groups continuously exposed to lactate-buffered PDF, PD4, 40 mm lactate pH 5.2 for 6 weeks). Open bars represent the trial phase, patients continuously exposed either to lactate or bicarbonate/lactate (25 mm bicarbonate/15 mm lactate pH 7.3) for 12 weeks. Data are presented as the mean ($\pm$ SEM) for each phase, $n = 5$ patients/group. Asterisk represents a significant reduction compared to the run-in phase.

from studies on peritoneal cell functions, and more recently from *ex-vivo* studies and PD effluent measurements in clinical trials, suggest, along with some *in-vivo* studies in rodents, that solution components can modulate the peritoneum [121–127]. Whilst these studies were initially aimed at providing the rationale for the peritoneal cavity's increased susceptibility to infection, they have more recently provided the basis for our understanding of the potential of PDF components in modulating peritoneal membrane structure and function in long-term PD. Part of the rationale for these studies is based on clinical evidence that loss of ultrafiltration can also occur in patients without a significant history of peritoneal infection, leading to the suggestion that 'other factors' such as continuous exposure to PDF components might play an important role in the process.

A contemporary view of our understanding of PDF biocompatibility issues suggests that their effects can be divided into:

1. 'Acute' effects which have a predominantly inhibitory outcome and result from short-term (minutes to hours) exposure to specific PDF components.
2. 'Chronic' effects which result from prolonged or repeated exposure (hours to years) to PDF.

Interestingly, various PDF components can have both acute and chronic effects, indicating their potential to modify peritoneal homeostasis by several mechanisms.

Acute effects of PDF: potential impact on peritoneal host defence

As mentioned previously, laboratory-based *in-vitro* experiments, as well as more limited animal experiments and *ex-vivo* studies in PD patients, have clearly identified that almost all components of conventional PDF levels (acidic lactate-buffered PDF containing 1.36% or 3.86% glucose) which are present at unphysiological concentrations modulate cell function [123, 127–134].

These include its pH (5.2–5.5), necessary to prevent the caramelization of glucose during its heat sterilization; its lactate concentration (40 mM) which is used as the buffering system; and its glucose concentration (75–214 mM) and associated hyperosmolality (350–500 mOsm/kg) necessary to produce an osmotic gradient for ultrafiltration. Additional studies have also identified that the heat sterilization of glucose-containing solutions gives rise to bioactive metabolites resulting from the chemical breakdown of glucose [135–138]. *In vitro* these glucose degradation products (GPD) have been shown to modulate cell functions [139, 140]. In addition to their direct modulatory effects on cell function these highly biologically active compounds are also important intermediates, particularly 3-deoxy glucasone, glyoxal and methylglyoxal in the formation of AGE. The impact of AGE formation on peritoneal membrane structure and function will be discussed later.

Chronic effects of PDF: impact on the structure of the peritoneal membrane

Whilst the link between structural and functional alterations in the peritoneal membrane is still largely hypothetical (see earlier), examination of peritoneal biopsies indicates that structural changes do occur in the dialysed membrane; it is therefore a logical step to suggest that these are linked to functional changes that are observed clinically. In the same manner the bioincompatible nature of PDF, together with evidence of the effects of glucose in other systems, suggests that it is very likely that it does have an impact *in vivo*.

PD patients are exposed to unphysiological levels of PDF components throughout their time on dialysis (approximately 3000 L/year), although its equilibration following infusion results in some PDF components reaching physiological levels at some stage during the dwell. Many, however, do not, and are at unphysiological levels for the whole dwell period. For example, glucose is infused at between 75 and 214 mM and at the end of a standard 4-h dwell will have reached 20–30 and 75–90 mM [123]. As the physiological glucose concentration is between 5 and 10 mM the potential impact is clear both in the short and long term. In addition, repeated infusion of solutions could theoretically lead to the accumulation of non-metabolizable compounds in the tissues of the peritoneal membrane or systemically (as occurs with maltose following polyglucose infusion) [141].

There is increasing evidence of chronic effects of PDF components on cell function which at least provide some rationale for the argument that solution biocompatibility might impact on the structure/function of the peritoneal membrane. The most compelling of this evidence relates to the effects of glucose on peritoneal cell function *in vitro* and *in vivo*, and is closely related to studies in diabetes and diabetic nephropathy on the modulating influence of glucose on cell and organ function [142, 143].

Initial studies in cultured mesothelial cells exposed to D-glucose demonstrated reduced cellular proliferation and viability [144, 145]. Subsequent studies demonstrated that prolonged exposure to D-glucose was associated with increased mesothelial cell expression of fibronectin mRNA, an effect which was D-glucose specific and independent of osmolality [33]. More recently, high concentrations of glucose have been shown to induce TGF-β_1 expression in cultured mesothelial cells [146]. Interestingly, spent dialysate isolated after a 4-h dwell contained significant latent TGF-β_1-inducing activity, an observa-

tion that suggests the profibrotic activity might potentially be present throughout the dwell period. Additionally these authors demonstrated that pro-inflammatory cytokines (1L-1β and TNF-α) augmented the effects of glucose and spent dialysate. Whilst it must be remembered that TGF-β_1 is secreted in a latent biologically inactive form, substances are also present in PD effluent capable of its activation [147].

Effects of chronic glucose exposure have also been observed in the peritoneal cavity of the experimental animals and in PD patients. Using the 'imprint' model, Gotloib *et al.* have clearly demonstrated that long-term exposure to glucose alters mesothelial cell structure and function [129–131]. *In vivo* the stimulatory effects of glucose may occur over an even shorter time scale, Fujimori *et al.* have recently demonstrated that intraperitoneal IL-6 levels correlate directly with the glucose content in the infused PDF [148]. The implication of these latter findings is unclear, but continuous modulation or activation of IL-6 synthesis might have long-term consequences for the control of inflammation within the peritoneal cavity [18, 40, 105, 107].

As mentioned earlier, continuous exposure of tissues to high concentrations of glucose (such as those present in PDF) can result in the formation of AGE, a process that is facilitated in PDF by the presence of GDP, many of which are intermediates in, or catalyse, AGE formation reactions [135–138, 149]. Examination of biopsies from the peritoneal membrane of PD patients clearly demonstrates the presence of AGE-modified proteins [47, 150, 151]. These could be due to *in-situ* formation due to high concentrations of glucose in the dialysate. Alternatively they could have been deposited (trapped) by diffusion from the blood, since increased levels of AGE are found in the serum of uraemic subjects. Although their functional significance remains to be precisely determined, data from other cell systems suggest that AGE modification of proteins modifies their metabolic fate (e.g. reduces collagen turnover) and can in some cases cause direct cell activation [152]. The implication of increased cellular activation and decreased extracellular matrix turnover for the development of fibrotic changes within the peritoneal cavity is clear [153]. In the past few years it has been suggested that 'carbonyl stress' in uraemia and AGE deposition may also be related to involving autoxidation products of carbohydrates and lipids, suggesting that both uraemia and glucose exposure may be important in AGE deposition in the peritoneal membrane [154]. It has also been reported that with increasing time on PD there is more AGE deposition in the peritoneum, particularly in vascular walls [155].

Honda *et al.* [47] examined peritoneal biopsies of patients with varying degrees of ultrafiltration for evidence of interstitial and vascular changes and AGE deposition. As mentioned earlier, they correlated changes in the peritoneal vasculature with the accumulation of the advanced glycosylation endproducts in patients with low ultrafiltration. The extent of AGE accumulation correlated with the progression of interstitial fibrosis and vascular sclerosis in this small study. Whilst these correlations do not represent causality, they certainly provide strong evidence for the role of AGE deposition in the generation of structural and functional defects in the peritoneal membrane [153].

Recently data have become available, as will be discussed below, from both long-term clinical trials and animal studies of PDF designed specifically to address biocompatibility issues, in particular pH and the levels of glucose degradation products [120, 156, 157]. Whilst neither of these factors has so far been directly implicated in structural alterations in the peritoneal membrane, a large body of information suggests that they have modulatory effects on cell function *in vitro* and *in vivo* [139, 140, 156–162]. Recent *ex-vivo* data clearly suggest, despite the large inter- and intra-patient variability, that these modified solutions might have a positive impact on membrane longevity [119, 120]. Further work is clearly required to substantiate these results.

Enhancing biocompatibility of PD

Whilst much of the biocompatibility evidence is very suggestive of *in-vivo* effects, in many cases proof based on *in-vivo* observation is lacking. Thus although *ex-vivo* studies suggest the bioincompatible nature of conventional lactate-buffered PDF containing glucose [132–134, 163], data from long-term observations in PD patients are required to definitively identify which PDF components impact (or not) on peritoneal host defence and the structure or function of the peritoneal membrane. The data from the recent clinical trials of PD-Bio® and Physioneal® are very suggestive of true *in-vivo* effects, but further information is required [119, 120].

Despite this lack of real *in-vivo* evidence that PDF components impact directly on peritoneal host defence, or contribute to loss of membrane function, the weight of *in-vitro* and *ex-vivo* evidence, together

with our increased understanding of the potential chronic effects of exposure to supra-physiological concentrations of PDF components, have resulted in the search for alternative solution formulations. These alternative solution formulations can be divided into those that replace or reduce glucose concentration with an alternative osmotic agent, e.g. polyglucose, glycerol, amino acids or a combination of these, and those that create a neutral or nearneutral pH solution either by replacing lactate as a buffer and/or preparing the solutions in dual-chamber bags such that the glucose can be sterilized separately, e.g. bicarbonate, bicarbonate in combination with glycyl-glycine or lactate, or conventional lactate solution at pH 6.8 [157, 164] (these solutions, as mentioned previously, have the added advantage of reduced GDP content as a result of the sterilizations of glucose at low pH).

Many of these solutions have undergone phase I or phase III trials and some have been introduced into clinical practice over the past few years. At present it is too early to assess whether any of these will impact on peritoneal membrane function. *In-vivo* and *ex-vivo* and animal studies, however, suggest that many of these formulations show significantly improved parameters of host defence compared to conventional acidic lactate buffered solutions [131, 134, 165–173]. It will be years, however, before the long-term effects of potentially more biocompatible PDF on peritoneal structure and function are definitively identified. Their introduction, however, allows us a unique opportunity to assess their impact compared to conventional solutions on peritoneal membrane longevity.

Whilst there is strong theoretical, circumstantial and *in-vitro* evidence linking peritoneal damage to toxic or unphysiological constituents within dialysis fluid, proving direct cause and effect has been difficult. This is in part due to the relatively long period over which peritoneal changes occur. It does seem likely, however, that strategies designed to avoid excessive glucose and GDP exposure and neutral pH solutions may have the potential to arrest, prevent or reverse (ongoing) peritoneal damage.

Potential measures to preserve the peritoneal membrane

At present it would appear that two factors are largely responsible for peritoneal membrane damage; namely, inflammation and the dialysate. It is therefore hoped that dealing with these influences will lead to improved longevity of the peritoneum with stable function. With respect to inflammation it is clearly important to prevent peritonitis. The Y set, incorporating flush-before-fill, is proven to be the best CAPD system at present in this respect. The possible regular use of pericatheter mupirocin may further cut the peritonitis rate [174], though the long-term effects, including the possibility of bacterial resistance, remain unknown. Once inflammation occurs it is critical to treat promptly, since there is some evidence that the cumulative inflammatory response correlates with subsequent changes in function [79]. Thus a possibly more aggressive approach to removing the cannula if the bags do not rapidly clear may be beneficial. Whether the use of anti-inflammatory molecules or agents will have a role is still unclear.

The major detrimental factor in the dialysate appears to be the glucose and/or its degradation products. Glucose polymer (icodextrin) produces less AGE *in vitro*. At present, though, only one bag of this substance can be used each day, because it produces high plasma levels of oligosaccharides, especially maltose. Bicarbonate-based dialysates contain less GDP [162] because of the way they are manufactured. Amino acid dialysate is by definition free of all glucose or its products. Once again, only one bag a day can be used because of the possibility of acidosis. Glycerol has been tried as an alternative, and one report suggests that using a combination of glucose-free bags including glycerol allows impaired aquaporin function to recover [175]. The long-term safety of glycerol is unknown. One possible way to avoid GDP would be to sterilize the fluid by cold filtration. This would, however, require a change in the procedures approved by the Drug Regulatory Authorities.

There is thus a case for restricting the amount of glucose exposure incurred by the peritoneum. This must start by educating the patient to maintain fluid balance by restricting intake and not by using 3.86% glucose bags. Furthermore, every effort should be made to maintain urine volume. Availability of bicarbonate-based dialysate may further reduce peritoneal damage. It is possible that glucose polymer should be used from an early stage in treatment. Both the latter suggestions will, however, be critically dependent on the prices charged by manufacturers, since all health-care systems worldwide are under financial pressure. A less acidic fluid than conventional dialysate which contains reduced levels of GDP has also been developed [176]. Use of this solution might reduce the number of patients developing problems with fluid removal. It must be pointed out that, to prove that a reduced glucose exposure will lead to less structural and functional peritoneal changes, will require a very large controlled trial of several years duration [177]. Table 2 summarizes potential methods for reducing membrane damage.

Conclusions

In summary, this chapter has attempted to link what is currently known about peritoneal structure and function to the clinical problems experienced in the management of PD patients. As our understanding of this membrane improves it provides us with an ever-increasing rational approach to therapeutic manipulation. Hopefully this, combined with the increasing number of treatment options available, should make it possible to enhance treatment quality, and improve patient and technique survival on this modality.

References

1. Maiorca R, Cancarini GC, Camerini C *et al.* Is CAPD competitive with haemodialysis for long-term treatment of uraemic patients? Nephrol Dial Transplant 1989; 4: 244–53.
2. Maiorca R, Vonesh E, Cavalli PL *et al.* A multi-centre, selection adjusted comparison of patient and technique survivals on CAPD and hemodialysis. Perit Dial Int 1990; 11: 118–27.
3. Fenton, SSA, Schaubel DE, Desmeules M *et al.* Hemodialysis versus peritoneal dialysis: a comparison of adjusted mortality rates. Am J Kidney Dis 1997; 30: 334–42.
4. Lupo A, Tarchini R, Cancarini GC *et al.* Long-term outcome in continuous ambulatory peritoneal dialysis: a 10-year survey by the Italian Cooperative Peritoneal Dialysis Study Group. Am J Kidney Dis 1994; 24: 826–37.
5. Davies SJ, Phillips L, Griffiths AM *et al.* What really happens to people on long-term peritoneal dialysis? Kidney Int 1998; 54: 2207–17.

Table 2. Potential measures to reduce peritoneal membrane damage

Reduce peritonitis	Y set
	Pericatheter mupirocin (NB resistance)
Reduce glucose degradation exposure	Use less 3.86% (4.25%) glucose
	Use icodextrin (glucose polymer)
	Use neutral or near-neutral PD fluid
	Use amino acid dialysate
	Cold filtration (if approved)
Reduce glucose exposure	Restrict sodium and water intake
	Use less 3.86% (4.25%) glucose
	Use icodextrin (glucose polymer)
	Use amino acid dialysate

6. Gotloib L, Shostack A. Ultrastructural morphology of the peritoneum: new findings and speculations on transfer of solutes and water during peritoneal dialysis. Perit Dial Bull 1987; 7: 119–29.

7. Gotloib L, Shostack A. The functional anatomy of the peritoneum as a dialysing membrane. In: Twardowski ZJ, Nolph KD, Khanna R, eds. Peritoneal Dialysis. New York: Churchill Livingstone, 1990, pp. 1–27.

8. Di Paolo N, Sacchi G, De Mia M *et al.* Morphology of the peritoneal membrane during continuous ambulatory peritoneal dialysis. Nephron 1986; 44: 204–11.

9. Di Paolo N, Sacchi G, Buoncristiani V. The morphology of the human peritoneum in CAPD patients. In: Maher J, ed. Frontiers in Peritoneal Dialysis. New York: Field Rich, 1985, pp. 11–19.

10. Satoh K, Prescott SM. Culture of mesothelial cells from bovine pericardium and characterisation of their arachidonate metabolism. Biochim Biophys Acta 1987; 930: 283–96.

11. Rennard SI, Jaurand M-C, Bignon J *et al.* Role of pleural mesothelial cells in the production of the submesothelial connective tissue matrix of lung. Am Rev Respir Dis 1984; 130: 267–74.

12. Gotloib L, Shostack A, Jaichenko J. Ruthenium-red-stained anionic charges of rat and mice mesothelial cells and basal lamina: the peritoneum is a negatively charged dialyzing membrane. Nephron 1988; 48: 65–70.

13. Gotloib L, Shostack A, Jaichenko J. Loss of mesothelial electronegative fixed charges during murine septic peritonitis. Nephron 1989; 51: 77–83.

14. Beavis J, Harwood JL, Coles GA, Williams JD. Intraperitoneal phosphatidyl choline levels in patients on continuous ambulatory peritoneal dialysis do not correlate with adequacy of ultrafiltration. J Am Soc Nephrol 1993; 3: 1954–60.

15. Beavis MJ, Harwood JL, Coles GA, Williams JD. Synthesis of phospholipids by human peritoneal mesothelial cells. Perit Dial Int 1994; 14: 348–55.

16. Dobbie JW, Pavlina T, Lloyd J, Johnson RC. Phosphatidylcholine synthesis by peritoneal mesothelium: its implication for peritoneal dialysis. Am J Kidney Dis 1988; 12: 31–6.

17. Stylianou E, Jenner LA, Davies M, Coles GA, Williams JD. Isolation, culture and characterisation of human peritoneal mesothelial cells. Kidney Int 1990; 37: 1563–70.

18. Topley N, Jörres A, Luttmann W *et al.* Human peritoneal mesothelial cells synthesize IL-6: induction by IL-1β and TNFα. Kidney Int 1993; 43: 226–33.

19. Topley N, Brown Z, Jörres A *et al.* Human peritoneal mesothelial cells synthesize IL-8: synergistic induction by interleukin-1β and tumor necrosis factor α. Am J Pathol 1993; 142: 1876–86.

20. Betjes MGH, Tuk CW, Struijk DG *et al.* Interleukin-8 production by human peritoneal mesothelial cells in response to tumor necrosis factor α, interleukin-1, and medium conditioned by macrophages co-cultured with *Staphylococcus epidermidis*. J Infect Dis 1993; 168: 1202–10.

21. Douvdevani A, Rapoport J, Konforty A *et al.* Human peritoneal mesothelial cells synthesize IL-1α and β. Kidney Int 1994; 46: 993–1001.

22. Andreoli SP, Mallett C, Williams K *et al.* Mechanisms of polymorphonuclear leukocyte mediated peritoneal mesothelial cell injury. Kidney Int 1994; 46: 1100–9.

23. Bermudez E, Everitt J, Walker C. Expression of growth factor and growth factor receptor RNA in rat pleural mesothelial cells in culture. Exp Cell Res 1990; 190: 91–8.

24. Bittinger F, Klein CL, Skarke C *et al.* PECAM-1 expression in human mesothelial cells: an *in vitro* study. Pathobiology 1996; 64: 320–7.

25. Boylan AM, Rüegg C, Jin KK *et al.* Evidence of a role for mesothelial cell-derived interleukin 8 in the pathogenesis of asbestos-induced pleurisy in rabbits. J Clin Invest 1992; 89: 1257–67.

26. Bult H, Coene MC, Rampart M, Herman AG. Complement derived factors and prostacyclin formation by isolated rabbit peritoneum and cultured mesothelial cells. Agents Actions 1984; 14: 237–47.

27. Cannistra SA, Ottensmeier C, Tidy J, DeFranzo B. Vascular cell adhesion molecule-1 expressed by peritoneal mesothelial partly mediates the binding of activated human T lymphocytes. Exp Haem 1994; 22: 996–1002.

28. Cantor J, Willhite M, Bray B *et al.* Synthesis of crosslinked elastin by a mesothelial cell culture. Proc Soc Exp Biol Med 1986; 181: 387–91.

29. Coene MC, Solheid C, Claeys M, Herman AG. Prostaglandin production by cultured mesothelial cells. Arch Int Pharmacodyn 1981; 249: 316–18.

30. Douvdevani A, Yulzari R, Zilberman M, Rukshin V, Chaimovitz C. TNF receptor in human peritoneal mesothelial cells: shedding of soluble TNF receptor after exposure to interleukin-1α. J Am Soc Nephrol 1995; 5: 444.

31. Harvey W, Amlot PL. Collagen production by human mesothelial cells *in vitro*. J Pathol 1983; 139: 337–47.

32. Jonjic N, Peri G, Bernasconi S *et al.* Expression of adhesion molecules and chemotactic cytokines in cultured human mesothelial cells. J Exp Med 1992; 176: 1165–74.

33. Kumano K, Schiller B, Hjelle JT, Moran J. Effect of osmotic solutes on fibronectin mRNA expression in rat peritoneal mesothelial cells. Blood Purif 1996; 14: 165–9.

34. Leavesley DI, Stanley JM, Faull RJ. Epidermal growth factor modifies the expression and function of extracellular matrix adhesion receptors expressed by peritoneal mesothelial cells from patients on CAPD. Nephrol Dial Transplant 1999; 14: 1208–16.

35. Liberek T, Topley N, Luttmann W, Williams JD. Adherence of neutrophils to human peritoneal mesothelial cells: role of intercellular adhesion molecule-1. J Am Soc Nephrol 1996; 7: 208–17.

36. Mackay AM, Tracy RP, Craighead JE, Cytokeratin expression in rat mesothelial cells *in vitro* is controlled by the extracellular matrix. J Cell Sci 1990; 95: 97–107.

37. Marshall BC, Santana A, Xu Q-P *et al.* Metalloproteinases and tissue inhibitor of metalloproteinases in mesothelial cells: cellular differentiation influences expression. J Clin Invest 1993; 91: 1792–9.

38. Topley N, Jörres A, Petersen MM *et al.* Human peritoneal mesothelial cell prostaglandin (PG) metabolism: induction by cytokines and peritoneal macrophage conditioned medium. J Am Soc Nephrol 1991; 2: 432.

39. Visser CE, Tekstra J, Brouwer-Steenbergen JJE *et al.* Chemokines produced by mesothelial cells: huGRO-α, IFN-γ inducible protein-10, monocyte chemotactic protein-1 and RANTES. Clin Exp Immunol 1998; 112: 270–5.

40. Witowski J, Jörres A, Williams JD, Topley N. Superinduction of IL-6 synthesis in human peritoneal mesothelial cells is related to induction and stabilization of IL-6 mRNA. Kidney Int 1996; 50: 1212–23.

41. Yung S, Thomas GJ, Stylianou E *et al.* Source of peritoneal proteoglycans: human peritoneal mesothelial cells synthesize and secrete mainly small dermatan sulphate proteoglycans. Am J Pathol 1995; 146: 520–9.

42. Yung S, Coles GA, Davies M. IL-1β, a major stimulator of hyaluronan synthesis *in vitro* of human peritoneal mesothelial cells: relevance to peritonitis in CAPD. Kidney Int 1996; 50: 1337–43.

43. Zeillemaker AM, Mul FPJ, Hoynck van Papendrecht AAGM *et al.* Polarized secretion of interleukin-8 by human mesothelial cells: a role in neutrophil migration. Immunology 1995; 84: 227–32.

44. Jörres A, Ludat K, Lang J *et al.* Establishment and functional characterisation of human peritoneal fibroblasts in culture: regulation of interleukin-6 production by proinflammatory cytokines. J Am Soc Nephrol 1996; 7: 2192–201.

45. Beavis MJ, Williams JD, Hoppe J, Topley N. Human peritoneal fibroblast proliferation in 3-dimensional culture: modulation by cytokines, growth factors and peritoneal dialysis effluent. Kidney Int 1997; 51: 205–15.

46. Honda K, Nitta K, Horita H, Yumura W, Nihei H. Morphological changes in the peritoneal vasculature of patients on CAPD with ultrafiltration failure. Nephron 1996; 72: 171–6.

47. Honda K, Nitta K, Horita S et al. Accumulation of advanced glycation end products in the peritoneal vasculature of continuous ambulatory peritoneal dialysis patients with low ultrafiltration. Nephrol Dial Transplant 1999; 14: 1541–9.

48. Mateijsen MAM, van der Wal AC, Hendriks PMEM et al. Vascular and interstitial changes in the peritoneum of CAPD patients with peritoneal sclerosis. J Am Soc Nephrol 1997; 8: 268–9.

49. Topley N, Craig JJ, Fallon M et al. Morphological changes in the peritoneal membrane of patients on peritoneal dialysis (PD) are related to time on treatment. J Am Soc Nephrol 1999; 10: 324A.

50. Rubin J, Herrara GA, Collins D. An autopsy study of the peritoneal cavity from patients on continuous ambulatory peritoneal dialysis. Am J Kidney Dis 1991; 17: 97–102.

51. Verger C, Luger A, Moore HL, Nolph KD. Acute changes in peritoneal morphology and transport properties with infectious peritonitis and mechanical injury. Kidney Int 1983; 23: 823–31.

52. Di Paolo N, Sacchi G. Peritoneal vascular changes in continuous ambulatory peritoneal dialysis (CAPD): an in vivo model for the study of the diabetic microangiopathy. Perit Dial Int 1989; 9: 41–5.

53. Gotloib L, bar-Sella P, Shostack A. Reduplicated basal lamina of small venules and mesothelium of human parietal peritoneum: ultrastructural changes of reduplicated peritoneal basement membrane. Perit Dial Bull 1985; 5: 212–14.

54. Dobbie J, Zaki M, Wilson L. Ultrafiltration studies on the peritoneum with special reference to chronic ambulatory peritoneal dialysis. Scott Med J 1981; 26: 213–23.

55. Dobbie JW, Lloyd JK, Gall CA. Categorization of ultrastructural changes in peritoneal mesothelium, stroma and blood vessels in uremia and CAPD patients. Adv Perit Dial 1990; 6: 3–12.

56. Dobbie JW. Pathogenesis of peritoneal fibrosing syndromes (sclerosing peritonitis) in peritoneal dialysis. Perit Dial Int 1992; 12: 14–27.

57. Dobbie JW. Peritoneal ultrastructure and changes with continuous ambulatory peritoneal dialysis. Perit Dial Int 1993; 13: S585–7.

58. Dobbie JW, Anderson JD, Hind C. Long-term effects of peritoneal dialysis on peritoneal morphology. *Perit Dial Int* 1994; 14: S16–20.

59. Dobbie JW. Ultrastructure and pathology of the peritoneum in peritoneal dialysis. In: Gokal R, Nolph KD, eds. The Textbook of Peritoneal Dialysis. Lancaster: Kluwer, 1994, pp. 17–44.

60. Pollock CA, Ibels LS, Eckstein RP et al. Peritoneal morphology on maintenance dialysis. Am J Nephrol 1989; 9: 198–204.

61. Selgas R, Fernandez-Reyes MJ, Bosque E et al. Functional longevity of the human peritoneum: how long is continuous peritoneal dialysis possible? Results of a prospective medium long-term study. Am J Kidney Dis 1994; 23: 64–73.

62. Davies SJ, Bryan J, Phillips L, Russell GI. Longitudinal changes in peritoneal kinetics: the effects of peritoneal dialysis and peritonitis. Nephrol Dial Transplant 1996; 11: 498–506.

63. Dobbie JW. Morphology of the peritoneum in CAPD. Blood Purif 1989; 7: 74–85.

64. Rigby RJ, Hawley CM. Sclerosing peritonitis: the experience in Australia. Nephrol Dial Transplant 1998; 13: 154–9.

65. Holland P. Sclerosing encapsulating peritonitis in chronic ambulatory peritoneal dialysis. Clin Radiol 1990; 41: 19–23.

66. Nomoto Y, Kawaguchi Y, Kubo H et al. Sclerosing encapsulating peritonitis in patients undergoing continuous ambulatory peritoneal dialysis: a report on the Japanese sclerosing encapsulating peritonitis study group. Am J Kidney Dis 1996; 28: 420–7.

67. Campbell S, Clarke P, Hawley C et al. Sclerosing peritonitis: identification of diagnostic, clinical, and radiological features. Am J Kidney Dis 1994; 24: 819–25.

68. Peltonen J, Kähäri L, Jaakkola S et al. Evaluation of transforming growth factor-β and type I procollagen gene expression in fibrotic skin diseases by in situ hybridisation. J Invest Dermatol 1990; 94: 365–71.

69. Wahl SM. Fibrosis: bacterial cell wall induced hepatic granulomas. In: Gallin JI, Goldstein IM, Snyderman R, eds. Basic Principles and Clinical Correlates. New York: Raven Press, 1988; pp. 841–59.

70. Elias JA, Freundlich B, Kern JA, Rosenbloom J. Cytokine networks in the regulation of inflammation and fibrosis in the lung. Chest 1990; 97: 1439–45.

71. Mauch C, Krieg T. Fibroblast–matrix interactions and their role in the pathogenesis of fibrosis. Rheum Dis Clin N Am 1990; 16: 93–107.

72. Mauch C, Hatamachi A, Scharffetter K, Kreig T. Regulation of collagen synthesis in fibroblasts within a three-dimensional collagen gel. Exp Cell Res 1988; 178: 493–503.

73. Kunico GS, Neilson EG, Haverty T. Mechanisms of tubulointerstitial fibrosis. Kidney Int 1991; 39: 550–6.

74. Freundlich B, Bomalaski JS, Neilson E, Jiminez SA. Regulation of fibroblast proliferation and collagen synthesis by cytokines. Immunol Today 1986; 7: 303–7.

75. Beavis MJ, Williams JD, Topley N. Repeated activation of human peritoneal fibroblasts results in sustained cell proliferation and collagen III mRNA expression. J Am Soc Nephrol 1997; 8: 512.

76. Selgas R, Bajo MA, Paiva A et al. Stability of the peritoneal membrane in long-term peritoneal dialysis patients. Adv Renal Replace Ther 1998; 5: 168–78.

77. Churchill DN, Thorpe KE, Nolph KD et al. Increased peritoneal membrane transport is associated with decreased patient and technique survival for continuous peritoneal dialysis patients. The Canada–USA (CANUSA) Peritoneal Dialysis Study Group. J Am Soc Nephrol 1998; 9: 1285–92.

78. Wang T, Heimburger O, Waniewski J, Bergstrom J, Lindholm B. Increased peritoneal permeability is associated with decreased fluid and small-solute removal and higher mortality in CAPD patients. Nephrol Dial Transplant 1998; 13: 1242–9.

79. Davies SJ, Brown B, Bryan J, Russell GI, Clinical evaluation of the peritoneal equilibration test: a population-based study. Nephrol Dial Transplant 1993; 8: 64–70.

80. Heimburger O, Waniewski J, Werynski A, Tranaeus A, Lindholm B. Peritoneal transport in CAPD patients with permanent loss of ultrafiltration capacity. Kidney Int 1990; 38: 495–506.

81. Kawaguchi Y, Hasegawa T, Nakayama M, Kubo H, Shigematu T. Issues affecting the longevity of the continuous dialysis therapy. Kidney Int Suppl 1997; 62: S105–7.

82. Bos WJW, Struijk DG, van Olden RW, Arisz, L, Krediet RT. Elevated ambulatory blood pressure in patients with ultrafiltration failure. Perit Dial Int 1998; 18: S12.

83. Ho-dac-Pannekeet MM, Atasever B, Struijk DG, Krediet RT. Analysis of ultrafiltration failure in peritoneal dialysis patients by means of standard peritoneal permeability analysis. Perit Dial Int 1997; 17: 144–50.

84. Monquil MC, Imholz AL, Struijk DG, Krediet RT. Does impaired transcellular water transport contribute to net ultrafiltration failure during CAPD? Perit Dial Int 1995; 15: 42–8.

85. Ho-dac-Pannekeet MM, Koopmans JG, Struijk DG, Krediet RT. Restriction coefficients of low molecular weight solutes and macromolecules during peritoneal dialysis. Adv Perit Dial 1997; 13: 72–6.

86. NKF-DOQI clinical practice guidelines for peritoneal dialysis adequacy. National Kidney Foundation. Am J Kidney Dis 1997; 30: S67–136.

87. Twardowski ZJ, Nolph KD, Khanna R et al. Peritoneal equilibration test. Perit Dial Bull 1987; 6: 131–7.

88. Garred LJ, Canaud B, Farrell PC. A simple kinetic model for assessing peritoneal mass transfer in continuous ambulatory peritoneal dialysis. J Artif Intern Org 1983; 6: 131–7.

89. Pannekeet MM, Imholz AL, Struijk DG et al. The standard peritoneal permeability analysis: a tool for the assessment of peritoneal permeability characteristics in CAPD patients. Kidney Int 1995; 48: 866–75.

90. Haraldsson B. Assessing the peritoneal dialysis capacities of individual patients. Kidney Int 1995; 47: 1187–98.

91. Verger C, Larpent L, Veniez BM. Mathematical determination of PET. Perit Dial Int 1990; 10: S181.

92. Cichocki T, Hanicki Z, Sulowicz W et al. Output of peritoneal cells into peritoneal dialysate. Nephron 1983; 35: 175–82.

93. Alobaidi H. Host defence in CAPD: a laboratory and clinical investigation. PhD thesis, University of Wales, 1986.

94. Visser CE, Steenbergen JJE, Betjes MGH et al. Interleukin-8 production by human mesothelial cells after direct stimulation with staphylococci. Infect Immun 1995; 10: 4206–9.

95. Visser CE, Brouer-Steenbergen JJE, Schadee-Eestermans IL et al. Ingestion of Staphylococcus aureus, Staphylococcus epidermidis and Escherichia coli by human peritoneal mesothelial cells. Infect Immun 1996; 64: 3425–8.

96. Topley N, Petersen MM, Mackenzie R et al. Human peritoneal mesothelial cell prostaglandin synthesis: induction of cyclooxygenase mRNA by peritoneal macrophage derived cytokines. Kidney Int 1994; 46: 900–9.

97. Suassuna JHR, Das Neves FC, Hartley RB, Ogg CS, Cameron JS. Immunohistochemical studies of the peritoneal membrane and infiltrating cells in normal subjects and in patients on CAPD. Kidney Int 1994; 46: 443–54.

98. Brauner A, Hylander B, Wretlind B. Interleukin-6 and interleukin-8 in dialysate and serum from patients on continuous ambulatory peritoneal dialysis. Am J Kidney Dis 1993; 22: 430–5.

99. Robson RL, Witowski J, Loetscher P, Topley N. Differential regulation of C-C and C-x-C chemokine synthesis in cytokine-activated human peritoneal mesothelial cells by INF-γ. Kidney Int 1997; 52: 1123.

100. Holmes CJ. Peritoneal host defense mechanisms in peritoneal dialysis. Kidney Int 1994; 46: S58–70.

101. Hollman AS, McMillan MA, Briggs JD, Junor BJ, Morley P. Ultrasound changes in sclerosing peritonitis following continuous ambulatory peritoneal dialysis. Clin Radiol 1991; 43: 176–9.

102. Krestin GP, Kacl G, Hauser M et al. Imaging diagnosis of sclerosing peritonitis and relation of radiologic signs to the extent of the disease. Abdom Imaging 1995; 20: 414–20.

103. Faller U, Stegen P, Klaus G, Mehls O, Troger J. Sonographic determination of the thickness of the peritoneum in healthy children and paediatric patients on CAPD. Nephrol Dial Transplant 1998; 13: 3172–7.

104. Zemel D, Betjes MGH, Dinkla C, Struijk DG, Krediet RT. Analysis of inflammatory mediators and peritoneal permeability to macromolecules shortly before the onset of overt peritonitis in patients treated with CAPD. Perit Dial Int 1994; 15: 134–41.

105. Zemel D, Koomen GCM, Hart AAM et al. Relationship of TNFα, interleukin-6, and prostaglandins to peritoneal permeability for macromolecules during longitudinal follow-up of peritonitis in continuous ambulatory peritoneal dialysis. J Lab Clin Med 1994; 122: 686–96.

106. Zemel D, Imholz ALT, de Wart DR et al. The appearance of tumor necrosis factor-α and soluble TNF-receptors I and II in peritoneal effluent during stable and infectious CAPD. Kidney Int 1994; 46: 1422–30.

107. Zemel D, ten Berge RJM, Struijk DG et al. Interleukin-6 in CAPD patients without peritonitis: relationship to the intrinsic permeability of the peritoneal membrane. Clin Nephrol 1992; 37: 97–103.

108. Zemel D, ten Berge RJM, Koomen GCM, Struijk DG, Krediet RT. Serum interleukin-6 in continuous ambulatory peritoneal dialysis patients. Nephron 1993; 64: 320–1.

109. Brauner A, Hylander B, Wretlind B. Tumor necrosis factor-α, interleukin-1β, and interleukin-1 receptor antagonist in dialysate and serum from patients on continuous ambulatory peritoneal dialysis. Am J Kidney Dis 1996; 27: 402–8.

110. Goldman M, Vandenabeele P, Moulart J et al. Intraperitoneal secretion of interleukin-6 during continuous ambulatory peritoneal dialysis. Nephron 1990; 56: 277–80.

111. Moutabarrik A, Nakanishi I, Namiki M, Tsubakihara Y. Interleukin-1 and its naturally occurring inhibitor in peritoneal dialysis patients. Clin Nephrol 1995; 43: 243–8.

112. Visser CE, Brouwer-Steenbergen JJE, Betjes MGH et al. Cancer antigen 125: a bulk marker for mesothelial cell mass in stable peritoneal dialysis patients. Nephrol Dial Transplant 1995; 10: 64–9.

113. Ho-dac-Pannekeet MM, Hiralall JK, Struijk DG, Krediet RT. Longitudinal follow-up of CA125 in peritoneal effluent. Kidney Int 1997; 51: 888–93.

114. Pannekeet MM, Koomen GCM, Struijk DG, Krediet RT. Dialysate CA125 in stable CAPD patients: no relation to transport parameters. Clin Nephrol 1995; 44: 248–54.

115. Yamagata K, Tomida C, Koyama A. Intraperitoneal hyaluronan production in stable continuous ambulatory peritoneal dialysis patients. Perit Dial Int 1999; 19: 131–7.

116. Pannekeet MM, Zemel D, Koomen GCM, Struijk DG, Krediet RT. Dialysate markers of peritoneal tissue during peritonitis and in stable CAPD. Perit Dial Int 1995; 15: 217–25.

117. Zweers MM, de Waart DR, Smit W, Struijk DG, Krediet RT. Growth factors VEGF and TGF-beta1 in peritoneal dialysis [see comments]. J Lab Clin Med 1999; 134: 124–32.

118. Lai KN, Lai KB, Szeto CC et al. Dialysate cell population and cancer antigen 125 in stable continuous ambulatory peritoneal dialysis patients: their relationship with transport parameters. Am J Kidney Dis 1997; 29: 699–705.

119. Simonsen O, Rippe B, Christensson A et al. Long-term clinical effects of a peritoneal dialysis fluid with less glucose degradation products. J Am Soc Nephrol 1999; 10: 322A.

120. Topley N, Krediet RT, Jones S et al. Peritoneal dialysate CA125, hyaluronan, TGF-b1 and pro-collagen I peptide in a randomized, controlled study of bicarbonate/lactate based CAPD solution. J Am Soc Nephrol 1999; 10: 230A.

121. Topley N, Alobaidi HM, Davies M et al. The effect of dialysate on peritoneal phagocyte oxidative metabolism. Kidney Int 1988; 34: 404–11.

122. Topley N, Coles GA, Williams JD. Biocompatibility studies on peritoneal cells. Perit Dial Int 1994; 14: S21–8.

123. Topley N. What is the ideal technique for testing the biocompatibility of peritoneal dialysis solutions? Perit Dial Int 1995; 205–9.

124. Topley N. Biocompatibility of peritoneal dialysis solutions and host defence. Adv Renal Rep Ther 1996; 3: 1–3.

125. Topley N, Davenport A, Li F-K, Fear H, Williams JD. Peritoneal defence in peritoneal dialysis. Nephrology 1996; 2: S167–72.

126. Jörres A, Williams JD, Topley N. Peritoneal dialysis solution biocompatibility: inhibitory mechanisms and recent studies with bicarbonate-buffered peritoneal dialysis solutions. Perit Dial Int 1997; 17: S42–6.

127. Jörres A, Gahl GM, Frei U. Peritoneal dialysis fluid biocompatibility: does it really matter? Kidney Int 1994; 46: S79–86.

128. Topley N, Williams JD. Effect of peritoneal dialysis on cytokine production by peritoneal cells. Blood Purif 1996; 14: 188–97.

129. Gotloib L, Waisbrut V, Shostak A, Kushnier R. Biocompatibility of dialysis solutions evaluated by histochemical techniques applied to mesothelial cell imprints. Perit Dial Int 1993; 13: 201–7.

130. Gotloib L, Waisbrut V, Shostak A, Kushnier R. Acute and long-term changes observed in imprints of mouse mesothe-

lium exposed to glucose-enriched, lactated, buffered dialysis solutions. Nephron 1995; 70: 466–77.

131. Gotloib L, Wajsbrot V, Shostak A, Kushnier R. Population analysis of mesothelium *in situ* and *in vivo* exposed to bicarbonate-buffered peritoneal dialysis fluid. Nephron 1996; 73: 219–27.

132. de Fijter CWH, Oe LP, Heezius ECJM, Donker AJM, Verbrugh HA. Low-calcium peritoneal dialysis fluid should not impact peritonitis rates in continuous ambulatory peritoneal dialysis. Am J Kidney Dis 1996; 27: 409–15.

133. de Fijter CWH, Verbrugh HA, Peters EDJ et al. *In vivo* exposure to the currently available peritoneal dialysis fluids decreases the function of peritoneal macrophages in CAPD. Clin Nephrol 1993; 39: 75–80.

134. de Fijter CWH, Verbrugh HA, Oe LP et al. Biocompatibility of a glucose polymer-containing peritoneal dialysis fluid. Am J Kidney Dis 1993; 4: 411–18.

135. Griffin JC, Marie SC. Glucose degradation in the presence of sodium lactate during autoclaving at 121 °C. Am J Hosp Pharm 1958; 15: 893–5.

136. Taylor RB, Jappy BM, Neil JM. Kinetics of dextrose degradation under autoclaving conditions. J Pharm Pharmacol 1971; 23: 121–9.

137. Heimlich KR, Martin AN. A kinetic study of glucose degradation in acid solution. J Am Pharm Assoc 1960; 49: 592–7.

138. Webb NE, Sperandio GJ, Martin AN. A study of the composition of glucose solutions. J Am Pharm Assoc 1958; 47: 101–3.

139. Weislander AP, Nordin MK, Kjellstrand PTT, Boberg UC. Toxicity of peritoneal dialysis fluids on cultured fibroblasts, L-929. Kidney Int 1991; 40: 77–9.

140. Wieslander AP, Nordin MK, Martinson E, Kjellstrand PTT, Boberg UC. Heat sterilised PD-fluids impair growth and inflammatory responses of cultured cell lines and human leukocytes. Clin Nephrol 1993; 39: 343–8.

141. Mistry CD, Gokal R, Peers A and the Midas Study Group. A randomised multicentre clinical trial comparing isoosmolar Icodextrin with hyperosmolar glucose solutions in CAPD. Kidney Int 1994; 46: 496–503.

142. Ruderman NB, Williamson JR, Brownlee M. Glucose and diabetic vascular disease. FASEB J 1992; 6: 2905–14.

143. Tilton RG, Baier LD, Harlow JE et al. Diabetes-induced glomerular dysfunction: links to a more reduced cytosolic ratio of NADH/NAD+. Kidney Int 1992; 41: 778–88.

144. Breborowicz A, Rodela H, Oreopoulos DG. Toxicity of osmotic solutes on human mesothelial cells *in vitro*. Kidney Int 1992; 41: 1280–5.

145. Liberek T, Topley N, Jörres A et al. Peritoneal dialysis fluid inhibition of phagocyte function: effects of osmolality and glucose concentration. J Am Soc Nephrol 1993; 3: 1508–15.

146. Kang DH, Hong YS, Lim HJ et al. High glucose solution and spent dialysate stimulate the synthesis of transforming growth factor-beta1 of human peritoneal mesothelial cells: effect of cytokine costimulation. Perit Dial Int 1999; 19: 221–30.

147. Phillips AO. Diabetic nephropathy: the modulation influence of glucose on transforming growth factor β production. Histol Histopathol 1998; 13: 565–74.

148. Fujimori A, Naito H, Miyazaki T et al. Elevation of interleukin-6 in the dialysate reflects peritoneal stimuli and deteriation of peritoneal function. Nephron 1996; 74: 471–2.

149. Lamb EJ, Cattell WR, Dawnay ABSJ. *In vitro* formation of advanced glycation end products in peritoneal dialysis fluid. Kidney Int 1995; 47: 1768–74.

150. Yamada K, Miyahara Y, Hamaguchi K et al. Immunohistochemical study of human advanced glycosylation end-products (AGE) in chronic renal failure. Clin Nephrol 1994; 42: 354–61.

151. Friedlander MA, Wu YC, Elgawish A, Monnier VM. Early and advanced glycosylation end products: kinetics of formation and clearance in peritoneal dialysis. J Clin Invest 1996; 97: 728–35.

152. Vlassara H. Recent progress on the biologic and clinical significance of advanced glycosylation end products. J Lab Clin Med 1994; 124: 19–30.

153. Miyata T, van Ypersele de Strihou C, Kurokawa K, Baynes JW. Alterations in nonenzymatic biochemistry in uremia: origin and significance of 'carbonyl stress' in long-term uremic complications. Kidney Int 1999; 55: 389–99.

154. Miyata T, Kurokawa K. Carbonyl stress: increased carbonyl modification of proteins by autoxidation products of carbohydrates and lipids in uremia [editorial]. Int J Artif Organs 1999; 22: 195–8.

155. Nakayama M, Kawaguchi M, Yamada K et al. Immunological detection of advanced glycosylation end products in the peritoneum and its possible pathophysiological role in CAPD. Kidney Int 1997; 51: 182–8.

156. Musi B, Carlsson O, Rippe A, Wieslander A, Rippe B. Effects of acidity, glucose degradation products, and dialysis fluid buffer choice on peritoneal solute and fluid transport in rats. Perit Dial Int 1998; 18: 303–10.

157. Rippe B, Simonsen O, Wieslander A, Landgren C. Clinical and physiological effects of a new, less toxic and less acidic fluid for peritoneal dialysis. Perit Dial Int 1997; 17: 27–34.

158. Wieslander A, Andren AHG, Nilsson-Thorell C et al. Are aldehydes in heat-sterilised peritoneal dialysis fluids toxic *in vitro*. Perit Dial Int 1995; 15: 348–52.

159. Wieslander A. Cytotoxicity of glucose degradation products in PD-fluids. PhD thesis, Lund: University of Lund, Sweden, 1995.

160. Wieslander AP, Andren AHG, Nilsson-Thorell C et al. Are aldehydes in heat sterilised peritoneal dialysis fluids toxic *in vitro*? Perit Dial Int 1995; 15: 348–52.

161. Wieslander AP. Cytotoxicity of peritoneal dialysis fluids – is it related to glucose breakdown products? Nephrol Dial Transplant 1996; 11: 958–9.

162. Cooker LA, Luneburg P, Faict D, Choo C, Holmes CJ. Reduced glucose degradation products in bicarbonate/lactate-buffered peritoneal dialysis solutions produced in two-chambered bags. Perit Dial Int 1997; 17: 373–8.

163. de Fijter CWH, Verbrugh HA, Oe LP et al. Peritoneal defence in continuous ambulatory versus continuous cyclic peritoneal dialysis. Kidney Int 1992; 42: 947–50.

164. Mackenzie RK, Jones S, Moseley A et al. *In vivo* exposure to bicarbonate/lactate and bicarbonate-buffered-peritoneal dialysis fluids (PDF) improves *ex vivo* peritoneal macrophage (PMØ) function. Am J Kidney Dis (In press).

165. Topley N, Kaur D, Petersen MM et al. *In vivo* effects of bicarbonate and bicarbonate-lactate buffered peritoneal dialysis solutions on mesothelial cell and neutrophil function. J Am Soc Nephrol 1996; 7: 218–24.

166. Topley N, Kaur D, Petersen MM et al. Bio-compatibility of bicarbonate-buffered peritoneal dialysis fluids: influence on mesothelial cell and neutrophil function. Kidney Int 1996; 49: 1447–56.

167. Fischer H-P, Schenk U, Kiefer T et al. *In vitro* effects of bicarbonate- versus lactate-buffered continuous ambulatory peritoneal dialysis fluids on peritoneal macrophage function. Am J Kidney Dis 1995; 26: 924–33.

168. Dobos GJ, Böhler J, Kuhlmann J et al. Bicarbonate-based dialysis solutions preserves granulocyte functions. Perit Dial Int 1994; 14: 366–70.

169. Jörres A, Gahl GM, Topley N et al. *In vitro* biocompatibility of alternative CAPD fluids; comparison of bicarbonate buffered and glucose polymer based solutions. Nephrol Dial Transplant 1994; 9: 785–90.

170. Manahan FJ, Int BL, Chan JC et al. Effects of bicarbonate-containing versus lactate-containing peritoneal dialysis solutions on superoxide production by human neutrophils. Artif Organs 1989; 13: 495–7.

171. Plum J, Fusshöller A, Schoenicke G et al. *In vivo* and *in vitro* effects of amino-acid-based and bicarbonate-buffered peritoneal dialysis solutions with regard to peritoneal transport

and cytokines/prostanoids dialysate concentrations. Nephrol Dial Transplant 1997; 12: 1625–60.

172. Schambye HT, Flesner P, Pedersen RB *et al.* Bicarbonate-versus lactate-based CAPD fluids: a biocompatibility study in rabbits. Perit Dial Int 1992; 12: 281–6.

173. Yatzidis H. Enhanced ultrafiltration in rabbits with bicarbonate glycylglycine peritoneal dialysis solution. Perit Dial Int 1993; 13: 302–6.

174. Thodis E, Bhaskaran S, Pasadakis P *et al.* Decrease in *Staphylococcus aureus* exit-site infections and peritonitis in CAPD patients by local application of mupirocin ointment at the catheter exit site [see comments]. Perit Dial Int 1998; 18: 261–70.

175. Ho-dac-Pannekeet MM, Struijk DG, Krediet RT. Improvement of transcellular water transport by treatment with glucose free dialysate in patients with ultrafiltration failure. Nephrol Dial Transplant 1996; 11: A255.

176. Rippe B, Simonsen O, Wieslander A, Landgren C. Clinical and physiological effects of a new, less toxic and less acidic fluid for peritoneal dialysis [see comments]. Perit Dial Int 1997; 17: 27–34.

177. Coles GA. Are solutions presently used bioincompatible? Perit Dial Int 1995; 15: S109–10.

19 Calcium, phosphate and renal osteodystrophy

A. J. HUTCHISON

Introduction

The first association between uraemia and bone disease was made by Lucas and reported in *Lancet* of 1883 [1]. However, it was not until nearly 40 years later that the major clinical and radiological manifestations of the skeletal changes were accurately defined [2, 3]. In 1943 the histopathology of osteitis fibrosa and osteomalacia was described [4], and in the same year the term 'renal osteodystrophy' was coined by Liu and Chu [5]. Subsequently the abnormalities of bone mass that occur in osteopenia and osteosclerosis were also described [6]. Following the research of Stanbury and Lumb [7, 8], there began a period of rapid advance in the understanding of the processes behind altered divalent ion metabolism, and the abnormalities of parathyroid hormone and vitamin D3 production that are seen in end-stage renal disease. Despite these advances, and the introduction of vitamin D3 replacement therapy, osteodystrophy remains a common complication of end-stage renal failure, and continues to pose diagnostic and therapeutic dilemmas for clinical nephrologists. It has become apparent that the spectrum of bone lesions seen in dialysis patients is changing, with hyperparathyroid disease becoming less common [9, 10], and furthermore, a different pattern of bone lesions is found in CAPD and haemodialysis patients [9–11]. In a histological study of 259 chronic dialysis patients in Canada the commonest bone lesion was found to be hyperparathyroid disease (50%) in haemodialysis patients, and adynamic bone (61%) in peritoneal dialysis patients [10]. In contrast, Malluche and Monier-Faugere (Kentucky, USA) reported that in a retrospective survey of 602 patients from 1982 to 1991 the mixed lesion was the commonest diagnosis [9], regardless of mode of dialysis (56% in CAPD and 49% in haemodialysis). The difference between these reports is noteworthy in itself, since both are large and reliable studies, but from centres many hundreds of miles apart. Whilst differing diagnostic criteria may account for some of the difference, it emphasizes the fact that, in dialysis patients, histomorphometric data represent the result of pathological processes, treatment regimes and environmental effects that have been on-going for many years.

Classification of renal osteodystrophy

In this chapter the term *renal osteodystrophy* is used to encompass all its skeletal manifestations such as osteitis fibrosa, osteomalacia, mixed lesions, the adynamic bone lesion, osteoporosis, osteosclerosis, and (in children) retardation of growth. However, renal osteodystrophy also includes a variety of extra-skeletal problems including myopathy, vascular and visceral calcification, and peripheral ischaemic necrosis.

Since the introduction of the undecalcified bone biopsy, significant advances have been made in the understanding of the histological changes underlying all forms of renal osteodystrophy. Renal bone disease has its origins early in the course of renal failure [12, 13], so that by the time GFR has fallen to 50% of normal, at least 50% of the patients exhibit abnormal bone histology [14, 15]. In a study of 16 patients with creatinine clearances between 20 and 59 ml/min, Baker *et al.* found all of them to have abnormal bone histology [16]. The classification of renal osteodystrophy is simplified by the recognition that there are essentially two groups of histological lesions: high and low turnover bone lesions.

High turnover bone lesions

Osteitis fibrosa cystica – the characteristic findings include a marked increase in bone resorption, osteoblastic and osteoclastic activity, and endosteal fibrosis (Fig. 1). In particular, the number of osteo-

R. Gokal, R. Khanna, R.Th. Krediet and K.D. Nolph (eds.), Textbook of Peritoneal Dialysis, 2nd Edition, 585–608.
© 2000 *Kluwer Academic Publishers. Printed in Great Britain.*

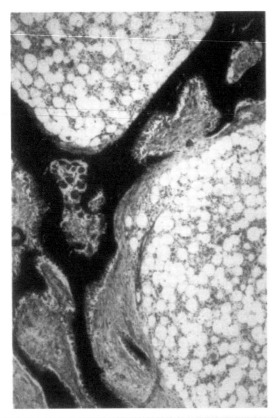

Figure 1. Bone histology in severe hyperparathyroid disease. Numerous large, multinucleate osteoclasts can be seen tunnelling into mineralized trabecular bone. Osteoblasts are also numerous, and peritrabecular fibrous tissue has been deposited in the marrow cavity (toluidine blue stain; original magnification ×100).

clasts is markedly increased, and they may be larger than normal with multiple nuclei. There may be a large increase in surface resorption with dissecting cavities where the osteoclasts have tunnelled through the trabecular bone. This results in deposition of fibrous tissue in the marrow spaces (peritrabecular fibrosis), and the formation of so-called 'woven bone', new bone matrix which is not lamellar but disorganized in structure. Although the bone may show increased osteoid, the use of tetracycline labelling prior to biopsy demonstrates that mineralization proceeds relatively normally. Skeletal mass may diminish as the rate of resorption exceeds that of formation.

The term '*osteitis*' implies inflammation of bone, which is not present, so that is it preferable to refer to this lesion as '*severe*' or '*predominant hyperparathyroid bone disease*' [9].

Mild hyperparathyroidism – here elevated parathyroid hormone levels increase bone turnover but peritrabecular fibrosis is minimal or absent.

Low turnover bone lesions

Osteomalacia – defective mineralization of bone, due to deficiency of 1,25-dihydroxyvitamin D3, results in a relative increase in the amount of osteoid or unmineralized bone matrix (Fig. 2). Osteitis fibrosa can also increase osteoid mass, simply as a result of increased bone turnover, but bone biopsy with dual tetracycline labelling will reliably distinguish these diseases. Aluminium accumulation can also lead to an osteomalacic-type osteodystrophy even in the presence of adequate 1,25-dihydroxyvitamin D3 levels [17]. In bone, the site of aluminium deposition is at the interface between mineralized bone and unmineralized osteoid. Here it appears to reduce osteoblast numbers and delay the process of mineralization, as demonstrated by diminished uptake of tetracycline into trabecular bone [18]. Studies have established an inverse relationship between bone aluminium accumulation and the rate of bone formation [19] and, even in cell-free laboratory

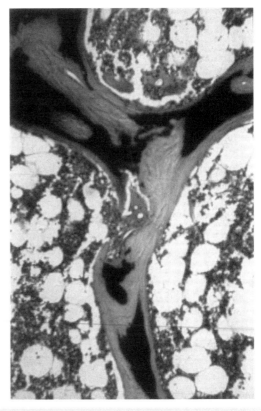

Figure 2. Bone histology in osteomalacia (not aluminium-related). Broad lamellar osteoid seams surround the calcified trabecular bone. In some areas the failure of mineralization has resulted in 'islands' of calcified bone so that the mechanical strength of the trabeculum is greatly reduced (toluidine blue stain; original magnification ×100).

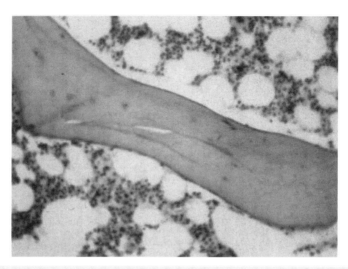

Figure 3. Bone histology in the adynamic lesion. Osteoid seams are very thin or almost absent. Numbers of osteoclasts and osteoblasts are greatly reduced and unrepaired microfractures can be seen within the mineralized bone (H & E stain; original magnification, ×100).

studies, aluminium has been shown to reduce both the formation and growth of hydroxyapatite crystals [20].

Adynamic bone lesion (Fig. 3), previously thought to be a result of aluminium accumulation in bone, this entity has now been shown also to occur in the absence of stainable bone aluminium and is characterized by an abnormally low bone formation rate, a defect of bone mineralization, normal or decreased osteoid thickness, decreased osteoblastic surfaces, and normal or decreased osteoclastic surfaces [15, 21]. This appearance is sometimes referred to as *aplastic*, a term usually reserved for structures that are congenitally absent, whereas *adynamic* more accurately conveys the inactivity of bone cells in this lesion. Little is known about its aetiology, and even less about its natural history, although there is some evidence to suggest that it is commoner in patients with diabetes [10, 22], elderly dialysis patients [23], and those on CAPD [9, 10]. Mixed bone disease – hyperparathyroidism and defective mineralization can often coexist in chronic renal failure with variable bone volume and rates of bone turnover.

Pathogenesis of renal osteodystrophy

Renal osteodystrophy is recognized to be a common complication of end-stage renal failure and is believed to have its origins early in the onset of renal impairment [24]. The mechanism of its development is both multifactorial and controversial, but since normal kidneys maintain calcium, phosphorus, magnesium and bicarbonate balance, synthesise 1,25- and 24,25-dihydroxyvitamin D3, act as a major target organ and excretory organ for parathyroid hormone, and also excrete aluminium, it is self-evident that renal failure will have numerous profound effects on mineral metabolism. These various factors all interact to a greater or lesser extent, but for simplicity are considered separately in the following sections.

Parathyroid hormone and calcium metabolism

Bone is continually being remodelled, and in health a balance is maintained between synthesis of bone matrix (osteoid formation), its mineralization, and subsequent resorption. This balance is governed by the relative activity of osteoblasts, osteoclasts and osteocytes. Increased secretion of parathyroid hormone (PTH) increases both the activity and numbers of these bone cells, causing an overall increase in bone turnover. Excessive production may result in deposition of fibrous tissue in the marrow spaces (osteitis fibrosa), endosteal fibrosis, and the formation of so-called 'woven bone', new bone matrix which is not lamellar but disorganized in structure. Skeletal mass may diminish as the rate of resorption exceeds that of formation, and recent results from the European Dialysis and Transplant Association Registry [25] show that in patients dialysed for up to 15 years, parathyroidectomy is still required in up to 40%. Similarly there is increasing evidence to suggest that, in the uraemic patient, low/normal levels of PTH may result in excessively low bone cell activity and overall bone turnover with or without the presence of aluminium [9, 10, 21, 23, 26–28].

PTH is a single-chain protein of 84 amino acids, the sequence of which was established by Keutmann et al. in 1978 [29]. It is synthesized in the parathyroid chief cell via two precursors, pre-pro-PTH and pro-PTH (115 and 90 amino acids respectively). PTH secretion occurs approximately 20 min after synthesis of the original pre-pro-PTH [30].

Significant elevations of serum parathyroid hormone have been reported in patients with only moderately abnormal glomerular filtration rates of 60–80 ml/min [16, 31, 32]. The secretion of PTH is controlled by many factors, but in renal impairment the most important stimulus is thought to be reduction in the level of serum-ionized calcium (Fig. 4). Factors which contribute to hypocalcaemia and elevation of serum PTH are phosphate retention, defective vitamin D metabolism, skeletal resistance to the calcaemic action of PTH, elevation of the 'set point' at which serum calcium suppresses PTH release and impaired degradation of circulating PTH [32].

Secretion of PTH is primarily controlled by the concentration of ionized calcium in the extracellular space so that hypocalcaemia stimulates, and hyper-

calcaemia suppresses PTH release [33]. This relationship between PTH and serum calcium can be represented as a sigmoidal curve, with a basal rate of secretion persisting even during hypercalcaemia [34]. In normal individuals the basal PTH level is approximately 20–25% of the maximally stimulated PTH level and is positioned in the initial part of the steep ascent of the sigmoidal curve. Therefore, a small decrease in serum calcium produces a large increase in serum PTH secretion. Felsenfeld observed that for the same ionized calcium level, serum PTH was higher during the induction of hypocalcaemia than during the recovery from hypocalcaemia [35]. Conversely, the PTH level was greater when hypercalcaemia was induced from the nadir of hypocalcaemia than when hypercalcaemia was induced from basal serum calcium. Furthermore the set point of calcium was greater during the induction of hypocalcaemia than during the recovery from hypocalcaemia. This differential response of PTH to the direction of change of serum calcium is known as 'hysteresis', and there is evidence that the PTH–calcium curves may differ in different forms of renal osteodystrophy or after a specific form of therapy such as desferrioxamine or calcitriol [35–37].

As well as suppressing PTH secretion, hypercalcaemia is also known to decrease parathyroid cell cyclic adenosine monophosphate (cAMP) but it is not clear whether this is the means by which PTH

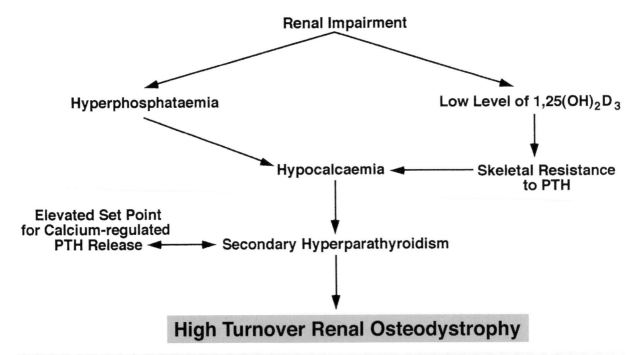

Figure 4. Factors contributing to the production of excess parathyroid hormone in dialysis patients.

is controlled or whether it is a secondary phenomenon [38].

Hyperplastic parathyroid glands are less sensitive to ionized calcium levels than are normal glands, suggesting that one cause of elevated PTH in chronic renal failure may be a shift in the 'set point' for calcium-regulated PTH secretion, in addition to the increase in parathyroid mass. The set point is defined as a calcium ion concentration necessary to suppress the secretion of PTH by 50%. Furthermore the degree of responsiveness across the calcium-sensitive range is altered so that hyperparathyroidism is a product of the increase in tissue mass (because the non-suppressible, basal secretion is increased) and the lack of suppression by calcium in the normocalcaemic range. Thus normal concentrations of ionized calcium may not be sufficient to suppress hyperplastic parathyroid glands, and serum levels have to be increased to the upper limits of normal to control the release of PTH in patients with secondary hyperparathyroidism [34]. However, there is evidence that once the parathyroid gland size exceeds a certain limit, the non-suppressible basal secretion alone becomes sufficient to increase serum parathyroid hormone to hyperparathyroid levels [39]. When this occurs parathyroidectomy is required.

Firm evidence now exists that parathyroid cells possess specific nuclear receptors for 1,25-dihydroxyvitamin D3 [39, 40]. When given intravenously to a group of 20 haemodialysis patients calcitriol produced a marked suppression ($70.1 \pm 3.2\%$) of PTH levels without a significant change in serum calcium, confirming that it is an important regulator of PTH secretion at least in states of calcitriol depletion [41]. Substantial degradation of calcitriol occurs in the intestine so that oral vitamin D increases intestinal calcium absorption but the delivery of calcitriol to peripheral target organs is limited [42]. This could explain the much greater effect of intravenous, compared to oral, calcitriol. PTH secretion is also affected by ionized magnesium; however only severe hypomagnesaemia seems to have any clinical relevance in that it has been shown to inhibit PTH secretion [43].

In addition to the abnormalities of secretion that occur in chronic renal failure, the process of degradation is incomplete. Normally, intact PTH is degraded by the liver and kidneys, resulting in the production of amino (N)- and carboxy (C)-terminal fragments. The fragments are further metabolized by the kidney, so that in the absence of renal function they will accumulate. C-terminal fragments are detectable up to 2 weeks after parathyroidectomy in chronic renal failure, yet decrease by 80% within 24 h of a successful renal transplant. Various portions of the PTH molecule may be measured by radioimmunoassay but it has been shown that the results of sandwich assays specific to the whole, or intact, 1–84 PTH molecule correlate best with the biological effects of PTH on bone in chronic renal failure [44, 45].

Vitamin D metabolism

The similarity between the bone disease caused by simple vitamin D deficiency and that which occurs in chronic renal failure has been recognized for many years, both at clinical [1] and histological levels [4]. It was also known that renal failure was associated with impaired intestinal absorption of calcium [5]. In renal failure both the bone lesions and the defect in calcium absorption were shown to be correctable by oral calciferol, but the amount required to have an effect is much larger than in simple deficiency states. The disease is 'vitamin D resistant'. Vitamin D3 (calciferol) circulates in the blood bound to vitamin D-binding protein, after having been synthesized in the skin or absorbed from the diet. In the liver it is metabolized by the enzyme vitamin-D-25-hydroxylase to form 25-hydroxyvitamin D (calcidiol; 25-OH–D). In most patients with chronic renal failure 25-OH–D levels are normal if they eat a balanced diet and their skin is not completely covered from the sun.

In the kidney 25-OH–D is further metabolized by a mitochondrial cytochrome P–450 oxidase, 25-OH–D-1α-hydroxylase, to form 1,25-dihydroxyvitamin D3 (calcitriol), the biologically active form of vitamin D. The exact location of the 1α-hydroxylase enzyme in human kidney is unknown. In 1973 Mawer *et al.* showed that calcitriol could not be detected in the serum of patients with chronic renal failure, after injection of radioactive cholecalciferol, and suggested that it was the inability to form this metabolite that was the cause of the vitamin D resistance [46]. This is now known to be the case, and is a result of reduced renal 1α-hydroxylase activity caused by loss of renal mass, hyperphosphataemia and possibly by uraemic toxins [47]. In addition to renal production of 1,25-OH–D3 humans can, in certain pathological states, produce it extrarenally. In sarcoidosis cultured alveolar macrophages and lymph node homogenates can convert 25-OH–D to 1,25-OH–D3 and a similar process probably accounts for the hypercalcaemia and hypercalciuria sometimes seen in other granulomatous diseases such as tuberculosis, silicosis, beryl-liosis and fungal diseases. In CAPD patients who have had one or more episodes of peritonitis cultured peritoneal macrophages are also able to convert 25-OH–D3 to 1,25-OH–D3 [48].

Once synthesized in the kidney, 1,25-OH–D3 is transported by vitamin D-binding protein to its target cells. It enters the cell by a mechanism that is poorly understood and is then transported to the nucleus. Here it interacts with its nuclear receptor, phosphorylating it to bring about interaction with chromatin and transcription of specific genes. In the small intestine this results in expression of the gene coding for calbindin, the calcium-binding protein. The activity of other proteins is also affected, with the net result that calcium and phosphate absorption from the intestine is stimulated. The effect of 1,25-OH–D3 on bone is to increase removal of calcium. A small decrease in serum ionized calcium stimulates PTH production which in turn stimulates the kidney to produce 1,25-OH–D3; 1,25-OH–D3 in conjunction with PTH increases osteoclastic activity and release of calcium, returning the ionized calcium level to normal.

1,25-OH–D3 has been conclusively shown to suppress PTH secretion in dialysis patients when administered orally or intravenously [41, 49–55]. It undoubtedly also has important immunoregulatory functions and is able to decrease the rate of proliferation of certain tumour cells, such as the HL-60 (human promyelocytic) cell, and even transform them into mature macrophages. 1,25-OH–D3 can also inhibit the proliferation of cultured human keratinocytes, an ability which has important clinical implications in that it has been shown to dramatically improve psoriasis in 75% of a group of patients given up to 2 μg/day [56]. It has recently been suggested that vitamin D deficiency may be an important factor in the pathogenesis of hypertension and insulin resistance in end-stage renal failure [57].

Phosphate metabolism

In the past, overactivity of the parathyroid glands in renal failure was explained by the trade-off hypothesis of Bricker [58]. He postulated that as renal failure progresses there is a tendency for serum phosphate levels to rise and ionized calcium levels to fall, resulting in a compensatory rise in PTH. The increase in PTH reduces tubular reabsorption of phosphate in the remaining nephrons and increases serum calcium. Thus serum values of phosphate and calcium may be kept within, or near, the normal

range at the expense of rising PTH levels and its resultant effects on the skeleton. However, more recent work has cast doubt on this, with the observations that hyperparathyroidism can develop even in the presence of a high serum calcium [59], and that hyperphosphataemia stimulates PTH secretion independent of serum calcium concentration [60–62]. However, increased phosphate excretion results in decreased activity of 25-OH–D-1α-hydroxylase, and consequently decreased production of 1,25-dihydroxyvitamin D3 [56]. This in turn stimulates increased synthesis and secretion of PTH in an attempt to stimulate renal production of 1,25-dihydroxyvitamin D3. As renal failure progresses the compensatory effect of PTH on 1,25-dihydroxyvitamin D3 deficiency is overcome and an absolute deficiency develops [15]. This further stimulates PTH levels and decreases gastrointestinal calcium absorption [63]. With further progression of renal failure, to a glomerular filtration rate of around 10 ml/min, phosphate excretion can no longer be increased and hyperphosphataemia occurs, exacerbating the hypocalcaemia. At this stage hypocalcaemia further stimulates PTH secretion, although doubt remains as to its role in the earlier stages of renal failure. In addition hyperphosphataemia can lead to extraskeletal calcification in soft tissues and, perhaps more worryingly, in blood vessels.

Magnesium metabolism

Although magnesium metabolism is affected by decreasing renal function, the clinical relevance of this is unknown. In normal subjects magnesium is absorbed from the small intestine and excreted in the urine, so that elevated serum levels are seen in renal failure [64, 65]. *In vitro*, magnesium is an inhibitor of crystallization and may increase bone levels of pyrophosphate – another inhibitor of mineralization [66]. In uraemia, bone magnesium is correlated with serum magnesium, and serum pyrophosphate is increased [67]. Hence it is theoretically possible that elevated serum magnesium could play a role in the development of osteomalacia, but there is no evidence in the literature that this is the case.

Moderate hypomagnesaemia can contribute to elevation of serum PTH [68], whereas severe hypomagnesaemia has been shown to inhibit PTH secretion [43].

Aluminium and osteodystrophy

In 1978 Ward *et al.* made the association between aluminium and bone disease in dialysis patients

[17]. Since then the importance attached to reducing exposure to aluminium has gradually increased, but the use of aluminium hydroxide as a phosphate binder is still quite widespread.

A normal human daily intake of aluminium ranges from 2 to 20 mg but gastrointestinal uptake is estimated to be only 0.5–1% of this. Normal urinary aluminium excretion varies between 20 and 50 mg/day but was shown to increase to 200–400 mg/day when normal individuals were given aluminium hydroxide in amounts commonly given to dialysis patients [69]. In end-stage renal failure the loss of urinary excretion plus exposure to aluminium in dialysate solutions, phosphate binders, and volume replacement fluids can result in the total body content rising by a factor of up to 20. Serum levels are a poor guide to total body load, since it is strongly protein-bound and largely deposited quickly in tissues such as bone, liver and spleen.

Aluminium accumulates at the interface between mineralized bone and unmineralized osteoid, where it delays the process of mineralization. Aluminium also accumulates in parathyroid glands and suppresses their secretion of PTH. In patients with aluminium-related bone disease and renal failure, PTH levels are commonly lower than would be expected and may be suppressed to normal levels, giving some degree of protection from hyperparathyroid bone disease [70], but possibly resulting in development of the adynamic bone lesion [44].

It is to be hoped that aluminium-related bone disease will gradually disappear as more physicians change to calcium-based phosphate binders, and exposure from other sources is sought out and reduced to minimal levels.

Acid–base balance

The role of acidosis in the pathogenesis of renal osteodystrophy is unclear. However, acidosis is involved in both calcium balance and PTH release. Acidotic azotaemic patients show increased losses of urinary and faecal calcium which can be reduced by alkali treatment, resulting in restoration of a neutral calcium balance [71]. In a study of 54 uraemic patients, infusion of sodium bicarbonate produced a rise in arterialysed capillary blood pH and a proportional fall of around 20% in serum PTH [72]. No significant change in serum ionized calcium was observed during the study. The clinical significance of these findings remains to be elucidated but it seems likely that, as with changes in magnesium

metabolism, the effects are of much less importance than those associated with PTH and Vitamin D.

Calcitonin

Calcitonin is a 32-amino acid single-chain peptide, and the major stimulus for its secretion is hypercalcaemia. Circulating calcitonin has a short half-life (around 10 min) and depends on renal function for degradation and excretion, so that high circulating levels are found in patients with renal failure [73]. Its role in normal human subjects is debated, since neither the absence of this hormone (as in completely thyroidectomized patients) nor its thousand-fold excess (as in patients with thyroid medullary carcinoma) is generally associated with any abnormality of calcium homeostasis or skeletal integrity [74]. However, there is around 40% structural homology between PTH and calcitonin receptors, the latter being found in bone, kidney, central nervous system, testis, placenta and on some tumour cells.

Clinical and radiological features of renal osteodystrophy

Clinical features of the altered mineral and skeletal metabolism that occurs in renal failure may be considered under two broad headings: extraskeletal and skeletal manifestations (Table 1).

Extraskeletal manifestations

Extraskeletal manifestations are mainly a result of deposition of calcium in soft tissues. Hyperphosphataemia can cause an increase in the calcium–phosphate product, to a point where its solubility product is exceeded and precipitation can occur in many sites. It has been suggested that calcium deposition in the skin may contribute to the pruritus that in severe cases can be quite disabling for dialysis patients, preventing sleep and resulting in widespread excoriations with skin sepsis.

Calcification in the conjunctiva is another common problem leading to the intensely painful 'red-eye', with flecks of calcium often clearly visible on examination.

A study of the calcium–phosphate product in a large number of haemodialysis patients demonstrated that the relative risk of death for those with a serum phosphate level greater than 6.5 mg/dl was 1.27 relative to those with a lower level [75]. The increased risk was not reduced by statistical adjust-

Table 1. Clinical and radiological features of renal osteodystrophy

Clinical manifestations
Skeletal
  Bone tenderness
  Bone pain
  Joint pains
  Spontaneous fracture
  Growth retardation

Extraskeletal
  Renal 'red-eye'
  Pruritus
  Myopathy
  Tumoral calcification
  Peripheral ischaemic necrosis

Radiological manifestations
Hyperparathyroidism
Erosion of tips of terminal phalanges, radial aspects of middle
  phalanges, distal ends of clavicles
'Pepper-pot' skull
Thinning of cortex in tubular bones
Osteopenic vertebral bodies with sclerotic upper and lower surfaces,
  results in 'rugger-jersey spine' appearance
Visceral/vascular calcification
Osteomalacia
Looser's zones (most often in pubic bones or femur), otherwise no
  specific features in milder cases
Adynamic lesion
No specific features, but associated with increased risk of vascular
  calcification

ment for coexisting medical conditions, delivered dose of dialysis, PTH level, nutritional parameters or markers of non-compliance. The calcium–phosphate product showed a mortality trend similar to phosphate alone, with those patients having products greater than $72 \text{ mg}^2/\text{dl}^2$ showing a relative mortality risk of 1.34 compared to those with products less than $52 \text{ mg}^2/\text{dl}^2$. There is no doubt that tight control of serum phosphate is vitally important for any dialysis patient.

Perhaps the most important extraskeletal manifestation is calcification of the vascular tree which frequently becomes visible on plain X-rays. Most commonly the calcification is localized to the medial layer of small and medium-sized arteries (Monckeberg's sclerosis). However, the abdominal aorta, femoral and digital arteries are often clearly outlined on films taken for skeletal survey, but the same process is undoubtedly occurring in the mesenteric, cerebral and coronary vasculature, resulting in considerable morbidity and mortality in dialysis and transplant patients [23, 76]. In severe cases, vascular calcification in the iliac and femoral vessels may render a patient untransplantable because anastomosis of the

vessels becomes impossible. Furthermore the risk of per-operative myocardial infarction is greatly increased, and heart failure, controlled by strict attention to fluid balance while on dialysis, may be unmasked by renal transplantation.

Skeletal manifestations

Skeletal signs and symptoms of renal osteodystrophy include bone pain, bone tenderness, spontaneous fractures, retardation of growth and joint disease. With the exception of adolescents with tubulo-interstitial pathology, symptoms are unusual in patients with end-stage renal disease, unless the decline in renal function has been particularly slow. However, those with tubulo-interstitial disease and adolescent patients are more prone to overt bone disease. The prevalence of symptoms among dialysis patients varies greatly from unit to unit, which may reflect differences in reporting or true differences due to a dialysis-induced cause such as aluminium intake [77, 78]. Both osteomalacia and osteitis fibrosa may be associated with bone pain, tenderness and proximal muscle weakness. In addition lower back and lower limb pain contribute to the reduced exercise ability that is common in dialysis patients. This in turn worsens muscle weakness and loss of skeletal mass. Periosteal new bone growth and osteosclerosis are usually asymptomatic but may often be seen on skeletal radiography.

Radiological features

Although regular radiological assessment, using plain radiographs, is the most frequently used method of monitoring renal osteodystrophy it is undoubtedly insensitive, and only reliably detects advanced cases. Malluche and Faugere state that information obtained from skeletal X-rays is limited and often misleading, and that most radiological signs considered to be pathognomonic of severe osteitis fibrosa can be found in any of the three histological types of renal osteodystrophy [15].

The earliest radiological feature of hyperparathyroidism is subperiosteal erosion occurring at the tufts of the terminal phalanges, the radial aspect of the middle phalanges and the distal ends of the clavicles. In a study of 30 end-stage renal failure patients, performed immediately prior to commencing dialysis, erosion of the terminal phalanges was seen in five of the eight patients who had severe hyperparathyroid disease on bone biopsy [45]. However, plain radiographs did not identify patients with mild hyperparathyroid disease, and the majority of patients were judged to have essentially normal skeletal surveys. These findings are in agreement with those of Owen *et al.*, who compared plain skeletal radiology with bone histology in 82 patients with renal failure, and found no correlation between radiological and histological indices [79]. We would therefore agree with the previously quoted statements of Malluche and Faugere [15], and question the need for the traditional annual skeletal survey which provides a significant dose of ionizing radiation. Apart from a generalized increase in radiolucency, radiological signs are uncommon in osteomalacia. However, Looser's zones may sometimes be seen and are characteristic of this condition.

In recent years other radiological techniques have been developed for examining bone in a more quantitative fashion, including skeletal scintigraphy, measurement of bone density and mineral content by single or dual photon densitometry, plus single and dual energy quantitative computed tomography (QCT) scan [80, 81]. These techniques are discussed later in the chapter.

Renal osteodystrophy and CAPD

The introduction of CAPD in the 1970s has provided new opportunities for the investigation and management of renal osteodystrophy. However, reports of its control and development in CAPD remain confusing, with some showing improvement [77, 82, 83] and others showing deterioration [84–86].

The different pattern of bone lesions seen in CAPD and haemodialysis is now well described [9–11, 87]. There are several differences between the dialysis modalities which may affect mineral metabolism [11]. CAPD is associated with far greater losses of middle and large molecular weight protein fractions, thereby removing more transferrin-bound aluminium, as well as 25-hydroxyvitamin D3. With CAPD, weekly phosphate removal is greater than haemodialysis, and it provides a steady-state biochemical profile unlike the 'saw-tooth' pattern of haemodialysis. Furthermore, the high calcium concentration in standard peritoneal dialysis fluids may have a significantly suppressive effect on PTH levels, contributing to the higher incidence of low-turnover bone disease seen in CAPD. In contrast, a haemodialysis patient will experience episodes of relative hypocalcaemia two or three times each week, and this may well stimulate PTH production.

Calcium and phosphorus balance in CAPD

In end-stage renal disease serum phosphate levels begin to rise and ionized calcium levels begin to fall once the GFR is less than 20 ml/min. These abnormalities can be at least partially corrected by the administration of oral calcium carbonate. However, ionized calcium levels may still below (0.9–1.1 mmol/L) when patients start CAPD, even though total serum calcium levels are normal [88]. Serum levels usually rise once CAPD has begun, since the majority of dialysis fluids currently in use have a calcium concentration of 1.75 mmol/L. Gastrointestinal absorption and peritoneal flux of calcium during dialysis are the two major determinants of overall calcium mass balance in peritoneal dialysis patients.

Gastrointestinal absorption

The gastrointestinal absorption of calcium has been studied by several groups and is known to be dependent on many factors including the degree of uraemia, serum phosphate level, PTH level, 1,25-dihydroxyvitamin D3 level and total calcium intake. In uraemic subjects Recker and Saville [89] found that calcium absorption ranged from 5% to 59%, whilst Clarkson and colleagues [90] and Ramirez *et al.* [91] reported figures of 8% and 28%, respectively. In a study of CAPD patients in our own unit, calcium absorption rate was subnormal in 18 of 19 subjects, although significant variation existed between patients. Percentage absorption ranged from 3.2% to 23.9%, results not dissimilar from those in uraemics [92]. Blumenkrantz examined absorption of dietary calcium in CAPD patients over the range 500–2500 mg/day [93] and suggested that it can be represented by the empirical relationship $Y = 0.42X - 277$ (where Y = amount absorbed, X = intake in mg/day). Therefore if the intake is around 730 mg/day, approximately 30 mg of calcium is absorbed by the patient.

If calcium salts are to be used as first-line therapy for hyperphosphataemia then oral intake and gastrointestinal absorption will be necessarily high. Once a patient is established on dialysis, control of hyperphosphataemia is very important, not only to minimize further stimulation of PTH secretion, but also to keep the calcium–phosphate product within the normal range. Failure to do this can result in rapid progression of vascular and soft-tissue calcification. The CAPD patient's high-protein diet (recommended minimum protein intake 1.2 g/kg/day) provides an obligatory phosphate intake of up to 1200 mg daily [93, 94]. Although peritoneal dialysis controls the hyperphosphataemia of end-stage renal disease more effectively than does haemodialysis [86, 95, 96], it removes only 310–320 mg/day [93, 97] – rather less than one-third of the amount required to bring phosphate levels into the normal range. Therefore if a neutral phosphate balance is to be achieved, the gastrointestinal elimination of phosphorus needs to be around 700 mg/day [98]. Since 40–80% of dietary phosphorus is absorbed by patients with renal failure [96] the fraction of phosphate absorbed must be reduced, and hence gastrointestinal elimination increased, by oral phosphate-binding agents.

The role of calcium salts in renal osteodystrophy

Established phosphate binders, avilable for clinical use, include aluminium hydroxide and carbonate, calcium carbonate, acetate and citrate, magnesium carbonate, keto-analogues of amino acids, and finally polyuronic acids (Table 2). Each of these binders has advantages and disadvantages, but only three are in widespread use – aluminium hydroxide, calcium carbonate and calcium acetate. Calcium carbonate is probably the most commonly used phosphate binder in CAPD patients, where maintenance of optimal serum calcium and phosphate levels is central to the treatment of hyperparathyroidism. Calcium ketoglutarate is also in use, particularly in certain European countries [99].

When CAPD was first introduced aluminium gels were the standard phosphate binders, and a high calcium concentration in the dialysis fluid (1.75 mmol/L–3.5 mEq/L) was therefore beneficial, rapidly bringing serum calcium levels into the normal range. Now that the dangers of aluminium accumulation have become apparent [70, 100], aluminium-containing phosphate binders have been replaced by calcium salts as first-line therapy for hyperphosphataemia in most renal units. Unfortunately calcium salts frequently result in hypercalcae-

mia when given in sufficiently large oral doses to control serum phosphate [101–103], so that aluminium-containing phosphate binders continue to be used. It has been suggested that, when used in low doses, with careful monitoring of serum aluminium, these binders are safe [15]. However, although only about 1% of the oral dose of aluminium is absorbed [104], even on modest doses this represents between 5 and 10 mg of elemental aluminium daily. Since CAPD removes only 40–50 mg daily [105] it is evident that tissue accumulation is inevitable and significant. If aluminium salts are to be completely avoided, then the hypercalcaemia associated with calcium salts must be prevented. Reduction of dialysis fluid calcium concentration is one means of achieving this end and has been studied in haemodialysis [106, 107] and peritoneal dialysis patients [108–114].

Maintenance of a high/normal serum ionized calcium and control of hyperphosphataemia can be beneficially employed to suppress PTH production, even in patients not taking vitamin D3 supplements. This is obviously desirable in patients with significantly elevated PTH levels, but in patients with normal or only mildly elevated levels, it is not necessarily so. Many of these patients will have the adynamic bone lesion, and a small rise in PTH levels may be beneficial. One method of achieving this would be to allow the serum ionized calcium to fall below the 'set point' for calcium-mediated PTH release, but at the same time one would want to maintain strict control of serum phosphate. This is not easy when the calcium supplement and phosphate binder are one and the same tablet, but such manoeuvres are undoubtedly facilitated by the availability of reduced calcium dialysis fluids. In this way, hypercalcaemic over-suppression of PTH can be minimized, whilst still allowing the ingestion of sufficiently large doses of calcium carbonate to enable good control of serum phosphate.

Control of serum phosphate is not only important in terms of its effect on PTH, but also for prevention, and sometimes treatment, of extraskeletal calcification. This potentially lethal aspect of renal osteodystrophy is a particular hazard in patients who have persistent hypercalcaemia and hyperphosphataemia. It is traditional to prescribe aluminium-containing binders for such patients on the grounds that the aluminium absorbed is likely to be less harmful than allowing the process of vascular calcification to continue unchecked. Utilization of reduced calcium dialysis fluid offers a better alternative for a least 50% of patients, with the other 50% achieving a

Table 2. Available compounds for use as phosphate binders in dialysis patients

Calcium-based	Others
Calcium carbonate	Aluminium carbonate
Calcium acetate	Magnesium carbonate
Calcium citrate	Aluminium hydroxide
Calcium gluconate	Magnesium hydroxide
Calcium alginate	Polyuronic acids
Calcium-ketovalin	Poly[allyamine hydrochloride]

reduction in aluminium intake although no change in the calcium–phosphate product (see below).

Novel non-calcaemic phosphate binders

A more efficient dialysis fluid is an attractive way of improving phosphate clearance, and this was tried in the early 1980s in an experimental rat model [115]. Polyethylenimine was utilized as an osmotic agent, and demonstrated measurable binding to phosphate. Unfortunately it was toxic to the rats and produced gross morphological changes in the visceral mesothelium and associated organs. A variety of other oral phosphate-binding agents have been tested and some are in clinical use [116]. However, none has achieved widespread acceptance because of problems of efficacy, palatability or solubility.

Two new compounds which have recently been tested in human phase III studies are poly[allyamine hydrochloride] (RenaGel; Geltex Pharmaceuticals, Waltham, Mass., USA) and lanthanum carbonate (Lambda; Shire Pharmaceuticals, Andover, UK). Poly-[allyamine hydrochloride] is a non-absorbable calcium- and aluminium-free compound which is reported to be as effective as calcium carbonate in an 8-week, placebo-controlled trial of 36 haemodialysis patients [117]. It also appeared to have a beneficial effect on the patients' lipid profile with a reduction in serum total and LDL cholesterol.

Lanthanum was first reported as a potential oral phosphate binder by Graff and Burnel [118]. Phosphate binding was estimated by the reduction of urinary excretion and increase in faecal excretion, and lanthanum citrate was found to be as effective as aluminium chloride, with less (but not zero) systemic absorption. Traces of lanthanum were detected in various tissues but the authors suggested that lanthanum could provide an alternative non-calcaemic binder. Human studies have confirmed its phosphate binding properties *in vivo* [119]. A third recently reported non-calcaemic phosphate binder is stabilized polynuclear iron hydroxide [120]. This has been shown to bind phosphate effectively in patients with preterminal renal failure over a 4-week period.

Peritoneal flux and reduced calcium dialysis fluid

During an exchange of 2 L of 1.36% glucose solution there is a net influx of calcium to the patient, although the amount varies from one study to the next (84 ± 18 mg/day [93]; 300 mg/day [121]. The transfer of calcium is also influenced by ultrafiltration rate and volume [122], so that a 1.36% glucose solution results in a 10 mg calcium uptake by the patient but the greater ultrafiltration from a 3.86% solution leads to a loss of 20 mg. This gives a net daily absorption of 10 mg if one hypertonic bag is used per day [122]. In another study, Kwong et al. [123] found an uptake of 29 mg per 1.36% exchange and a loss of 6 mg per 3.86% exchange, suggesting a larger net gain of around 80 mg daily. However, a lower PD fluid calcium concentration of 1.5 mmol/L causes the balance to become negative with a loss of 50 ± 36 mg/day [78]. These findings suggest that patients using dialysis solutions containing 1.75 mmol/L of calcium are in a significantly positive calcium balance even before considering the additional gut absorption from oral calcium carbonate and vitamin D therapy.

The theoretical work by Martis et al. [98] formed the basis for the commercial production of a peritoneal dialysis fluid with a calcium concentration of 1.25 mmol/L, in an attempt to decrease the incidence of hypercalcaemia in CAPD patients taking oral calcium salt phosphate binders. Clinical studies have now confirmed this theoretical work [113, 124]. Although dialysis fluids with other concentrations of calcium can be obtained (0, 0.60, 1.00, 1.45 mmol/L), 1.25 mmol/L would appear to be the logical choice for a new standard CAPD fluid because it is so close to normal serum ionized calcium levels. This results in a homeostatic effect, with calcium being lost into the peritoneum when serum levels are above 1.25 mmol/L, but being absorbed from the peritoneum during times of relative hypocalcaemia. All other proposed calcium concentrations are outside the normal range of serum ionized calcium and therefore cannot exert this homeostatic effect.

Convective effects of ultrafiltration increase the removal of calcium from the peritoneum so that patients using one or more 3.86% glucose exchanges per day will have a significantly greater negative peritoneal calcium balance than patients using only 1.36% exchanges. Whilst in theory this could result in some degree of hypocalcaemia, in practice it rarely occurs, as calcium absorption from oral phosphate binders is usually sufficient to compensate.

A 2-year prospective biochemical, radiological and histological study of 1.25 mmol/L calcium PD fluid showed it to be safe in compliant, well-monitored patients [125]. It allowed administration of larger doses of calcium carbonate and achievement of good control of serum phosphate and calcium–phosphate product. Parathyroid hormone levels were suppressed in the majority of patients, and bone histology and density did not deteriorate. By utilizing this more physiological dialysis fluid, aluminium-containing phosphate binders may be completely avoided in most CAPD patients.

In a smaller study of 1.25 mmol/L calcium dialysis solution, 11 CAPD patients were selected on the basis of persistent hypercalcaemia and uncontrolled hyperphosphataemia [110]. After 3 months these patients were changed from standard 1.75 mmol/L calcium, to 1.25 mmol/L calcium solution and followed for a further 6 months. Overall mean calcium–phosphate product changed little; however, in a subgroup of six patients it fell significantly, while in the other five it tended to rise. The group's mean serum aluminium fell significantly and although geometric mean iPTH rose slightly (but non-significantly) there was an association between phosphate control and iPTH at 6 months. In the subgroup of patients whose calcium–phosphate product fell, there was a much smaller rise in iPTH than in the others (57.3 to 73.2 vs 52.8 to 167.1 pg/ml). This suggests that in those patients using standard solutions, with apparently poor calcium and phosphate control, around 50% of them may, by changing to 1.25 mmol/L calcium solution, achieve a normal calcium–phosphate product whilst still avoiding aluminium salts. In this group of patients a lower calcium solution (0.75–1.00 mmol/L) may well prove appropriate.

Cunningham *et al.* [114] have used a similar low-calcium dialysis fluid to enable the use of calcium carbonate plus alphacalcidol in a group of CAPD patients. In 17 CAPD patients taking oral calcium carbonate, reductions in dialysis fluid calcium concentration to 1.45 mmol/L or 1.00 mmol/L enabled most of the patients to also take oral alphacalcidol. Parathyroid hormone, serum aluminium and alkaline phosphatase levels were all decreased during the 11 months of the study, with the authors concluding that a dialysate calcium concentration of 1.75 mmol/L is too high for the majority of calcium carbonate-treated patients, and that substantial reductions of the dialysate calcium concentration are required. Other workers have used 1.0 mmol/L calcium fluid in hypercalcaemic CAPD patients, again with similar results [28, 126]. Utilization of solutions with calcium concentrations of 1.00 mmol/L and below put the patient into a permanent negative calcium balance, so that very close attention must be given to PTH levels and compliance with oral calcium and vitamin D therapy.

Serum magnesium in CAPD

Magnesium levels are consistently elevated in CAPD patients managed with standard dialysate containing 0.75 mmol/L of magnesium [88, 121]. No toxicity has been reported at these levels; indeed hypermagnesaemia may have a suppressive effect on PTH release and retard the development of arterial calcification in CAPD patients [127]. Hypermagnesaemia may therefore be beneficial, but it has also been shown that normalization of serum magnesium is associated with an improvement in bone histology in haemodialysis patients [128]. Reducing the magnesium content to 0.25 mmol/L normalizes serum magnesium levels in CAPD patients [95, 124]. Parsons *et al.* [129, 130] have described the use of a low-calcium/zero magnesium CAPD fluid with a combination of calcium carbonate and magnesium carbonate in liquid form as the phosphate binder. Using this approach, mean serum phosphate levels of 1.4–1.5 mmol/L were obtained without causing hypermagnesaemia, although hypomagnesaemia was seen in two of 32 patients. Zero magnesium fluids have also been studied by Shah *et al.* [131], and offer the advantage of permitting larger doses of magnesium salt phosphate binders, but there are two disadvantages. First, patients may experience gastrointestinal upset, since magnesium salts have a laxative effect [132], and secondly monitoring of compliance and serum magnesium levels becomes obligatory, as hypomagnesaemia has been associated with cardiac rhythm disturbances [133–135] and electrocardiographic abnormalities [136].

Acid–base balance and 40 mmol/L lactate PD fluid

There is considerable evidence that as renal mechanisms for acid excretion fail, bone mineral stores become an important source of buffer [137, 138]. Acetazolamide produces a metabolic acidosis in normal subjects by inhibiting carbonic anhydrase in the proximal tubular epithelium, resulting in a bicarbonate diuresis. In virtually anuric haemodialysis patients it might therefore be expected to have little effect, but in fact produces a severe metabolic acidosis [139], suggesting that it is interfering with extrarenal buffering. Carbonic anhydrase is present in osteoclasts [140], and may be activated by PTH to promote bone resorption by release of H^+ ions [141]. The availability of bone buffers and bicarbonate would therefore depend on the activity of PTH, and could be inhibited by acetazolamide. It can therefore be seen that during a time of prolonged metabolic acidosis, such as exists in many CAPD patients using PD fluid with only 35 mmol/L lactate

[142], buffering by bone would be linked to bone resorption and increased PTH levels.

The use of PD fluid containing 40 mmol/L lactate corrects the mild acidosis experienced by most CAPD patients using the lower lactate concentration that is common in most European countries. Optimal correction of acidosis has been shown to change the progression of osteodystrophy in haemodialysis patients by Lefebvre et al. who, over 18 months, prospectively studied two groups of patients, dialysed against either standard dialysis fluid (32–24 mmol/L), or against fluid supplemented with 7–15 mmol/L of bicarbonate to achieve a predialysis plasma bicarbonate of 24 mmol/L. The supplemented group had a decreased rate of progression of secondary hyperparathyroidism in patients with high bone turnover, and stimulated bone turnover in those with low bone formation rates [143].

Parathyroid hormone in CAPD

Although the prevalence of symptomatic bone disease has decreased in recent years, the 1989 EDTA Registry report showed that around 40% of all patients dialysed for up to 15 years still required parathyroidectomy [25]. This partly reflects the poor understanding of the pathogenesis of secondary hyperparathyroidism that existed in the 1970s and 1980s, and partly the difficulty of monitoring vitamin D and PTH levels.

In the past 5 years considerable progress has been made with the introduction of sensitive and specific assays for calcium-regulating hormones [44, 144]. This has resulted in new concepts for prophylaxis and treatment of renal osteodystrophy, which hopefully will further improve long-term results.

CAPD has been shown to clear significant amounts of PTH from the serum. Using a C-terminal assay Delmez et al. [122] found a clearance rate of 1.5 ml/min or $13.6 \pm 3.2\%$ of the estimated total extracellular iPTH. Despite this, there is no clear-cut consensus on the effect of CAPD on PTH levels, although the weight of evidence is in favour of a steady decline with time [77, 82, 145–147]. However, other reports show no change [122], an increase in the levels [84, 148] or a variable response [85]. The reason for these differences lies in the widely varying practices between centres with regard to the use of calcium carbonate, aluminium hydroxide, vitamin D3 treatment and also the different radioimmunoassays used for measurement of iPTH and its fragments.

Until recently CAPD tended to be seen as a prescription in itself, with a standard set of guidelines that were suitable for every patient. As a result, the majority were treated with four 2-L exchanges, a phosphate binder, vitamin supplements and a small oral dose of 1,25-dihydroxyvitamin D3. PTH levels were rarely measured, and the dosage of calcitriol was changed only if hypercalcaemia occurred or evidence of osteitis fibrosa appeared on plain radiology of the hands.

Maintenance of a high serum ionized calcium (1.2–1.3 mmol/L) and strict control of serum phosphate, from the time of first starting dialysis, has been shown to decrease PTH levels in CAPD patients without the addition of vitamin D3 therapy [111, 125] but Hercz et al. [10, 28] have shown that such suppression can result in a hitherto infrequently recognized form of renal osteodystrophy, the non-aluminium-related, or 'idiopathic', adynamic bone disease. Hence the question now is not only 'what is the best way to suppress PTH', but also 'can PTH be over-suppressed?'.

Vitamin D in CAPD

Vitamin D metabolism is well known to be abnormal in uraemia, with very low levels of 1,25-dihydroxyvitamin D3 [46]. However, there are additional factors affecting vitamin D levels relating to the CAPD itself. Levels of 1,25-dihydroxyvitamin D3 are known to be very low, and sometimes undetectable, at the start of CAPD [45, 147]. 25-Hydroxyvitamin D3 levels are usually within the normal range at the start of CAPD but begin to decline thereafter [77, 97]. This is not unexpected since peritoneal dialysis effluent contains significant amounts of vitamin D binding protein, an α_2-globulin of molecular weight 59 kDa, which binds all three vitamin D metabolites (1,25-dihydroxyvitamin D3, 25-hydroxyvitamin D3 and 24,25-hydroxyvitamin D3). Losses of 1,25-dihydroxyvitamin D3 and 24,25-dihydroxyvitamin D3 have been shown to average approximately 6–8% of the plasma pool per day [149]. Thus, CAPD patients probably require 2–3 times the maintenance doses used in haemodialysis patients if it is thought necessary to bring serum levels of 1,25-dihydroxyvitamin D3 into the normal range. These doses frequently produce the problem of hypercalcaemia.

In England a seasonal variation in 25-hydroxyvitamin D3 levels was found by Cassidy et al. [150], and in sunnier climates patients may be able to maintain 25-hydroxyvitamin D3 levels within the normal range throughout the year. Whether 24,25-dihydroxyvitamin D3 plays an important role in bone mineralization remains to be proved, but Dunstan *et al.* [151] have shown that the combination of 1,25-dihydroxyvitamin D3 and 24,25-dihydroxyvitamin D3 given orally did not appear to confer any additional benefit compared with 1,25-dihydroxyvitamin D3 alone. This result is challenged by the work of Chaimovitz and colleagues, who suggest that 24,25-dihydroxyvitamin D3 plays a role in the regulation of PTH levels [152], and when given in conjunction with 1,25-dihydroxyvitamin D3 suppressed osteoclastic parameters without causing hypercalcaemia.

The role of calcitriol therapy in CAPD

In CAPD patients with serum PTH levels of greater than 400 pg/ml there is increasing evidence that the best way to administer oral vitamin D3 is in once- or twice-weekly pulses to reduce the incidence of hypercalcaemia [55, 153], a technique now being adopted in many centres. The idea of pulse therapy was initially investigated in haemodialysis patients, where thrice-weekly intravenous pulses of 1,25-(OH)2D3 were administered at the end of a haemodialysis session [41]. This regime resulted in marked suppression of iPTH levels with a mean decrement of around 70%, although Slatopolsky surmised that this was largely as a result of the rise in serum ionized calcium that occurred during the study. Furthermore, this study also demonstrated that when equal doses of intravenous or oral calcitriol were given, the serum concentration of calcitriol was six to eight times higher with the intravenous preparation, resulting in a greater delivery to non-intestinal target tissues and allowing greater expression of its biological effect on the parathyroid glands. However, even this degree of suppression was insufficient to restore iPTH to satisfactory levels, because of the large non-suppressible basal secretion rate of hypertrophied glands. Interestingly, it has also been shown that administering calcitriol at night reduces both the incidence and severity of hypercalcaemia in haemodialysis patients [154]!

Korkor demonstrated that the parathyroid glands from patients with chronic renal failure contained only one-third as many calcitriol receptors as are found in parathyroid adenomas [155], and in animal studies it is known that uraemia results in a two- to four-fold decrease in receptor numbers as compared to normal values [156, 157]. Thus it is likely that reduced receptor numbers in the parathyroid glands of uraemic patients render them less responsive to the inhibitory effects of calcitriol, so that suppression requires high peak serum levels.

Since the initial work of Slatopolsky several other workers have confirmed that both pulse intravenous 1,25-dihydroxyvitamin D3 and alpha-calcidol are effective in reducing serum PTH levels in haemodialysis patients [49, 51, 54], although all found difficulty in distinguishing direct effects on parathyroid secretion from indirect effects mediated by raising serum calcium. Subsequent studies in CAPD patients have tended to confirm this work, but some controversy still exists over the ideal regime of administration [158–160]. It is however, clear that 1,25-dihydroxyvitamin D3 does have a direct suppressive effect on parathyroid cells by influencing transcription of the parathyroid gene [40, 161]. Delmez *et al.* demonstrated that calcitriol could also be given intraperitoneally in CAPD patients where again it produced a rise in serum ionized calcium levels and a significant fall in serum PTH [83]. However, continued control of serum phosphate is also required, since hyperphosphataemia will significantly blunt the effect of calcitriol therapy [162].

Oral pulse calcitriol therapy

The discovery that intermittent dosage of 1,25-dihydroxyvitamin D3 was very effective in suppressing PTH levels led to a Japanese group trying oral pulse therapy in haemodialysis patients. Nineteen patients received 4.0 mg of oral calcitriol twice weekly after dialysis, which resulted in a fall of more than 45% in PTH levels after 6 months of treatment, despite a small fall in serum ionized calcium [52]. Similar results were then reported by Martin *et al.* in CAPD patients, using an initial twice-weekly oral dose of 5 mg of calcitriol [55]. Once again the decrease in PTH levels was not associated with any rise in serum calcium, and this mode of administration would appear to be the most appropriate to CAPD patients.

Calcitriol analogues

In rats with normal renal function 22-oxa-calcitriol has been shown to have very little calcaemic activity [163], yet it suppresses PTH mRNA levels equally as effectively as 1,25-(OH)2D3 [164]. A similar effect is reported in seven of eight nephrectomized rats [40], and in dogs with over 12 months of renal failure administration of a single intravenous dose of 5 mg of 22-oxa-calcitriol decreased PTH by 80% over 24 h without any change in serum calcium or phosphate levels [164]. However, Drueke and co-workers found similar degrees of hypercalcaemia in rats with chronic renal failure treated with either 1,25-(OH)2D3 or 22-oxa-calcitriol [165], and this observation has been confirmed in a study of 82 hyperparathyroid haemodialysis patients, where PTH suppression was associated with a rise in serum calcium [166, 167]. Other analogues, such as 2b-3-hydroxypropoxy calcitriol, EB 1089 and KH 1060 are under investigation as immunosuppressive agents, as well as for their effects on divalent ion metabolism [168].

Calcimimetics

Compounds that act as calcium receptor agonists are called calcimimetics because they mimic or potentiate the effects of extracellular calcium on parathyroid cell function. The discovery of such compounds with potent and selective activity, but no effect on serum calcium levels, enables a pharmacological approach to regulating plasma levels of PTH. Calcimimetic compounds could conceivably provide a specific medical therapy for hyperparathyroidism in renal disease, but substantive clinical trial reports are awaited [169–171].

Renal osteodystrophy in diabetic patients

A number of reports over the past 12 years have suggested that insulin-dependent diabetes mellitus is associated with lower serum levels of PTH [87, 172, 173], and decreased responsiveness to acute hypocalcaemia [174]. Therefore it has been suggested that diabetic patients may be more prone to low-turnover bone disease, and relatively protected from severe hyperparathyroidism. However, until recently it has been difficult to separate the effects of diabetes from those of aluminium accumulation, but Pei et al. [87] have now shown that diabetes mellitus is an important risk factor for both aluminium-related bone disease and the non-aluminium-related idiopathic adynamic bone lesion. These authors also noted that diabetes appears to enhance the risk of developing aluminium bone disease, possibly by increasing gastrointestinal absorption and bone surface accumulation of aluminium. This finding adds further impetus to the drive to eliminate use of aluminium-based phosphate binders wherever possible.

The idiopathic adynamic bone lesion in CAPD

The spectrum of bone disease has changed over the past 10 years with the emergence of the adynamic bone lesion, now present in over 20% of dialysis patients [9, 10, 21, 23], and the welcome decline in the usage of aluminium-containing phosphate binders. The association of adynamic bone with low PTH levels has resulted in a reassessment of attempts to suppress serum PTH to 'normal' levels in both predialysis and dialysis patients [21, 175] and acknowledgement that blanket prescription of continuous low-dose oral calcitriol therapy for all dialysis patients is unwise [176].

This lesion occurs more commonly in patients aged over 50 years at start of dialysis (Table 3), in those with a longer duration of predialysis renal failure [23], and in diabetic patients [87]. In a longitudinal histological study of bone disease in CAPD [125], five of eight patients who completed a full 2 years of follow-up were found to have developed the adynamic lesion (Fig. 5). None of the patients reported symptoms attributable to the lesion, and it has no characteristic radiological findings. Bone mineral density did not decline over the 2 years, but even longer follow-up may be required for signs and symptoms to appear. It is associated with normal or suppressed levels of parathyroid hormone [9, 10, 44, 45], and high or high/normal levels of ionized calcium. Sherrard et al. noted that the adynamic bone lesion was the commonest histological diagnosis in their study of 267 dialysis patients [10], and that it occurred more frequently in PD (61%) than in haemodialysis patients (36%). They suggest that this may be due to the more sustained and higher calcium levels associated with PD, which may result in more effective suppression of PTH than the intermittent calcium load of haemodialysis.

Table 3. Associations of the idiopathic a dynamic bone lesion

Clinical
Age >50 years
Diabetes mellitus
Commoner in CAPD than haemodialysis patients

Biochemical
Low/normal parathyroid hormone
High/normal ionized calcium
Low/normal bone alkaline phosphatase and other markers of bone turnover

Radiological
Increased incidence of vascular calcification

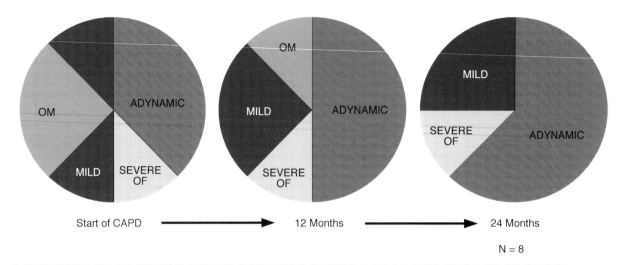

Figure 5. Changes in bone histology in eight patients over 24 months of continuous ambulatory peritoneal dialysis.

In a 10-year retrospective study of 1803 patients on chronic maintenance dialysis Malluche and Faugere report a gradual increase in the incidence of the adynamic bone lesion, so that in 1991 it affected 20% of patients. The primary factors associated with the occurrence of this lesion were found to be aluminium accumulation, increased age, diabetes mellitus, and possibly CAPD. In addition these authors noted a tendency towards hypercalcaemia, and accumulation of microfractures which they suggest might ultimately lead to clinical bone fracture.

In our own patients we have found an association between adynamic bone and the presence of significant vascular calcification, which may be related to the higher serum calcium levels found in patients with this lesion. This is a worrying association since many of these patients will be hoping for renal transplantation, which may become impossible when vascular calcification is severe. Furthermore it seems likely that adynamic bone would be significantly more prone to the osteoporotic effects of high-dose steroid immunosuppression, as well as avascular necrosis of the femoral head. Under normal circumstances the skeleton provides a large buffering capacity for both serum calcium and phosphate. If the bone is adynamic its buffering ability may be significantly reduced, and serum levels are therefore much more easily influenced by dietary intake or absorption from the dialysis fluid. Under these conditions there is a greater likelihood of the calcium–phosphate product being exceeded, and the process of metastatic calcification beginning. If this is the case then it would be very important to allow PTH levels

to rise slightly and stimulate bone turnover, whilst maintaining strict control of serum phosphate. In this way one would also hope to induce resorption of vascular calcium deposits. It is evident that the use of calcitriol, a powerful modulator of calcium and PTH, should be tailored to the individual patient's clinical situation, not merely prescribed in an unthinking fashion as a 'vitamin supplement'. Tailoring of any therapy requires the clinician to gather certain data in order to determine appropriate management. In this case one needs to examine the patient's serum calcium, phosphate and parathyroid hormone levels, in conjunction with bone histology data in certain cases. On the basis of these findings one can plan individual treatment along the lines of the clinical algorithm shown in Fig. 6.

Recommendations for management of osteodystrophy in CAPD

Techniques for monitoring renal osteodystrophy in CAPD patients are still evolving. In the past different units have approached the problem in widely differing ways, with some only monitoring serum calcium, phosphate and alkaline phosphatase plus annual skeletal surveys, and others performing much more detailed (and expensive) investigations, sometimes including bone biopsy. If we consider the available techniques under three broad headings – biochemical, radiological and histological – certain recom-

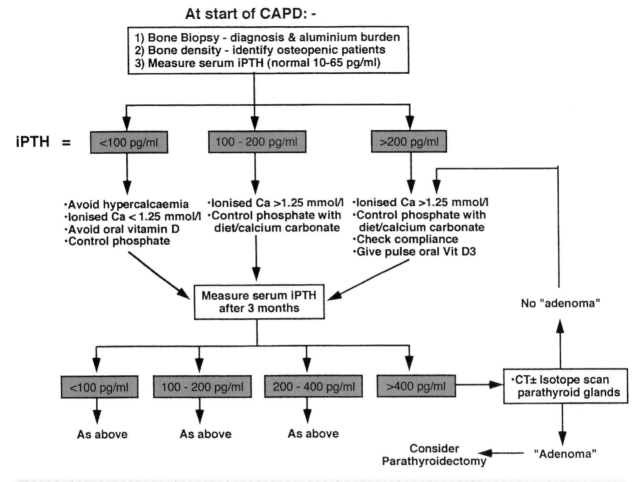

Figure 6. Clinical algorithm for the monitoring and management of renal osteodystrophy in CAPD patients.

mendations can be made, given the present state of understanding (Table 4).

Biochemical monitoring

In dialysis patients, changes in serum calcium and phosphate do not reflect disease processes within the skeleton as they may do in patients with normal renal function. They are primarily influenced by the patient's diet and oral intake of phosphate binders plus the amount of dialysis that patient is receiving. A rise in serum alkaline phosphatase is more indicative of increased bone turnover, but is seen only in advanced hyperparathyroidism. A rising level is generally associated with histologically severe osteitis fibrosa. The bone isoenzyme of alkaline phosphatase is a more sensitive indicator and low levels are associated with a greater likelihood of adynamic bone histology [23]. However, regular estimation of intact molecule PTH remains the most useful biochemical investigation. More recently measurement

Table 4. Recommendations for the management of renal osteodystrophy in adult CAPD patients (see also Fig. 6)

1. Restrict dietary phosphate, as far as possible within the confines of a 1.2 g/kg/day protein diet.
2. Use 1.25 mmol/L (2.5 mEq/L) calcium dialysis fluid to minimize hypercalcaemia. Individual patients may require higher or lower concentrations depending on serum ionized calcium (or total corrected calcium) and phosphate levels.
3. Calcium carbonate/acetate given twice daily with main meals. Dose titrated to serum calcium and phosphate levels. Educate patients to distribute dose according to phosphate intake.
4. Measure serum parathyroid hormone every 3 months (see Fig. 6) and use pulse oral vitamin D3 therapy if necessary. Replace 25-hydroxyvitamin D3 if serum levels are low.
5. Measure serum magnesium and aluminium every 6 months, unless patient is taking oral aluminium (then measure every 3 months).

of serum osteocalcin has become possible, providing a marker of osteoblast activity, but the very short half-life of the molecule means that unless the serum is spun and frozen within 20 min any subsequent assay is likely to be invalid. For this reason it seems unlikely to be helpful in clinical practice, and in any case reports show a close correlation with intact PTH levels in dialysis patients [177]. Another marker of hyperparathyroid bone disease, tartrate-resistant acid phosphatase (TRAP), has recently been reported to be a sensitive indicator of high- and low-turnover bone states [178, 179]. This enzyme is produced by actively resorbing osteo-clasts, and can be measured in serum by immuno-assay or colorimetrically. Experience with this marker is limited at present.

The most widely available, and generally useful, marker at present, is intact PTH, which should be measured every 3 or 4 months in all CAPD patients. Regular measurement of total alkaline phosphatase is unnecessary, although it will continue to be per-formed as part of the 'liver screen'.

Radiological monitoring

Routine, full skeletal surveys are unnecessary, and could be replaced by regular monitoring of serum PTH with plain X-rays of the hands plus a single lateral view of the lumbar spine [125, 180, 181]. This would greatly reduce the dose of radiation received by CAPD patients without detriment to patient care. In addition significant financial savings could be made. Some measurement of skeletal bone density should be made at the time of starting dialy-sis in all patients, so that those with subnormal bone density can be identified and special efforts made to improve the situation. Whether this measurement is best performed by QCT, SPA, DPA or DEXA scan would depend on local facilities and expertise.

Skeletal scintigraphy may be performed using technetium labelled 99m-methylene diphosphonate, but correlation of scan results with bone histology is poor, although increased uptake has been demon-strated in severe hyperparathyroid bone disease [182–184].

Single-photon absorptiometry (SPA): this is the most widely used method of quantifying bone min-eral density in renal osteodystrophy. A highly colli-mated beam of photons is used with 125I as a source. However, the single-energy beam requires a constant thickness of soft tissue around the bone to produce reliable results, and it cannot distinguish between trabecular and cortical bone. Studies have found that mineral content tends to be lower than normal in patients with renal failure [45, 185–187], but it does not allow differentiation between different types of osteodystrophy.

Dual photon absorptiometry (DPA): DPA utilizes an isotope with two energies (153 Gd), thereby over-coming the requirement of SPA for a constant thick-ness of soft tissue around the bone. It can therefore be used to measure bone mineral density in any skeletal site, but normal scan results have been seen in haemodialysis patients with histologically proven osteodystrophy [181].

Quantitative computed tomography (QCT): the principle of this technique is the same as for standard CT scanning, and a calibration phantom placed under the patient is used to relate bone mineral density to Hounsfield units. True bone density is measured in g/cm^3 and it is less affected by artefacts such as soft tissue calcification. However, it delivers a relatively high radiation dose.

In our own experience, bone density measure-ments are, if anything, less helpful than plain radio-graphs, since there is no correlation with histological diagnosis. Although end-stage renal failure patients were found to have reduced bone density, compared to age- and sex-matched normal values, the majority of patients had both QCT and SPA results within 2 SD of normal. Piraino *et al.* used QCT to measure bone mineral density in a group of 31 patients who had been on dialysis (19 peritoneal dialysis, 10 haemodialysis) for a mean of 5.3 years [188]. It is now known that the type of dialysis influences bone histology [11]; therefore it may be misleading to consider peritoneal dialysis and haemodialysis patients together. However, as in our study, Piraino *et al.* found that serum PTH was a better indicator of the type of bone disease present than was QCT-determined bone density, and concluded that the usefulness of this technique in patients with renal failure is limited.

Dual-energy X-ray absorptiometry (DEXA): less experience is available with the more recently devel-oped DEXA scan. It has several theoretical advan-tages over the other techniques, including low radiation dose, greater precision and rapidity of scanning. Despite this, measurements can be dis-torted by several artefacts such as ostephytes, calci-fication of the aorta or other soft tissues, and previous vertebral collapse. In 25 dialysis patients no correlation was found between QCT and DEXA measurements of vertebral bone mineral density [189].

Whilst single bone density measurements may be unhelpful, sequential studies might be more helpful, having initially established the hsitological diagnosis by biopsy. Decreasing bone density in a patient known to previously have osteitis fibrosa would suggest deterioration, especially if associated with a high iPTH.

Transiliac bone biopsy

Bone biopsy with tetracycline labelling is undoubtedly the only reliable method of diagnosing the type and severity of renal osteodystrophy. This is rarely performed in clinical practice because of patients' and doctors' perceptions of its painfulness and invasiveness. In our experience it is no more painful than Jamshidi marrow biopsies, which are routinely performed in many clinical situations if the blood film suggests it is necessary.

Local expertise permitting, CAPD patients ought to undergo a tetracycline-labelled bone biopsy at the time of starting dialysis, to establish the exact histology of their bone plus the degree of aluminium accumulation. In many cases this could be performed under general anaesthetic by the surgeon as the Tenckhoff catheter is inserted. Thereafter, one can probably surmise what is happening to the histology on the basis of regular PTH measurements once the initial histology is known.

These recommendations can be formed into a clinical algorithm (Fig. 6). The implementation of this scheme depends first on maximal restriction of dietary phosphate, within the limitations of a diet providing 1.2 g protein/kg body weight per day, and secondly on the routine use of CAPD fluid with a calcium concentration of 1.25 mmol/L, magnesium of 0.25 mmol/L and lactate of 40 mmol/L. Calcium carbonate should be given in doses adequate to maintain serum phosphate below 1.8 mmol/L and aluminium-containing binders should be avoided. If hypercalcaemia occurs calcium carbonate could be partially or completely replaced by poly[allyamine hydrochloride] (RenaGel; Geltex Pharmaceuticals, Waltham, Mass., USA) [117] . At present this non-calcaemic phosphate binder is available only in the USA, but it will soon become more widely available. Serum ionized calcium and iPTH should be measured every 3 months to provide a guide for treatment with oral calcitriol. If iPTH is less than 200 pg/ml vitamin D3 is not required. If iPTH exceeds 200 pg/ml then attention should be paid to maintenance of a high/normal ionized calcium level and tighter dietary control of phosphate where possible. Calcitriol should be given as intermittent-pulse doses [55], and iPTH remeasured after 3 months. If the level remains significantly elevated, or is rising, then appropriate scans should be ordered to search for a parathyroid adenoma with a view to possible para-

thyroidectomy (provided the patient does not have significant aluminium deposition).

Serum magnesium levels should be measured once every 6 months, especially in those patients whose dietary intake may be low, to check for hypomagnesaemia. Plasma aluminium levels should also be monitored every 6 months, even in patients not taking aluminium-containing phosphate binders, since there are other sources of this metal such as drugs and drinking-water. It must be remembered that aluminium uptake can be significantly enhanced by citrate ingestion and oral vitamin D3.

Utilization of these guidelines should enable good control of divalent ion metabolism, and prevention or amelioration of osteodystrophy in the majority of CAPD patients. Further advances will hinge on a greater understanding of the vitamin D/parathyroid axis in renal failure, along with the development of safe, non-calcaemic analogues of vitamin D3 plus more efficient phosphate binders, possibly based on substances other than aluminium or calcium.

Summary

Disorders of calcium, magnesium, phosphate, vitamin D3, and parathyroid hormone can combine to produce a variety of skeletal and extraskeletal pathologies in CAPD patients. The recognition of the long-term toxicity of aluminium-containing phosphate binders, and their withdrawal, is a significant step in the drive towards combating renal osteodystrophy. However, the replacement of aluminium by calcium-containing phosphate binders has been primarily hampered by the occurrence of hypercalcaemia in many patients. This problem is further compounded by the increased gastrointestinal absorption brought about by oral vitamin D3, and the probably unnecessary peritoneal absorption of calcium from PD fluid. An increasing range of dialysis solutions is becoming available, so that in the future it will be possible to tailor peritoneal dialysis treatment to the needs of the individual patient. New non-calcaemic phosphate binders are now entering clinical use, and will further increase the options available to clinicians. Calcimimetic agents are currently experimental, but may in the future provide an effective means of controlling PTH independently of serum calcium levels.

The judicious use of a variety of biochemical and radiological investigations, plus bone histomorphometry where appropriate, can provide a rational basis for the monitoring and management of divalent ion metabolism and renal osteodystrophy in CAPD patients.

References

1. Lucas R. On a form of late rickets associated with albuminuria, rickets of adolescence. Lancet 1883; 1: 993–4.
2. Fletcher H. Case of infantilism with polyuria and chronic renal disease. Proc R Soc Med Lond 1911; 95–7.
3. Barber H. The bone deformities of renal dwarfism. Lancet 1920; 1: 18–20.
4. Follis R, Jackson D. Renal osteomalacia and osteitis fibrosa. Bull Johns Hopkins Hosp 1943; 72: 232–4.
5. Liu S, Chu H. Studies of calcium and phosphorus metabolism with special reference to pathogenesis and effects of dihydrotachysterol (A.T. 10) and iron. Medicine 1943; 22: 103–7.
6. Garner A, Ball J. Quantitative observations on mineralised and unmineralised bone in chronic renal azotaemia and intestinal malabsorption syndrome. J Pathol Bacteriol 1966; 91: 545–9.
7. Stanbury S, Lumb G. Metabolic studies of renal osteodystrophy. Medicine 1962; 41: 1–28.
8. Stanbury S, Lumb G. Parathyroid function in chronic renal failure: a statistical survey of the plasma biochemistry in azotaemic renal osteodystrophy. Q J Med 1966; 35: 1–12.
9. Malluche H, Monier-Faugere M. Risk of adynamic bone disease in dialyzed patients. Kidney Int 1992; 42 (suppl. 38): S62–7.
10. Sherrard D, Hercz G, Pei Y et al. The spectrum of bone disease in end-stage renal failure – an evolving disorder. Kidney Int 1993; 43: 436–42.
11. Coburn J. Mineral metabolism and renal bone disease: effects of CAPD versus hemodialysis. Kidney Int 1993; 43 (suppl. 40): S92–100.
12. Llach F, Massry S, Singer F, Yurokawa K, Kaye J, Coburn J. Skeletal resistance to endogenous parathyroid hormone in patients with early renal failure. A possible cause of secondary hyperparathyroidism. J Clin Endocrinol Metab 1975; 41: 339–45.
13. Avioli L. The renal osteodystrophies. In: Brenner BFCR, ed. The Kidney. Philadelphia: Saunders, 1986, pp. 1542–80.
14. Malluche H, Ritz E, Kutschera J et al. Calcium metabolism and impaired mineralization in various stages or renal insufficiency. In: Normal A, Schaeffer K, Grigoleit H, Herrath D, Ritz E, eds. Vitamin D and Problems Related to Uremic Bone Disease. Berlin: Walter de Gruyter, 1975, pp. 513–22.
15. Malluche H, Faugere M. Renal bone disease 1990: an unmet challenge for the nephrologist. Kidney Int 1990; 38: 193–211.
16. Baker L, Abrams S, Roe C, Faugere M, Fanti P, Subayti Y, Malluche H. 1,25-dihydroxyvitamin D3 administration in moderate renal failure: a prospective double-blind trial. Kidney Int 1989; 35: 661–9.
17. Ward M, Feest T, Ellis H et al. Osteomalacic dialysis osteodystrophy: evidence for a water-borne aetiological agent, probably aluminium. Lancet 1978; 1: 841–5.
18. Cournot-Witmer G, Plachot J, Borudeau A et al. Effect of aluminum on bone and cell localization. Kidney Int 1986; 29 (suppl. 18): S37–40.
19. Ott S, Maloney N, Coburn J, Alfrey A, Sherrard D. The prevalence of bone aluminum deposition in renal osteodystrophy and its relation to the response to calcitriol therapy. N Engl J Med 1982; 307: 709–14.
20. Posner A, Blumenthal N, Boskey A. Model of aluminum-induced osteomalacia: inhibition of apatite formation and growth. Kidney Int 1986; 29 (suppl. 18): S17–19.
21. Fournier A, Moriniere P, Cohen-Solal M et al. Adynamic bone disease in uremia: may it be idiopathic? Is it an actual disease? Nephron 1991; 58: 1–12.
22. Cuevas X, Aubia J, Bosch J et al. Histomorphometric bone patterns of diabetic–uremic patients on dialysis are established in pre-dialysis stage already. Nephrol Dial Transplant 1992; 7: 756 (abstract).
23. Hutchison A, Whitehouse R, Boulton H et al. Histological, radiological and biochemical features of the adynamic bone lesion in CAPD patients. Am J Nephrol 1994; 14: 19–29.
24. Coburn J. Renal osteodystrophy. Kidney Int 1980; 17: 677–93.
25. Fassbinder W, Brunner F, Brynger H et al. Combined report on regular dialysis and transplantation in Europe, XX, 1989. Nephrol Dial Transplant 1991; 6 (suppl. 1): 5–35.
26. Dunstan C, Evans R, Hills E, Wong S, Alfrey A. Effect of aluminum and parathyroid hormone on osteoblasts and bone mineralization in chronic renal failure. Calc Tissue Int 1984; 36: 133–8.
27. Charhon S, Chavassieux P, Chapuy M, Boivin G, Meunier P. Low rate of bone formation with or without histologic appearance of osteomalacia in patients with aluminum intoxication. J Lab Clin Med 1985; 106: 123–31.
28. Hercz G, Pei Y, Manuel A et al. Aplastic osteodystrophy without aluminum staining in dialysis patients. Kidney Int 1990; 37: 449 (abstract).
29. Keutmann H, Sauer M, Hendry G et al. Complete amino-acid sequence of human parathyroid hormone. Biochemistry 1978; 17: 5723–9.
30. Chu L, MacGregor R, Hamilton J et al. Conversion of proparathyroid hormone to parathyroid hormone: the use of amines as specific inhibitors. Endocrinology 1974; 95: 1431–8.
31. Arnaud C. Hyperparathyroidism and renal failure. Kidney Int 1973; 4: 89–92.
32. Slatopolsky E, Martin K, Morrissey J, Hruska K. Parathyroid hormone: alterations in chronic renal failure. In: Robinson R, ed. Nephrology. New York: Springer, 1985, pp. 1292–304.
33. Sherwood L, Mayer G, Ramberg C et al. Regulation of parathyroid hormone secretion: proportional control by calcium, lack of effect of phosphate. Endocrinology 1968; 83: 1043–51.
34. Slatopolsky E, Lopez-Hilker S, Dusso A et al. The interrelationship between vitamin D and parathyroid hormone secretion in health and disease. In: Davison, A, ed. Nephrology. London: Baillière Tindall, 1988, vol. 2, pp. 1067–75.
35. Felsenfeld A, Ross D, Rodriguez M. Hysteresis of the parathyroid hormone response to hypocalcemia in haemodialysis patients with low turnover aluminum bone disease. J Am Soc Nephrol 1991; 6: 1136–43.
36. Dunlay R, Rodriguez M, Felsenfeld A, Llach F. Direct inhibitory effect of calcitriol on parathyroid function (sigmoidal curve) in dialysis patients. Kidney Int 1989; 36: 1093–8.
37. Cunningham J, Altmann P, Gleed J, Butter K, Marsh F, O'Riordan J. Effect of direction and rate of change of calcium on parathyroid hormone secretion in uraemia. Nephrol Dial Transplant 1989; 4: 339–44.
38. Brown E, Gardener D, Windeck R et al. Relationship of intracellular 3',5'-adenosine monophosphate accumulation to parathyroid hormone release from dispersed bovine parathyroid cells. Endocrinology 1978; 103: 2323–33.
39. Kitaoka M, Fukagawa M, Tanaka Y, Ogata E, Kurokawa K. Parathyroid gland size is critical for long-term prognosis of calcitriol pulse therapy in chronic dialysis patients. J Am Soc Nephrol 1991; 2: 637 (abstract).
40. Fukagawa M, Kaname S, Igarashi T, Ogata E, Kurokawa K. Regulation of parathyroid hormone synthesis in chronic renal failure in rats. Kidney Int 1991; 39: 874–81.
41. Slatopolsky E, Weerts C, Thielan J et al. Marked suppression of secondary hyperparathyroidism by intravenous administration of 1,25-dihydroxycholecalciferol in uremic patients. J Clin Invest 1984; 74: 2136–43.
42. Salusky I, Goodman W, Norris K, Horst N, Fine R, Coburn J. Bioavailability of calcitriol after oral, intravenous, and intraperitoneal doses in dialysis patients. In: Norman A, Schaefer K, Griroleit H, Herrath D, eds. Vitamin D. Molecu-

lar, Cellular and Clinical Endocrinology. Berlin: Walter de Gruyter, 1988, pp. 783–4.

43. Chase L, Slatopolsky E. Secretion and metabolic efficiency of parathyroid hormone in patients with severe hypomagnesemia. J Endocrinol Metab 1974; 38: 363–71.

44. Cohen-Solal M, Sebert J, Boudailliez B et al. Comparison of intact, midregion, and carboxy terminal assays of parathyroid hormone for the diagnosis of bone disease in hemodialyzed patients. J Clin Endocrinol Metab 1991; 73: 516–24.

45. Hutchison A, Whitehouse R, Boulton H et al. Correlation of bone histology with parathyroid hormone, vitamin D, and radiology in end-stage renal disease. Kidney Int 1994; 44: 1071–7.

46. Mawer E, Taylor C, Backhouse J, Lumb G, Stanbury S. Failure of formation of 1,25-dihydroxycholecalciferol in chronic renal insufficiency. Lancet 1973; 1: 626–8.

47. Rapoport J, Shany S, Chaimovitz C. Continuous ambulatory peritoneal dialysis and vitamin D. Nephron 1988; 48: 1–3.

48. Hayes M, O'Donoghue D, Ballardie F, Mawer E. Peritonitis induces the synthesis of 1-a-25, dihydroxyvitamin D3 in macrophages from CAPD patients. FEBS 1987; 220: 307–10.

49. Lind L, Wengle B, Wide L, Wrege U, Ljunghall S. Suppression of serum parathyroid hormone levels by intravenous alpha-calcidol in uremic patients on maintenance hemodialysis. Nephron 1988; 48: 296–9.

50. Andress D, Norris K, Coburn J, Saltopolsky E, Sherrard D. Intravenous calcitriol in the treatment of refractory osteitis fibrosa of chronic renal failure. N Engl J Med 1989; 321: 274–9.

51. Ljunghall S, Althoff P, Fellstrom B et al. Effects on serum parathyroid hormone of intravenous treatment with alphacalcidol in patients on chronic hemodialysis. Nephron 1990; 55: 380–5.

52. Tsukamoto Y, Nomura M, Takahashi Y et al. The 'oral 1,25-dihydroxyvitamin D3 pulse therapy' in hemodialysis patients with severe secondary hyperparathyroidism. Nephron 1991; 57: 23–8.

53. Gallieni M, Brancaccio D, Padovese P et al. Low-dose intravenous calcitriol treatment of secondary hyperparathyroidism in hemodialysis patients. Kidney Int 1992; 42: 1191–8.

54. Moriniere P, Maurouard C, Boudailiez B et al. Prevention of hyperparathyroidism in patients on maintenance dialysis by intravenous 1-alpha-hydroxyvitamin D3 in association with Mg(OH)₂ as sole phosphate binder. Nephron 1992; 60: 154–63.

55. Martin K, Ballal H, Domoto D, Blalock S, Weindel M. Pulse oral calcitriol for the treatment of hyperparathyroidism in patients on continuous ambulatory peritoneal dialysis: preliminary observations. Am J Kidney Dis 1992; 19: 540–5.

56. Holick M. Vitamin D and the kidney. Kidney Int 1987; 32: 912–29.

57. Mak R, Wong J. The vitamin D–parathyroid hormone axis in the pathogenesis of hypertension and insulin resistance in uremia. Miner Electrolyte Metab 1992; 18: 156–9.

58. Bricker N. On the pathogenesis of the uremic state. An exposition of the 'trade-off' hypothesis. N Engl J Med 1972; 286: 1093–9.

59. Faugere MC, Friedler R, Fanti P, Malluche H. Lack of histologic signs of Vit D deficiency in early development of renal osteodystrophy. J Bone Miner Res 1988; 3 (suppl. 1): S95.

60. Lopez-Hilker S, Galceran T, Chan UL, Rapp N, Martin K, Slatopolsky E. Hypocalcaemia may not be essential for the development of secondary hyperparathyroidism in chronic renal failure. J Clin Invest 1986; 78: 1097–102.

61. Ritz E, Matthias S, Seidel A, Reichel H, Szabo A, Horl W. Disturbed calcium metabolism in renal failure – pathogenesis and therapeutic strategies. Kidney Int 1992; 42 (suppl. 38): S37–42.

62. Nielsen PK, Feldt-Rasmussen U, Olgaard K. A direct effect *in vitro* of phosphate on PTH release from bovine parathyroid tissue slices but not from dispersed parathyroid cells. Nephrol Dial Transplant 1996; 9: 1762–9.

63. Massry S, Tuma S, Dua S, Goldstein D. Reversal of skeletal resistance to parathyroid hormone in uremia by vitamin D metabolites. J Lab Clin Med 1979; 94: 152–7.

64. Brookfield R. The magnesium content of serum in renal insufficiency. Q J Med 1937; 6: 87–90.

65. Randall R, Cohen M, Spray C, Rossmeisl E. Hypermagnesaemia in renal failure. Ann Internal Med 1964; 61: 73–88.

66. Moriniere P, Vinatier I, Westeel P et al. Magnesium hydroxide as a complementary aluminium-free phosphate binder to moderate doses of oral calcium carbonate in uraemic patients on chronic haemodialysis: lack of deleterious effect on bone mineralization. Nephrol Dial Transplant 1988; 3: 651–6.

67. Alfrey A, Solomons C. Bone pyrophosphate in uremia and its association with extraosseous calcification. J Clin Invest 1976; 57: 700–5.

68. MacIntyre I, Davidsson D. The production of secondary potassium depletion, sodium retention, nephrocalcinosis and hypercalcaemia by magnesium deficiency. Biochem J 1958; 70: 456–62.

69. Kaehny W, Hegg A, Alfrey A. Gastrointestinal absorption of aluminium from aluminium-containing antacids. N Engl J Med 1977; 296: 1389–90.

70. de Broe M, D'Hasse P, Elseviers M, Clement J, Visser W, van de Vyver F. Aluminium and end-stage renal failure. In: Davidson A, ed. Nephrology: Proceedings of the X ICN. Cambridge: Baillière Tindall, 1988, vol. 2, pp. 1086–116.

71. Litzow J, Lemann J, Lennon E. The effect of treatment of acidosis on calcium balance in patients with chronic azotemic renal disease. J Clin Invest 1967; 46: 280–4.

72. Kuster S, Ritz E, Horl W. A role for metabolic acidosis in the genesis of renal secondary hyperparathyroidism. In: Israel Eliahou H, Iaina A, Bar-Khayim Y, eds. Abstract Book, XIIth International Congress of Nephrology, Jerusalem, 1993, p. 467.

73. Lee J, Parthemore J, Deftos L. Immunochemical heterogeneity of calcitonin in renal failure. J Clin Endocrinol Metab 1977; 45: 528–33.

74. Marcus R. Endocrine control of bone and mineral metabolism. In: Olefsky M, ed. Metabolic Bone and Mineral Disorders. Contemporary Issues in Endocrinology and Metabolism; vol. 5. New York: Churchill Livingstone, 1988, pp. 21–2.

75. Block GA, Hulbert-Shearon TE, Levin NW, Port FK. Association of serum phosphorus and calcium × phosphate product with mortality risk in chronic hemodialysis patients: a national study. Am J Kidney Dis 1998; 31: 607–17.

76. Goldsmith DJ, Covic A, Sambrook PA, Ackrill P. Vascular calcification in long-term haemodialysis patients in a single unit: a retrospective analysis. Nephron 1997; 77: 37–43.

77. Gokal R, Ramos J, Ellis H, Parkinson I, Sweetman V, Dewar J, Ward M, Kerr D. Histological renal osteodystrophy, and 25-hydroxycholecalciferol and aluminium levels in patients on CAPD. Kidney Int 1983; 23: 15–21.

78. Calderaro V, Oreopoulos D, Meema H et al. The evolution of renal osteodystrophy in patients undergoing continuous ambulatory peritoneal dialysis. Proc EDTA 1980; 533–42.

79. Owen J, Parnell A, Keir M et al. Critical analysis of the use of skeletal surveys in patients with chronic renal failure. Clin Radiol 1988; 39: 578–82.

80. Adams J, Chen S, Adams P, Isherwood I. Measurement of trabecular bone mineral by dual energy computed tomography. J Comput Assist Tomogr 1982; 6: 601–7.

81. Genant H, Block J, Steiger P, Glueer C, Ettinger B, Harris S. Appropriate use of bone densitometry. Radiology 1989; 170: 817–22.

82. Rahman R, Heaton A, Goodship T et al. Renal osteodystrophy in patients on CAPD: a five year study. Perit Dial Bull 1987; 7: 1–4.

83. Delmez J, Dougan C, Gearing B et al. effects of intraperitoneal calcitriol on calcium and parathyroid hormone. Kidney Int 1987; 31: 795–9.

84. Digenis G, Khanna R, Pierratos A *et al.* Renal osteodystrophy in patients managed on CAPD for more than three years. Perit Dial Bull 1983; 3: 81–6.

85. Kurtz S. Clinical parameters of renal bone disease: a comparison of CAPD and haemodialysis. Dial Transplant 1985; 14: 30–6.

86. Bucciante G, Biachi M, Valenti G. Progress of renal osteodystrophy during CAPD. Clin Nephrol 1984; 6: 279–83.

87. Pei Y, Hercz G, Greenwood C *et al.* Renal osteodystrophy in diabetic patients. Kidney Int 1993; 44: 159–64.

88. Gokal R, Fryer R, McHugh M *et al.* Calcium and phosphate control in CAPD patients. In: Legrain M, ed. Amsterdam: Excerpta Medica, 1980, pp. 283–91.

89. Recker R, Saville P. Calcium absorption in renal failure: its relationship to blood urea nitrogen, dietary calcium intake, time on dialysis, and other variables. J Lab Clin Med 1971; 78: 380–8.

90. Clarkson E, Eastwood J, Koutsaimanis K *et al.* Net intestinal absorption of calcium in patients with chronic renal failure. Kidney Int 1973; 3: 258–63.

91. Ramirez J, Emmett M, White M *et al.* The absorption of dietary phosphorus and calcium in haemodialysis patients. Kidney Int 1986; 30: 753–9.

92. Hutchison A, Boulton H, Herman K, Prescott M, Gokal R. The use of oral stable strontium to provide an index of intestinal calcium absorption in chronic ambulatory peritoneal dialysis patients. Miner Electrolyte Metab 1992; 18: 160–5.

93. Blumenkrantz M, Kopple J, Moran J, Coburn J. Metabolic balance studies and dietary protein requirements in patients undergoing CAPD. Kidney Int 1982; 21: 849–61.

94. Lindholm B, Bergstrom J. Nutritional aspects of CAPD. In: Gokal R, ed. Continuous Ambulatory Peritoneal Dialysis. Edinburgh: Churchill Livingstone, 1986, pp. 228–55.

95. Nolph K, Prowant B, Serkes K *et al.* Multicenter evaluation of a new peritoneal dialysis solution with a high lactate and a low magnesium concentration. Perit Dial Bull 1983; 3: 63–6.

96. Hercz G, Coburn J. Prevention of phosphate retention and hyperphosphatemia in uremia. Kidney Int 1987; 32 (suppl. 22): S215–20.

97. Delmez J, Fallon M, Bergfeld M, Gearing B, Dougan C, Teitelbaum S. Continuous ambulatory peritoneal dialysis and bone. Kidney Int 1986; 30: 379–84.

98. Martis L, Serkes K, Nolph K. Calcium carbonate as a phosphate binder: is there a need to adjust peritoneal calcium concentrations for patients using calcium carbonate? Perit Dial Int 1989; 9: 325–8.

99. Bro S, Rasmussen RA, Handberg J, Olgaard K, Feldt-Rasmussen B. Randomized crossover study comparing the phosphate binding efficacy of calcium ketoglutarate versus calcium carbonate in patients on chronic hemodialysis. Am J Kidney Dis 1998; 31: 257–62.

100. Andreoli S, Briggs J, Junor B. Aluminium intoxication from aluminium-containing phosphate binders in children with azotemia not undergoing dialysis. N Engl J Med 1984; 310: 1079–84.

101. Salusky I, Coburn J, Foley J, Nelson P, Fine R. Effects of oral calcium carbonate on control of serum phosphorus and changes in plasma aluminium levels after discontinuation of aluminium-containing gels in children receiving dialysis. J Pediatr 1986; 108: 767–70.

102. Slatopolsky E, Weerts C, Lopez-Hilker S *et al.* Calcium carbonate as a phosphate binder in patients with chronic renal failure undergoing dialysis. N Engl J Med 1986; 315: 157–61.

103. Stein H, Yudis M, Sirota R. Calcium carbonate as a phosphate binder. N Engl J Med 1987; 316: 109–10.

104. Ott S. Aluminum accumulation in individuals with normal renal function. Am J Kidney Dis 1985; 4: 297–301.

105. Joffe P, Olsen F, Heaf J, Gammelgaard B, Podenphant J. Aluminium concentrations in serum, dialysate, urine and bone among patients undergoing continuous ambulatory peritoneal dialysis. Clin Nephrol 1989; 32: 133–8.

106. Slatopolsky E, Weerts C, Norwood K *et al.* Long-term effects of calcium carbonate and 2.5 mEq/liter calcium dialysate on mineral metabolism. Kidney Int 1989; 36: 897–903.

107. Van der Merwe W, Rodger R, Grant A *et al.* Low calcium dialysate and high-dose oral calcitriol in the treatment of secondary hyperparathyroidism in haemodialysis patients. Nephrol Dial Transplant 1990; 5: 874–7.

108. Gokal R, Hutchison A. Calcium, phosphorus, aluminium and bone disease in continuous ambulatory peritoneal dialysis patients. In: Hatano M, ed. Nephrology. Tokyo: Spinger, 1991, vol. 2, pp. 1602–9.

109. Hutchison A, Gokal R. Towards tailored dialysis fluids in CAPD: the role of reduced calcium and magnesium dialysis fluids. Perit Dial Int 1992; 12: 199–203.

110. Hutchison A, Were A, Boulton H, Mawer E, Laing I, Gokal R. Control of hypercalcaemia, hyperphosphataemia and hyperaluminaemia in CAPD by reduction in dialysate calcium concentration. Nephrol Dial Transplant 1992; 7: 1143 (abstract).

111. Hutchison A, Freemont A, Boulton H, Gokal R. Low-calcium dialysis fluid and oral calcium carbonate in CAPD: a method of controlling hyperphosphataemia whilst minimizing aluminium exposure and hypercalcaemia. Nephrol Dial Transplant 1992; 7: 1219–25.

112. Hutchison A, Gokal R. Improved solutions for peritoneal dialysis: physiological calcium solutions, osmotic agents and buffers. Kidney Int 1992; 42 (suppl. 38): S152–9.

113. Piraino B, Perlmutter J, Holley J, Johnston J, Bernardini J. The use of dialysate containing 2.5 mEq/L calcium in peritoneal dialysis patients. Perit Dial Int 1992; 12: 75–6.

114. Cunningham J, Beer J, Coldwell R, Noonan K, Sawyer N, Makin H. Dialysate calcium reduction in CAPD patients treated with calcium carbonate and alfacalcidol. Nephrol Dial Transplant 1992; 7: 63–8.

115. McGary TJ, Nolph KD, Moore HL, Kartinos NJ. Polycation as an alternative osmotic agent and phosphate binder in peritoneal dialysis. Uremia Invest 1984–5; 8: 79–84.

116. Hutchison AJ. Calcitriol, lanthanum carbonate and other new phosphate binders in the management of renal osteodystrophy. Perit Dial Int 1999; 19 (suppl. 2): S408–12.

117. Chertow GM, Burke SK, Lazarus JM *et al.* Poly[allyamine hydrochloride] (RenaGel): a noncalcaemic phosphate binder for the treatment of hyperphosphatemia in chronic renal failure. Am J Kidney Dis 1997; 29: 66–71.

118. Graff L, Burnel D. A possible non-aluminum oral phosphate binder? A comparative study on dietary phosphorus absorption. Res Commun Mol Pathol Pharmacol 1995; 90: 373–88.

119. Dewberry K, Fox JS, Stewart J, Murray JR, Hutchison AJ. Lanthanum carbonate: a novel non-calcium containing phosphate binder. J Am Soc Nephrol 1997; 8: A2610.

120. Hergesell O, Ritz E. Stabilized polynuclear iron hydroxide is an efficient oral phosphate binder in uraemic patients. Nephrol Dial Transplant 1999; 14: 863–7.

121. Parker A, Nolph K. Magnesium and calcium transfer during continuous ambulatory peritoneal dialysis. Trans Am Soc Artif Intern Organs 1980; 26: 194–6.

122. Delmez J, Slatopolsky E, Martin K, Gearing B, Herschel R. Minerals, vitamin D, and parathyroid hormone in continuous ambulatory peritoneal dialysis. Kidney Int 1982; 21: 862–7.

123. Kwong M, Lee J, Chan M. Transperitoneal calcium and magnesium transfer during an eight hour dialysis. Perit Dial Bull 1987; 7: 85–9.

124. Hutchison A, Merchant M, Boulton H, Hinchcliffe R, Gokal R. Calcium and magnesium mass transfer in peritoneal dialysis patients using 1.25 mmol/L calcium, 0.25 mmol/L magnesium dialysis fluid. Perit Dial Int 1993; 13: 219–23.

125. Hutchison A, Boulton H, Freemont A, Gokal R. Effective control of phosphate, intact PTH and osteodystrophy by

low-calcium dialysate and oral CaCO₃ in CAPD. (Abstract). Nephrol Dial Transplant 1992; 7: 759.

126. Hamdy N, Brown C, Boletis J *et al.* Mineral metabolism in CAPD. In: Berlyne G, Giovanetti S, eds. CAPD: Host Defence, Nutrition and Ultrafiltration. Contributions to Nephrology, vol. 85. Basel: Karger, 1990, pp. 73–8.

127. Meema H, Oreopoulos D, Rapoport A. Serum magnesium level and arterial calcification in end-stage renal disease. Kidney Int 1987; 32: 388–94.

128. Gonella M, Ballanti P, Della Rocca C *et al.* Improved bone morphology by normalizing serum magnesium in chronically hemodialyzed patients. Miner Electrolyte Metab 1988; 14: 240–5.

129. Breuer J, Moniz C, Baldwin D, Parsons V. The effects of zero magnesium dialysate and magnesium supplements on ionized calcium concentration in patients on regular dialysis treatment. Nephrol Dial Transplant 1987; 2: 347–50.

130. Parsons V, Baldwin D, Moniz C, Marsden J, Ball E, Rifkin I. Successful control of hyperparathyroidism in patients on continuous ambulatory peritoneal dialysis using magnesium carbonate and calcium carbonate as phosphate binders. Nephron 1993; 63: 379–83.

131. Shah G, Winer R, Cutler R *et al.* Effects of a magnesium-free dialysate on magnesium metabolism during continuous ambulatory peritoneal dialysis. Am J Kidney Dis 1987; 10: 268–75.

132. Aitken J, Allison S, Arkell D *et al.* Gastro-intestinal system. In: Mehta D, ed. British National Formulary. Published by the British Medical Association, London, 1999, p. 52.

133. Dyckner T, Wester P. Relation between potassium and magnesium in cardiac arrhythmias. Acta Med Scand 1981; 647 (suppl.): 163–9.

134. Whang R. Magnesium deficiency: pathogenesis, prevalence, and clinical implications. Am J Med 1987; 82 (suppl. 3A): 24–9.

135. Hollifield J. Magnesium depletion, diuretics, and arrhythmias. Am J Med 1987; 82 (suppl. 3A): 30–7.

136. Seelig M. Electrocardiographic patterns of magnesium depletion appearing in alcoholic heart disease. Ann NY Acad Sci 1969; 162: 906–17.

137. Lemann J, Lennon E. Role of diet, gastrointestinal tract and bone in acid–base homeostasis. Kidney Int 1972; 1: 275–9.

138. Kaye M, Frueh A, Silverman M. A study of vertebral bone powder from patients with chronic renal failure. J Clin Invest 1978; 49: 442–53.

139. De Marchi S, Cecchin E. Severe metabolic acidosis and disturbances of calcium metabolism induced by acetazolamide in patients on haemodialysis. Clin Sci 1990; 78: 295–302.

140. Maren T. Carbonic anhydrase. N Engl J Med 1985; 313: 179–81.

141. Waite L. Carbonic anhydrase inhibitors, parathyroid hormone and calcium metabolism. Endocrinology 1972; 91: 1160–5.

142. Nolph K, Sorkin M, Rubin J *et al.* Continuous ambulatory peritoneal dialysis: three-year experience at one center. Ann Intern Med 1980; 92: 609–13.

143. Lefebvre A, de Vernejoul M, Gueris J, Goldfarb B, Graulet A, Morieux C. Optimal correction of acidosis changes progression of dialysis osteodystrophy. Kidney Int 1989; 36: 1112–8.

144. Mawer E, Hann J, Berry J, Davies M. Vitamin D metabolism in patients intoxicated with ergocalciferol. Clin Sci 1985; 68: 135–41.

145. de Fremont J, Moriniere P, Roussel J. Control of hyperparathyroidism by CAPD. Kidney Int 1982; 21: 122–6.

146. Teitelbaum S, Fallon M, Gearing G, Dougan C, Delmez J. The effects of CAPD on bone histomorphometry. Kidney Int 1982; 21: 180–4.

147. Loschiavo C, Fabris A, Adami S *et al.* The effects of CAPD on renal osteodystrophy. Perit Dial Bull 1985; 5: 53–5.

148. Nolph K, Ryan L, Prowant B, Twardowski Z. A cross sectional assessment of serum vitamin D and triglycerides in a CAPD population. Perit Dial Bull 1984; 4: 232.

149. Aloni Y, Shany S, Chaimovitz C. Losses of 25-hydroxy-vitamin D in peritoneal fluid: possible mechanism for bone disease in uraemic patients treated with CAPD. Miner Electrolyte Metab 1983; 9: 82–6.

150. Cassidy M, Owen J, Ellis H *et al.* Renal osteodystrophy and metastatic calcification in long term CAPD. Q J Med 1983; 213: 29–48.

151. Dunstan C, Hills E, Norman A *et al.* Treatment of haemodialysis bone disease with 24,25-dihydroxyvitamin D₃ and 1,25-dihydroxyvitamin D₃ alone or in combination. Miner Electrolyte Metab 1985; 11: 358–68.

152. Burbea Z, Gibor Y, Ladkani D *et al.* Combined oral treatment with 24,25(OH)₂D₃ and 1alpha(OH)D₃ regulates PTH level in secondary HPT of hemodialysis patients. Nephrol Dial Transplant 1992; 7: 755.

153. Gonzalez E, Bander S, Thieland B, Martin K. Comparison of intravenous and pulse oral calcitriol for suppression of PTH in patients on haemodialysis. J Am Soc Nephrol 1991; 2: 636 (abstract).

154. Schaefer K, Umlauf E, von Herrath D. Reduced risk of hypercalcaemia for hemodialysis patients by administering calcitriol at night. Am J Kidney Dis 1992; 19: 460–4.

155. Korkor A. Reduced binding of [3H] 1,25-dihydroxyvitamin D3 in the parathyroid glands of patients with renal failure. N Engl J Med 1987; 316: 1573–7.

156. Merke J, Hugel U, Zlotkowski A *et al.* Diminished parathyroid 1,25-(OH)2D3 receptors in experimental uremia. Kidney Int 1987; 32: 350–3.

157. Brown A, Dusso A, Lopez-Hilker S, Lewis-Finch J, Grooms P, Slatopolsky E. 1,25-(OH)2D3 receptors are decreased in parathyroid glands from chronically uremic dogs. Kidney Int 1989; 35: 19–23.

158. Scanziani R, Dozio B, Bonforte G, Surian M. Effects of calcitriol pulse therapy per os in CAPD patients. Adv Perit Dial 1994; 10: 270–4.

159. Bechtel U, Mucke C, Feucht HE, Schiffl H, Sitter T, Held E. Limitations of pulse oral calcitriol therapy in CAPD. Am J Kidney Dis 1995; 25: 291–6/.

160. Romanini D, Gazo A, Bellazzi R, Vincenzi A, Nai M, Santagostino M. Long term effect of oral calcitriol single weekly pulse in CAPD and HD. Adv Perit Dial 1994; 10: 267–9.

161. Fockens P, Hillen P, van Boven W, van Buchem-Ramakers T, Juttman J. Treatment of secondary hyperparathyroidism in haemodialysis patients by intravenous administration of vitamin D one-alpha derivatives. Calcif Tissue Int 1986; 39: A117.

162. Shoji S, Nishizawa Y, Tabata T *et al.* Influence of serum phosphate on the efficacy of oral 1,25 dihydroxyvitamin D3 pulse therapy. Miner Electrolyte Metab 1995; 21: 223–8.

163. Brown A, Ritter C, Finch J *et al.* The noncalcaemic analogue of vitamin D, 22-oxacalcitriol, suppresses parathyroid hormone synthesis and secretion. J Clin Invest 1989; 84: 728–32.

164. Brown A, Finch J, Lopez-Hilker S *et al.* New active analogues of vitamin D with low calcemic activity. Kidney Int 1990; 38 (suppl. 29): S22–7.

165. Kubrusly M, Gagne E, Hanrotel C, Lacour B, Drueke T. Effect of calcitriol versus 22-oxa-calcitriol on intestinal calcium transport in rats with severe chronic renal failure. Nephrol Dial Transplant 1992; 7: 761.

166. Kurokawa K, Akizawa T, Suzuki M, Akiba T, Ogata E, Slatopolsky E. Suppression of PTH by 22-oxacalcitriol in hemodialysis patients with secondary hyperparathyroidism. J Am Soc Nephrol 1995; 6: 966 (abstract).

167. Kurokawa K, Akizawa T, Suzuki M, Akiba T, Ogata E, Slatopolsky E. Effect of 22-oxacalcitriol on hyperparathyroidism of dialysis patients: results of a preliminary study. Nephrol Dial Transplant 1996; 11 (suppl. 3): 121–4.

168. Posner GH. New vitamin D analogues. Nephrol Dial Transplant 1996; 11 (suppl. 3): 32–6.

169. Sherrard DJ. Calcimimetics in action. Kidney Int 1998; 53: 510–11.

170. Ott SM. Calcimimetics – new drugs with the potential to control hyperparathyroidism. J Clin Endocrinol Metab 1998; 83: 1080–2.

171. Nemeth EF, Bennett SA. Tricking the parathyroid gland with novel calcimimetic agents. Neprol Dial Transplant 1998; 13: 1923–5.

172. McNair P, Christensen M, Madsbad S, Christensen C, Transbol I. Hypoparathyroidism in diabetes mellitus. Acta Endocrinol 1981; 96: 81–6.

173. Andress D, Hercz G, Kopp J *et al.* Bone histomorphometry of renal osteodystrophy in diabetic patients. J Bone Miner Res 1987; 2: 525–31.

174. Heidbreder E, Gotz R, Schafferhans K, Heidland A. Diminished parathyroid gland responsiveness to hypocalcemia in diabetic patients with uremia. Nephron 1986; 42: 285–9.

175. Cohen Solal M, Sebert J, Boudalliez B *et al.* Non-aluminic adynamic bone disease in non-dialyzed uremic patients: a new type of osteopathy due to over treatment? Bone 1992; 13: 1–5.

176. Fournier A, Moriniere P, Ben Hamidi F *et al.* Use of alkaline calcium salts as phosphate binder in uremic patients. Kidney Int 1992; 42 (suppl. 38): S50–61.

177. Mazzaferro S, Coen G, Ballanti P *et al.* Osteocalcin, iPTH, alkaline phosphatase and hand X-ray scores as predictive indices of histomorphometric parameters in renal osteodystrophy. Nephron 1990; 56: 261–6.

178. Maruyama Y, Arai K, Yoshida K *et al.* Study of tartrate resistant acid phosphatase in patients with chronic renal failure on maintenance hemodialysis. Nippon Jinzo Gakkai Shi 1991; 33: 297–302.

179. Stamatiades D, Stathakis C, Boletis J *et al.* Serum tartrate resistant acid phosphatase: a simple index for the evaluation of secondary hyperparathyroidism of patients on hemodialysis and CAPD. Perit Dial Int 1992; 12 (suppl. 2): 82.

180. Mohini R, Dumler F, Rao D. Skeletal surveys in renal osteodystrophy. ASAIO Trans 1991; 37: 635–7.

181. DeVita M, Rasenas L, Bansal M *et al.* Assessment of renal osteodystrophy in hemodialysis patients. Medicine 1992; 71: 284–90.

182. Olgaard K, Heerfordt J, Madsen S. Scintigraphic skeletal changes in uremic patients on regular hemodialysis. Nephron 1976; 17: 325–34.

183. Hodson E, Howman Giles R, Evans R *et al.* The diagnosis of renal osteodystrophy: a comparison of technetium 99m-pyrophosphate bone scintigraphy with other techniques. Clin Nephrol 1981; 16: 24–8.

184. Karsenty G, Vigneron N, Jogetti V *et al.* Value of the 99mTc-methylene diphosphonate bone scan in renal osteodystrophy. Kidney Int 1986; 29: 1058–65.

185. Heaf J, Nielsen L, Mogensen N. Use of bone mineral content determination in the evaluation of osteodystrophy among hemodialysis patients. Nephron 1983; 35: 103–7.

186. Rickers H, Christensen M, Rodbro P. Bone mineral content in patients on prolonged maintenance hemodialysis: a three-year follow-up study. Clin Nephrol 1983; 20: 302–7.

187. Lindergard B, Johnell O, Nilsson B, Wiklund P. Studies of bone morphology, bone densitometry and laboratory data in patients on maintenance hemodialysis treatment. Nephron 1985; 39: 122–9.

188. Piraino B, Chen T, Cooperstein L, Segre G, Puschett J. Fractures and vertebral bone mineral density in patients with renal osteodystrophy. Clin Nephrol 1988; 30: 57–62.

189. Funke M, Maurer J, Grabbe E, Scheler F. Comparitive studies with quantitative computed tomography and dual-energy X-ray absorptiometry on bone density in renal osteopathy. Rofo Fortschr Geb Rontgenstr Neuen Bildgeb Verfahr 1992; 157: 145–9.

20 Non-infectious complications of peritoneal dialysis

J. M. BARGMAN

Introduction

Peritoneal dialysis is associated with a collection of unique complications apart from peritonitis and those involving the catheter, exit site and tunnel. Some complications are related to increased intra-abdominal pressure, such as abdominal hernias and leaks of dialysis fluid. Other complications are similar to those encountered in haemodialysis patients. Examples of these include dialysis-associated amyloidosis and acquired cystic disease of the kidney. Finally, the long-term presence of dialysis fluid in the peritoneal cavity can result in a rare syndrome of sclerosing encapsulating peritonitis. This chapter will address these and other non-infectious complications of peritoneal dialysis.

Hernias

The presence of dialysis fluid in the peritoneal cavity leads to increased intra-abdominal pressure (IAP). Pressure within the abdomen rises in proportion to the volume of dialysate instilled [1, 2]. The supine patient generates the lowest IAP for a given volume of intraperitoneal fluid. Even in the supine patient on automated peritoneal dialysis, intraperitoneal pressure is closely correlated with the volume of instilled dialysate [3]. Coughing and straining in the sitting and upright positions result in the highest pressures. In addition, patients who are older, and those who are more obese, generate higher IAP for a given activity [2].

In accordance with Laplace's law, the tension on the abdominal wall increases with the instillation of dialysate, as a result of the rise in IAP and the larger radius of the abdomen. Increased abdominal pressure and abdominal wall tension lead to hernia formation in those with congenital or acquired defects in or around the abdomen. The areas of weakness are probably very important in the pathogenesis of

hernias. Indeed, the IAP in patients with hernias is no different from the pressure measured in those without hernias [4]. A host of hernias has been described in peritoneal dialysis (PD) patients (Table 1). The most common hernia is incisional or through the catheter placement site [5, 6]; in other reports inguinal [7–10] or umbilical [11–13] (Fig. 1) hernias occur most frequently. Asymptomatic hernias are probably quite common and may not be detected until some complication such as bowel strangulation occur. Different centres report a cumulative incidence of 10–15% of hernias in their PD patients [6, 14]. Patients with hernias tend to be older, female, multiparous, those who have experienced a higher frequency of postoperative leak at the time of catheter insertion [6], and those who have undergone a previous hernia repair [5]. The mean time for development of hernia is 1 year and the risk increases by 20% for each year on continuous ambulatory peritoneal dialysis (CAPD) [5]. Patients with polycystic kidney disease may be predisposed to hernia formation and leaks either as a result of higher IAP caused by the large kidneys or as a manifestation of a generalized disorder of collagen [15, 16].

A major potential area of weakness is the abdominal incision for the implantation of the dialysis catheter. When this incision is made in the midline there is a predilection for incisional hernia to develop because this is an anatomically weak area [17]. Change to a paramedian incision through the rectus

Table 1. Hernias in patients on peritoneal dialysis

Umbilical [5–7, 9–13]	Incisional [5–7, 9, 11, 18]
Inguinal [5–11, 13]	Cystocoele [6] Foramen of Morgagni [20, 21]
Catheter incision site [4, 7, 10, 23, 25]	Richter's [24, 33]
	Enterocoele [6, 34]
Ventral [7, 10, 13]	Spigelian [35]
Catheter exit site	Obturator [22, 36]
Epigastric [5, 6, 9]	

R. Gokal, R. Khanna, R.Th. Krediet and K.D. Nolph (eds.), Textbook of Peritoneal Dialysis, 2nd Edition, 609–646.
© 2000 Kluwer Academic Publishers. Printed in Great Britain.

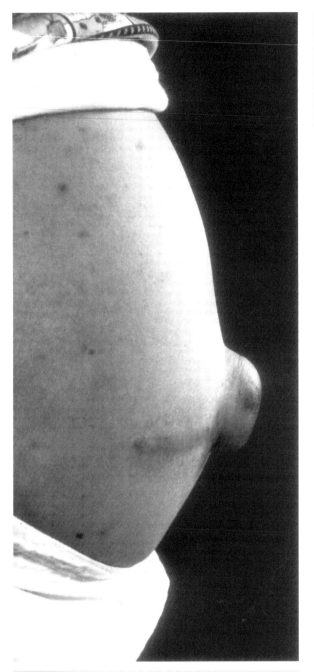

Figure 1. Umbilical hernia in a peritoneal dialysis patient.

muscle has resulted in less perioperative leaks and hernia formation [18].

Another area of potential weakness for herniation is the processus viginalis. After the migration of the testes in fetal life, the processus viginalis normally undergoes obliteration. Frequently this does not occur, and the increased abdominal pressure during CAPD may push bowel into the processus viginalis, resulting in an indirect inguinal hernia. Male paedi-

atric patients may be predisposed to this complication, and if they develop a unilateral inguinal hernia, both sides should probably be repaired prophylactically [19].

Most hernias present as a painless swelling [6]. Bowel has been reported to herniate through the diaphragm at the foramen of Morgagni and present as a retrosternal air–fluid level or juxtacardiac mass [21, 21]. The rate obturator hernia can present with increasing paraesthesia and hyperaesthesia in the thigh [22].

The most worrisome complications are incarceration and strangulation of bowel. This can occur through almost any kind of hernia, but especially a small one. Umbilical hernias may have a particular predilection for bowel strangulation [14]. Hernias may present as a tender lump [23, 24], recurrent Gram-negative peritonitis, bowel obstruction or perforation [6, 25, 26]. Bowel incarceration or strangulation can mimic peritonitis [9, 24, 25] and this complication must be kept in mind, particularly if the site of herniation itself is not obvious.

With the recent trend of emphasis on adequacy of small-solute transport, many patients are being prescribed larger volumes of dialysate such as 2.5 and 3.0 L fill volumes. As discussed, increased fill volumes are associated with increased IAP. It remains to be seen whether the higher fill volumes will lead to an increased incidence of hernias and dialysate leaks. The higher pressures secondary to the bigger volumes may possibly be offset by the growing trend of automated dialysis, wherein the patient dialyses mostly in the supine position. Two recent reports found no increase in the incidence of hernia with larger dialysis volumes, although there was an increase in the use of cyclers, which may have confounded the effect [27, 28].

Treatment of hernias

Hernias warrant surgical repair. Although large ventral hernias carry little measurable risk of bowel incarceration [29] they are unsightly and prone to enlarge. The other types of hernias should be repaired because of the risk of bowel incarceration and strangulation. The patient can be maintained temporarily on low-volume PD preoperatively to allow time for wound healing. Conventional hernioplasty may be followed by the insertion of an overlying polypropylene mesh to reinforce the hernia repair [30]. The addition of the mesh may afford a quicker return to full-volume dialysis [31]. Subsequent development of peritonitis does not appear to be complicated by mesh infection [30]. In the mal-nourished patient, even low-tension repair with a mesh can fail with recurrence of hernia [32]. If hernias recur, other options include changing the patient to night-time cycler dialysis, in which the patient dialyses supine (and hence under lower IAP) or using lower volumes of dialysate but with more frequent exchanges.

Genital oedema

Oedema of the labia majora or scrotum and penis is a distressing complication of PD. Early reports suggested that up to 10% of CAPD patients could experience genital oedema [37–42], although more recent reports document a lower incidence of this complication [43, 44]. It appears that women have a much lower incidence of genital oedema compared to men [43, 44]. This disparity may be the result of the processus viginalis being patent more often in males; alternatively, labial swelling may not be as noticeable compared to swelling over the penis and scrotum. On the other hand, rarely dialysate can dissect through the pouch of Douglas, the vaginal vault, or even travel through the Fallopian tubes and present with leakage through the vagina [45–49].

Two mechanisms have been suggested to explain genital oedema [37]. First, dialysate can track through the soft-tissue plane from the catheter inser-tion site, from a soft-tissue defect within a hernia, or from a peritoneo-fascial defect. In any of these cases, genital oedema can be associated with oedema of the anterior abdominal wall [38]. Secondly, dialysis fluid can travel through a patent processus vaginalis to the labia or scrotum where it may leak into the surrounding soft tissue. This has been particularly described in young boys on PD [50, 51]. If bowel accompanies the dialysate through the processus viginalis, there will be an associated inguinal hernia; in fact, the presence of scrotal oedema may suggest a clinically occult indirect inguinal hernia [39].

The presence of abdominal wall oedema suggests that the origin of the peritoneal leak is proximal to the inguinal region in one of the potential sites listed above. On clinical examination the patient should stand. Asymmetry of the abdomen may indicate dialysis leak into the abdominal wall. Moreover, when the dialysate has dissected superficially, the abdominal wall can look pale and boggy. The skin indentations made by an elastic waistband, underwear or by the catheter lying across the abdo-men look deeper and more prominent than usual.

Treatment of genital oedema

Treatment of actual genital oedema includes bed rest, scrotal elevation if symptomatic, and the use of frequent low-volume exchanges by cycler, if possible [37]. In the case of abdominal wall leaks, cessation of PD for a week or two, or conversion of nocturnal PD (with dry days), for 2 weeks may be sufficient to allow healing of the leak [52]. Many or most patients can resume CAPD [38]. It is unclear whether antibiotics should be given prophylactically in the case of pericatheter leaks, but they are recom-mended in some centres [53].

There is some experience with infiltration of the catheter cuff *in situ* with fibrin glue to stop pericath-eter leakage [54]. Preliminary results suggest that infiltration of the deep cuff with fibrin glue at cath-eter implantation may prevent subsequent pericath-eter leakage of dialysate [55].

Radiological and isotopic diagnosis of hernias and genital oedema

Abdominal scintigraphy with technetium 99m has proven successful in identifying and locating the site of abdominal leaks or a patent processus viginalis. Different radioligands have been used with the tracer including DTPA, albumin colloid and tin colloid. One to five millicuries are injected into 0.5 to 2 L of dialysate [37, 42, 56, 57]. It has been suggested that the patient sit up and lean forward to encourage the radiolabelled dialysate into the leaking sites [58]. Delayed images after ambulation may be necessary to detect the leak [59, 60]. In addition, multiple projections should be taken in order to separate an abdominal wall leak from the peritoneal dialysate directly posterior to it [59]. While the dose of iso-tope may seem hefty, much of the radiation is drained out of the body with the dialysate after the study. Therefore, the net dose of radiation is only a fraction of that originally instilled in the peritoneal cavity [58].

Computerized tomographic (CT) scanning can be helpful in diagnosing leaks and the cause of genital oedema. Different agents (iopamidol, diatrizoate) have been employed in various volumes of dialysis fluid. It makes sense to use the largest volume tolera-ble in conjunction with manoeuvres to raise the IAP in order to facilitate fluid egress from the peritoneal cavity [61]. Peritoneal installation of radiocontrast dye with CT scanning detects more leaks and hernias compared to plain peritoneography without CT scanning [61–64]. CT scanning can demonstrate collections of dialysate/dye in the anterior abdominal wall which can track inferiorly and collect in the scrotum. Alternatively, dye can be visualized in the processus vaginalis as a cord-like structure and subsequent cuts can follow this inferiorly to the genitalia. Within the scrotal sac it can often be discerned whether the contrast/dialysate forms a hydrocoele or whether the fluid has dissected through the tunica vaginalis into the scrotal wall itself.

Hydrothorax

Increased IAP can result in leak of dialysis fluid from the peritoneal cavity, across the diaphragm, and into the pleural space. The accumulation of dialysis fluid in the pleural cavity is called hydrothorax. It is not clear how often hydrothorax occurs in patients receiving PD. Most studies estimate that the incidence is less than 5%, which would make it a less frequent consequence of raised IAP than abdominal hernias [65–70]. In one study the incidence was as high as 10% [71]. However, it is possible that hydrothorax does occur even more frequently, but does not come to medical attention if the patient is asymptomatic or if minor complaints of shortness of breath are overlooked.

Pathogenesis of hydrothorax

A defect in the diaphragm must be present to allow flux of dialysis fluid from the peritoneal into the pleural cavity. Autopsy studies have revealed localized absence of muscle fibres in the hemidiaphragm [72, 73]. These missing muscle fibres are replaced with a disordered network of collagen. One or more defects in the tendinous part of the hemidiaphragm have been observed [72–75].

When hydrothorax has been investigated by surgery or pleuroscopy, 'blisters' or 'blebs' have sometimes been noted on the pleural surface of the diaphragm. Presumably these represent the areas of deficiency in the usual support structures of the diaphragm described at autopsy [75]. With the installation of dialysis fluid into the peritoneal cavity these blebs can be seen to swell, weep and even rupture, thus providing the pathway for the movement of dialysate into the pleural space.

In paediatric patients receiving PD who develop hydrothorax, diaphragmatic eventration rather than hernia has been described at surgery [76].

It is likely that these defects in the musculotendinous part of the diaphragm are not rare occurrences

but, in a manner similar to patent processus vaginalis, come to medical attention only when there is fluid in the abdominal cavity under increased pressure. This explains why hydrothorax has been described in patients on PD and in those with liver disease or with ovarian cancer and ascites.

The extent of the deficiency in the hemidiaphragm varies among patients. Those with a preexistent clear connection between peritoneal and pleural space probably correspond to those patients who develop hydrothorax with their first-ever infusion of dialysis fluid. In contrast, there are patients who develop hydrothorax months to years after starting PD. Presumably those patients have attenuated tissue separating pleural from peritoneal space, and it may take repeated exposure to raised IAP or an episode of peritonitis to remove the barrier between the two cavities.

It has been suggested that in a subset of patients with hydrothorax there is a one-way passage between peritoneal and pleural cavities. This phenomenon might explain the persistence of hydrothorax after drainage of dialysis effluent. Postulated mechanisms for one-way flow include a valve-like defect in the diaphragm, or the action of the hepatic capsule to tamponade backflow of dialysate from the pleural to the peritoneal space [77].

In rare instances dialysis fluid may flux into the pericardial space, particularly if communication between the two cavities had been established by previous pericardiocentesis [78–80].

Diagnosis of hydrothorax

The majority of patients with hydrothorax are women. The reason for this sexual predominance is not clear, although stretching of the hemidiaphragm from previous pregnancy has been suggested [75]. The pleural collection is almost always on the right side, a phenomenon also noted with Meigs syndrome and hepatic ascites. It may be that the presence of the heart and pericardium prevent flux of fluid across the left hemidiaphragm [75].

Finally, patients whose renal failure is the result of autosomal dominant polycystic kidney disease may have a higher risk of developing hydrothorax on PD. Possible explanations include higher than average IAP resulting from the space occupied by the large kidneys, or perhaps greater inherent weakness of the diaphragm as a part of a generalized membrane defect seen in this condition [81, 82].

Small pleural effusions can be asymptomatic and are detected by routine chest radiographs. Larger pleural effusions can lead to respiratory embarrassment.

The shortness of breath which results from the pleural effusion can be mistaken for congestive heart failure. The patient may choose more hypertonic dialysis solutions in an effort to increase ultrafiltration. In the patient with hydrothorax, however, increased ultrafiltration will lead to even greater IAP with further flux of dialysate into the pleural space, worsening the symptoms. Therefore, a history of a patient complaining of dyspnoea that appears to worsen with hypertonic dialysate should suggest the possibility of hydrothorax, particularly if effluent returns are less than normal (i.e. they are trapped in the pleural space).

Physical examination is consistent with pleural effusion, with absent breath sounds and stony dullness to percussion in the lung base. Tension hydrothorax has rarely been reported [83].

Chest X-ray shows a pleural effusion which occurs on the right side in most patients. Clearly other causes for pleural effusion should be ruled out, including local parenchymal lung disease, congestive heart failure or pleuritis. The scenario wherein a patient develops a large right-sided pleural effusion with the first few dialyses is strongly suggestive of hydrothorax. However, in a patient on CAPD for months who develops peritonitis, fluid overload and pleural effusion, making the correct diagnosis can be more difficult.

In the patient in whom the aetiology of the pleural effusion is uncertain, a thoracentesis can be helpful in making the correct diagnosis. If the pleural fluid is composed of dialysate, the glucose concentration is very high (usually greater than 40 mmol/L) and the fluid has a low protein concentration consistent with a transudate. Some investigators have pointed out that the *dextro* isomer of lactate is present in dialysis fluid but not in 'endogenous' pleural effusions, and this is another way of identifying dialysate in the pleural fluid [84]. However, most laboratories are not equipped to rapidly detect D-lactate, and certainly glucose concentration remains an easier and cheaper way to look for dialysis fluid.

It has been suggested that the dye methylene blue can be instilled in the periotoneal cavity before the pleural tap, and blue staining of the pleural fluid provides evidence of peritoneal–pleural communication. However, intraperitoneal methylene blue can lead to chemical peritonitis; furthermore, the blue staining may be so faint as not to be appreciated in the pleural fluid, leading to a false-negative result [85].

Even when the diagnosis is certain, thoracentesis should also be used in patients who are short of breath from the hydrothorax. Evacuation of one or more litres of fluid should lead to significant improvement in the patient's respiratory status.

In the absence of thoracentesis, the presence of a peritoneal–pleural communication can be confirmed by isotopic scanning. In different studies, between 3 and 10 mCi of technetium-labelled macro-aggregated albumin or sulphur colloid has been instilled into the peritoneal cavity along with the usual volume of dialysis fluid. The patient should move around to ensure mixing of the radioisotope and dialysate and to raise the IAP. Subsequent scanning detects movement of the isotope above the hemidiaphragm. This usually is detectable in the first few minutes, but sometimes late pictures (up to 6 h) need to be taken. This method is convenient but not absolutely foolproof. Defects have been found in the diaphragm at surgery in patients in whom isotopic scanning was negative [86–89].

Other studies have reported the use of contrast peritoneography using diatrizoate and iopamidol, but experience with these non-isotopic methods is limited [90].

Treatment of hydrothorax

Thoracentesis is recommended for the immediate treatment of hydrothorax if respiratory compromise is present. Otherwise, simply discontinuing PD often leads to rapid and dramatic resolution of the pleural effusion [69, 70, 91, 92]. In a small number of patients the effusion is slow to resolve, suggesting that there may be a one-way or ball-valve type communication between peritoneal and pleural space, as previously discussed. In this instance, thoracentesis may be helpful to hasten the resolution of the pleural effusion.

Subsequent treatment depends on whether the patient is going to continue on peritoneal dialysis. The occurrence of hydrothorax occasionally is so distressing to the patient that he or she may request transfer to haemodialysis. In this case the communication between peritoneal and pleural space should be of no consequence and nothing further needs to be done once the effusion has resolved.

If the patient is going to continue with PD there are a number of different options:

Temporary haemodialysis (2–4 weeks) with subsequent return to CAPD

Especially in the presence of peritonitis, there may be a transient loss of the integrity of the cell layers overlying a diaphragmatic defect. If PD is temporarily discontinued and the mesothelium allowed to reconstitute itself over the defect, it is possible that the peritoneo–pleural communication may become re-sealed. It is less likely that this would be effective in those patients demonstrating pleural leak with the first dialysis, but even this phenomenon has been reported after a 2-month hiatus on haemodialysis. It has been suggested that the dialysate in the pleural space may act as a sclerosing agent and prevent subsequent leaks [93].

Temporary haemodialysis with a return to a PD regimen with lower IAP

Patients who experience hydrothorax on CAPD are sometimes able to resume PD by cycler. Even though the supine position might be thought of as conducive to the movement of fluid into the pleural cavity, it appears to be more than compensated by the reduction in IAP afforded by this posture [94]. The use of smaller dialysis volumes with more frequent exchanges is helpful in minimizing the increment in IAP [95, 96].

Obliteration of the pleural space ('pleurodesis')

Previous studies have reported the successful obliteration of the pleural cavity. In this instance the leaves of the pleura stick together and prevent the re-accumulation of pleural fluid.

There are various agents used to induce pleurodesis. Oxytetracycline (20 mg/kg) has been administered via a thoracostomy tube [70, 71, 84, 91]. It is important that the patient remain supine, up to 24 h, and assume different positions, including head-down, to ensure exposure of the agent to all the pleural surfaces. The patient should also receive analgesia, as this procedure can be painful. Talc has also been reported as a successful agent for pleurodesis [97–99].

Obliteration of the pleural cavity has also been accomplished by the instillation of 40–100 ml of autologous blood. The patient should be maintained, if possible, on haemodialysis for a few weeks to allow the pleurodesis to take place. More than one installation of blood may be necessary, but the benefit of the blood is that it appears to be a relatively painless procedure compared to the use of talc or tetracycline [100–102]. There are reports from Japan of the use of OK-432, a haemolytic streptococcal preparation, and the use of *Nocardia rubra* cell wall skeleton to effect pleurodesis [70].

Finally, a combination of aprotinin–calcium-chloride–thrombin and 'fibrin glue' instilled in the drained pleural cavity was reported to successfully prevent recurrent hydrothorax in a patient who had previously failed treatment with other agents [103].

Operative repair

At thoracotomy a communication between peritoneal and pleural space may be visualized. Sometimes the 'blebs' or blisters are quickly recognized and these can be sutured and reinforced with Teflon felt patches [75]. It is recommended that 2–3 L of dialysate be infused into the peritoneal cavity through the dialysis catheter. The diaphragm is inspected from the pleural side for seepage of dialysate through holes or blisters. It is important that the surgeon be patient as it may take time for the seepage to be recognized [104, 105].

In the case of eventration of the diaphragm, as reported in the paediatric literature, surgical repair can be effected by plication with non-absorbable suture. These patients are able to return to PD successfully [76, 106].

In summary, hydrothorax is a well-described but relatively uncommon complication of PD. Diagnosis is relatively simple once the possibility of peritoneal–pleural communication has been entertained. Thoracentesis may be necessary to confirm the diagnosis and is mandated by respiratory embarrassment. If the patient is willing to continue with PD, several treatment options are available.

Respiratory complications

The effects of CAPD on respiration can be divided into those related to the physical presence of dialysis fluid in the peritoneal cavity, and its effect on the mechanics of breathing, and those resulting from the carbohydrate loading of dialysate glucose absorption, which can affect intermediary metabolism and change respiration in a substrate-driven manner. Sleep apnoea is increasingly recognized in end-stage renal disease patients and will be discussed separately.

Changes in pulmonary function resulting from altered mechanics of breathing

Early studies of PD suggested that this procedure compromised respiratory function [107]. However, these and other studies were reported in acutely ill subjects, and many other factors could have affected the integrity of the lungs, pleura and respiratory muscles. Later studies of stable patients on chronic

PD demonstrated that 2 L of dialysis fluid in the abdomen resulted in reduction of most lung volumes, including the functional residual capacity (FRC) [108–113]. These changes can persist [112] or normalize after only 2 weeks on CAPD [110].

It has been suggested that as the FRC decreases to less than the closing volume, small airways will collapse and cause ventilation–perfusion mismatch and arterial hypoxaemia [114]. At the outset of dialysis, instillation of dialysate is associated with an average 5 mmHg fall in arterial p_{O_2} in the sitting position and an average 8 mmHg decrease when the patient is supine. These changes are seen in association with a fall in FRC. When these patients are re-studied a few months later, there is no longer a decrement in arterial P_{O_2}, despite a similar fall in FRC. It has been suggested that some long-term adjustment takes place, such as redistribution of blood away from the more poorly ventilated lower segments of the lungs [111]. Other studies have not confirmed arterial hypoxaemia in patients on PD [108, 110, 115], although arterial hypoxaemia has recently been reported in both haemodialysis and PD patients with polycystic kidney disease while ambulatory, which was improved in assuming the supine position [116].

The changes in lung volumes have not been found to be any more severe in patients with chronic obstructive airways disease [110], and it has been advised that obstructive airways disease should not be regarded as a contraindication to the use of PD [117]. In the case of severe pulmonary disease the advice is to perform a trial of instillation of PD fluid with monitoring of pulmonary function before committing the patient to peritoneal access surgery [118]. It has been demonstrated by total-body plethysmography that the presence of 2 L of dialysis fluid has no effect on airways resistance [112]. Indeed, it is conceivable that the presence of dialysis fluid in the abdomen can facilitate pulmonary function. This change may be explainable by altered diaphragmatic contractility secondary to stretch of the diaphragm caused by the dialysate [109]; that is, with increased length of the muscle fibres there is improved muscle function. Explained in another way, the presence of the intraperitoneal fluid increases the upward curvature of the diaphragm. The radius of the new curve is smaller. Laplace's law dictates that the diaphragm generates more pressure for a given amount of muscle tension when the radius is smaller. Therefore, the contractility of the diaphragm may increase in the presence of intraperitoneal fluid [119]. This effect is analogous to

the benefit which the patient with obstructive airways disease achieves by holding a pillow tightly against the abdomen. However, there is an upper limit to this relationship, after which the diaphragm loses efficiency and compromise of ventilation occurs [119]. More sophisticated testing, including electromyographic recording of the diaphragm using intragastric and intra-oesophageal catheters, has confirmed that diaphragmatic strength is significantly improved when the abdomen is filled with dialysate. This parameter was measured as the maximum transdiaphragmatic pressure. The improvement in strength again was suggested to be a result of an adaptive change in the diaphragm's force–length ratio as a result of tonic stretch from the intra-abdominal dialysate [120].

A study of pulmonary function in predialysis, PD, haemodialysis and renal transplant patients showed that the diffusion factor for carbon monoxide, while reduced in all the groups, was significantly lower in the group of patients on CAPD, with a mean DLCO just under 70% of predicted value. The authors postulated that this surprising finding was most likely the result of subclinical pulmonary oedema (potentiated by the low serum albumin in the CAPD group) or else the result of interstitial fibrosis caused by repeated episodes of pulmonary oedema [121]. However, another intriguing possibility is that the raised IAP leads to reflux, chronic aspiration, and the consequent development of restrictive lung disease [122]. In a related way, reflux has been implicated as a cause of chronic cough in patients on PD [123].

Substrate-induced changes in respiration

The nature and availability of energy substrate can alter intermediary metabolism and affect ventilation. This relationship has been described in patients undergoing total parenteral nutrition, where hypercaloric glucose and amino acid solutions produce significant increase in minute ventilation, carbon dioxide excretion and oxygen consumption [124]. A theoretical treatment of substrate absorption during CAPD predicts that the absorption of glucose and, to a lesser extent, lactate would drive intermediary metabolism and lead to the changes in respiration described above. The increase in metabolically driven ventilation could prove dangerous to the patient with lung disease [124].

Studies in patients on CAPD confirm increased minute volume, oxygen consumption and carbon dioxide excretion compared to controls [125]. This suggests that the lactate and glucose absorbed are incorporated into the Krebs cycle. Moreover, because some of the glucose is metabolized in a manner that does not require oxygen, but does produce carbon dioxide, the respiratory quotient increases. In the normal situation, however, the arterial P_{CO_2} does not increase, because the patient is stimulated to hyperventilate and 'blow off' the extra carbon dioxide. In the patient who is too ill to hyperventilate, this may not be the case. Cohn and co-workers described a patient with systemic lupus erythematosus and renal and respiratory failure who developed acute respiratory acidosis each time a high-glucose dialysis solution was used. The acidosis would abate when the dialysis was changed to one with a lower concentration of glucose. The authors suggested that the carbohydrate loading led to lipogenesis, a process associated with a respiratory quotient (CO_2 produced per O_2 used) as great as 8. In the patient with compromised ventilatory status and respiratory muscle dysfunction, the extra carbon dioxide could not be exhaled quickly enough, and so hypercapnoea ensued. The use of dialysis solutions with lower glucose concentration resulted in less net glucose absorption and hence less substrate-driven carbon dioxide production [126].

Sleep apnoea

Obstructive sleep opnoea is characterized by repeated bouts of apnoea which each last for 10 s or more. Often the apnoea is recognized by snoring with the resumption of breathing, and by its sequela of excessive daytime somnolence. The apnoeas can result in arterial hypoxaemia and hypercapnoea, which in turn can lead to pulmonary arterial and systemic hypertension. The apnoeic periods are broken by the arousal reaction, accompanied by sympathetic outflow. This sympathetic response or other responses are probably responsible for the association between cardiovascular and cerebrovascular disease and sleep apnoea [127, 128].

Both haemodialysis and PD patients often report disturbances of sleep, including non-restorative sleep, early wakening and daytime sleepiness. The contribution of sleep disturbances in general, and obstructive sleep apnoea in particular, to these symptoms is unknown. In addition, whether PD confers an additional insult to sleep by the presence of dialysate (or dialysate exchange by automated cyclers) during sleeping time is unknown. Unlike conventional haemodialysis, PD effects solute flux during the sleeping hours. Besides the potential disturbance of 2 or more litres of dialysate in the peritoneal cavity, potential sleep-enhancing molecules might be dialysed out during a long overnight dwell [129].

Studies on sleeping patterns in patients on PD suffer from small numbers, and the patients who are recruited report significant sleep disturbances. Therefore, results from these studies are probably not generalizable to the PD population as a whole. In the subset of patients reporting these disturbances, polysomnography demonstrates a high prevalence ($> 50\%$) of obstructive sleep apnoea [127, 130, 131]. This prevalence is comparable to that of a cohort of self-selected haemodialysis patients with sleep disturbances [127, 130]. While the prevalence appears excessive, it is in a self-referred group with sleep disturbances. It is still not clear whether there is a truly higher general prevalence of sleep apnoea in dialysis patients, and if so, what it is about the renal failure that should lead to this association.

Studies in PD patients suggest that the presence of the dialysate in the peritoneal cavity does not confer additional disturbance of sleep unless that patient has obstructive sleep apnoea. In the small numbers of apnoeic patients there was striking arterial hypoxaemia when the patients slept with dialysate *in situ* (P_{O_2} 78 ± 7 mmHg) than when they slept without dialysis fluid (P_{O_2} 92 ± 4 mmHg). Sleep as a whole was also more disturbed with dialysate in the peritoneal cavity [130]. Again, whether the difference is the result of the physical presence of the dialysate, with attendant changes in intra-abdominal or diaphragmatic pressures, or a metabolic effect of the dialysis fluid is unclear.

Acid–base and electrolyte disorders

Disorders of water metabolism

In patients on PD the serum sodium concentration will depend on the relative amount of salt and water ingested and the net salt and water flux across the peritoneal membrane. Renal excretion may contribute in those with residual renal function. Sodium flux into the peritoneal cavity in the PD patient is caused by diffusion and convection. Because sodium is sieved by the peritoneal membrane, the fluid entering the peritoneal cavity by osmotically driven flow is hyponatraemic, that is, more water than salt flows from plasma to peritoneal compartment [132, 133]. In theory this flux should leave the patient with a relative water deficit; the patient should become hypernatraemic. However, hypertonicity is a powerful stimulant of ADH secretion, which in turn stimulates thirst. The patient will drink water or some other hypotonic fluid until tonicity is restored. In fact, patients on CAPD may actually demonstrate plasma sodium concentrations slightly lower than normal. There are a number of reasons for the relative water excess, including increased water intake or low sodium concentration in the dialysis solution [134]. Infants undergoing PD and fed normal infant formula may be prone to hyponatraemia because sodium losses from ultrafiltration are greater than sodium gained from ingestion of formula. Moreover, the proprietary infant formulas have a high water to sodium ratio, leading to water accumulation and hyponatraemia [135].

In a study of insulin-dependent diabetics with hyperglycaemia, those on haemodialysis were able to nearly normalize the serum tonicity, whereas PD patients remained hypertonic owing to continued loss of water in excess of solute into the dialysate. In hyperglycaemia the increased extracellular glucose effects osmotic flux of water from the intracellular compartment to the extracellular fluid compartment, which brings the extracellular osmolality towards normal. The fall in serum sodium concentration resulting from this movement of water into the extracellular compartment can be predicted. Patients on haemodialysis, however, demonstrate a greater fall in serum sodium concentration than do hyperglycaemic patients not on dialysis. On the other hand, patients on PD behave more like the non-dialysis patients. One explanation is that the haemodialysis patient drinks water in response to increased plasma osmolality, and in the absence of ongoing osmotic diuresis, is able to lower plasma tonicity. In contrast, the patient on PD undergoes continuous loss of water in excess of sodium (see above), and in this way mimics the effect of the osmotic diuresis seen in hyperglycaemia with normal renal function. The excess loss of water can perpetuate the hyperosmolar state [136].

Another cause of hyponatraemia is intracellular potassium depletion. In this instance sodium fluxes into the cell to replete the intracellular cation balance. Whether hyponatraemia is a surrogate for potassium depletion (and malnutrition) in the dialysis patient remains to be determined.

Disorders of potassium metabolism

Hypokalaemia is found in 10–36% OF CAPD patients [137–139]. Hypokalaemia can be pro-

found, as reported in a diabetic CAPD patient with vomiting and diarrhoea [140]. Ongoing losses of potassium in the dialysate may contribute to hypokalaemia in some patients. This may be compounded by poor nutritional intake, particularly of potassium-replete foods such as fruits and vegetables. A recent examination of hypokalaemia in a single PD unit concluded that black race was the strongest predictor of hypokalaemia. This finding was ascribed to avoidance of fruit and vegetables as the result of ethnocultural food preferences [139]. However, in general, other factors such as cellular uptake and bowel losses play a role. Muscle biopsy studies show that the muscle potassium content is increased in CAPD patients, presumably reflecting intracellular uptake [134].

The abnormal potassium metabolism of end-stage renal disease may contribute to the increased cardiac morbidity and mortality seen in dialysis patients [141]. It is recommended that the serum potassium concentration be maintained at greater than 3.0 mmol/L in the asymptomatic patient, and greater than 3.5 mmol/L in the patient on digoxin or with a history of cardiac arrhythmias [142]. Potassium supplementation should be monitored in dialysis patients because of the absence of renal reserve to excrete excess potassium. Potassium chloride can be added to the dialysate to diminish the concentration gradient for diffusion of potassium into the dialysis fluid. In the acute setting, up to 20 mmol/L of KCl can be added to the dialysate with a low incidence of side-effects. This dose has been reported to increase the plasma potassium concentration by an average 0.44 mmol/L over 2–3 h. However, the effect of this hyperkalaemic solution on the peritoneal membrane is unknown, so this treatment should be used only in urgent settings [137].

Hyperkalaemia is occasionally seen in acute PD and CAPD patients. It has been noted to occur after acute renal failure [143, 144] and has been attributed to breakdown of glycogen with consequent release of potassium. Other factors which affect extrarenal potassium disposal, such as insulin deficiency, converting enzyme inhibitors and beta-blockers, should be considered.

Acid–base balance

In health the kidneys help to maintain acid–base balance via excretion of acid and generation of new bicarbonate. As the kidneys fail, however, net acid excretion diminishes and metabolic acidosis develops. It is important, therefore, that any form of dialysis provide replenishment of buffer.

In the early years of PD, bicarbonate, the obvious choice, was employed as a buffer. However, bicarbonate reacts with calcium chloride, leading to precipitation of calcium carbonate. Therefore, other less reactive buffers had to be used, and experience has accumulated with lactate and acetate. Dialysate containing glucose must be kept at pH 5–6 to prevent caramelization. At equimolar concentrations of acetate and lactate, acetate demonstrates higher titratable acidity. Therefore, when instilled into the peritoneal cavity, solutions containing acetate remain acidic longer than to lactate-based solutions [145]. The prolonged acidity of the solution may explain reports of abdominal pain and chemical peritonitis with the use of acetate-based dialysate [145, 146] (other long-term effects of acetate are discussed in the section on sclerosing peritonitis). Serum lactate remains low in patients receiving lactate-containing dialysate. Patients receiving equimolar amounts of acetate-containing dialysate, on the other hand, demonstrate abnormally high levels of plasma acetate [147]. This finding suggests that less lactate is absorbed, or it is more efficiently metabolized than acetate. The patient receiving lactate shows normal serum bicarbonate levels [147, 148] suggesting that adequate amounts of lactate are being absorbed and converted to bicarbonate. In PD patients, gain of alkali from ingested food and absorption from the dialysate just matches daily acid production, so that these patients are in acid–base balance [149]. The dialysate lactate is composed of both the easily metabolized L isomer and the slowly metabolized D isomer. Both isomers are absorbed from dialysate in equal amounts. The lack of accumulation of the D isomer in blood suggests that it is indeed metabolized to a significant extent [150, 151], although previous investigations have suggested otherwise [152]. The fate of absorbed D-lactate is of concern because of reports of cerebral dysfunction in patients with high blood levels of this isomer [153]. During intermittent PD there is a net gain in body buffer of about 80 mmol, the result of lactate absorption surpassing bicarbonate loss from plasma to dialysate. High rates of ultrafiltration mitigate this effect via both increased loss of bicarbonate and diminished absorption of lactate. Presumably this is on the basis of convective forces [150, 154]. Indeed, this is consistent with a recent report in which high transporters (who ultrafilter less well) had higher systemic pH and plasma bicarbonate concentration compared to low transporters. How-

ever, the authors suggested that the higher transporters also had greater net gain of lactate which was subsequently utilized as buffer [155].

Ammonium chloride loading has demonstrated that patients on CAPD tolerate an acid load better than patients receiving haemodialysis. The tolerance does not seem to increase with time on CAPD [156].

Use of lactate does have its drawbacks. Its use in patients with lactic acidosis may worsen the metabolic derangement [157, 158]. In this setting, specially prepared bicarbonate-based solutions are recommended [159], or the use of a proportioning system similar to that used in bicarbonate-based haemodialysis [160]. Lactate may be an inappropriate buffer in patients with hepatic failure. In this setting lactate may not be sufficiently converted to bicarbonate, leading to acidosis and lactate accumulation [144, 161]. In this context metformin, an oral hypoglycaemic agent, should not be used in PD patients, because of the risk of lactic acidosis [162, 163]. Future PD solutions which are bicarbonate-based should mitigate these problems [164].

Optimal correction of metabolic acidosis may be important to prevent negative protein balance. Both short-term and long-term studies suggest that correcting metabolic acidosis is associated with diminished protein catabolism and increased body weight and midarm circumference, an index of nutrition [165, 166]. Cross-sectional surveys of serum pH or bicarbonate levels compared to nutritional state are confounded by the observation that patients with high protein intake may be more acidaemic as a result of metabolism of these proteins. Therefore, the relationship between acidosis and nutritional state may not be obvious [167, 168]. In other words, metabolic acidosis may lead to body protein breakdown, but high protein intake and good nutritional status may be associated with a mild metabolic acidosis. Surveys and cross-sectional analyses of patients need to take this seeming paradox into account.

Patients on PD may develop metabolic or respiratory alkalosis. The metabolic alkalosis can result from contraction of the extracellular fluid volume, as reported in the treatment phase of hyperglycaemia [169, 170] or with the frequent use of hypertonic dialysis solutions [171]. In patients with respiratory alkalosis the normally functioning kidneys defend against alkalaemia by excreting bicarbonate. The CAPD patient has no such mechanism. Furthermore, the constant infusion of buffer in the patient with respiratory alkalosis can lead to serious alkalaemia [172, 173].

Respiratory alkalosis may appear during the initial stages of dialysis. In the acidotic patient commencing dialysis the infusion of buffer will correct the extracellular acidosis. However, because the bicarbonate anion crosses the blood–brain barrier relatively slowly, the cerebrospinal fluid bathing the respiratory centre will remain relatively acid. This cerebrospinal fluid acidosis will continue to stimulate respiratory drive and maintain hyperventilation in the face of now-normal extracellular fluid pH. Therefore, respiratory alkalosis will develop as a PD because the conversion of lactate to bicarbonate occurs slowly enough to allow cerebrospinal fluid equilibration with extracellular fluid.

Cardiovascular complications

The development of left ventricular hypertrophy (LVH) in non-uraemic hypertensives confers a negative prognosis for cardiovascular morbidity and mortality [175]. The relationship also appears to hold in the uraemic population [176]. The pathogenesis of myocardial hypertrophy in uraemic patients is varied and includes putative factors such as hypertension, chronic anaemia, and extracellular fluid volume overload [117]. In addition, the uraemic state is associated with intermyocardiocytic fibrosis, which further compromises ventricular compliance [178]. Echocardiographic studies have documented a decrease in left ventricular mass in many CAPD patients in whom it was increased at the beginning of dialysis. These patients experienced near-normalization of the end-diastolic dimension, left ventricular frictional shortening, and ejection fraction [179]. These changes were thought to be the result of improved control of systemic blood pressure. However, not all studies have confirmed regression of LVH in patients on PD. The discrepancy may be the result of different degrees of control of the extracellular fluid volume, different methodological approaches to the assessment of LVH, and the different pharmacological approaches to the control of systemic hypertension [177, 180].

The reduction in blood pressure seen in many PD patients can also have deleterious effects. Diabetic patients have been reported to experience exacerbation of peripheral vascular disease during CAPD. Risk factors for the worsening of peripheral perfusion include smoking, previous symptoms of peripheral vascular disease, and absent limb pulses. It has been suggested that the lowered blood pressure on CAPD compromises blood flow to the ischaemic limbs [181]. The use of erythropoietin in diabetic PD patients has recently been identified as a particular risk for the development of peripheral vascular disease [182]. It is not clear whether this complication also holds for diabetic patients on haemodialysis or whether it is unique to PD.

Persistent hypocalcaemia after parathyroidectomy has been implicated as a cause of congestive cardiomyopathy in CAPD patients. It has been suggested that concomitant reduction in intracellular calcium compromises the force developed by the contractile elements of the heart. Cardiac function and dilation improve with calcium repletion [183]. Hypocalcaemia is a significant and important predictor of morbidity and mortality in a cohort of haemodialysis and PD patients, although the relationship to parathyroid hormone levels is not clear [184].

Although it is not well documented, valvular disease, especially valvular sclerosis, may progress in an accelerated fashion in dialysis patients [185]. This may be the result of altered calcium–phosphorus product or other unknown factors [186]. Valve replacement is feasible in dialysis patients, although the outcome is better with bioprosthetic compared to mechanical valves [187].

The elevated IAP caused by the presence of dialysis fluid in the peritoneal cavity has the potential to affect cardiac function. In cirrhotic patients, drainage of ascitic fluid produces a fall in right and left atrial pressure with improvement in cardiac function [188]. There is no consensus on the influence of peritoneal dialysate on cardiac function. Studies have been unable to document a decrease in cardiac function with infusions of as much as 3 L of dialysate [189], whereas others have reported up to a 20% decrease in cardiac index with 2 L of intraperitoneal fluid [190, 191]. Perhaps what makes the most sense physiologically was a study that found that it was the subgroup of patients with LVH who showed echocardiographically-detectable changes in function with the infusion of large (3 L or more) volumes of dialysate [192]. The reduction in LV systolic function was felt to be the result of reduction in preload, because a significant decrease in the LV internal diameter in diastole was found. It is predicted that the subgroup of patients with LVH are the patients in whom cardiac function is affected by preload reduction [177]. In other words, the patients with LVH and diminished LV compliance would be vulnerable to a decrease in LV preload resulting from decreased venous return [192]. However, decreased venous return could not explain the reduced cardiac output in all the patients. Some of these patients had no change in right heart pressure. In these patients increased cardiac surface pressure from the bulging of the diaphragm into the thoracic cavity may have compromised cardiac function [192]. In this regard it is interesting to note that inferior attenuation on cardiac thallium-201 imaging has been noted in patients holding 2 L of PD fluid. The elevation of the diaphragm as a result of increased IAP was thought to be the cause of the abnormal scan, as opposed to myocardial disease [193]. In summary, it appears that the presence of intraperitoneal dialysate usually does not exert a clinically significant effect on the cardiovascular system, although there is a potential for such an effect with the use of large (3 L or more) volumes in patients with diminished cardiac compliance.

A discussion of coronary artery disease and the CAPD patient is beyond the scope of this chapter. However, ischaemic heart disease and its complications remain a very significant cause of death in this population. Hypertension, altered calcium and phosphorus metabolism, unfavourable lipid profiles [194], and glucose intolerance may all contribute to the development of, or worsening of, coronary artery disease in the patient on CAPD.

Gastrointestinal complications of PD

Pancreatitis

Risk of pancreatitis in PD patients

Patients on PD may be at risk for the development of pancreatitis. Peritoneal dialysate can gain access to the lesser sac of the peritoneal cavity via the epiploic foramen. The posterior surface of the lesser sac serves as the anterior surface of the pancreas. Therefore, any constituent of the dialysate has the potential to irritate the pancreas. Proposed irritants include the high glucose concentration of dialysis fluid, unidentified toxic byproducts of the dialysate, bags, or tubing [195], acidity of the dialysate [196] and, of course, the infected dialysate of peritonitis [196, 197]. Rechallenge with peritoneal dialysate after an episode of pancreatitis has resulted in a recurrent episode of pancreatitis [198]. In addition, there may be a predilection for pseudocyst formation [196].

Other risk factors for pancreatic inflammation in patients on CAPD include hypertriglyceridaemia,

which is prevalent in these patients. In addition, patients with aplastic bone disease are prone to hypercalcaemia when given calcium supplements with vitamin D, and the elevated serum calcium is another risk factor for acute pancreatitis [199].

Despite all the potential risk factors outlined above, it still remains controversial whether acute pancreatitis occurs more frequently in CAPD patients compared to those on haemodialysis. In a review of the literature, Gupta *et al.* concluded that, in fact, acute pancreatitis was not more common in CAPD patients, and that previous reports to the contrary were the result of reporting bias [200]. However, given the potential for contact between PD fluid and the pancreas, and the frequency of at least transient episodes of hypercalcaemia in CAPD patients, there remains a strong theoretical risk for a predisposition toward acute pancreatitis in this population compared to those of haemodialysis. In this regard a recent review of pancreatitis among dialysis and transplant patients concluded that this complication was more common in PD patients. The occurrence rate was 4.3 episodes per 100 treatment-years, compared to 1.4 episodes per 100 treatment-years in the haemodialysis cohort [201].

Diagnosis of pancreatitis

Diagnosis of acute pancreatitis may be difficult. It should be considered in cases of culture-negative peritonitis, especially if the abdominal pain fails to resolve or localizes in the epigastrium. Hiccoughs may be present [202]. The serum amylase will rise with pancreatitis. However, because patients with chronic renal failure can have elevated serum amylase levels, there is overlap between the elevated levels seen in patients with renal failure and pancreatitis and those with renal failure alone [196]. Serum amylase values greater than three times the upper limit of normal are suggestive of acute pancreatitis [203]. A reivew of the literature concerning pancreatitis in CAPD patients shows that the amylase level was elevated in 18 of 23 patients. In the 18 the mean increase was 8.5 times the upper limit of normal [200]. In the other five patients, however, the serum amylase was normal. In summary, it seems that a markedly elevated serum amylase is strongly suggestive of acute pancreatitis, but normal levels do not rule out this diagnosis.

It has been reported that an increased amylase level in the dialysis effluent (greater than 100 U/L) indicates acute pancreatitis or other intra-abdominal pathology compared to the lower levels seen with dialysis-associated peritonitis [204]. However this has not been confirmed in other centres [197, 200].

The dialysis fluid is usually clear with pancreatitis, and the lack of cloudy fluid should suggest a cause of the abdominal pain other than peritonitis [205]. Dialysate leukocytosis with sterile culture has occasionally been described in pancreatitis [206]. Pancreatitis may also occur simultaneously or as a complication of PD peritonitis [195, 196, 291].

Ultrasound and CT scanning can demonstrate an engorged, oedematous pancreas [196, 198], or pseudocyst formation. Unfortunately, these radiological studies are also frequently normal [195, 196]. The mortality is high and part of the reason may be that time to diagnosis may be delayed on the assumption that the abdominal pain is the result of bacterial peritonitis. In fact, the diagnosis may be made for the first time at post-mortem examination. Mortality is higher in patients with acute haemorrhagic pancreatitis (in which case the presentation may be with haemoperitoneum and abdominal pain), and conversely, the persistence of clear dialysis fluid throughout the course of pancreatitis is a good prognostic sign [207].

Hepatic complications

In CAPD patients receiving intraperitoneal insulin a unique hepatic lesion can develop. A layer of fat may be deposited under the hepatic capsule exposed to the peritoneal cavity [208–210]. The thickness of this fatty layer correlates with the degree of obesity, as well as the size of the dose of intraperitoneal insulin. It has been proposed that the insulin in the peritoneal dialysate causes increased concentration of this hormone at the capsule and at the level of the subcapsular hepatocytes. In the face of relative peripheral insulin deficiency, free fatty acids are delivered to the liver where they are re-esterified in the presence of the high insulin levels under the hepatic capsule. Pathologically, there may be associated steatonecrosis, but liver function remains normal [208]. However, it is important that this complication be kept in mind. One of our CAPD patients on intraperitoneal insulin underwent CT scanning for abdominal pain and was reported to have metastatic carcinoma of the liver. However, the abnormality was distributed just under the liver capsule across the surface of the liver exposed to the dialysate. A needle biopsy confirmed that the lesion was not cancer, but the above-described subcapsular steatosis.

The liver is at risk for abscess formation as a result of dialysis-associated peritonitis. This diagnosis should be considered in cases of persistent peritonitis. Ultrasound of the liver may be normal and exploratory laparotomy may be necessary [211]. Needle aspiration and drainage under CT guidance is a less invasive alternative.

Other rare complications reported include portal vein thrombosis as a complication of *Staphylococcus aureus* peritonitis in a patient with alcoholic cirrhosis [212] and ascites after discontinuation of PD. In the latter case, infection of the dialysis fluid should be ruled out with paracentesis. Another suggested cause for post-PD ascites includes portal hypertension, although in other instances the pathogenesis remains obscure [213].

Other gastrointestinal complications

Many patients on CAPD complain of abdominal bloating and reflux. It has been assumed that the cause of these symptoms is the increased IAP and volume. It might be expected that the increased abdominal pressure dynamics across the oesophageal–gastric junction and leads to oesophageal reflux or spasm. One study using manometry to measure oesophageal pressures and peristalsis found no increase in oesophageal pressure or pressure at the lower oesophageal sphincter when 1.5–2.5 L of dialysate was instilled in the peritoneal cavity [214]. Symptomatic patients (nausea, vomiting, epigastric fullness) were found in another study to have reduced lower oesophageal sphincter pressure compared to asymptomatic CAPD controls [215]. The combination of increased IAP seen in PD, diminished lower oesophageal sphincter pressure, and delayed gastric emptying [216] is certainly a risk for the development of reflux symptoms. Collection of dialysis fluid in the lesser sac of the peritoneal cavity can push on the stomach and aggravate gastro-oesophageal symptomatology further [217].

Treatment includes small frequent meals, avoidance of foods which reduce sphincter pressure (chocolate, alcohol), decreased dialysis volumes, and the use of histamine-2 blockers and proton-pump inhibitors. Pro-motility agents may be helpful, including cisapride and erythromycin [218].

The small bowel is vulnerable to catheter-related perforation. This complication results from pressure necrosis from the dialysis catheter. Small bowel perforation of this type has been reported not only in patients with an unused PD catheter, but also in patients actively receiving CAPD [219]. Perforation of the jejunum unrelated to the PD catheter has also been reported [220].

There are rare reports of ischaemic colitis and necrotizing enteritis as complications of PD [205, 221–223]. The likeliest cause is hypotension with consequent hypoperfusion of the bowel. However, the development of ischaemic bowel in a normotensive 6-year-old child on PD with improvement upon transfer to haemodialysis suggests PD itself may play a role in the bowel ischaemia [222]. Marked gastrointestinal bleeding from dilated submucosal vessels in the bowel have been reported in association with the use of hypertonic dextrose solutions. No such bleeding occurred when the patient changed to haemodialysis. It was suggested that PD provoked mesenteric vasodilation which promoted the gastrointestinal bleeding [224]. Conversely, angiodysplastic bleeding has been reported to stop when haemodialysis patients are transferred to PD [225, 226].

Finally, free air in the peritoneal cavity, or pneumoperitoneum, usually presents as free air under the diaphragm. In non-dialysis patients, this radiological sign suggests perforation of an abdominal viscus and usually leads to laporatomy. However, air can be infused along with dialysis fluid, particularly with 'flush before fill' systems. Therefore, many PD patients have the incidental finding of pneumoperitoneum [227, 228]. If the finding is the result of the concomitant accidental infusion of air along with dialysis fluid, the outcome is benign and the air should gradually resorb. However, in the PD patient who presents with abdominal pain, pneumoperitoneum is hard to interpret. Previous reports suggest that the larger the volume of free air, the greater the likelihood of viscus perforation [227, 229]. Unfortunately, this relationship has not been substantiated in other reports [228, 230]. Clearly the interpretation of the free air must be taken in clinical context: free air under the diaphragm on a chest X-ray in a well PD patient is little cause for concern, but even a small amount of free air in a patient with abdominal pain must at least suggest the possibility of perforation of an abdominal viscus, and not automatically be dismissed as air infused during a dialysis exchange.

Sclerosing encapsulating peritonitis

Incidence and clinical presentation

This rare and devastating complication consists of progressive inanition, vomiting, intermittent bowel obstruction, and decreased peritoneal transport of water and solutes [221, 231–235]. The small intestine is bound or encapsulated by a thick fibrous layer, rendering the peritoneal surface opaque. The fibrous layer resembles a 'thick shaggy membrane' [221], 'marble' [236], 'cocoon' or a 'fruit rind' which may or may not peel off the bowel relatively easily [237]. The bowel so exposed may appear normal [237]. A different form of sclerosing peritonitis has been described in which the diffuse sclerosing process extends transmurally with incorporation of the inner circular muscular layer and myenteric plexus of the small bowel in the fibrosing process [238].

The prevalence of sclerosing peritonitis varies among different units, with rates reported from 0.7% [239] to 3.7% of patients under study [240]. Put another way, the incidence reported varied from 2.6/1000 patient-years [240], 3.5/1000 patient-years [241] and 4.2/1000 patient-years [239]. The incidence appears to increase in patients on PD for several years [239, 240, 242]. As will be discussed below, some variability in the data may be accounted for by the definition used for sclerosing peritonitis in each centre. For example, a recent study described 16 patients with peritoneal sclerosis, but only half of them had true sclerotic encapsulation [241].

Patients with this syndrome have a generally poor outcome, with at least 50% mortality [236, 239], probably on the basis of severe malnutrition and recurrent bowel obstruction. The diagnosis of bowel obstruction may be delayed because the fibrosing process does not allow the bowel to distend and display the typical radiological findings [232].

Sclerosing encapsulating peritonitis (SEP) appears to be a distinct and devastating syndrome and the name should not be used interchangeably with 'peritoneal sclerosis'. The latter term should be reserved for the finding of non-encapsulating sclerosis and fibrous adhesions associated with ultrafiltration failure. This condition is seen in patients who have had prolonged PD or recurrent episodes of peritonitis, but may be present at the initiation of dialysis. Indeed, the lack of rigorous differentiation between these two entities may confuse any attempt to define aetiological factors, particularly among different dialysis centres.

Pathogenesis of sclerosing peritonitis

The cause of SEP is uncertain. There are numerous possibilities (see Table 2). The original reports came from centres where the dialysate buffer was primarily acetate rather than lactate [221, 235]. It has been suggested that acetate may be irritating to the peritoneal membrane and perhaps initiate the fibrosing process [221, 243]. Acetate-containing dialysate

Table 2. Postulated causes of sclerosing encapsulating peritonitis

Acetate-containing dialysate [221, 235, 243]
Recurrent peritonitis [221, 232, 245]
Plastic particles [235, 272]
Formaldehyde [235]
Bacterial filter causing upstream multiplication of bacteria with pyrogen release into peritoneum stimulating interluekin-1 production [248]
Multiple abdominal surgeries [245]
Unrecognized subclinical peritonitis with fastidious bacteria or fungi [247]
Intraperitoneal contamination with chlorhexidine in alcohol sprayed on connector [246, 266]
Hypertonic acidic dialysate [235]
Catheter [235, 254, 273]
Beta-blockers [231, 235, 243]
High interdialytic peritoneal content of fibrinogen [237]

exposes mesothelium to concentrations of this buffer anion that are 350–450 times that normally found in the peritoneal cavity [244]. However, SEP has also been reported in patients dialysing with lactate [245, 246], although in some cases the disease in question may be peritoneal sclerosis [245] or transmural bowel fibrosis [238].

Recurrent peritonitis or subclinical 'grumbling' peritonitis [247] has been suggested as a cause of this syndrome, although clearly many patients have never had peritonitis (detectable clinically) or had a relatively low incidence of peritonitis [235, 241, 242]. Alternatively, it is possible that one severe episode of peritonitis may condition the peritoneal milieu for the development of this syndrome.

Shaldon and colleagues have postulated that the use of a bacterial filter in the dialysis tubing may be linked to the high incidence of SEP. They suggested that bacteria trapped upstream of the filter secrete pyrogen, which crosses the filter and enters the peritoneal cavity where it stimulates macrophages to secrete interleukin-1 [248]. This lymphokine stimulates fibroblast proliferation and so could accelerate the fibrosing process. Once again, however, only some patients with SEP have used bacterial filters.

As suggested by Dobbie, however, the large molecular weight of interleukin-1 would impede its transport through or around mesothelium to affect the more deeply situated fibroblasts. In addition, histologically, loss of the normal cellular constituents appears to be more important than fibroblast proliferation in the pathogenesis of peritoneal fibrosis and sclerosis [244]. Indeed, rather than fibroblast proliferation, it may be the loss of plasminogen activation from the damaged mesothelial cells that impairs normal fibrinolysis and allows fibrosis [244, 249].

Markedly elevated levels of type I and type III procollagen propeptides have been found in the peritoneal fluid of a patient who subsequently developed peritoneal fibrosis [250]. Relatedly, a rodent model of sclerosing peritonitis or abdominal cocoon has been developed by the intraperitoneal instillation of bleach to produce inflammation, followed by instillation of blood. The clot retraction process brings the loops of bowel together into an abdominal mass. The authors suggest that intraperitoneal haemorrhage, such as during surgery, may contribute to the pathogenesis of this syndrome [251]. In this regard Hendriks and co-workers noted that the subset of patients with 'peritoneal sclerosis' had a greater number of catheter-related surgeries compared to the cohort without sclerosis [241]. However, primacy must be given to the induction of an intraperitoneal fibrinous exudate from any cause as the final common pathway in this syndrome [249].

A retrospective analysis in one dialysis unit demonstrated that all the patients who developed SEP were members of a subgroup who sprayed their connectors at each exchange with 0.5% chlorhexidine in 70% alcohol [246]. The authors studied the effect of this antiseptic over the short term in a rat model and demonstrated inflammation in submesothelial tissues. The incidence of SEP in this unit has diminished since changing the antiseptic protocol. On the other hand, a study in Y-set patients observed no difference in peritoneal transport characteristics in patients with or without accidental hypochlorite infusion, or in the same patient before and after this infusion [252]. However, in the first study the patients had regular exposure to the potential contaminant, chlorhexidine, as part of their connector care, whereas in the latter study there was a one-time exposure to the disinfectant. Therefore the studies are not comparable.

The presence of the dialysis catheter in the peritoneal cavity could promote an inflammatory or foreign-body response. In this regard a similar encapsulating peritoneal sclerosis has been described in patients with ascites in whom LeVeen shunts have been implanted [253]. Given all the patients with implanted silastic catheters, the SEP-type response is very rare. In addition, it would not explain the predilection for European centres. It is interesting, however, that localized fibrosis and peritoneal pseudocyst formation may develop in relation to the PD catheter. This phenomenon has also been observed in patients with a ventriculoperitoneal shunt [254].

Other factors include the use of beta-blockers, which have been linked to peritoneal sclerosis [255,

256]. Finally, there are many potentially toxic factors related to the dialysis itself, including hypertonicity and acidity of the dialysate. Interestingly, SEP has been reported in a haemodialysis patient never on PD [257].

Taken in sum, there is no single factor which can be incriminated in the pathogenesis of SEP. It is likely that the aetiology is multifactorial. Because of the association with the use of acetate in the dialysis solution most centres avoid its use.

The radiological picture may be suggestive. While extensive plaque-like or eggshell calcification may be seen, it may be more indicative of the more benign calcifying peritonitis (see below). By ultrasound, changes that have been noted in SEP include increased small bowel peristalsis, tethering of the bowel to the posterior abdominal wall, echogenic strands and new membrane formation [258]. A characteristic trilaminar appearance of the bowel wall may suggest this diagnosis [259]. With CT scanning the advanced picture is characteristic (see Fig. 2). In the early stages loculated ascites, adherent bowel loops, narrowing of the bowel lumen and thickening of the peritoneal membrane may be a marker of the subsequent development of SEP, although these changes may also be seen with peritoneal fibrosis [260–262].

Even though a causal relationship has never been established with certainty, most centres have abandoned the use of acetate as dialysis buffers because of its association with the sclerosing syndrome. Similarly, after the report of the potential relationship of chlorhexidine with development of SEP, use of this antiseptic declined rapidly. Indeed, as emphasized by Dobbie [244], the peritoneal mesothelium is sensitive to cytotoxic and even carcinogenic effects of a wide variety of substances. The use of any agent that might enter the peritoneum must be tempered with consideration of its long-term effects on this delicate membrane.

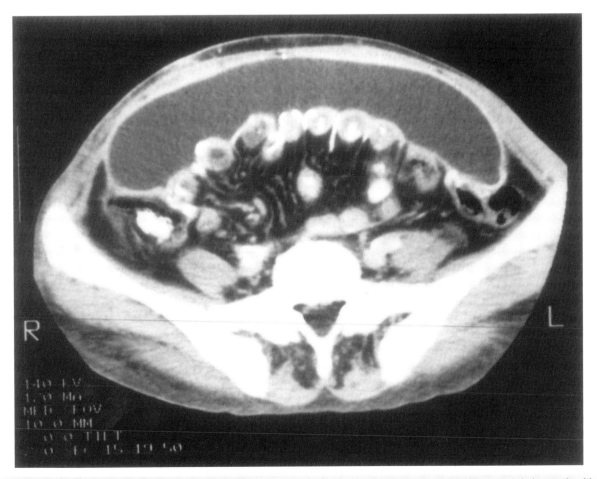

Figure 2. Computerized tomographic (CT) scan of the abdomen in a patient with advanced sclerosing encapsulating peritonitis. Note the thickened, dense peritoneal membrane binding the bowel to the posterior aspect of the peritoneal cavity.

Management of patients with sclerosing peritonitis

Surgical treatment of SEP is fraught with hazard and can lead to severe bleeding. In cases of life-threatening obstruction or necrosis of bowel, however, the surgeon may have no other choice but to operate. Postoperative mortality is high. It has been suggested that in cases of bowel resection primary anastomosis is best avoided. Instead, one suggestion is that the bowel be put to rest and the patient receive parenteral alimentation before anastomosis is attempted [263]. Careful surgical removal of the encapsulating membrane after a course of parenteral nutrition has led to good results in some cases [264]. However, avoidance of surgical intervention has been advised, if conservative measures are successful [265].

A very important but as yet unsolved management problem is whether the patient with early but definite SEP should be transferred to haemodialysis or deliberately maintained on PD. The rationale for the latter decision is to keep bowel loops separate from one another 'afloat' in dialysate so there is no opportunity for the bowel and peritoneal membrane to become matted down in the posterior peritoneum. Two of our patients with SEP appeared to develop their disease after they were transferred to haemodialysis. Others have noted that patients with chlorhexidine-associated SEP who were maintained on CAPD survived, whereas almost all of those transferred to haemodialysis died of progressive disease. The one patient who received a transplant, and presumably immunosuppression, died from intestinal obstruction (see below) [266]. Similarly, it has been noted that the onset of symptomatic SEP appears soon after transfer to another treatment modality [267]. Therefore, while the first response would be to stop PD, it is possible that the dry peritoneum can accelerate the encapsulating process. If peritoneal transport is sufficient, a case could be made to continue PD instead. However, there are too few cases documented to put forth firm recommendations.

A provocative report suggested that the use of prednisone and azathioprine in patients with chlorhexidine-associated SEP led to improved outcome with recovery of bowel function [268]. This report has been followed by other case reports of improvement with corticosteroids [269], or with corticosteroids and azathioprine followed by surgical release of the intra-abdominal fibrous tissue [270]. The occasional case of recovery following renal transplantation has been attributed to the use of immunosuppresive drugs for the transplant, but progression of sclerosis has been reported even after successful renal transplantation [271].

In summary, in order to standardize reporting among different centres, 'sclerosing peritonitis' should be reserved for the distinct syndrome involving fibrous encapsulation of bowel. It is important that the diagnosis be suspected in a PD patient (or a former PD patient now on haemodialysis or with a kidney transplant) with weight loss and recurrent bowel obstruction. Many surgeons and gastroenterologists may not be familiar with this syndrome because it is not prominently reported in the non-dialysis literature. Management includes careful attention to nutrition, including the use of total parenteral nutrition, and judicious surgical technique, preferably by a surgeon with experience in this complication. Corticosteroids and other immunosuppressive agents may have a role in the management of this syndrome, but they cannot be recommended at this time because of the paucity of reports and the high incidence of side-effects from these medications.

Calcifying peritonitis

Marichal *et al.* [274] described two patients on CAPD who developed recurrent abdominal pain and incomplete bowel obstruction. Radiographs revealed multiple calcifications which had an eggshell pattern on the loops of the small bowel. One of the patients came to laparotomy, where the intestinal loops were found to be free, in contrast to the appearance in SEP. Pathologically the parietal peritoneum showed fibrous thickening and few cells. Also seen were bands of ossification and calcium deposits. The authors called this entity 'progressive calcifying peritonitis'. Other interesting aspects of these patients included the fact that they dialysed with acetate buffers, and one of the patients had hyperparathyroidism and recurrent haemoperitoneum. The patients had a benign course compared to that of SEP, and once PD was discontinued bowel function improved [274].

The relatively benign outcome was substantiated by a report from Australia of a long-term CAPD patient with similar features, extensive plaque-like calcification on visceral and parietal peritoneum, and again haemoperitoneum. This patient had elevated levels of parathyroid hormone and increased calcium–phosphate product. After surgical excision of some of the plaques the patient was able to return to PD [275].

However, the optimistic outlook for calcifying peritonitis has been tempered by a report of a long-term CAPD patient who developed extensive peritoneal calcification but whose course was more typical of SEP. This patient had recurrent ileus which did not improve with transfer to haemodialysis. She ultimately sustained bowel infarction and died [276].

The aetiology of calcifying peritonitis remains obscure. In the original report acetate was implicated as a cause [274] but subsequent patients dialysed with lactate buffer. As in the more sinister SEP, it is possible that the calcification is a reaction to multiple episodes of bacterial peritonitis. It has been suggested that haemoperitoneum could accelerate the calcification, because iron in the peritoneal cavity can serve as a nidus for precipitation of calcium [277]. Not all the patients had haemoperitoneum, however.

Perhaps the likeliest cause is a disorder in the phosphate–calcium–parathyroid hormone axis. Some of the patients had markedly increased levels of parathyroid hormone, and it is conceivable that the peritoneal calcification was a manifestation of calciphylaxis or calcinosis [278, 279]. On the other hand, calcifying peritonitis has been reported in patients years after parathyroidectomy. In this setting it has been suggested that after parathyroidectomy the bone reverts to a low-turnover state. Administration of calcium and vitamin D analogues results in extraosseous or metastatic calcification, one consequence of which is the peritoneal calcification [280].

Calcifying peritonitis has been reported so infrequently that it is difficult to provide any recommendations for management. Clearly it is advisable to avoid hypercalcaemia or marked elevations of the calcium–phosphate product. It is possible that the development of calcifying peritonitis may be an indication for parathyroidectomy if the level of hormone is markedly increased, particularly if there is uncontrolled hypercalcaemia.

From the available reports it is not clear whether calcifying peritonitis is in itself an indication for transfer to haemodialysis, although the original report implied that bowel motility improved once PD was stopped [274].

Haemoperitoneum

Presentation and aetiology of haemoperitoneum

Peritoneal dialysis affords a 'window' into the peritoneal cavity. Intraperitoneal bleeding is likely to occur frequently in physiological and pathological settings, but is not detected. With drainage of the dialysis effluent, peritoneal bleeding will be readily apparent by the appearance of bloody effluent, known as haemoperitoneum.

The presence of blood in the dialysis effluent can be distressing to the patient and a source of concern to the physician. As little as 2 ml of blood can render 1 L of dialysis fluid noticeably blood-tinged [281].

Haemoperitoneum has a wide differential diagnosis, as shown in Table 3. A common and benign cause of blood in the peritoneal cavity is menstruation. In a recent review of haemoperitoneum, menstrual bleeding was the single cost common cause, accounting for one-third of the benign episodes [282]. The majority of regularly menstruating women on CAPD experience recurrent haemoperitoneum [283].

Table 3. Reported causes of haemoperitoneum

Gynecological
Menstruation [284, 285, 288]
Ovulation [285]
Ovarian cysts [282, 285–287]

Neoplastic
Renal cell carcinoma [299]
Adenocarcinoma of colon [299]

Polycystic diseases
Polycystic kidney disease [294]
Polycystic liver disease [300]

Gastrointestinal
Catheter-induced splenic injury [289, 302]
Hepatic metastases [290]
Hepatoma [291, 292]
Spontaneous splenic rupture in chronic myelogenous leukaemia [303]
Colonic perforation in dialysis amyloid [304]
Spontaneous rupture of splenic infarct [305]
Acute cholecystitis [281]
Post-colonoscopy [281, 282]
Intraperitoneal connective tissue pouch [306]
Pancreatitis [282]

Haematological
Idiopathic thrombocytopenic purpura [282, 293]
Anticoagulation therapy [282]

Diseases of the peritoneal membrane
Sclerosing peritonitis [282, 298]
Peritoneal calcification [275]
Radiation-induced peritoneal fibrosis [297]

Miscellaneous
Leakage from extraperitoneal haematoma [282, 295, 307]
Post-pericardiocentesis [308]
Angiomyolipoma of kidney [309]
IgA nephritis [310]
Mixed connective tissue disease [311]
Extracorporeal lithotripsy [296]
Spontaneous rupture of umbilical vein [312]

There are two mechanisms by which menstruation could lead to haemoperitoneum. If there is endometrial tissue in the peritoneal cavity it will shed simultaneously with the intrauterine endometrium, and so bloody dialysate will occur simultaneously with menstrual flow. The alternative mechanism is that the shed uterine tissue and blood both moves out of the uterine cervix and refluxes in retrograde fashion through the Fallopian tubes into the peritoneal cavity. The peritoneal bleeding may start a few days prior to the appearance of blood per vagina [284]. It has been suggested that the timing of menstrual pain matches the appearance of peritoneal blood rather than vaginal menstrual flow, so that the peritoneal blood may be an important cause of dysmenorrhoea [284].

Women of reproductive age may also experience haemoperitoneum coincident with ovulation at mid-cycle [282, 285]. It is suggested that the source of blood is bleeding from the ovary with the rupture and release of the ovum. Other ovarian sources of bleeding include ruptured cysts, which can bleed sufficiently to necessitate transfusion [286, 287].

The episodes of haemoperitoneum associated with menstruation and ovulation are recognized by their periodicity and occurrence in women of reproductive age. While this cause of blood in the dialysate is considered benign, there are potential complications. The blood loss can exacerbate the anaemia of chronic renal failure, and for this reason alone anovulant therapy may be indicated. A reported association between haemoperitoneum and *Staphylococcus epidermidis* peritonitis suggests that the bloody dialysate may provide a rich growth medium for intraperitoneal bacteria. Moreover, the retrograde movement of blood from the uterine cavity through the Fallopian tubes may passively carry bacteria into the peritoneum and lead to peritonitis [45, 288]. Other investigators, however, have been unable to document an increased frequency of peritonitis in relation to menstruation-generated haemoperitoneum [282].

In the patient who is not menstruating, haemoperitoneum must be carefully investigated. There are a number of surgical causes of blood in the peritoneal cavity, including cholecystitis [281], rupture of the spleen [289] and pancreatitis [282]. In these instances it should be apparent that the patient has a painful abdomen, and the localized tenderness in concert with the bloody effluent should mandate an urgent surgical consultation. Surgical causes of haemoperitoneum may also present less acutely. We recently managed an elderly man with asymptomatic haemoperitoneum who upon investigation had adenocarcinoma of the colon with serosal invasion. Primary and metastatic tumours of the liver can present with haemoperitoneum [290–292].

Haemoperitoneum has been observed in patients with coagulation disorders [282, 293], polycystic kidney disease [294], post-colonoscopy [281, 282], leakage from a haematoma outside the peritoneal cavity [282, 295] and that seen after extracorporeal lithotripsy for kidney stones [296].

Recurrent haemoperitoneum may be a harbinger of disease of the peritoneal membrane itself. Bloody effluent has been described in patients with peritoneal calcification in association with hyperparathyroidism [275], in patients with radiation-induced peritoneal injury [297], and as the presenting abnormality in patients who develop sclerosing peritonitis [282, 298].

In patients with polycystic kidney disease, bleeding into a cyst can be associated with haematuria or haemoperitoneum [294]. A patient with polycystic kidney disease on peritoneal dialysis was described with bloody effluent [299]. In this case, however, the bleeding was painless, which is unusual if a kidney cyst had ruptured into the peritoneal cavity. Moreover, there was associated leukocytosis of the dialysis effluent. These unusual features led to further investigations, which revealed that the patient had renal cell carcinoma [299]. Rupture of hepatic cysts can also result in haemoperitoneum [300].

Management of haemoperitoneum

The patient with haemoperitoneum is at risk of the intraperitoneal blood coagulating in the catheter lumen. Therefore, use of intraperitoneal heparin 500–1000 U/L has been recommended for as long as the dialysate still has visible blood or fibrin. In our experience the intraperitoneal heparin does not worsen the bleeding or lead to systemic anticoagulation. In some instances of haemoperitoneum the use of rapid exchanges with dialysate at room temperature leads to rapid resolution of the bleeding. It is postulated that the relatively cool dialysate induces peritoneal vasoconstriction, and this leads to haemostasis [301].

Women of reproductive age should be instructed about haemoperitoneum, because it is a common occurrence in this group and can be very frightening if it is not anticipated. All other cases of haemoperitoneum warrant appropriate investigation, including imaging procedures and surgical consultation if indicated.

Chyloperitoneum

The pathological influx of chylomicrons rich in triglycerides into the peritoneal cavity is referred to as chylous ascites, or as chyloperitoneum in the patient on PD. This phenomenon results from the interruption of the lymphatic drainage from the gut to the main lymphatic trunks. Compromise of the integrity of these lymphatic channels is most commonly the result of neoplasm, particularly lymphoma [313–315].

After a fatty meal, long-chain fatty acids are incorporated into chylomicrons, which enter the lymphatic circulation. Therefore chyloperitoneum is an intermittent event occurring after the ingestion of fat and clearing some time afterwards. Because medium-chain triglycerides are not absorbed through the lymphatic channels, chylous ascites has been treated by prescribing a diet in which fat is delivered in this form [316], thus obviating the need for lymphatic drainage of triglyceride.

In the patient not on PD, chylous ascites is likely to present as increasing abdominal girth and peripheral oedema [313]. For the patient on PD, chyloperitoneum presents as milky-white effluent which can be mistaken for peritonitis.

The diagnosis is suggested by the white, milky appearance of the dialysate in conjunction with the absence of any indication of peritonitis. Lipoprotein electrophoresis shows lipid staining at the origin, characteristic of chylomicrons [317]. When the dialysate is separated into layers upon standing, the supernatant stains positively for fat with Sudan black, and dissolves with ether [317, 318]. The triglyceride level of the dialysate is greater than the plasma triglyceride level, a characteristic of intestinal lymph [315].

The aetiology of chyloperitoneum is obscure. In every case there must be communication between the peritoneal lymphatics and peritoneal cavity. The dialysis catheter or its trochar could sever a lymph vessel. In the non-dialysis patient bacterial peritonitis has been incriminated in the pathogenesis of chylous ascites and encapsulating periotonitis [319]. In patients on PD, chyloperitoneum has been reported spontaneously in the neonate [320] as a complication of tuberculous peritonitis [321] and around peritoneal catheter insertion [317, 318, 322]. Interestingly, chyloperitoneum was reported in five Japan-

ese patients given a calcium channel-blocker called manidipine [323]. We puzzled over a CAPD patient who presented with recurrent episodes of cloudy peritoneal dialysate associated with low peritoneal cell counts and sterile bacteriological cultures. Investigation revealed extensive retroperitoneal lymphoma and the episodes of cloudy dialysate represented chyloperitoneum [324].

Chyloperitoneum should be part of the differential diagnosis of recurrent cloudy fluid or 'culture-negative' peritonitis. Its diagnosis warrants further investigation into the cause. Temporary cessation of PD and a diet of medium-chain fatty acids may be helpful until its resolution [317, 320].

Acquired cystic disease of the kidney

Incidence and pathogenesis

Acquired cystic disease of the kidney is the term used to describe the progressive replacement of renal parenchyma by cysts in patients with chronic renal failure. This phenomenon was initially described in patients receiving chronic haemodialysis [325]. It had been suggested that a retained uraemic toxin or one unique to haemodialysis stimulated cystic transformation in the end-stage kidney [326]. It has become clear that acquired cystic disease of the kidney is not unique to the subset of the population with chronic renal failure that receives haemodialysis. This complication has been reported in patients with renal failure who have never undergone dialysis, and in patients on PD who were never exposed to haemodialysis [327–329]. Indeed, the acquired cystic disease in patients who have received only PD can be so prominent it can be mistaken for polycystic kidney disease [330] (Fig. 3). These observations suggest that factor(s) in the uraemic milieu are probably responsible for cystic transformation, rather than something particular to the dialysis process itself.

At present there have been reports of acquired cystic disease in approximately 200 CAPD patients [331]. As in the haemodialysis literature, there is great variation reported for the prevalence of this condition. This variation is the result of the method used to diagnose the cysts, i.e. post-mortem examination of the kidneys versus ultrasound, the particular population being studied, and the criteria used for making the diagnosis. In a review by Ishikawa the reported prevalence of this condition in CAPD

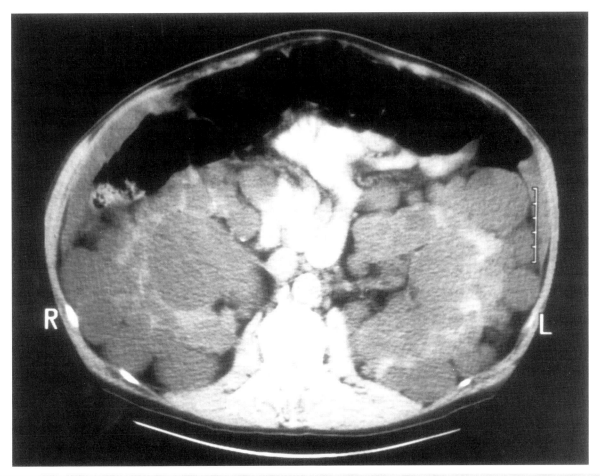

Figure 3. Advanced acquired cystic disease of the kidneys shown by CT scan. This long-term PD patient had small, shrunken kidneys at the start of dialysis. (Reproduced from ref. 330, with permission.)

patients varied from 3% to 100% with a mean prevalence of 41%. Methods of diagnosis included ultrasound, CT scanning, magnetic resonance imaging and post-mortem studies [331]. In comparing the prevalence of acquired cysts in haemodialysis and CAPD patients, a number of confounding factors need to be recoginzed. Cystic transformation has been reported to be more common in males than in females [332, 333]. Moreover, it has been associated with increasing age [332, 334] and with longer duration of dialysis [333, 335]. (The latter factor explains why acquired cysts were described earlier in haemodialysis than in PD patients, because there is a greater prevalence of long-term haemodialysis patients.) When corrected for the duration of dialysis there appears to be no difference in the prevalence of cysts [336]. Therefore, any comparison must take into account the patients' age and sex and duration of dialysis before the actual mode of dialysis can be implicated in facilitating cystic change. With these

limitations in mind surveys of dialysis patients suggest that the prevalence of acquired cystic disease of the kidneys averages about 40–50% and is independent of the mode of dialysis [331, 332, 334].

Risk of neoplastic transformation

In dialysis patients with acquired renal cysts, there is a small but significant risk of the development of renal malignancy. The prevalence of renal cancer will again vary depending on the method of detection. A recent review noted a prevalence of 1.3% for renal malignancy in a dialysis population with acquired cysts [337], which is a two-fold risk compared to renal failure patients without cysts [338]. In CAPD patients, however, the incidence was 0.4%, or two out of 475 patients examined in one group analysis [331]. Overall, there are few reports of renal cell malignancy complicating acquired cysts in patients, and two rare instances of metastatic disease.

In one case the renal neoplasm was a poorly differentiated transitional cell carcinoma, and analgesic abuse could not be effectively ruled out as a causative factor [339]. In another instance, however, renal cell carcinoma was confirmed in a nephrectomy specimen with acquired cystic disease and subsequently hepatic metastases occurred [338].

The lower incidence of renal neoplasia in PD patients with acquired cystic disease, when viewed in an optimistic light, might reflect the better-preserved immune function seen in these patients compared to those receiving haemodialysis. In other words, tumour surveillance may be more effective as a result of improved immune function. This is suggested by the observation that transplant patients (on immunosuppression) have a greater propensity to metastatic disease of renal cell carcinoma than patients on dialysis [340], and that acquired cystic disease of the native kidneys may more readily undergo neoplastic transformation in patients who have received a kidney transplant [341]. On the other hand, it may simply be that the index of suspicion is lower in those managing patients on PD consequent to the paucity of reports of renal neoplasms in this group [338–344].

Many reports of neoplastic transformation in dialysis patients with acquired renal cysts conclude by advising 'regular' or annual surveillance by ultrasound. However, this approach must be tempered by consideration of the enormous cost involved to do this compared to the low incidence of renal cancer and even lower incidence of metastatic disease in the population of PD patients. Perhaps, as suggested by Ishikawa [331], only those at high risk should be screened; that is, men on long-term CAPD with extensive cystic transformation of the kidneys.

There have been reports of spontaneous haemorrhage into the cysts of PD patients with acquired cystic disease of the kidneys [343, 344]. This may occur less frequently than in haemodialysis because of the reduced need for systemic anticoagulation [331].

Pruritus

More than half of dialysis patients have pruritus during their time on renal replacement therapy [345]. The itch is severe in only a small minority of dialysis patients, but can be distracting enough as to be an unacceptable burden. Dialysis patients have committed suicide because of intractable itch. There appears to be no significant difference in the preva-

lence of pruritus between patients on haemodialysis and PD [346].

The aetiology of uraemic pruritus remains obscure. Hyperparathyroidism and abnormalities in divalent iron metabolism have been implicated in uraemic pruritus. It has been observed that itching will often dramatically improve in hyperparathyroid dialysis patients after removal of the parathyroid glands [347]. However, the correlation between parathyroid gland hypersecretion and pruritus is not tight; although studies have demonstrated that patients with itch overall have higher levels of parathyroid hormone, there is no correlation between the severity of pruritus and levels of the hormone [345]. Moreover, studies of skin mineral content in pruritic and non-pruritic dialysis patients have been conflicting [345].

The role of histamine is also not well elucidated. It is recognized to cause itching and allergic skin reactions and has long been suspected to play a role in uraemic pruritus. Mast cells, which release histamine, have been found in increased numbers in the skin of uraemic patients [348, 349]. However, other studies could not confirm the increase in skin mast cells, or the relationship between plasma histamine levels and itch [350]. Examination of the use of erythropoietin for uraemic itch in haemodialysis patients found a correlation between symptomatology and plasma histamine levels [351].

There are theoretical reasons why pruritus might be less prevalent and less severe in patients on CAPD compared to those on haemodialysis. Reactions with the extracorporeal circuit, including the sterilizers and plasticizers, are known to be immunogenic and can sometimes produce hypersensitivity reactions. If middle molecule retention is important in the pathogenesis of pruritus, it might be anticipated that the better clearance of these molecules by PD may afford protection against pruritus [349]. Finally, improved divalent ion metabolism and control of hyperparathyroidism with CAPD might also be expected to correlate with a reduced prevalence of pruritus. A study of severe pruritus in dialysis patients found a lower prevalence in CAPD compared to haemodialysis [352]. However, other surveys have been unable to document any difference in this complaint between the two dialysis modalities [350, 353]. Plasma histamine levels were not different among CAPD, haemodialysis or predialysis patients, and there was no correlation between these levels and the extent of itch [350]. Perhaps the intervening appearance of high-flux dialysers and more careful management of calcium and phosphate have resulted in a more equal distribution of pruritic complaints among haemodialysis and PD patients related to other, as yet unknown, factors.

Patients with chronic renal failure often have dry skin, and this can contribute to pruritus [354]. A recent study reported a correlation between hydration of the stratum corneum of the skin and complaints of itch in haemodialysis and PD patients. The dryness may be amenable to treatment with skin emollients [355].

Trying to study the treatment of pruritus is fraught with hazard. Measurement is confounded by its subjective nature, the absence of animal models, and the lack of validated measurements. The effect of treatment is subjected to bias on the part of investigator and patient [356]. It is likely that the placebo effect is significant.

Measures to relieve pruritus include skin moisturizers [355], activated oral charcoal, cholestyramine, intravenous lidocaine, antihistamines, ketotifen (which stabilizes mast cells) and erythropoietin [345, 351]. Parthyroidectomy may be helpful in those with advanced hyperparathyroidism.

Many studies have reported relief of pruritus with ultraviolet phototherapy. the mechanism of action is unknown, but is confined to the ultraviolet B spectrum. Postulated mechanisms of action include inactivation of pruritogens, reduction of skin phosphorus content, or alternation of signalling in cutaneous nerves [346]. A meta-analysis of published trials of therapy for uraemic pruritus found that only ultraviolet B phototherapy fulfilled the criteria for clinically significant improvement [356]. While noting that many of the studies were flawed, the authors concluded that this phototherapy was the treatment of choice in moderate to severe uraemic pruritus. The effects of lidocaine, charcoal and nicergoline were statistically, but not clinically, significant, and the effect of the bile acid sequestrant cholestyramine was clinically insignificant [356].

Insofar as pruritus may be a surrogate for underdialysis or impaired middle molecular clearance, it has been observed that pruritic patients have a worse outcome than patients without itch [357, 358]. Therefore parameters of dialysis adequacy should be closely monitored in these patients.

Calciphylaxis

This rare and unusual skin condition has been reported in end-stage renal disease patients, including those on PD [359–362].

This syndrome usually presents with livedo reticularis and progresses to the formation of cutaneous ulcers and necrotic eschars. There may be simultaneous development of lesions around several areas of the body. There is a predilection for the torso and thighs. Women appear to be affected more frequently than men. This syndrome is different from slowly progressive gangrene of the digits secondary to vascular calcification [363].

The aetiology is obscure, although it occurs most frequently in patients with renal failure. Many patients have severe hyperparathyroidism and an abnormal calcium–phosphorus product. It is held that the calcium and parathyroid abnormalities sensitize the patient, and when a 'challenging agent' is introduced the patient responds with vascular and soft-tissue calcification [278]. Treatment includes meticulous local care of the skin and subcutaneous lesions with timely debridement. There are anecdotal reports that urgent parathyroidectomy may be lifesaving in the subset of patients with hyperparathyroidism [364]. Careful attention to calcium and phosphorus levels is a reasonable strategy. Hyperbaric oxygen therapy has been helpful in one report [359].

Dialysis-associated amyloidosis

Amyloid deposits in the bones and joints of longterm haemodialysis patients were described in the 1980s. This interesting syndrome of 'haemodialysisassociated amyloidosis included carpal tunnel syndrome, subchondral bone cysts, spondyloarthropathy and pathological fractures [365]. This amyloid is composed of β_2-microglobulin (B_2M) [366, 367]. Since then, pathological studies have revealed that B_2M amyloid can deposit in tissues outside the musculoskeletal system, including skin, soft tissue and viscera [368–371].

This protein is a B cell product and is present on almost all cell membranes. It is measurable in plasma. These levels may be the result of production by lymphocytes, or from normal cell turnover and release of membrane constituents. It is freely filtered at the glomerulus and absorbed and catabolized in the proximal tubule. With renal insufficiency the filtration and catabolism of B_2M decreases and plasma levels increase.

Since the musculoskeletal syndrome was originally described exclusively in long-term haemodialysis patients, many factors related to haemodialysis were postulated to play a role in the formation of

B_2M amyloid. First, B_2M levels were markedly elevated in long-term haemodialysis patients, especially in those patients using small-pore membranes and those with negligible endogenous renal function. Secondly, the stimulation of the immune system by the repeated interface of blood with artificial membranes was postulated to lead to increased production of B_2M [365].

Serum levels of B_2M are also very high in patients receiving peritoneal dialysis, although not as high as levels in haemodialysis patients using conventional membranes [372–374]. Explanations put forth to explain the discrepancy include better clearance of this middle molecule by the peritoneal than by the haemodialysis membrane [375], the lack of immune stimulation using the peritoneal membrane and, in long-term patients, better preservation of endogeneous renal function [376].

However, by the mid-1980s presumptive evidence of B_2M amyloidosis in CAPD patients began to emerge. The prevalence of carpal tunnel syndrome, subclinical median mononeuropathy, bone cysts, discitis and cervical spondyloarthropathy suggested that PD patients were not protected from this articular complication [374, 377–380]. Subsequently B_2M amyloid was isolated from the tensoynovium of a long-term CAPD patient undergoing surgical release for carpal tunnel syndrome [381]. Large interstitial B_2M amyloid deposits were also isolated from the synovial tissue of the hip of a long-term CAPD patient undergoing prosthetic hip replacement [382]. Finally, post-mortem studies in long-term PD patients have confirmed the deposition of this type of amyloid in the intervertebral discs of the lumbosacral spine [383], the synovium of the scapulohumeral joint, hip and wrist [384] and the capsules of the shoulder joint and periarticular tissues [385].

The prevalence of dialysis-associated amyloidosis is difficult to reconcile among various surveys. Some studies report the prevalence of carpal tunnel syndrome or bone cysts as a surrogate for amyloid deposition, which may not necessarily be accurate and could underestimate the true prevalence of this condition [377, 378, 380, 386–388]. The most accurate way to diagnose B_2M amyloidosis is at postmorten, although in this case the amyloidosis, while present, may not have been associated with morbidity during life. A recent post-mortem analysis has demonstrated a high prevalence of B_2M amyloid deposition in CAPD patients [389]. In this study eight of 26 CAPD patients and 13 of 26 haeomdialysis patients had tissue evidence of B_2M amyloid.

When adjusted for duration of dialysis there was no statistical difference between the two modalities, although the trend was still for more amyloid in the haemodialysis patients [389]. Unfortunately, no data were available about the residual renal function in these patients.

A worrisome manifestation of B_2M amyloidosis is destructive cervical spondyloarthropathy. Again this complication had hitherto been documented only in long-term haemodialysis patients [390]. However, in our institution a patient who had received CAPD for 13 years developed this spondyloarthropathy, complicated by a compressive myelopathy. The cartilage removed at the time of fusion grafting was positive for amyloid composed of B_2M (Fig. 4) [391].

In summary, levels of B_2M in patients on PD are lower than those in patients receiving haemodialysis with conventional membranes. However, these levels are still much higher than those seen in controls. The relative paucity of reports of dialysis-associated amyloid in CAPD patients does not necessarily reflect a proportionately lower incidence of this arthropathy. There are fewer long-term PD patients compared to haemodialysis patients. The level of suspicion for this complication may not be as high in those treating CAPD patients. When adjusted for duration of dialysis the prevalence will probably be higher than previously thought [389].

Tendonitis, tendon rupture and calcific periarthritis

Spontaneous tendon rupture can occur in dialysis patients and may be associated with hyperparathyroidism and osteodystrophy [392]. This complication has been described mainly in patients undergoing haemodialysis. However, we have seen a young patient on CAPD with rupture of the quadriceps femoris tendon. Bilateral rupture of the tendon of the long head of the bicep muscle has also been described [393] and was attributed to the strain of the spiking and hanging of the 2-L bag.

Lateral epicondylitis or 'spike elbow' has also been described in CAPD [394]. This inflammation may be an overuse syndrome caused by the repetitive insertion of the spike with a twisting and pushing motion.

Calcific periarthritis has also been well described in patients on dialysis, although again it has been more frequently reported in patients on haemodialysis. Deposits of hydroxyapatite, calcium pyrophos-

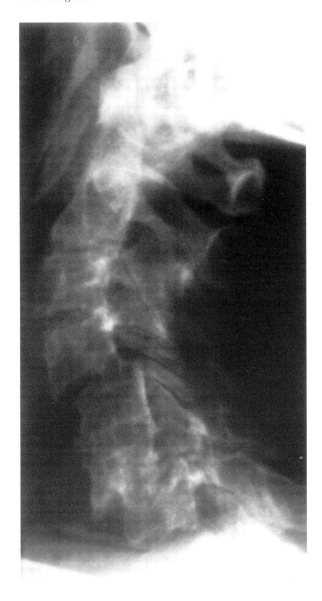

Figure 4. Radiograph of the cervical spine in a long-term CAPD patient who developed destructive spondyloarthropathy. Analysis of resected vertebral tissue revealed amyloid composed of β_2-microglobulin.

phate dihydrate (CPPD) or calcium oxalate [395] can accumulate around the joints and lead to acute attacks of synovitis or periarticular inflammation. This syndrome has been associated with an elevated calcium–phosphorus product and hyperparathyroidism [396]. In CAPD patients there is no association between inflammatory arthritis or periarthritis and PTH-induced subperiosteal resorption. Furthermore, changing patients from intermittent to continuous PD with improvement in the calcium–

phosphorus product has no salutary effect on the arthritis or periarthritis [397]. These findings suggest that the calcific periarthritis may be related to factors other than parathyroid overactivity or increased calcium–phosphorus product. A young lupus patient on CAPD with only modest elevation in the calcium–phosphorus product developed severe progressive calcific periarthritis resembling tumoural calcinosis which had to be surgically excised [398].

Back pain

The instillation of dialysis fluid into the peritoneal cavity can lead to alteration in spinal mechanics in the upright posture. In the patient with lax abdominal musculature the abdomen protrudes under the weight and volume of dialysate, and this swings the centre of gravity anteriorly. The normal lumbar lordosis is inappropriately accentuated.

Many patients entering PD programmes are elderly or have been deconditioned by years of illness and poor nutrition. Moreover, some patients have had treatment with corticosteroids or have undergone previous abdominal surgery. It is not surprising, therefore, that the abdominal musculature is often weak, leading to the alteration in spinal mechanics outlined above. In addition, the elderly uraemic patient may be at risk of degenerative disc disease, spondylolysis, spondylolisthesis and osteoporosis. Therefore the combination of intraperitoneal fluid, poor abdominal muscle tone, and intrinsic disease of the spinal column may culminate in back pain. This pain may be the result of paraspinal muscle spasm, posterior facet disease or sciatica [399]. With the recent emphasis on adequacy of small-solute clearance, many centres are using higher instilled volumes of dialysate, such as 2.5 L and 3.0 L [400]. The trend may be expected to aggravate posterior facet syndromes in predisposed individuals, especially if they are ambulatory with these larger volumes.

Treatment includes simple back education, where the patient learns the appropriate way to stand, bend over, and so on, to minimize strain on the back. Pelvic tilt exercises are simple and can be performed by patients on PD [399]. Judicious use of skeletal muscle relaxants or anti-inflammatory agents may be necessary for short-term relief of symptoms.

In the patient complaining of persistent back pain, further evaluation is warranted. This includes vertebral radiographs to evaluate the bony structures.

The opinion of a rheumatologist or physiotherapist may be necessary.

The dialysis regimen can be changed to APD. Dialysis in the supine position removes the lordotic stress on the lumbar vertebrae and paraspinal support tissues. Moreover, larger dialysis volumes can be used overnight. It is advisable to keep some fluid in the day dwell for adequacy considerations, but that will depend on the individual patient and circumstances. With this regimen the adverse effect of intraperitoneal fluid on spinal mechanics is minimized and the patient may be able to perform PD despite abnormal spinal mechanics.

Oxalate metabolism and kidney stones

Oxalate is freely filtered at the glomerulus and secreted in the proximal tubule. As renal function deteriorates, oxalate retention and hyperoxalaemia supervene [401]. The retained oxalate is deposited as the poorly soluble calcium salt in kidney, bone, hyaline and fibrocartilage, myocardium, lungs, central nervous system and blood vessels (reviewed in ref. 392). Chondrocalcinosis and pseudogout can be caused by calcium oxalate as well as calcium phrophosphate dihydrate in patients with end-stage renal disease [395].

In patients on CAPD, plasma levels of oxalate are three to five times higher than in controls [402] and are equivalent to predialysis levels in haemodialysis patients [403]. Because of its low molecular weight (90 Da) it is rapidly cleared during haemodialysis and levels fall about 40%. On the other hand, CAPD clears about 300 $\mu mol/day$, which approximates the amount synthesized daily. Therefore, CAPD can maintain steady-state plasma levels of oxalate, but at levels much higher than normal [403–405]. Previous studies of oxalate removal by PD should be interpreted in the light of the recent finding of rising oxalate levels in the drained effluent, suggesting ongoing production of oxalate *ex vivo* in the dialysate [405]. Detailed studies on two patients determined that dialysate levels of oxalate were approximately 40–50% of plasma levels after a 3–4 h dwell, but there was almost total equilibration after a 12 h dwell [406]. Furthermore, although clearance of oxalate is greater per unit time with haemodialysis, total weekly elimination is similar with CAPD because of the longer time of dialysis [407]. In young patients with oxalosis, a combination of haemodialysis and equilibration (long dwell) PD

may be the best combination to keep blood oxalate levels under control until liver/kidney transplantation can be arranged [406].

Ascorbic acid supplements cause a further increase in plasma oxalate levels. One hundred milligrams of oral ascorbic acid resulted in nearly a 20% increase in plasma levels of oxalate [405]. In patients on CAPD taking vitamins, the benefit of vitamin C supplements should be weighed against the potential hazard of further elevating plasma oxalate values. These patients have normal plasma levels of ascorbic acid before receiving supplementation, so there may not be a need for vitamin C treatment. Concurrent treatment with 10 mg of vitamin B6 results in a 17% decrease in oxalate levels in patients already taking ascorbic acid, but these levels remain markedly elevated [405]. Pyridoxine supplementation does not appear to lower significantly the plasma oxalate or oxalate generation rate in PD patients not taking vitamin C either [408].

A significant number of patients on CAPD will pass kidney stones. In one survey [409], 10 of 186 CAPD patients (5.4%) passed renal calculi after 6–9 months on CAPD. Half of these stones were composed of calcium oxalate monohydrate and the rest were made of protein matrix alone or calcium apatite. Metabolic investigation of CAPD patients has demonstrated that, while the total excretion of calcium and oxalate is necessarily diminished, the urinary concentration of oxalate is significantly elevated compared to normals, and the ionic calcium concentration in the urine is lower than normal. However, the calcium oxalate activity product is in the 'labile' region and varies according to the urinary ionized calcium concentration. This dependence upon urinary calcium is different from normals, where the calcium oxalate activity product depends upon the concentration of both urinary oxalate and calcium. Therefore, although the urine ionic calcium concentration is low in renal failure, relative increases in this level will significantly influence the activity product and lead to crystallization. The administration of 1,25-dihydroxy vitamin D3 correlates with the urine ionized calcium concentration [409] and could be considered a risk factor for stone formation. With the move from aluminium-containing to calcium-containing phosphate binders, it will be interesting to see whether the incidence of calcium-containing stones increases in CAPD patients.

Interestingly, intraluminal lithiasis should be kept in mind as a rare cause of obstruction of the PD catheter. Impaction of a calcium-struvite calculus in the intraperitoneal tip of the catheter lumen has been described. The authors suggested that a fibrin clot could have adhered to the catheter and served as a nidus for mineralization in this patient with an elevated calcium–phosphate product [410].

Transplantation

Outcome of allografts in PD patients

As CAPD grew in popularity, more data became available on the outcome of renal transplantation in these patients. Two reports from the early 1980s led to concern. A significant increase in the helper to suppressor T lymphocyte ratio in patients on long-term CAPD was associated with an increased incidence of graft rejection when compared to haemodialysis patients [411]. Similarly, a second study found decreased graft survival in patients previously receiving CAPD when compared to those on haemodialysis. This decreased survival was apparent as early as 1 month post-transplant. Again, the patients who had been on PD had a higher ratio of circulating helper T lymphocytes and did not display the T-cell lymphopenia found in the haemodialysis patients [412]. Although the implication is that the increased ratio of circulating T lymphocytes is linked with graft rejection, it has not been demonstrated that the ratio of helper to suppressor T lymphocytes bears any consistent relationship to graft outcome [413]. Unlike haemodialsyis patients, CAPD patients did not benefit from pretransplant blood transfusions [412]. Indeed, a fall in panel reactive antibodies was noted in three children with their conversion from haemodialysis to PD, which was attributed to a reduced need for blood transfusion during the latter treatment [414].

Since these two reports, many centres have compared patient and graft outcome in their PD and haemodialysis patients. While there is some variation from centre to centre, there does not appear to be any consistent trend in the survival of either graft or patients between the two modalities of dialysis [415–427]. Many of the studies consisted of small numbers of PD patients, which limits the power of statistical analysis and increases the chance of beta error. However, as pointed out [428], even the studies involving large numbers of PD patients have shown similar, if not identical, graft and patient survival. It is conceivable that the intense immunosuppressive therapy given to transplant patients negates any modest innate difference in immuno-

competence between the two dialysis modalities. A recent analysis of more than 500 patients who survived the first 6 months after transplant demonstrated that duration of dialysis prior to transplant was an important predictor of survival (the more years of dialysis, the higher the mortality), but that modality of dialysis could not predict patient survival [429]. Interestingly, Spanish investigators reported that patients receiving a kidney transplant had a higher incidence of delayed graft function if they were on haemodialysis rather than peritoneal dialysis [430]. The haemodialysis patients had received more blood transfusions beforehand and the kidneys they received had longer cold ischaemia time, and both these factors may have contributed to the delayed graft function. Moreover, the haemodialysis cohort received more immunosuppresisve therapy and suffered more late infections compared to those on CAPD pretransplant [430].

Two centres in Europe have observed a higher incidence of arterial and venous thrombosis of the renal allograft in the perioperative period in patients who were on CAPD compared to those on haemodialysis. Murphy et al. [431] reported graft thrombosis in nine of 97 CAPD patients compared to one of 99 haemodialysis patients. Three of the nine had a risk for hypercoagulability such as nephrotic syndrome. Subsequent reports from the Netherlands documented graft thrombosis in 7.3% of CAPD patients receiving kidneys compared to 3.6% of haemodialysis patients [432]. No obvious reason could be found for the increased thrombosis. In contrast, a recent review of more than 800 kidney transplants conduced that, if anything, there was a trend towards a higher rate of thrombosis of the allograft in haemodialysis patients [430].

Other risks unique to the PD patient

The PD patient may face extra risk of infection from the peritoneal cavity and catheter. Previous episodes of peritonitis have been postulated to leave a nucleus of infection which could develop into overwhelming sepsis. The development of peritonitis could pose a life-threatening complication in patients receiving immunosuppressive drugs [415]. The incidence of peritonitis in the post-transplant period does appear to be significant, varying from 5% to 35% if the patient needs to resume PD because of graft non-function [419, 422, 425]. Peritonitis is easily managed by antibiotics, lavage, and catheter removal if necessary [415, 417, 433], although in one patient it led to death from sepsis [420]. The simultaneous administration of cytotoxic agents does not hamper the response of bacterial peritonitis to antibiotic therapy.

Most centres electively remove the PD catheter about 2–3 months post-transplant [416, 417, 419, 433–435], although some remove it at the time of transplant and haemodialyse the patient as needed thereafter [436]. Because of the risk of bowel perforation, an unused catheter should be flushed regularly and removed no later than 2–3 months after successful transplantation.

Post-transplant ascites has been reported in children [437] and adults [438] who were on CAPD before the transplant. In adults the ascites lasted up to 50 days, but ultimately resolved [438].

Finally, there is the risk of mechanical problems in the PD patient undergoing transplant. The catheter exit site can be close to the transplant bed. (Initial implantation sites of PD catheters should be chosen with this potential problem in mind.) If the PD peritoneum has not been disrupted during transplant surgery, PD can be performed postoperatively, if necessary. There have been reports of drainage of dialysate through the transplant incision [420, 422] and through the site of a transplant nephrectomy [421]. This complication is managed by temporarily stopping PD and proving antibiotic coverage.

Cancer

While cardiovascular and infectious complications comprise the major causes of death in dialysis patients, it is unclear whether there is a higher incidence of cancer and cancer-related deaths in this population. It is possible that, as part of a change in immune function in the dialysis population [438, 440], there is impaired tumour surveillance. Unfortunately, many of these studies are hampered by small sample size, selection bias, and perhaps a bias in favour of increased diagnosis in a more closely monitored population [441, 442]. For example, a survey of haemodialysis patients in Japan showed a higher incidence of cancer in patients dialysing at university-affiliated hospitals rather than private hospitals. The authors suggested that closer follow-up and higher autopsy rates were responsible for this difference [441]. Studies in haemodialysis patients on the whole demonstrate no real consensus as to whether there is a greater risk of malignancy [443].

Cancer appears to be a relatively rare cause of death in dialysis patients, according to North American registry data. This is because cardiovascular and infectious aetiologies eclipse malignancy in this population. There may be some exceptions. Patients with failed renal transplants have a higher incidence of skin cancers, lymphoma, and other malignancies secondary to chronic immunosuppression. Dialysis patients with lupus nephritis who also received immunosuppression with drugs such as cyclophosphamide or chlorambucil may be at increased risk for neoplasia. The risk of cancerous transformation of acquired renal cysts has already been discussed.

A recent analysis of cancer screening of dialysis patients notes that many of the commonly used tests may have diminished yield in dialysis patients [444]. In combination with the accelerated death rate from cardiovascular disease, the authors suggest that routine cancer screening would not extend the life expectancy of a dialysis patient. Their theoretical treatment using optimal, inexpensive screening tests resulted in a net gain in life expectancy of 5 days or less from screening for breast, cervical, colorectal and prostate cancer [445].

As a public health policy issue cancer screening may not be worthwhile, especially in the elderly patient with significant comorbidity. It still may be good medical practice to employ screening in young, high-risk patients such as those with a failed kidney transplant, or those who have received chronic immunosuppressive therapy for other reasons.

Acknowledgements

The author thanks V. Brown for secretarial assistance, and S. and M. Silverman for their forbearance.

References

1. Gotloib L, Mines M, Garmizo L, Varka I. Hemodynamic effects of increasing intra-abdominal pressure in peritoneal dialysis. Perit Dial Bull 1981; 1: 41–4.
2. Twardowski Z, Khanna R, Nolph K *et al.* Intra-abdominal pressures during natural activities in patients treated with continuous ambulatory peritoneal dialysis. Nephron 1986; 44: 129–35.
3. Durand PY, Chanliau J, Gamberoni J, Hestin D, Kessler M. APD: clinical measurement of the maximal acceptable intra-peritoneal volume. Adv Perit Dial. 1994; 10: 63–7.
4. Durand PY, Chanliau J, Gamberoni J, Hestin D, Kessler M. Routine measurement of hydrostatic intra-peritoneal pressure. Adv Perit Dial 1992; 8: 108–12.
5. O'Connor J, Rigby R, Hardie I *et al.* Abdominal hernias complicating continuous ambulatory peritoneal dialysis. Am J Nephrol 1986; 6: 271–4.
6. Digenis G, Khanna R, Mathews R, Oreopoulos DG. Abdominal hernias in patients undergoing continuous ambulatory peritoneal dialysis. Perit Dial Bull 1982; 2: 115–17.

7. Rubin J, Raju S, Teal N, Hellems E, Bower J. Abdominal hernia in patients undergoing continuous ambulatory peritoneal dialysis. Arch Intern Med 1982; 142: 1453–5.

8. Kauffman H, Adams M. Indirect inguinal hernia in patients undergoing peritoneal dialysis. Surgery 1986; 99: 254–5.

9. Engeset J, Youngson G. Ambulatory peritoneal dialysis and hernial complications. Surg Clin N Am 1984; 64: 385–92.

10. Rocco M, Stone W. Abdominal hernias in chronic peritoneal dialysis patients: a review. Perit Dial Bull 1985; 5: 171–4.

11. Tzamaloukas A, Bevan M, Cox B *et al.* Clinical associations and effects of hernias in CAPD patients. Perit Dial Bull 1986; 6 (suppl.): S21 (abstract).

12. Wise M, Manos J, Gokal R. Small umbilical hernias in patients on CAPD (letter). Perit Dial Bull 1984; 4: 270–1.

13. Wetherington G, Leapman S, Robinson R, Filo RS. Abdominal wall and inguinal hernias in continuous ambulatory peritoneal dialysis patients. Am J Surg 1985; 150: 357–60.

14. Suh H, Wadhwa NK, Cabralda T, Sokunbi D, Pinard B. Abdominal wall hernias in ESRD patients receiving peritoneal dialysis. Adv Perit Dial 1994; 10: 85–8.

15. Modi KB, Grant AC, Garret A, Rodger RSC. Indirect inguinal hernia in CAPD patients with polycystic kidney disease. Adv Perit Dial 1989; 5: 84–6.

16. Sorensen VR, Joffe P. Subcutaneous swelling during CAPD. Perit Dial Int 1998; 18: 232–5.

17. Apostolidis NS, Tzardis PJ, Manouras AJ, Kosenidou MD, Katirtzoglou AN. The incidence of postoperative hernia as related to the site of insertion of permanent peritoneal catheter. Am Surg 1988; 54: 318–19.

18. Spence P, Mathews R, Khanna R, Oreopoulos DG. Improved results with a paramedian technique for the insertion of peritoneal dialysis catheters. Surg Gynecol Obstet 1985; 161: 585–7.

19. Khoury AE, Charendoff J, Balfe JW, McLorie GA, Churchill BM. Hernias associated with CAPD in children. Adv Perit Dial 1991; 7: 279–82.

20. Ramos J, Burke D, Veitch P. Hernia of Morgagni in patients on continuous ambulatory peritoneal dialysis (letter). Lancet 1982; 1: 161–2.

21. Polk D, Madden RL, Lipkowitz GS *et al.* Use of computerized tomography in the evaluation of a CAPD patient with a foramen of Morgagni hernia: a case report. Perit Dial Int 1996; 16: 318–20.

22. Grossi C, Faiolo S, Tettamanzi F, Zani B, Mangano S, Scalia P. Obturator hernia, a rare complication in a CAPD patient: report of a case. Perit Dial Int 1993; 13 (suppl. 1): S11 (abstract).

23. Griffin P, Coles G. Strangulated hernias through Tenckhoff cannula sites. Br Med J 1982; 284: 1837.

24. Power D, Edward N, Catto G, Muirhead N, MacLeod A, Engeset J. Richter's hernia: an unrecognized complication of chronic ambulatory peritoneal dialysis. Br Med J 1981; 283: 528.

25. Shohat J, Shapira Z, Shmueli D, Boner G. Intestinal incarceration in occult abdominal wall herniae in continuous ambulatory peritoneal dialysis. Isr J Med Sci 1985; 21: 985–7.

26. Steiner RW, Halasz NA. Abdominal catastrophes and other unusual events in continuous ambulatory peritoneal dialysis patients. Am J Kidney Dis 1990; 15: 1–7.

27. Bleyer AJ, Casey MJ, Russell GB, Kandt M, Burkart JM. Peritoneal dialysate fill-volumes and hernia development in a cohort of peritoneal dialysis patients. Adv Perit Dial 1998; 14: 102–4.

28. Hussain SI, Bernardini J, Piraino B. The risk of hernia with large exchange volumes. Adv Perit Dial 1998; 14: 105–7.

29. Moffat F, Deitel M, Thompson D. Abdominal surgery in patients undergoing long-term peritoneal dialysis. Surgery 1982; 92: 598–604.

30. Imvrios G, Tsakiris D, Gakis D *et al.* Prosthetic mesh repair of multiple recurrent and large abdominal hernias in continuous ambulatory peritoneal dialysis patients. Perit Dial Int 1994; 14: 338–43.

31. Lewis DM, Bingham C, Beaman M, Nicholls AJ, Riad HN. Polypropylene mesh hernia repair – an alternative permitting rapid return to peritoneal dialysis. Nephrol Dial Transplant 1998; 13: 2488–9.

32. Abraham G, Nallathambi MN, Bhaskaran S, Srinivasan L. Recurrence of abdominal wall hernias due to failure of mesh repair in a peritoneal dialysis patient. Perit Dial Int 1997; 17: 89–91.

33. Madden M, Beirne G, Zimmerman S, Sollinger H. Acute bowel obstruction: an unusual complication of chronic peritoneal dialysis. Am J Kidney Dis 1982; 1: 219–21.

34. Nassberger L. Enterocele due to continuous ambulatory peritoneal dialysis (CAPD). Acta Obstet Gynecol Scand 1984; 63: 283.

35. Francis D, Schofield I, Veitch P. Abdominal hernias in patients treated with continuous ambulatory peritoneal dialysis. Br J Surg 1982; 69: 409.

36. Lee A, Waffle C, Trebbin W. Clostridial myonecrosis. Origin from an obturator hernia in a dialysis patient. JAMA 1983; 246: 1232–3.

37. Kopecky R, Funk M, Kreitzer P. Localized genital edema in patients undergoing continuous ambulatory peritoneal dialysis. J Urol 1985; 134: 880–4.

38. Beaman M, Feehally J, Smith B, Walls J. Anterior abdominal wall leakage in CAPD patients: management by intermittent peritoneal dialysis (letter). Perit Dial Bull 1985; 5: 81–2.

39. Cooper JC, Nicholls AJ, Simms JM, Platts MM, Brown CB, Johnson AG. Genital oedema in patients treated by continuous ambulatory peritoneal dialysis: an unusual presentation of inguinal hernia. Br Med J 1983; 286: 1923–4.

40. Orfei R, Seybold K, Blumberg A. Genital edema in patients undergoing continuous ambulatory peritoneal dialysis (CAPD). Perit Dial Bull 1984; 4: 251–2.

41. Twardowski Z, Tully R, Nichols W, Sunderranjan S. Computerized tomography (CT) in the diagnosis of subcutaneous leak sites during continuous ambulatory peritoneal dialysis (CAPD). Perit Dial Bull 1984; 4: 163–6.

42. Schurgers M, Boelaert J, Daneels R, Robbens E, Vandelanotte M. Open processus vaginalis. Perit Dial Bull 1983; 3: 30–1.

43. Tzamaloukas AH, Gibel LJ, Eisenberg B *et al.* Scrotal edema in patients on CAPD: causes, differential diagnosis and management. Dial Transplant 1992; 21: 581–90.

44. Abraham G, Blake PG, Mathews RE, Bargman JM, Izatt S, Oreopoulos DG. Genital swelling as a surgical complication of continuous ambulatory peritoneal dialysis. Surg Gynecol Obstet 1990; 170: 306–8.

45. Coward R, Gokal R, Wise M, Mallick NP, Warrell D. Peritonitis associated with vaginal leakage of dialysis fluid in continuous ambulatory peritoneal dialysis. Br Med J 1982; 284: 1529.

46. Caporale N, Perez D, Alegre S. Vaginal leak of peritoneal dialysate liquid. Perit Dial Int 1991; 11: 284–5.

47. Ogunc G, Oygur N. Vaginal fistula: a new complication in CAPD (letter). Perit Dial Int 1995; 15: 84–5.

48. Whiting M, Smith N, Agar J. Vaginal peritoneal dialysate leakage per fallopian tubes (letter). Perit Dial Int 1995; 15: 85.

49. Bradley A, Mamtora, Pritchard N. Transvaginal leak of peritoneal dialysate demonstrated by CT peritoneography. Br J Radiol 1997; 70: 652–3.

50. Ralph-Edwards A, Maziak D, Deitel M, Thompson DA, Kucey DS, Bayley TA. Sudden rupture of an indirect inguinal hernial sac with extravasation in two patients on continuous ambulatory peritoneal dialysis. Canal J Surg 1993; 37: 70–2.

51. Sackey AH, Cook RC, Judd BA. Rupture of hernial sac in an infant after CAPD (letter). Perit Dial Int 1994; 14: 92–3.

52. Litherland J, Gibson M, Sambrook P, Lupton E, Beaman M, Ackrill P. Investigation and treatment of poor drains of dialysate fluid associated with anterior abdominal wall leaks in patients on chronic ambulatory peritoneal dialysis. Nephrol Dial Transplant 1992; 7: 1030–4.

53. Holley JL, Bernardini J, Piraino B. Characteristics and outcome of peritoneal dialysate leaks and associated infections. Adv Perit Dial 1993; 9: 240–3.

54. Joffe P. Peritoneal dialysis catheter leakage treated with fibrin glue. Nephrol Dial Transplant 1993; 8: 474–6.

55. Sojo E, Bisigniano L, Turconi A *et al.* Is fibrin glue useful in preventing dialysate leakage in children on CAPD? Preliminary results of a prospective randomized study. Adv Perit Dial 1997; 13: 277–80.

56. Mandel P, Faegenburg D, Imbriano L. The use of technetium-99m sulfur colloid in the detection of patent processus vaginalis in patients on continuous ambulatory peritoneal dialysis. Clin Nucl Med 1985; 10: 553–5.

57. Dubin L, Froelich J. Evaluation of scrotal edema in a patients on peritoneal dialysis. Clin Nucl Med 1985; 10: 173–4.

58. Johnson BF, Segasby CA, Holroyd AM, Brown CB, Cohen GL, Raftery AT. A method for demonstrating subclinical inguinal herniae in patients undergoing peritoneal dialysis: the isotope 'peritoneoscrotogram'. Nephrol Dial Transplant 1987; 2: 254–7.

59. Berman C, Velchik MG, Shusterman N, Alavi A. The clinical utility of the Tc-99m SC intraperitoneal scan in CAPD patients. Clin Nucl Med 1989; 14: 405–9.

60. Sissons GRJ, Meecham Jones SM, Evans C, Richards AR. Scintigraphic detection of abdominal hernias associated with continuous ambulatory peritoneal dialysis. Br J Radiol 1991; 53: 1158–61.

61. Twardowski ZJ, Tully RJ, Ersoy FF, Dedhia NM. Computerized tomography with and without intraperitoneal contrast for determination of intra-abdominal fluid distribution and diagnosis of complications in peritoneal dialysis patients. ASAIO Trans 1990; 36: 95–103.

62. Caimi F, Roveroe G, Phillipson M, Battaglia E. Contribution of peritoneography combined with computerized tomography, in the assessment of abdominal complications in patients undergoing continuous peritoneal dialysis. Radiol Med 1991; 81: 656–9.

63. Litherland J, Lupton EW, Ackrill PA, Venning M, Sambrook P. Computed tomographic peritoneography: CT manifestations in the investigation of leaks and abnormal collections in patients on CAPD. Nephrol Dial Transplant 1994; 9: 1449–52.

64. Camsari T, Celik A, Ozaksoy D, Salman S, Cavdar C, Sifil A. Non-infectious complications of continuous ambulatory peritoneal dialysis: evaluation with peritoneal computed tomography. Scand J Urol Nephrol 1997; 31: 377–80.

65. Maher J, Schreiner G. Hazards and complications of dialysis. N Engl J Med 1965; 273: 370–7.

66. Edwards S, Unger A. Acute hydrothorax: a new complication of peritoneal dialysis. JAMA 1967; 199: 189–91.

67. Bunchman T, Wood E, Lynch R. Hydrothorax as a complication of peritoneal dialysis. Perit Dial Bull 1987; 7: 237–9.

68. Scheldewaert R, Bogaerts Y, Pauwels R, Van DerStraeten M, Ringoir S, Lameire N. Management of a massive hydrothorax in a CAPD patient: a case report and a review of the literature. Perit Dial Bull 1982; 2: 69–72.

69. Abraham G, Shoker A, Blake P, Oreopoulos D. Massive hydrothorax in patients on peritoneal dialysis: a literature review. Adv Perit Dial 1988; 4: 121–5.

70. Nomoto Y, Suga T, Nakajima A *et al.* Acute hydrothorax in continuous ambulatory peritoneal dialysis – a collaborative study of 161 centers. Am J Nephrol 1989; 9: 363–7.

71. Chow CC, Sung JY, Cheung CK, Hamilton-Wood C, Lai KN. Massive hydrothorax in continuous ambulatory peritoneal dialysis: diagnosis, management and review of the literature. NZ Med J 1988; 101: 475–7.

72. Lieberman F, Hidemura R, Peters R, Reynolds T. Pathogenesis and treatment of hydrothorax complicating cirrhosis with ascites. Ann Intern Med 1966; 64: 341–51.

73. Johnston R, Loo R. Hepatic hydrothorax. Studies to determine the source of fluid and report of thirteen cases. Ann Intern Med 1964; 61: 385–401.

74. Grefberg N, Danielson B, Benson L *et al.* Right-sided hydrothorax complicating peritoneal dialysis. Nephron 1983; 34: 130–4.

75. Boeschoten EW, Krediet RT, Roos CM, Kloek JJ, Schipper MEI, Arisz L. Leakage of dialysate across the diaphragm: an important complication of continuous ambulatory peritoneal dialysis. Neth J Med 1986; 29: 242–6.

76. Bjerki HS, Adkins ES, Foglia RP. Surgical correction of hydrothorax from diaphragmatic eventration in children on peritoneal dialysis. Surgery 1991; 109: 550–4.

77. Ramon RC, Carrasco AM. Hydrothorax in peritoneal dialysis. Perit Dial Int 1998; 18: 5–10.

78. Hou C-H, Tsai T-J, Hsu K-L. Peritoneopericardial communication after pericardiocentesis in a patient on continuous ambulatory peritoneal dialysis with dialysis pericarditis. Nephron 1994; 68: 125–7.

79. Nather S, Anger H, Koall W *et al.* Peritoneal leak and chronic pericardial effusion in a CAPD patient. Nephrol Dial Transplant 1996; 11: 1155–8.

80. Joseph UA, Jhingran SG, Olivero JJ. Scintigraphic assessment of pericardio-peritoneal window patency: relevance to peritoneal dialysis. Clin Nucl Med 1995; 20: 613–14.

81. Fletcher S, Turney JH, Brownjohn AM. Increased incidence of hydrothorax complicating peritoneal dialysis in patients with adult polycystic kidney disease. Nephrol Dial Transplant 1994; 9: 832–3.

82. Vareesangthip K, Wilkinson R, Thomas T. Lack of function of an N-ethylmaleimide-sensitive thiol protein in erythrocyte membrane of autosomal dominant polycystic kidney disease. J Am Soc Nephrol 1998; 9: 1–8.

83. Trust A, Rossoff LJ. Tension hydrothorax in a patient with renal failure. Chest 1990; 97: 1254–5.

84. Benz R, Schleifer CR. Hydrothorax in CAPD. Successful treatment with intrapleural tetracycline and a review of the literature. Am J Kidney Dis 1985; 2: 136–40.

85. Macia M, Gallego E, Garcia-Cobaleda I, Chahin J, Garcia J. Methylene blue as a cause of chemical peritonitis in a patient on peritoneal dialysis (letter). Clin Nephrol 1995; 43: 136.

86. Adam W, Arkies L, Gill G, Meagher E, Thomas G. Hydrothorax with peritoneal dialysis: radionuclide detection of a pleuro-peritoneal connection. Austr NZ J Med 1980; 10: 330–2.

87. Gibbons G, Baumert J. Unilateral hydrothorax complicating peritoneal dialysis. Use of radionuclide imaging. Clin Nucl Med 1983; 3: 83–4.

88. Kennedy J. Procedures used to demonstrate a pleuroperitoneal communication: a review. Perit Dial Bull 1985; 5: 168–70.

89. Mestas D, Wauquier JP, Escande G, Baquet JC, Veyr A. Diagnosis of hydrothorax complicating CAPD and demonstration of successful therapy by scintigraphy (letter). Perit Dial Int 1991; 11: 283–5.

90. Walker F, McAllister C, McKee P, McNulty J. Intra-peritoneal lopamidol, a new radiocontrast agent in the diagnosis of a pleuroperitoneal communication (letter). Perit Dial Int 1986; 6: 108–9.

91. Green A, Logan M, Medawar W *et al.* The management of hydrothorax in continuous ambulatory peritoneal dialysis (CAPD). Perit Dial Int 1990; 10: 271–4.

92. Vezina D, Winchester JF, Rakowski TA. Spontaneous resolution of massive hydrothorax in a CAPD patient (letter). Perit Dial Bull 1987; 7: 212–13.

93. Ing A, Rutland J, Kalowski S. Spontaneous resolution of hydrothorax in continuous ambulatory peritoneal dialysis (letter). Nephron 1992; 61: 247–8.

94. Townsent R, Fragola JA. Hydrothorax in a patient receiving continuous ambulatory peritoneal dialysis – successful treatment with intermittent peritoneal dialysis. Arch Intern Med 1982; 142: 1571–2.

95. Christidou F, Vayonas G. Recurrent acute hydrothorax in a CAPD patient: successful management with small volumes of dialysate (letter). Perit Dial Int 1995; 15: 389.

96. Simmons LE, Mir AR. A review of management of pleuro-peritoneal communication in five CAPD patients. Adv Dial 1989; 5: 81–3.

97. Posen G, Sachs H. Treatment of recurrent pleural effusions in dialysis patients by talc insufflation. Am Soc Artif Intern Organs, 25th Annual Meeting, New York, 1979, p. 75 (abstract).

98. Jagasia MH, Cole FH, Stegman MH, Deaton P, Kennedy L. Video-assisted talc pleurodesis in the management of pleural effusion secondary to continuous ambulatory peritoneal dialysis: a report of three cases. Am J Kidney Dis 1996; 28: 772–4.

99. Mak S-K, Chan MWK, Tai Y-P *et al.* Thoracoscopic pleurodesis for massive hydrothorax complicating CAPD. Perit Dial Int 1996; 16: 421–5.

100. Hidai H, Takatsu S, Chiba T. Intrathoracic instillation of autologous blood in treating massive hydrothorax following CAPD (letter). Perit Dial Int 1989; 9: 221–2.

101. Catizone L, Zuchelli A, Zuchelli P. Hydrothorax in a PD patient: successful treatment with intrapleural autologous blood instillation. Adv Perit Dial 1991; 7: 86–90.

102. Okada K, Takahashi S, Kinoshita Y. Effect of pleurodesis with autoblood on hydrothorax due to continuous ambulatory peritoneal dialysis-induced diaphragmatic communication (letter). Nephron 1993; 65: 153–4.

103. Vlachojannis J, Bloettcher I, Brandt L, Schoeppe W. A new treatment for unilateral recurrent hydrothorax during CAPD. Perit Dial Bull 1985; 5: 180–1.

104. Pattison C, Rodger R, Adu D *et al.* Surgical treatment of hydrothorax complicating CAPD. Clin Nephrol 1984; 21: 191–3.

105. Allen SM, Matthews HR. Surgical treatment of massive hydrothorax complicating continuous ambulatory peritoneal dialysis. Clin Nephrol 1991; 36: 299–301.

106. Kawaguchi AL, Dunn JC, Fonkalsrud EW. Management of peritoneal dialysis-induced hydrothorax in children. Am Surg 1996; 62: 820–4.

107. Derlyne G, Lee H, Ralston A, Woolcock JA. Pulmonary complications of peritoneal dialysis. Lancet 1966; 2: 75–8.

108. Ahluwalia M, Ishikawa S, Gellman M *et al.* Pulmonary functions during peritoneal dialysis. Clin Nephrol 1982; 18: 251–6.

109. Gomez-Fernandez P, Sanchez Agudo L, Calatrava J *et al.* Respiratory muscle weakness in uremic patients under continuous ambulatory peritoneal dialysis. Nephron 1984; 36: 219–23.

110. Singh S, Dale A, Morgan B, Sahebjami H. Serial studies of pulmonary function in continuous ambulatory peritoneal dialysis. Chest 1984; 86: 874–7.

111. Taveira da Silva A, Davis W, Winchester J, Coleman DE, Weir CW. Peritonitis, dialysate infusion and lung function in continuous ambulatory peritoneal dialysis (CAPD). Clin Nephrol 1985; 24: 79–83.

112. O'Brien AA, Power J, O'Brien L, Clancy L, Keogh JA. The effect of peritoneal dialysate on pulmonary function and blood gases in CAPD patients. Irish J Med Sci 1990; 159: 215–16.

113. Gokbel H, Yeksan M, Dogan E, Gundogan F, Uzun K. Effect of CAPD applications on pulmonary function (letter). Perit Dial Int 1998; 18: 344–5.

114. Freedman S, Maberly D. Gas exchange in renal failure (letter). Br Med J 1971; 3: 48.

115. Blumberg A, Keller R, Marti H. Oxygen affinity of erythrocytes and pulmonary gas exchange in patients on continuous ambulatory peritoneal dialysis. Nephron 1984; 38: 248–52.

116. Korzets Z, Golan E, Ben-Chitrit S, Smorjik Y, Os P, Bernheim J. Orthostatic hypoxaemia in dialysed adult polycystic kidney disease patients. Nephrol Dial Transplant 1997; 12: 733–5.

117. Oreopoulos D, Rebuck A. Risks and benefits of peritoneal dialysis. Chest 1985; 88: 6742.

118. Leblanc M, Ouimet D, Tremblay C, Nolin L. Peritoneal instillation test before CAPD in a case of severe pulmonary disease. Perit Dial Int 1995; 15: 384–7.

119. Rebuck A. Peritoneal dialysis and the mechanics of the diaphragm (editorial). Perit Dial Bull 1982; 2: 109–10.

120. Wanke T, Auinger M, Lahrmann H *et al.* Diaphragmatic function in patients on continuous ambulatory peritoneal dialysis. Lung 1994; 172: 231–40.

121. Bush A, Gabriel R. Pulmonary function in chronic renal failure: effects of dialysis and transplantation. Thorax 1991; 46: 424–8.

122. Smith S, Goldberg M. Pulmonary insufficiency as a result of chronic aspiration secondary to CAPD therapy. Am J Kidney Dis 1985; 6: A19 (abstract).

123. Holley JL, Piraino B. CAPD-associated cough (letter). Perit Dial Int 1995; 15: 392–3.

124. Eiser A. Pulmonary gas exchange during hemodialysis and peritoneal dialysis: interaction between respiration and metabolism. Am J Kidney Dis 1985; 6: 131–42.

125. Fabris A, Biasioli S, Chiaramonte C *et al.* Buffer metabolism in continuous ambulatory peritoneal dialysis (CAPD): relationship with respiratory dynamics. Trans Am Soc Artif Intern Organs 1982; 28: 270–5.

126. Cohn J, Balik RA, Bone RC. Dialysis-induced respiratoryacidosis. Chest 1990; 98: 1285–8.

127. Hallett M, Burdens, Stewart D, Mahony J, Farrell PC. Sleep apnea in ESRD patients on HD and CAPD. Perit Dial Int 1996 (suppl. 1): S429–33.

128. Kraus MA, Hamburger RJ. Sleep apnea in renal failure. Adv Perit Dial 1997; 13: 88–92.

129. Moldofsky H, Krueger J, Walter J *et al.* Sleep-promoting material extracted from peritoneal dialysate of patients with end stage renal disease and insomnia. Perit Dial Bull 1985; 5: 189–93.

130. Wadhwa NK, Seliger M, Greenberg HE, Bergofsky E, Mendelson WB. Sleep related respiratory disorders in end-stage renal disease patients on peritoneal dialysis. Perit Dial Int 1992; 12: 51–6.

131. Stepanski E, Faber M, Zorick F, Basner R, Roth T. Sleep disorders in patients on continuous ambulatory peritoneal dialysis. J Am Soc Nephrol 1995; 6: 192–7.

132. Ahearn DJ, Nolph KD. Controlled sodium removal with peritoneal dialysis. Trans Am Soc Artif Organs 1972; 18: 423–8.

133. Ho-dac-Pannekeet MM, Atasever B, Strujik D, Krediet R. Analysis of ultrafiltration failure in peritoneal dialysis patients by means of standard peritoneal permeability analysis. Perit Dial Int 1997; 17: 144–50.

134. Lindholm B, Alvestrand A, Hultman E, Bergstrom J. Muscle water and electrolytes in patients undergoing continuous ambulatory peritoneal dialysis. Acta Med Scand 1986; 219: 323–30.

135. Paulson WD, Bock GH, Nelson AP, Moxey-Mims MM, Crim LM. Hyponatremia in the very young chronic peritoneal dialysis patient. Am J Kidney Dis 1989; 14: 196–9.

136. Tzamaloukas A, Avasthi P. Effect of hyperglycemia on serum sodium concentration and tonicity in out-patients on chronic dialysis. Am J Kidney Dis 1986; 7: 477–82.

137. Spital A, Sterns R. Potassium supplementation via the dialysate in continuous ambulatory peritoneal dialysis. Am J Kidney Dis 1985; 6: 173–6.

138. Oreopoulos D, Khanna R, Williams P, Vas S. Continuous ambulatory peritoneal dialysis – 1981. Nephron 1982; 30: 293–303.

139. Khan A, Bernardini J, Johnston J, Piraino B. Hypokalemia in peritoneal dialysis patients (letter). Perit Dial Int 1996; 16: 652.

140. Rostand S. Profound hypokalemia in continuous ambulatory peritoneal dialysis. Arch Intern Med 1983; 143: 377–8.

141. Dolson GM. Do potassium deficient diets and K removal by dialysis contribute to the cardiovascular morbidity and mor-

tality of patients with end-stage renal disease? (editorial). Int J Artif Organs 1997; 20: 134–5.

142. Bargman J, Jamison R. Disorders of potassium homeostasis. In: Sutton R, Dirks J, eds. Diuretics: Physiology, Pharmacology and Clinical Use. Philadelphia, PA: W.B. Saunders, 1986, pp. 296–319.

143. Boen S. Peritoneal Dialysis in Clinical Medicine. Springfield, IL: Charles C. Thomas, 1974.

144. Vaamonde C, Michael V, Metzger R et al. Complications of acute peritoneal dialysis. J Chron Dis 1975; 28: 637–59.

145. Pedersen F, Ryttov N, Deleuran P, Dragsholt C, Kildeberg P. Acetate versus lactate in peritoneal dialysis solutions. Nephron 1985; 39: 55–8.

146. Ahlmen J, Stelin G. Abdominal pains during CAPD with acetate buffered dialysate (letter). Lancet 1983; 2: 1247.

147. LaGreca G, Biasioli S, Chiaramonte S et al. Acid–base balance on peritoneal dialysis. Clin Nephrol 1981; 16: 1–7.

148. Nissenson A. Acid–base homeostasis in peritoneal dialysis patients. Int J Artif Organs 1984; 7: 175–6.

149. Uribarri J, Buquing J, Oh M. Acid–base balance in chronic peritoneal dialysis patients. Kidney Int 1995; 47: 269–73.

150. Richardson R, Roscoe J. Bicarbonate, L-lactate and D-lactate balance in intermittent peritoneal dialysis. Perit Dial Bull 1986; 6: 178–85.

151. Yasuda T, Ozawa S, Shiba C et al. D-lactate metabolism in patients with chronic renal failure undergoing CAPD. Nephron 1993; 63: 416–22.

152. Rubin J, Adair C, Johnson B, Bower JD. Stereospecific lactate absorption during peritoneal dialysis. Nephron 1982; 31: 224–8.

153. Veech R, Fowler R. Cerebral dysfunction and respiratory alkalosis during peritoneal dialysis with D-lactate-containing dialysis fluids (letter). Am J Med 1987; 82: 572–3.

154. Feriani M, Ronco C, La Greca G. Acid–base balance with different CAPD solutions. Perit Dial Int 1996; 1: S126–9.

155. Kang D-H, Yoon K-I, Lee H-Y, Han D-S. Impact of peritoneal membrane transport characteristics on acid–base status in CAPD patients. Perit Dial Int 1998; 18: 294–302.

156. Singh S, Hong C, Dale A, Morgan B. Comparison of buffering capacity in patients on hemodialysis and continuous ambulatory peritoneal dialysis. Nephron 1986; 42: 29–33.

157. Naparstek Y, Friedlaender M, Rubinger D, Popovtzer MM. Lactic acidosis and peritoneal dialysis. Isr J Med Sci 1982; 18: 513–14.

158. Conte F, Tommasi A, Battini G et al. Lactic acidosis coma in continuous ambulatory peritoneal dialysis (letter). Nephron 1986; 43: 148.

159. Foulks C, Wright L. Successful repletion of bicarbonate stores in ongoing lactic acidosis: a role for bicarbonate-buffered peritoneal dialysis. South Med J 1981; 74: 1162–3.

160. Feriani M, Biasioli S, Borin D et al. Bicarbonate buffer for CAPD solution. Trans Am Soc Artif Intern Organs 1985; 31: 668–72.

161. Lee H, Hill L, Hewill V et al. Lactic acidemia in peritoneal dialysis. Proc Eur Dial Transplant Assoc 1967; 4: 150–5.

162. Khan IH, Catto GRD, MacLeod AM. Severe lactic acidosis in patient receiving continuous ambulatory peritoneal dialysis. Br Med J 1993; 307: 1056–7.

163. Schmidt R, Horn E, Richards J, Stamatakis M, Pharm D. Survival after Metformin-associated lactic acidosis in peritoneal dialysis-dependent renal failure. Am J Med 1997; 102: 486–8.

164. Feriani M, Carobi C, LeGreca G, Buoncristiani U, Passlick-Deetjen J. Clinical experience with a 39 mmol/L bicarbonate-buffered peritoneal dialysis solution. Perit Dial Int 1997; 17: 17–21.

165. Graham KA, Reaich D, Channon SM et al. Correction of acidosis in CAPD decreases whole body protein degradation. Kidney Int 1996; 49: 1396–400.

166. Stein A, Moorhouse J, Iles-Smith H et al. Role of an improvement in acid–base status and nutrition in CAPD patients. Kidney Int 1997; 52: 1089–95.

167. Dumler F, Galan M. Impact of acidosis on nutritional status in chronic peritoneal dialysis patients. Adv Perit Dial 1996; 12: 307–10.

168. Kang SW, Lee SW, Lee IH et al. Impact of metabolic acidosis in serum albumin and other nutritional parameters in long-term CAPD patients. Adv Perit Dial 1997; 13: 249–52.

169. Tzamaloukas A. 'Contraction' alkalosis during treatment of hyperglycemia in CAPD patients. Perit Dial Bull 1983; 3: 196–9.

170. Garella S. Contraction alkalosis in patients on CAPD (letter). Perit Dial Bull 1984; 4: 187–8.

171. Gault M, Ferguson E, Sidhu J et al. Fluid and electrolyte complications of peritoneal dialysis. Ann Intern Med 1971; 75: 253–62.

172. Kenamond T, Graves J, Lempert K, Moss A, Whittier F. Severe recurrent alkalemia in a patient undergoing continuous cyclic peritoneal dialysis. Am J Med 1986; 81: 548–50.

173. Wuthrich RP. Occurrence of respiratory alkalosis in continuous ambulatory peritoneal dialysis patients with pulmonary disease. Am J Kidney Dis 1995; 25: 79–81.

174. Posner J, Plum F. Spinal fluid pH and neurological symptoms in systemic acidosis. N Engl J Med 1967; 277: 605–13.

175. Levy D, Anderson K, Savage D, Balkus S, Kannel W, Castelli W. Echocardiographically detected left ventricular hypertrophy: prevalence and risk factors. The Framingham Heart Study. Ann Intern Med 1988; 108: 7–13.

176. Silberberg DS, Barre P, Prichard S, Sniderman AD. Left ventricular hypertrophy: an independent determinant of survival in end stage renal failure. Kidney Int 1989; 36: 286–90.

177. Wizemann V, Timio M, Alpert MA, Kramer W. Options in dialysis therapy: significance of cardiovascular findings. Kidney Int Suppl 1993; 43: 585–91.

178. Mall G, Huther W, Schneider J, Lundin P, Ritz E. Diffuse intermyocardiocytic fibrosis in uremic patients. Nephrol Dial Transplant 1990; 5: 39–44.

179. Leenen F, Smith D, Khanna R, Oreopoulos DG. Changes in left ventricular anatomy and function on CAPD. Perit Dial Bull Suppl 1983; 3: S26–8.

180. Alpert MA, Huting J, Twardowski ZJ, Khanna R, Nolph KD. Continuous ambulatory peritoneal dialysis and the heart. Perit Dial Int 1995; 15: 6–11.

181. Brown P, Johnston K, Fenton S, Cattran DC. Symptomatic exacerbation of peripheral vascular disease with chronic ambulatory peritoneal dialysis. Clin Nephrol 1981; 16: 258–61.

182. Wakeen M, Zimmerman SW. Association between human recombinant EPO and peripheral vascular disease in diabetic patients receiving peritoneal dialysis. Am J Kidney Dis 1998; 33: 488–93.

183. Feldman AM, Fivush B, Zahka KG, Ouyang P, Baughman KL. Congestive cardiomyopathy in patients on continuous ambulatory peritoneal dialysis. Am J Kidney Dis 1988; 11: 76–9.

184. Foley RN, Parfrey P, Harnett J et al. Hypocalcemia, morbidity and mortality in end stage renal disease. Am J Nephrol 1996; 16: 386–93.

185. Huting J. Progression of valvular sclerosis in end-stage renal disease treated by long-term peritoneal dialysis. Clin Cardiol 1992; 15: 745–50.

186. Huting J. Mitral valve calcification as an index of left ventricular dysfunction in patients with end-stage renal disease on peritoneal dialysis. Chest 1994; 105: 383–8.

187. Lucke J, Samy R, Atkins B et al. Results of valve replacement with mechanical and biological prosthesis in chronic renal dialysis patients. Ann Thorac Surg 1997; 64: 129–32.

188. Guazzi M, Polese A, Magrini F, Fiorentini C, Olivari M. Negative influences of ascites on cardiac function of cirrhotic patients. Am J Med 1975; 59: 165–70.

189. Schurig R, Gahl G, Schartl M et al. Central and peripheral hemodynamics in long-term peritoneal dialysis patients. Proc Eur Dial Transplant Assoc 1979; 16: 165–9.

190. Swartz C, Onesti G, Mailloux L *et al.* The acute hemodynamic and pulmonary perfusion effects of peritoneal dialysis. Trans Am Soc Artif Intern Organs 1969; 15: 367–72.

191. Acquatella H, Perez-Rozas M, Burger B *et al.* Left ventricular function in uremia: a hemodynamic and echocardiographic study. Nephron 1978; 22: 160–74.

192. Franklin JO, Alpert MA, Twardowski ZJ *et al.* Effect of increasing intra-abdominal pressure and volume on left ventricular function in continuous ambulatory peritoneal dialysis (CAPD). Am J Kidney Dis 1988; 12: 291–8.

193. Rab ST, Alazraki NP, Guertler-Krawczynska E. Peritoneal fluid causing inferior attenuation on SPECT thallium-201 myocardial imaging in women. J Nucl Med 1988; 29: 1860–4.

194. Bartens W, Nauck M, Scholimeyer P, Wanner C. Elevated lipoprotein(a) and fibrinogen serum levels increase the cardiovascular risk in continuous ambulatory peritoneal dialysis patients. Perit Dial Int 1996; 16: 27–33.

195. Caruana R, Wolfman N, Karstaedt N, Wilson D. Pancreatitis: an important cause of abdominal symptoms in patients on peritoneal dialysis. Am J Kidney Dis 1986; 7: 135–40.

196. Rutsky E, Robards M, Van Dyke J, Rostand S. Acute pancreatitis in patients with end stage renal disease without transplantation. Arch Intern Med 1986; 146: 1741–5.

197. Singh S, Wadhwa N. Peritonitis, pancreatitis and infected pseudocyst in a continuous ambulatory peritoneal dialysis patient. Am J Kidney Dis 1987; 9: 84–6.

198. Flynn C, Chandran P, Shadur C. Recurrent pancreatitis in a patient on CAPD (letter). Perit Dial Bull 1986; 6: 106.

199. Donnelly S, Levy M, Prichard S. Acute pancreatitis in continuous ambulatory peritoneal dialysis. Perit Dial Int 1988; 8: 187–90.

200. Gupta A, Yuan ZY, Balaskas EV, Khanna R, Oreopoulos DG. CAPD and pancreatitis: no connection. Perit Dial Int 1992; 12: 309–16.

201. Padilla B, Pollak V, Pesce A, Kant K, Gilinsky N, Deddens J. Pancreatitis in patients with end-stage renal disease. Medicine 1994; 73: 8–20.

202. Pitrone F, Pelligrino E, Mileto G, Consolo F. May pancreatitis represent a CAPD complication? Report of two cases with a rapid evolution to death (letter). Int J Artif Organs 1985; 8: 235–6.

203. Royse VL, Jensen DM, Corwin HL. Pancreatic enzymes in chronic renal failure. Arch Intern Med 1987; 147: 537–9.

204. Burkart J, Haigler S, Caruana R, Hylander B. Usefulness of peritoneal fluid amylase levels in the differential diagnosis of peritonitis in peritoneal dialysis patients. J Am Soc Nephrol 1991; 1: 1186–91.

205. Steiner RW, Halasz NA. Abdominal catastrophes and other unusual events in continuous ambulatory peritoneal dialysis patients. Am J Kidney Dis 1990; 15: 1–7.

206. Rambausek M, Ziegler T, Ritz E. Incipient pancreatitis causing cloudy effluent in a patient on CAPD (letter). Perit Dial Bull 1986; 6: 160.

207. Pannekeet M, Krediet R, Boeschoten E, Arisz L. Acute pancreatitis during CAPD in the Netherlands. Nephrol Dial Transplant 1993; 8: 1376–81.

208. Wanless IR, Bargman JM, Oreopoulos DG, Vas SL. Subcapsular steatonecrosis in obesity. Mod Pathol 1989; 2: 69–74.

209. Grove A, Vyberg B, Vyberg M. Focal fatty change of the liver. Virchows Arch A Pathol Anat 1991; 419: 69–75.

210. Burrows C, Jones A. Hepatic subcapsular steatosis in a patient with insulin dependent diabetes receiving dialysis. J Clin Pathol 1994; 47: 274–5.

211. Luciani L, Gentile M, Scarduelli B, Sinico R, D'Amico G, Samori G. Multiple hepatic abscesses complicating continuous ambulatory peritoneal dialysis. Br Med J 1982; 285: 543.

212. Lambrecht GLY, Malbrain MLNG, Zachee P, Daelemans R, Lins RL. Portal vein thrombosis complicating peritonitis in a patient on chronic ambulatory peritoneal dialysis. Perit Dial Int 1994; 14: 282–3.

213. Haz MZ, Tzamaloukas AH, Malhotra D, Gibel LJ. Symptomatic ascites after discontinuous of continuous peritoneal dialysis. Perit Dial Int 1997; 17: 568–72.

214. Hylander BI, Dalton CB, Castel DO, Burkart J, Rossner S. Effect of intraperitoneal fluid volume changes on esophageal pressures: studies in patients on continuous ambulatory peritoneal dialysis. Am J Kidney Dis 1991; 17: 307–10.

215. Kim M-J, Kwon KH, Lee SW. Gastroesophageal reflux disease in CAPD patients. Adv Perit Dial 1998; 14: 98–101.

216. Bird NJ, Streather CP, O'Doherty MJ, Barton IK, Gaunt JE, Nunan TO. Gastric emptying in patients with chronic renal failure on continuous ambulatory peritoneal dialysis. Nephrol Dial Transplant 1994; 9: 287–90.

217. Redwood NFW, Wilkinson R, Jones NAG. Vomiting caused by a dialysis fluid 'pseudocyst'. Br J Surg 1993; 80: 224.

218. deGraaf-Strukowska L, van Hees C, Ferwerda J, Schut N, van Dorp W. Two non-diabetic patients with delayed gastric emptying during CAPD effectively treated with erythromycin. Nephrol Dial Transplant 1995; 10: 2349–50.

219. Korzets Z, Golan E, Ben-Dahan J, Neufeld D, Bernheim J. Decubitus small-bowel perforation in ongoing continuous ambulatory peritoneal dialysis. Nephrol Dial Transplant 1992; 7: 79–81.

220. Yamamoto Y, Mure T, Sano K, Hirano H, Osawa G. Spontaneous jejunal perforation in continuous ambulatory peritoneal dialysis. Nephron 1993; 64: 161–2.

221. Rottembourg J, Gahl G, Poignet J *et al.* Severe abdominal complications in patients undergoing continuous ambulatory peritoneal dialysis. Eur Dial Transplant Assoc Proc 1983; 20: 236–42.

222. Koren G, Aladjem M, Militiano J, Seegal B, Jonash A, Boichis H. Ischemic colitis in chronic intermittent peritoneal dialysis. Nephron 1984; 36: 272–4.

223. Wehling M, Jenni R, Steurer J. Buhler H, Siegenthaler W, Kuhlmann U. Ischemic colitis in a patient undergoing continuous ambulatory peritoneal dialysis. Perit Dial Bull 1982; 2: 123–4.

224. Tomson C, Morgan A. Bleeding from small intestinal telangiectases complicating CAPD (letter). Perit Dial Bull 1985; 5: 258.

225. Yorioka K, Hamaguchi N, Taniguchi Y *et al.* Gastric antral vascular ectasia in a patient on hemodialysis improved with CAPD. Perit Dial Int 1996; 16: 177–8.

226. Chang I, Chen T, Ng Y, Yang W. Recurrent intestinal angioplastic bleeding in a patient on hemodialysis ceasing spontaneously with CAPD (letter). Perit Dial Int 1998; 18: 342–3.

227. Suresh K, Port F. Air under the diaphragm in patients undergoing continuous ambulatory peritoneal dialysis. Perit Dial Int 1989; 9: 309–11.

228. Kiefer T, Schenk U, Weber J, Hubel E, Kuhlmann U. Incidence and significance of pneumoperitoneum in continuous ambulatory peritoneal dialysis. Am J Kidney Dis 1993; 22: 30–5.

229. Lampainen E, Khanna R, Schaefer R, Twardowski Z, Nolph K. Is air under the diaphragm a significant finding in CAPD patients? ASAIO Trans 1986; 32: 581–2.

230. Spence P, Mathews R, Khanna R, Oreopoulos D. Indications for operation when peritonitis occurs in patients on chronic ambulatory peritoneal dialysis. Surg Gynecol Obstet 1985; 161: 450–2.

231. Grefberg N, Nilsson P, Andreen T. Sclerosing obstructive peritonitis, beta-blockers, and continuous ambulatory peritoneal dialysis (letter). Lancet 1983; 2: 733–4.

232. Bradley J, McWhinnie D, Hamilton D *et al.* Sclerosing obstructive peritonitis after continuous ambulatory peritoneal dialysis (letter). Lancet 1983; 2: 113–14.

233. Hauglustaine D, Monballyu J, Van Meerbeek J, Goddeeris P, Lauwarijns J, Pichielsen P. Sclerosing obstructive peritonitis, beta-blockers, and continuous ambulatory peritoneal dialysis (letter). Lancet 1983; 2: 734.

234. Verger C, Celicout B, Larpent L, Goupil A. Sclerosing encapsulating peritonitis during continuous ambulatory peritoneal dialysis. Presse Med 1986; 15: 1311–140.

235. Slingeneyer A, Mion C, Mourad G, Canaud B, Faller B, Beraud JJ. Progressive sclerosing peritonitis: a late and severe complication of maintenance peritoneal dialysis. Trans Am Soc Artif Intern Organs 1983; 29: 633–40.

236. Pusateri R, Ross R, Marshall R, Meredith J, Hamilton RW. Sclerosing encapsulating peritonitis: report of a case with small bowel obstruction managed by long-term home parental hyperalimentation, and a review of the literature. Am J Kidney Dis 1986; 8: 56–60.

237. Ing T, Daugirdas J, Gandhi V. Peritoneal Sclerosis in peritoneal dialysis patients. Am J Nephrol 1984; 4: 173–6.

238. Hauglustaine D, Van Meerbeek J, Monballyu J, Goddeeris P, Lauwerijns J, Michielsen P. Sclerosing peritonitis with mural bowel fibrosis in a patient on long-term CAPD. Clin Nephrol 1984; 22: 158–62.

239. Rigby RJ, Hawley CM. Sclerosing peritonitis: the experience in Australia. Nephrol Dial Transplant 1998; 13: 154–9.

240. Yokota S, Kumano K, Sakai T. Prognosis for patients with sclerosing encapsulating peritonitis following CAPD. Adv Perit Dial 1997; 13: 221–3.

241. Hendriks PMEM, Ho-dac-Pannekeet MM, van Gulik TM. Peritoneal sclerosis in peritoneal dialysis patients: analysis of clinical presentation, risk factors, and peritoneal transport kinetics. Perit Dial Int 1997; 17: 136–43.

242. Nomoto Y, Kawaguchi Y, Kubo H, Hirano H, Sakai S, Kurokawa K. Sclerosing encapsulating peritonitis in patients undergoing continuous ambulatory peritoneal dialysis: a report of the Japanese Sclerosing Encapsulating Peritonitis Study Group. Am J Kidney Dis 1996; 28: 420–7.

243. Oreopoulos D, Khanna R, Wu G. Sclerosing obstructive peritonitis after CAPD (letter). Lancet 1983; 2: 409.

244. Dobbie JW. Pathogenesis of peritoneal fibrosing syndromes (sclerosing peritonitis) in peritoneal dialysis. Perit Dial Int 1992; 12: 14–27.

245. Daugirdas J, Gandhi V, McShane A et al. Peritoneal sclerosis in continuous ambulatory peritoneal dialysis patients dialyzed exclusively with lactate-buffered dialysate. Int J Artif Organ 1986; 9: 413–16.

246. Junor B, Briggs J, Forwell M, Dobbie J, Henderson I. Sclerosing peritonitis – the contribution of chlorhexidine in alcohol. Perit Dial Bull 1985; 4: 101–4.

247. Ing T, Daugirdas J, Gandhi V, Leehey D. Sclerosing peritonitis after peritoneal dialysis (letter). Lancet 1983; 2: 1080.

248. Shaldon S, Koch K, Quellhorst E, Dinarello CA. Pathogenesis of sclerosing peritonitis in CAPD. Trans Am Soc Artif Intern Organs 1984; 30: 193–4.

249. Dobbie JW, Jasani MK. Role of imbalance of intracavity fibrin formation and removal in the pathogenesis of peritoneal lesions in CAPD. Perit Dial Int 1997; 17: 121–4.

250. Joffe P, Jensen LT. Type I and III procollagens in CAPD: markers of peritoneal fibrosis. Adv Perit 1991; 7: 158–60.

251. Levine S, Saltzman A. Abdominal cocoon: an animal model for a complication of peritoneal dialysis. Perit Dial Int 1996; 16: 613–16.

252. DeVecchi AF, Castelnovo C, Scalamogna A, Paparella M. Symptomatic accidental introduction of disinfectant electrolytic chlorhexidizer solution into the peritoneal cavity of CAPD patients. Clin Nephrol 1992; 37: 204–8.

253. Greenlee H, Stanley M, Reinhardt G et al. Small bowel obstruction from compression and kinking of intestine by thickened peritoneum in cirrhotics with ascites treated with LeVeen shunt. Gastroenterology 1979; 76: 1282–5.

254. Namasivayam J. Intraperitoneal pseudocyst formation as a complication of continuous ambulatory peritoneal dialysis. Br J Radiol 1991; 64: 463–4.

255. Brown P, Baddeley H, Read A et al. Sclerosing peritonitis, an unusual reaction of a B-adrenergic-blocking drug (practolol). Lancet 1974; 2: 1477–81.

256. Clark C, Terris R. Sclerosing peritonitis associated with metaprolol. Lancet 1983; 1: 937.

257. McLaughlin K, Butt G, Madi A, McMillan M, Mactier R. Sclerosing peritonitis occurring in a hemodialysis patient. Am J Kidney Dis 1996; 27: 729–32.

258. Hollman AS, McMillan MA, Briggs JD, Junor BJ, Morley P. Ultrasound changes in sclerosing peritonitis following continuous ambulatory peritoneal dialysis. Clin Radiol 1991; 43: 176–9.

259. Campbell S, Clarke P, Hawley C et al. Sclerosing peritonitis: identification of diagnostic, clinical, and radiological features. Am J Kidney Dis 1994; 24: 819–25.

260. Korzets A, Korzets Z, Peer G et al. Sclerosing peritonitis. Possible early diagnosis by computerized tomography of the abdomen. Am J Nephrol 1988; 8: 143–6.

261. Krestin GP, Kacl G, Hauser M, Keusch G, Burger HR, Hoffmann R. Imaging diagnosis of sclerosing peritonitis and relation of radiologic signs to the extent of the disease. Abdom Imaging 1995; 20: 414–20.

262. Stafford-Johnson DB, Wilson TE, Francis IR, Swartz R. CT appearance of sclerosing peritonitis in patients on chronic ambulatory peritoneal dialysis. J Comput Assist Tomogr 1998; 22: 295–9.

263. Kittur DS, Korpe SW, Raytch RE, Smith GW. Surgical aspects of sclerosing encapsulating peritonitis. Arch Surg 1990; 125: 1626–8.

264. Smith L, Collins JF, Morris M, Teele RL. Sclerosing encapsulating peritonitis associated with continuous ambulatory peritoneal dialysis: surgical management. Am J Kidney Dis 1997; 29: 456–60.

265. Assalia A, Schein M, Hashmonai M. Problems in the surgical management of sclerosing encapsulating peritonitis. Isr J Med Sci 1993; 29: 686–8.

266. Lo W-K, Chan K-T, Leung ACT, Pang S-W, Tse C-Y. Sclerosing peritonitis complicating continuous ambulatory peritoneal dialysis with the use of chlorhexidine in alcohol. Adv Perit Dial 1990; 6: 79–84.

267. Slingeneyer A. Preliminary report on a cooperative international study on sclerosing encapsulating peritonitis. Contrib Nephrol 1987; 57: 239–47.

268. Junor BJR, McMillan MA. Immunosuppression in sclerosing peritonitis. Perit Dial Int Suppl 1993; 13: S64 (abstract).

269. Mori Y, Matsuo S, Sutoh H, Toriyama T, Kawahara H, Hotta N. A case of a dialysis patient with sclerosing peritonitis successfully treated with corticosteroid therapy alone. Am J Kidney Dis 1997; 30: 275–8.

270. Bhandari S, Wilkinson A, Sellars L. Sclerosing peritonitis: value of immunosuppression prior to surgery. Nephrol Dial Transplant 1994; 9: 436–7.

271. Bowers VD, Ackermann JR, Richardson W, Carey LC. Sclerosing peritonitis. Clin Transplant 1994; 8: 369–72.

272. Lasker N, Burke J, Patchefsky A. Peritoneal reactions to particulate matter in peritoneal dialysis solutions. Trans Am Soc Artif Intern Organs 1975; 21: 342–5.

273. Novello A, Port F. Sclerosing encapsulating peritonitis (editorial). Int J Artif Organs 1986; 9: 393–6.

274. Marichal JF, Faller B, Brignon P, Wagner D, Straub P. Progressive calcifying peritonitis: a new complication of CAPD? Nephron 1987; 45: 229–32.

275. Francis DMA, Busmanis I, Becker G. Peritoneal calcification in a peritoneal dialysis patient: a case report. Perit Dial Int 1990; 10: 237–40.

276. Cox SV, Lai J, Suranyi M, Walker N. Sclerosing peritonitis with gross peritoneal calcification: a case report. Am J Kidney Dis 1992; 20: 637–42.

277. Klemm G. Peritoneal calcification and calciphylaxis. Nephron 1989; 51: 124.

278. Seyle H, Gabbiani G, Strebel R. Sensitization to calciphylaxis by endogenous parathyroid hormone. Endocrinology 1962; 71: 554–8.

279. Fletcher S, Gibson J, Brownjohn AM. Peritoneal calcification secondary to severe hyperparathyroidism. Nephrol Dial Transplant 1995; 10: 277–9.

280. Wakabayashi Y, Kawaguchi Y, Shigematsu T *et al.* Three cases of extensive peritoneal calcification (ECP) in patients with long-term CAPD. Perit Dial Int Suppl 1993; 13: S99 (abstract).

281. Nace G, George A Jr, Stone W. Hemoperitoneum: a red flag in CAPD. Perit Dial Dubb 1985; 5: 42–4.

282. Greenberg A, Bernardini J, Piraino BM, Johnston JR, Perlmutter JA. Hemoperitoneum complicating chronic peritoneal dialysis: single-centre experience and literature review. Am J Kidney Dis 1992; 19: 252–6.

283. Holley JL, Schiff M, Schmidt RJ, Bender FH, Dumler F. Hemoperitoneum occurs in over half of menstruating women on peritoneal dialysis. Perit Dial Int 1996; 16: 650.

284. Blumenkrantz M, Gallagher N, Bashore R *et al.* Retrograde menstruation in women undergoing chronic peritoneal dialysis. Obstet Gynecol 1981; 57: 667–70.

285. Harnett J, Gill D, Corbett L, Parfrey PS, Gault H. Recurrent hemoperitoneum in women receiving continuous ambulatory peritoneal dialysis. Ann Intern Med 1987; 107: 341–3.

286. Fraley DS, Johnston JR, Bruns FJ, Adler S, Segel DP. Rupture of ovarian cyst: massive hemoperitoneum in continuous ambulatory peritoneal dialysis patients: diagnosis and treatment. Am J Kidney Dis 1988; 12: 69–71.

287. Fenton S. Recurrent hemoperitoneum in a middle-aged woman on CAPD. Perit Dial Int 1998; 18: 88–93.

288. Coronel F, Maranjo P, Torrente J, Prats D. The risk of retrograde menstruation in CAPD patients (letter). Perit Dial Bull 1984; 4: 190–1.

289. de los Santos CA, von Eye O, d'Avila D, Mottin CC. Rupture of the spleen: a complication of continuous ambulatory peritoneal dialysis. Perit Dial Bull 1986; 6: 203–4.

290. Fine A, Novak C. Hemoperitoneum due to carcinomatosis in the liver of a CAPD patient. Perit Dial Int 1996; 16: 181–3.

291. Peng S-J, Yang C-S. Hemoperitoneum in CAPD patients with hepatic tumors. Perit Dial Int 1996; 16: 84–6.

292. Posthuma N, van Eps RS, ter Wee PM. Hemoperitoneum due to (hepatocellular) adenoma. Perit Dial Int 1998; 18: 446–7.

293. Williams PF, Beer S. Hemoperitoneum in a patient with idiopathic thrombocytopenic purpura (ITP) and renal failure (letter). Perit Dial Bull 1985; 5: 258–9.

294. Blake P, Abraham G. Bloody effluent during CAPD in a patient with polycystic kidneys (letter). Perit Dial Int 1988; 8: 167.

295. Campisi S, Cavatorta F, DeLucia E. Iliopsoas spontaneous hematoma: an unusual cause of hemoperitoneum in CAPD patients (letter). Perit Dial Int 1992; 12: 78.

296. Huserl F, Tapia N. Peritoneal bleeding in a CAPD patient after extracorporeal lithotripsy (letter). Perit Dial Bull 1987; 7: 262.

297. Hassell L, Moore J Jr, Conklin J. Hemoperitoneum during continuous ambulatory peritoneal dialysis: a possible complication of radiation induced peritoneal injury. Clin Nephrol 1984; 21: 241–3.

298. Modi K, Henderson I. fatal massive hemoperitoneum after cessation of CAPD (letter). Clin Nephrol 1987; 27: 47.

299. Twardowski ZJ, Schreiber MJ. Peritoneal dialysis case forum: a 55 year old man with hematuria and blood-tinged dialysate. Perit Dial Int 1992; 12: 61–6.

300. Rutecki GW, Asfoura JY, Whittier FC. Autosomal dominant polycystic liver disease as an etiology of hemoperitoneum during CCPD. Perit Dial Int 1995; 15: 367–87.

301. Goodkin DA, Benning MH. An outpatient maneuver to treat bloody effluent during continuous ambulatory peritoneal dialysis (CAPD). Perit Dial Int 1990; 10: 227–9.

302. Van der Niepen P, Sennesael JJ, Verbeelen DL. Massive hemoperitoneum due to spleen injury by a dislocated Tenckhoff catheter. Perit Dial Int 1994; 14: 90–3.

303. Wang JY, Lin YF, Lin SH, Tsao TY. Hemoperitoneum due to splenic rupture in a CAPD patient with chronic myelogenous leukemia. Perit Dial Int 1998; 18: 334–7.

304. Min CH, Park JH, Ahn JH *et al.* Dialysis-related amyloidosis (DRA) in a patient on CAPD presenting as haemoperioneum with colon perforation. Nephrol Dial Transplant 1997; 12: 2761–3.

305. Karlagasundaram NS, Macdougall IC, Turney JH. Massive haemoperitoneum due to rupture of splenic infarct during CAPD. Nephrol Dial Transplant 1998; 13: 2380–1.

306. Shohat J, Shapira Z, Yussim A, Boner G. An unusual cause of massive intraperitoneal bleeding in CAPD. Perit Dial Bull 1984; 4: 257–8.

307. Giron FF, Sanchez FH, Alcalde MP, Martinez JG. Hemoperitoneum in peritoneal dialysis secondary to retroperitoneal hematoma. Perit Dial Int 1996; 16: 644.

308. Bender F. Hemoperitoneum after pericardiocentesis in a CAPD patient. Perit Dial Int 1996; 16: 330.

309. Ramon G, Miguel A, Caridad A, Colomer B. Bloody peritoneal fluid in a patient with tuberous sclerosis in a CAPD program (letter). Perit Dial Int 1989; 9: 353.

310. Rambausek M, Waldherr R, Ritz E. Recurrent episodes of bloody dialysate in mesangial IgA-glomerulonephritis (IgA-GN) during upper respiratory tract infections. Perit Dial Bull 1987; 7: S62 (abstract).

311. Ohtomo Y, Higasi Y. A case of MCTD patient with recurrent hemoperitoneum receiving CAPD who had a successful recovery with an increase in steroids. Nippon Jinzo Gakkai Shi 1992; 34: 325–9.

312. Goldstein AM, Gorlick N, Gibbs D, Fernandez-del Castillo C. Hemoperitoneum due to spontaneous rupture of the umbilical vein. Am J Gastroenterol 1995; 90: 315–17.

313. Press OW, Press NO, Kaufman SD. Evaluation and management of chylous ascites. Ann Intern Med 1982; 96: 358–64.

314. Vasko J, Tapper R. The surgical significance of chylous ascites. Arch Surg 1967; 95: 355–68.

315. Kelley M Jr, Butt H. Chylous ascites: an analysis of etiology. Gastroenterology 1960; 39: 161–70.

316. Haskim SA, Rohold HB, Babayan JK *et al.* Treatment of chyluria and chylothorax with medium-chain triglyceride. N Engl J Med 1964; 270: 756–61.

317. Porter J, Wang WH, Oliveria DBG. Chylous ascites and continuous ambulatory peritoneal dialysis. Nephrol Dial Transplant 1991; 6: 659–61.

318. Humayun H, Daugirdas J, Int T *et al.* Chylous ascites in a patient treated with intermittent peritoneal dialysis. Artif Organs 1984; 8: 358–60.

319. Leport J, Devars Du Mayne J-F, Hay J-M, Cerf M. Chylous ascites and encapsulating peritonitis: unusual complications of spontaneous bacterial peritonitis. Am J Gastroenterol 1987; 82: 463–5.

320. Melnick JZ, McCarty CM, Hunchik MP, Alexander SR. Chylous ascites complicating neonatal peritoneal dialysis. Pediatr Nephrol 1995; 9: 753–5.

321. Huang C-H, Chen H⁻S, Chen Y-M, Tsai T-J. Fibroadhesive form of tuberculous peritonitis: chyloperitoneum in a patient undergoing automated peritoneal dialysis. Nephron 1996; 72: 708–11.

322. Pomeranz A, Reichenberg Y, Schurr D, Drukker A. Chyloperitoneum: a rare complication of peritoneal dialysis. Perit Dial Bull 1984; 4: 35–7.

323. Yoshimoto K, Saima S, Eschizen H, Nakamura Y, Ishizaki T. A drug-induced turbid peritoneal dialysate in five patients treated with continuous ambulatory peritoneal dialysis. Clin Nephrol 1993; 40: 114–17.

324. Bargman JM, Zent R, Ellis P, Auger M, Wilson S. Diagnosis of lymphoma in a CAPD patient by peritoneal fluid cytology. Am J Kidney Dis 1994; 23: 747–50.

325. Dunnill MS, Millard PR, Oliver D. Acquired cystic disease of the kidneys: a hazard of long-term intermittent maintenance hemodialysis. J Clin Pathol 1977; 30: 868–77.

326. Crocker JFS, Safe SH. An animal model of hemodialysis induced polycystic kidney disease (PKD). Kidney Int 1984; 25: 183 (abstract).

327. Bommer J, Waldherr R, VanKaick G, Strauss L, Ritz E. Acquired renal cysts in uremic patients – *in vivo* demonstration by computed tomography. Clin Nephrol 1980; 14: 299–303.

328. Mickisch O, Bommer J, Bachman S, Waldherr R, Mann JFE, Ritz E. Multicystic transformation of kidneys in chronic renal failure. Nephron 1984; 38: 93–9.

329. Beardsworth SF, Goldsmith HJ, Ahmad R, Lamb G. Acquisition of renal cysts during peritoneal dialysis. Lancet 1984; 2: 1482.

330. Poulopoulos V, Bargman JM. Acquired cystic disease mimicking polycystic kidney disease in long-term CAPD patients. Perit Dial Int 1995; 15: 75–6.

331. Ishikawa I. Acquired renal cystic disease and its complications in continuous ambulatory peritoneal dialysis patients. Perit Dial Int 1992; 12: 292–7.

332. Miller LR, Soffer O, Nassar VH, Kutner MH. Acquired renal cystic disease in end-stage renal disease: an autopsy study of 155 cases. Am J Nephrol 1989; 9: 322–8.

333. Mollofre C, Almirall J, Campistol JM, Andreu J, Cardesa A, Revert L. Acquired renal cystic disease in HD: a study of 82 nephrectomies in young patients. Clin Nephrol 1992; 7: 297–302.

334. Frifelt JJ, Larsen C, Elle B, Dyreborg U. Multicystic transformation of the kidneys in dialysis patients. Scand J Urol Nephrol 1989; 23: 51–4.

335. Ishikawa I, Shikura N, Nagahara M, Shinoda A, Saito Y. Comparison of severity of acquired renal cysts between CAPD and hemodialysis. Adv Perit Dial 1991; 7: 91–5.

336. Sasaki H, Terasawa Y, Taguma Y, Hotta O, Suzuki K, Nakamura K. Comparative study of cystic variations of the kidneys in haemodialysis and continuous ambulatory peritoneal dialysis patients. Int Urol Nephrol 1996; 28: 247–54.

337. Glicklich D. Acquired cystic kidney disease and renal cell carcinoma: a review. Semin Dial 1991; 4: 273–83.

338. Master U, Cruz C, Schmidt R, Dumler F, Babiarz J. Renal malignancy in peritonelsa dialysis patients with acquired cystic kidney disease. Adv Perit Dial 1992; 7: 145–9.

339. Spencer SJW, Philips ME. Transitional cell carcinoma in acquired cystic disease of the kidney in a patient on CAPD. Nephrol Dial Transplant 1990; 5: 464–5.

340. Pope JC, Koch MO, Bluth RF. Renal cell carcinoma in patients with end-stage renal disease: a comparison of clinical significance in patients receiving hemodialysis and those with renal transplants. Urology 1994; 44: 497–501.

341. Levine LA, Gburek BM. Acquired cystic disease and renal adenocarcinoma following renal transplantation. J Urol 1994; 151: 129–32.

342. Smith JW, Sallman AL, Williamson MR, Lott CG. Acquired renal cystic disease: two cases of associated adenocarcinoma and a renal ultrasound survey of a peritoneal dialysis population. Am J Kidney Dis 1987; 10: 41–6.

343. Trabucco AF, Johansson SL, Egan JD, Taylor RJ. Neoplasia and acquired renal cystic disease in patients undergoing chronic ambulatory peritoneal dialysis. Urology 1990; 35: 1–4.

344. Cotterell L, Egan JD, Wells IC et al. Significant incidence of ACKD in CAPD patients. Perit Dial Bull 1986; 6: S5 (abstract).

345. Balaskas EV, Oreopoulos DG. Uremic pruritus (part I). Dial Transplant 1992; 21: 192–244.

346. Balaskas E. Uremic pruritis in CAPD patients. Perit Dial Int 1997; 17: 440–1.

347. Massry SG, Popovtzer MM, Coburn JW et al. Intractable pruritus as a manifestation of secondary hyperparathyroidism in uremia. Disappearance of itching after subtotal parathyroidectomy. N Engl J Med 1968; 279: 698–700.

348. Matsumoto M, Ishimaru K, Horie A. Pruritus and mast cell proliferation of the skin in end stage renal failure. Clin Nephrol 1985; 23: 285–8.

349. Dimkovic N, Djukanovic L, Radmilovic A, Bojic P, Juloski T. Uremic Pruritus and skin mast cells. Nephron 1992; 61: 5–9.

350. Mettang T, Fritz P, Weber J, Machleidt C, Hubel E, Kuhlmann U. Uremic pruritus in patients on hemodialysis or continuous ambulatory peritoneal dialysis (CAPD). The role of plasma histamine and skin mast cells. Clin Nephrol 1990; 34: 136–41.

351. DeMarchi S, Cecchin E, Villalta D, Sepiacci G, Santini G, Bartoli E. Relief of pruritis and decreases in plasma histamine concentrations during erythropoietin therapy in patients with uremia. N ENgl J Med 1992; 326–969–74.

352. Bencini PL, Montagnino G, Citterio A, Graziani G, Crosti C, Ponticelli C. Cutaneous abnormalities in uremic patients. Nephron 1985; 40: 316–21.

353. Albert C, Michel C, Ikeni A et al. Pruritus in patients on hemodialysis (HD) or peritoneal dialysis (PD). Perit Dial Int Suppl 1, 1991; Abstracts of the XI Annual CAPD Conference, abstract 5.

354. Francos GC. Uremic pruritus. Semin Dial 1988; 1: 209–12.

355. Morton C, Lafferty M, Hau C, Henderson I, Jones M, Lowe J. Pruritus and skin hydration during dialysis. Nephrol Dial Transplant 1996; 11: 2031–6.

356. Tan JKL, Haberman HF, Coldman AJ. Identifying effective treatments for uremic pruritus. J Am Acad Dermatol 1991; 25: 811–18.

357. Carmichael A, McHugh M, Martin A. Renal itch as an indicator of poor outcome. Lancet 1991; 333: 1225–6.

358. Balaskas E, Grapsa E. Uremic pruritus is a poor prognostic factor of outcome (letter). Perit Dial Int 1995; 15: 177.

359. Vassa N, Twardowski Z, Campbell J. Hyperbaric oxygen therapy in calciphylaxis-induced skin necrosis in a peritoneal dialysis patient. Am J Kidney Dis 1994; 23: 878–81.

360. Fine A, Fleming S, Leslie W. Calciphylaxis presenting with calf pain and placques in four continuous ambulatory peritoneal dialysis patients and in one predialysis patient. Am J Kidney Dis 1995; 25: 498–502.

361. McAuley K, Devereux F, Walker R. Calciphylaxis in two non-compliant patients with end-stage renal failure. Nephrol Dial Transplant 1997; 12: 1061–3.

362. Bleyer A, Choi M, Igwemezie B, de la Torre E, White W. A case control study of proximal calciphylaxis. Am J Kidney Dis 1998; 32: 376–83.

363. Bargman J, Prichard S. A usual peritoneal dialysis patient with an unusual skin disease. Perit Dial Int 1995; 15: 252–258.

364. Duh Q-Y, Lim R, Clark O. Calciphylaxis in secondary hyperparathyroidism. Arch Surg 1991; 126: 1213–19.

365. Kleinman KS, Coburn JW. Amyloid syndromes associated with hemodialysis (editorial). Kidney Int 1989; 35: 567–75.

366. Gejyo F, Yamada T, Odani S et al. A new form of amyloid protein associated with chronic hemodialysis was identified as beta-2-microglobulin. Biochem Biophys Res Commun 1985; 129: 701–6.

367. Shirahama T, Skinner M, Cohen AS et al. Histochemical and immunohistochemical characterization of amyloid associated with chronic hemodialysis as beta-2-microglobulin. Lab Invest 1985; 53: 705–7.

368. Sato KC, Kumakiri M, Koizume H et al. Lichenoid skin lesions as a sign of B_2-microglobulin-induced amyloidosis in a long-term haemodialysis patient. Br J Dermatol 1993; 128: 686–9.

369. Tam Y, Htwe M, Chandra R, Smith-Behn J. Bilateral B_2-microglobulin amyloidomas of the buttocks in a long-term hemodialysis patient. Arch Pathol Lab Med 1994; 118: 651–3.

370. Lutz AE, Schneider U, Ehlerding G, Frenzel H, Koch KM, Kuhn K. Right ventricular cardiac failure and pulmonary

hypertension in a long-term dialysis patient – unusual presentation of visceral B₂-microglobulin amyloidosis. Nephrol Dial Transplant 1995; 10: 555–8.

371. Matsuo K, Nakamoto M, Tasunaga C, Goya T, Sugimachi K. Dialysis-related amyloidosis of the tongue in long-term hemodialysis patients. Kidney Int 1997; 52: 832–8.

372. Tielemans C, Dratwa M, Bergmann P et al. Continuous ambulatory peritoneal dialysis vs. hemodialysis: a lesser risk of amyloidosis? Nephrol Dial Transplant 1988; 3: 291–4.

373. Sethi D, Gower PE. Dialysis arthropathy, B₂-microglobulin and the effect of dialyser membrane. Nephrol Dial Transplant 1988; 3: 768–72.

374. Miguel Alonso JL, Cruz A, Lopez Revuelta K et al. Continuous ambulatory peritoneal dialysis does not prevent the development of dialysis-associated amyloidosis. Nephron 1989; 53: 389–90.

375. Lysaght MJ, Pollock CA, Moran JE, Ibels LS, Farrell PC. Beta-2 microglobulin removal during continuous ambulatory peritoneal dialysis (CAPD). Perit Dial Int 1989; 9: 29–35.

376. Montenegro J, Martinez I, Saracho R, Gonzalez R. B₂ microglobulin in CAPD. Adv Perit Dial 1992; 8: 369–72.

377. Benz RL, Siegfried JW, Teehan BP. Carpal tunnel syndrome in dialysis patients: comparison between continuous ambulatory peritoneal dialysis and hemodialysis populations. Am J Kidney Dis 1988; 11: 473–6.

378. Cornelia F, Bardin T, Faller B et al. Rheumatic syndromes and B₂-microglobulin amyloidosis in patients receiving long-term peritoneal dialysis. Arthritis Rheum 1989; 32: 785–8.

379. Cruz A, Gonzalez T, Balsa A et al. Destructive spondylo-arthropathy in long-term CAPD and hemodialysis (letter). J Rheum 1989; 16: 1169–70.

380. Bicknell JM, Lim AC, Raroque HG, Tzamaloukas A. Carpal tunnel syndrome, subclinical median mononeuropathy, and peripheral polyneuropathy: common early complications of chronic peritoneal dialysis and hemodialysis. Arch Phys Med Rehabil 1991; 72: 378–81.

381. Gagnon RF, Lough JO, Bourgouin PA. Carpal tunnel syndrome and amyloidosis associated with continuous ambulatory peritoneal dialysis. Can Med Assoc J 1988; 139: 753–5.

382. Benhamou CL, Bardin T, Noel LH et al. Beta-2 microglobulin amyloidosis as a complication of peritoneal dialysis treatment (letter). Clin Nephrol 1988; 30: 346.

383. Athanasou NA, Ayers D, Raine AJ, Oliver DO, Duthie RB. Joint and systemic distribution of dialysis amyloid. Q J Med 1991; 78: 205–14.

384. Jadoul M, Noel H, van Ypersele de Strihou C. B₂-microglobulin amyloidosis in a patient treated exclusively by continuous ambulatory peritoneal dialysis. Am J Kidney Dis 1990; 15: 86–8.

385. Colombi A, Wegmann W. Beta-2 microglobulin amyloidosis in a patient on long-term continuous ambulatory peritoneal dialysis (CAPD). Perit Dial Int 1989; 9: 321–4.

386. Jadoul M, Malghem J, Vande Berg B, van Ypersele de Strihou C. Ultrasonographic detection of thickened joint capsules and tendons as marker of dialysis-related amyloidosis: a cross-sectional and longitudinal study. Nephrol Dial Transplant 1993; 8: 1104–9.

387. Catizone L, Cocchi R, De Vecchi A et al. Dialysis-related amyloidoss in a large CAPd population. Adv Perit Dial 1995; 11: 213–17.

388. Nomoto Y, Kawaguchi Y, Ohira S et al. Carpal tunnel syndrome in patients undergoing CAPD: a collaborative study in 143 centers. Am J Nephrol 1995; 15: 295–9.

389. Jadoul M, Garbar C, Vanholder R et al. Prevalence of histological B₂-microglobulin amyloidosis in CAPD patients compared with hemodialysis patients. Kidney Int 1998; 54: 956–9.

390. Allard JC, Artze ME, Porter G, Ghandurmnaymneh L, de Velasco R, Perez GO. Fatal destructive cervical spondyloarthropathy in two patients on long-term dialysis. Am J Kidney Dis 1992; 19: 81–5.

391. Digenis G, Davidson G, Dombros N, Katz A, Bookman A, Oreopoulos DG. Destructive spondyloarthropathy in a patient on CAPD for 13 years. Perit Dial Int 1993; 13: 228–31.

392. Ramsay AG. Joint disease in end stage renal disease. Semin Dial 1988; 1: 21–7.

393. Lustig S, Morduchowicz G, Rosenfeld J, Boner G. Bilateral rupture of the tendon of the long head of the biceps muscle in continuous ambulatory peritoneal dialysis (letter). Perit Dial Bull 1986; 6: 42–3.

394. Baum J, Cestero R, Jain V. Peritoneal dialysis spike elbow (letter). N Engl J Med 1983; 308: 1541.

395. Hoffman GS, Schumacher HR, Paul H et al. Calcium oxalate microcrystalline-associated arthritis in end stage renal disease. Ann Intern Med 1982; 97: 36–42.

396. Cassidy MJD, Owen JP, Ellis HA et al. Renal osteodystrophy and metastatic calcification in long-term continuous ambulatory peritoneal dialysis. Q J Med 1985; 54: 29–48.

397. Chalmers A, Reynolds WJ, Oreopoulos DG, Meema HE, Meindok H, deVeber GA. The arthropathy of maintenance intermittent peritoneal dialysis. Can Med Assoc J 1980; 123: 635–8.

398. Grinlinton FM, Vuletic JC, Gow PJ. Rapidly progressive calcific periarthritis occurring in a patient with lupus nephritis receiving chronic ambulatory peritoneal dialysis. J Rheum 1990; 17: 1100–3.

399. Hamodraka-Mailis A. Pathogenesis and treatment of back pain in peritoneal dialysis patients. Perit Dial Bull Suppl 1983; 3: S41–3.

400. Hussain SI, Bernardini J, Piraino B. The risk of hernia with large exchange volumes. Adv Perit Dial 1998; 14: 105–7.

401. Constable AR, Joekes AM, Kasidas GP et al. Plasma level and renal clearance of oxalate in normal subjects and in patients with primary hyperoxaluria or chronic renal failure or both. Clin Sci 1979; 56: 299–304.

402. Mitwalli A, Oreopoulos D. Hyperoxaluria and hyperoxalemia: one more concern for the nephrologist (editorial). Int J Artif Organs 1985; 8: 71–4.

403. Yamauchi A, Fujii M, Shirai D et al. Plasma concentration and peritoneal clearance of oxalate in patients on continuous ambulatory peritoneal dialysis (CAPD). Clin Nephrol 1986; 25: 181–5.

404. Tomson CRV, Channon SM, Parkinson IS et al. Plasma oxalate in patients receiving continuous ambulatory peritoneal dialysis. Nephrol Dial Transplant 1988; 3: 295–9.

405. Shah GM, Ross EA, Sabo A, Pichon M, Reynolds RD, Bhagavan H. Effects of ascorbic acid and pyridoxine supplmentation on oxalate metabolism in peritoneal dialysis patients. Am J Kidney Dis 1992; 20: 42–9.

406. Bunchman T, Swartz R. Oxalate removal in type I hyperoxaluria or acquired oxalosis using HD and equilibration PD. Perit Dial Int 1994; 14: 81–4.

407. Hoppe E, Graf D, Offner G, Latta K, Byrd D, Michalk D, Brodehl J. Oxalate elimination via hemodialysis or peritoneal dialysis in children with chronic renal failure. Pediatr Nephrol 1996; 10: 488–92.

408. Marangella M, Bagnis C, Bruno M, Petrarulo M, Gabella P, Linari F. Determinants of oxalate balance in patients on chronic peritoneal dialysis. Am J Kidney Dis 1993; 21: 419–26.

409. Oren A, Husdan H, Cheng P-T et al. Calcium oxalate kidney stones in patients on continuous ambulatory peritoneal dialysis. Kidney Int 1984; 25: 534–8.

410. Antoniou S, Syreggelas D, Papadopoulos C, Dimitriadis A. Intraluminal lithiasis of a peritoneal catheter. Perit Dial Int 1991; 11: 358–60.

411. Gelfand M, Kois J, Quillin G et al. CAPD yields inferior transplant results compared to hemodialysis. Perit Dial Bull 1984; 4: 526 (abstract).

412. Guillou P, Will E, Davidson A et al. CAPD – a risk factor in renal transplantation? Br J Surg 1984; 71: 878–80.

413. Cardella C. Peritoneal dialysis and renal transplantation (editorial). Perit Dial Bull 1985; 5: 149–51.

414. Latta K, Offner G, Hoyer PF, Brodehl J. Reduction of cytotoxic antibodies after continuous ambulatory peritoneal dialysis in highly sensitized patients (letter). Lancet 1988; 2: 847–8.

415. Gokal R, Ramos J, Veitch P et al. Renal transplantation in patients on CAPD. Dial Transplant 1982; 11: 125–55.

416. Shapiro Z, Shnueli D, Yussim A, Boner G, Haimovitz C, Servadio C. Kidney transplantation in patients on continuous ambulatory peritoneal dialysis. Proc Eur Dial Transplant Assoc 1984; 21: 932–5.

417. Evangelista J, Bennett-Jones D, Cameron J et al. Renal transplantation in patients treated with hemodialysis and short-term and long-term continuous ambulatory peritoneal dialysis. Br Med J 1985; 291: 1004–7.

418. Donnelly P, Lenhard T, Proud G et al. Continuous ambulatory peritoneal dialysis and renal transplantation: a five year experience. Br Med J 1985; 291: 1001–4.

419. Tsakiris D, Bramwell S, Briggs J, Junor BJR. Transplantation in patients undergoing CAPD. Perit Dial Bull 1985; 5: 161–4.

420. Diaz-Buxo J, Walker P, Burgess W et al. The influence of peritoneal dialysis on the outcome of transplantation. Int J Artif Organs 1986; 9: 359–62.

421. Glass N, Miller D, Sollinger H, Zimmerman SW, Simpson D, Belzer FO. Renal transplantation in patients on peritoneal dialysis. Perit Dial Bull 1985; 5: 157–60.

422. Rubin J, Kirchner K, Raju S, Krueger RP, Bower JD. CAPD patients as renal transplant patients. Am J Med Sci 1987; 294: 175–80.

423. Cardella C. Renal transplantation in patients on peritoneal dialysis. Perit Dial Bull 1980; 1: 12–14.

424. Fries D, Brocard JF, Plaisant B et al. Continuous ambulatory peritoneal dialysis and renal transplantation. Nephrologie 1989; 10 (suppl.): 18–21.

425. O'Donoghue D, Manos J, Pearson R et al. Continuous ambulatory peritoneal dialysis and renal transplantation: a 10 year experience in one center. Perit Dial Int 1992; 12: 242–9.

426. Hurault de Ligny B, Ryckelynck J Ph, Batho JM, Cardineau E, Lavaltier B. Renal transplantation in patients on continuous ambulatory peritoneal dialysis (CAPD). Perit Dial Int 1993; 12 (suppl. 1): S22 (abstract).

427. Kyllonen L, Helantera A, Salmela K, Ahonen J. Dialysis method and kidney graft survival. Transplant Proc 1992; 24: 354.

428. Winchester JF, Rotellar C, Goggins M et al. Transplantation in peritoneal dialysis and hemodialysis. Kidney Int 1993; 43 (suppl. 40): S101–5.

429. Cosio FG, Alamir A, Yim S et al. Patient survival after renal transplantation: I. The impact of dialysis pre-transplant. Kidney Int 1998; 53: 767–72.

430. Perez Fontan M, Rodriguez-Carmona A, Bouza P et al. Delayed graft function after renal transplantation in patients undergoint peritoneal dialysis and hemodialysis. Adv Perit Dial 1996; 12: 101–4.

431. Murphy BG, Hill CM, Middleton D et al. Increased renal allograft thrombosis in CAPD patients. Nephrol Dial Transplant 1994; 9: 1166–9.

432. van der Vliet JA, Barendregt WB, Hoitsma AJ, Buskens FG. Increased incidence of renal allograft thrombosis after continuous ambulatory peritoneal dialysis. Clin Transplant 1996; 10: 51–4.

433. Rigby R, Petrie J. Transplantation in patients on continuous ambulatory peritoneal dialysis (letter). Transplantation 1984; 37: 533.

434. Ryckelynck J-P, Verger C, Pierre D, Sabatier J-C, Faller B, Beaud J-M. Early post transplantation infections in CAPD patints. Perit Dial Bull 1984; 4: 40–1.

435. Andreetta B, Verrina E, Sorino P et al. Complications linked to chronic peritoneal dialysis in children after kidney transplantation: experience of the Italian Registry of Pediatric Chronic Peritoneal Dialysis. Perit Dial Int 1996; 16: S570–3.

436. Steinmuller D, Novick A, Braun W et al. Renal transplantation of patients on chronic peritoneal dialysis. Am J Kidney Dis 1984; 3: 436–9.

437. Stephanidis C, Balfe J, Arbus G, Hardy BE, Churchill BM, Rance CP. Renal transplantation in children treated with continuous ambulator peritoneal dialysis. Perit Dial Bull 1983; 3: 5–8.

438. Dutton S. Transient post-transplant ascites in CAPD patients (letter). Perit Dial Bull 1983; 3: 164.

439. Webb D, Smith C, Lee G, Wallington TB. Does continuous ambulatory peritoneal dialysis alter immune function? Clin Sci 1984; 66: 14 (abstract).

440. Shohat B, Boner G, Waller A, Rosenfeld JB. Cell-mediated immunity in uremic patients prior to and after 6 months' treatment with continuous ambulatory peritoneal dialysis. Isr J Med Sci 1986; 22: 551–5.

441. Inamoto H, Ozaki R, Matsuzaki T, Wakui M, Saruta T, Osawa A. Incidence and mortality pattern of malignancy and factors affecting the risk of malignancy in dialysis patients. Nephron 1991; 59: 611–17.

442. Digenis G, Pierratos A, Ayiomamitis A, Dombros N, Sombolos K, Oreopoulos DG. Cancer in patients on CAPD. Perit Dial Bull 1986; 6: 122–4.

443. Marple B, MacDougall M. Development of malignancy in the end-stage renal disease patient. Semin Nephrol 1993; 13: 306–14.

444. Gornik H, Lazarus J, Chertow G. Cancer screening and detection in patients with end-stage renal disease (editorial). Int J Artif Organs 1998; 21: 495–500.

445. Chertow G, Paltiel A, Owen W, Lazarus J. Cost-effectiveness of cancer screening in end-stage renal disease. Arch Intern Med 1996; 156: 1345–50.

21 | Peritoneal dialysis in diabetic end-stage renal disease

M. MISRA AND R. KHANNA

Introduction

The management of diabetic patients with end-stage renal disease (ESRD) has undergone significant changes over the past 20 years. In countries with adequate socioeconomic conditions, even diabetics with extensive comorbid diseases refused renal transplantation are generally accepted for chronic dialysis despite the inevitably poor long-term prognosis [1–4]. As a result, diabetes has become the most prevalent cause of ESRD in the USA; on average about one-third of new dialysis patients have diabetes as the cause of renal disease [5]. Renal transplantation is the generally preferred treatment for diabetic patients with end-stage renal failure because it leads to better quality of life than any form of dialysis [6]. Though the first year mortality in diabetic patients on dialysis (haemodialysis or peritoneal dialysis) has decreased dramatically between 1985 and 1995, diabetic renal disease still has one of the highest mortality rates at the end of first year of dialysis when compared to renal transplantation and dialysis in non-diabetics [7]. Nearly half of the diabetic patients begun on dialysis do not survive beyond 2 years, and less than one in five diabetic patients undergoing maintenance dialysis is capable of any activity beyond personal care [8]. In such a setting, choosing a dialytic mode which has a better potential for survival, and that promotes better quality of life, is extremely important. However, choosing a dialysis therapy at present is subject to the strong personal biases of both physician and patient. This is because a clear difference between the outcomes of haemodialysis and peritoneal dialysis for diabetic patients has not been observed. In the 1960s and early 1970s intermittent peritoneal dialysis (IPD) performed on diabetic ESRD patients, either in hospital or at home, with a cycler over 30–40 h/week, showed a promising decline or even arrest of uraemic neuropathy and retinopathy. However, possibilities for patient survival beyond 2–3 years were dismal

[9–13]. Thus, it appears that with the loss of residual-renal function, which takes about 2–3 years in PD patients, the amount of dialysis provided with IPD was not adequate, and the majority of patients were dying from either electrolytic abnormalities or progressive uraemia. The introduction of continuous ambulatory and continuous cyclic peritoneal dialysis (CAPD/CCPD) during the late 1970s allowed both diabetic and non-diabetic patients to be treated adequately, and was quickly established as a viable alternative renal replacement therapy to haemodialysis [14–22].

The proposed benefits of CAPD/CCPD

There are both medical and social benefits of CAPD/CCPD [23]. Since it is essentially a home therapy, and allows flexibility in treatment, CAPD/CCPD has several social benefits: it allows home dialysis at a lower cost, permits long-distance travel, permits uninterrupted job-related activity, etc. However, in choosing a dialysis therapy both medical and social benefits should be taken into consideration. The proposed medical benefits of CAPD/CCPD that make it a preferred therapy over haemodialysis are listed in Table 1. During the course of this chapter we will attempt to examine these issues in more detail, to determine whether there is sufficient evidence to make such claims.

Table 1. Proposed benefits of CAPD

1. Slow and sustained ultrafiltration and a relative lack of rapid fluid and electrolyte changes compared to haemodialysis
2. Ease of blood-pressure control
3. Preservation of residual renal function for a period longer than haemodialysis
4. Access for dialysis is easier
5. Blood sugar control is possible through intraperitoneal route
6. Steady-state biochemical parameters

R. Gokal, R. Khanna, R.Th. Krediet and K.D. Nolph (eds.), Textbook of Peritoneal Dialysis, 2nd Edition, 647–665.
© 2000 Kluwer Academic Publishers. Printed in Great Britain.

Drawbacks of CAPD

Despite the many attractive advantages of CAPD, some of its drawbacks are of significant consequence and, therefore, may limit its widespread application. CAPD-related episodes of peritonitis, although less frequent with the use of devices that employ the 'flush-before-fill' technique, and no higher in incidence than in non-diabetic CAPD patients, are one of the major causes of morbidity and therapy failure. Continuous loss of protein through the dialysate may aggravate nutritional problems of some of the chronically ill patients. Long-term integrity of the peritoneum, a biological membrane, has not been unequivocally established. Some of the social problems related to CAPD, such as distorted body image and burnout due to continuous therapy, may also limit its long-term use. Normalization of blood pressure in some diabetic patients with autonomic dysfunction and orthostatic hypotension may pose problems with maintaining fluid balance, and may aggravate ischaemic complications. Excessive weight gain and hyperlipidaemia as a consequence of continuous glucose absorption in some patients can be causes for concern. Ultrafiltration failure may be a troublesome problem, particularly in diabetics. During the past few years, advances in the field have enabled us to address some of these concerns and propose remedial measures to improve the risk–benefit ratio of this therapy. These aspects will be discussed in more detail later in this chapter.

When is the ideal time to initiate dialysis in diabetics?

Nearly every diabetic patient approaching end-stage renal failure has hypertension [24]. Additionally, the relative or absolute lack of insulin causes hyperglycaemia, ketosis and changes in transmembrane electrical potential in diabetics [25]. These problems lead to a higher frequency of fluid retention, electrolyte and acid–base disturbances in diabetics at a glomerular filtration rate higher than non-diabetics. Keeping this concern in mind, since April 1995 the United States Health Care Financing Administration's (HCFA) guidelines for diabetic patients with ESRD initiating dialysis have been revised. The HCFA now recommends that such patients may be started on dialysis at a C_{Cr} of less than 15 ml/min or a serum creatinine of 6.0 mg/dl (the respective comparable figures for non-diabetic patients being 10 ml/min and 8 mg/dl). Nevertheless, the average

creatinine clearance at which dialysis is initiated was 4.9 ml/min [26]. The correlation betwen early initiation of dialysis and better patient outcome was reported as early as 1985 [27], later confirmed by several other studies [28, 29].

Theoretically at least, optimal pre-ESRD care and timely initiation of dialysis (before renal Kt/V falls below 2.0) seem attractive options. However, issues such as cost, patient burnout and access-related morbidity need to be addressed in a controlled trial [30]. The recently released dialysis outcomes quality initiative (DOQI) guidelines of the National Kidney Foundation make a strong case for such a timely start of dialysis in both diabetic as well as non-diabetic ESRD patients [31].

Peritoneal access

One of the advantages of peritoneal dialysis is the ease with which the peritoneum can be accessed. It is possible to use the catheter for supine peritoneal dialysis immediately after its insertion. This avoids the need for temporary access or preplanned-access surgery that is so often necessary in haemodialysis. Access to the peritoneal cavity is obtained through the use of either a Tenckhoff catheter or one of its newer modifications [32, 33]. The technique of catheter insertion, break-in procedure, and postoperative catheter care in diabetics is similar to that used in non-diabetic patients and described in detail in Chapter 9 of this book.

The common catheter complications are exit/tunnel infection, catheter-cuff extrusion, poor dialysate flow, dialysate solution leak, pain in association with fluid flow, and peritonitis. CAPD experience over 10 years has confirmed the earlier observations that catheter survival rates, infectious and non-infectious complications of peritoneal access are no different for diabetic patients than non-diabetic patients on peritoneal dialysis [34]. The spectrum of microorganisms causing peritonitis in diabetics is no different; the earlier feared predilection for fungal infection in diabetics has turned out to be ill-founded. Although a cause-and-effect relationship is not established, the route of insulin delivery seems to influence the incidence of exit-site and/or tunnel infection; in an exhaustive survey of CAPD/CCPD patients with ESRD attributed to diabetes mellitus, performed by the USA NIH CAPD Registry [34], exit-site and/or tunnel infection rates per patient-year by route of insulin administration were calculated. Although differences in rates were small, diabetics never using insulin had the lowest rate of exit-site/tunnel infection per patient-year (0.47), while patients using subcutaneous insulin reported the highest rate (0.65). The exit-site/tunnel infection rate per patient-year for patients using intraperitoneally administered insulin (0.60) was similar to the rate reported for patients using a combination of subcutaneous and intraperitoneal insulin (0.54). Blind patients using subcutaneously administered versus blind patients using intraperitoneal insulin reported similar rates per patient-year of exit-site/tunnel infection. Catheter replacement rates per patient year were similar for all patient groups (0.16–0.20).

Dialysis schedules

Intermittent peritoneal dialysis

During the 1970s the recommended scheme of peritoneal dialysis was intermittent peritoneal dialysis (IPD) with an automated peritoneal dialysis cycler providing 40 h of dialysis a week, divided into one or two sittings [9]. Blood sugar control while on IPD was achieved with insulin administered both subcutaneously and intraperitoneally. The amount of insulin administered was adjusted to individual requirements. On dialysis days the patients were given the usual daily dose of insulin by subcutaneous injection; an additional amount of regular insulin was added to the dialysis solution until the last five exchanges of dialysis to compensate for the glucose absorbed from the peritoneal cavity during the dialysis solution exchanges. Insulin was omitted from the last few exchanges to prevent post-dialysis hypoglycaemia. Insulin requirements were determined at the initiation of each patient's first few treatments. The amount of insulin required was directly proportional to the amount of glucose load instilled during dialysis to achieve ultrafiltration. It took up to 2 weeks after initiation of dialysis to determine the exact amount of insulin required by an individual patient. Once established, the insulin requirements did not generally change unless new complications were encountered. In these patients, retinopathy and neuropathy seemed to stabilize during the course of IPD treatment. Haemoglobin and haematocrit were maintained at satisfactory levels without blood transfusions. Compared to non-diabetics on IPD, these patients experienced

a higher incidence of fibrin-clot formation in dialysis effluent and a higher incidence of peritonitis. The patients also experienced higher rates of arterial calcification and hypertension. The majority of patients died from cardiac and cerebrovascular complications. Significant percentages of patients died suddenly at home, presumably due to a coronary event or from an electrolyte abnormality. The probability of patient survival at 1 and 2 years was 44% and 20%, respectively [9]. Outcomes of IPD in other centres with smaller numbers of patients were similar [10–13]. The main reason for the low survival rate may have related to inadequate dialysis, since this IPD scheme as advocated in the past provided (under the best circumstances) a dialysis creatinine clearance of 20 L/week or less. Presumably most patients were under-dialysed and became more uraemic with the gradual loss of renal function. Since the advent of CAPD the use of such a scheme of IPD has declined. In any case, due to its inadequacies, such a prescription is no longer recommended or acceptable as an effective renal replacement therapy.

Automated peritoneal dialysis (APD)

A variant of IPD with a much longer weekly duration and a larger amount of dialysis, daily night-time IPD (NIPD), is now used for home treatment in patients who are unsuitable for CAPD [35–38]. Other than the patient's preference, the indications for NIPD include those patients having high peritoneal membrane solute transport characteristics and those who develop complications as a result of increased intra-abdominal pressure during CAPD. The rise in intra-abdominal pressure in the supine position is considerably lower than in the upright position [39]. During the NIPD treatment at home the patient is confined to bed, and sleeps during most of the therapy time. In order to provide the recommended amount of dialysis of 66 L/week of creatinine clearance or 2.2 of Kt/V_{urea}, NIPD needs to be carried out, depending on the peritoneal solute transport rate, 8–12 h/day using dialysis solution flow rates ranging from 12 to 17 L/day. A typical NIPD prescription is for a 1.5–2.5 L fill volume and 1 h cycles for 8–10 h of treatment time. In patients with low peritoneal transport characteristics, additional dialysis may be provided by the last bag fill option and leaving the solution dwelling in the peritoneal cavity during the day. Like IPD, the major benefit of NIPD is the lower, incidence of complications related to high intra-abdominal pressure compared to CAPD. Importantly, the peritonitis rate is considerably lower probably due to a reduced number of connections and improved host-defence mechanisms [40].

Continuous cyclic peritoneal dialysis (CCPD)

CCPD is a reversal of the CAPD schedule [41]. It uses multiple short cycles during the night with an automated cycler and a long day time exchange while the patient is ambulatory. With this technique, variable volumes of dialysis solution are delivered for a prescribed dwell time with the aid of an automated cycler during the night (three or four 2 L commercial dialysis solution infusions are generally administered during the night, each dwelling for 2–3 h) and then are drained by gravity at the end of the dwell. An additional 2 L of dialysis solution is infused in the morning and is allowed to dwell intraperitoneally for the next 14–15 h with the catheter capped. Hypertonic dialysis solution containing 2.5–4.25% dextrose is recommended for the daytime exchange in order to prevent significant absorption of the solution. Diaz-Buxo [41] observed that it is difficult to design a uniform method for intraperitoneal insulin administration for blood glucose control in CCPD patients due to the fact that during the day, when most of the dietary caloric load is consumed, they carry out only one peritoneal dialysis exchange for 12–14 h and essentially no food is eaten during the night, when several dialysis exchanges are carried out. Nevertheless, Diaz-Buxo claims excellent glycaemic control can be obtained in the majority of patients if time is spent to individualize the precise dose of insulin required, and if a regular and predictable caloric intake is maintained with little day-to-day variation. He recommends that the insulin dose be appropriately divided among all the dialysis solution bags, depending upon the caloric load. Such a distribution avoids sudden and massive infusions of insulin and consequent hypoglycaemia or hyperglycaemia. The average intraperitoneal insulin dose required for good control of glycaemia has been about three times the pre-dialysis total subcutaneous dose. In most cases 50% of the intraperitoneal dose is used for the long-dwell daytime exchange, with the remaining 50% equally divided among the nocturnal exchanges. For more detailed instructions readers are advised to refer to the protocol recommended by Diaz-Buxo [41]. The 1-year patient survival for diabetic patients on CCPD is reported to be 76% [41]. The main indications for

CCPD in diabetics include: patient preference; young diabetics awaiting cadaver or living-related renal transplantations; and older, blind and dependent diabetics requiring partner support for the dialysis technique. The medical circumstances under which CCPD is often recommended over CAPD are in CAPD patients who have shown a tendency to develop complications related to increased intra-abdominal pressure. Another group of patients who may benefit from CCPD are those who complain of chronic low-back pain on CAPD.

Continuous ambulatory peritoneal dialysis (CAPD)

The standard CAPD technique has been previously reported [14]. In short, in the past the technique usually consisted of exchanging four 2 L dialysis solution bags/day using appropriate glucose concentrations from the range available (0.5, 1.5, 2.5, 4.25 g%) to achieve adequate ultrafiltration. Patients are taught to add insulin into the dialysis solution according to the protocol to be discussed later. The technique of CAPD is usually modified to accommodate the handicapped diabetic patient's desire to self-perform dialysis at home. Visual impairment, peripheral vascular disease with amputation of a part or entire limb, and peripheral neuropathy with sensory and/or motor function impairment are some of the physical disabilities observed in these diabetic populations. Devices such as the Ultraviolet box [42], Splicer [43], Oreopoulos-Zellerman connector [44], Y-system [45], and Injecta aid [46] are used with success in many patients. These devices have enabled a number of blind diabetics to self-perform CAPD. Although published reports of usage of such devices are scarce, anecdotal experiences of their usefulness are encouraging. In our centre the training period averages 5 working days while a complex patient may take as much as 20 working days.

Theoretical modelling [47, 48], later confirmed by studies using multivariate analyses [49], convincingly demonstrate an association between urea and/or creatinine clearance and survival in dialysis patients. For example, a weekly Kt/V_{urea} of 2.1 (corresponding to a creatinine clearance of 70 ml/min) predicted a 2-year survival of 78% in the CANUSA study [49]. No particular target value of creatinine clearance or Kt/V_{urea} for diabetes is currently available. However, based on a review of the available data, the recently released DOQI guidelines recommend that an adequate amount of dialysis should achieve at least a combined (dialysis and residual-renal function) creatinine clearance of 60 L/week or a Kt/V_{urea} of 2.0 [50] in all patients. Many CAPD patients must use 2.5–3.0 L exchanges to achieve these targets.

Glucose as an osmotic agent

Several years of experience with peritoneal dialysis has indicated that glucose has proved to be an effective osmotic agent for inducing ultrafiltration during peritoneal dialysis. However, use of glucose has been identified with numerous undesirable metabolic effects, which necessitate a search for alternative osmotic agents. An average CAPD patient typically absorbs 100–150 g of glucose per day during the course of CAPD with glucose-based PD solutions. This inevitably large amount of carbohydrate absorption unavoidably leads to unwanted metabolic problems such as obesity, hypertriglyceridaemia, and premature atherosclerosis [51]. There is also concern that continuous contact of the peritoneum with glucose may induce peritoneal mesothelial damage by non-enzymatic glycosylation leading to formation of advanced glycosylation end-products (AGE). Both *in-vitro* and *ex-vivo* evidence points towards AGE formation in conventional dextrose-containing dialysate [52–54]. The accumulation of AGE products may be a significant factor in the treatment failure of the long-term peritoneal dialysis patient by their effect on peritoneal membrane function and morphology [55]. In addition, higher doses of insulin required to maintain the blood sugar at normal levels may cause hyperinsulinaemia which, even in healthy persons, has been shown to be a risk factor for atherosclerotic heart disease [56, 57]. To obviate the unacceptable metabolic consequences of glucose absorption, efforts have been made to substitute glucose with xylitol [58], amino acids [59], gelatin [60], polyglucose [61], glycerol [62], or polypeptide [63]. Although every agent tried has been found to be an effective osmotic agent, and also prevented or minimized the unwanted metabolic effect of glucose, none has been found to have the favourable metabolic profile of glucose. As a result of unacceptable toxicity or metabolic profiles, or prohibitively higher cost, compared to glucose, their use as osmotic agents has been limited. Amino acid mixtures of 1–2% in the dialysis solution have been used effectively to induce ultrafiltration in non-diabetic CAPD patients [59]. In four diabetic patients followed for >12 months on a 1% amino acid solution, serum albumin and cholesterol increased when compared with the control group [64]. The absorbed amino acids cause significant increases in total body nitrogen and transferrin, reduce the inevitable glucose load and lower serum triglyceride levels. Use of such mixtures in diabetic CAPD patients has the potential to reduce many of the undesirable effects of glucose. However, their effectiveness over long periods has not been established. Furthermore, the high cost of amino acid mixtures could be a major limiting factor in their general use. Glycerol-containing dialysis solution has been used successfully in diabetic CAPD patients. This agent was well tolerated by the patients, was non-toxic to the peritoneal membrane, did not cause hepatotoxicity, and did not increase protein losses in the dialysate [62, 65]. Blood sugar was easily controlled with insulin. Some patients did develop signs and symptoms of hyperosmolality. However, glycerol showed no benefits over glucose because it delivered similar amounts of total caloric load and the problem with hyperlipidaemia was unaltered. Larger molecular-weight polyglucose (Icodextrin) appears to be a safe and effective osmotic agent providing sustained ultrafiltration by a mechanism resembling 'colloid' osmosis [66]. A total of 240 patient-years experience, ranging from single dwell to full-scale multicentre studies, has thus far been accumulated with the use of Icodextrin. Its ability to provide sustained ultrafiltration over prolonged dwells, and absence of any significant long-term effect on peritoneal permeability, make it a viable alternative osmotic agent as compared to dextrose in diabetic CAPD patients [67]. However, to date no specific studies using Icodextrin have been performed in diabetic patients. Polypeptides as an osmotic agent have been found to be safe in CAPD patients during an acute study [63]. However, long-term studies are needed to evaluate its usefulness, and also to study whether it has nutritional value in addition to its osmotic effect. Overall, at least for now, glucose remains the most widely used osmotic agent for peritoneal dialysis although Icodextrin may be used as an alternative agent in specific situations as a part of the peritoneal dialysis fluid regimen.

Blood sugar control during peritoneal dialysis

The aim of blood sugar control during peritoneal dialysis is to maintain a state of euglycaemia throughout the dwell time, control post-meal glycaemia, and avoid morning hypoglycaemia. Uraemia alters the insulin responsiveness; hence the amount required to control blood sugar in a dialysis patient becomes unpredictable [68]. Glycosylated haemoglobin C (HbA$_1$C) is widely used as an indicator of monitoring glycaemic control in peritoneal dialysis. HbA$_1$C metabolism is unaltered in renal failure. Although carbamylation of Hb is known to interfere with a particular HbA$_1$C assay, when immunological or other chemical methods of assay are utilized, this problem is easily overcome. Increasing HbA$_1$C levels usually imply worsening control (regardless of the method used) and correlate with glycaemic control [69]. Several methods have been used for blood glucose control during peritoneal dialysis, especially during CAPD. The survey of the USA NIH CAPD Registry [34] in 499 patients with ESRD attributed to diabetic nephropathy found five different treatment regimens for blood sugar control during CAPD therapy; 86% of the surveyed patients were taking insulin only, 2% took insulin with an oral hypoglycaemic agent, 4% were on an oral agent only, 6% were on diet therapy alone and the remaining 2% were on no specific therapy at all. Of the 434 patients taking insulin, 36% received it through subcutaneous injections only, 54% through intraperitoneal delivery only, and 10% through a combination of subcutaneous injections and intraperitoneal delivery. Although there are no studies that show one regimen of insulin administration clearly superior to others for CAPD patients, for reasons discussed below, if insulin is required to control blood sugar, attempts should be made to administer it intraperitoneally.

Kinetics of intraperitoneal insulin

There is evidence to suggest that intraperitoneal insulin delivery allows more rapid and consistent absorption of insulin; when absorbed, insulin preferentially enters the hepatic portal venous circulation and this hepatic delivery may beneficially affect lipid metabolism and peripheral insulin levels.

There are several similarities between the absorption kinetics of intraperitoneally administered insulin and the normal secretion of insulin by the islet cells. Insulin release in a normal person is a complex coordinated interplay of food absorbed from the gut, gastrointestinal hormones, and other hormonal and neural stimuli. Insulin secreted by the islet cells is taken into the portal vein, and, thereafter, the liver removes 50–60% of the secreted insulin presented

to it [70]. In the basal state the portal/peripheral ratio of insulin is 3:1. Following bursts of secretion in response to glucose or amino acids, the portal/peripheral ratio may reach a value of 9:1. Insulin administered into the peritoneal cavity is absorbed preferentially by diffusion across the visceral peritoneum into the portal venous circulation. Additionally, direct absorption through the capsule of the liver has also been reported [71]. Once in the liver, a significant fraction of insulin is cleared by the liver during its first pass. Initial delivery of insulin to the liver simulates physiological insulin secretion more closely; absorption is continuous until the end of the dwell [72–78].

Some of the causes for glycaemic lability in diabetic patients taking subcutaneous insulin injections [79, 80] are degradation of insulin in the subcutaneous tissues and variations in absorption due to factors such as depth and location of injection, exercise, or regional blood flow. Peritoneal delivery of insulin alleviates these variables and allows for predictable metabolic management [70, 81, 82].

Benefits of intraperitoneal insulin

There are benefits when insulin is delivered to the liver during its first pass. Relatively few studies have carefully examined this issue. Studies in dogs show that insulin delivery via the portal route may be necessary to maintain normal levels of hormones and metabolites [83, 84]. However, both portal and peripheral insulin delivery have similar effects on hepatic and extrahepatic carbohydrate metabolism [85].

Excessive basal hepatic glucose output is the principal cause of elevated fasting plasma glucose levels in non-insulin-dependent diabetes mellitus (NIDDM) [86, 87]; in normal and NIDDM subjects, hepatic glucose output is much more sensitive to suppression by insulin than is stimulation of peripheral glucose uptake [88]. While reviewing the benefits of intraperitoneal insulin, Duckworth and colleagues argue in favour of treating NIDDM with intraperitoneal insulin because intraperitoneal insulin delivery can selectively inhibit increased hepatic glucose output with a relatively lower degree of hyperinsulinaemia in NIDDM compared to subcutaneous insulin injections [89]. Duckworth [70] stresses that, for any given dose of insulin, the amount that reaches the peripheral circulation is considerably less when the insulin is delivered intraperitoneally rather than subcutaneously. This observation is all the more important in view of the increasing evidence suggesting that circulating insulin levels may be directly related to the risk of atherosclerosis [90–92].

In normal subjects a low basal level of insulin is maintained between ingestion of meals [93]. Peritoneal delivery of insulin results in rapid and consistent absorption and allows for maintaining a low basal level between meals. The significance of maintaining a basal level of insulin was clearly shown by studies showing that programmed insulin-infusion systems, which provide insulin in basal as well as pre-meal doses, are far more effective in normalizing blood glucose concentrations in type I diabetes than pre-meal insulin doses alone [94]. Persistent hyperinsulinaemia, a rare occurrence in normal subjects, occurs frequently when insulin is subcutaneously injected. One study suggests that intraperitoneal insulin is necessary to normalize lactate levels [95].

A number of studies suggest that intraperitoneal insulin therapy is associated with lipoprotein profiles of lower atherogenic potential [96–98]. These studies demonstrated a reduction in the cholesterol content of high-density lipoprotein (HDL) in patients treated with intraperitoneal insulin compared with subcutaneous insulin, with no change in apolipoproteins A-I and A-II. Moreover, intraperitoneal insulin was associated with lower very-low-density lipoprotein (VLDL) triglycerides, VLDL apolipoprotein B and near-normal levels of cholesterol ester transfer. The conclusion of these studies was that intraperitoneal insulin was more physiological and corrected a key step in reverse cholesterol transport in patients with IDDM. Hepatic functions, other than carbohydrate and lipid metabolism, that are dependent on insulin may also be improved with intraperitoneal administration [70]. For example, intraperitoneal insulin results in higher levels of plasma hydroxyvitamin D levels than subcutaneous insulin, even with comparable glucose control [99].

Both intensive subcutaneous insulin therapy and peritoneal insulin delivery can return the blood glucose levels and glycosylated haemoglobin values to normal. But the benefit of peritoneal delivery is fewer glycaemic excursions, so that the difference between low and high glucose values during a day are lower compared to subcutaneous insulin [100]. Moreover, frequency of hypoglycaemic episodes is reduced with peritoneal insulin.

A three-step euglycaemic clamp in six matched groups (healthy subjects, insulin-dependent diabetics with normal kidney function, non-diabetic uraemics, non-dialysed uraemic diabetics, and diabetics on haemodialysis and CAPD) showed that the insulin-mediated glucose uptake is closer to normal in CAPD patients taking intraperitoneal insulin than in subjects on haemodialysis taking subcutaneous insulin [101]. In another retrospective study [102], insulin requirements were examined in two groups of dialysed and non-dialysed diabetic patients, one treated with subcutaneous insulin and the other with intraperitoneal insulin. The blood glucose levels were significantly lower with the CAPD/intraperitoneal group compared to both CAPD/subcutaneous and HD/subcutaneous groups at every time interval for as long as 15 months.

Because of the similarities between the effects of intraperitoneally administered insulin and the physiologically secreted insulin, glycaemic and metabolic control during CAPD is more physiological than during haemodialysis. Such an advantage should impact on the overall long-term progression of diabetic complications in patients on dialysis. The effects of intraperitoneal insulin in the progression of target organ diseases in CAPD patients are difficult to ascertain because of the high prevalence of end-stage multi-organ damage at the time of initiation of dialysis; nearly half the patients do not survive 2 years on the therapy. Moreover, young patients with early target organ damage, appropriately, are very quickly transplanted and do not stay on the therapy long enough to observe the impact of therapy. Unless observations in diabetic CAPD patients extending over 5–10 years are carried out, we will not know intraperitoneal insulin's effect on the slowing of the progression of target organ diseases. For now, it is clear that short-term metabolic control with intraperitoneal insulin is better than that achieved with subcutaneous insulin and, therefore, should favour CAPD over haemodialysis.

Problems of intraperitoneal insulin therapy

Some anecdotal experiences suggest increased incidence of peritonitis in patients receiving intraperitoneal insulin [103]. Contrary to this observation, the National CAPD Registry survey of peritonitis rates per patient-year by route of insulin administration and type of diabetes management revealed patients using a combination of subcutaneous and intraperitoneal insulin experienced the lowest rate (0.93 episodes per patient-year) of peritonitis [34]. The peritonitis rate per patient-year for patients using subcutaneously administered insulin (1.03) was similar to the rate reported for patients using intra-peritoneal insulin (1.06). Blind patients using subcutaneously administered versus blind patients using intraperitoneal insulin reported similar rates of peritonitis. It has been suggested that insulin may have a bactericidal effect.

The other problem observed with the use of intra-peritoneal insulin is subcapsular liver steatonecrosis [104] and malignant omentum syndrome [105]. Steatosis in a unique subcapsular distribution was observed during autopsy in 10 of 11 CAPD patients treated with intraperitoneal insulin and in none of the nine control CAPD patients receiving no insulin. More studies are needed to understand the impor-tance of this focal lesion in the livers of CAPD patients receiving intraperitoneal insulin. In patients with malignant omentum syndrome, insulin is trapped in the omentum, probably in response to foreign protein.

From the above discussion it is evident that there are a number of metabolic and long-term benefits to peritoneal delivery of insulin for diabetic patients. Diabetic dialysis patients, despite the far-advanced target organ damage, should be given the benefit of peritoneal delivery of insulin for better metabolic control and to derive the antiatherogenic benefit, however small.

Steps of blood sugar control in a new CAPD patient using the intraperitoneal route

Several protocols of blood sugar control with intra-peritoneal insulin have been published [16, 20, 106–109]. These protocols were designed based on the vast experiences of the individual centres. There are no studies that compare the effectiveness of different methods, but from a clinical perspective they all seem effective in achieving the goal of good metabolic control. The method described below is the one practised at our centre.

The goal of therapy is to maintain blood sugar at about 150 mg/dl throughout the day and achieve a HbA_1C level of 7% or below without the hypogly-caemic symptoms. During and for a week or two after the initiation of CAPD, blood sugar is con-trolled with daily multiple subcutaneous injections of regular insulin as per the standard practice of blood sugar control. This interval allows for CAPD to be established and the dialysis dose to be deter-mined. An attempt is made to switch to the intra-peritoneal route of insulin administration after

explaining the practice to the patient. It is not uncommon for patients to refuse the intraperitoneal approach for fear of the unknown. On the first day of the switch, 100% of the CAPD daily subcutaneous insulin dose is divided among all four exchanges, with a reduced insulin dose (50–70%) added to the overnight dwell. Although many patients may need more than 100% of subcutaneous dose of insulin when switched to the intraperitoneal route, it is recommended to use caution initially in order to avoid severe hypoglycaemia. Although the amount of insulin required to control blood sugar intra-peritoneally is comparatively smaller than in the subcutaneous route, when the liver is insulinized during the first pass of exogenous insulin through the intraperitoneal route, only about half the injected amount is absorbed through the peritoneal route during a 6 h dialysis exchange [78]. Therefore, it is appropriate to initiate intraperitoneal mode with 100% of the subcutaneous dose.

Review of fasting, 2 h postprandial and/or pre-exchange blood glucose results of the previous day allows stepwise changes in insulin added to each cycle until the desired blood glucose control is achieved. Below are some helpful hints for the use of intraperitoneal insulin. The dialysis exchanges are performed during the day to coincide with the major meals, i.e. breakfast, lunch, and supper. The fourth exchange is made at around 2300 h, at which time a small snack may be taken. The patient is advised to consume a diet providing 20–25 Kcal/kg body weight/day and containing protein of 1.2–1.5 g/kg body weight. During the initial control, blood sugar by the finger-stick method is estimated four times a day, pre-exchange. After cleaning the blood port of the dialysis solution bag with a sterilizing solution, using a syringe with a long needle, regular insulin is added to each dialysis solution bag. The time of insulin injection into the bag, prior to solution infu-sion, should be standardized. The bag is inverted two or three times to aid mixing. Increments in insulin are required for each additional hypertonic dialysis cycle incorporated into the daily routine. Increments differ among patients. Individual patient requirements are determined during training. Patients are trained to check their blood sugar levels with the finger-prick method. This method, which gives quick results and correlates well with venous blood sugar levels, helps the patient monitor unex-pected fluctuations in blood sugar. The finger-prick test is performed 5–10 min before each bag exchange and, whenever necessary, the dose of insulin added to the next bag is adjusted according to the guide-lines taught the patient at the time of training.

Intraperitoneal insulin requirements during episodes of peritonitis are widely believed to be increased, but hypoglycaemia has recently been reported when the usual dose of intraperitoneal insulin was continued during peritonitis [110]. Also, in diabetic rats it has been shown that peritonitis does not change intraperitoneal requirements during standardized peritoneal dialysis exhanges [111]. Blood glucose during peritonitis is likely to be determined by the relative importance of increased insulin absorption and reduced carbohydrate intake due to anorexia versus increased glucose absorption and the infection-related catabolic state. If care is not exercised, severe fatal hypoglycaemia may be encountered with intraperitoneal insulin administration.

In diabetic CAPD patients such treatment objectives as maintaining morning-fasting glucose less than 140 mg/dl, post-meal hyperglycaemia less than 200 mg/dl, and HbA_1C levels less than 9% is easily achieved with intraperitoneal insulin administration. Insulin injected into the tubing and flushed into the peritoneal cavity with a small volume of dialysis solution reduces the total amount of insulin needed to normalize blood sugar compared to mixing insulin with the dialysis solution prior to infusion [112]. Some type II diabetic patients have difficulty maintaining satisfactory blood sugar levels even with very large doses of insulin. The reason for such refractoriness to intraperitoneal injection of insulin is not clear, but is believed to be due to the trapping of insulin in the mesenteric or omental lymphatics [105].

Site of intraperitoneal delivery

Most protocols recommend mixing insulin with the dialysis solution before delivery into the peritoneal cavity. This way, insulin is diluted nearly 2000 times and a very low insulin concentration is achieved in the solution. Due to the low concentration gradient, insulin diffusion is slow and continuous. On the other hand, when insulin is injected into the connecting tube through a special injection port, a high concentration of insulin is achieved in the first 50 ml of dialysis solution that gets infused into the peritoneal cavity [106]. This approach may reduce the amount of insulin required.

Blood sugar control during APD

Blood-sugar control while on NIPD is achieved with insulin administered either subcutaneously or both subcutaneously and intraperitoneally. The amount of insulin administered is adjusted to individual requirements. During the day, patients are given the daily dose of insulin, usually long-acting, by subcutaneous injection, the dose determined both by patient's dietary caloric intake and insulin sensitivity An additional amount of long-acting insulin is given subcutaneously or regular insulin intraperitoneally at the initiation of cycler therapy. The amount of insulin needed is dependent on the patient's insulin sensitiveness and the amount of glucose absorbed during the dialysis. Type I diabetics typically need considerably less insulin compared to type II diabetics. During the first few treatments, blood sugar is determined several times and insulin dose is titrated to maintain the desired blood sugar level. It takes several treatment days to determine the exact amount of insulin required by an individual patient. Once stable, blood sugar may be checked periodically during treatment.

Clinical results

Blood pressure control

Blood pressure control on CAPD is simple, due to continuous sustained ultrafiltration and sodium removal, which maintains patients at their dry body weight [113, 114]. The reduction in blood pressure is most marked during the initial weeks of therapy and additional decreases occur over the next few months [114]. The blood pressure response to CAPD correlates well with the reduction in fluid body weight, emphasizing the importance of fluid volume in the pathogenesis of hypertension in ESRD. Hypertension can often be controlled without drug therapy, even when plasma renin and aldosterone levels are observed to be increased [115].

During CAPD exchanges, net water as well as sodium is removed. A typical CAPD patient loses about 1–1.5 L/day of ultrafiltrate with a sodium concentration of about 132 mEq/L since the dialysate equilibrates with serum sodium during a 4–6 h exchange [116, 117]. The total sodium loss during a day can also be readily calculated as the sum of (drain volume × drained dialysate sodium concentration) − (infusion volume × infused dialysate sodium concentration) for each day. Thus, a typical CAPD patient could easily lose up to 132–198 mEq/day of sodium through the ultrafiltrate. A patient accustomed to restricted sodium intake during the course of chronic renal failure continues his/her low-sodium diet during CAPD therapy. Consequently, CAPD patients become sodium-depleted over the course of therapy due to the combination of dialysate sodium loss and restricted consumption. Initially, such sodium depletion is beneficial in controlling hypertension. Most CAPD patients, requiring multiple antihypertensive agents for control of hypertension prior to starting CAPD, gradually need fewer and fewer drugs, eventually discontinuing them altogether [114]. If, at this time, dietary sodium intake is not liberalized, severe sodium depletion could lead to hypotension, especially in patients with primary cardiac disease. Total body sodium depletion results in decreased vascular response to infusions of pressor agents such as norepinephrine [118]. Salt repletion in such patients results in restoration of the vascular pressure response, extracellular fluid volume, and blood pressure.

In certain CAPD patients, such as those with diabetic autonomic neuropathy or cardiac dysfunction, hypotension may occur readily and very early after initiating CAPD. Surprisingly, many patients are asymptomatic, despite a severe degree of hypotension (possibly due to a lack of renin response from the kidneys, since most patients are functionally anephric).

On the other hand, during intermittent dialysis therapies the dialysate sodium concentration decreases due to solute sieving with ultrafiltration, hence sodium loss is considerably diminished [116]. Consequently, hypertension control in patients on intermittent dialysis therapies is not readily achieved. Most patients require fluid and dietary salt restriction and very many need antihypertensive medications. Hypotension, if it occurs in these patients, is generally transient and is a result of rapid ultrafiltration during treatment. From the above discussion it is apparent that, due to its effect on salt and water balance, CAPD controls blood pressure readily and a significant number of such patients do not require medication.

Benefits of slow and continuous ultrafiltration during CAPD

Rapid ultrafiltration, i.e. 3–4 L of fluid removal during a typical 3–4 h haemodialysis, three times a week, causes intravascular fluid volume depletion leading to hypotension in many diabetic patients. In most of these patients this acute transient hypotension is usually managed by infusion of saline or colloid solution to restore intravascular volume and

maintain blood pressure. In patients with significant coronary, carotid, or peripheral artery disease, ischaemic symptoms, or in some instances irreversible ischaemic complications such as myocardial infarction or stroke, may ensue if hypotension is sustained. Fluid infused to correct hypotension essentially negates the purpose of ultrafiltration and, more importantly, adds to the cost of dialysis. Contrary to haemodialysis, patients on CAPD do not need this rapid rate of ultrafiltration; typically these patients require 1–2 L of fluid removal over a 24 h period. Unless the patient is clearly dehydrated, transient acute hypotension during CAPD is infrequent. There are no data in the literature that compare in a prospective manner the impact of dialysis therapy on the ischaemic complications of vascular diseases of similar severity in patients on haemodialysis and CAPD. Nevertheless, analysis of death rates by cause of death for all diabetic ESRD patients on haemodialysis (35 683 patient-years at risk) and CAPD (5254 patient-years at risk) during 1987–89 in the USA showed mortality from myocardial infarction and cerebrovascular events was greater among diabetic patients on CAPD/CCPD (151.6 deaths per 1000 patient-years at risk) compared to diabetic patients on haemodialysis (129.7 deaths per 1000 patient-years at risk) [8]. This higher death rate from cardiac causes in CAPD diabetic patients may in part be a reflection of selection bias, i.e. preferential use of CAPD/CCPD for patients known to have severe cardiovascular disease.

Residual-renal function

The importance of residual-renal function in the management of dialysis patients has been under-recognized; 1 ml/min of residual renal creatinine clearance adds 10 L/week to total (dialysis and renal) weekly clearance. Residual-renal function contributes to the overall clearance of small and middle molecular weight solutes and fluid removal. In addition, substantial amounts of sodium, potassium, phosphate and acid excretion permit liberal fluid and dietary intake. Due to the contribution of renal function to solute clearance, the dialysis prescription may be modified to reduce the dose of dialysis and, in some, time spent on dialysis per treatment.

There are indications that the rates of decline of residual-renal function in patients on haemodialysis and CAPD may be different. Since the original publication of Rottembourg and colleagues in 1983 [119], which showed a stable residual-renal function (assessed by creatinine clearance) over a period of 18 months in 22 insulin-dependent diabetic patients on CAPD compared to 56 insulin-dependent diabetic patients treated with haemodialysis, several more studies have confirmed the observation that residual-renal function in CAPD patients is preserved for a longer period, in some up to 60 months, compared to haemodialysis patients [120–130]. If, indeed, residual-renal function decays faster in haemodialysis patients than in CAPD patients, on a theoretical ground several potential mechanisms could be operating in combination to make haemodialysis nephrotoxic:

1. As discussed earlier, patients on haemodialysis frequently experience rapid changes in extracellular fluid volumes during aggressive ultrafiltration. The result is an acute fall in blood pressure and, most likely, an acute fall in renal blood flow and glomerular capillary pressure, resulting in ischaemia of remaining functioning nephrons.
2. There is evidence to suggest that the passage of blood through extracorporeal circulation triggers the secretion of interleukin 1 and tumour necrosis factor [131]. Levels of tumour necrosis factor alpha are increased in uraemic patients; dialysis further increases these levels. Circulating cytokines may directly or indirectly generate vascular and immune injury *in vivo* [132]. Alternatively, blood membrane contact may trigger the release of reactive oxygen metabolites into circulation that may damage residual renal tissue [133]. Shah has suggested that reactive oxygen metabolites generated by neutrophils enhance glomerular basement membrane degradation by proteolytic enzymes and may cause a profound constrictive response in the glomerular capillaries [133]. The evidence cited above suggests that haemodialysis could be nephrotoxic and, hence, could cause deterioration of residual-renal function at a rate faster than the natural progression of the primary renal disease. Absence of such nephrotoxic effect in patients on CAPD may permit natural progression of renal disease and, in many, preservation of native kidney function for a longer period.

It is important to point out that the evidence cited above is only suggestive of a trend, because many cited studies were retrospective, were not matched for glomerular filtration rate (GFR) between two therapies at the initiation of dialysis, for frequency of complicating events such as severe hypotension and were not controlled for administration of other nephrotoxic drugs. Moreover, reliance on creatinine clearance as an estimate of GFR has always been questioned. In research studies measurement of residual GFR after administration of cimetidine in doses of 800 mg/day to CAPD patients closely approximates inulin clearance. In clinical practice however, estimation of residual-renal function by calculating the mean of urea and creatinine clearance seems a practical way of circumventing this problem [134].

Visual problems

Most insulin-dependent diabetics have irreversible retinal lesions before they start dialysis, especially during the terminal phase of renal failure when hypertension tends to be severe. In the great majority, by the time they reach the stage of dialysis, ocular lesions are far too advanced to expect any useful recovery. However, attempts should be made to preserve any useful vision the patient has. Specialized eye care is essential for all these patients. Many patients benefit from vitrectomy and panretinal photocoagulation, even with advanced retinal lesions [135–137]. The common lesions seen at the time of initiating CAPD are background retinopathy, proliferative retinopathy, and vitreous haemorrhage. Retinal detachment may also be seen in some cases. Therefore, better preservation of ocular function depends on the more aggressive approach to blood pressure and glucose control during the predialysis phase. Retinal ischaemia may be made worse by the rapid fluctuations in intervascular volume during the intermittent therapy. CAPD avoids many of the problems inherent in the intermittent forms of dialysis. Stabilization or even improvement of ocular function in diabetic patients maintained on CAPD has been reported by several centres [20, 46, 135, 137].

Cardiac and vascular diseases

Morbidity and mortality due to atherosclerotic heart disease and microangiopathy remain the main cause of death among diabetics undergoing peritoneal dialysis. Small-vessel disease leading to ischaemic gangrene of the extremities is a common complication of type I diabetes. Short-term experience with CAPD in diabetics does not suggest that ischaemic complications occur any more frequently in diabetics than in non-diabetics. In the only long-term experience, reported by Zimmerman *et al.* [138], the incidence of ischaemic and/or gangrenous complication was extremely low. The keys to preserving adequate circulation to extremities include avoidance of smoking and hypotensive episode and lipid regulation.

Metabolic and nutritional problems

Loss of proteins, amino acids, polypeptides, and vitamins in the dialysate contribute to the morbidity and slow rehabilitation of diabetic patients on CAPD. Such losses pose a special problem in those diabetics who may be wasted and malnourished because of poor food intake, vomiting, catabolic stresses, and intercurrent illness. Twenty-four hour amino acid losses in the dialysate average about 2.25 g/day, with about 8 g/day of proteins [139]. In uncomplicated cases, dialysate daily protein losses correlate with serum-protein concentration and body-surface area. During peritonitis, the protein losses are excessive, and in combination with inadequate food intake due to poor appetite or inability to eat, may produce severe hypoproteinaemia, hypoalbuminaemia, and hypoimmunoglobulinaemia. Therefore, during the course of a prolonged peritonitis episode, physicians should consider early parenteral nutrition.

Continuous absorption of glucose during CAPD may aggravate the pre-existing hypertriglyceridaemia, a frequently seen lipid problem in both dialysed and non-dialysed uraemics [20, 140–146]. The prevalence of hypertriglyceridaemia in long-term CAPD patients is reported to be about 80% [147, 148] and hypercholesterolaemia prevalence to be about 15–30% [147, 149]. Insulin levels correlate directly with the level of serum triglycerides [150], hence it is not surprising to find that diabetics who have hyperinsulinaemia either due to exogenous or endogenous insulin have a significant problem of hypertriglyceridaemia. At the start of therapy most patients have either normal or low cholesterol levels. During the initial months after the initiation of therapy, both serum cholesterol and triglycerides increase [51, 142, 151–154]. The increase in cholesterol is predominantly due to the increase in the fractions of VLDL and LDL, and, to a lesser extent, the increase in HDL fraction [51, 149]. The HDL fractions are being lost in the dialysate during CAPD [155], hence, the serum levels can be lower than normals. Nevertheless, due to increased intake of energy, CAPD patients are reported to have high levels of HDL [156–158]. The lipid disorders are more marked in those with pre-existing lipid disorders, especially in diabetics.

Peritonitis

CAPD-related peritonitis is one of the major causes of morbidity in CAPD patients. Experiences over 10 years have indicated that the spectrum of pathology, clinical manifestations and management of peritonitis in diabetics and non-diabetics are similar. The earlier fear that diabetic-CAPD patients would contract peritonitis with unusual organisms more often than non-diabetic patients has proved unfounded [159]. As in non-diabetics, peritonitis in diabetics is caused predominantly by skin bacteria. About 40% of bacterial peritonitis is due to *Staphylococcus epidermidis*. While this organism is a weak pathogen, in recent years it has been recognized with increasing frequency as the cause of wound infections and endocarditis. *Staphylococcus epidermidis* does not produce toxins, and pathogenicity depends entirely on its ability to initiate a pyogenic process. The clinical illness is usually mild, and the disease responds well to antibiotic treatment. Other organisms isolated during episodes of peritonitis include *Staph. aureus*, *Streptococcus viridans*, Gram-negative enteric organisms, and, very rarely, anaerobic organisms. A very small fraction of peritonitis is caused by fungi. Insulin administration into the dialysis solution bag breaks the sterility of the system and could potentially contaminate the peritoneal cavity and cause peritonitis. However, clinical experience has shown this not to be a significant problem. The incidence of peritonitis in diabetics is no more than the incidence of peritonitis in non-diabetics on CAPD [160]. More recently a large single-centre prospective study has shown significantly higher peritonitis rates in diabetics (1.2 versus 0.8 episodes/patient-year). However, there was no difference between the diabetic and non-diabetic patients in the first episode in terms of catheter-related infection and exit-site infection [161]. The National CAPD Registry surveyed peritonitis rates per patient-year by route of insulin administration and type of diabetes management [34]. Although differences in the rates were not large, diabetics never using insulin had the highest rate of peritonitis per patient-year (1.31), while patients using a combination of subcutaneous and intraperitoneal insulin experienced the lowest rate (0.93). The reason for such a protective effect in patients using insulin is unclear; it is suggested that insulin may have a bactericidal effect. The recent trend has been to use devices meant to facilitate exchange procedures or protect against peritoneal contamination, especially the Y-set system, the introduction of which has significantly lowered the incidence of peritonitis [162].

Treatment of CAPD-related peritonitis including the right selection of antibiotics and duration of treatment, appropriate time for catheter removal, etc. is similar for diabetic and non-diabetic patients alike, and has been reported extensively elsewhere [159]. Due to the enhanced absorption of glucose during peritonitis, hyperglycaemia is frequently observed in diabetics, and insulin requirements may increase. However, some patients may experience hypoglycaemia if they are unable to eat, and insulin administration is continued at the same dosage as that prior to peritonitis. Close monitoring of blood glucose during the episode of peritonitis is essential to prevent either hypoglycaemia or hyperglycaemia. Due to increased protein losses during peritonitis, the patient's nutrition must be watched closely during the acute phase and, in some, parenteral nutrition should be considered. Generally, the outcome of peritonitis treatment is good. Most patients continue on CAPD after the peritonitis is cured. A small percentage (2–5%) will drop out of the CAPD programme, for a variety of reasons, including loss of membrane efficiency.

Patient and technique survival on CAPD

The 3-year cumulative patient survival rates on CAPD are significantly better than those achieved with intermittent peritoneal dialysis [14]. However, the actuarial survival and technique success rates for diabetics are lower than in non-diabetics of comparable age on CAPD. The reported 3-year survival rates for diabetics range from 40% to 60%, depending on the ages of patients [163–165]. These results were not statistically different from 115 diabetic patients treated at the same centre during the same period with haemodialysis. Data from the USRDS show a lower survival for diabetic patients on peritoneal dialysis *vis-à-vis* haemodialysis [166–168]. However, in all these studies dialysis dose was not adjusted for in the analysis. As long as the therapy dose is matched between two therapies, comparable survival is achieved between diabetic patients on peritoneal dialysis and haemodialysis [169, 170]. In contrast to USRDS data, lower adjusted mortality rates in diabetic patients on peritoneal dialysis as compared to haemodialysis have been reported by a Canadian Registry [171]. The USRDS Annual Report of 1991 compared the 1-year survival rates, adjusted for age, sex and race, for diabetics on haemodialysis and CAPD/CCPD from day 90 of dialysis [172]. The 1-year survival for the haemodialysis group was slightly better than for CAPD/CCPD (69.6% versus 65.7%). Interestingly, 1-year survival for non-diabetic patients was almost identical in the two groups. However, these results are unadjusted for severity of coexisting diseases such

as coronary artery diseases and cerebrovascular conditions. The median age for diabetic patients was 53 years for CAPD and 55 years for haemodialysis patients. However, when the mortality was analysed according to the age of patient, mortality rates tended to be higher for haemodialysis patients than for CAPD patients among younger patients (age 40 years or below), while the opposite was the case among older patients (age over 40 years). Another study by the Michigan Kidney Registry [173] in the cohort initiating dialysis in 1989 with Cox's proportional hazards analysis showed diabetic patients age 20–59 years had a 38% lower relative risk of death on CAPD ($p = 0.01$) compared to haemodialysis. Diabetics aged 60 years and older had a 19% higher risk on CAPD versus haemodialysis, but this difference was statistically not significant ($p = 0.08$). By showing a better survival rate on CAPD compared to haemodialysis, younger patients, who as a group tended to be relatively free from cardiac disease compared to older patients, may be displaying the beneficial effects of CAPD, i.e. better blood-pressure control, use of intraperitoneal insulin, etc. on diabetic patients. On the other hand, the higher mortality rate for older patients on CAPD is probably a reflection of selection bias regarding treatment modality for diabetic patients; older diabetic patients with severe cardiac and peripheral vascular diseases are preferentially chosen for CAPD/CCPD treatment.

The lower technique survival rate for CAPD is a reflection of peritonitis as the major problem of CAPD; peritonitis used to be the major cause of drop-out from CAPD [8]. Since the introduction of the Y-set system the peritonitis rate has improved significantly [174]; the rate of peritonitis in the past 2 or 3 years is about one episode every 16–24 patient-months compared to one episode every 12 patient-months before the introduction of the Y-set system. This improvement in peritonitis rates will have a favourable impact on the drop-out rate from CAPD. Moreover, during the past 2 years, adequacy standards for CAPD patients have received more attention [50, 175]. This also favourably influences the drop-out rates due to inadequate dialysis, which accounts for nearly 15–20% of CAPD drop-outs. In the next 3–5 years these two improvements in technique are expected to improve CAPD/CCPD survival rates.

Technique-related complications

Complications which are a direct result of increased intra-abdominal pressures, such as dialysate leaks, hernia, haemorrhoids, and a compromised cardiac pulmonary status, occur with the same frequency in diabetics as in non-diabetics. As discussed earlier, peritoneal membrane function as assessed by serum chemistries, and based on a peritoneal equilibration test (N. Lameire, personal communication) in the absence of peritonitis, remains stable over a period of time. Transient loss of ultrafiltration during an episode of peritonitis is frequent, but full recovery is expected when peritonitis is resolved. Irreversible loss of ultrafiltration, as in non-diabetic patients, may occur in diabetic CAPD patients mainly as a sequela of severe peritonitis and due to sclerosing peritonitis [176–178]. Although the exact aetiology of sclerosing peritonitis has not been established, its occurrence, once most prevalent in Europe, has been almost eliminated since acetate buffer in the dialysis solution has been replaced by lactate.

Hospitalization rates

Because of the numerous complications associated with diabetes, diabetic patients on CAPD tend to have increased morbidity and require more frequent hospitalization than non-diabetic patients. For type I and type II diabetics the rate of hospitalization (33 days per patient-year of treatment) appears to be similar. Hospitalization due to causes directly related to CAPD technique are progressively decreasing. The rate of hospitalization for diabetics on CAPD is comparable to diabetics on haemodialysis.

Can peritoneal dialysis be a long-term therapy for ESRD patients?

During the early years of CAPD it was feared that long-term CAPD in diabetics may not have been feasible because of extensive microvascular disease. Lower solute and water clearance was predicted for diabetics compared to non-diabetics [179]. In addition, concerns of membrane injury from high rates of peritonitis led most to believe there would be a short life for the peritoneal membrane and a high drop-out from the therapy after a short period. However, contrary to earlier expectations, a recent study in a group of 130 CAPD patients reported similar peritoneal transport characteristics for both diabetics and non-diabetics [180], and peritoneal membrane function for solute and water transfer remained stable for up to 60 months [181, 182]. Although experience with long-term survival of diabetics on CAPD is very limited, there are now

reports of diabetic patients who have been successfully managed on CAPD for longer than 5 years [138, 183]. Characteristically, the patients who survive for a long period tend to be free from associated cardiac disease and are non-smokers. Actuarial survival was 44% at 5 years (26 patients at risk) in one of the series [138]. The NIH CAPD registry survey reported that, of the 7161 CAPD patients surveyed, 19% were on treatment for 3 years or more [34]. These long-term patients included a smaller percentage (18%) of patients with diabetes than short-term cohorts (26%).

Thus, it is becoming apparent that, compared to non-diabetics, diabetic patients on CAPD tend to have lower patient survival results because they tend to have significantly more cardiovascular complications than their counterparts. Compared to diabetic patients on haemodialysis the younger diabetic patients with a relative lack of coexisting diseases tend to have a lower mortality on CAPD/CCPD. Increased mortality and morbidity of older diabetic patients on CAPD is a reflection of the impact of comorbid conditions. Improvements in peritonitis rates during CAPD and establishment of adequacy standards will have a favourable impact on drop-out rates from CAPD/CCPD.

Can CAPD/CCPD be recommended over haemodialysis for diabetic patients?

Diabetes is an exceedingly complex disease, and the management of diabetic patients is exceptionally challenging. While acknowledging that both dialysis modalities, CAPD and haemodialysis, have unique advantages and disadvantages for managing diabetic ESRD patients, there is a need to individualize dialysis therapy to derive maximum benefit from a therapy. Based on the available evidence it is clear that there are some unique features of CAPD that are conducive to better long-term outcomes in diabetic patients. For example, maintenance of residual-renal function for 5 years or more after initiating dialysis should have a great impact on patient management. Residual-renal function allows for liberal diet intake, including fluid. The presence of significant residual-renal function also gives one the flexibility to modify the dialysis prescription, to adjust better to a patient's needs. Lastly, the benefits of intraperitoneal insulin have not been emphasized enough. Besides being convenient, peritoneal delivery of insulin during CAPD achieves better metabolic control compared to subcutaneous injections and, in the long run, produces several effects which are antiatherogenic. Indeed, this is an added advantage in the management of a diabetic patient. Besides these medical benefits, patients with severe coronary or carotid artery diseases may find slow but continuous peritoneal dialysis more tolerable than intermittent haemodialysis. In conclusion, there are several reasons to recommend CAPD/CCPD over haemodialysis for diabetic ESRD patients who cannot be transplanted, and who choose chronic dialysis as the mode of renal replacement therapy.

Summary

It is becoming apparent that, with proper selection of patients, diabetic patients can survive for a long period on CAPD. Variances in reported mortality for diabetic peritoneal dialysis patients are primarily due to the failure to include variables such as dialysis adequacy in statistical analysis. The morbidity and mortality observed on CAPD therapy is primarily related to associated-risk factors such as cardiovascular disease, atherosclerotic complications, and infection. Ability to administer intraperitoneal insulin during CAPD enables simulation of normal insulin secretion by the islet cells. There is no conclusive evidence that CAPD patients tend to retain residual-renal function for a longer period of time. The incidence of peritonitis is decreasing and will affect the CAPD drop-out rate. Introduction of Icodextrin peritoneal dialysis solution will allow better preservation of peritoneal membrane and minimize dropouts from ultrafiltration failure.

References

1. Friedman EA. Clinical imperatives in diabetic nephropathy. Kidney Int 1982; 23 (suppl.): S16–19.
2. Friedman EA. Overview of diabetic nephropathy. In: Keen H, Legrain M, eds. Prevention and Treatment of Diabetic Nephropathy. Lancaster: MTP, 1983, pp. 3–19.
3. Friedman EA. Clinical strategy in diabetic nephropathy. In: Friedman E, l'Esperance F, eds. Diabetic Renal-Retinal Syndrome. New York: Grune & Stratton, 1986, vol. 3, pp. 331–7.
4. Legrain M. Diabetics with end-stage renal disease: the best buy (Editorial). Diabet Nephro 1983; 2: 1–3.
5. Markell MS, Friedman EA. Care of the diabetic patient with end stage renal disease. Semin Nephrol 1990; 10: 274–86.
6. Friedman EA. How can the care of diabetic ESRD patients be improved? Semin Dial 1991; 4: 13–14.
7. Patient mortality and survival, Unites States Renal Data System 1998 Annual Report. Am J Kidney Dis 1998; 32: S69–80.

8. US Renal Data Systems. USRDS 1989 Annual Data Report. Bethesda, MD: National Institutes of Health, National Institute of Diabetes and Digestive and Kidney Diseases, August 1989.
9. Katirtzoglou A, Izatt S, Oreopoulos DG. Chronic peritoneal dialysis in diabetics with end-stage renal failure. In: Friedman EA, ed. Diabetic Renal-Retinal Syndrome. Orlando. FL: Grune & Stratton, 1982, pp. 317–32.
10. Blumenkrantz MJ, Shapiro DJ, Minura N et al. Maintenance peritoneal dialysis as an alternative in the patients with diabetes mellitus and end-stage uremia. Kidney Int 1974; 6 (suppl. 1): S108.
11. Quelhorst E, Schuenemann B, Mietzsch G, Jacob I. Hemo and peritoneal dialysis treatment of patients with diabetic nephropathy. A comparative study. Proc Eur Dial Transplant Assoc 1978; 15: 205.
12. Mion C, Slingeneyer A, Salem JL, Oules R, Mirouze J. Home peritoneal dialysis in end stage diabetic nephropathy. J Dial 1978; 2: 426–7.
13. Warden GS, Maxwell JG, Stephen RL. The use of reciprocating peritoneal dialysis with a subcutaneous peritoneal dialysis in end stage renal failure in diabetes mellitus. J Surg Res 1978; 24: 495–500.
14. Amair P, Khanna R, Leibel B et al. Continuous ambulatory peritoneal dialysis in diabetics with end-stage renal disease. N Engl J Med 1982; 306: 625–30.
15. Legrain M, Rottembourg J, Bentchikou A et al. Dialysis treatment of insulin dependent diabetic patients. A ten year experience. Clin Nephrol 1984; 21: 72–81.
16. Lameire N, Dhaene M, Mattthys E et al. Experience with CAPD in diabetic patients. In: Keen H, Legrain M, eds. Prevention and Treatment of Diabetic Nephropathy. Lancaster: MTP, 1983, pp. 289–97.
17. Polla-Imhoof B, Pirson Y, Lafontaine JJ et al. Resultats de l'hémodialyse chronique et de la transplantation rénale dans le traitement de l'urémie terminale du diabétique. Néphrologie 1982; 3: 80–4.
18. Thompson NM, Simpson RW, Hooke D, Atkins RC. Peritoneal dialysis in the treatment of diabetic end stage renal failure. In: Atkins R, Thomson NM, Farell PC, eds. Peritoneal Dialysis. New York: Churchill Livingstone, 1981, pp. 345–55.
19. Khanna R, Wu G, Chisholm L, Oreopoulos DG. Update: Further experience with CAPD in diabetics with end stage disease. Diabet Nephro 1983; 2: 8–12.
20. Khanna R, Wu G, Prowant B, Jastrzebska J, Nolph KD, Oreopoulos DG. Continuous ambulatory peritoneal dialysis in diabetics with end stage renal disease: a combined experience of two North American centers. In: Friedman E, l'Esperance F, eds. Diabetic Renal Retinal Syndrome. New York: Grüne & Stratton, 1986, vol. 3, pp. 363–81.
21. Rottembourg J. Le traitement de l'insuffisance rénale du diabétique. Presse Med 1987; 46: 437–40.
22. Shapiro FL. Haemodialysis in diabetic patients. In: Keen H, Legrain M, eds. Prevention and Treatment of Diabetic Nephropathy. Lancaster: MTP, 1983, pp. 247–59.
23. Khanna R, Oreopoulos DG. Continuous ambulatory peritoneal dialysis in diabetics. In: Brenner BM, Stein JH, eds. The Kidney in Diabetes Mellitus. New York: Churchill Livingstone, 1989, pp. 185–202.
24. Mauer SM, Morgensen CE, Kjellstrand CM. Diabetic nephropathy. In: Schrier RW, Gottschalk CW, eds. Diseases of the Kidney. Boston: Little, Brown, 1993, pp. 2153–88.
25. Narins RG, Krishna GG, Kopyt NP. Fluid–electrolyte and acid–base disorders complicating diabetes mellitus. In: Schrier RW, Gottschalk CW, eds. Diseases of the Kidney. Boston: Little, Brown, 1993, pp. 2563–97.
26. United States Renal Data System. The USRDS Dialysis Morbidity and Mortality Study, Wave 2. Am J Kidney Dis 1997; 30 (suppl. 1): S67–85.
27. Bonomini V, Feletti C, Scolari MP, Stefoni S. Benefits of early initiation of dialysis. Kidney Int 1985; 28: S57–9.

28. Tattersal J, Greenwood R, Farrington K. Urea kinetics and when to commence dialysis. Am J Nephrol 1995; 15: 283–9.
29. Churchill DN. An evidence based approach to initiation of dialysis. Am J Kidney Dis 1997; 30: 899–906.
30. Mehrotra R, Nolph D. Argument for timely initiation of dialysis. J Am Soc Nephrol 1998; 9: S96–9.
31. Initiation of dialysis, Dialysis Outcomes Quality Initiative. Am J Kidney Dis 1997; 30 (suppl. 2): S70–3.
32. Tenckhoff H, Schechter H. A bacteriologically safe peritoneal access device. Trans Am Soc Artif Intern Organs 1968; 14: 181.
33. Khanna R, Twardowski ZJ. Peritoneal dialysis. In: Nolph KD, ed. Peritoneal Dialysis. Dordrecht; Kluwer, 1989, pp. 319–43.
34. Lindblad AS, Novak JW, Nolph KD et al. A survey of diabetics in the CAPD/CCPD population. In: Lindblad, Novak, Nolph, eds. Continuous Ambulatory Peritoneal Dialysis in the USA. Dordrecht: Kluwer, 1989, pp. 63–74.
35. Twardowski ZJ, Nolph KD, Khanna R, Gluck Z, Prowant BF, Ryan LP. Daily clearances with continuous ambulatory peritoneal dialysis and nightly peritoneal dialysis. Trans Am Soc Artif Intern Organs 1986; 32: 575–80.
36. Khanna R, Twardowski ZJ, Gluck Z, Ryan LP, Nolph KD. Is nightly peritoneal dialysis (NPD) an effective peritoneal dialysis schedule? Abstracts, American Society of Nephrology – Kidney Int 1986; 29: 233.
37. Nolph KD, Twardowski ZJ, Khanna R. Clinical pathology conference: peritoneal dialysis. Trans Am Soc Artif Intern Organs 1986; 32: 11–16.
38. Scribner BH. Foreword to second edition. In: Nolph KD, ed. Peritoneal Dialysis. Boston: Martinus Nijhoff Publishers, 1985, pp. xi–xii.
39. Twardowski ZJ, Khanna R, Nolph KD et al. Intraabdominal pressure during natural activities in patients treated with continuous ambulatory peritoneal dialysis. Nephron 1986; 44: 129–35.
40. Twardowski ZJ. New approaches to intermittent peritoneal dialysis therapies. In: Nolph KD, ed. Peritoneal Dialysis. Dordrecht: Kluwer, 1988, pp. 133–51.
41. Diaz-Buxo JA. Continuous cyclic peritoneal dialysis. In: Nolph KD, ed. Peritoneal Dialysis. Dordrecht: Kluwer, 1989, pp. 169–83.
42. Perras ST, Zappacosta AR. Reduction of peritonitis with patients education and Travenol CAPD germicidal exchange system. Am Nephrol Nurses Assoc 1986; 13: 219.
43. Hamilton RW. The sterile connection device: a review of its development and status report – 1986. In: Khanna R, Nolph KD, Prowant BF et al., eds. Advances in Continuous Ambulatory Peritoneal Dialysis. Toronto: Peritoneal Dialysis Bulletin, Inc., 1986, pp. 186–9.
44. Fenton SSA, Wu G, Bowman C et al. The reduction in the peritonitis rate among high-risk CAPD patients with the use of the Oreopoulos–Zellerman connector. Trans Am Soc Artif Intern Organs 1985; 31: 560.
45. Buoncristiani U, Quintalinani G, Cozzari M, Carobia C. Current status of the Y-set. In: Khanna R, Nolph KD, Powant BF et al., eds. Advances in Continuous Ambulatory Peritoneal Dialysis. Toronto: Peritoneal Dialysis Bulletin, Inc., 1986, pp. 165–71.
46. Flynn CT. The diabetics on CAPD. In: Friedman EA, ed. Diabetic Renal-Retinal Syndrome. Orlando, FL: Grune & Stratton, 1982, pp. 321–30.
47. Popovich RP, Moncrief JW. Kinetic modeling of peritoneal transport. Contrib Nephrol 1979; 17: 59–72.
48. Keshaviah PR, Nolph KD, Prowant B et al. Defining adequacy of CAPD with urea kinetics. Adv Perit Dial 1990; 6: 173–7.
49. Churchill DN, Taylor DW, Keshaviah PR. Adequacy of dialysis and nutrition in continuous peritoneal dialysis: association with clinical outcomes. J Am Soc Nephrol 1996; 7: 198–207.
50. Adequate dose of peritoneal dialysis. Dialysis Outcomes Quality Initiative. Am J Kidney Dis 1997; 30 (suppl. 2): S86–92, 41–3.
51. Lindholm B, Bergström J. Nutritional management of patients undergoing peritoneal dialysis. In: Nolph KD, ed. Peritoneal Dialysis. Dordrecht: Kluwer, 1988, pp. 230–60.
52. Lamb E, Catell WR, Dawnay AB. Glycated albumin in serum and dialysate of patients on continuous ambulatory peritoneal dialysis. Clin Sci 1993; 84: 619–26.
53. Lamb E, Catell WR, Dawnay AB. In vitro formation of advanced glycation end products in peritoneal dialysis fluid. Kidney Int 1995; 47: 1768–74.
54. Friedlander MA, Wu YC, Elgawish A, Monnier V. Early and advanced glycation end products. Kinetics of formation and clearance in peritoneal dialysis fluid. J Clin Invest 1996; 97: 728–35.
55. Mahiout A, Ehlerding G, Brunkhorst R. Advanced glycation end products in the peritoneal fluid and in the peritoneal membrane of continuous ambulatory peritoneal dialysis patients. Nephrol Dial Transplant 1996; 11 (suppl. 5): 2–6.
56. Stout RW. Diabetes and atherosclerosis – the role of insulin. Diabetologia 1979; 16: 141.
57. Zavaroni A, Bonora E, Pagliara M et al. Risk factor for coronary artery disease in healthy persons with hyperinsulinemia and normal glucose tolerance. N Engl J Med 1989; 320: 702–6.
58. Bazzato G, Coli U, Landini S. Xylitol and low doses of insulin: new perspectives for diabetic uremic patients on CAPD. Perit Dial Bull 1982; 2: 161.
59. Williams FP, Marliss EB, Anderson GH et al. Amino acids absorption following intraperitoneal administration in CAPD patients. Perit Dial Bull 1982; 2: 124.
60. Twardowski ZJ, Khanna R, Nolph KD. Osmotic agents and ultrafiltration in peritoneal dialysis. Nephron 1986; 42: 93.
61. Mistry CD, Mallick NP, Gokal R. The use of large molecular weight glucose polymer as an osmotic agent in CAPD. In: Khanna R, Nolph KD, Prowant BF et al., eds. Advances in Continuous Ambulatory Peritoneal Dialysis. Toronto: Peritoneal Dialysis Bulletin, Inc., 1986, pp. 7–11.
62. Matthys E, Dolkart R, Lameire N. Extended use of a glycerol containing dialysate in the treatment of diabetic CAPD patients. Perit Dial Bull 1987; 7: 10.
63. Imholz ALT, Lameire N, Faict D, Koomen GCM, Krediet RT, Martis L. Evaluation of short-chain polypeptides as an osmotic agent in CAPD patients. Perit Dial Int 1993; 13: S62.
64. Scanziani R, Dozio B, Iacuitti G. CAPD in diabetics: use of aminoacids. In: Ota K, Maher J, Winchester J, Hirszel P, eds. Current Concepts in Peritoneal Dialysis. Amsterdam: Excerpta Medica, 1993, pp. 628–32.
65. Goodship THJ, Heaton A, Wilkinson R, Ward MK. The use of glycerol as an osmotic agent in continuous ambulatory peritoneal dialysis. In: Ota K, Maher J, Winchester J, Hirszel P, eds. Current Concepts in Peritoneal Dialysis. Amsterdam: Excerpta Medica, 1992, pp. 143–7.
66. Mistry CD, Gokal R. The use of glucose polymer in CAPD: essential physiological and clinical conclusions. In: Oka K, Maher J, Winchester J, Hirszel P, eds. Current Concepts in Peritoneal Dialysis. Amsterdam: Excerpta Medica, 1992, pp. 138–42.
67. Peers E, Gokal R. Icodextrin: overview of clinical experience. Perit Dial Int 1997; 17: 22–6.
68. Avram MM, Paik SK, Okanya D, Rajpal K. The natural history of diabetic nephropathy: unpredictable insulin requirements. A further clue. Clin Nephrol 1984; 21: 36–8.
69. Tzamaloukas AH. Interpreting glycosylated hemoglobin in diabetic patients on peritoneal dialysis. Adv Perit Dial 1996; 12: 170–5.
70. Duckworth WC. Insulin degradation: mechanisms, products and significance. Endocr Rev 1988; 9: 319–45.
71. Zingg W, Shirriff JM, Liebel B. Experimental routes of insulin administration. Perit Dial Bull 1982; 2: S24–7.
72. Felig P, Wahren J. The liver as site of insulin and glucagon action in normal, diabetic and obese humans. Israel J Med Sci 1975; 11: 528.

73. Rubin J, Reed V, Adair C, Bower J, Klein E. Effect of intraperitoneal insulin on solute kinetics in CAPD: Insulin kinetics in CAPD. Am J Med Sci 1986; 291: 81.

74. Rubin J, Bell AH, Andrews M, Jones Q, Planch A. Intraperitoneal insulin – a dose–response curve. Trans Am Soc Artif Intern Organs 1989; 35: 17–21.

75. Micossi P, Crostallo M, Librenti MC et al. Free-insulin profiles after intraperitoneal, intramuscular and subcutaneous insulin administration. Diabet Care 1986; 9: 575–8.

76. Schade DS, Eaton RP. The peritoneum – a potential insulin delivery route for a mechanical pancreas. Diabet Care 1980; 3: 229.

77. Shapiro DJ, Blumenkrantz MJ, Levin SR, Coburn W. Absorption and action of insulin added to peritoneal dialysate in dogs. Nephron 1979; 23: 174.

78. Wideroe T, Smeby LC, Berg KJ, Jorstad S, Svartas IM. Intraperitoneal insulin absorption during intermittent and continuous peritoneal dialysis. Kidney Int 1983; 23: 22.

79. Paulsen EP, Courtney JW III, Duckworth WC. Insulin resistance caused by massive degradation of subcutaneous insulin. Diabetes 1979; 28: 640–5.

80. Schade DS, Duckworth WC. In search of the subcutaneous insulin degradation syndrome. N Engl J Med 1986; 315: 147–53.

81. Campbell IC, Kritz H, Najemnic C, Hagmueller G, Irsigler K. Treatment of Type I diabetic with subcutaneous insulin resistance by a totally implantable insulin infusion device ('Infusaid'). Diabet Res 1984; 1: 83–8.

82. Wood DF, Goodchild K, Guillou P, Thomas DJ, Johnston DG. Management of 'brittle diabetes' with a preprogrammable implanted insulin pump delivering intraperitoneal insulin. Br Med J 1990; 301: 1143–4.

83. Albisser AM, Normura M, Greenberg GR, McPhedran NT. Metabolic control in diabetic dogs treated with pancreatic autotransplants and insulin pumps. Diabetes 1986; 35: 97.

84. Ishida T, Chap Z, Chou J et al. Effects of portal and peripheral venous insulin infusion on glucose production and utilization in depancreatized conscious dogs. Diabetes 1984; 33: 984–90.

85. Kryshak EJ, Butler PD, Marsh C et al. Pattern of postprandial carbohydrate metabolism and effects of portal and peripheral insulin delivery. Diabetes 1990; 39: 142.

86. Olefsky J. Pathogenesis of insulin resistance and hyperglycemia in non-insulin dependent diabetes mellitus. Am J Med 1990; 79: 1–7.

87. DeFronzo RA. Lilly lecture 1987. The triumvirate: B-cell, muscle, liver: a collusion responsible for NIDDM. Diabetes 1988; 3: 667–87.

88. Campbell PJ, Mandarino LJ, Gerich JE. Quantification of the relative impairment in actions of insulin on hepatic glucose production and peripheral glucose uptake in non-insulin dependent diabetes mellitus. Metabolism 1988; 37: 15–21.

89. Duckworth WC, Saudek CD, Henry RR. Why intraperitoneal delivery of insulin with implantable pump in NIDDM? Diabetes 1992; 41: 657–61.

90. Cullen K, Steinhouse NS, Wearne KL, Welborn TA. Multiple regression analysis of risk factors for cardiovascular and cancer mortality in Busselton, Western Australia: thirteen year study. J Chron Dis 1983; 36: 371–7.

91. Fuller JH, Shipley MJ, Rose G, Jarrett RJ, Heen H. Coronaryheart disease risk and impaired glucose tolerance: the White-Hall study. Lancet 1983; 1: 1373–6.

92. Pyorala K. Relationship of glucose tolerance and plasma insulin to the incidence of coronary heart disease: results from two population studies in Finland. Diabet Care 1979; 2: 131–41.

93. Shafrir E, Bergman M, Felig P. The endocrine pancreas; diabetes mellitus. In: Felig P, Baxter JD, Broadus AE, Froahman LA, eds. Endocrinology and Metabolism. New York: McGraw-Hill, 1987, pp. 1043–78.

94. Tamborlane WV, Sherwin RS, Genel M, Felig P. Reduction to normal of plasma glucose in juvenile diabetes by subcuta-neous administration of insulin with a portable pump. N Engl J Med 1979; 300: 573.

95. Selam JL, Kashyap M, Alberti KGM et al. Comparison of intraperitoneal and subcutaneous insulin administration on lipids apolipoproteins, fuel metabolites, and hormones in Type I diabetes mellitus. Metabolism 1989; 38: 908–12.

96. Kashyap ML, Gupta AK, Selam JL et al. Improvement in reverse cholesterol transport associated with programmable implantable intraperitoneal insulin delivery. Diabetes 1991; 40 (suppl. 1): 3A (abstract).

97. Ruotolo G, Micossi P, Galimberti G et al. Effects of intraperitoneal versus subcutaneous insulin administration on lipoprotein metabolism in Type I diabetes. Metabolism 1990; 38: 598.

98. Bagdade JD, Subbaiah PV, Ritter M, Dunn FL. Intraperitoneal insulin delivery normalizes cholesteryl ester transfer in IDDM. Diabetes 1991; 40 (suppl.): 269A (abstract).

99. Colettte C, Pares-Herbute N, Monnier L, Swlam JL, Thomas N, Mirouze J. Effect of different insulin administration modalities on vitamin D metabolism of IDDM patients. Horm Metab Res 1989; 21: 37–41.

100. Saudek CD, Salem JL, Pitt HA et al. A preliminary trial of the programmable implantable medication system for insulin delivery. N Engl J Med 1989; 321: 574–9.

101. Schmitz O. Insulin-mediated glucose uptake in nondialyzed and dialyzed uremic insulin-dependent diabetic subjects. Diabetes 1985; 34: 1152–9.

102. Grefberg N, Danielson BG, Nilsson P, Berne C. Decreasing insulin requirements in CAPD patients given intraperitoneal insulin. J Diabet Complic 1987; 1: 16–19.

103. Scalamogna A, Castelnova C, Crepaldi M et al. Incidence of peritonitis in diabetic patients on CAPD: intraperitoneal vs. subcutaneous insulin therapy. In: Khanna R, Nolph KD, Prowant BF, Twardowski ZJ, Oreopoulos DG, eds. Advances in CAPD. Toronto: University of Toronto Press, 1987, pp. 166–70.

104. Wanless IR, Bargman JM, Oreopoulos DG, Vas SI. Subcapsular steatonecrosis in response to peritoneal insulin delivery: a clue to the pathogenesis of steatonecrosis in obesity. Mod Pathol 1989; 2: 69–74.

105. Harrison NA, Rainford DJ. Intraperitoneal insulin and the malignant omentum syndrome. Nephrol Dial transplant 1988; 3: 103.

106. Rottembourg J. Peritoneal dialysis in diabetics. In: Nolph KD, ed. Peritoneal Dialysis. Dordrecht: Kluwer, 1988, pp. 365–79.

107. Khanna R, Oreopoulos DG. CAPD in patients with diabetes mellitus. In: Gokal R, ed. Continuous Ambulatory Peritoneal Dialysis. Edinburgh: Churchill Livingstone, 1986, pp. 291–305.

108. Carta Q, Monge L, Triolo G et al. Continuous insulin infusion in the management of uremic diabetic patients on dialysis: clinical experience with subcutaneous and intraperitoneal delivery. Diabet Nephro 1987; 4: 83–7.

109. Groop LC, van Bonsdorff MC. Intraperitoneal insulin administration does not promote insulin antibody production in insulin dependent patients on dialysis. Diabet Nephro 1985; 4: 80–2.

110. Henderson IS, Patterson KR, Leung ACT. Decreased intraperitoneal insulin requirements during peritonitis on continuous ambulatory peritoneal dialysis. Br Med J 1985; 290: 474.

111. Mactier RA, Moore H, Khanna R, Shah J. Effect of peritonitis on insulin and glucose absorption during peritoneal dialysis in diabetic rats. Nephron 1990; 54: 240–4.

112. Rottembourg J, El Shahat Y, Agrafiotis A et al. Continuous ambulatory peritoneal dialysis in insulin dependent diabetics: a 40 months experience. Kidney Int 1983; 23: 40.

113. Nolph KD, Sorkin M, Rubin J et al. Continuous ambulatory peritoneal dialysis: Three-year experience at one center. Ann Intern Med 1983; 92: 609–13.

114. Young MA, Nolph KD, Dutton S, Prowant BF. Anti-hypertensive drug requirements in continuous ambulatory peritoneal dialysis. Perit Dial Bull 1984; 4: 85–8.

115. Glasson PH, Favre H, Valloton MB. Response of blood pressure and the renin–angiotensin–aldosterone system to chronic ambulatory peritoneal dialysis in hypertensive end-stage renal failure. Clin Sci 1982; 63: S207–9.

116. Nolph KD, Hano JE, Teschan PE. Peritoneal sodium transport during hypertonic peritoneal dialysis: physiologic mechanisms and clinical implications. Ann Intern Med 1969; 70: 931–41.

117. Nolph KD, Sorkin M, Moore H. Autoregulation of sodium and potassium removal during continuous ambulatory peritoneal dialysis. ASAIO Trans 1980; 6: 334–7.

118. Leenen FHH, Shah P, Boer WH, Khanna R, Oreopoulos DG. Hypotension on CAPD: an approach to treatment. Perit Dial Bull 1983; 3: S33–5.

119. Rottembourg J, Issad B, Poignet JL et al. Residual renal function and control of blood glucose levels in insulin-dependent diabetic patients treated by CAPD. In: Keen H, Legrain M, eds. Prevention and Treatment of Diabetic Nephropathy. Boston: MTP, 1983, pp. 339–59.

120. Cancarini GC, Brunori G, Camerini C, Brasa S, Manili L, Maiorca R. Renal function recovery and maintenance of residual diuresis in CAPD and hemodialysis. Perit Dial Bull 1986; 6: 77–9.

121. Lysaght M, Vonesh E, Ibels L et al. Decline of residual renal function in hemodialysis and CAPD patients; a risk adjusted growth function analysis. Nephrol Dial Transplant 1989; 4: 499 (abstract).

122. Lysaght M, Pollock C, Schindaglm K, Ibeles L, Farrell P. The relevance of urea kinetic modeling to CAPD. ASAIO Trans 1988; 34: 84.

123. Slingeneyer A, Mion C. Five year follow-up of 155 patients treated by CaPD in European–French speaking countries. Perit Dial Int 1989; 9 (suppl. 1): 176 (abstract).

124. Rottembourg J, Issad B, Allouache M, Jacobs C. Recovery of renal function in patients treated by CAPD. In: Khanna R, Nolph KD, Prowant BF, Twardowski ZJ, Oreopoulos DG, eds. Advances in Peritoneal Dialysis. Toronto: University of Toronto Press, 1989, pp. 63–6.

125. Michael C, Bindi P, Kareche M, Mignon F. Renal function on recovery on chronic dialysis: what is best, CAPD or hemodialysis? Nephrol Dial Transplant 1989; 4: 499–500 (abstract).

126. Nunan To, Wing AJ, Brunner FB, Selwood NH. Native kidneys sometimes recover after prolonged dialysis and transplantation. In: Giovanetti C, ed. Proceedings of the V International Capri Conference on Uremia. Capri, 1986, pp. 132–49.

127. Nolph KD. Is residual renal function preserved better with CAPD than hemodialysis? AKF Nephrol Letter 1990; 7: 1–4.

128. Shekkarie MA, Port FK, Wolfe RA et al. Recovery from end-stage renal disease. Am J Kidney Dis 1990; 15: 61–5.

129. Mourad G, Mimram A, Mion C. Recovery of renal function in patients with accelerated malignant nephrosclerosis on maintenance dialysis with management of blood pressure by captopril. Nephron 1985; 41: 166–9.

130. Wauters JP, Brunner HR. Discontinuation of chronic hemodialysis after control of arterial hypertension: long-term follow-up. Proc Eur Dial Transplant Assoc 1982; 19: 182–6.

131. Herbelin A, Nguyen AT, Zingraft J, Urena P, Descamps-Latscha B. Influence of uremia and hemodialysis on circulating interleukin-1 and tumor necrosis factor alpha. Kidney Int 1990; 37: 116–25.

132. Cotran RS, Pober JS. Effects of cytokines on vascular endothelium; their role in vascular and immune injury. Kidney Int 1989; 35: 969–75.

133. Shah AH. Role of reactive oxygen metabolites in experimental glomerular disease. Kidney Int 1989; 35: 1093–106.

134. Van Olden RW, Krediet RT, Struijk DG, Arisz L. Measurement of residual renal function in patients treated with continuous ambulatory peritoneal dialysis. J Am Soc Nephrol 1995; 7: 745–50.

135. Rottembourg J, Bellio P, Maiga K, Remaoun M, Rousselie F, Legrain M. Visual function, blood pressure and blood glucose in diabetic patients undergoing continuous ambulatory peritoneal dialysis. Proc Eur Dial Transplant Assoc 1984; 21: 330–4.

136. Kohner E, Chahal P. Retinopathy in diabetic nephropathy. In: Keen H, Legrain M, eds. Prevention and Treatment of Diabetic Nephropathy. Lancaster: MTP, 1983, pp. 191–6.

137. Diaz-Buxo JA, Burgess WP, Greenman M, Chandler JT, Farmer CD, Walker PJ. Visual function in diabetic patients undergoing dialysis: comparison of peritoneal and hemodialysis. Int J Artif Organs 1984; 7: 257–62.

138. Zimmerman SW, Johnson CA, O'Brien M. Survival of diabetic patients on continuous ambulatory peritoneal dialysis for over five years. Perit Dial Bull 1987; 7: 26.

139. Dombros N, Oren A, Marliss EB et al. Plasma amino acids profiles and amino acid losses in patients undergoing CAPD. Perit Dial Bull 1982; 2: 32–7.

140. Norbeck H. Lipid abnormalities in continuous ambulatory peritoneal dialysis patients. In: Legrain M, ed. Continuous Ambulatory Peritoneal Dialysis. Amsterdam: Excerpta Medica, 1979, pp. 298–301.

141. Khanna R, Brechenridge C, Roncari D, Digenis G, Oreopoulos DG. Lipid abnormalities in patients undergoing continuous ambulatory peritoneal dialysis. Perit Dial Bull 1983; 3: 13–16.

142. Gokal, R, Ramos JM, McGurk JG, Ward MK, Kerr DNS. Hyperlipidemia in a patient on continuous ambulatory peritoneal dialysis. In: Gahl G, Kessel M, Nolph KD, eds. Advances in Peritoneal Dialysis. Amsterdam: Excerpta Medica, 1981, pp. 430–33.

143. Moncrief JW, Pyle WK, Simon P, Popovich RP. Hypertriglyceridemia, diabetes mellitus and insulin administration in patient undergoing continuous ambulatory peritoneal dialysis. In: Moncrief J, Popovich R, eds. CAPD Update. New York: Masson, 1981, pp. 143–65.

144. Sorge F, Castro LA, Nagel A Kessel M. Serum glucose, insulin growth hormone, free fatty acids and lipids responses to high carbohydrate and to high fat isocaloric diets in patients with chronic, non-nephrotic renal failure. Horm Metab Res 1975; 7: 118–27.

145. Sanfelippo ML, Swenson RS, Reavan GM. Response of plasma triglycerides to dietary change in patients on hemodialysis. Kidney Int 1978; 14: 180–6.

146. Cattran DC, Steiner GS, Fenton SSA, Ampil M. Dialysis hyperlipemia: response to dietary manipulations. Clin Nephrol 1980; 13: 177–82.

147. Ramos JM, Heaton A, McGurk GJ, Wark MK, Kerr DNS. Sequential changes in serum lipids and their subfractions in patients receiving continuous ambulatory peritoneal dialysis. Nephron 1983; 353: 20–3.

148. Nolph KD, Ryan KL, Prowant B, Twardowski Z. A cross sectional assessment of serum vitamin D and triglyceride concentrations in a CAPD population. Perit Dial Bull 1984; 4: 232–7.

149. Lindholm B, Norbeck HE. Serum lipids and lipoproteins during continuous ambulatory peritoneal dialysis. Acta Med Scand 1986; 220: 143–51.

150. Heaton A, Johnston DG, Haigh JW, Ward MK, Alberti KGMM, Kerr DNS. Twenty-four hour hormonal and metabolic profiles in uraemic patients before and during treatment with continuous ambulatory peritoneal dialysis. Clin Sci 1985; 69: 449–57.

151. Keusch G, Bammatter F, Mordasini R, Binswanger U. Serum lipoprotein concentrations during continuous ambulatory peritoneal dialysis (CAPD). In: Gahl GM, Kessel M, Nolph KD, eds. Advances in Peritoneal Dialysis. Amsterdam: Excerpta Medica, 1981, pp. 427–9.

152. Lindholm B, Karlander SG, Norbeck HE, Fürst P, Bergström J. Carbohydrate and lipid metabolism in CAPD patients. In: Atkins R, Thomson N, Farrell P, eds. Peritoneal Dialysis. Edinburgh: Churchill Livingstone, 1981, pp. 198–210.

153. Lindholm B, Alvestrand A, Fürst P *et al.* Metabolic effects of continuous ambulatory peritoneal dialysis. Proc EDTA 1980; 17: 283–9.

154. Lindholm B, Karlander SG, Norbeck HE, Bergström J. Glucose and lipid metabolism in peritoneal dialysis. In: La Greca G, Biasoli S, Ronco C, eds. Peritoneal Dialysis. Milano: Whichtig Editore, 1982, pp. 219–30.

155. Kagan A, Barkhayim Y, Schafer Z, Fainaru, M. Low level of plasma HDL in CAPD patients may be due to HDL loss in dialysate. Perit Dial Int 1988; A79 (abstract).

156. Roncari DAK, Breckenridge WC, Khanna R, Oreopoulos DG. Rise in high-density lipoprotein-cholesterol in some patients treated with CAPD. Perit Dial Bull 1987; 1: 136–7.

157. Breckenridge WC, Roncari DAK, Khanna R, Oreopoulos DG. The influence of continuous ambulatory peritoneal dialysis on plasma lipoproteins. Atherosclerosis 1982; 45: 249–58.

158. Tsukamoto Y, Okubo M, Yoneda T, Marumo F, Nakamura H. Effects of a polyunsaturated fatty acid-rich diet on serum lipids in patients with chronic renal failure. Nephron 1982; 31: 236–41.

159. Vas SI. Peritonitis. In: Nolph KD, ed. Peritoneal Dialysis. Dordrecht: Kluwer, 1989, pp. 261–88.

160. Nolph KD, Cutler SJ, Steinberg SM, Novak JW. Special studies from the NIH USA CAPD Registry. Perit Dial Bull 1986; 6: 28–35.

161. Lye WC, Leong SO, van der Straaten JC, Lee EJC. A prospective study of peritoneal dialysis related infections in CAPD patients with diabetes mellitus. Adv Perit Dial 1993; 9: 195–7.

162. Rottembourg J, Brouard R, Issad B, Allouache M, Jacobs C. Prospective randomized study about Y connectors in CAPD patients. In: Khanna R, Nolph KD, Prowant BF, Twardowski ZJ, Oreopoulos DG, eds. Advances in Continuous Ambulatory Peritoneal Dialysis. Toronto: Peritoneal Dialysis Bulletin, Inc., 1987, pp. 107–13.

163. Madden MA, Zimmerman SW, Simpson DP. CAPD in diabetes mellitus – the risks and benefits of intraperitoneal insulin. Am J Nephrol 1982; 2: 133 (abstract).

164. Wing AF, Broyer M, Brunner FP *et al.* Combined report on regular dialysis and transplantation in Europe 1982. Proc Eur Dial Transplant Assoc – ERA 1983; 20: 5–75.

165. Williams C and the University of Toronto Collaborative Dialysis Group. CAPD in Toronto – an overview. Perit Dial Bull 1983; 35: 2.

166. Bloembergen WE, Port FK, Mauger EA *et al.* A comparison of mortality between patients treated with hemodialysis and peritoneal dialysis. J Am Soc Nephrol 1995; 6: 177–83.

167. Bloembergen WE, Port FK, Mauger EA *et al.* A comparison of cause of death between patients treated with hemodialysis and peritoneal dialysis. J Am Soc Nephrol 1995; 6: 184–91.

168. Port FK, Turenne MN *et al.* Continuous ambulatory peritoneal dialysis and hemodialysis: comparison of patient mortality with adjustment for comorbid conditions. Kidney Int 1994; 45: 1163–9.

169. Keshaviah P, Ma J, Thorpe K, Churchill D, Collins A. Comparison of 2 year survival on hemodialysis (HD) and peritoneal dialysis (PD) with dose of dialysis matched using the peak concentration hypothesis. J Am Soc Nephrol 1995; 6: 540 (abstract).

170. Marcelli D, Spotti D, Conte F *et al.* Survival of diabetic patients on peritoneal dialysis or hemodialysis. Perit Dial Int 1996; 16 (suppl. 1): S283–7 (abstract).

171. Fenton SSA, Schaubel DE, Desmeules M *et al.* Hemodialysis versus peritoneal dialysis: a comparison of adjusted mortality rates. Am J Kidney Dis 1997; 30: 334–42.

172. US Renal Data System, USRDS 1991 Annual Data Report. Bethesda, MD: National Institutes of Health, National Institute of Diabetes and Digestive and Kidney Diseases, August 1991.

173. Nelson CB, Port FK, Wolfe RA, Guire KE. Dialysis patient survival: evaluation of CAPD vs. HD using 3 techniques. Perit Dial Int 1992; 12 (suppl. 1): 144 (abstract).

174. Port FK, Held PJ, Nolph KD, Turenne MN, Wolfe RA. Risk of peritonitis and technique failure by CAPD technique: a national study. Kidney Int (In press).

175. Keshaviah P, Nolph KD, Prowant BF *et al.* Defining adequacy of CAPD with urea kinetics. In: Khanna R, Nolph KD, Prowant BF, Twardowski ZJ, Oreopoulos DG, eds. Advances in Peritoneal Dialysis. Toronto: University of Toronto Press, 1990, pp. 173–7.

176. Faller B, Marichal JD. Loss of ultrafiltration in CAPD. Clinical Data. In: Gahl G, Kessel M, Nolph KD, eds. Advances in Peritoneal Dialysis. Amsterdam: Excerpta Medica, 1981, pp. 227–32.

177. Slingeneyer A, Mion C, Mourad G, Canaud B, Faller B, Beraud JJ. Progressive sclerosing peritonitis: a late and severe complications of maintenance peritoneal dialysis. Trans Am Soc Artif Intern Organs, 1983; 29: 633.

178. Rottembourg J, Brouard R, Issad B, Allouache M, Ghali B, Boudjemaa A. Role of acetate in loss of ultrafiltration during CAPD. In: Berlyne GM, Giovannetti S, eds. Contribution to Nephrology. Basel: Karger, 1987, p. 197.

179. Nolph KD, Stolta M, Maher JF. Altered peritoneal permeability in patients with systemic vasculitis. Ann Intern Med 1973; 78: 891.

180. Twardowski ZJ, Nolph KD, Khanna R *et al.* Peritoneal equilibration test. Perit Dial Bull 1987; 7: 138.

181. Hallett MD, Kush RD, Lysaght MJ, Farrell PC. The stability and kinetics of peritoneal mass transfer. In: Nolph KD, ed. Peritoneal Dialysis. Dordrecht; Kluwer, 1989, pp. 380–8.

182. Struijk DG, Krediet RT, Koomen GCM *et al.* Functional characteristics of the peritoneal membrane in long-term continuous ambulatory peritoneal dialysis. Nephron 1991; 59: 213–20.

183. Gilmore J, Wu G, Khanna R, Oreopoulos DG. Long term CAPD. Perit Dial Bull 1985; 5: 112.

22 | Peritoneal dialysis in children

B. A. WARADY, S. R. ALEXANDER, J. W. BALFE AND E. HARVEY

Introduction and personal notes

Like many chapters in this book, the origins of the present chapter can be traced to the 1976 discovery of continuous ambulatory peritoneal dialysis (CAPD) by Moncrief, Popovich and their associates [1]. Early on, PD was widely considered to be the renal replacement therapy (RRT) of choice for acute renal failure in paediatric patients, primarily because PD is intrinsically simple, safe and easily adapted for use in patients of all ages and sizes. However, following on the heels of the seminal work of Moncrief and Popovich, it became apparent that CAPD was a method of chronic RRT that was ideally suited to the needs of the paediatric patient with end-stage renal disease (ESRD), as well.

In the first edition of this book and chapter, the practical aspects of providing chronic peritoneal dialysis (CPD) to children were highlighted, in large part reflecting the vast clinical experience of two of the current authors (S.R.A. and J.W.B.) who helped pioneer the use of CAPD for children. In this edition our goal has been to build on that foundation. Once again, we have made every effort to include the most current information considered vital to the provision of 'optimal' dialytic care in the paediatric clinical arena. In doing so we have incorporated what we believe are the most noteworthy clinical experiences published by our paediatric nephrology colleagues from around the globe. In addition, we have purposely made reference to a variety of research efforts pertinent to PD because of their impact on the clinical needs of patients and to serve as a stimulus for future research in this area of paediatric ESRD care. In the end we hope that the chapter we have created provides valuable practical assistance to those of you who are dedicated to caring for children requiring PD, and their families.

Notes on the history of PD use in children

The peritoneal cavity has been used in the treatment of serious illness in children for at least 75 years. In 1918 Blackfan and Maxcy described the successful use of intraperitoneal injections of saline solution in dehydrated infants [2], a method that is still used in rural areas of some developing countries. The initial reports describing the use of PD to treat children suffering from acute renal failure were published by Bloxsom and Powell in 1948 (in the premier issue of the journal, *Pediatrics*) and by Swan and Gordon in 1949 [3, 4]. These reports appeared at a time when worldwide published clinical experience with PD did not total 100 patients [5].

The experience of Swan and Gordon was the more successful of the two initial paediatric PD reports [4]. The technique ('continuous peritoneal lavage') and apparatus used by these pioneering Denver paediatric surgeons allowed large volumes of dialysate to flow continuously by gravity from 20-L carboys through a rigid metal catheter that had been surgically implanted into the upper abdomen. Dialysate was constantly drained by water suction through an identical catheter implanted in the pelvis. Fluid balance was maintained by adjusting dialysate dextrose content between 2 g% and 4 g%, and excellent solute clearances were achieved by providing an average dialysate delivery of 33 L/day. Dialysate temperature was regulated by adjusting the number of illuminated 60 W incandescent light bulbs in a box placed over the dialysate inflow path.

Although two of the three children treated by Swan and Gordon survived after 9 and 12 days of continuous peritoneal lavage, it was more than a decade before the use of PD in children was again reported. During the 1950s the development of disposable nylon catheters and commercially prepared dialysate made PD a practical short-term treatment for acute renal failure [6]. The adaptation of this

R. Gokal, R. Khanna, R.Th. Krediet and K.D. Nolph (eds.), Textbook of Peritoneal Dialysis, 2nd Edition, 667–708.
© 2000 *Kluwer Academic Publishers. Printed in Great Britain.*

technique for use in children was described in 1961 by Segar and associates in Indianapolis [7] and in 1962 by Ettledorf and associates in Memphis [8]. Both groups later demonstrated the effectiveness of PD as a treatment for boric acid and salicylate intoxication, two of the most common intoxications in small children during the 1960s [9, 10].

Subsequent reports established PD as the most frequently employed RRT for acute renal failure in paediatric patients [11–17]. PD appeared ideally suited for use in children. As compared to haemodialysis (HD), PD was intrinsically simple, safe, and easily adapted for use in patients of all ages and sizes, from newborn infants to fully grown adolescents. In contrast, HD at this early stage of development required large extracorporeal blood circuits that were either poorly tolerated or frankly impossible to achieve in many children. The widespread popularity of PD as the acute RRT of choice for children was enhanced by the prevalent notion that the peritoneum was 'more efficient' in the child, a concept addressed later in this chapter.

While successful as a treatment for acute renal failure, PD appeared to have much less to offer the child with ESRD. Initial chronic PD techniques required reinsertion of the dialysis catheter for each treatment, making prolonged use in small patients difficult, and routinely resulted in inadequate dialysis [18]. The development of a permanent peritoneal catheter, first proposed by Palmer and associates [19, 20] and later refined by Tenckhoff and Schecter [21] made long-term PD an accessible form of RRT for paediatric patients. When Boen [22] and then Tenckhoff [23] devised an automated dialysate delivery system that could be used in the home, chronic intermittent peritoneal dialysis (IPD) became a practical alternative to chronic HD for children. Largely as a result of the pioneering efforts of the paediatric ESRD treatment team in Seattle [24, 25], paediatric chronic IPD programmes were established in a few prominent paediatric dialysis centers [26–29]. However, there was little enthusiasm for chronic IPD among paediatric nephrologists during this period, because it was associated with many of the least desirable features of chronic HD (e.g. substantial fluid and dietary restrictions, immobility during treatments, and the need for complex machinery), without providing the efficiency of HD.

A new era in the history of PD for children was heralded by the description of CAPD in 1976 by Moncrief, Popovich and associates [1]. CAPD appeared particularly well suited for use in children. Advantages over HD and of special importance to children included near steady-state biochemical control, no disequilibrium syndrome, greatly reduced fluid and dietary restrictions, and freedom from repeated dialysis needle punctures. CAPD also allowed children of all ages to receive dialysis at home, offering them the opportunity to experience more normal childhoods. Finally, CAPD made possible the routine treatment of very young infants, thereby extending the option of RRT to an entire population of patients previously considered too young for chronic dialysis.

CAPD was first used in a child in 1978 in Toronto [30, 31] and soon became available in other paediatric dialysis programmes in North America and Western Europe [32–37]. In Canada, dialysate was available in small-volume plastic containers soon after the first paediatric CAPD patients were trained, but in the United States, early efforts to adapt CAPD for paediatric patients were hampered by the commercial availability of dialysate only in 2000 ml containers. Parents were taught to discard surplus fluid from the 2000 ml containers and infuse the remainder [34], or to prepare small-volume bags at home by filling blood bank transfer packs [32]. Hospital pharmacies would periodically prepare small-volume dialysate bags for individual families [33]. These wasteful, expensive, and potentially risky methods became unnecessary in July 1980, when dialysate in 500 and 1000 ml plastic containers became commercially available in the United States [38]. The subsequent addition of 250, 750, and 1500 ml containers completed a range of standardized dialysate containers that accommodated most paediatric CAPD patients.

The next step in the resurgence of CPD for children was the reintroduction of the automated cycler. Continuous cycler peritoneal dialysis (CCPD) was first used in a child by Price and Suki in 1981 [39]. Cycler dialysis subsequently became extremely popular among paediatric PD programmes in North America [40]. Further modifications of the CCPD regimen focused on elimination of most of the daytime exchange (i.e., nightly intermittent peritoneal dialysis [NIPD]). During the past 15 years the growth of CAPD, CCPD, NIPD and other CPD variations has been spectacular [40]. Before 1982, fewer than 100 paediatric patients had been treated with CAPD worldwide, and CCPD for children was virtually unknown [39]. By the end of 1998, CPD remained the most frequently prescribed chronic dialysis modality for children in the United States, Canada, Australia, New Zealand [40] and in many other parts of the world as well.

Demographic issues

Incidence of ESRD in children

ESRD is not a common paediatric disorder. In the United States from 1987 to 1996 there were only 11 to 15 new paediatric ESRD cases per million children of similar age reported each year [41]. This contrasts sharply with the incidence of congenital heart disease (8000 per million children) and childhood leukaemia (40 per million) [42, 43]. Published information on the incidence of ESRD in paediatric patients reveals marked geographic variability. Using reports from single paediatric ESRD treatment centres, national surveys and national and multinational registries, Gusmano and Perfumo documented an incidence ranging from 2.1 to >10 new cases per million children per year [44]. Such differences are more likely to reflect regional economic and social conditions rather than actual geographic differences in the prevalence of diseases that result in renal failure.

ESRD incidence also varies according to age, as shown in Table 1, which provides data from the United States Renal Data System (USRDS) for 1977, 1987, and 1996 [41, 45]. Note that ESRD incidence increases with increasing age. Note also that ESRD incidence is much greater in adults than it is in any paediatric age group.

Table 1 also shows the differences in ESRD incidence rates over time. Of interest is the relative increase in ESRD incidence seen in the younger paediatric age groups, compared to older paediatric patients. While these data could be interpreted as showing an absolute increase in the disorders leading to ESRD in children <10 years of age between 1977 and 1996, it seems more likely that during this period renal replacement therapy was provided to an increasing number of very young children who previously would have been excluded from many ESRD treatment programmes.

The variability in ESRD incidence seen among different geographic areas, age groups and observation periods serves to emphasize that these are not true incidence figures, but rather the incidence of the decision to treat children with RRT. That decision has been influenced by economic and social conditions, as well as by developing technologies.

Prevalence of ESRD in children

Children account for only a small fraction of the total ESRD patient population. Of the 28,064 registered PD patients receiving treatment in the United States on 31 December 1996, only 737 (2.6%) were less than 20 years of age (ref. 41, p. C.5). Table 2 displays USRDS ESRD patient counts for 31 December of 1992 and 1996 by age group and treatment modality. Total paediatric dialysis (HD + PD) patient counts are small and increased by 24% between 1992 and 1996, compared to a 38% increase for adults during the same period. However, the relative importance of PD for children in the United States is clearly shown in Table 2. In 1996 PD was used to treat 34% of all paediatric dialysis patients 0–19 years old and 60% of children <15 years of age. In contrast, only 13% of registered adult dialysis patients were treated with PD in 1996. Between 1992 and 1996 the paediatric PD population increased by 27%, keeping pace with the overall increase in the paediatric dialysis population. During the same period the adult PD population increased by 22%, while the total adult dialysis patient population increased at nearly twice that rate.

Table 1. ESRD incidence in the United States in 1977, 1987 and 1996 by age at start of ESRD therapy

Age group (years)	New patients 1977	PMP/year 1987	PMP/year 1996
0–4	2	6	10
5–9	4	5	7
10–14	11	12	13
15–19	21	23	30
20–44	–	76	125
45–64	–	272	473
64–74	–	520	1042

P = Per million population, age-adjusted.
Data from USRDS 1987 and 1996 [41, 45].

Table 2. Living United States ESRD patients on 31 December of 1992 and 1996 by patient age and treatment modality

Age group (years)	1992 HD	1992 PD	1992 Tx	1996 HD	1996 PD	1996 Tx
0–4	19	76	150	63	150	207
5–9	47	62	474	63	97	551
10–14	131	157	775	152	175	1055
15–19	548	295	1217	633	326	1682
0–19	745	590	2616	911	748	3495
20–85 +	125 940	22 421	52 791	177 267	27 316	75 315

HD = In-centre, in-centre self and home haemodialysis.
PD = CAPD, CCPD and other PD modalities.
TX = Functioning transplant.
Data from ref. 41, p. C.5.

The data in Table 2 also demonstrate the importance of transplantation to paediatric ESRD management. Patients with functioning transplants accounted for nearly 70% of paediatric ESRD patients in 1996, compared to 27% of adults.

Causes of ESRD in children

Approximately one-half of children requiring RRT have a congenital or hereditary renal disorder and one-half an acquired renal lesion. This is in contrast to the adult ESRD population in which over 80% of patients have an acquired renal disease. Table 3 lists the primary renal disorders of 2828 paediatric dialysis patients (HD and PD patients combined) reported between 1 January 1992 and 16 January 1997 to the dialysis patient database of the North American Pediatric Renal Transplant Cooperative Study (NAPRTCS) [46]. The most frequently identified primary renal diseases were aplastic/hypoplastic/dysplastic kidneys (15.0%), focal segmental glomerulosclerosis (14.8%) and obstructive uropathy (13.1%).

Table 3. Primary reneal disease diagnosis in paediatric dialysis patients

Diagnosis	No.	Percentage
Aplastic/hypoplastic/dysplastic kidneys	425	15.0
Focal segmental glomerulosclerosis	418	14.8
Obstructive uropathy	371	13.1
Systemic immunological disease	210	7.4
Chronic glomerulonephritis	110	3.9
Reflux nephropathy	100	3.5
Haemolytic uraemic syndrome	92	3.3
Polycystic kidney disease	89	3.1
Syndrome of agenesis of abdominal musculature	66	2.3
Congenital nephrotic syndrome	65	2.3
Medullary cystic disease/juvenile nephronophthisis	61	2.2
Idiopathic crescentic glomerulonephritis	60	2.1
Pyelonephritis/interstitial nephritis	56	2.0
Familial nephritis	53	1.9
Renal infarct	48	1.7
Membranoproliferative glomerulonephritis type I	46	1.6
Cystinosis	44	1.6
Membranoproliferative glomerulonephritis type II	29	1.0
Wilms' tumour	22	0.8
Drash syndrome	21	0.7
Oxalosis	18	0.6
Membranous nephropathy	13	0.5
Sickle-cell nephropathy	11	0.4
Diabetic glomerulosclerosis	4	0.1
Other	285	8.3
Unknown	161	5.7

Adapted from ref. 46.

The frequency with which structural anomalies of the urinary tract occur among children with ESRD has important implications for paediatric ESRD programmes. PD techniques must be made compatible with a wide variety of urinary diversions. Close collaboration with paediatric urologists and surgeons is essential to the successful integration of PD with reconstruction or revision of these urinary tracts prior to transplantation.

Principles of peritoneal membrane solute and fluid transport

The peritoneal exchange process is the sum of two simultaneous and interrelated transport mechanisms: diffusion and convection. Diffusion refers to the movement of solute down a concentration (electrochemical) gradient, while convection refers to movement of solutes that are 'trapped' in a fluid flux, the magnitude of which is determined by the ultrafiltration rate [47]. A variety of studies have provided evidence that it is the functional and not the anatomical peritoneal surface area that participates in this solute and water exchange, the functional component accounting for only 25–30% of total peritoneal surface area [48].

Effective membrane surface area and solute permeability: diffusive transport

In an early example of the peritoneal equilibration test (PET) in paediatric patients, Gruskin and associates examined time-related changes in dialysate-to-blood concentration ratios for seven different solutes in children, 4 months to 18.5 years of age [49]. By rigidly controlling dialysis mechanics in these studies, Gruskin demonstrated the distortions created by even minor perturbations in exchange volume and dwell time. Diffusion curves constructed for each solute were found to be fundamentally similar to adult reference curves. Gruskin concluded that apparent age-related differences in PD 'efficiency' described in previous reports were probably the result of differences in dialysis mechanics employed in those studies [50–56].

Subsequent studies of diffusive transport made use of the fact that, in the absence of an osmotic gradient between blood and dialysate, the rate of diffusive transfer is directly related to the mass transfer area coefficient (MTAC), the membrane size and the concentration gradient of the solute across the peritoneal membrane [57]. The MTAC is a single parameter that is essentially independent of dialysis mechanics (e.g. exchange volume, dialysate dextrose concentration) and represents the peritoneal surface area and the diffusive permeability of the membrane. It has also been characterized as the clearance rate which can be expected in the absence of ultrafiltration or solute accumulation in the dialysate. In an early study in which MTAC values were measured in paediatric patients, Morgenstern et al. found the MTACs for urea, creatinine, uric acid and glucose in eight children, 1.5–18 years of age, to be similar to adult reference values [58]. Geary et al. determined MTAC values in 28 paediatric patients and suggested that solute transport capacity varies with age and does not approach adult values until later childhood [59]. In the most recent study Warady et al. determined the MTACs for urea, creatinine, glucose and potassium in 83 children <1–18 years of age who were evaluated in a standardized manner with the test exchange volume scaled to body surface area (BSA) (e.g. 1100 ml/m^2) [60]. The mean normalized (to BSA) MTAC values for creatinine, glucose and potassium significantly decreased with age and suggested either an inverse relationship between patient age and functional peritoneal surface area or an age-related difference in peritoneal permeability.

In addition to the MTAC, the rate of dissipation of the solute gradient between blood and dialysate also has a significant impact on diffusive transfer. This rate is influenced by a host of factors including cycle frequency and dialysate volume. The impact of dialysate volume is a result of the principle of geometry of diffusion [61]. This principle suggests that the larger the dialysate volume, the greater the amount of solute transfer that can occur before the dialysate solute concentration begins to rise significantly, and the longer the transperitoneal concentration gradient will persist to drive diffusion. This principle is particularly important when studies of diffusive transport, such as the PET, are conducted. The infant's peritoneal membrane surface area is twice that of an adult when scaled to body weight. Accordingly, historical attempts to devise a paediatric PET to evaluate peritoneal solute transport, in which test exchange volumes were scaled to body weight, resulted in relatively small dialysate volumes being used in the youngest patients [50]. In turn, there was rapid equilibration of solute and the inaccurate perception of enhanced membrane transport capacity [50–56]. On the other hand, scaling the test exchange volume by BSA allows for an equivalent relationship between dialysate volume and peri-

toneal membrane surface area for children of all ages and sizes so that any detectable differences in solute equilibration rates in this setting are the result of true differences in diffusive transport [60, 62, 63]. The use of BSA as the most appropriate 'scaling factor' has been validated in studies conducted by Kohaut et al. [50], de Boer et al. [64], Warady et al. [60], and most recently, Schaefer et al. [65]. Studying their patients in accordance with the three-pore model of peritoneal transport developed by Rippe et al. [66, 67], Schaefer and colleagues [65] clearly demonstrated that the functional peritoneal exchange surface is a linear function of BSA and independent of patient age.

Convective mass transfer and ultrafiltration

The removal of fluid during a CPD exchange reflects the interaction of the hydraulic permeability of the peritoneal membrane with the permeability of the peritoneum to the osmotically active solutes on either side of the membrane. Convective mass transfer has its greatest influence on large solute removal in contrast to the mass transfer of small solutes. Studies conducted by Pyle have demonstrated that the contribution of convection to urea transport in a 4-h CAPD exchange with 4.25% glucose is 12%, 45% for inulin and 86% for total protein [68].

Early studies and much clinical experience suggested that adequate ultrafiltration could be difficult to achieve in infants and younger children. A more rapid decline in dialysate dextrose concentration and osmolality was observed in the youngest patients and the inadequate ultrafiltration was attributed to this mechanism [69, 70]. Later, Kohaut et al. demonstrated that apparent differences in the ultrafiltration capacity in children from infancy to adolescence disappear when the exchange volume is scaled to BSA rather than body weight [50]. Nevertheless, the infant's BSA to body mass ratio is so much greater than that of older patients, it can be difficult to achieve comparable exchange volumes in the clinical setting. For example, an exchange volume of 1100 ml/m^2 BSA that equates to a volume of 35 ml/kg body weight in an older child often represents an 'intolerable' volume of >50 ml/kg body weight in a very young infant. The latter situation often necessitates the use of relatively smaller exchange volumes in infants and young children, which have a negative impact on ultrafiltration capacity and necessitate an alteration of the dialysis prescription. Finally, recent data suggest that the body size-normalized fluid reabsorption rate may be slightly increased in young infants compared to older children and adults, and have an impact on net ultrafiltration [65]. Whereas this finding may be a manifestation of a greater lymphatic absorption rate in the youngest children (see below), it is more likely the result of a reversed movement of fluid along hydrostatic and oncotic pressure gradients as a result of greater intraperitoneal pressures being generated in the smallest patients [71].

Peritoneal lymphatic absorption

Studies of ultrafiltration in children have to some extent been hindered by the absence of information on the contribution of lymphatic absorption to net ultrafiltration. Mactier and associates suggested that children have relatively greater rates of lymphatic fluid absorption than adults, which results in a reduced mean ultrafiltration by 27% [72]. However, the lymphatic absorption rates of the children were similar to adult reference values when the rates were scaled for BSA. Similarly, Schröder *et al.* studied 17 children on PD and found that net transcapillary ultrafiltration and lymphatic absorption were not dependent upon patient age [73]. While additional investigative efforts are surely needed on this topic, lymphatic flow most likely accounts for only 20–30% of dialysate uptake by the body [74].

Summary

In summary, a great deal of progress has been made characterizing the contributions of diffusive and convective transport to peritoneal membrane mass transfer in children following the acceptance of BSA as the uniformed scaling factor in kinetic studies. Whereas minor age-related differences in solute and water transport may exist, the previous reports of substantial differences between children and adults can be accounted for by perturbations in the dialysis mechanics used for the test exchanges and the reliance on body weight as the scaling factor. These pitfalls must be avoided when studies of peritoneal transport function are used to guide therapy, as will be discussed below in the section on the PET in children.

Peritoneal dialysis for acute renal failure

Indications and contraindications

The conservative management of acute renal failure (ARF) in paediatric patients requires meticulous attention to fluid and electrolyte balance. Minor

errors can have severe consequences. Dietary restrictions, phosphate binders, diuretics, sodium bicarbonate, calcium salts, antihypertensive medications, and sodium–potassium exchange resins all play important roles in delaying or avoiding dialysis in some children, although such tactics are not likely to be successful in oligo-anuric children. Several factors are at work in the paediatric patient that tend to defeat even the most carefully conceived conservative management plans. Children with ARF are profoundly catabolic, resulting in accumulation of uraemic solutes at surprisingly rapid rates. In the oliguric child it is difficult to meet energy requirements while abiding by stringent limitations on allowable fluid intake. As a result, dialysis and ultrafiltration tend to be promptly employed in paediatric patients with ARF.

Widely accepted clinical indications for RRT in children with ARF are listed in Table 4. Such lists may not adequately portray the need to consider the rate at which conditions lead to a deteriorating clinical condition in the individual child. A marginal clinical situation should not be tolerated in any child when prompt institution of RRT will control fluid and solute derangements and allow adequate nutrition.

The convenience, simplicity and relative safety of PD have allowed the nephrologist to begin dialysis in the child as soon as it is needed, without undue anxiety over potential complications from the procedure itself. The popularity of PD over HD for critically ill paediatric patients has traditionally rested on two important features: ready access to the peritoneum (vs. typically more difficult vascular access), and better tolerance of PD by unstable children. Recent advances in vascular access techniques and equipment, along with improvements in haemo-

Table 4. Indications for dialysis in children with acute renal failure

Hyperkalaemia (serum $[K^+] > 7.0$ mEq/L)
Intractable acidosis
Fluid overload; often with hypertension, congestive heart failure, or pulmonary oedema
Severe azotaemia (BUN > 150 mg/dl)
Symptomatic uraemia (encephalopathy, pericarditis, intractable vomiting, haemorrhage)
Hyponatraemia, hypocalcaemia, hyperphosphataemia (severe symptomatic)
Fluid removal for optimal nutrition, transfusions, infusions of medications, etc.

These are general guidelines. Each case must be individualized (see text).

dialysis (primarily bicarbonate buffers and ultrafiltration control modules) have narrowed the choice between dialysis modalities in many paediatric centres. Moreover, the introduction of continuous haemofiltration techniques for children has begun to challenge the pre-eminence of PD for the most critically ill paediatric patients [75, 76]. Although vascular access is required, continuous haemofiltration is well tolerated by haemodynamically unstable children. Clear indications for one RRT modality over the others are now rarely present, and often it is the experience of the centre that dictates the selection of the RRT modality.

There are few contraindications to acute PD. Absolute contraindications all relate to the lack of an adequate peritoneal cavity. Neonates with an omphalocoele, diaphragmatic hernia or gastroschisis cannot be treated with PD. Recent abdominal surgery is not an absolute contraindication, as long as there are no draining abdominal wounds. Children with vesicostomies and other urinary diversions, polycystic kidneys, colostomies, gastrostomies, prune-belly syndrome and recent bowel anastomoses have been successfully treated with PD. Peritoneal dialysis can be used to treat acute allograft dysfunction immediately following renal transplantation, as long as the allograft has been placed in an extraperitoneal location. Extensive intra-abdominal adhesions may prevent PD in some patients. Surgical lysis of such adhesions often results in prolonged intraperitoneal haemorrhage.

Technical considerations

Catheters

Acute catheters: temporary vs permanent. A reliable catheter is the cornerstone of successful acute PD. The choice between a percutaneously placed temporary catheter and a surgically placed 'permanent' catheter is usually somewhat arbitrary, reflecting local practice. An increased incidence of peritonitis has been associated historically with the use of the same temporary catheter for longer than 72 h [77].

Surgical placement of a cuffed permanent catheter in the setting of ARF has the advantage of assuring good immediate function, but must be weighed against the risks and delays incurred by an operative procedure requiring general anaesthesia. Anaesthesiologists may be reluctant to administer general anaesthesia to a child with the metabolic derangements of ARF. In patients considered high-risk for general anaesthesia, initial placement of a percutaneous catheter under local analgesia allows immediate dialysis. A surgical catheter can then be placed once the child is stable and it is clear that more than 5 days of dialysis will be needed. Surgical catheter placement at the bedside is readily performed in unstable intensive-care unit (ICU) patients [78, 79].

Temporary catheters for acute peritoneal dialysis. The familiar paediatric Trocath (McGaw, Irvine, CA) has been replaced in most paediatric centres by a percutaneously inserted silastic or Teflon catheter that is placed using the Seldinger technique and a peel-away sheath (Cook Critical Care, Bloomington, IN). The advantages of these catheters were described by Murphy and associates [80]. Poor drainage is a common problem with percutaneous catheters that is usually caused by omental envelopment [81]. When this occurs, it is best to avoid repeated abdominal punctures and proceed to surgical catheter placement.

Temporary catheters for infants. When treating small infants (e.g. those weighing < 1500 g) such commonly found ICU items as 14-gauge plastic intravenous catheters can serve as dialysis catheters. A small curled catheter designed to drain pleural effusions without a water seal (the Starzl Pleural Catheter®, Cook) can also be used. This catheter is inserted over a guidewire and can be placed flat just beneath the anterior abdominal wall. Multiple fenestrations in the curled intraperitoneal segment increase drainage and reduce obstructions. A neonatal acute catheter is also available from Cook.

Permanent catheters for ARF. Standard, single-cuff Tenckhoff catheters (straight or curled) can be used to treat ARF. There is no difference in the techniques used to place permanent catheters, whether the patient is to receive acute or chronic PD. (Permanent catheters will be discussed later in this chapter in the section on chronic peritoneal dialysis.) The use of fibrin glue at the entrance of the catheter to the peritoneum may decrease the incidence of dialysate leakage [82].

Peritoneal dialysis solutions

Peritoneal dialysis solutions (PDS) are commercially available in standard dextrose concentrations of 1.5%, 2.5%, and 4.25%. Acute dialysis is usually begun with the 2.5% solution in order to obtain better ultrafiltration at the outset when fluid overload is frequently present and the exchange volume

Table 5. Peritoneal dialysis solution containing bicarbonate for use in infants intolerant of lactate dialysate

NaCl (0.45%)	896.0 ml
NaCl (2.5 mEq/ml)	12.0 ml
NaHCO$_3$ (1.0 mEq/ml)	40.0 ml
MgSO$_4$ (10%)	1.8 ml
D$_{50}$ W	50.0 ml

Final composition: Na = 139 mEq/L; Cl = 99 mEq/L; Mg = 1.5 mEq/L; SO$_4$ = 1.5 mEq/L; HCO$_3$ = 40 mEq/L; hydrous dextrose = 2.5 g/dl. Calculated osmolality = 423 mOsm/kg H$_2$O.
Modified from ref. 82.

must be kept relatively low to avoid leaks from the new catheter insertion site. PD solutions must be warmed to body temperature before infusion. Adults usually complain of discomfort during the infusion of cool PDS, but infants may respond to unwarmed PDS with a fall in blood pressure. The heater platform of the automated cycler or blood transfusion warming devices placed in the PDS inflow path may be used. Alternatively, water-filled heating pads may be wrapped around the hanging bags of fresh PDS.

Some infants do not tolerate the lactate that is absorbed from standard PDS [83]. These babies are often hypoxaemic with an ongoing metabolic acidosis. Such infants will do better if they are treated from the outset with a PDS that has been prepared by the hospital pharmacy containing bicarbonate instead of lactate. A bicarbonate PDS formula is shown in Table 5. Note that calcium must be given by an alternative route and serum ionized calcium levels must be closely monitored when bicarbonate dialysis is used.

The acute PD prescription

The PD prescription must specify dialysate composition, exchange volume, exchange inflow, dwell and drain times and the number of exchanges to be performed in 24 h. During the initial 24 h after catheter placement, the exchange volume is kept low, usually 15–20 ml/kg, to reduce the risk of dialysate leakage. Over the ensuing 3–5 days the exchange volume is increased gradually, to reach a maximum of 40–45 ml/kg. Respiratory embarrassment and hydrothorax have been reported with the use of exchange volumes approaching 50 ml/kg [84, 85].

Initial stabilization on PD requires 24–48 h of frequent exchanges, 40–60 min each, in order to remove the accumulated solutes and excess fluid. This corresponds to a traditional acute IPD regimen. Once stabilized, dialysis can proceed indefinitely. By gradually extending dwell times and increasing

exchange volumes toward 40–45 ml/kg, a typical maintenance PD regimen can be reached in a few days. Familiarity with CPD regimens used in the treatment of ESRD has led to the popularity of standard CPD regimens for the treatment of ARF [86, 87]. There is no need to periodically suspend PD in order to see if renal function will return; kidneys seem to begin performing again when ready to do so, independent of ongoing PD. While there have been no systematic studies of this approach to the acute PD prescription, the advantages of the near steady-state biochemical and fluid control achievable with CPD are compelling.

PD for ESRD in children

The NAPRTCS database has demonstrated that PD accounts for 64–69% of all registered chronic dialysis patients since the inception of the dialysis registry in 1992 [88, 89]. Until recently, firm guidelines did not exist as to when to initiate RRT in children with ESRD. The decision to start dialysis was based on a combination of factors including urea and creatinine levels (which vary with age), potassium and acid–base balance, growth, and the patient's general well-being. In general, dialysis has been felt to be necessary once the glomerular filtration rate falls below 10 ml/min/1.73 m^2, but may be required sooner in individual patients.

In 1997 the NKF-DOQI guidelines on peritoneal dialysis adequacy were published [90]. They suggest that dialysis should be initiated when the renal urea clearance per week normalized to total body water (Kt/V urea) falls below 2.0, especially if symptoms of uraemia are present, if lean body weight is decreasing or if dietary protein intake is voluntarily diminished. The validity of this guideline in children has not been established, but conventional wisdom suggests that earlier initiation of dialysis before symptoms of uraemia and malnutrition develop should be beneficial in the paediatric age group.

Indications and contraindications for CPD

The majority of paediatric patients can be managed with CPD. Thus, the choice of CPD over chronic HD is most often based on patient and family preference, centre philosophy, and availability of the desired modality. Absolute indications for CPD include [91–93]:

1. very small patients
2. lack of vascular access

3. contraindications to anticoagulation
4. cardiovascular instability.
5. lack of proximity to a paediatric HD centre.

There are a number of conditions that constitute absolute contraindications to CPD. These include the presence of the following [90]:

1. omphalocoele
2. gastroschisis
3. bladder extrophy
4. diaphragmatic hernia
5. obliterated peritoneal cavity and peritoneal membrane failure.

Relative contraindications include:

1. impending abdominal surgery
2. impending living-related renal transplantation
3. lack of an appropriate caregiver

The presence of a colostomy, gastrostomy, ureterostomy and/or pyelostomy does not preclude CPD. Patients with bladder augmentation, and prunebelly syndrome [94] have also been successfully managed with CPD. Controversy exists as to whether the presence of a ventriculoperitoneal cerebrospinal fluid shunt constitutes a contraindication to CPD. Limited experience suggests CPD is acceptable in this situation if no feasible alternative dialysis option exists, recognizing the risks of peritonitis in this patient population [95].

In the absence of a compelling indication, or a relative or absolute contraindication to CPD, the quality of life for both patient and family assumes great importance in dialysis modality selection [96, 97]. However, philosophically, CPD should be considered as merely one form of treatment in the continuum of RRT, and patients and families should understand that a switch in modality may be necessary at some point in the child's management.

Choice of dialysis modality

For most patients the choice of CPD as a dialytic modality is determined by personal preference, as well as by the dialysis centres' philosophy. CPD is the preferred modality for children in most centres as it allows for increased attendance at school and is less disruptive to the family's activity. When compared to HD, CPD is associated with better control of blood pressure and fluid balance and allows for a more liberal food and water intake [93]. Studies have shown that CPD is also associated with better rehabilitation and less depression than HD [98].

Recent data suggest that children cared for in paediatric centres are more likely to receive CPD than those cared for in combined paediatric and adult centres [99]. In the United States, adolescent children of black race appear to receive HD more frequently than PD [100].

In the majority of cases, children who receive CPD do so with some form of automated peritoneal dialysis (APD). The automated forms include NIPD, CCPD and tidal peritoneal dialysis (TPD). The preference for APD over CAPD is reflected in the 70% incidence of APD usage in CPD patients registered in the 1995 NAPRTCS database [88]. Despite the benefits of APD, many adolescents prefer the greater freedom of CAPD. The average 10 h nocturnal APD session may prohibit social activities, or result in late attendance at school.

Certain medical considerations may also dictate a particular therapy. In oliguric or anephric patients who are 'high transporters' based on their peritoneal equilibration test (PET) [101], ultrafiltration is insufficient with the long dwell times of CAPD, making APD the treatment of choice. In particular, NIPD with a dry abdomen during waking hours avoids absorption of dialysate which must then be ultrafiltered at night. For patients with high urinary output renal failure in whom substantial ultrafiltration by dialysis is not necessary, the extra solute clearance provided by the daytime dwell of CCPD, even when partially absorbed, is beneficial. TPD is reserved for patients with ultrafiltration failure or inadequate solute removal when a switch to HD or CAPD, respectively, is not feasible. Patients who are 'slow transporters' are best dialysed by CAPD. Use of APD in these patients results in inadequate solute removal and symptomatic uraemia, while ultrafiltration is well maintained.

PD catheters

Peritoneal access is a key factor in the success and longevity of CPD. Goals for the PD access include the attainment of rapid dialysate flow rates, no fluid leaks, minimal catheter movement at the skin exit site (ES), a low incidence of catheter-related infections, and placement of the catheter at a site that is both reachable and visible to the child or caregivers.

A multitude of PD catheters have appeared since Tenckhoff's original catheter in 1968, and no consensus yet exists as to the optimal catheter for paediatric CPD. A decision regarding catheter choice and usage should take into account the following factors:

1. catheter design
2. number of cuffs
3. exit-site orientation
4. implantation.

Catheter design

The straight internal portion of PD catheters have largely been replaced with coil catheters; the latter design eliminates infusion pain and pain related to catheter tip pressure on the peritoneum. They also have a lower failure rate in terms of poor dialysate flow due to catheter migration [102]. A 1995 survey of the North American Pediatric Peritoneal Dialysis Study Consortium (PPDSC) documented the use of coil catheters by 88% of centres [103], while the 1995 NAPRTCS database recorded a 57.6% incidence of coil catheters [88].

Number of cuffs

In 1985 Twardowski provided evidence that exit-site infection (ESI) rates in adults were lower with double-cuff catheters [104] vs. single-cuff catheters amidst a number of other studies supporting this finding [104–106]. However, three subsequent prospective studies have failed to show a difference in ESI rates for single- and double-cuff catheters [107–109]. Despite conflicting data and the lack of randomized controlled trials, most adult nephrologists are convinced of the superiority of double-cuff catheters, with their use representing more than 70% of catheters in a 1994 survey [110].

When two cuffs are used with a straight tunnel configuration, external cuff extrusion is a frequent complication. Early experience with a high rate of external cuff extrusion in children resulted in a preference for single-cuff catheters in paediatric patients [111–117]. This is reflected in the 1995 data from both the PPDSC and NAPRTCS, which documented a 64–69% incidence of single-cuff catheters [88, 103, 118]. However, single-cuff catheters are associated with a significantly higher rate of peritonitis and a shorter interval to first peritonitis episode in children when compared to the experience with double-cuff catheters [118, 119]. In a paediatric study of 20 single-cuff vs. 20 double-cuff catheters [120, 121], Lewis noted a higher incidence of ESI and peritonitis with single-cuff catheters. Paediatric data from Italy document a preference for double-cuff catheters (82.5%) with only an 8.3% incidence of cuff extrusion [122]. This rate of cuff extrusion is higher than the 3% incidence reported from one large adult series [123]. Paediatric data from Japan

suggest that catheter survival is improved with double-cuff vs. single-cuff catheters at both 1 and 3 years post-catheter implantation [124]. Perhaps in response to this type of data, the NAPRTCS database shows an increase in the percentage of double-cuff catheters from 29.9% in 1993 to 34% in 1997 [89].

Exit-site orientation

Early data in adults demonstrated a lower rate of ESI with downward-pointing exit sites compared to upward-pointing ones, and a trend towards lower ESI rates when compared to lateral-pointing exit sites [104]. However, a subsequent study of single-cuff catheters did not demonstrate a difference in ESI rates for upward- vs. downward-pointing exit sites [125].

In children, data correlating exit-site orientation to ESI rate have, until recently, been virtually non-existent [126]. However, more recent information has provided evidence that the direction of the catheter exit site strongly influences the peritonitis rate. Although 69% of paediatric centres within the PPDSC, and only 25.7% of NAPRTCS centres, reported using a downward-pointing exit site, the NAPRTCS demonstrated a peritonitis rate of one infection per 18.8 patient-months with a downward-pointing exit site compared to an infection rate of one infection per 10.6 patient-months with an upward-facing exit site [88, 103, 118, 119]. As expected, swan-neck catheters, which are characterized by a permanent bend of the subcutaneous portion and an arcuate tunnel, were associated with a lower incidence of peritonitis than catheters with straight tunnels.

Proximity of the PD catheter exit site to diapers and gastrostomy tube/button exit sites are paediatric-specific risk factors for infection. Additionally, catheter trauma may occur during crawling. The swan-neck presternal catheter, developed by Twardowski [127], may be useful in selected paediatric patients who are still in diapers, have gastrostomies, vesicostomies or ureterostomies, are obese, crawling or subject to recurrent ESI [128, 129]. It also allows for tub bathing. A 5-year follow-up of this catheter in 10 children documented an extremely low ESI rate of one infection per 162 patient-months [130]. However, trauma to the exit site was not reduced, catheter disconnection in the subcutaneous tunnel occurred in two children, and catheter survival greater than 1 year occurred in only 36% of patients.

Catheter implantation and postoperative care

The catheter insertion site, exit site and tunnel configuration should be determined well in advance of the surgical procedure, taking into account patient preference, previous surgical scars, abdominal configuration including skin folds and belt line [131–133]. Midline catheter insertion has been associated with a significant incidence of catheter leakage [104]. Adoption of a lateral placement technique through the body of the rectus muscle has resulted in a decrease in catheter leakage [131, 134–137]. Avoidance of leakage is essential since it not only delays ingrowth of fibrous tissue into the cuffs, but also provides a medium for bacterial growth. Lewis has found that placement of the catheter cuff in a superficial (just below the subcutaneous fascia) location vs. a deep (in the rectus sheath) location is associated with a higher (60% vs. 38%) loss of catheters to infection [121]. The exit site should afford easy visual access and should not be compromised by bending movements of the patient. For children, ensuring the exit site is out of the diaper area and away from other ostomy sites, such as gastrostomy tubes, is critical to avoid contamination of the exit site.

Prospective trials on the effectiveness of prophylactic antibiotics for insertion of PD catheters are scant [132]. Bennett-Jones et al. [138] studied the effect of a single preoperative dose of gentamicin compared with no antibiotics, and found a significant reduction in the rate of ESI and peritonitis in the gentamicin-treated group. A recent retrospective paediatric study by Sardegna et al. [139] found a significant reduction in peritonitis occurring in the first 2 weeks post-catheter insertion in patients given preoperative antibiotics, regardless of the antibiotic type. Studies evaluating the healing of exit sites postoperatively suggest that early bacterial colonization with both Gram-positive and Gram-negative organisms is associated with impaired wound healing and is a risk factor for subsequent ESI and catheter loss [140]. Accordingly, current recommendations suggest the use of a first-generation cephalosporin in adults and children at the time of catheter placement [131]. This will require a change of practice in some centres as a 1993 North American survey documented the use of prophylactic antibiotics at the time of catheter insertion in only 61% of paediatric centres [141].

The role of omentectomy remains controversial, although it is recognized that catheter occlusion by omentum is more common in children than adults. Only 53% of centres surveyed by the PPDSC routinely perform an omentectomy [103]. Lewis [142] found a 4.5% catheter occlusion rate in children subjected to omentectomy compared to a 22.7% occlusion rate in those without an omentectomy, a difference that did not reach statistical significance. He suggested that the use of a partial omentectomy be reserved for patients who did not require immediate catheter function, due to the increased risk of leaking post-omentectomy.

Following catheter insertion, the catheter should be flushed with 10 ml/kg of heparinized dialysate until the effluent is clear, to ensure patency. The usual heparin concentration is 500 units/L of dialysate. During the postoperative healing period, stress on the surgical wound due to high intra-abdominal pressure may disrupt the healing process and lead to dialysate leakage [140]. Attention to the prevention of vomiting and straining, and the use of adequate analgesia, is essential. Where possible, a delay of 10–15 days prior to using the chronic catheter is desirable, although only 24% of paediatric centres surveyed in 1995 practised this routinely [103]. When delaying catheter usage is not feasible, the use of lower volume exchanges initially is advisable [134, 133, 143]. Protocols for initiation of dialysis are highly variable, but generally involve some fraction of the full dialysis volume which is increased over time.

To prevent early catheter colonization, sterile, non-occlusive dressings should be utilized until the catheter exit site is well healed. Catheter immobilization is imperative to prevent trauma to the healing exit site. A detailed review of acute and chronic exit site care for paediatric patients is available [144].

Finally, current recommendations do not call for routine flushing of catheters after the initial postoperative break-in period [131]. Where practised, flushing protocols vary widely from centre to centre.

Specialized equipment for paediatric patients

In the early years of paediatric CPD, adult solutions and equipment were adapted for paediatric use. With the realization that CPD was ideally suited to the paediatric population, and with the expanding use of CPD, newer equipment was developed with specific paediatric capabilities.

Paediatric catheters

Almost all adult PD catheter configurations (straight, coil, swan-neck, single- and double-cuff) are available in infant and paediatric sizes and differ primarily in their length. Small transfer sets for paediatric patients are also available.

Dialysate bag size

Early in the course of paediatric CPD, most patients were maintained on CAPD. The availability of dialysate in small bags (300, 500 and 750 ml bags) was considered a major advance in the care of children on CPD. However, over the past two decades there has been an overwhelming move toward APD with nearly 70% of PD patients in the NAPRTCS database receiving APD and only 25% receiving CAPD [101]. As a result, production of small-volume bags is not feasible economically and only 1.0, 1.5, 2.0, 2.5, 3.0 and 5.0 L bags are available for APD. In addition, the development of 'disconnect' systems, such as Twin Bag® (Baxter Healthcare Corp, Deerfield, IL) and Freedom Set® (Fresenius USA, Concord, CA) has circumvented the problem of having to carry unused dialysate from larger volume bags. The smallest Twin Bag® available is 1500 ml. Small patients on CAPD must either weigh their bag during infusion or approximate the appropriate volume. The Twin Bag® also comes in 2.0 L, 2.5 L and 3.0 L volumes.

Paediatric cyclers

The major improvement in cycler technology over the past 5 years has been the development of portable cyclers. The previously used Pac-X® and Pac-Xtra® (Baxter Healthcare Corp) cyclers are large and the calibration mechanisms very sensitive, precluding movement of the cycler even within the home setting.

The Home Choice® (Baxter Healthcare Corp) cycler is a small and extremely portable cycler that is being used by the vast majority of paediatric APD patients in North America. The range of delivered volumes inherent to this cycler make it suitable for paediatric use in all but the smallest patients. The minimum and maximum delivered volumes are 100 and 3000 ml, respectively. Delivered dialysate volumes can be increased by 10 ml increments to 500 ml, by 50 ml increments up to 1000 ml and by 100 ml increments thereafter. The total therapy volume, ranges from a minimum volume of 200 ml to a maximum 80 L. Total volume can be increased by increments of 50 ml to 2.0 L, by 100 ml increments to 5.0 L and by 500 ml increments thereafter. Unfortunately, paediatric-specific tubing is not

available for the Home Choice® cycler. The standard adult tubing has a 40 ml dead space, which potentially causes significant recirculation in very small infants and precludes the use of this cycler for dialysis in most children less than 5kg body weight.

An additional portable and easy-to-use cycler is the Fresenius Delmed 90/2® (Fresenius USA, Concord, CA). This cycler has a range of delivered volumes from 25 ml to 3000 ml which can be prescribed in 10 ml increments. The tubing 'dead space' is only that of the PD catheter and transfer set due to the cycler tubing 'Y' configuration. It can be specifically programmed for paediatric dialysis with only a 10 ml recirculation volume. This cycler is ideal for APD and in particular TPD for infants and small children. The Pac-Xtra®, while not portable, has a minimum dwell volume of 50 ml and also has paediatric TPD capabilities.

Choosing among commercially available PD solutions

Currently, the composition of commercially available PD solutions (PDS) is the same for children and adults. The majority of PDS are bio-incompatible in that they are hyperosmolar, use glucose as the osmotic agent and use lactate buffered at a low pH of 5.5. Evidence is strong that these factors contribute to impaired functioning of the peritoneal immune system and may interfere with peritoneal repair. As a result, newer solutions utilizing alternative osmotic agents and buffer sources are being developed and tested [145]. Characteristics of the ideal PDS include the following [146, 147]:

1. provides optimal ultrafiltration and solute clearance
2. does not impair peritoneal defence mechanisms
3. allows for maintenance of long-term peritoneal membrane integrity
4. supplements nutritional deficiencies
5. iso-osmolar
6. physiological pH using bicarbonate as a buffer
7. contains antimicrobial and antifungal properties.

Buffers

Acidosis is common in ESRD and can be offset by the provision of alkali in the dialysate. Currently used PD solutions contain lactate in concentrations of 35–40 mmol/L with pH of approximately 5.5. This acid pH is known to be toxic to peritoneal cells.

Sodium bicarbonate appears to be the ideal buffer for PDS. However, insoluble calcium salts form in solutions containing bicarbonate, calcium and glucose. Additionally, an acid pH is necessary to prevent caramelization of glucose during heat sterilization. To circumvent these problems, two approaches have been employed: large-scale filter sterilization of pH-neutral bicarbonate solutions or manufacture of the solution in a two-chambered bag, with mixing immediately prior to infusion [148].

Studies to date show that bicarbonate-buffered solutions, regardless of formulation, are more biocompatible than conventional lactate-buffered solutions [148]. Preliminary clinical experience in adults with bicarbonate (38 mmol/L) and bicarbonate-lactate (25 mmol/L and 15 mmol/L respectively) solutions demonstrate equally adequate correction of uraemic acidosis, without adverse effects [149]. However, the ideal concentration of bicarbonate in PDS has not yet been determined. Higher concentrations of bicarbonate (39 mmol/L) in the PDS may be associated with alkalosis [150], and decreased biocompatibility [151, 152]. The effect of improved biocompatibility on peritonitis rates must also be determined [147]. No paediatric experience with bicarbonate-buffered solutions has been published, and their use in paediatrics will probably await further clarification of the ideal solution in adult patients.

Osmotic agents

The most widely used osmotic agent in PDS has been glucose. While glucose is safe and inexpensive, its ultrafiltration (UF) effects are short-lived and it is generally felt to be toxic to the peritoneum, especially in high concentrations and when used long-term. In addition, its use has been associated with the development of hyperglycaemia, hyperlipidaemia, hyperinsulinism and obesity. Of the variety of alternative osmotic agents investigated, the two most successful are glucose polymers (Icodextrin) and amino acids [146]. The paediatric experience with the latter will be discussed later in this chapter.

Glucose polymers are large molecular weight oligosaccharides. Currently, PDS contain Icodextrin at a concentration of 7.5% with an average molecular weight of 20 kDa. Glucose polymers are isosmotic and produce ultrafiltration by colloid osmosis. More than 10 years of clinical experience (none with children) have been accumulated with Icodextrin, with the following observations [153, 154]:

1. UF with Icodextrin is equivalent to that obtained with 4.25% glucose solutions, and is sustained over dwell periods as long as 12 h

2. Icodextrin maintains UF during peritonitis
3. Icodextrin is less able to glycate proteins compared to glucose-based PD solutions
4. single daily exchanges of Icodextrin have been used successfully in adults with type 1 UF failure, prolonging CAPD by an average of 12–16 months in one study [153] and 22 months in another [155]
5. single daily exchanges with Icodextrin have been used for the daytime dwell for patients on APD, with resultant sustained UF and improved solute clearance
6. Icodextrin has been used in patients with diabetes
7. Icodextrin increases convective flow through the small-pore system, improves clearance of β_2-microgloblin, and has no effects on the peritoneal permeability characteristics [156].

The main disadvantage of solutions containing Icodextrin is the accumulation of maltose, although no related adverse clinical effects have yet been described. Maltose levels reach steady state within 2 weeks of commencing a single daily dose of Icodextrin, fall to normal levels within 2 weeks of ceasing Icodextrin and do not accumulate in tissue stores. There is a single published report of hypersensitivity to Icodextrin manifested by exfoliative dermatitis [157], although three additional patients experienced a transient eczematoid rash which resolved spontaneously [155].

Other solutions, such as PD-Bio, a glucose- and lactate-based solution with higher pH (6.3) and no glucose degradation products, are currently under investigation with promising preliminary biocompatibility and UF results [158]. Use in paediatrics will again await further clinical studies in adults.

Calcium

The use of calcium-containing phosphate binders is now standard practice following recognition that aluminium accumulates in ESRD and has multiple toxicities. The combination of supplemental calcium and PDS containing 1.75 mmol/L calcium resulted in frequent hypercalcaemia. As a result, lower calcium solutions containing 1.25 mmol/L calcium were developed and are now widely used [147, 159, 160].

Paediatric data have demonstrated a significantly more negative calcium mass transfer during exchanges with dialysate containing 1.25 mmol/L of calcium as compared to 1.75 mmol/L [161]. Thus, supplemental calcium is generally necessary in patients receiving dialysis with PDS containing low concentrations of calcium to prevent the development of a negative calcium balance. Additionally, negative calcium mass transfer may stimulate parathyroid hormone secretion which influences the need for supplemental vitamin D in this patient population [162]. While dialysate with 1.25 mmol/L calcium is probably acceptable in the majority of paediatric patients, selected patients with refractory hypocalcaemia and/or hyperparathyroidism without hypercalcaemia may benefit from a higher calcium concentration in the dialysate.

Magnesium

Hypermagnesaemia is common in patients with ESRD and on CPD, in the absence of tubulointerstitial diseases of the kidney [163]. Currently available PDS have magnesium concentrations of 0.75, 0.5 and 0.25 mmol/L. Dialysis against a solution with 0.75 mmol/L magnesium results in a net magnesium gain and, in some cases, hypermagnesaemia. The adverse effects of hypermagnesaemia are not entirely known. However, studies have shown that hypomagnesaemia stimulates parathyroid hormone (PTH) secretion, while hypermagnesaemia suppresses PTH secretion. In adults, a significant inverse correlation between serum magnesium and PTH levels has been documented, and suggests that hypermagnesaemia may also be a risk factor for adynamic bone disease [164]. Dialysis against the 0.25 mmol/L or a zero magnesium solution has been shown to result in a normal serum magnesium level in most cases, although hypomagnesaemia has occasionally been reported. The optimal dialysate magnesium concentration for both adults and children is not known. The 0.5 mmol/L solution may represent a 'happy medium', but will probably not be suitable for all patients. Monitoring of serum magnesium levels, with the goal of maintaining a normal serum magnesium level, should dictate the magnesium content of the PDS for a specific patient.

Recommendations for dialysis solutions

Of the currently available PDS, the most 'physiological' solution is one containing 1.25 mmol/L of calcium and either 0.25 or 0.5 mmol/L magnesium. Lactate values of 35 mmol/L will correct acidosis in the majority of patients. Paediatric experience is required before Icodextrin can be recommended as a routine solution, but extensive adult experience in Europe holds promise. More data on bicarbonate-based, neutral pH solutions are required in adults before use of the solutions can be implemented in children.

Chronic PD prescription

The PD prescription for children has evolved empirically from guidelines that adapted adult CAPD for paediatric patients [32–37]. A CAPD regimen of four or five exchanges/day with an exchange volume of 900–1100 ml/m^2 BSA (35–45 ml/kg) of 2.5% dextrose dialysis solution has routinely yielded net UF volumes of up to 1100 ml/m^2 with acceptable biochemical control. Using similar exchange volumes, the greatest percentage of children on CPD receive cycler dialysis with a regimen consisting of six to eight exchanges over 8–10 h per night.

The current goal of achieving dialysis adequacy (see below) in terms of solute clearance in the most cost-effective manner has highlighted the need to be cognizant of a patient's BSA, peritoneal membrane solute transport capacity and residual renal function (RRF) when designing the dialysis prescription [165–167]. In most patients (except for the rapid transporter), the most effective way to increase solute clearance is to increase the exchange volume and not the exchange frequency. In addition, some clinicians advocate a direct assessment of a patient's maximum tolerated intraperitoneal volume as part of the prescription process [168]. Measurement of RRF assumes greatest significance in those situations in which target solute clearances fail to be achieved solely by the dialysis process. Calculated as the average of residual creatinine clearance and residual urea clearance as a means of taking the tubular secretion of creatinine and reabsorption of urea into consideration, the contribution of RRF towards a target goal may be substantial early in the course of dialysis. Subsequently, a progressive loss of RRF usually occurs and mandates modification of the dialysis prescription if target clearances are to be attained [169–171]. As discussed below, categorization of a patient's peritoneal membrane transport capacity can best be determined by the performance of a PET.

The most recent development in the prescription process, the use of computer-based dialysis modeling to achieve target PD doses, has now been successfully applied to the paediatric CPD population [172–174]. In contrast to instituting the CPD prescription based on PET transport categorization only, with subsequent empirical prescription changes guided by clinical experience alone, the use of computerized modeling makes it possible to tailor the CPD prescription to an individual patient in an efficient manner using computer calculations. Prescription recommendations are made with the 'PD Adequest' (Baxter Healthcare) program using PET data to generate MTAC values, whereas the 'Pack PD' (Fresenius) and the 'PDC' (Gambro) program use data generated from the personal dialysis capacity test.

Principles of the PET and its role in prescription management

The peritoneal equilibration test or PET was developed by Twardowski et al. as a clinically applicable means of characterizing solute transport across the peritoneum [101]. The procedure yields data necessary to determine the fractional equilibration of creatinine and glucose between dialysate and blood expressed as a dialysate to plasma (D/P) ratio for creatinine and a ratio of dialysate glucose to initial dialysate glucose (D/D_0). Since the transport capacity of a patient's peritoneal membrane is such an important factor to consider when determining the dialysis prescription, a PET evaluation should be conducted soon after the initiation of dialysis [165, 166, 175]. However, since there is evidence that a PET performed within the first week of CPD may yield higher transport results than a PET performed several weeks later, the National Kidney Foundation–Dialysis Outcomes Quality Initiative (NKF-DOQI) has recommended that the PET be conducted $\geqslant 1$ month following the initiation of CPD [90, 167]. The PET evaluation should be repeated when knowledge of the patient's current membrane transport capacity is necessary for the determination of the CPD prescription, especially when clinical events have occurred (e.g. repeated peritonitis) which may have altered transport characteristics.

Whereas a test exchange volume of 2000 ml is used in all adult PET studies, irrespective of patient size, current recommendations in children are for the use of a BSA standardized PET exchange volume of $1000–1100 \text{ ml/m}^2$, which takes into consideration the previously mentioned age-independent relationship between BSA and peritoneal surface area. It also allows for comparison of individual patient data to population norms determined with a comparable test procedure. The Pediatric Peritoneal Dialysis Study Consortium (PPDSC) and the Mid-European Pediatric Peritoneal Dialysis Study Group (MEPPS) have both conducted large multicentre trials and have established reference curves for solute equilibration in children [176, 177].

The availability of the PET makes it possible to predict a patient's likely response to a specific PD schedule. Thus, children who are classified as rapid transporters based on their 4-h D/P creatinine or their 4-h D/D_0 glucose value are likely to dialyse most efficiently using short, frequent dialysis cycles as in CCPD or NIPD. On the other hand, a low-average transporter may benefit most from a schedule which includes longer dwell times as in classical CAPD. The PET data can also be used to determine the APEX time, an additional index used to determine the optimum contact time between the functional peritoneal membrane surface area and dialysate [168, 178, 179]. The APEX time is defined as the intersection time of the dialytic urea saturation and glucose desaturation curves with typical times in children ranging from 18 to 71 min.

Proper use of the data derived from the PET requires that dialysate creatinine values are corrected for glucose interference when a photometric method of creatinine determination is used since falsely elevated creatinine values may result [101]. This situation can be avoided by the use of the enzymatic assay method of creatinine determination. In addition, measured plasma solute concentrations should be divided by 0.9 to account for their presence in plasma water only and not in whole plasma. Failure to do so has resulted in solute D/P ratios greater than unity [180].

The presence of residual dialysate volumes has been noted in several adult and paediatric PET studies, and can complicate the interpretation of results [176, 181]. A large residual volume containing solute that is equilibrated with serum during the long overnight dwell that precedes the PET can artificially inflate solute D/P ratios. This is especially true during the initial 1–2 h of the PET, and can thereby influence the categorization of solute transport capacity.

Finally, the personal dialysis capacity (PDC) test has recently been validated as an alternative to the PET to assess individual peritoneal transport characteristics in children and adults [182]. The PDC test is based upon the three-pore model of peritoneal mass transport developed by Rippe et al. that assumes peritoneal fluid and water transport occurs across three types of pores of varying size. The paediatric experience has been published by Schaefer et al. [172].

PD adequacy

Reference to PD adequacy in children should rightly take into account the dialysis process, growth, nutrition, management of anaemia and osteodystrophy and a variety of other topics covered in this chapter. However, PD adequacy and solute clearance have been used almost interchangeably since the performance of the National Cooperative Dialysis Study in the adult HD population [183]. As part of the NKF-DOQI project, studies of adult CPD patients, in which clinical outcome parameters (e.g. frequency of hospitalization, patient morbidity and mortality) and solute clearance have been monitored were reviewed. In turn, dialysis adequacy was characterized in terms of small-solute clearance as a total (residual renal plus peritoneal dialysis) weekly Kt/V urea $\geqslant 2.0$ and a total weekly creatinine clearance $\geqslant 60$ L/1.73 m^2 for the patient receiving CAPD [90]. The recommended target clearances were slightly greater for patients receiving cycler dialysis. Since very few data coupling dialysis dose to outcome are available in paediatrics, making it impossible to define PD adequacy in children with confidence, the current clinical experience suggests that the paediatric population should use clearance goals that are similar to or greater than those recommended by DOQI. Whereas it had been hoped that growth would be the ideal outcome parameter to measure in children, preliminary data from the MEPPS have revealed the absence of any correlation between total solute clearance and longitudinal change in height standard deviation score (SDS) [177]. Further evaluation of these data is vitally important.

It is noteworthy that there are few data to support the preference of one solute clearance measure (Kt/V urea vs. creatinine clearance) over another and discrepancies in the results (e.g. target clearance met by Kt/V urea criteria but not by creatinine clearance) may occur in as many as 20% of patients [184]. The reasons for the discrepancies are multifactorial and include the amount of RRF present and the differences that exist in peritoneal transport of urea and creatinine. Automated PD prescriptions using frequent short exchanges favour a higher Kt/V urea, whereas long dwell times favour creatinine clearance. Accordingly, initial outcome studies in adults have used both measures of adequacy, as well as an ongoing assessment of the patient's clinical condition. An additional assessment of adequacy, the Solute Removal Index (SRI) may also prove to be valuable in paediatric patients receiving cycler dialysis [185].

As mentioned above, Kt/V urea has found wide acceptance as a marker of small-solute clearance and is calculated as the urea clearance normalized for the volume of urea distribution or total body water

(TBW). Unfortunately, a method for the determination of V has not been validated in children receiving CPD, although some investigators have recommended the use of bioelectric impedance [186]. At present it is recommended that the formulas of Mellits and Cheek (that were derived from healthy subjects aged 1 month to approximately 30 years of age) be used to estimate TBW [187]. The specific formulas are as follows:

For Boys:

$$V \text{ (litres)} = -1.927 + 0.465 \times \text{Wt (kg)}$$
$$+ 0.045 \times \text{Ht (cm)}$$

when Ht $\leqslant 132.7$ cm

$$V = -21.993 + 0.406 \times \text{Wt} + 0.209 \times \text{Ht}$$

when height is $\geqslant 132.7$ cm

For Girls:

$$V \text{ (litres)} = 0.076 + 0.507 \times \text{Wt} + 0.013 \times \text{Ht}$$

when height is $\leqslant 110.8$ cm

$$V = -10.313 + 0.252 \times \text{Wt} + 0.154 \times \text{Ht}$$

when height is $\geqslant 110.8$ cm.

Ideally, UF capacity should also be considered a component of adequate PD and a patient's membrane transport capacity may be particularly important in this context. Recent studies in adult CPD patients have revealed that the relative risks of technique failure and patient mortality are significantly increased in patients categorized as high transporters by the PET [188]. While the reasons for the increased risk noted in this population of patients are unknown, it has been postulated that the rapid glucose absorption that characterizes the high transport state may predispose patients to chronic fluid overload and cardiovascular morbidity [189].

Implicit in the approach to achieve and maintain dialysis adequacy is the need to repeatedly measure total solute clearance. Ideally, 24-h collections of urine and dialysis fluid should be obtained three times per year, or when there has been a significant change in the patient's clinical status that may influence dialysis performance. Computer-generated estimates of solute removal are not an adequate substitute for a collected specimen [176, 190]. Recognizing the difficulty of accurately collecting urine in infants and young children, many clinicians attempt to achieve the adequacy targets through the contribution of CPD clearance alone.

Nutritional management of children on CPD

Nutritional goals

The goal of nutritional management of children on CPD is to maximize nutrition and normalize growth parameters, while minimizing the metabolic consequences of uraemia. This is frequently accomplished in the face of anorexia, and often necessitates enteral feeding, which may have adverse effects on motor skills and social development. The achievement of a normal nutritional status is uncommon among children treated with CPD, despite access to an essentially unlimited diet. Several reviews of the nutritional approach to paediatric patients on CPD are available and are summarized below and in Table 6 [191–193]. Recommendations must take into account both losses and absorption of nutrients in the dialysis fluid [194, 195].

Optimal energy requirements have not been established, but consensus recommends that prepubertal children on CPD receive 100% of the recommended daily allowances (RDAs) of the National Academy of Sciences for children of the same height–age and sex [196]. In addition, glucose absorption from dialysate can provide up to 12% of the daily caloric intake [197]. Obesity due in part to dialysate glucose absorption is a common problem in adults treated with CPD. The caloric intake should be adjusted accordingly if obesity develops in children on CPD. Carbohydrates should be complex in nature and provide at least 35% of dietary energy intake.

Protein intake must be carefully controlled avoiding protein malnutrition from an excessively restrictive diet while avoiding toxicity from nitrogenous waste products from an excessively generous diet. At least 50% of dietary protein intake should be of high biological value due to the higher percentage of essential amino acids, which are beneficial in promoting muscle anabolism and decreasing muscle wasting [198]. If the BUN exceeds 70 mg/dl (30 mmol/L) in a child who is eating more than the prescribed protein intake, in the absence of other causative factors, reduction of protein intake should be considered. Alternatively, the amount of dialysis can be increased. Before limiting protein intake in a child on CPD, care should be taken to ensure that sufficient dialysis is being prescribed for the protein intake and that sufficient non-protein calories are being offered. Monitoring of the protein intake can be accomplished by measuring urea nitrogen appearance in dialysate and urine. The DOQI guidelines [90] suggest the nutritional status of paediatric CPD patients be assessed at least every 6 months by standard clinical nutritional evaluations and by the modified Borah equation [199]:

$$PNA \ (g/day) = (6.49 \times UNA) + (0.294 \times V)$$
$$+ \ protein \ losses \ (g/day)$$

where:

UNA = urea nitrogen appearance (g/day)

V = total body water [200].

To avoid a persistent negative nitrogen balance, protein supplementation may be necessary for children in whom an *ad-lib* diet is unsatisfactory, or for those with recurrent peritonitis [201, 202].

In infants and young children, approximately 50% of the dietary energy intake should come from fat, with a polyunsaturated:saturated fatty acid ratio of 1.5:1.0. Although serum lipids levels are elevated in patients on CPD, they remain stable on such a regimen [203, 204]. Dietary fat should be less in older children, but the age at which intake should

Table 6. Guidelines for nutritional therapy for children receiving chronic peritoneal dialysis

Nutrient	Infant	Pre-puberty	Puberty	Post-puberty
Energy (kcal/kg/day)	110–150	70–100	Males, 60 Females, 48	Males, 60 Females, 48
Protein (g/kg/day)	2.5–3.0	2.5	2.0	1.5
Fat		50% dietary energy intake		
Vitamins: Pyridoxine (B6) Ascorbic acid Folic acid		5–10 mg/day 75–100 mg/day 1.0 mg/day		

be curtailed is controversial as inappropriate restriction could result in growth impairment [205, 206].

Supplementation of water-soluble vitamins is mandatory for children on CPD (Table 6). Provision of 100% of the RDA is probably sufficient for all of these vitamins. Vitamin D should be provided in the active form either as calcitriol or calcidiol. Iron supplementation is necessary in most children on CPD since most are receiving recombinant human erythropoietin. Carnitine levels are frequently reduced in children on CPD for more than 4 months and carnitine supplementation is indicated in children who are in turn symptomatic with findings such as a myopathy [207, 208]. Zinc deficiency has been reported in children on CPD and some centres recommend routine supplementation [209, 210].

In general, fluid, sodium and potassium intake in the child on CPD can be substantially greater than in HD patients. Fluid intake varies widely in children, depending mainly on residual urine output. Restriction of fluid intake is usually necessary only in small anephric or oligoanuric patients, or those with poor ultrafiltration from membrane failure. An inappropriately high dietary sodium intake will stimulate thirst and consequently increase fluid intake. It is usual to prescribe a no-added-salt diet and only rarely a low-salt diet for the severely hypertensive patient. Infants, especially those with renal dysplasia, frequently require sodium supplementation to avoid hyponatraemia and even hypotension. Hyperkalaemia is not uncommon during the initiation of CPD. Potassium restriction is warranted at this time along with the use of exchange resins when indicated. Constipation should be avoided since stool potassium excretion helps maintain potassium balance. Later on, children tend not to require potassium restriction; however, they are cautioned about eating excessive amounts of high-potassium foods. Phosphate restriction is important, although compliance is difficult and most patients are taking phosphate binders in the form of calcium carbonate.

Monitoring nutritional management requires tracking of growth and other anthropometric parameters (e.g. mid-arm circumference, skinfold thickness), serum protein, albumin, serum transferrin, and 3-day dietary intake recalls. The Subjective Global Assessment (SGA) is recommended for monitoring the nutritional status of adults on CPD [211]. It addresses four items, namely weight change, anorexia, subcutaneous tissue, and muscle mass. Unfortunately, there is not a similar standardized assessment tool for children. CPD patients may gain fat and water weight while losing lean body mass, making the assessment tools less reliable as determinants of nutritional status [202, 212]. Studies in adults using bioelectrical impedance have uncovered subtle changes in lean body mass that were not detected by anthropometrics [213]. In adults, fat-free, oedema-free body mass can be calculated by measuring creatinine excretion [214]. These techniques have not been systematically tested in children.

Controlled enteral nutrition

In the infant and young child on CPD, optimal feeding is necessary for growth and neurological development. Unfortunately, the anorexia of chronic renal failure results in inadequate spontaneous dietary intake. Abdominal fullness from the dialysate, peritoneal dextrose absorption, gastro-oesophageal reflux, and behaviour problems may contribute to poor nutrition. In addition, when formulas are fortified with various fat, carbohydrate and protein additives they become viscous and unpalatable, precluding oral acceptance by the infant. These factors, plus the extensive time commitment and negative parent–child interaction that frequently accompany attempts to get these children to eat have led to widespread reliance on controlled enteral nutritional feeding (tube feeding). Tube feeding is accomplished using a nasogastric (NG), gastrostomy (G), nasojejunal (NJ), or gastrojejunal (GJ) tube [215–220]. In patients on NIPD or CCPD, continuous overnight tube feedings have the advantage of providing nutrients during the period of most intensive dialysis by innocuously consolidating the feeding routine. Night-time tube feeding also allows the stomach to be empty during the day, which may permit spontaneous oral eating. It is usually necessary to combine night-time tube feeding with daytime boluses to reach nutritional goals.

While most paediatric centres are quick to use tube feeding in children unable to attain adequate nutrition spontaneously, opinions differ regarding the optimal tube feeding regimen. Each has its advantages and disadvantages. Gastrostomy tubes offer convenience and cosmetic advantages and avoid the struggle of tube insertion. Complications of G-tube feeding include: nausea, vomiting and diarrhoea, which usually respond to reduction in volume and/or formula density; gastritis from the irritation of the tube, which can be managed by antacids or histamine H_2-receptor antagonist therapy; displacement of the tube which is easily replaced at home by the parent; G-tube obstruction; G-tube exit site infection; and gastrocutaneous fistula which requires surgical closure. Care of the exit site is necessary to avoid peritonitis.

NG-tube feedings avoid the trauma of surgical or percutaneous G-tube placement and the risks of dialysate leaks and G-tube exit-site infections. Patient acceptance has improved with the use of small (8 Fr), soft silastic tubes. However, tube placement remains an unpleasant experience and vomiting is a universal complication. Routine replacement of an NG-tube is done once each month, at which time the other nostril is used. The cosmetic effect is noticed by grandparents for infants and schoolmates for children. Sinusitis and otitis have not increased in these children [221, 222].

As mentioned above, both G-tube and NG-tube feedings are associated with vomiting and the risk of aspiration. Fortunately, serious aspiration is rare in these children, possibly because they have a good gag reflex and overzealous feeding is avoided. Children should be evaluated for the presence of gastro-oesophageal reflux disease (GERD) prior to the initiation of tube feeding, and may require a surgical anti-reflux procedure if severe reflux is demonstrated. Medical GERD therapy (e.g. ranitidine, metoclopramide, and other agents) can be effectively employed in those whose reflux is not severe. GJ- and NJ-tubes are used to overcome vomiting [221]. Maintaining fixation of the tube in the jejunum is difficult and it is frequently displaced into the stomach.

Both G-tube and NG-tube feeding can interfere with the natural learning process for swallowing. Exclusively tube-fed infants shun solid foods as a consequence of a hyperactive gag reflex [219, 222]. Tube feeding must sometimes be continued for months after a successful kidney transplant in these infants while they learn to chew and swallow solids without gagging. Speech development may also be delayed in some NG-tube fed infants as the tube may interfere with phonation [222].

Regardless of the route of enteral feeding, time must be provided for oral stimulation and gratification in order to encourage development of oral motor skills and speech performance. Pacifiers and gum massage encourage non-nutritive sucking during tube-feeding sessions and at other times during the day. Oral intake of food prior to tube feeding is encouraged, even when most of the intake is via the tube. A multidisciplinary behavioural team approach is often useful in managing these children [198, 202, 205, 222].

No nutritionally complete commercial formula for children on CPD is currently available. Therapy consists of a basic formula (e.g. Similac PM 60/40 [Ross]; S-29 [Wyeth]; Pediasure [Ross]; Nepro [Abbott]) with added modules of carbohydrate (glucose polymers), fat (emulsified fat, or corn or safflower oil), and protein (casein or whey) customized to meet the needs of the particular child. Whey modules are lower in phosphorus and are more soluble. Emulsified fat is more expensive than vegetable oils, but is preferable in continuous feedings because of better mixing and suspension.

Intraperitoneal amino acids

While CPD utilizing glucose-based dialysis solutions is effective in controlling uraemia and fluid balance, glucose absorption from the dialysis solution with a consequent increase in the blood glucose concentration may contribute to obesity, and has been implicated in hypertriglyceridaemia and anorexia. Additionally, losses of protein and amino acids into the dialysate may contribute to the hypoalbuminaemia, protein malnutrition, and abnormal plasma amino acid profiles seen in CPD patients. Greater dialysate losses of protein have been seen in younger patients [194, 195, 223]. Thus, amino acid dialysis solutions have been investigated both in adults and children as an alternative dialysis solution, and have been well tolerated and successful in managing CPD patients [194, 224–230].

There are many short-term and long-term studies of amino acid dialysis which demonstrate adequate removal of urea, creatinine and fluid. There are conflicting reports on the nutritional value of amino acid dialysis. Kopple et al. conducted a carefully controlled multicentre study of 18 adults on CPD and demonstrated a significantly positive nitrogen balance from amino acid dialysis. Total serum protein increased; however, serum albumin did not. These patients became acidotic on amino acid dialysis, yet this was not treated and could have adversely affected the study. Acidosis can have a major deleterious effect on protein nutrition in patients on CPD which can be reversed when the acidosis is treated [231]. Amino acid dialysis solutions are now commercially available (i.e. Nutrineal, Baxter Healthcare, Deerfield, IL) [232]. It is hopefully anticipated that this new therapy will improve the nutrition of children on CPD. The fact that recombinant human growth hormone (r-HuGH) given to adults on CPD reduces plasma essential amino acids and promotes a net anabolic process [233] emphasizes the need for more studies on amino acid dialysis and the role of r-HuGH in the nutritional management of children.

Management of the very young infant: special considerations

The 1995 NAPRTCS database reveals that 90% of infants below 1 year of age are managed with CPD, rather than HD [88]. Infants with ESRD present a special challenge to the paediatric nephrologist since successful management includes aggressive nutritional support, careful attention to metabolic abnormalities and bone disease, delivery of adequate dialysis, and the use of r-HuGH. Using this aggressive approach along with nocturnal APD, Becker *et al.* [234] recently reported an excellent outcome in 19 infants, 10 of whom commenced CPD at or below 1 year of age. There was no mortality in this patient population, and those reaching school age were in age-appropriate grades. Catch-up growth was achieved in those treated with r-HuGH. This study serves to illustrate the considerable improvement in outcome over the past decade for this subpopulation of children on CPD. It also highlighted those areas where ongoing research and improvement are still needed, especially related to growth, cognitive development, infectious complications and mortality. A number of problems are especially pertinent to infants on CPD, as outlined below.

Growth failure

Growth failure in infants on CPD has been well documented in the setting of conservative management. While some improvement in growth has been achieved with aggressive nutritional support (usually with tube feedings), careful attention to correction of acidosis and electrolyte imbalance, treatment of renal osteodystrophy and tailoring of CPD to achieve adequate dialysis, growth often remains suboptimal and growth lost during infancy is rarely recovered [89, 235–248]. We have now entered a new 'era', with increasingly widespread use of r-HuGH in children with chronic renal insufficiency (CRI) and those with ESRD on dialysis. Growth rates of children on dialysis have been improved with the use of r-HuGH, but continue to be inferior to the rates enjoyed by children with CRI [249]. The impact of r-HuGH on the growth rates of infants on CPD remains to be seen, although reports such as that from Becker *et al.* are encouraging [234].

Development

Developmental delay was previously reported as a significant and serious complication associated with conservative management and CPD in infants with renal insufficiency. Developmental outcome has improved, however, with aggressive dietary management, early institution of PD, control of hyperparathyroidism, and avoidance of aluminium-containing phosphate binders [239, 241–243, 246, 250–252]. Gross motor delay is relatively common and may be related to prolonged hospitalization and abdominal distension from PD fluid. Mild hypotonia is also common, some of which may be associated with carnitine deficiency [207].

The intellectual status of older children on CPD has recently been reported and 76.7% had an intelligence quotient (IQ) in the average range [253]. Unfortunately, the duration of dialysis was not reported, precluding any evaluation of the impact of dialysis delivery. In a Japanese series of 15 infants who commenced CAPD under 2 years of age, and who received aggressive nutritional support, the developmental quotient was low but stable and the IQ was normal in most patients at 5–6 years of age [246]. Warady *et al.* assessed global intelligence in 19 children (mean age 6.6 ± 1.3 years) who started CPD at $\leqslant 3$ months of age and found it to be impaired in only one (5%) patient [252].

Nutrition

The nutritional management of the infant on CPD represents a special challenge as the optimal requirements are poorly defined. Using the RDAs as a basis the following recommendations have been made: energy intake, 110–150 kcal/kg/day, with 35–50% from carbohydrate and 50% from fat; protein intake, 2.5–3.0 g/kg/day with protein of high biological value, to account for both required intake and dialysate protein losses [91, 191, 254, 255]. Vitamin requirements are similar to older children [256, 257]. Mean plasma fluoride concentrations in infants on CPD are significantly greater than controls during the first 18 months of life. Whereas no fluorosis in deciduous teeth has been observed, the effect on permanent teeth remains unreported. Since infants on CPD are at risk for markedly elevated fluoride levels, they should not be fluoride supplemented [258]. Gastro-oesophageal reflux may occur in up to 73% of infants with ESRD, especially those less than 12 months of age, and may complicate the provision of adequate nutrition [259]. The achievement of adequate caloric intake in the anuric or oliguric infant represents an additional challenge. Highly concentrated formulas, with the addition of 'modules' of protein, carbohydrate and/or lipid to base formulas, must be employed.

Hyponatraemia

Hyponatraemia is commonly present, especially in infants with high-output renal insufficiency, and may contribute to growth failure. The hyponatraemia is due to multiple factors, including the low sodium content of infant formulas, high ultrafiltration requirements relative to body weight with obligate sodium losses in the dialysate, renal sodium losses in non-oliguric patients and inadequate ultrafiltration. Oral sodium supplementation with sodium chloride or bicarbonate may be necessary to achieve a normal sodium status and optimize growth [239, 243, 253, 260, 261]. Required sodium supplementation averages 3–5 mmol/kg/day, but may be as high as 5–10 mmol/kg/day [261].

Hypophosphatemia

Similac PM 60/40® (Ross Laboratories, Montreal, Quebec), is commonly used in infants with ESRD to minimize phosphate intake. Its phosphate content is 6 mmol/L compared to most standard infant formulas which contain 9–13 mmol/L of phosphate. Carnation Good Start® (Carnation Nestle Food Company, Glendale, CA) has an intermediate phosphate content of 8 mmol/L, providing a substantially cheaper alternative to PM 60/40®. As a result, hypophosphataemia is common in infants on CPD and receiving phosphate binders. It may be as deleterious to bone integrity as hyperphosphataemia [262]. Its occurrence requires the cessation of phosphate binders if they are being used, and/or an increase in dietary phosphate content.

Poor ultrafiltration

Equilibration of glucose across the peritoneal membrane is faster in young children than in adults when exchange volumes are scaled to body weight rather than BSA [52]. Using volumes scaled to BSA, glucose equilibration in infants is similar in children and adults [50, 263, 264]. Clinically and probably as a result of the use of relatively smaller exchange volumes, many infants demonstrate type 1 ultrafiltration 'failure' with long dwell times. This is of concern in a population whose caloric intake is primarily in liquid form. Ultrafiltration can be maximized by using appropriate exchange volumes scaled to BSA and/or nocturnal APD with short dwell times (45–60 min). Tidal PD should be considered when UF is inadequate, particularly in oliguric or anuric infants. Tidal PD has also recently been used successfully as 'rescue' therapy for poorly functioning catheters in infants [265].

Infectious complications

The frequency of infectious complications remains higher in infants on dialysis than in older children and adults, although the use of automated cyclers [242], and disconnect systems [266] has reduced paediatric peritonitis rates overall. Possible explanations for the infant experience include the proximity of the PD catheter exit site to the diaper area and gastrostomy tube, as well as the greater use of single-cuff catheters with an upward-facing exit site [119, 122, 131, 245]. The NAPRTCS database shows peritonitis rates of 1.19 episodes per patient-year for infants 0–1 years of age compared to 0.97 per patient-year for 2–5-year-olds and 0.77 per year for children > 12 years of age [119]. Multiple patient data registries also document shorter catheter survival in infants compared to older children [119, 122, 124, 131] in association with the elevated infection rates.

Hypogammaglobulinaemia

Hypogammaglobulinaemia has been reported in infants on PD, and is postulated to be associated with increased infection rates [267, 268]. However, a recent prospective study of 17 infants on CPD [269] has shown that while hypogammaglobulinaemia is common (71%), it may be transient and generally does not interfere with the development of a protective antibody response to vaccination. Furthermore, there was no association between hypogammaglobulinaemia and an increased risk of sepsis or peritonitis.

Mortality

Whereas reported mortality rates in infants on CPD vary widely, and may reflect patient selection, the rates are routinely higher than those reported in older children [119, 239, 245]. Mortality rates in infants commencing dialysis under 1 year of age range from 13.8–16% in the NAPRTCS database [119, 261], to 43% in the series of Ellis et al. [244]. Risk factors for death in the latter study included oliguria and the presence of other major organ system abnormalities. Verrina et al. reported mortality rates of 10.9% after 1 year and 17.8% after 2 years on dialysis [245]. In addition to mortality, morbidity as measured by the need for hospitalization for complications related to CPD is significantly higher in younger children compared to older children on CPD or CHD [270].

Dialysis considerations

The widely used Home Choice® cycler has a minimum delivered dialysate volume of 100 ml and a tubing dead space of 40 ml. This may preclude its use in very small infants because of reduced dialysis efficiency with small exchange volumes and significant recirculation in the cycler tubing. Other cyclers with smaller tubing dead space and smaller delivered volumes, such as the Fresenius Delmed 90/2®, and the Pac-Xtra® may be more appropriate for this select patient population.

Polyuric infants may absorb significant amounts of dialysate resulting in repeated low drain alarms. This can be overcome by reducing the drain alarm limit [261]. Polyuric infants are also prone to volume contraction with significant amounts of ultrafiltration. This can be circumvented by the use of combinations of 0.5% and 1.5% dextrose PDS during cycling, or with high-volume, low-caloric density feedings with salt supplementation [271]. Unfortunately, the 0.5% solution is generally available only in Canada. This latter solution is particularly useful in infants and children on CPD to prevent volume contraction during episodes of gastroenteritis.

No paediatric standards for dialysis adequacy exist. Current DOQI guidelines are extrapolated from the adult literature and have not been validated for children [90]. Whether parameters for dialysis adequacy in infancy will be the same as for older children awaits a systematic study with appropriate paediatric outcome measures.

Transplantation

The final goal of ESRD management is a functioning transplant. Infants may be an ideal group for transplantation as they have a greater capacity for growth and healing and are often less malnourished, growth-retarded and chronically ill than older children with a longer period of ESRD. In addition, recent data show significantly improved growth rates post-transplantation compared to CPD in the 6-month to 4-year age group [248]. However, controversy exists as to the optimal timing of transplantation. Traditionally, infants were maintained on CPD until they reached an appropriate size (approximately 10 kg) to optimize surgical outcome, the major complication being vascular thrombosis [272, 273]. More recently, numerous authors have reported patient and graft survival rates similar to older children and improved growth and neurological development in infants transplanted at less than 1 year of age [239, 242, 251, 275–278]. Living-related transplantation

appears particularly successful in infants, with superior graft survival compared to cadaveric grafts [88, 240, 242, 274, 276–278]. However, it is important to recognize that the 1995 NAPRTCS database documents that 0–1-year-olds account for only 6.2% of paediatric transplants, for a total of 51 transplants from 1987 to 1995 [88], and that the registry documents a relative risk of graft failure of 2.03 for recipients under 2 years of age. Clearly, additional multicentre data are necessary to supplement the encouraging single-centre reports.

Transplantation requires an intensive multidisciplinary approach and should be undertaken at the 'optimal' time for each patient, taking into account parental wishes, availability of dialysis and donors, nutritional status, growth, and surgical experience and outcome for the particular institution [277]. Some infants will require time on dialysis to allow necessary surgical intervention or to correct malnutrition, while others may proceed directly to transplantation without dialysis. The risks of transplantation and prolonged immunosuppression must be weighed against the risks and outcome of prolonged PD in the developing infant.

In summary, caring for an infant on CPD can be very successful when there is attention to detail. However, it should also be mentioned that the care necessary for this population is associated with a physical, financial and emotional cost that may on occasion be overwhelming for a family [279]. A recent multinational survey of paediatric nephrologists revealed that 41% offer RRT to all infants under 1 month of age, and 53% to all infants between 1 and 12 months of age [280]. Eighty per cent and 62% of nephrologists surveyed felt it was sometimes acceptable for parents to refuse renal replacement for infants <1 month old and 1–12 months old, respectively. Thus, the prevailing opinion among physicians who routinely care for these infants is that it is still acceptable, with informed consent, for parents to elect conservative therapy or withdrawal of therapy, if the burden of care outweighs the benefits of dialysis and transplantation for an individual child and family [280–282].

Renal anaemia and its treatment in children on CPD

Recombinant human erythropoietin (r-HuEPO) corrects the anaemia of chronic renal failure and eliminates the need for red blood cell transfusions in almost all adult [283–285] and paediatric [286–288] dialysis patients. Improvements in exercise tolerance, cognitive function, work capacity, sexual function, and overall sense of well-being have been consistently described in adult dialysis patients treated with r-HuEPO [289, 290]. Paediatric dialysis patients may enjoy even greater benefits from r-HuEPO therapy. While 25–60% of adult dialysis patients were transfusion-dependent prior to the availability of r-HuEPO, virtually all children treated with HD required transfusions from the earliest months of dialytic therapy and over 75% of children treated with CPD for more than 12 months also became transfusion-dependent [35, 291, 292]. Repeated red blood cell transfusions had profoundly adverse effects in children, including frequent exposure to infectious agents, sensitization to human HLA antigens, and chronic iron intoxication. Of these, perhaps the most consistently damaging to children was the development of high titres of preformed anti-HLA antibodies. This resulted in increased waiting time on the cadaver transplant list and decreased overall allograft survival, both of which have been shown to be associated with a history of only six or more transfusions prior to cadaveric transplantation [293]. Initiation of r-HuEPO therapy and consequent cessation of transfusions has been shown to decrease titres of panel-reactive antibodies in multiply-transfused children [294].

Children with ESRD have additional problems unique to the paediatric patient that may be ameliorated by correction of renal anaemia. Poor growth is a consistent feature of uraemia in children to which severe anaemia may contribute [295, 296], although consistently beneficial effects of r-HuEPO on growth in dialysed children have not been demonstrated [297]. Cognitive function is diminished in uraemic children, a problem that is not improved by dialysis, but does improve following successful renal transplantation [298]. Correction of anaemia has been associated with improved cognitive function in adults on PD [299] and with improvement in brainstem auditory evoked response in children [300]. The limited energy and exercise capacity of uraemic children are closely related to the degree of renal anaemia [301] and adversely affect the capacity of these children to study and play normally with other children. It is a critical task of childhood to develop adequate self-esteem for psychosocial independence in adult life; thus, although difficult to measure, the harmful effects of renal anaemia during childhood may be felt for a lifetime.

Pretreatment concerns

Experience with the use of r-HuEPO in paediatric dialysis patients has been detailed in recent reviews [288, 302, 303]. How anaemic should a child on CPD be before r-HuEPO is started? The NKF-DOQI guidelines on the treatment of anaemia have recommended a target range for haematocrit of 33% (haemoglobin 11 g/dl) to 36% (haemoglobin 12 g/dl) for both adults and children [304]. While these levels are below the normal ranges, available data from paediatric trials of r-HuEPO therapy is almost exclusively derived from patients who have achieved no more than these mildly anaemic haematocrit/haemoglobin levels [286, 287, 305, 306]. Higher haematocrit/haemoglobin targets for adults have been advocated by some [307], but have not been studied in children.

Hypertension develops or worsens in one-fourth to one-third of children treated with r-HuEPO [288, 303]. It seems prudent to insist on superbly controlled hypertension as a prerequisite for initiating therapy. Particular attention should be paid to maintaining children at their dry weights during initiation of r-HuEPO therapy. Blood pressure must be carefully monitored in all treated patients, but especially those not receiving antihypertensive therapy when r-HuEPO is begun.

Iron deficiency will inhibit r-HuEPO effectiveness [308]. Prior to initiating r-HuEPO treatment, a patient's iron status should be assessed by measuring serum iron, total iron binding capacity (TIBC), and serum ferritin levels. Transferrin saturation (TS) $\geqslant 20\%$ and serum ferritin level > 100 ng/ml are indirect, yet usually reliable, indicators of adequate iron stores to support vigorous erythropoiesis [308].

$$TS(\%) = (\text{serum iron}/TIBC) \times 100$$

Correction of iron deficiency at the outset of CPD may delay the need for r-HuEPO therapy in some children and will increase the efficacy of r-HuEPO in all.

Early concerns about an increased risk of seizures in treated patients have not been substantiated [283, 309]. Initial reports of seizures may have actually been describing hypertensive encephalopathy rather than a primary neuroelectric event. r-HuEPO should not be withheld from children with stable, well-controlled seizure disorders.

Dosing

r-HuEPO is effective when given intravenously, intraperitoneally, or subcutaneously. Over 90% of paediatric PD patients followed by the dialysis patient database of the NAPRTCS receive r-HuEPO via the subcutaneous route [310]. Intraperitoneal administration of r-HuEPO has been proposed as way to improve compliance [311], a more serious issue several years ago when citrate-buffered preparations of r-HuEPO were associated with significant pain at the subcutaneous injection site [312, 313]. Intraperitoneal administration is safe [311], but to be effective it must be given in a small-volume of dialysate (50 ml) [314].

A reasonable starting subcutaneous dose is 80–120 U/kg per week given in one to three divided doses [305]. Infants and young children require higher doses and should be started at 300 U/kg per week, usually in three divided doses [305, 315]. There is no need to begin at a higher dose, then reduce to 'maintenance' dosing levels. The primary goal of therapy is to select a dose that increases the haematocrit steadily at about 1–2% per week, generally considered to be a rate at which adjustments in volume status and antihypertensive medications can be safely made to maintain normal blood pressure [302].

A patient's haematocrit should be measured weekly during the initial 2–3 months of therapy, or until a new steady-state haematocrit level has been achieved. The rate of rise of the haematocrit is linear and will reflect the difference between the new and old rates of erythropoiesis, with the period of increasing haematocrit lasting for one erythrocyte survival time [316]. The survival time is decreased in uraemic children and varies from patient to patient, averaging about 60 days [317]. When a new steady state is achieved, the haematocrit stabilizes. If the new level is below target, an increase in dose is needed, but further adjustments in dose should be infrequent, since the steady-state haematocrit resulting from any given dose is not going to be seen for at least 6 weeks in most children. Similarly, it makes little sense to ever completely discontinue r-HuEPO in response to a haematocrit that is too high. The full effects of a stoppage of r-HuEPO will not be fully apparent for at least one erythrocyte life time, at which point the haematocrit may fall precipitously. Better to reduce the dose and follow haematocrits weekly until the new steady state is achieved. Once the haematocrit stabilizes within the target range, monthly haematocrits and serum iron, TIBC and ferritin measurements performed every 3 months are sufficient to monitor r-HuEPO therapy.

Iron supplementation

Almost all children on CPD receiving r-HuEPO require iron supplements. Oral iron preparations differ in tolerability and absorption with the most potent preparation, ferrous sulphate, also the one most often associated with gastrointestinal side effects [318]. Absorption of oral iron is enhanced by increased gastric acidity, as is seen when iron is taken before or several hours after a meal or with small doses of vitamin C. Absorption is diminished by phosphate binders, tannins (tea, coffee) and green leafy vegetables. The usual starting dose of oral iron is 2–3 mg elemental iron/kg per day.

When oral iron supplements are unsuccessful, intravenous iron is indicated. Experience in North America is limited to iron dextran [305, 319]. Newer preparations (ferric sodium gluconate, ferric saccharate) are available in Europe [320, 321]. The protocol for iron dextran therapy used in the United States paediatric multicentre r-HuEPO trial is given in Table 7.

r-HuEPO 'resistance'

A suboptimal response to r-HuEPO can occur as a consequence of iron deficiency, infection (e.g. peritonitis) or other inflammatory processes [322], hyperparathyroidism [323], aluminium intoxication [324], and vitamin B12 or folate deficiency. Of these, iron deficiency is the most common.

Immune status and vaccine responsiveness

The propensity for infection that characterizes children on CPD has led to a number of studies that have evaluated the immune status of this population. Abnormalities of humoral immunity including hypogammaglobulinaemia, deficiencies of IgG2 and abnormal responses to childhood immunization have all been noted [267, 269, 325–327].

Katz *et al.* first described hypogammaglobulinaemia in infants receiving CAPD [267]. Whereas immunoglobulin losses into the effluent were present, these losses could not fully explain the low serum IgG levels seen. It was hypothesized that 'uraemic toxins' might suppress immunoglobulin synthesis. Recently, Neu *et al.* described hypogammaglobulinaemia in 12 of 17 (71%) patients <42 months of age and maintained on cycler PD [325]. No cause-and-effect relationship between low serum IgG levels and infection was evident in this study. Similar clinical observations will need to be conducted in the future to determine if patients on CPD

Table 7. Iron dextran administration in paediatric peritoneal dialysis patients

Indication
Parenteral iron is indicated for patients with low iron stores (transferrin saturation <20%). A trial of oral iron may be attempted before initiation of parenteral iron in those patients with borderline iron stores who are able to tolerate oral iron.

Risks
Side-effects are uncommon and include fever, urticaria, headache, malaise, and arthralgias. Anaphylaxis has been reported in <1% of patients given intravenous iron dextran. Recent experience in centres treating adult dialysis patients has shown a much lower incidence if smaller doses are given over a prolonged treatment course. Due to the risk of anaphylaxis each patient is given a test dose prior to initiation of treatment.

Administration of test dose
The test dose is:
  0.5 ml (25 mg) in patients >20 kg
  0.3 ml (15 mg) in patients 10–20 kg
  0.2 ml (10 mg) in patients <10 kg
Administer dose intravenously over 1 min. Adverse effects should occur within a few minutes. Observe for 1 h before giving therapeutic dose or discharging patient from unit.

Administration of dose
Iron dextran will be diluted in normal saline and administered as an intravenous infusion over 2 h. The patient's Fe and TIBC will be repeated 2 weeks after the dose. If the patient's iron stores are still low the dose will be repeated.

Dose
The dose is adjusted for patient weight.

Weight	Dose	Volume of normal saline infusion
<20 kg	500 mg	250 ml
10–20 kg	250 mg	125 ml
<10 kg	125 mg	75 ml

who are found to have low serum immunoglobulin levels by routine screening should receive prophylactic intravenous immunoglobulin therapy.

Current recommendations are that children on dialysis should receive all of the standard childhood immunizations in addition to the influenza and pneumococcal vaccines [328]. While it is hoped that this approach will help alleviate the risk of vaccine-preventable disease, it should be noted that very few studies have specifically evaluated vaccination response in children immunized while on dialysis. Most of the studies that have been conducted involved relatively small numbers of patients. Based on the information that has been collected to date, guidelines for immunizing patients on CPD are as follows [328, 329]:

1. Patients should receive all standard immunizations according to the recommended immunization schedule of the American Academy of Pediatrics [330–332].
2. Older patients who have not had natural varicella may receive the varicella vaccine if not previously immunized. Transplantation should be delayed for >8 weeks following this live viral vaccine.
3. Patients should receive supplemental immunization with the influenza and pneumococcal vaccines. The influenza vaccine should be provided yearly and booster inoculations of the pneumococcal vaccine will be required [333, 334].
4. Antibody response to the measles–mumps–rubella (MMR) vaccine and varicella should be evaluated prior to transplantation [328]. Re-immunization is recommended if the patient is unprotected.
5. Doubling of the recommended dose of hepatitis B vaccine should be considered [335, 336]. Antibody levels to hepatitis B should be monitored every other year.

r-HuGH therapy

Progressive growth retardation is an almost universal characteristic of children on dialysis such that a substantial percentage of patients who develop ESRD during childhood attain a final adult height that is less than the third percentile on the growth chart (Height Standard Deviation Score [SDS] of < -1.88) [248, 337]. While there are a host of factors that may contribute to the subnormal height velocity experienced in association with impaired renal function, disorders of the growth hormone (GH)/insulin-like growth factor (IGF) access is undoubtedly the major factor [338]. Additional aetiological factors include: (1) age at onset of renal disease; (2) protein and calorie malnutrition; (3) acid–base disturbances; (4) water and electrolyte disturbances and (5) renal osteodystrophy [339].

It has been recognized for some time that GH levels are elevated in patients with ESRD despite evidence of growth retardation in the same patients. The elevated levels seem to be a manifestation of impaired degradation of GH by the kidney with a resultant significantly higher GH half-life in patients with renal insufficiency. The findings are compatible with end-organ hyporesponsiveness to GH [340]. In contrast to the elevated GH levels it appears that there are excessive quantities of one or more of six insulin growth factor binding proteins (IGFBPs) in comparison to the quantity of IGFs. The resultant decreased IGF bioactivity plays a significant pathogenic role in the ESRD-associated growth failure

[338, 340, 341]. In addition, the density of GH receptors in growth hormone target organs appears to be decreased [342, 343].

Treatment with recombinant human growth hormone (r-HuGH) may accelerate the growth of patients with renal insufficiency by increasing the IGF-1 levels to overcome the growth-inhibiting effects of IGFBPs and by restoring the IGF bioactivity [340]. r-HuGH has been shown to be safe and effective in controlled studies of children with chronic renal insufficiency prior to ESRD and in uncontrolled observations on a small number of children on CPD [344]. Using a r-HuGH dose of 1 IU/kg/day (Europe) or 0.05 mg/kg/day (United States), first-year growth velocity is enhanced in children on CPD, but less than in patients with pre-terminal renal insufficiency [341]. Whether this is a dose-related phenomenon or a manifestation of growth factor loss into peritoneal effluent is unknown [345]. When used, r-HuGH should be continued until the time of transplantation, until the patient reaches the 50th percentile for mid-parental height or until the final adult height is achieved. However, r-HuGH-stimulated growth during the second and subsequent years of treatment is typically less than that seen during the initial year of therapy. If r-HuGH is discontinued prior to transplantation, a subsequent fall in height velocity may indicate the need to reinitiate therapy [346]. Monitoring of renal osteodystrophy is particularly important in children receiving r-HuGH therapy [347].

Renal osteodystrophy

Renal osteodystrophy represents a spectrum of skeletal disorders ranging from high-turnover lesions of secondary hyperparathyroidism to low-turnover lesions and adynamic bone disease [348]. Whereas factors related to the development of the former lesion include phosphate retention, hypocalcaemia, decreased levels of 1,25-dihydroxyvitamin D, skeletal resistance to parathyroid hormone and reduced vitamin D receptor expression in the parathyroid glands, pathogenic factors responsible for the latter lesion include treatment with CPD, calcium carbonate therapy and vitamin D therapy [349]. The clinical presentation of renal osteodystrophy is generally insidious, although it may be manifested by renal bone pain, bony deformities, muscle weakness and extraskeletal calcification. Although renal osteodystrophy is considered one of the major determinants of growth retardation in children with ESRD, treat-

ment of osteodystrophy does not regularly result in normal growth velocity [350].

The hallmark of treatment includes the achievement of age-appropriate serum phosphorus levels with dietary modification and non-aluminium-containing phosphate binding agents, as well as vitamin D therapy. Dietary phosphorus should be restricted to 400–800 mg/day to help achieve serum phosphorus levels of 4.8–7.4 mg/dl during the first 3 months of life, 4.5–5.8 mg/dl at 1–2 years and 4.0–5.5 mg/dl in older children [351]. When used as a phosphate binder, doses of calcium carbonate range from 2.5 to 7.5 g/day. Doses of 1,25-dihydroxyvitamin D or calcitriol usually range from 0.25 to 0.75 µg/day [352]. Since both calcium carbonate and calcitriol can result in hypercalcaemia, the use of low-calcium dialysate may be advisable. While intermittent oral or intraperitoneal calcitriol therapy are both effective, the former therapy when used in large doses has been associated with the development of the adynamic bone lesion and poor growth in children on APD [353, 354]. Although controversial, calcitriol therapy should be prescribed with a target intact PTH level 3–4 times the upper limit of normal for patients receiving daily therapy [346, 349]. Serum PTH values < 150 pg/ml are typically present in children with the adynamic lesion. Whereas the histological impact of r-HuGH on renal osteodystrophy continues to be studied in children on CPD, close monitoring for bony deformities in this setting is necessary if early detection and treatment are to occur.

Complications

Peritonitis

The single most serious complication which occurs in children on CPD is peritonitis [355–360]. Present data suggest that children have a significantly greater tendency to develop peritonitis than adults, with an increased number of children experiencing an episode of peritonitis during the first year of therapy. Reductions in peritonitis rates have been reported in both adults and children in association with treatment of *Staphylococcus aureus* nasal carriage, as well as with recent technical developments such as newer disconnect systems and flush-before-fill techniques [356, 360, 361]. Preliminary results have been reported from a large multicentre trial to evaluate this new technology in children [362].

Recent evaluation of the NAPRTCS database showed a total of 1078 reported episodes of peritonitis in 1198 treatment-years, resulting in an annualized peritonitis rate of 0.9 episodes or 1 infection every 13.3 patient-months [355, 363]. The rate of peritonitis was higher in patients during their first year of life with an annualized rate of 1.19 or 1 infection every 10.1 months versus an annualized rate of 0.8 or 1 episode every 15.7 patient-months in children > 12 years of age. In addition, Gram-positive infections accounted for approximately 50% of the episodes of peritonitis, and Gram-negative infections slightly more than 20%. Fungal peritonitis represented < 2% of the episodes of peritonitis.

The current approach to treatment of peritonitis primarily relies on the intraperitoneal administration of antibiotics. Antibiotics frequently employed include cephalosporins, aminoglycosides and vancomycin, although recent recommendations discourage the indiscriminant use of vancomycin because of the emergence of strains of vancomycin-resistant enterococci [VRE] [363, 364]. The vestibular and ototoxic side-effects of aminoglycosides continue to be a concern [365]. Although recommendations have been proposed for the treatment of CPD-related peritonitis, further clarification is required with respect to the optimal treatment for children [366, 367].

Exit-site and tunnel infections

Exit-site and tunnel infections are a continuing problem for paediatric CPD programmes. The NIH National CAPD Registry has reported an increased incidence of exit-site/tunnel infections in children compared to adults (0.8 vs. 0.6 episode/year, respectively), and an increased probability of experiencing a first infection during the initial 12 months of therapy [368].

Exit-site infections (ESI) in children may present with only slight erythema to a purulent ulcerated erosion. The pathogenesis is multifactorial. Many potential contributing factors are proposed including mechanical irritation, hypersensitivity to silicone rubber, excessive sweating, and local granulation tissue formation. Levy and associates retrospectively reviewed their experience with 157 episodes of ESI occurring in 50 children treated with CPD at a single centre during 950 patient-months of dialysis [369]. The ESI was characterized as purulent in 39 and non-purulent in 71 episodes. *Staphylococcus aureus* was the most frequently observed (nearly 50%) organism in both purulent and non-purulent infections. *Pseudomonas aeruginosa* was the most common Gram-negative organism (10.6%). Patient age, gender and primary renal disease were not correlated with ESI incidence nor did the presence of

gastrostomy tube exit sites, diaper use or pyelostomies favour the development of an ESI in these children. Exit-site infections in diapered infants were more often due to Gram-positive organisms than enteric organisms.

Catheter exit site care is felt to be pivotal in the prevention of infection. Routine management has undergone many changes through the years, reflecting the failure to find a satisfactory approach. Initially, a sterile dressing technique using an occlusive 'giant bandaid' was prescribed. Subsequently, a sterile gauze dressing changed weekly for the first month after catheter insertion was used. After the first month, patients were taught to scrub the exit site with povidone-iodine solution when they showered (at least every other day). Patients are now instructed to shower with plain soap and water, dry with a clean towel, paint a circle of povidone-iodine solution around the exit site and let it dry. Any crusting is removed with 3% hydrogen peroxide before applying the iodine. The adult experience has suggested benefits associated with the use of Mupirocin ointment at the exit site in *S. aureus* nasal carriers [370]. The importance of catheter fixation is stressed. Infants are bathed in a tub of shallow water to avoid soaking the exit site. The gauze dressing is left on during the bathing and changed afterwards with the exit site gently cleaned with a povidone-iodine swab.

Exit-site infections are routinely treated with oral antibiotics [366]. Only if improvement is not seen promptly are intraperitoneal antibiotics used, the specific agent chosen based on culture results. Medical management of ESIs due to *Pseudomonas* organisms are frequently refractory to therapy and catheter replacement may be required.

Hernias, leaks and hydrothorax

Hernias. Abdominal wall hernias are common in children on CPD, occurring in 22–40% of paediatric patients [372, 373]. Multiple hernias are seen. Khoury *et al.* described 28 hernias in 18 children on CPD [372]. There were 18 inguinal hernias (64%) that occurred in 12 children (11 males), whose average age was 5.2 years. Increased intra-abdominal pressure associated with CPD has the potential of converting an asymptomatic patent processus vaginalis into a clinically significant inguinal hernia. It is important to note that the incidence of a patent processus vaginalis is higher in infants. Von Lillien *et al.* reported 60 hernias in 37 children treated with CPD [373]. Incarceration is uncommon.

Prevention and management of hernias varies among centres. Hernias in children are likely to occur early in the course of CPD. Poor nutrition, prior abdominal surgery, and corticosteroid therapy are risk factors. Young males are at the greatest risk for inguinal hernias. In these infants, demonstration of a patent processus vaginalis by peritoneography [113] or ultrasound at the time of catheter placement allows pre-emptive repair and prevention of an inguinal hernia. The use of CCPD with a reduced daytime exchange volume should be considered for patients felt to be at risk.

Most hernias can be repaired electively. Patients should be monitored for development of hernias both before catheter placement and during CPD therapy. If a hernia is diagnosed, elective repair is scheduled promptly. Parents are instructed to observe the child for signs and symptoms of hernia incarceration while awaiting surgery. In most cases of inguinal hernias in males <2 years of age, a bilateral repair is recommended.

Leaks. Dialysate leakage from the catheter exit site can complicate the placement of newly inserted catheters. Dialysate can also leak from the peritoneal cavity into various tissue planes, most often into subcutaneous tissue around a previous surgical incision or into the genital area. The subcutaneous fluid expands because it is hypertonic dialysate and consequently absorbs water. Conservative management, occasionally including temporary suspension of CPD, is usually sufficient to allow these leaks to resolve. Aspiration of the subcutaneous fluid is not helpful and should be avoided.

A leak into the genital area can be difficult to distinguish from an inguinal hernia. Both CT scan [374] and scintigraphy [375] have been used for this purpose. Most of these patients can be managed conservatively by reducing the exchange volume and bedrest, or switching from CAPD/CCPD to temporary NIPD with a dry day. If a patent processus vaginalis is present, it may require ligation to prevent recurrence of a genital leak.

Hydrothorax. Hydrothorax is an uncommon complication of CPD in children [376] and adults [377, 378]. It is usually right-sided. The prevalence of pleuroperitoneal connections in the general population is unknown, since they are not challenged with PD. It is suggested that the leaks occur because of the effect of raised intra-abdominal pressure on small defects in the pleuroperitoneum covering the diaphragm [379]. It is believed that a tiny bleb arises on the surface of the diaphragm and then ruptures, forming a one-way valve leading to a tension hydro-

thorax. Alternatively, the potential pleuroperitoneal connection is present as a congenital defect in the diaphragm.

It is important to consider other causes of pleural effusion in CPD patients, including congestive heart failure, fluid overload, and hypoalbuminaemia. In patients in whom the cause is uncertain, tests are necessary to prove the pleuroperitoneal connection. There are various techniques, including thoracentesis to measure the pleural fluid for dextrose or to detect the presence of intraperitoneally infused dye by colorimetric testing (indigo carmine) [380] or direct visualization (methylene blue), and chest fluoroscopy after infusing dilute radioopaque contrast media or radioisotope [381] into the peritoneal cavity.

Transfer to haemodialysis will resolve the problem. For patients who need to return to CPD, sealing of the pleuroperitoneal connection with an intrathoracic sclerosing agent (i.e. autologous haemoglobin) or surgical patch-grafting have been reported [377, 378, 382, 383].

Abdominal catastrophes

Compared to adults on CPD, children rarely experience dialysis-related abdominal catastrophes; however, such events do exist in children and thus age should not be considered as a barrier.

Sclerosing encapsulating peritonitis

Sclerosing encapsulating peritonitis is uncommon in children [384]. The bowel becomes encapsulated in a fibrous cocoon which is extremely difficult to surgically dissect free. It can occur in patients who have been exposed to short-term dialysis although the length of time on CPD is a recognized risk factor. The use of acetate dialysis solutions was incriminated in a report from Europe [385]. The problem is frequently fatal, although there are reports of treatment with immunosuppressive drugs and surgery being helpful. However, surgery is dangerous and should be avoided if possible [386].

Other major disorders of the gastrointestinal tract

Diverticulitis is a frequent source of bowel perforation and faecal peritonitis in adults which fortunately has not been reported in children. In contrast, appendicitis must be considered in all children on CPD who present with fever and abdominal pain, the same symptoms seen with peritonitis. After an appendectomy, CPD should be suspended until the stump has healed.

Pancreatitis has been described in adults and rarely in children on CPD [387, 388]. Concerns that CPD predisposes a patient to develop pancreatitis have been disputed [389]. Cessation of CPD and transfer to haemodialysis may be indicated in some cases.

Neoplasia

Wilms tumour is a common paediatric malignancy that has an association with ESRD (i.e. Denys–Drash syndrome: Wilms tumour, pseudohermaphroditism, nephropathy) [390]. Wilms tumours rapidly increase in size and are usually diagnosed by palpation of an abdominal mass. Younger children must be examined intermittently with the abdomen empty of dialysate. Rarely, suspicious cells in the dialysate may be identified as malignant using flow cytometry.

Miscellaneous complications

It is not possible to list all the complications. However, a brief review of some of the more important or uniquely paediatric complications are provided.

Hypogammaglobulinaemia. Hypogammaglobulinaemia has been reported in infants and younger children on CPD [391]. This may be particularly significant since mortality rates are highest in this age group of CPD children [267], and the majority of the deaths are from infection. This complication should be monitored and treatment considered with intravenous gammaglobulin when hypogammaglobulinaemia is detected, especially in the setting of an active infection.

Prune-belly syndrome. Children with prune-belly syndrome can be treated with CPD, despite their deficient abdominal musculature [94]. To prevent leaks the percutaneous catheter insertion technique can be helpful in achieving a watertight seal at the thin abdominal wall. A slow break-in period to permit healing is advised Although CAPD is not possible for these boys, CCPD is possible, limiting the daytime volumes to increase patient comfort. Although huge exchange volumes can be accommodated by these children, this should be avoided.

Hydrocephalus. Children with myelomeningocoele typically have a neurogenic bladder which may lead to ESRD. In addition, these children often have hydrocephalus requiring ventriculoperitoneal (VP)

shunting. When children with VP shunts require dialysis, the option of CPD is commonly entertained. Recurrent peritonitis is a risk for all CPD patients; however, the consequences of peritonitis are greater for these children. The risk of a simple peritonitis episode involving the VP shunt has led some but not all to consider the presence of a VP shunt as an absolute or relative contra-indication to CPD [392]. If haemodialysis is not possible, converting the VP shunt to a ventriculoatrial or venticulopleural shunt prior to starting CPD are options.

Genitourinary surgery. Children with inadequate bladders are treated with a bladder augmentation procedure using bowel, stomach or dilated ureter [393]. Creation of the augmented bladder requires extensive surgery with attendant risks for the development of adhesions. In addition, the augmented bladder segment is attached to a vascular pedicle which resides in the peritoneal cavity. Despite the magnitude of the surgery, and potential for complications, these children do well on CPD.

Many children on CPD require elective nephrectomies, usually for hypertension or to remove a potential focus of infection prior to renal transplantation. If it is necessary only to remove kidneys, the use of a posterior lumbotomy approach avoids invasion of the peritoneal cavity and allows CPD to continue postoperatively. For patients requiring nephroureterectomy via a transperitoneal approach, CPD must often be suspended for a brief period, relying on temporary HD.

CPD can also be offered to children who require a vesicostomy or pyeloureterostomy. Few dialysis complications related to these forms of urinary diversion occur.

Bloody dialysate. Children on CPD will occasionally experience bloody dialysate following minor trauma. The bleeding is probably due to catheter trauma in most cases. Mild bleeding can mimic the cloudy fluid of peritonitis. Conservative management is usually successful. The peritoneal cavity is flushed with dialysate with the option of adding low-dose heparin to reduce the risk of clot obstructing the catheter. Patients, parents, teachers and coaches often need reassurance that such episodes are of little consequence, and should not interfere with the normal physical or sporting activities.

Bloody dialysate can occur in postmenarchal girls secondary to retrograde menstruation. Conservative management as above is all that is needed.

Quality of life and other psychosocial issues

Some authors claim that the survival of patients with ESRD depends on factors other than the mode of treatment. Therefore, determination of the quality of life for ESRD patients is important for clinical decision making and also for allocation of resources. Careful studies in adults using time trade-off measurements show that successful transplantation is the preferred treatment, providing the best quality of life, with no difference between the various dialysis modalities [394, 395].

One study of 73 children and adolescents compared psychosocial adjustment to ESRD for patients on HD, CPD and following transplantation [396]. Significant advantages of transplantation over dialysis, and of CPD over HD, were found. Children with transplants exhibited less social and functional impairment and fewer treatment-associated practical difficulties. Parents of transplanted children also had fewer practical difficulties. Children on CPD had less social impairment, less depression, better adjustment, less behavioural disturbance, and fewer practical problems related to treatment than their HD counterparts. Depression and anxiety scores were lower in parents of children on CPD. While this study suggests better-adjusted parents of CPD children, possibly due to greater involvement in their child's care, the potential for parental 'burn-out' exists with prolonged CPD. It is difficult for parents to meet the medical, psychological and social needs of the child on CPD and still have sufficient time to meet the needs of other family members [397].

The real success of advances in transplantation and dialysis therapy must be judged by the patient's rehabilitation. Children with ESRD differ from those with many chronic disorders by the persistence of their disease, the reliance on technology despite successful transplantation, and a much higher incidence of multiple disabilities as compared to the general population. A large multicentre study of children and adolescents with ESRD noted school attendance was good during the first years, but subsequent education was frequently disrupted and inadequate [398]. Attendance at schools providing opportunity for a university career was low, and only 52% of eligible patients attended vocational school. Only 14% of adolescents over 18 years of age achieved independent living. Factors which appear to contribute to this poor outcome include delays in social and sexual maturation, retardation of growth, and psychological and behaviour disturbances such as depression, anxiety, withdrawal and denial, which have their roots in chronic illness during childhood.

The outcome of children with renal insufficiency since infancy remains less than optimal. However, adolescents with later-onset renal failure show better potential for rehabilitation, as demonstrated in a study of 118 patients with onset of renal failure at 10–20 years of age [399]. The cumulative survival rate of transplanted patients was 80.1% after 18 years. Functional status was good or excellent in 73.5% of transplant patients, but in only 45% of dialysis patients, with HD patients functioning poorly compared to CPD patients. Most patients achieved an appropriate level of formal education, but more slowly than their unaffected counterparts. Twenty-nine per cent were living independently or with a spouse, and four patients had become parents. Significant linear growth retardation was seen in 35.6% of patients, primarily in those with growth retardation prior to transplantation.

Short stature, combined with alterations in body image related to the need for CPD catheters, central venous lines, feeding tubes or fistulas, may contribute to psychological maladjustment in children with ESRD. While parents can ensure the compliance of younger children for dialysis and medications, adolescents present a particular challenge with respect to compliance. Peer pressure often results in dietary indiscretion, and fear of being labelled different may cause a child to forgo dialysis exchanges at school. Embarrassment about catheters, fatigue or the dialysis *per se* may result in failure to participate in physical-fitness classes, which results in poor levels of physical activity with attendant health risks.

In summary, it appears that CPD offers most children and their families a better quality of life than HD. The ability to attend school every day may be one of the most beneficial features of CPD for children. Among patients on PD, 77% were attending school full-time and 15% part-time or at home [363], as compared to children receiving HD (46% and 41%, respectively). Few restrictions to physical activities are necessary. Swimming is permitted, although attention must be paid to securing the catheter while in the water, and only chlorinated swimming pools (rather than rivers and lakes) are recommended. Summer camping experiences are encouraged for the CPD patient in order to encourage them to achieve their full potential [400].

Transplantation

Improving patient and allograft survival rates in children have confirmed the long-standing impression that renal transplantation is the treatment of choice for all paediatric dialysis patients [88]. Thus, dialysis is best considered a bridge to get children safely to or between renal transplants. To be a successful dialysis modality for children, CAPD/CCPD has to be readily compatible with transplantation. However, when CAPD was first developed for children, in the early 1980s, some nephrologists and transplant surgeons were hesitant to transplant children on CAPD, primarily because of a perceived risk of peritonitis under immunosuppression and a fear of increased graft and patient loss [401]. These fears have proved unfounded. Nearly two decades of experience with transplantation in children maintained on CAPD/CCPD has failed to demonstrate any adverse impact of CAPD/CCPD on transplant outcome. Currently two-thirds of children receiving transplants in North America are maintained pre-transplant on CAPD/CCPD [310].

Preoperative management

Preoperative evaluation of the child on CPD includes assessment for evidence of a tunnel or exit site infection and for peritonitis. Dialysate is sent for cell count, differential, Gram's stain and culture. When dialysate studies indicate bacterial peritonitis the transplant should be postponed. A localized exit site infection does not mandate postponement as long as the catheter is removed at the time of transplant surgery, using a separate drape and scrub of the abdomen. However, the presence of a significant tunnel infection is a contraindication to transplantation.

While dialysis the night before transplant surgery is customary, not all children need it. For small children the volume depletion associated with CPD immediately prior to transplantation can make intraoperative fluid loading more difficult [402].

Dialysis catheter

An extensive literature review by Chavers revealed that the reported time of routine PD catheter removal in children varied widely, from immediately at the time of transplant to up to 4 months post-transplant [403]. Local experience and custom seem to drive these policies, rather than the demonstrated superiority of any particular approach. When the allograft is placed in an intraperitoneal location in infants and small children, the catheter typically is removed during transplant surgery [402, 404]. Later removal in patients receiving retroperitoneal transplants allows for use of PD post-transplant in cases of primary allograft non-function or early acute

rejection. Post-transplant ascites can also be drained if necessary using the PD catheter. When these problems are infrequently encountered in a centre, the PD catheter is more likely to be removed early. Because such problems typically occur during the first post-transplant days, if a patient is doing well there seems little reason to leave the catheter in place beyond the initial hospitalization [402, 403].

Patient and graft survival

A randomized comparison of PD and HD in children has not been performed. However, several series from single centres have compared outcomes following transplantation of paediatric HD and PD patients, and have found no significant differences in patient and graft survival rates [404, 405]. Reports of patient and graft survival rates >90% at 1 year among children maintained on PD prior to transplantation have become commonplace [402, 404, 406, 407].

Complications post-transplant related to PD

Peritonitis following transplantation is an infrequent complication, occurring in 1–11% of transplanted children [405, 408–410] in centres where PD catheters are routinely removed 2 weeks to 3 months post-transplant. No correlation has been found between the number of pretransplant peritonitis episodes and the incidence of post-transplant peritonitis [410]. Fever in an immuno-suppressed child with an indwelling PD catheter mandates a work-up for peritonitis. Management of post-transplant peritonitis has not been studied systematically. Most centres remove the PD catheter and treat with parenteral antibiotics.

Cellulitis of the PD catheter exit site and/or tunnel has occurred in some series more often than peritonitis [409, 411]. Recent treatment for acute rejection has been cited as a risk factor for PD catheter exit-site/tunnel infection. The care of the exit site post-transplant has not been studied. High rates of exit-site/tunnel infection have been reported by centres employing daily cleansing regimens using povidone-iodine [409, 411].

Post-transplant ascites occurs in up to one-third of paediatric PD patients [403]. Ascitic fluid volumes can be substantial and can result in uncomfortable abdominal distension, respiratory distress and traction on the incompletely healed transplant incision. The cause is unknown, although fluid loading post-transplant, especially in infants, may play a role [412]. Drainage may be required, but repeated drainage may contribute to re-formation of ascitic fluid.

Choice of HD or PD as a chronic renal replacement therapy in children

Renal transplantation has been widely recognized as the treatment of choice for children with ESRD. It can relieve the burden of continuous and repetitive treatments while simultaneously restoring the child to a virtually normal metabolic homeostasis and permit near-normal growth and development [413, 414]. Despite this preference for renal transplantation, large-scale registry data indicate that a large proportion of children with ESRD require a prolonged period of treatment with chronic dialysis. The choice of the optimum chronic dialysis modality, HD or PD, for the individual paediatric patient can be difficult.

There are few studies directly comparing the efficacy of chronic HD and PD in children, and those that have attempted to do so have either compared historically different patient groups or failed to randomly assign treatment modalities. The proposed advantages of HD include the minimal technical assistance required of the patient and family, decreased treatment times and the relative security associated with the long-term experience of successful HD treatment in children. The proposed advantages of PD include decreased dependence on the treatment centre, the ability to perform dialysis in the home, reduced dietary restrictions, easier control of hypertension, reduced r-HuEPO requirements, near-elimination of painful venipunctures and relatively easier adaptation for use in infants.

In one comparison of the two modalities in a single paediatric centre, PD appeared to be associated with lower transfusion rates, improved rehabilitation and better metabolic control [292], although these conclusions were subsequently disputed [415]. At present it is impossible to find convincing evidence that either form of dialysis is clearly preferable for the majority of children with ESRD, although clear preferences may exist in individual cases. More often, the choice of dialysis treatment is influenced by the preference of the centre or by its technical capabilities. Whenever possible, patient and family choice should be considered a major component to the ultimate success of either modality.

Congenital hyperammonaemia and other inborn errors of metabolism

Congential urea cycle enzymopathies are characterized by a reduced capacity to synthesize urea, which leads to accumulation of ammonium and other nitrogenous urea precursors [416]. Severely affected neonates develop vomiting, lethargy, seizures and coma within the first few days of life. The central nervous system symptomatology is thought to be primarily due to the effects of increased blood ammonium concentration. Emergency treatment is aimed at rapid and sustained removal of accumulated ammonium. Exchange transfusion, acute PD, haemofiltration (continuous arteriovenous haemofiltration/continuous venovenous haemofiltration [CAVH/CVVH]) and HD have all been employed [417, 419].

Haemodialysis is the most effective method for removal of ammonia, being at least 10 times more effective than PD [418, 420]. However, the institution of HD in small infants can be technically difficult. In some centres PD continues to be used for the treatment of infants with congenital hyperammonaemia. The superiority of PD over exchange transfusion in this setting has been demonstrated [421]. In studies performed in 53 episodes of hyperammonaemic coma, ammonium was removed more rapidly with PD than with exchange transfusion, and the rebound hyperammonaemia that followed treatment with exchange transfusion did not occur in babies treated with PD. Recently, the use of CAVH/CVVH has been shown to be particularly beneficial in the setting of hyperammonaemia. In one report ammonia clearance with CAVH exceeded that achieved with PD [422].

Intoxications

Treatment of intoxications in small children remains an important if infrequently tested area of expertise for the nephrologist who is likely to be consulted regarding the advisability of dialysis in these situations. For many years PD played an important role in the treatment of small children who had been poisoned with substances removable by dialysis [423]. However, the use of PD to treat intoxications in children has nearly disappeared in most centres. Several factors seem to be responsible for this phenomenon. Improvements in acute HD techniques and equipment specifically developed for use in small children have made HD the initial choice for intoxications. Haemoperfusion techniques and devices are also readily adapted for use in children of almost any size. Reliable percutaneous vascular access procedures and catheters designed for use in small children have become widely available. As a result of these and other developments, emergency HD is available for infants and children in paediatric dialysis centres throughout North America and Europe. Regardless of a patient's size, HD is many more times effective than PD at removing dialysable drugs and poisons [424, 425]. Peritoneal dialysis is an acceptable alternative only for those children too small to receive HD at the facility at which they are being treated, and too unstable to be safely transported to a paediatric dialysis centre for emergency HD.

References

1. Popovich RP, Moncrief JW, Decherd JW et al. The definition of a novel wearable/portable equilibrium dialysis technique. Trans Am Soc Artif Intern Organs 1976; 5: 64 (abstract).
2. Blackfan KD, Maxcy KF. The intraperitoneal injection of saline solution. Am J Dis Child 1918; 15: 19–28.
3. Bloxsum A, Powell N. The treatment of acute temporary dysfunction of the kidneys by peritoneal irrigation. Pediatrics 1948; 1: 52–7.
4. Swan H, Gordon HH. Peritoneal lavage in the treatment of anuria in children. Pediatrics 1949; 4: 586–95.
5. Odel HM, Ferris DO, Power MH. Peritoneal lavage as an effective means of extra-renal excretion. Am J Med 1950; 9: 63–77.
6. Maxwell MH, Rockney RB, Kleeman CR et al. Peritoneal dialysis: I. Technique and applications. JAMA 1959; 170: 917–24.
7. Segar WE, Gibson RK, Rhamy R. Peritoneal dialysis in infants and small children. Pediatrics 1961; 27: 602–13.
8. Ettledorf JN, Dobbins WT, Sweeney MJ et al. Intermittent peritoneal dialysis in the management of acute renal failure in children. J Pediatr 1962; 60: 327–39.
9. Segar WE. Peritoneal dialysis in the treatment of boric acid poisoning. N Engl J Med 1960; 262: 798–800.
10. Ettledorf NJ, Dobbins WT, Summit RL et al. Intermittent peritoneal dialysis using 5 per cent albumin in the treatment of salicylate intoxication in children. J Pediatr 1961; 58: 226–36.
11. Lloyd-Still JD, Atwell JD. Renal failure in infancy, with special reference to the use of peritoneal dialysis. J Pediatr Surg 1966; 1: 466–75.
12. Manley GL, Collip PJ. Renal failure in the newborn: treatment with peritoneal dialysis. Am J Dis Child 1968; 115: 107–10.
13. Lugo G, Ceballos R, Brown W et al. Acute renal failure in the neonate managed by peritoneal dialysis. Am J Dis Child 1969; 118: 655–9.
14. Gianantonio CA, Vitacco M, Mendelbarzee J et al. Acute renal failure in infancy and childhood. J Pediatr 1962; 61: 660–78.
15. Wiggelinkhuizen J. Peritoneal dialysis in children. S Afr Med J 1971; 45: 1047–54.
16. Day RE, White RHR. Peritoneal dialysis in children: review of 8 years' experience. Arch Dis Child 1977; 52: 56–61.
17. Chan JCM. Peritoneal dialysis for renal failure in childhood. Clin Pediatr 1978; 17: 349–54.
18. Feldman W, Baliah T, Drummond KN. Intermittent peritoneal dialysis in the management of chronic renal failure in children. Am J Dis Child 1968; 116: 30–6.
19. Palmer RA, Quinton WE, Gray JF et al. Prolonged peritoneal dialysis for chronic renal failure. Lancet 1964; 1: 700–2.
20. Palmer RA, Newell JE, Gray JF et al. Treatment of chronic renal failure by prolonged peritoneal dialysis. N Engl J Med 1966; 274: 248–54.
21. Tenckhoff H, Schecter H. A bacteriologically safe peritoneal access device. Trans Am Soc Artif Intern Organs 1966; 14: 181–6.
22. Boen ST, Mion CM, Curtin FK et al. Periodic peritoneal dialysis using the repeated puncture technique and an automated cycling machine. Trans Am Soc Artif Intern Organs 1964; 10: 409–14.
23. Tenckhoff H, Meston B, Shilipetar G. A simplified automatic peritoneal dialysis system. Trans Am Soc Artif Intern Organs 1972; 18: 436–40.
24. Counts S, Hickman R, Garbaccio A et al. Chronic home peritoneal dialysis in children. Trans Am Soc Artif Intern Organs 1973; 19: 157–67.
25. Hickman RO. Nine years' experience with chronic peritoneal dialysis in childhood. Dial Transplant 1978; 7: 803.
26. Brouhard BH, Berger M, Cunningham RJ et al. Home peritoneal dialysis in children. Trans Am Soc Artif Intern Organs 1979; 25: 90–4.
27. Baluarte HJ, Grossman MS, Polinsky MD et al. Experience with intermittent home peritoneal dialysis (IHPD) in children. Pediatr Res 1980; 14: 994 (abstract).
28. Lorentz WB, Hamilton RW, Disher B et al. Home peritoneal dialysis during infancy. Clin Nephrol 1981; 15: 194–7.
29. Potter DE, McDaid TK, Ramirez JA et al. Peritoneal dialysis in children. In: Atkins RC, Thomson NM, Farrell PC, eds. Peritoneal Dialysis. New York: Churchill Livingstone, 1981, pp. 356–61.
30. Oreopoulos DG, Katirtzoglou A, Arbus G et al. Dialysis and transplantation in young children (Letter). Brit Med J 1979; 1: 1628–9.
31. Balfe JW, Irwin MA. Continuous ambulatory peritoneal dialysis in children. In: Legrain, M, ed. Continuous Ambulatory Peritoneal Dialysis. Amsterdam: Excerpta Medica, 1980, pp. 131–6.
32. Alexander SR, Tseng CH, Maksym KA et al. Clinical parameters in continuous ambulatory peritoneal dialysis for infants and young children. In: Moncrief JW, Popovich RP, eds. CAPD Update. New York: Masson, 1981, pp. 195–209.
33. Kohaut ED. Continuous ambulatory peritoneal dialysis: a preliminary pediatric experience. Am J Dis Child 1981; 135: 270–1.
34. Potter DE, McDaid TK. McHenry K et al. Continuous ambulatory peritoneal dialysis (CAPD) in children. Trans Am Soc Artif Intern Organs 1981; 27: 64–7.
35. Salusky IB, Lucullo L, Nelson P et al. Continuous ambulatory peritoneal dialysis in children. Pediatr Clin N Am 1982; 29: 1005–12.
36. Guillot M, Clermont J-J, Gagnadoux M-F, Broyer M. Nineteen months' experience with continuous ambulatory peritoneal dialysis in children: main clinical and biological results. In: Gahl GM, Kessel M, Nolph KD, eds. Advances in Peritoneal Dialysis. Amsterdam: Excerpta Medica, 1981, pp. 203–7.
37. Eastham EJ, Kirplani H, Francis D et al. Pediatric continuous ambulatory peritoneal dialysis. Arch Dis Child 1982; 57: 677–80.
38. Alexander SR. Pediatric CAPD update – 1983. Perit Dial Bull 1983; 3 (suppl.): S15–22.
39. Price CG, Suki WN. Newer modifications of peritoneal dialysis: options in the treatment of patients with renal failure. Am J Nephrol 1980; 1: 97–104.
40. Alexander SR, Honda M. Continuous peritoneal dialysis for children: a decade of worldwide growth and development. Kidney Int 1993; 43 (suppl. 40): S65–74.
41. US Renal Data System. USRDS 1998 Annual Data Report, National Institutes of Health, National Institute of Diabetes and Digestive and Kidney Diseases, Bethesda, MD, April 1998, p. A3.
42. Hoffman JIE. Congenital heart disease. Pediatr Clin N Am 1990; 37: 25–44.
43. Poplack DG. Acute lymphoblastic leukemia. In: Pizzo PA, Poplack DG, eds. Principles and Practice of Pediatric Oncology. New York: Lippincott, 1989, p. 323.

44. Gusmano R, Perfumo F. Worldwide demographic aspects of chronic renal failure in children. Kidney Int 1993; 43 (suppl. 41): S31–5.

45. US Renal Data System. USRDS 1989 Annual Data Report, National Institutes of Health, National Institute of Diabetes and Digestive and Kidney Diseases, Bethesda, MD, August 1989.

46. North American Pediatric Renal Transplant Cooperative Study 1997 Annual Data Report. Potomac, MD: EMMES Corporation, May 1997, p. 75.

47. Rippe B, Stelin G. Simulations of peritoneal transport during CAPD. Application of two-pore formalism. Kidney Int 1989; 35: 1234–44.

48. Morgenstern B. Structure and function of the pediatric peritoneal membrane. In: Fine RN, Alexander SR, Warady BA, eds. CAPD/CCPD in Children. Norwell: Kluwer, 1998, pp. 73–85.

49. Gruskin AB, Cote ML, Baluarte HJ. Peritoneal diffusion curves, peritoneal clearances, and scaling factors in children of differing ages. Int J Pediatr Nephrol 1982; 3: 271–8.

50. Kohaut EC, Waldo FB, Benfield MR. The effect of changes in dialysate volume on glucose and urea equilibration. Perit Dial Int 1994; 14: 236–9.

51. Schroder CH, van Dreumel JM, Reddingius R et al. Peritoneal transport kinetics of glucose, urea, and creatinine during infancy and childhood. Perit Dial Int 1991; 12: 322–5.

52. Geary DF, Harvey EA, MacMillan JH et al. The peritoneal equilibration test in children. Kidney Int 1992; 42: 102–5.

53. Ellis EN, Watts K, Wells TG et al. Use of the peritoneal equilibration test in pediatric dialysis patients. Adv Perit Dial 1991; 7: 259–61.

54. Edefonti A, Picca M, Galato R et al. Evaluation of the peritoneal equilibration test in children on chronic peritoneal dialysis. Perit Dial Int 1993; 13 (suppl. 2): S260–2.

55. Mendley SR, Umans JG, Majkowski NL. Measurement of peritoneal dialysis delivery in children. Pediatr Nephrol 1993; 7: 284–9.

56. Hanna JD, Foreman JW, Gehr TWB et al. The peritoneal equilibration test in children. Pediatr Nephrol 1993; 7: 731–4.

57. Vonesh EF, Lysaght MJ, Moran J et al. Kinetic modeling as a prescription aid in peritoneal dialysis. Blood Purif 1991; 9: 246–70.

58. Morgenstern BZ, Pyle WK, Gurskin AB et al. Transport characteristics of the pediatric peritoneal membrane. Kidney Int 1984; 25: 259–64.

59. Geary DF, Harvey EA, Balfe JW. Mass transfer area coefficients in children. Perit Dial Int 1994; 14: 30–3.

60. Warady BA, Alexander SR, Hossli S et al. Peritoneal membrane transport function in children receiving long-term dialysis. J Am Soc Nephrol 1996; 7: 2385–91.

61. Morgenstern BZ. Equilibration testing: close but not quite right. Pediatr Nephrol 1993; 7: 290–1.

62. Schaefer F, Langenbeck D, Heckert KH et al. Evaluation of peritoneal solute transfer by the peritoneal equilibration test in children. Adv Perit Dial 1992; 8: 410–15.

63. Sliman GA, Klee KM, Gall-Holden B et al. Peritoneal equilibration test curves and adequacy of dialysis in children on automated peritoneal dialysis. Am J Kidney Dis 1994; 24: 813–18.

64. de Boer AW, van Schaijk TC, Willems HL et al. The necessity of adjusting dialysate volume to body surface area in pediatric peritoneal equilibration tests. Perit Dial Int 1997; 17: 199–202.

65. Schaefer F, Haraldsson B, Haas S et al. Estimation of peritoneal mass transport by three-pore model in children. Kidney Int 1998; 54: 1372–9.

66. Rippe B, Stelin G Haraldsson B. Computer simulations of peritoneal fluid transport in CAPD. Kidney Int 1991; 40: 315–25.

67. Rippe B. A three-pore model of peritoneal transport. Perit Dial Int 1993; 13 (suppl. 2): S35–8.

68. Pyle WK. Mass transfer in peritoneal dialysis. PhD dissertation, University of Texas, 1981.

69. Kohaut EC, Alexander SR. Ultrafiltration in the young patient on CAPD. In: Moncrief JW, Popovich RP, eds. CAPD Update. New York: Masson, 1981, pp. 221–6.

70. Balfe JW, Hanning RM, Vigneux A et al. A comparison of peritoneal water and solute movement in younger and older children on CAPD. In: Fine RN, Scharer K, Mehls O, eds. CAPD in Children. New York: Springer-Verlag, 1985, pp. 14–19.

71. Schaefer F, Fischbach M, Heckert KH et al. Hydrostatic intraperitoneal pressure in children on peritoneal dialysis. Perit Dial Int 1996; 16 (suppl. 2): S79 (abstract).

72. Mactier RA, Khanna R, Moore H et al. Kinetics of peritoneal dialysis in children: role of lymphatics. Kidney Int 1988; 34: 82–8.

73. Schröder CH, Reddingius RE, van Dreumel JA et al. Transcapillary ultrafiltration and lymphatic absorption during childhood continuous ambulatory peritoneal dialysis (CAPD). Nephrol Dial Transplant 1991; 6: 571–3.

74. Rippe B. Is lymphatic absorption important for ultrafiltration? Perit Dial Int 1995; 15: 203–4.

75. Leone MR, Jenkins RD, Golper TA et al. Early experience with continuous arteriovenous hemofiltration in critically ill pediatric patients. Crit Care Med 1986; 14: 1058–63.

76. Ronco C, Brendolan A, Bragantini L et al. Treatment of acute renal failure in newborns by continuous arteriovenous hemofiltration. Kidney Int 1986; 29: 908–15.

77. Day RE, White RHR. Peritoneal dialysis in children. Review of 8 years' experience. Arch Dis Child 1977; 52: 56–61.

78. Leumann EP, Knecht B, Dangel P et al. Peritoneal dialysis is newborns: Technical improvements. In: Bulla M, ed. Renal Insufficiency in Children. New York: Springer-Verlag, 1982, pp. 147–50.

79. Borzotta A, Harrison HL, Groff DB. Technique of peritoneal dialysis cannulation in neonates. Surg Gynecol Obstet 1983; 157: 73–4.

80. Murphy JLM, Reznik VM, Mendoza SA et al. Use of a guide wire inserted catheter for acute peritoneal dialysis. Int J Pediatr Nephrol 1987; 8: 199–202.

81. Lewis MA, Nycyk JA. Practical peritoneal dialysis – the Tenckhoff catheter in acute renal failure. Pediatr Nephrol 1992; 5: 715–7.

82. Sojo ET, Bisigniano L, Grosman M et al. Ten years' experience with CAPD catheters. In: Fine RN, Alexander SR, Warady BA (eds), CAPD/CCPD in children, 2nd ed. Kluwer Academic Publishers, Boston 1998: 263–79.

83. Nash MA, Russo JC. Neonatal lactic acidosis and renal failure: the role of peritoneal dialysis. J Pediatr 1977; 91: 101–5.

84. Lorentz WB. Acute hydrothorax during peritoneal dialysis. J Pediatr 1979; 94: 417–9.

85. Groshong T. Dialysis in infants and children. In: Van Stone JC, ed. Dialysis in the Treatment of Renal Insufficiency. New York: Grune & Stratten, 1983, pp. 234–6.

86. Posen GA, Luisello J. Continuous equilibration peritoneal dialysis in treatment of acute renal failure. Perit Dial Bull 1980; 1: 6–7.

87. Abbad FCB, Ploos van Amstel SLB. Continuous ambulatory peritoneal dialysis in small children with acute renal failure. Proc EDTA 1982; 19: 607–13.

88. Warady BA, Hebert D, Sullivan EK, Alexander SR, Tejani A. Renal transplantation, chronic dialysis, and chronic renal insufficiency in children and adolescents. The 1995 Annual Report of the North American Pediatric Renal Transplant Cooperative Study. Pediatr Nephrol 1997; 11: 49–64.

89. Alexander SR, Donaldson LA, Sullivan EK. CAPD/CCPD for children in North America: The NAPRTCS experience. In: Fine RN, Alexander SR, Warady BA, eds. CAPD/CCPD in Children, 2nd edn. Boston: Kluwer, 1998: 1–16.

90. Golper T, Churchill D, Burkhart J et al. Clinical Practice Guidelines for Peritoneal Dialysis Adequacy. National Kidney Foundation Dialysis Outcomes Quality Initiative. New York: National Kidney Foundation, 1997.

91. Alexander SR, Salusky IB, Warady BA *et al.* Peritoneal Dialysis Workshop: Pediatrics Recommendations. Perit Dial Int 1997; 17 (suppl. 3): S25–7.

92. Salusky IB, Holloway M. Selection of peritoneal dialysis for pediatric patients. Perit Dial Int 1997; 17 (suppl. 3): S35–7.

93. Lingens N, Soergel M, Loirat C *et al.* Ambulatory blood pressure monitoring in paediatric patients treated by regular haemodialysis and peritoneal dialysis. Pediatr Nephrol 1995; 9: 167–72.

94. Crompton CH, Balfe JW, Khoury A. Peritoneal dialysis in the prune belly syndrome. Perit Dial Int 1994; 14: 17–21.

95. Warady BA, Hellerstein S, Alon U. Advisability of initiating chronic peritoneal dialysis in the presence of a ventriculoperitoneal shunt (Letter). Pediatric Nephrol 1990; 4: 96.

96. Dunne S, Lewis S, Bonner P *et al.* Quality of life for spouses of CAPD patients. ANNA J 1994; 21: 237–46.

97. Reynolds JM, Postlethwaite RJ. Psychosocial burdens of dialysis treatment modalities: Do they differ and does it matter? Perit Dial Int 1996; 16 (suppl.): S548–50.

98. Kaiser BA, Polinsky MS, Stover J *et al.* Growth of children following the initiation of dialysis: a comparison of three modalities. Pediatr Nephrol 1994; 8: 733–8.

99. Furth SL, Powe NR, Hwang W *et al.* Does greater pediatric experience influence treatment choices in chronic disease management? Dialysis modality choice for children with end-stage renal disease. Arch Pediatr Adolesc Med 1997; 151: 545–50.

100. Furth SL, Powe NR, Hwang W *et al.* Racial differences in choice of dialysis modality for children with end-stage renal disease. Pediatrics 1997; 99: E6.

101. Twardowski ZJ, Nolph KD, Khanna R *et al.* Peritoneal equilibration test. Perit Dial Bull 1986; 7: 138–47.

102. Nielsen PK, Hemmingsen C, Friis SU *et al.* Comparison of straight and curled Tenckhoff peritoneal dialysis catheters implanted by percutaneous technique: a prospective randomized study. Perit Dial Int 1995; 15: 18–21.

103. Neu AM, Kohaut EC, Warady BA. Current approach to peritoneal access in North American children: a report of the Pediatric Peritoneal Dialysis Study Consortium. Adv Perit Dial 1995; 11: 289–292.

104. Twardowski ZJ, Nolph KD, Khanna R *et al.* The need for a 'swan neck' permanently bent, arcuate peritoneal dialysis catheter. Perit Dial Bull 1985; 4: 219–23.

105. Lindblad AS, Hamilton RW, Nolph KD *et al.* A retrospective analysis of catheter configuration and cuff type: a national CAPD registry report. Perit Dial Int 1988; 8: 129–33.

106. Lee HB, Park MS, Cha MK *et al.* The peritoneal access. Perit Dial Int 1996; 16 (suppl. 1): S322–6.

107. Diaz-Buxo J, Gessinger W. Single-cuff versus double-cuff Tenckhoff catheter. Perit Dial Bull 1984; 4 (suppl.): S100–2.

108. Kim D, Burke D, Izatt S *et al.* Single- or double-cuff peritoneal catheters? A prospective comparison. Trans Am Soc Artif Intern Organs 1984; 30: 232–5.

109. Mitwalli A, Kim D, Wu G *et al.* Single vs. double-cuff peritoneal catheters: a prospective controlled trial. Adv Perit Dial 1985; 1: 35–40.

110. Twardowski ZJ, Nolph KD, Khanna R *et al.* Computer interaction: catheters. Adv Perit Dial 1994; 10: 11–18.

111. Balfe JW, Vigneux A, Willumsen J *et al.* The use of CAPD in the treatment of children with end-stage renal disease. Perit Dial Bull 1981; 1: 35–8.

112. Vigneux A, Hardy BE, Balfe JW. Chronic peritoneal catheter in children – one or two dacron cuffs? Perit Dial Bull 1981; 1: 151.

113. Alexander SR, Tank ES. Surgical aspects of continuous ambulatory peritoneal dialysis in infants, children and adolescents. J Urol 1982; 127: 501–4.

114. Watson AR, Vigneux A, Hardy BE *et al.* Six-year experience with CAPD catheters in children. Perit Dial Bull 1985; 5: 119–22.

115. Watson AR, Vigneux A, Balfe JW *et al.* Chronic peritoneal catheters in a pediatric population. Adv Perit Dial 1985; 1: 41–4.

116. Warady BA, Jackson MA, Millspaugh J *et al.* Prevention and treatment of catheter-related infections in children. Perit Dial Bull 1987; 7: 34–36.

117. Verrina E, Bassi S, Perfumo F *et al.* Analysis of complications in a chronic peritoneal dialysis pediatric patient population. Perit Dial Int 1992; 13 (suppl. 3): S257–9.

118. Watkins S, Sullivan K. Risk factors for peritonitis in North American children receiving peritoneal dialysis. A Report of the North American Pediatric Renal Transplant Cooperative Study. 17th Annual Conference on Peritoneal Dialysis. Denver, Colorado, 1997.

119. Warady BA, Sullivan EK, Alexander SR. Lessons from the peritoneal dialysis patient database: A report of the North American Pediatric Renal Transplant Cooperative Study. Kidney Int 1996; 53 (suppl. 1) S68–71.

120. Lewis MA, Smith T, Postlethwaite RJ *et al.* A comparison of double-cuffed with single-cuffed Tenckhoff catheters in the prevention of infection in pediatric patients. Adv Perit Dial 1997; 13: 274–6.

121. Lewis MA, Smith T, Roberts D. Peritonitis, functional catheter loss and the sitting of the dacron cuff in chronic peritoneal dialysis catheters in children. Eur J Pediatr Surg 1996; 6: 285–7.

122. Rinaldi S, Sera F, Verrina E *et al.* The Italian Registry of Pediatric Chronic Peritoneal Dialysis: a ten-year experience with chronic peritoneal dialysis catheters. Perit Dial Int 1998; 18: 71–4.

123. Rugiu C, Lupo A, Bernich P *et al.* 14-year experience with the double-cuff straight Tenckhoff catheter. Perit Dial Int 1997; 17: 301–3.

124. Honda M. The Japanese experience with CAPD/CCPD in children. In: Fine RN, Alexander SR, Warady BA, eds. CAPD/CCPD in Children, 2nd edn. Boston: Kluwer, 1998, pp. 35–48.

125. Eklund BH, Honkanen EO, Kala AR *et al.* Catheter configuration and outcome in patients on continuous ambulatory peritoneal dialysis: a prospective comparison of two catheters. Perit Dial Int 1994; 14: 70–4.

126. Hymes LC, Clowers B, Mitchell C *et al.* Peritoneal catheter survival in children. Perit Dial Bull 1986; 6: 185–7.

127. Twardowski ZJ, Nichols WK, Nolph KD *et al.* Swan neck presternal ('bath tub') catheter for peritoneal dialysis. Adv Perit Dial 1992; 8: 316–24.

128. Sieniawska M, Roszkowska-Blaim M, Warchol S. Swan neck presternal catheter for continuous ambulatory peritoneal dialysis in children. Pediatr Nephrol 1993; 7: 557–8.

129. Sieniawska M, Roszkowska-Blaim M, Warchol S. Preliminary results with the swan neck presternal catheter for CAPD in children. Adv Perit Dial 1993; 9: 321–4.

130. Warchol S, Roszkowska-Blaim M, Sieniawska M. Swan neck presternal peritoneal dialysis catheter: Five-year experience in children. Perit Dial Int 1998; 18: 183–7.

131. Gokal R, Alexander S, Ash S *et al.* Peritoneal catheters and exit-site practices toward optimum peritoneal access: 1998 Update. Perit Dial Int 1998; 18: 11–33.

132. Cruz C. Implantation techniques for peritoneal dialysis catheters. Perit Dial Int 1996; 16 (suppl. 1): S319–21.

133. Lewis S, Prowant B, Douglas C *et al.* Nursing practice related to peritoneal catheter exit site care and infections. ANNA J 1996; 23: 609–15.

134. Khanna R, Nolph K, Oreopoulos D. Peritoneal access: the essentials of peritoneal dialysis. Boston: Kluwer, 1993.

135. Helfrich GB, Pechan BW, Alijani MR *et al.* Reduction of catheter complications with lateral placement. Perit Dial Bull 1983; 3 (suppl. 4): S2–4.

136. Stegmayr B, Hedberg B, Sandzen B *et al.* Absence of leakage by insertion of peritoneal dialysis catheter through the rectus muscle. Perit Dial Int 1990; 10: 53–5.

137. Stegmayr BG, Wikdahl AM, Arnerlov C *et al.* A modified lateral technique for the insertion of peritoneal dialysis catheters enabling immediate start of dialysis. Perit Dial Int 1998; 18: 329–31.

138. Bennett-Jones DN, Martin J, Barratt AJ et al. Prophylactic gentamicin in the prevention of early exit-site infections and peritonitis in CAPD. Adv Perit Dial 1988; 4: 147–50.

139. Sardegna K, Beck AM, Strife CF. Evaluation of perioperative antibiotics at the time of dialysis catheter placement. Pediatr Nephrol 1998; 12: 149–52.

140. Twardowski ZJ, Prowant BF. Exit-site healing post catheter implantation. Perit Dial Int 1996; 16 (suppl. 3): S51–70.

141. Prowant BF, Warady BA, Nolph KD. Peritoneal dialysis catheter exit-site care: results of an international survey. Perit Dial Int 1993; 13: 149–54.

142. Lewis M, Webb N, Smith T *et al.* Routine omentectomy is not required in children undergoing chronic peritoneal dialysis. Adv Perit Dial 1995; 11: 293–5.

143. Khanna R, Twardowski ZJ. Peritoneal catheter exit site (Editorial). Perit Dial Int 1988; 8: 119–23.

144. Harvey E, Braj B, Balfe JW. Prevention, diagnosis and treatment of PD catheter exit-site and tunnel infections in children. In: Fine RN, Alexander SR, Warady BA, eds. CAPD/CCPD in Children, 2nd edn. Boston: Kluwer, 1998, pp. 349–68.

145. Breborowicz A, Oreopoulos DG. Recent developments in peritoneal dialysis solutions. Perit Dial Int 1997; 17: 9–10.

146. Gokal R. Peritoneal dialysis solutions: Nutritional aspects. Perit Dial Int 1997; 17 (suppl. 3): S69–72.

147. Hutchison AJ, Gokal R. Improved solutions for peritoneal dialysis: physiological calcium solutions, osmotic agents and buffers. Kidney Int 1992; 38 (suppl.): S153–9.

148. Topley N. *In vitro* biocompatibility of bicarbonate-based peritoneal dialysis solutions. Perit Dial Int 1997; 17: 42–7.

149. Coles GA, Gokal R, Ogg C *et al.* A randomized controlled trial of a bicarbonate- and a bicarbonate/lactate-containing dialysis solution in CAPD. Perit Dial Int 1997; 17: 48–51.

150. Feriani M, Carobi C, La Greca G *et al.* Clinical experience with a 39 mmol/L bicarbonate-buffered peritoneal dialysis solution. Perit Dial Int 1997; 17: 17–21.

151. Schambye HT, Pedersen FB, Wang P. Bicarbonate is not the ultimate answer to the biocompatibility problems of CAPD solutions: a cytotoxicity test of CAPD solutions and effluents. Adv Perit Dial 1992; 8: 42–6.

152. Schambye HT, Pedersen FB, Christensen HK *et al.* The cytotoxicity of continuous ambulatory peritoneal dialysis solutions with different bicarbonate/lactate ratios. Perit Dial Int 1993; 13 (suppl. 2): S116–18.

153. Peers E, Gokal R. Icodextrin: overview of clinical experience. Perit Dial Int 1997; 17: 22–6.

154. Wilkie ME, Brown CB. Polyglucose solutions in CAPD. Perit Dial Int 1997; 17 (suppl. 2): S47–50.

155. Wilkie ME, Plant MJ, Edwards L *et al.* Icodextrin 7.5% dialysate solution (glucose polymer) in patients with ultrafiltration failure: extension of CAPD technique survival. Perit Dial Int 1997; 17: 84–7.

156. Krediet RT, Ho-dac-Pannekeet MM, Imholz AL *et al.* Icodextrin's effects on peritoneal transport. Perit Dial Int 1997; 17: 35–41.

157. Lam-Po-Tang MK-L, Bending MR, Kwan JT. Icodextrin hypersensitivity in a CAPD patient. Perit Dial Int 1997; 17: 82–4.

158. Rippe B, Simonsen O, Wieslander A *et al.* Clinical and physiological effects of a new, less toxic and less acidic fluid for peritoneal dialysis. Perit Dial Int 1997; 17: 27–34.

159. Hutchison AJ, Freemont AJ, Boulton HF *et al.* Low-calcium dialysis fluid and oral calcium carbonate in CAPD. A method of controlling hyperphosphataemia whilst minimizing aluminum exposure and hypercalcaemia. Nephrol Dial Transplant 1992; 7: 1219–25.

160. Bro S, Brandi L, Daugaard H *et al.* Calcium concentration in the CAPD dialysate: what is optimal and is there a need to individualize? Perit Dial Int 1997; 17: 554–9.

161. Sieniawska M, Roszkowska-Blaim M, Wojciechowska B. The influence of dialysate calcium concentration on the PTH level in children undergoing CAPD. Perit Dial Int 1996; 16 (suppl. 1): S567–9.

162. Ritz E, Passlick-Deetjen J, Zeier M *et al.* Prescription of calcium concentration and PTH control. Perit Dial Int 1996; 16 (suppl. 1): S300–4.

163. Hutchison AJ. Serum magnesium and end-stage renal disease. Perit Dial Int 1997; 17: 327–9.

164. Navarro J, Mora C, Garcia M *et al.* Hypermagnesemia in CAPD: relationship with parathyroid hormone levels. Perit Dial Int 1998; 18: 77–80.

165. Burkart JM, Schreiber M, Korbet SM *et al.* Solute clearance approach to adequacy of peritoneal dialysis. Perit Dial Int 1996; 16: 457–70.

166. Blake P, Burkart JM, Churchill DN *et al.* Recommended clinical practices for maximizing peritoneal dialysis clearances. Perit Dial Int 1996; 16: 448–56.

167. Rocco MV. Body surface area limitations in achieving adequate therapy in peritoneal dialysis patients. Perit Dial Int 1996; 16: 617–22.

168. Fischbach M, Terzic J, Becmeur F *et al.* Relationship between intraperitoneal hydrostatic pressure and dialysate volume in children on PD. Adv Perit Dial 1996; 12: 330–4.

169. Ferber J, Schärer K, Schaefer F *et al.* Residual renal function in children on haemodialysis and peritoneal dialysis therapy. Pediatr Nephrol 1994; 8: 579–83.

170. Canada–USA (CANUSA) Peritoneal Dialysis Study Group. Adequacy of dialysis and nutrition in continuous peritoneal dialysis: association with clinical outcomes. J Am Soc Nephrol 1996; 7: 198–207.

171. Lutes R, Perlmutter J, Holley JL *et al.* Loss of residual renal function in patients on peritoneal dialysis. Adv Perit Dial 1993; 9: 165–8.

172. Schaefer F, Haraldsson B, Haas S *et al.* Estimation of peritoneal mass transport by three-pore model in children. Kidney Int 1998; 54: 1372–79.

173. Verrina E, Amici G, Perfumo F *et al.* The use of the PD Adequest mathematical model in pediatric patients on chronic peritoneal dialysis. Perit Dial Int 1998; 18: 322–8.

174. Warady BA, Watkins S, Andreoli S *et al.* Assessment of kinetic modeling in children receiving peritoneal dialysis (PD): a report of the Pediatric Peritoneal Dialysis Study Consortium (PPDSC). J Am Soc Nephrol 1998; 9: 303A (abstract).

175. Warady BA. The use of the peritoneal equilibration test to modify peritoneal dialysis modality in children. Semin Dial 1994; 7: 403–8.

176. Warady BA, Alexander SR, Hossli S *et al.* Peritoneal membrane transport function in children receiving long-term dialysis. J Am Soc Nephrol 1996; 7: 2385–91.

177. Schaefer F. Adequacy of peritoneal dialysis in children. In: Fine RN, Alexander SR, Warady BA, eds. CAPD/CCPD in Children. Norwell: Kluwer, 1998, pp. 99–118.

178. Reznick VM, Lorr EJ, Collins M *et al.* The acute peritoneal equilibration test (APEX): optimizing acute peritoneal dialysis in children. Perit Dial Int 1993; 13 (suppl. 1): S65.

179. Fischbach M, Lahlou A, Eyer D *et al.* Determination of individual ultrafiltration time (APEX) and purification phosphate time (PPT) by peritoneal equilibration test (PPT). Application to individual peritoneal dialysis modality prescription in children. Perit Dial Int 1996; 16: S557–60.

180. Waniewski J, Heimburger D, Werynski A *et al.* Aqueous solute concentrations and evaluation of mass transport coefficients in peritoneal dialysis. Nephrol Dial Transplant 1992; 7: 50–6.

181. Fukuda M, Kawamura K, Okawa T *et al.* The peritoneal equilibration test variables in pediatric CAPD patients. Acta Paediatr Jpn 1994; 36: 57–61.

182. Haraldsson B. Assessing the peritoneal dialysis capacities of individual patients. Kidney Int 1995; 47: 1187–98.

183. Gotch FA, Sargent JA. A mechanistic analysis of the National Cooperative Dialysis Study (NCDS). Kidney Int 1985; 28: 526–34.

184. Chen HH, Shetty A, Afthentopoulos IE *et al.* Discrepancy between weekly *Kt/V* and weekly creatinine clearance in patients on CAPD. Adv Perit Dial 1995; 11: 83–7.

185. Verrina E, Alessandra B, Gusmano R *et al.* Chronic renal replacement therapy in children: which index is best for adequacy? Kidney Int 1998; 54: 1690–6.

186. Wühl E, Fusch C, Schärer K *et al.* Assessment of total body water in paediatric patients on dialysis. Nephrol Dial Transplant 1996; 11: 75–80.

187. Cheek DB, Mellits D, Elliott D. Body water, height, and weight during growth in normal children. Am J Dis Child 1966; 112: 312–17.

188. Churchill DN, Thorpe KE, Nolph KD *et al.* Increased peritoneal membrane transport is associated with decreased patient and technique survival for continuous peritoneal dialysis patients. J Am Soc Nephrol 1998; 9: 1285–92.

189. Heimburger O, Stenvinkel P, Berglund L *et al.* Increased plasma lipoprotein (a) in continuous ambulatory peritoneal dialysis is related to peritoneal transport of proteins and glucose. Nephron 1996; 72: 135–44.

190. Vonesh EF, Burkart J, McMurray SD *et al.* Peritoneal dialysis kinetic modeling: validation in a multicenter clinical study. Perit Dial Int 1996; 16: 471–81.

191. Nelson P, Stoker J. Principles of nutritional assessment and management of the child with ESRD. In: Fine RN, Gruskin AB, eds. End Stage Renal Disease in Children. Philadelphia: WB Saunders, 1984, pp. 209–26.

192. Hellerstein S, Holliday MA, Grupe WE *et al.* Nutritional management of children with chronic renal failure. Summary of the task force on nutritional management of children with chronic renal failure. Pediatr Nephrol 1987; 1: 195–211.

193. Salusky IB. Nutritional management of pediatric patients on chronic dialysis. In: Nissenson AR, Fine RN, Gentile DE, eds. Clinical Dialysis, 3rd edn. Norwalk: Appleton & Lange, 1995, pp. 535–48.

194. Hanning RH, Balfe JW, Zlotkin SH. Effectiveness and nutritional consequences of amino acid-based vs. glucose-based dialysis solutions in infants and children receiving CAPD. Am J Clin Nutr 1987; 46: 22–30.

195. Blumenkrantz MJ, Schmidt RW. Nutritional management of the CAPD patient. Perit Dial Bull 1981; 1: 22–4.

196. National Research Council. Recommended Dietary Allowances, 10th edn. Washington, DC: National Academy Press, 1989, pp. 1–284.

197. Salusky IB, Fine RN, Nelson P *et al.* Nutritional status of children undergoing continuous peritoneal dialysis. Am J Clin Nutr 1983; 38: 599–611.

198. Wassner SJ, Abitbol C, Alexander S *et al.* Nutritional requirements for infants with renal failure. Am J Kidney Dis 1986; 7: 300–5.

199. Kopple JD, Jones MR, Keshaviah *et al.* A proposed glossary for dialysis kinetics. Am J Kidney Dis 1995; 26: 963–81.

200. Mellits ED, Cheek DB. The assessment of body water and fatness from infancy to adulthood. Monogr Soc Res Child Dev 1970; 35: 12–26.

201. Elias RA, McArdle AH, Gagnon RF. The effectiveness of protein supplementation on the nutritional management of patients on CAPD. Adv Perit Dial 1989; 5: 177–80.

202. Buchwald R, Pena JC. Evaluation of nutritional status in patients on continuous ambulatory peritoneal dialysis (CAPD). Perit Dial Int 1989; 9: 295–301.

203. Querfeld U, Salusky IB, Nelson P *et al.* Hyperlipidemia in pediatric patients undergoing peritoneal dialysis. Pediatr Nephrol 1988; 2: 447–52.

204. Scolnik D, Balfe JW. Initial hypoalbuminemia and hyperlipidemia persist during chronic peritoneal dialysis in children. Perit Dial Int 1993; 13: 136–9.

205. Lifshitz F, Moses N. A complication of dietary treatment of hypercholesterolemia. Am J Dis Child 1989; 143: 537–42.

206. Workshop Proceedings. An evaluation of the 1990 Canadian Nutrition Recommendations for total fat/saturated fat intake for children between the ages of 12 and 18 years. In: Kubow S, ed. Workshop Proceedings. An evaluation of the 1990 Canadian Nutrition Requirements for Total Fat/Saturated Fat Intake for Children Between the Ages of 2 and 18 years. Kush Medical Communications, McGill University, 1990, pp. 1–52.

207. Warady BA, Borum P, Stall C *et al.* Carnitine status of pediatric patients on continuous ambulatory peritoneal dialysis. Am J Nephrol 1990; 10: 109–14.

208. Murakami R, Momota T, Yoshiya K *et al.* Serum carnitine and nutritional status in children treated with continuous ambulatory peritoneal dialysis. J Pediatr Gastroenterol Nutr 1990; 11: 371–4.

209. Tamura T, Vaughn WH, Waldo FB *et al.* Zinc and copper balance in children on continuous ambulatory peritoneal dialysis. Pediatr Nephrol 1989; 3: 309–13.

210. Zlotkin SH, Rundle MA, Hanning RM *et al.* Zinc absorption from the glucose and amino acid dialysates in children on continuos ambulatory peritoneal dialysis (CAPD). J Am Coll Nutr 1987; 6: 345–50.

211. Detsky AS, McLaughlin JR, Baker JP *et al.* What is subjective global assessment of nutritional status? J Parenter Enteral Nutr 1987; 11: 8–13.

212. Lindholm B, Bergstrom J. Nutritional aspects on peritoneal dialysis. Kidney Int Suppl 1992; 38: S165–71.

213. Schmidt R, Dumler F, Cruz C *et al.* Improved nutritional follow-up of peritoneal dialysis patients with bioelectrical impedance. Adv Perit Dial 1992; 8: 157–9.

214. Forbes GB, Bruning GJ: Urinary creatinine excretion and lean body mass. Am J Clin Nutr 1976; 29: 1359–66.

215. Levin L, Balfe JW, Geary D *et al.* Gastrostomy tube feeding in children on CAPD. Perit Dial Bull 1987; 7: 223–6.

216. Balfe JW, Secker DJ, Coulter PE *et al.* Tube feeding in children on chronic peritoneal dialysis. Adv Perit Dial 1990; 6: 257–61.

217. O'Regan S, Garel L. Percutaneous gastrojejunostomy for caloric supplementation in children on peritoneal dialysis. Adv Perit Dial 1990; 6: 273–5.

218. Warady BA, Kriley M, Belden B *et al.* Nutritional and behavioral aspects of nasogastric tube feedings in infants receiving chronic peritoneal dialysis. Adv Perit Dial 1990; 6: 265–8.

219. Wood EG, Bunchman TE, Khurana R *et al.* Complications of nasogastric and gastrostomy tube feeding in infants receiving chronic peritoneal dialysis. Adv Perit Dial 1990; 6: 162–4.

220. Brewer ED. Growth of small children managed with chronic peritoneal dialysis and nasogastric tube feedings: 203 months experience in 14 patients. Adv Perit Dial 1990; 6: 269–72.

221. Garel L, O'Regan S. Percutaneous gastrojejunostomy for enteral alimentation in children on chronic cycler peritoneal dialysis. Adv Perit Dial 1988; 4: 79–83.

222. Kamen RS. Impaired development of oral-motor functions required for normal oral feeding as a consequence of tube feeding during infancy. Adv Perit Dial 1990; 6: 276–8.

223. Dombros N, Oren A, Marliss E *et al.* Plasma amino acid profiles and amino acid losses in patients undergoing CAPD. Perit Dial Bull 1982; 2: 27–32.

224. Hanning RH, Balfe JW, Zlotkin SH. Effect of amino acid-containing dialysis solutions on plasma amino acid profiles in children with chronic renal failure. J Pediatr Gastroenterol Nutr 1987; 307: 1537–42.

225. Canepa A, Perfumo F, Carrea A *et al.* Long-term effect of amino-acid dialysis solution in children on continuous ambulatory peritoneal dialysis. Pediatr Nephrol 1991; 5: 215–9.

226. Honda M, Kamiyama Y, Hasegawa O et al. Effects of short-term essential amino acid-containing dialysate in young children on CAPD. Perit Dial Int 1991; 11: 76–80.

227. Young GA, Dibble JB, Hobson SM et al. The use of an amino acid-based CAPD fluid over 12 weeks. Nephrol Dial Transplant 1989; 4: 285–92.

228. Dombros N, Prutis K, Tong N et al. Six-month overnight intraperitoneal amino-acid infusion in continuous ambulatory peritoneal dialysis (CAPD) patients – no effect on nutritional status. Perit Dial Int 1990; 10: 79–84.

229. Qamar IU, Levin L, Balfe JW et al. Effects of three month amino acid dialysis compared to dextrose dialysis in children on CAPD. Perit Dial Int 1994; 14: 34–41.

230. Kopple JD, Bernard D, Messana J et al. Treatment of malnourished CAPD patients with an amino acid based dialysate. Kidney Int 1995; 47: 1148–57.

231. Stein A, Moorhouse J, Iles-Smith H et al. Role of an improvement in acid-base status and nutrition in CAPD patients. Kidney Int 1997; 52: 1089–95.

232. Jones M, Hagen T, Algrim-Boyle C et al. Treatment of malnutrition with 1.1% amino acid peritoneal dialysis solution: Results of a multicenter outpatient study. Am J Kidney Dis 1998; 32: 761–9.

233. Ikizler TA, Wingard R, Flakoll P et al. Effects of recombinant human growth hormone on plasma and dialysate amino acid profiles in CAPD patients. Kidney Int 1996; 50: 229–34.

234. Becker N, Brandt JR, Sutherland TA et al. Improved outcome of young children on nightly automated peritoneal dialysis. Pediatr Nephrol 1997; 11: 676–9.

235. Alexander SR. CAPD in infants less than one year of age. In: Fine RN, Gruskin AB, eds. End Stage Renal Disease in Children. Philadelphia: WB Saunders, 1984, pp. 149–71.

236. Kohaut EC. Growth in children with end-stage renal disease treated with continuous ambulatory peritoneal dialysis for at least one year. Perit Dial Bull 1982; 2: 159–61.

237. Watson AR, Taylor J, Balfe JW. Growth in children on CAPD: a reappraisal. Adv Perit Dial 1985; 1: 171–7.

238. Warady BA, Stall C, Paulsen J et al. A unique approach to peritoneal dialysis in infants. Am J Kidney Dis 1986; 7: 235–40.

239. Kohaut EC, Welchel J, Waldo FB et al. Aggressive therapy of infants with renal failure. Pediatr Nephrol 1987; 1: 150–3.

240. Fine RN. Renal transplantation of the infant and young child and the use of pediatric cadaver kidneys for transplantation in pediatric and adult populations. Am J Kidney Dis 1988; 12: 1–10.

241. Warady BA, Kriley M, Lovell H et al. Growth and development of infants with end-stage renal disease receiving long-term peritoneal dialysis. J Pediatr 1988; 112: 714–9.

242. Tapper D, Watkins S, Burns M et al. Comprehensive management of renal failure in infants. Arch Surg 1990; 125: 1276–81.

243. Qamar IU, Balfe JW. Experience with chronic peritoneal dialysis in infants. Child Nephrol Urol 1991; 11: 159–64.

244. Ellis EN, Pearson D, Champion B et al. Outcome of infants on chronic peritoneal dialysis. Adv Perit Dial 1995; 11: 266–9.

245. Verrina E, Zacchello G, Perfumo F et al. Clinical experience in the treatment of infants with chronic peritoneal dialysis. Adv Perit Dial 1995; 11: 281–4.

246. Honda M, Kamiyama Y, Kawamura K et al. Growth, development and nutritional status in Japanese children under 2 years on continuous ambulatory peritoneal dialysis. Pediatr Nephrol 1995; 9: 543–8.

247. Holtta TM, Ronnholm KA, Jalanko H et al. Peritoneal dialysis in children under 5 years of age. Perit Dial Int 1997; 17: 573–80.

248. Turenne MN, Port FK, Strawderman RL et al. Growth rates in pediatric dialysis patients and renal transplant recipients. Am J Kidney Dis 1997; 30: 193–203.

249. Wuhl E, Haffner D, Nissel R et al. Short dialyzed children respond less to growth hormone than patients prior to dialysis. Pediatr Nephrol 1996; 10: 294–8.

250. Polinsky MS, Kaiser BA, Stover JB et al. Neurologic development of children with severe chronic renal failure from infancy. Pediatr Nephrol 1987; 1: 157–65.

251. Tagge EP, Campbell DAJ, Dafoe DC et al. Pediatric renal transplantation with an emphasis on the prognosis of patients with chronic renal insufficiency since infancy. Surgery 1987; 102: 692–8.

252. Warady BA, Belden B, Kohaut E. Neurodevelopmental outcome of children initiating peritoneal dialysis in early infancy. Pediatr Nephrol 1998 (in press).

253. Jaramillo-Solorio RM, Menodoza-Guevara L, Garcia-Lopez E. Intellectual output of children with chronic renal failure on continuous ambulatory peritoneal dialysis. Perit Dial Int 1996; 16 (suppl. 1): S554–6.

254. Salusky IB. The nutritional approach for pediatric patients undergoing CAPD/CCPD. Adv Perit Dial 1990; 6: 245–51.

255. Kohaut EC. Nutrition in the pediatric ESRD patient on peritoneal dialysis. Perit Dial Int 1997; 17 (suppl. 3): S67–8.

256. Warady BA, Kriley M, Alon U et al. Vitamin status of infants receiving long-term peritoneal dialysis. Pediatr Nephrol 1994; 8: 354–6.

257. Kriley M, Warady BA. Vitamin status of pediatric patients receiving long-term peritoneal dialysis. Am J Clin Nutr 1991; 53: 1476–9.

258. Warady BA, Koch M, O'Neal DW et al. Plasma fluoride concentration in infants receiving long-term peritoneal dialysis. J Pediatr 1989; 115: 436–9.

259. Ruley EJ, Bock GH, Kerzner B et al. Feeding disorders and gastroesophageal reflux in infants with chronic renal failure. Pediatr Nephrol 1989; 3: 424–9.

260. Paulson WD, Bock GH, Nelson AP et al. Hyponatremia in the very young chronic peritoneal dialysis patient. Am J Kidney Dis 1989; 14: 196–9.

261. Bunchman TE. Chronic dialysis in the infant less than 1 year of age. Pediatr Nephrol 1995; 9 (suppl.): S18–22.

262. Roodhooft AM, Van Hoeck KJ, Van Acker KJ. Hypophosphatemia in infants on continuous ambulatory peritoneal dialysis. Clin Nephrol 1990; 34: 131–5.

263. Morgenstern BZ. Peritoneal equilibration in children. Perit Dial Int 1996; 16 (suppl. 1): S532–9.

264.. Geary DF. Performance and interpretation of the peritoneal equilibration test in children. Perit Dial Int 1996; 16 (suppl. 1): S540–2.

265. Ramage I, Bradbury MG, Braj B et al. Early continuous cycling peritoneal dialysis failure in infants: rescue tidal peritoneal dialysis. Perit Dial Int 1998; 18: 437–40.

266. Aguilar A, Mendoza L, Morales AM et al. Disconnect systems in children undergoing continuous ambulatory peritoneal dialysis. Transplant Proc 1996; 28: 3388.

267. Katz A, Kashtan CE, Greenberg LJ et al. Hypogammaglobulinemia in uremic infants receiving peritoneal dialysis. J Pediatr 1990; 117: 258–61.

268. Kuizon B, Melocoton TL, Holloway M et al. Infectious and catheter-related complications in pediatric patients treated with peritoneal dialysis at a single institution. Pediatr Nephrol 1995; 9 (suppl.): S12–17.

269. Neu AM, Warady BA, Lederman HM et al. Hypogammaglobulinemia in infants and young children maintained on peritoneal dialysis. Perit Dial Int 1998; 18: 440–3.

270. Verrina E, Perfumo F, Zacchello G et al. Comparison of patient hospitalization in chronic peritoneal dialysis and hemodialysis: a pediatric multicenter study. Perit Dial Int 1996; 16 (suppl. 1): S574–7.

271. Neu AM, Warady BA. Special considerations in the care of the infant CAPD/CCPD patient. In: Fine RN, Alexander SR, Warady BA, eds. CAPD/CCPD in Children, 2nd edn. Boston: Kluwer, 1998, pp. 169–82.

272. Brodehl J, Offner G, Pichlmayr R *et al.* Kidney transplantation in infants and young children. Transplant Proc 1986; XVIII (4 suppl. 3): 8–11.

273. Koffman CG, Rigden SP, Bewick M *et al.* Renal transplantation in children less than five years of age. Transplant Proc 1989; 21: 2001–2.

274. Nevins TE. Transplantation in infants less that 1 year of age. Pediatr Nephrol 1987; 1: 154–6.

275. Kalia A, Brouhard BH, Travis LB *et al.* Renal transplantation in the infant and young child. Am J Dis Child 1988; 142: 47–50.

276. McMahon Y, MacDonell RC, Richie RE *et al.* Is kidney transplantation in the very small child (<10 kg) worth it? Transplant Proc 1989; 21: 2003–5.

277. Nevins T. Treatment of very young infants with ESRD–renal transplantation as soon as possible (< 1 yr of age): controversy. Adv Perit Dial 1990; 6: 283–5.

278. Najarian JS, Frey DJ, Matas AJ *et al.* Successful kidney transplantation in Infants. Transplant Proc 1991; 23: 1382–3.

279. MacDonald H. Chronic renal disease: the mother's experience. Pediatr Nurs 1995; 21: 503–7, 574.

280. Geary DF. Attitudes of pediatric nephrologists to management of end-stage renal disease in infants. J Pediatr 1998; 133: 154–6.

281. Cohen C. Ethical and legal considerations in the care of the infant with end-stage renal disease whose parents elect conservative therapy. An American perspective. Pediatr Nephrol 1987; 1: 166–71.

282. Bunchman TE. The ethics of infant dialysis. Perit Dial Int 1996; 16 (suppl.): S505–8.

283. Eschbach JW, Abdulhadi MH, Browne JK *et al.* Recombinant human erythropoietin in anemic patients with end-stage renal disease: results of a phase III multicenter clinical trial. Ann Intern Med 1989; 111: 992–1000.

284. Winearls CG, Oliver DO, Pippard MJ *et al.* Effect of human erythropoietin derived from recombination DNA on the anemia of patients maintained by chronic hemodialysis. Lancet 1986; 2: 1175–8.

285. Bennett W. A multicenter clinical trial of Epoetin beta for anemia of end-stage renal disease. J Am Soc Nephrol 1991; 1: 990–8.

286. Sinai-Trieman L, Salusky IB, Fine RN. Use of subcutaneous recombinant human erythropoietin in children undergoing continuous cycling peritoneal dialysis. J Pediatr 1989; 114: 550–4.

287. Warady BA, Sabath RJ, Smith CA *et al.* Recombinant human erythropoietin in pediatric patients receiving long-term peritoneal dialysis. Pediatr Nephrol 1991; 5: 718–23.

288. Alexander SR. Pediatric uses of recombinant human erythropoietin: the outlook in 1991. Am J Kidney Dis 1991; 18 (suppl. 1): 42–53.

289. Evans RW, Rader B, Manninen DL. The quality of life of hemodialysis recipients treated with recombinant human erythropoietin. JAMA 1990; 263: 825–30.

290. Canadian Erythropoietin Study Group. Association between recombinant human erythropoietin and quality of life and exercise capacity of patients receiving hemodialysis. Br Med J 1990; 300: 573–8.

291. Eschbach JW. The anemia of chronic renal failure: pathophysiology and the effects of recombinant erythropoietin. Kidney Int 1989; 35: 134–48.

292. Baum M, Powell D, Calvin S *et al.* Continuous ambulatory peritoneal dialysis in children: Comparison with hemodialysis. N Engl J Med 1982; 307: 1537–42.

293. Chavers BM, Sullivan EK, Tejani A *et al.* Pre-transplant blood transfusion and renal allograft outcome: a report of the North American Pediatric Renal Transplant Cooperative Study. Pediatr Transplant 1997; 1: 122–8.

294. Grimm PC, Sinai-Trieman L, Sekiya NM *et al.* Effects of recombinant human erythropoietin on HLA sensitization and cell mediated immunity. Kidney Int 1990; 38: 12–18.

295. Rizzoni G, Broyer M, Guest G *et al.* Growth retardation in children with chronic renal disease: scope of the problem. Am J Kidney Dis 1986; 7: 256–61.

296. French CB, Genei M. Pathophysiology of growth failure in chronic renal insufficiency. Kidney Int 1984; 30: S59–64.

297. Stefanidis CJ, Koulieri A, Siapera D *et al.* Effect of correction of anemia with recombinant human erythropoietin on growth of children treated with CAPD. Adv Perit Dial 1992; 8: 460–3.

298. Fennell RS, Rasbury WC, Fennell EB *et al.* Effects of kidney transplantation on cognitive performance in a pediatric population. Pediatrics 1984; 74: 273–8.

299. Temple RM, Deary IJ, Winney RJ. Recombinant erythropoietin improves cognitive function in patients maintained in patients on chronic ambulatory peritoneal dialysis. Nephrol Dial Transplant 1995; 10: 1733–8.

300. Montini G, Zacchello G, Baraldi E *et al.* Benefits and risks of anemia correction with recombinant human erythropoietin in children maintained by hemodialysis. J Pediatr 1990; 117: 556–60.

301. Ulmer HE, Greiner H, Schuller HW *et al.* Cardiovascular impairment and physical working capacity in children with chronic renal failure. Acta Pediatr Scand 1987; 67: 43–9.

302. Jabs K, Harmon WE. Recombinant human erythropoietin therapy in children on dialysis. Adv Renal Replace Ther 1996; 3: 24–36.

303. Jabs K, Harmon W. Anemia and its treatment in children on CAPD/CCPD. In: Fine RN, Alexander SR, Warady BA, eds. CAPD/CCPD in Children, 2nd edn. Boston: Kluwer, 1998, pp. 183–98.

304. NKF-DOQI clinical practice guidelines for the treatment of anemia of chronic renal failure. National Kidney Foundation Dialysis Outcomes Quality Initiative. Am J Kidney Dis 1997; 30 (suppl. 3): S194–240.

305. Jabs K, Alexander S, McCabe D *et al.* Primary results from the US multicenter pediatric recombinant erythropoietin study. J Am Soc Nephrol 1994; 5: 456 (abstract).

306. Van Damme-Lombaerts R, Broyer M, Businger J *et al.* A study of recombinant human erythropoietin in the treatment of anemia of chronic renal failure in children on hemodialysis. Pediatr Nephrol 1994; 8: 338–42.

307. Eschbach JW, Gilenny R, Robertson T. Normalizing the hematocrit in hemodialysis patients with EPO improves quality of life and is safe. J Am Soc Nephrol 1993; 4: 425 (abstract).

308. van Wyck DB. Iron management during recombinant human erythropoietin therapy. Am J Kidney Dis 1989; 14 (suppl. 1): 9–13.

309. Edmunds ME, Walls J, Tucker B *et al.* Seizures in haemodialysis patients treated with recombinant human erythropoietin. Nephrol Dial Transplant 1989; 4: 1065–9.

310. The North American Pediatric Renal Transplant Cooperative Study 1997 Annual Data Report. Potomac, Maryland: EMMES Corporation, May 1997, p. 98.

311. Reddingus RE, Schroder CH, Monnens LAH. Intraperitoneal administration of recombinant human erythropoietin in children on continuous ambulatory peritoneal dialysis. Eur J Pediatr 1992; 151: 540–2.

312. Granolleras C, Leskopf W, Shaldon S *et al.* Experience of pain after subcutaneous administration at different preparations of recombinant human erythropoietin: a randomized, double-blind crossover study. Clin Nephrol 1991; 36: 294–8.

313. Frenken LA, Van Lier HJ, Jordans JG *et al.* Identification of the component part in an Epoietin alfa preparation that causes pain after subcutaneous injections. Am J Kidney Dis 1993; 22: 553–6.

314. Reddingus RE, Schroder CH, Koster AM *et al.* Pharmacokinetics of recombinant human erythropoietin in children treated with continuous ambulatory peritoneal dialysis. Eur J Pediatr 1994; 153: 850–4.

315. Scigalla P. Effect of recombinant human erythropoietin treatment on renal anemia and growth of children with end-

stage renal disease. In: Gurland HJ, Moran J, Samtleben W, Scigalla P, Wieczorek L, eds. Erythropoietin in Renal and Non-renal Anemias. Contributions to Nephrology. Basel: Karger, 1991, pp. 201–11.

316. Uehlinger DE, Gotch FA, Scheiner LB. A pharmacodynamic model of erythropoietin therapy for uremic anemia. Clin Pharmacol Ther 1992; 51: 76–89.

317. Muller-Wiefel DE, Sinn H, Gilli G et al. Hemolysis and blood loss in children with chronic renal failure. Clin Nephrol 1977; 8: 481–6.

318. Crosby WH. The rationale for treating iron deficiency anemia. Arch Intern Med 1984; 144: 471–2.

319. Reed MD, Bertino JS, Halpin TC Jr. Use of intravenous iron dextran injection in children receiving total parenteral nutrition. Am J Dis Child 1981; 135: 829–31.

320. Silverberg DS, Blum M, Peer G et al. Intravenous ferric saccharate as an iron supplement in dialysis patients. Nephron 1996; 72: 413–7.

321. Zanen AL, Adriaasen HJ, van Bommel EF et al. Oversaturation of transferrin after intravenous ferric gluconate (Ferrlecit) in hemodialysis patients. Nephrol Dial Transplant 1996; 11: 820–4.

322. Hymes LC, Hawthorne SM, Chavers BM. Impaired response to recombinant human erythropoietin therapy in children with peritonitis. Dial Transplant 1994; 23: 462–3.

323. Rad DS, Shih MS, Mohini R. Effect of serum parathyroid hormone and bone marrow fibrosis on the response to erythropoietin in uremia. N Engl J Med 1993; 328: 171–5.

324. Navarro M, Alonso A, Avilla JM. Anemia of chronic renal failure. Treatment with erythropoietin. Child Nephrol Urol 1991; 11: 146–51.

325. Neu AM, Warady BA, Lederman HM et al. Hypogammaglobulinemia in infants and young children maintained on peritoneal dialysis. Perit Dial Int 1998; 18: 440–3.

326. Neu AM, Lederman HM, Warady B et al. Humoral immunity in infants maintained on CPD. J Am Soc Nephrol 1994; 5: 467.

327. Schroeder CH, Bakkeren JA, Weemaes CM et al. IgG2 deficiency in young children treated with continuous ambulatory peritoneal dialysis (CAPD). Perit Dial Int 1989; 9: 261–5.

328. Fivush BA, Neu AM. Immunization guidelines for pediatric renal disease. Semin Nephrol 1998; 18: 256–63.

329. Fivush BA, Neu AM. Immunizations in pediatric CAPD/CCPD patients. In: Fine RN, Alexander SR, Warady BA, eds. CAPD/CCPD in Children. Norwell: Kluwer, 1998, pp. 219–28.

330. AAP Committee on Infectious Disease. Recommended childhood immunization schedule – United States, January–December 1999. Pediatrics 1999; 103: 182–5.

331. AAP Committee on Infectious Diseases. Recommendations for the use of live attenuated varicella vaccine. Pediatrics 1995; 95: 791–6.

332. Greenbaum LA, Salusky IB. Poor humoral response to the varicella vaccine in a pediatric dialysis population. J Am Soc Nephrol 1996; 7: 1447.

333. Furth SL, Neu AM, McColley SA et al. Immune response to influenza vaccination in children with renal disease. Pediatr Nephrol 1995; 9: 566–8.

334. Wadwa RP, Feigin RD. Pneumococcal vaccine: an update. Pediatrics 1999; 103: 1035–7.

335. Vazquez G, Alvarez T, Mendoza L et al. Comparison in the response to recombinant hepatitis B virus vaccine in children with chronic renal failure, with and without dialysis. Perit Dial Int 1997; 17 (suppl. 1): S90.

336. Watkins SL, Hoss RJ, Alexander AR et al. Response to recombinant hepatitis B vaccine (Recombivax HB) in children with chronic renal failure. J Am Soc Nephrol 1994; 5: 344.

337. Hokken-Koelega ACS, van Zaal MA, van Bergen W et al. Final height and its predictive factors after renal transplantation in childhood. Pediatr Res 1994; 36: 323–328.

338. Tönshoff B, Mehls O. Growth in children on CAPD/CCPD and the use of recombinant human growth hormone to treat growth delay in these children. In: Fine RN, Alexander SR, Warady BA, eds. CAPD/CCPD in Children. Norwell: Kluwer, 1998, pp. 143–67.

339. Warady BA, Jabs K. New hormones in the therapeutic arsenal of chronic renal failure. Pediatr Nephrol 1995; 42: 1551–77.

340. Powell DR, Liu F, Baker BK et al for the Southwest Pediatric Nephrology Study Group. Modulation of growth factors by growth hormone in children with chronic renal failure. Kidney Int 1997; 51: 1970–9.

341. Tönshoff B, Mehls O. Growth retardation in children with chronic renal insufficiency: current aspects of pathophysiology and treatment. J Nephrol 1995; 8: 133–42.

342. Leung DW, Spencer SA, Cachianes G et al. Growth hormone receptor and serum binding protein: purification, cloning and expression. Nature 1987; 330: 537–43.

343. Tönshoff B, Cronin MJ, Reichert M et al. Reduced concentration of serum growth hormone (GH)-grinding protein in children with chronic renal failure: Correlation with GH insensitivity. J Clin Endocrinol Metab 1997; 82: 1007–13.

344. Tönshoff B, Fine RN. Recombinant human growth hormone for children with renal failure. Adv Renal Replace Ther 1996; 3: 37–47.

345. Bereket G, Lin JJ, Bereket A et al. Peritoneal loss of insulin-like growth factor-I and binding proteins in end-stage renal disease. Pediatr Nephrol 1998; 12: 581–8.

346. Warady BA, Alexander SR, Watkins S et al. Optimal care of the pediatric end-stage renal disease (ESRD) patient on dialysis. Am J Kidney Dis 1999; 33: 1–18.

347. Kaufman DB. Growth hormone and renal osteodystrophy: a case report. Pediatr Nephrol 1998; 12: 157–9.

348. Salusky IB, Goodman WG. Growth hormone and calcitriol as modifiers of bone formation in renal osteodystrophy. Kidney Int 1995; 48: 657–65.

349. Kuizon BD, Salusky IB. Diagnosis and treatment of renal bone diseases in children undergoing CAPD/CCPD. In: Fine RN, Alexander SR, Warady BA, eds. CAPD/CCPD in Children. Norwell: Kluwer, 1998, pp. 199–217.

350. Chan JCM, McEnery PT, Chinchilli VM et al. A prospective, double-blind study of growth failure in children with chronic renal insufficiency and the effectiveness of treatment with calcitriol versus dihydrotachysterol. J Pediatr 1994; 124: 520–8.

351. Portale A. Calcium and phosphorus. In: Holliday MA, Barratt TM, Avner ED, eds. Pediatric Nephrology. Baltimore: Williams & Wilkins, 1994, p. 247.

352. Salusky IB, Ramirez JA, Goodman WG. Disorders of bone and mineral metabolism in chronic renal failure. In: Holliday MA, Barratt TM, Avner ED, eds. Pediatric Nephrology. Baltimore: Williams & Wilkins, 1994, p. 1287.

353. Salusky IB, Kuizon BD, Belin TR et al. Intermittent calcitriol therapy in secondary hyperparathyroidism: a comparison between oral and intraperitoneal administration. Kidney Int 1998; 54: 907–14.

354. Kuizon BD, Goodman WG, Jüppner H et al. Diminished linear growth during intermittent calcitriol therapy in children undergoing CCPD. Kidney Int 1998; 53: 205–11.

355. Warady BA, Sullivan EK, Alexander SR. Lessons from the peritoneal dialysis patient database: A Report of the North American Pediatric Renal Transplant Cooperative Study. Kidney Int 1996; 49 (suppl. 53): S68–71.

356. Port FK, Held PJ, Nolph KD et al. Risk of peritonitis and technique failure by CAPD connection technique: A national study. Kidney Int 1992; 41: 967–74.

357. Warady BA, Campoy SF, Gross SP et al. Peritonitis with continuous ambulatory peritoneal dialysis and continuous cycling peritoneal dialysis. J Pediatr 1984; 105: 726–30.

358. Watson AR, Vigneaux A, Bannatyne RM et al. Peritonitis during continuous ambulatory peritoneal dialysis in children. CMAJ 1986; 134: 1019–22.

359. Levy M, Balfe JW. Optimal approach to the prevention and treatment of peritonitis in children undergoing continuous ambulatory and continuous cycling peritoneal dialysis. Semin Dial 1994; 7: 442–9.

360. Harvey E, Secker D, Braj B et al. The team approach to the management of children on chronic peritoneal dialysis. Adv Ren Replace Ther 1996; 3: 3–13.

361. Kingwatanakul P, Warady BA. Staphylococcus aureus nasal carriage in children receiving long-term peritoneal dialysis. Adv Perit Dial 1997; 13: 280–3.

362. Watkins S, Warady BA, Ogrinc F, Schlichting L, for the Pediatric Dialysis Study Consortium. Impact on flush-before-fill methodology on frequency of peritonitis in patients receiving automated peritoneal dialysis. Pediatr Nephrol 1998; 12: 452 (abstract).

363. Vas SI. VRE and emperical vancomycin for CAPD peritonitis: use at your own/patient's risk (Letter). Perit Dial Int 1998; 18: 86–7.

364. Troidle L, Kliger AS, Gorban-Brennan N et al. Nine episodes of CPD-associated peritonitis with vancomycin resistant enterococci. Kidney Int 1996; 50: 1368–72.

365. Warady BA, Reed L, Murphy G et al. Aminoglycoside ototoxicity in pediatric patients receiving long-term peritoneal dialysis. Pediatr Nephrol 1993; 7: 178–81.

366. Keane WF, Alexander SR, Bailie GR et al. Peritoneal dialysis-related peritonitis treatment recommendations: 1996 update. Perit Dial Int 1996; 16: 557–73.

367. Schaefer F, Klaus G, Müller-Wiefel DE et al. Intermittent versus continuous intraperitoneal glycopeptide/ceftazidime treatment in children with peritoneal dialysis-associated peritonitis. J Am Soc Nephrol 1999; 10: 136–45.

368. Alexander SR, Linblad AS, Nolph KD, Novak JS. Pediatric CAPD/CCPD in the United States: a review of the National CAPD Registry's pediatric population for the period January 1, 1981 through August 31, 1986. In: Twardowski ZJ, Nolph KD, Khanna R, eds. Peritoneal Dialysis, New Concepts and Applications; vol. 22 in the series: Contemporary Issues in Nephrology (JH Stein series ed.). New York: Churchill Livingstone, 1990, pp. 231–55.

369. Levy M, Balfe JW, Geary D et al. Exit-site infection during continuous and cycling peritoneal dialysis in children. Perit Dial Int 1990; 10: 31–5.

370. Thodis E, Bhaskaran S, Pasadakis P et al. Decrease in *Staphylococcus aureus* exit-site infections and peritonitis in CAPD patients by local application of mupirocin ointment at the catheter exit-site. Perit Dial Int 1998; 18: 244–6.

371. Khanna R, Twardowski ZJ. Recommendations for treatment of exit-site pathology. Perit Dial Int 1996; 16: S100–4.

372. Khoury AE, Charendoff J, Balfe JW et al. Hernias associated with CAPD in children. Adv Perit Dial 1991; 7: 279–82.

373. von Lilien T, Salusky IB, Yap HK et al. Hernias: a frequent complication in children treated with continuous peritoneal dialysis. Am J Kidney Dis 1987; 10: 356–60.

374. Robson WL, Leung AK, Putnins RE et al. Genital edema in children on continuous ambulatory peritoneal dialysis. Child Nephrol Urol 1990; 10: 205–10.

375. Ducassou D, Vuillemin L, Wone C et al. Intraperitoneal injection of technetium-99m sulfur colloid in visualization of a peritoneo-vaginalis connection. J Nucl Med 1984; 25: 68–9.

376. Bunchman TE, Wood EG, Lynch RE. Hydrothorax as a complication of pediatric peritoneal dialysis. Perit Dial Bull 1987; 7: 237–9.

377. Townsend R, Fragula J. Hydrothorax in a patient receiving CAPD. Arch Intern Med 1982; 142: 1571–2.

378. Scheldewaert R, Rogaerts Y, Pauvels R et al. Management of massive hydrothorax in a CAPD patient. A case report and review of the literature. Perit Dial Bull 1987; 2: 69–72.

379. Leveen HH, Piccone VA, Hutto RB. Management of ascites with hydrothorax. Am J Surg 1984; 148: 210–3.

380. Hidai H, Takatsu S, Chiba T. Intrathoracic instillation of autologous blood in treating massive hydrothorax following CAPD. Perit Dial Int 1989; 9: 221–2.

381. Mestas D, Wauquier JP, Escande G et al. A diagnosis of hydrothorax-complicated CAPD and demonstrations of successful therapy by scintography (Letter). Perit Dial Int 1991; 11: 283–4.

382. Benz RL, Schleifer CR. Hydrothorax in continuous ambulatory peritoneal dialysis: successful treatment with intrapleural tetracycline and a review of the literature. Am J Kidney Dis 1985; 5: 136–40.

383. Simmons LE, Mir RA. A review of management of pleuro-peritoneal communication in five CAPD patients. Adv Perit Dial 1989; 5: 81–3.

384. Niaudet P. Loss of ultrafiltration and sclerosing encapsulating peritonitis in children undergoing CAPD/CCPD. In: Fine RN, ed. Chronic Ambulatory Peritoneal Dialysis (CAPD) and Chronic Cycling Peritoneal Dialysis (CCPD) in Children. Boston: Martinus Nijhoff, 1987, pp. 201–19.

385. Slingeneyer A. Preliminary report on cooperative international study in sclerosing peritonitis. Contrib Nephrol 1987; 57: 239–47.

386. Smith L, Collins JF, Morris M et al. Sclerosing encapsulating peritonitis associated with continuous ambulatory peritoneal dialysis: Surgical management. Am J Kidney Dis 1997; 29: 456–60.

387. Ford DM, Portman RJ, Lum GM. Pancreatitis in children on chronic dialysis treated with valproic acid. Pediatr Nephrol 1990; 4: 259–61.

388. Osorio A, Seidel FG, Warady BA. Hypercalcemia and pancreatitis in a child with adynamic bone disease. Pediatr Nephrol 1997; 11: 223–5.

389. Gupta A, Yuan ZY, Balaskas EV et al. CAPD and pancreatitis: No connection. Perit Dial Int 1992; 12: 309–16.

390. Drash A, Sherman F, Hartmann W et al. A syndrome of pseudohermaphroditism, Wilms' tumor, hypertension, and degenerative renal disease. J Pediatr 1970; 76: 585–93.

391. Fivush BA, Case B, May MW et al. Hypogammaglobulinemia in children undergoing continuous ambulatory peritoneal dialysis. Pediatr Nephrol 1989; 3: 186–8.

392. Warady BA, Hellerstein S, Alon U. Letter to the editor: Concerning peritoneal dialysis in the presence of ventriculo-peritoneal shunt. Pediatr Nephrol 1990; 4: 96.

393. Hendren WH, Hendren RB. Bladder augmentation: experience with 129 children and young adults. J Urol 1990; 144: 445.

394. Churchill DN, Morgan J, Torrance G. Quality of life in end-stage renal disease. Perit Dial Bull 1984; 4: 20–3.

395. Churchill DN. The effect of treatment modality on the quality of life for patients with end-stage renal disease (ESRD). Adv Perit Dial 1988; 4: 63–5.

396. Brownbridge G, Fielding DM. Psychosocial adjustment to end-stage renal failure: Comparing haemodialysis, continuous ambulatory peritoneal dialysis and transplantation. Pediatr Nephrol 1991; 5: 612–62.

397. LePontois J, Moel DI, Cohn RA. Family adjustment to pediatric ambulatory dialysis. Am J Orthopsychiatry 1987; 57: 78–83.

398. Rosenkranz J, Bonzel K-E, Bulla M et al. Psychosocial adaptation of children and adolescents with chronic renal failure. Pediatr Nephrol 1992; 6: 459–63.

399. Roscoe JM, Smith LF, Williams EA et al. Medical and social outcome in adolescents with end-stage renal disease. Pediatr Clin N Am 1987; 34: 789–801.

400. Warady BA. Therapeutic camping for children with end-stage renal disease. Pediatr Nephrol 1994; 8: 387–90.

401. Fine RN, Scharer K. Renal transplantation in children treated by CAPD. A report on a cooperative study. In: Fine RN, Scharer K, Mehls O, eds. CAPD in Children. Heidelberg: Springer-Verlag, 1985, pp. 212–20.

402. Salvatierra O Jr, Alexander S, Krensky A. Pediatric kidney transplantation at Stanford. Pediatr Transplant 1998; 2: 165–76.

403. Chavers B. Transplantation of the pediatric CAPD/CCPD patient. In: Fine RN, Alexander SR, Warady BA, eds.

CAPD/CCPD in Children, 2nd edn. Boston: Kluwer, 1998, pp. 57–72.

404. Nevins TE, Danielson G. Prior dialysis does not affect the outcome of pediatric renal transplantation. Pediatr Nephrol 1991; 5: 211–16.

405. Stefanidis CJ, Balfe JW, Arbus GS *et al.* Renal transplantation in children treated with continuous ambulatory peritoneal dialysis. Perit Dial Bull 1983; 3: 5–7.

406. Laine J, Holmberg C, Samela K *et al.* Renal transplantation in children with emphasis on young patients. Pediatr Nephrol 1994; 8: 313–16.

407. Ogawa O, Hoshinaga K, Hasegawa A *et al.* Successful transplantation in children treated with CAPD. Transplant Proc 1989; 21: 1997–9.

408. Watson AR, Vigneux A, Balfe JW. Renal transplantation in children on CAPD and post-transplant ascites. Perit Dial Bull 1984; 4: 189–91.

409. Leichter HE, Salusky IB, Ettenger RB *et al.* Experience with renal transplantation in children undergoing peritoneal dialysis (CAPD/CCPD). Am J Kidney Dis 1986; 8: 181–4.

410. Andreeta B, Verrina E, Sorino P. Complications linked to chronic peritoneal dialysis in children after kidney transplantation. Experience of the Italian Registry of Pediatric Chronic Peritoneal Dialysis. Perit Dial Int 1996; 16 (suppl. 1): S570–5.

411. Palmer J, Kaiser BA, Polinsky MS *et al.* Peritoneal dialysis catheter infections in children after renal transplantation. Choosing the time of removal. Pediatr Nephrol 1994; 8: 715–18.

412. Issad B, Mouquet C, Bitker M *et al.* Is overhydration in CAPD patients a contraindication to renal transplantation? Adv Perit Dial 1994; 10: 68–72.

413. Fine RN. Renal transplantation for children – the only realistic choice. Kidney Int 1985; 17: S15–17.

414. Harmon WE, Jabs K. Factors affecting growth after renal transplantation. J Am Soc Nephrol 1992; 2: S295–303.

415. Harmon WE. Continuous ambulatory peritoneal dialysis in children (Letter). N Engl J Med 1983; 308: 968.

416. Shih VE. Congential hyperammonemic syndromes. Clin Perinatol 1976; 3: 3–4.

417. Siegel NJ, Brown RS. Peritoneal clearance of ammonia and creatinine in a neonate. J Pediatr 1973; 82: 1044–6.

418. Wiegand C, Thompson T, Bock GH *et al.* The management of life-threatening hyperammonemia: A comparison of several therapeutic modalities. J Pediatr 1980; 96: 142–4.

419. Sperl W, Geiger R, Maurer H *et al.* Continuous arteriovenous haemofiltration in hyperammonaemia of newborn babies. Lancet 1990; 336: 1192–3.

420. Rutledge SL, Havens PL, Haymond MW *et al.* Neonatal hemodialysis: Effective therapy for the encephalopathy of inborn errors of metabolism. J Pediatr 1990; 116: 125–8.

421. Batshaw ML, Brusilow SW. Treatment of hyperammonemic coma caused by inborn errors of urea synthesis. J Pediatr 1980; 97: 893–900.

422. Wong KY, Wong SN, Lam SY *et al.* Ammonia clearance by peritoneal dialysis and continuous arteriovenous hemodiafiltration. Pediatr Nephrol 1998; 12: 589–91.

423. Chan JCM, Campbell RA. Peritoneal dialysis in children: a survey of its indications and applications. Clin Pediatr 1973; 12: 131–9.

424. Van Stone JC. Hemodialysis. In: Gonick HC, ed. Current Nephrology. New York: John Wiley, 1984, pp. 87–105.

425. Rubin J. Comments on dialysis solution composition, antibiotic transport, poisoning and novel uses of peritoneal dialysis. In: Nolph KD, ed. Peritoneal Dialysis. The Hague: Martinus Nijhoff, 1985, p. 253.

23 | Quality of life after peritoneal dialysis

T. APOSTOLOU AND R. GOKAL

Introduction

Interest in measuring quality of life in relation to health care has increased enormously [1, 2], and in the past two decades has emerged as an important attribute of clinical investigation and patient care [3]. Moreover, quality of life assessments are increasingly recognized as a major endpoint for phase III randomized controlled trials. Several clinical trial organizations have now introduced the notion of quality of life as a standard part of new trials. In the UK the Medical Research Council-funded trials in general are expected either to assess the impact of every new trial on quality of life or to justify not doing so [4, 5]. Just as introducing evidence-based medicine into clinical practice gathers momentum, so do quality of life assessments, which have to be considered against any gains in therapeutic efficacy resulting from current or new treatments.

This is equally true for end-stage renal disease (ESRD), where its importance lies in providing not only for absolute survival but also the quality of that survival. The main purpose, however, is to provide more accurate assessments of individuals' or populations' health and at the same time of the benefits and harms that may result from health care. This is even more important in renal failure care where advances are not uncommon and there are several alternative therapies available to manage patients; the relative effectiveness of these changes and therapies needs proper evaluation and assessment as regards quality of life [3, 6, 7]. Unquestionably, one of the goals of an ESRD programme (Table 1) is to achieve maximum psychosocial maturation and development, whilst at the same time adapting to the stresses of therapy [8].

Definition

The definition of quality of life is difficult as it embraces many dimensions, ranging from physical

Table 1. Ideal goals for a renal replacement programme as they relate to quality of life

1. Restoration of normal levels of biological, psychological and social adaptation and longevity
2. Minimal adverse effect of treatment as above
3. Maximum psychological and social maturation
4. Optimum family function and minimum treatment-related stress
5. Minimal patient care stresses on health professionals and high professional satisfaction

well-being and cognitive competence, to the establishment of satisfactory interrelationships, proper housing and its enjoyable occupation, and the possession of sufficient income to explore the world beyond that necessary for basic biological survival [9].

Before one talks about quality we must define the term. In the dictionary quality is defined as 'the degree of excellence of a thing' and 'life' as 'the ability to function and grow'. So, quality of life is the degree of worth of someone's life. It is the quality of the way that one is functioning in society and experiencing the events that characterize existence as a human being, both subjectively and objectively. But how do we know if a thing is 'excellent' or not? Thus, quality of life is a relative notion and significantly related to an individual's social background and political system of a given country. It is judged differently by individuals who compare one thing with a standard, which can be a personal one or a consensus one. In terms of medical care there is the quality that the doctor perceives, the quality that the patient perceives and the quality that (in a hospital setting) the management perceives; difficulties can arise because these perceptions may not coincide. From the physician's point of view this perspective may even be somewhat narrower; factors such as advancing age, income, and relationships are all outside a physician's control and hence they are principally concerned with measures of health related to quality of life. In terms of maintaining good health this can be

R. Gokal, R. Khanna, R.Th. Krediet and K.D. Nolph (eds.), Textbook of Peritoneal Dialysis, 2nd Edition, 709–735.
© 2000 Kluwer Academic Publishers. Printed in Great Britain.

divided into general, physical, mental and social aspects (Table 2) [10].

The term quality of life misleadingly suggests an abstract and philosophical approach but indeed should reflect the content and purpose of measures – health-related quality of life, subjective health status, functional status, i.e. an individual's level of functioning in relation to some measurements [11]. These words – health status, functional status and quality of life – are often used interchangeably to refer to the same domain of 'health'. Thus the health domain ranges from negatively valued aspects of life, such as death, to the more positively valued aspects such as happiness, prosperity and role functioning. In that respect more specific definitions have emerged. Alexander and Willems [12] state that the fundamental basis of quality of life involves continuously functioning reciprocal interactions between the patient and the environment, and encompasses such crucial areas as interrelationships, physical well-being, social activities, personal development, recreation and economic circumstances. Stout and Auer [13] identified several measures which include mobility, physical performance, employment (objective measures) and ability to lead a satisfactory social life and have sexual and affectionate relationships (subjective measures). Churchill [14] identified a global concept, which entailed an estimate of all reciprocal interactions between patients and the environment. Guyatt *et al.* [10] use the term health-related quality of life because many aspects of life that we do not consider as health (e.g. income, environment, freedom) may affect health; consequently almost all aspects of life can become health-related in case of a dismal situation. Another common definition in the literature is health-related quality of life (HRQOL). As a working definition of quality of life, this is the value assigned to the duration of life, as modified by the impairments, functional states, perceptions and social opportunities that are affected by disease, injury, treatment or policy [15].

Quality of life measures can be used in many ways in health care (Table 3) over and above those stated

Table 3. Applications of quality of life measures

Applications

Screening and monitoring psychosocial problems in individual patient care
Medical audit
Outcome in health services
Evaluation research
Clinical trials
Population surveys of perceived health problems
Cost-effective analysis

already. These aspects, especially those related to audit, achievement of standards, quality of patient care and cost-effective analysis, are assuming greater importance [16].

Thus, although there is not a universally agreed definition of quality of life, or an agreed standard for measuring it, consensus as to what should be measured, at the very least, revolves around general measures. These include physical health and symptoms, functional status and activities of daily life, mental well-being and social health, including social role functioning and social support networks. These need to be built into health care programmes. Indeed the 'appropriate health care and technology programme' of the World Health Organization had as target 31: 'by 1990 all member states should have built effective mechanisms for ensuring the quality of patient care'.

Consideration of quality of life, as well as of survival, always implicit in good clinical practice, has hitherto lacked explicit expression; it is important to do so now. Two important questions come to the fore.

1. Is individual quality of life open to quantitative assessment?
2. Can aggregated indices of quality of individual life be used as a component in deciding health services priorities?

These questions form the basis of a wider debate indirectly addressed here using available publications in the field of renal replacement therapy.

Table 2. Items of health divided into general, physical, mental and social domains

General	Physical	Mental	Social
Pain and suffering	Physical functioning	Positive well-being	Gets along well
Health concerns and distress	Mobility	Life satisfaction self-esteem	Sexuality
Energy and fatigue	Role functioning	Autonomy	Social contacts
Overall health current	Physical symptoms	Anxiety/depression	
	Disease state and severity	Cognitive function	

Dimension and instruments

Although the concept of quality of life is inherently subjective, and definitions vary, the contents of the various instruments used for measuring it show some similarity in terms of different dimensions or domains of quality of life that are intended for study. These dimensions or domains can be subdivided into physical functions (e.g. mobility, self-care), emotional functions (well-being, life satisfaction, autonomy, depression, anxiety), social function (intimacy, social support, social contact, sexuality), role performance (work, housework), and pain and other symptoms (fatigue and nausea, disease-specific symptoms) [11]. Hence dimensions or domains of quality of life include not only the physical condition of the patient, important though this is, but also how he/she feels about life and his/her relation to it. It also includes how patients react to a certain dismal condition, how they relate to the social environment and their capacity to continue working and achieve contentment. These are, of course, not independent variables and should all be taken into account in assessing quality of life. What is ethically desirable in choosing between all these aspects is difficult to ascertain, but Black [17] has set up three possible criteria.

1. Assessments made by sufferers from particular states are to be preferred to vicarious estimates (in the phrase 'experito credo', the 'expert' in the subjective content of the illness is the patient, not the doctor or nurse).
2. A method that takes into account several variables is preferable to uni- or bidimensional methods even at the expense of numerical complexity.
3. When several variables have been measured, some weighting should be made in favour of those which can be more rather than less objectively measured. Indeed fitness for work may be used in comparing the efficacy of different treatments for end-stage renal failure [18]. Although fitness for work combines the physical and psychological dimension, it is a simple measure but one devoid of practicality.

These above concepts thus imply that, since quality of life is multidimensional, it can be evaluated only from a multidimensional perspective. In addition, a more controversial issue is the need to include multiple items to assess each dimension of quality of life. For conceptual, psychometric and health policy-related reasons, multi-item assessments within a given dimension are necessary if there is going to be any progress in understanding the dimension and its relationship to patient illnesses, therapies and other life circumstances [7, 19]. However, as is the case in burgeoning research areas, many of the underlying conceptual models and research questions have outstripped the developments and evaluation of suitable measurement instruments.

Instruments

There are two basic types of instrument used to assess quality of life: generic and disease-specific. The latter have been developed to focus on one disease or a narrow range of a disease, e.g. arthritis impact measurement scale [20]. Generic instruments are intended to be applicable to a wide range of health problems, usually insensitive to changes in quality of life, but are particularly useful for surveys that attempt to document and compare the range of disability in a general population or a patient group [21]. Disease-specific instruments focus on aspects of health status that are influenced by the disease under investigation, and they have the potential for an increased responsiveness because they study the most relevant health-related aspects of quality of life for the patient [21]. Among the generic instruments that are commonly used are the Sickness Impact Profile (SIP) [22]. Nottingham Health Profile (NIP) [23] medical outcomes study short form-36 (SF-36) [24] while a number of disease-specific instruments are in use or under investigation.

Although some instruments are administered by clinicians or interviewers, increasingly the emphasis has been on self-completed questionnaires, for economy of use. This has some disadvantages, e.g. greater likelihood of low response rate, missing items and misunderstanding. The quantitative information provided also varies. Most of the instruments give a scoring system for the different dimensions or domains of quality of life under investigation, which usually do not combine. Others assess dimensions that may be summed to provide a single score, e.g. the quality of life index (QL index), developed for use in cancer, which consists of five elements (activity, daily living, health, support and outlook) which are summed to provide a single index total [25].

The preference-based measurement is another approach to evaluating quality of life, and these are techniques that try to assign numerical values from 0 to 1 to health states reflecting the individual's preference for health, where 1 corresponds to perfect health and 0 to death. The utility value can be used to weight the quantity of life, forming the quality-adjusted life years, an index which is used to prioritize resource and funding allocations among different services (see time-trade-off hypothesis instrument) [26].

Requirements for a measure

Reliability

All instruments must produce the same results on repeated use under the same conditions. This can be examined by test–retest reliability (although it may be difficult to distinguish measurement error from real changes in quality of life) or by examining the internal reliability (the degree of agreement of items addressing equivalent concepts). Inter-rater reliability needs to be established for interview-based instruments. Reliable instruments will generally show that stable patients have more or less the same results after repeated administrations [11, 21, 27].

Validity

Validity examines whether the instrument used is measuring what it is intended to measure. This is more difficult to assess because instruments are measuring an inherently subjective phenomenon. When there is a gold standard it is easy to assess the validity of the instrument. Hence, no gold standard for quality of life exists, but there are some instances in which a specific target for a quality of life measure exists that can be treated as a gold standard. This is called criterion validity (an instrument is valid if its results correspond to those of the criterion used as a standard) [10]. An informal approach is to examine 'face validity' – whether instruments cover a full range of relevant topics [28], the range of patient experiences [29], and the instrument appears to be measuring what it is intended to measure. A more formal approach is to examine construct validity, a theoretically derived notion of the dimensions or domains we want to measure. This involves comparisons between the patterns of relations of a quality of life instrument with other more established measures, e.g. laboratory vs clinical [30], and different health statuses [31]. Above all, once validity has been shown for one purpose it cannot be assumed for all possible populations or applications [32].

Sensitivity of change or responsiveness

This is an instrument's ability to detect changes during a period of time. Measures of quality of life that can distinguish between patients at a point in time are not necessarily as sensitive to changes in patients over time when repeated. This aspect is a crucial requirement for longitudinal studies, especially clinical trials [33].

Appropriateness

To ensure that the quality of life measure used is most appropriate, the health problem and likely range of impacts of other treatments need to be carefully considered. Investigators sometimes use a wide range of measures, such as a 'scatter-gun' approach, which has problems, and one approach may be to use instruments that let patients select dimensions of most concern which can be assessed over time [34,35].

Practicality

This is important and current quality of life measures are most practical for use in clinical trials and formal evaluation studies. For regular use the more detailed and comprehensive measures are impractical to administer, process, hard to interpret and incorporate into decision making [35].

Overall the design, analysis and interpretation of studies are crucial and are well reviewed by Fletcher *et al.* [21]. More specific to renal diseases, Deniston *et al.* [36] assessed quality of life in ESRD using 10 different multi-item indices and nine single-item measures. Correlations between these measures suggest that these indices tend to represent either functions or feeling with moderate relationships within the two clusters but little between them. These workers concluded that, depending on the measures chosen to assess quality of life, different conclusions about the relationship of quality of life to demographic characteristics are likely to be reached. Hence there is the need to think more critically about the nature of the quality of life in arriving at judgements, and the relative validity of these different measures.

Instruments used in quality of life assessment of ESRD patients

Renal diseases, especially renal replacement therapy, have a significant impact upon quality of life. In the past decade quality of life of ESRD patients has received considerable attention as a therapeutic outcome and as a useful consideration for therapeutic decision making. Many instruments are available and have been used (Table 4), for assessing quality of life in dialysis and transplant patients. Most of the measures that have been used were generic, providing broader outcome indicators with renal patients.

Two main approaches have been used to measure HRQOL: *health profile measurements* (generic and disease-specific instruments) or preference based measurements. Disease-specific instruments are those which include the HRQOL dimensions most relevant for patients affected by a particular condition. Disease-specific instruments are more sensitive to clinical changes, but do not allow HRQOL comparisons between patients with different pathologies. Generic instruments include different dimensions of quality of life considered generally important and broadly applicable. They enable comparisons among different population groups (healthy population groups and/or groups with different illnesses) to be made.

The *preference-based measurement* uses different techniques to assign numerical values (utilities) to health states. Several health state descriptions are presented to patients, health professionals or the general population. A value from 0 to 1 is assigned to each health state using different techniques, such as rating scale, standard gamble or time trade-off. The value assigned to each health state reflects the individual's preferences for health states, where one corresponds to perfect health and zero to death.

Generic instruments

The commonly used generic instruments have been the Nottingham Health Profile, the Karnofsky Performance Scale (KPS), the Sickness Impact Profile (SIP) and the SF-36. The KPS has been used extensively in measuring quality of life in renal disease, although there was scepticism regarding its use because it was developed to assess cancer patients. Anyway, it remains a valuable *objective* measure of physical condition. On this scale transplanted patients were found to do better than dialysis patients [3], erythropoietin improved the score of dialysis patients [37], and the KPS score on entry to dialysis was found to predict 2-year mortality [38].

The SIP has been found to be sensitive to changes in quality of life, and to distinguish between treatment modalities [39], but its main drawback is the length of the questionnaire.

The SF-36 has been used successfully as an outcome measure of quality of life in ESRD patients and has revealed quality of life improvements derived from treatment [40]. This instrument has shown dialysis patients to have worse and variable quality of life in comparison with the general population, and has shown good responsiveness in many studies [41, 42]; it has been accepted easily by ESRD patients.

Table 4. Various instruments used in assessing quality of life in ESRD patients. This is not a comprehensive list but lists the main ones utilized

Functional ability	Health status	Renal-specific	General–subjective	Psychological	Stressors and therapy satisfaction
Karnofsky Performance Index (KPI)	Sickness Impact Profile (SIP)	Parfrey's Uremic Index	Quality of life index	Psychological Well-Being	HD Stress Scale, Dialysis Stress Scale
Activities of daily living (ADL)	Time Trade-Off (TTO)	Kidney Disease Questionnaire	Well being Life satisfaction	Self Esteem	Simmons Multi-choice Items
Spitzer Quality of Life Index	MOS short form (SF-36)	Kidney Disease Quality of Life (KDQOL)	Cantrill's Ladder semantic differential	Profile of Mood States (POMS)	General Treatment Stress
	General Health Questionnaire	Renal Dependent Quality of Life (RDQoL)	Emotional Well-Being	Psychological Affect	Modality Specific Stress
	Nottingham Health Profile	Renal Quality of Life Profile (RQLP)	Social Well-Being	Psychological Adjustment to Physical Illness Scale (PAIS)	Stressor Assessment Scale
	EuroQol	HD Quality of Life Questionnaire	Campbell's Index of Well Being	Brief Symptom Inventory	

Renal-specific instruments

The Kidney Disease Questionnaire (KDQ) was developed in 1990 by Devins et al. [43], while the same instrument appears as an original paper in *Nephron* developed by Laupacis et al. in 1992 [44]. It contains 26 questions in five dimensions: physical symptoms, fatigue, depression, relationships with others, and frustration. The questionnaire demonstrated construct validity when compared with the SIP and time trade-off technique, and is reproducible [44]. Responsiveness was tested in detecting improvement in erythropoietin therapy in a randomized, placebo-controlled trial [45]. A limitation of the instrument is that it can be used only in haemodialysis (HD) patients.

The Kidney Disease Quality of Life (KDQOL) instrument was developed in 1994 by a working group with support from industry [46]. After release of the KDQOL Long Form, the group began work on the KDQOL-SF Short Form [47]. Currently KDQOL studies are under way at the University of Michigan as the Dialysis Outcomes and Practice Study (DOPPS) – a longitudinal study of treatment and outcomes for haemodialysis (HD) patients. A pilot test study in China is also under investigation, while a renal outcome study has been conducted in six countries using this questionnaire and KPS, with a primary purpose to determine the differences in mortality rates between CAPD and HD patients [48]. The KDQOL has been found to be reliable, and to display construct validity.

The Quality of Life Assessment, developed by Parfrey et al. in 1989 for use in ESRD patients [49], contains a mixture of measures, is brief, reproducible and responsive and it is validated. Its limitation resides in the need for a trained interviewer.

The Haemodialysis Quality of Life Questionnaire, developed by Churchill et al. [50], is another example of a self-administered specific questionnaire, sensitive and reliable.

The Renal-Dependent Quality of Life (RDQoL) questionnaire, developed by Bradley [51], is based on a diabetes-specific quality of life instrument and is an individualized one with face and content validity. It is currently being evaluated in research and clinical work.

The Renal Quality of Life Profile (RQLP), developed by Salek and co-workers [52, 53], is a self-completion measure specific to ESRD, easy to complete with good reliability and validity.

Other measures have also been, and are being, used in assessment of quality of life of ESRD patients. At present it is difficult to say which of them is the best for this purpose. It seems that specific instruments which are also treatment modality-specific, easy to complete, possibly self-administered and suitable for longitudinal studies should be adapted for use in these patients, combined with a generic instrument.

Multidisciplinary team in managing renal failure patients

A patient's quality of life is dependent not only on completion of all the technical aspects of the work of physicians and nurses, but also on his or her adaptation to dialysis treatment, which is a continuous process. There is a constant conflict between dependence on a machine or a catheter and the independence needed to maintain a normal life. Coping with dialysis is a matter of multidisciplinary approach, and this entails preparation of the patient before dialysis treatment is necessary. Since up to 40% of ESRD patients present for the first time in terminal renal failure, adequate preparation is impossible in all. McKevitt [54] defines the health care support system as a "Network of individuals in groups, who provide care and assistance – physical, medical, social, emotional and financial – and who are called on in various degrees, particularly when an individual or family's own resources are insufficient to cope with needs, problems and crisis. Support in the form of care and treatment, information and education, empathy and encouragement and reassurance, guidance and counselling and concrete resources are provided, based on sensitivity and an understanding to the individuals total situation and of their special concerns and needs." It is not surprising, considering the extent to which such support systems develop, that there are a variety of opinions on this elusive question of quality of life. What is well known is that where support systems break down, or do not exist, rehabilitation of the patient can be more difficult [55]. DeNour [56] stresses the importance of staff attitudes and the rehabilitation of HD patients, in particular the importance of working as a team to help the patient. Similar arguments would apply equally to CAPD patients. A key factor in the success of treatment is that communication within the health care and multidisciplinary team is good, and that treatment aims and expectations relayed to the patient and the family are consistent and realistic. Denial in the health care team, especially on the part of the physician, can lead to conflict and difficulty in adjustment for the patient [56]. Maintaining good communication within such a complex support system can be difficult. The importance of the team developing a consistent and positive philosophy towards treatment is further delineated by McKevitt [57]. Burton et al. [58] found CAPD patients were more satisfied with the support received from household members and from spouses than HD patients. This could be due to the fact that roles within the family appear less affected with CAPD than with HD [59].

Rasgon et al. [60] evaluated the benefits of a multidisciplinary, predialysis intervention to help home dialysis patients (28 CAPD and two home HD) maintain employment. They succeeded in maintaining employment in 74% of the patients. Sesso and Yoshihiro [61] evaluated the quality of life of 113 HD patients, who had a late or early referral to dialysis treatment. Using a number of instruments they demonstrated that late diagnosis of chronic renal failure and the consequent lack of predialysis care adversely affect the quality of life of these patients.

In the management of patients with ESRD, quality of life has a wide and varied definition, which is undoubtedly connected with the quality and the enthusiasm of the multidisciplinary health care team (nurses, doctors, social workers, physiotherapists, occupational therapists, dieticians, psychologists). They have to liaise closely with other important facets of the patient's total environment (family, social groups, community and society – the latter becoming more important especially as it concerns employment, health departments and local authorities) [13].

A social worker is indeed an important and effective member of the multidisciplinary team and does require special counselling skills, knowledge of group work, handy therapy techniques and an ability to work in difficult social situations and family environments.

Studies on quality of life in ESRD patients

History

It is apparent that all the published reports can be classified according to three study periods or eras: these consist of the early period 1966–72, the middle period 1973–80, and the contemporary period of 1980 onwards. The types of studies conducted have varied by period with the least amount of empirical work being published during the early period. This period tended to focus on the 'stress' of dialysis and its psychiatric morbidity. It was also related to the maximization of scarce dialysis and economic resources, and patient selection was a primary consideration with rehabilitation used as a selection criterion [62].

The middle period, up until 1980, was probably the least exciting. However, it was during this period that the economic issues surrounding dialysis were in large part resolved, especially in the United States [63] and in Europe. This, by and large, seemed to resolve the inherent patient selection/resource rationing problem and gave rise to a substantial increase in the size of the ESRD patient population. Nevertheless, several studies were published on various aspects of quality of life including psychosocial adaptation and employment, and how these varied according to dialysis modality [64, 65].

The contemporary period, over the past 15 years or so, has proven to be the most exciting. During this time transplantation clearly has come into its own with other interesting innovations including the development of peritoneal dialysis (and its various modifications) as a major mode of renal replacement therapy. It was during this period (1981) that Gutman et al. published a landmark study in the New England Journal of Medicine on the physical activity and employment status of maintenance HD patients [66] and this was accompanied by an editorial in the same issue of the journal [67]. Considerable doubt about the objective success of dialysis was raised by this survey, which showed few ESRD patients were truly rehabilitated; only 25% of hospital HD patients were capable of doing more than caring for themselves. Whilst this study may have been 'superficial' and suffered from 'sampling' errors, it reopened a debate on how good these treatments were related to the enormous cost. Rennie [67] argued that there was a need for a national database and debate to better understand this problem. Shortly afterwards the Health Care Financing Administration (HCFA) convened a task force to examine the problem associated with renal patient rehabilitation. At the same time the HCFA funded the National Kidney Dialysis and Kidney Transplantation Study [68, 69]. It was not until this contemporary period that a truly comprehensive appreciation of the quality of life of ESRD patients emerged. Many investigations from a wide variety of disciplinary backgrounds embarked upon quality of life assessments. It is also during this time that several innovative features and economic factors made their mark on renal replacement therapy. These included:

1. Establishment of CAPD and its subsequent growth in the treatment of ESRD patients.
2. Development of automated peritoneal dialysis (APD) and the need to monitor adequacy of PD.
3. Improving transplantation results with the introduction of cyclosporin and the newer immunosuppressive drugs.
4. The introduction of recombinant human erythropeoitin (EPO) for the treatment of anaemia of chronic renal failure. This very significant improvement does question the value of any study completed before the availability of EPO. The numerous and significant improvements in both subjective and objective aspects of quality of life following EPO have now been verified, including those at the energy level, appetite, exercise capability and cognitive function [37, 70–77]. Because previous studies did not usually control for level of anaemia, the results may reflect the adverse effects of anaemia rather than uraemia or its treatment.
5. Finally, there is the problem concerning the escalating costs of renal replacement therapy and the desire on the part of governments to ration health care. This has obviously raised a considerable amount of debate, even in countries such as the United States, where the treatment for patients with ESRD has been financed since 1973 by Medicare's ESRD programme [78–80].

Quality of life in PD: comparisons between PD and HD

Early studies

The advent of PD was a major addition to the therapeutic armamentarium available to treat ESRD patients. PD and HD are very different modality treatments in terms of technique, clearance of solutes, maintenance of residual renal function and life independence. A number of comparative studies between patients on CAPD and HD brought about conflicting results on survival and clinical outcomes that also reflected indirectly the quality of life in each mode of treatment. In a good editorial [81], Hamlet's agony has been paraphrased in 'PD or not PD? That Is the Question', indicating the nephrologist's agony for the future of renal replacement therapy and especially that of PD.

In 1981 a series of studies began at the Battelle Human Affairs Research Centres in Seattle, USA, concerning the quality of life of dialysis and transplant patients. These studies [7] in chronological order were:

1. the National Kidney Dialysis and Kidney Transplantation Study
2. the National Heart Transplantation Study
3. the Kidney Transplant Immunosuppressive Protocol Study
4. the Amgen Recombinant Human Erythropoietin Study.

These have been referred to as the 'Battelle' series. The first of these, by Evans *et al.* [6], was a cross-sectional study involving 11 dialysis and transplant centres from which 859 patients were randomly selected for interview. Of these patients 287 were on home HD, 347 on in-centre HD, 81 on CAPD, and 144 transplants. This study looked at objective (functional impairment Karnofsky index, and ability to work) and subjective indicators (life satisfaction, well-being and general affect). The overall results are summarized in Table 5, which shows the results for the Karnofsky index. This shows that normal physical activity was present in 79% of transplant patients, 59% of home HD and 48% of CAPD patients. On the three subjective measures, transplant patients again had a higher quality of life than dialysis patients, who nevertheless compared favourably with the general population. Hence the perceived quality of life of the various groups did not differ significantly. However, the study concluded that objective evidence of successful rehabilitation did not exist, except in the case of transplant recipients and some patients undergoing home dialysis.

In a similar study, Morris and Jones [82] compared 160 patients with ESRD managed by the same renal replacement modes; they endorsed transplantation as a method of improving the quality of life for

Table 5. Functional ability according to the Karnofsky index in the four groups of patients studied by Evans *et al.* (percentages)

	HHD (n = 287)	ICHD (n = 347)	CAPD (n = 81)	TP (n = 144)
Normal physical activity	59	44	48	79
Normal physical activity part of time	25	25	25	9
Self-care only	9	13	12	5
Requires assistance	7	18	15	7

the majority of patients with ESRD. This study also showed that for older patients with ESRD, CAPD is well tolerated and shows superiority over in-centre HD. However, moderately high levels of psychological distress were noted in all forms of ESRD treatments.

The 'Battelle' series of studies, referred to above, addressed similar subjective and objective measures to assess quality of life. Of the three studies that were compiled together for analysis (excluding the National Heart Transplantation Study), the subjective quality of life assessment in the various patient groups again highlighted the superiority of subjective indicators in the transplant group, as well as the improvement in HD patients following EPO therapy. CAPD patients in the Battelle series also demonstrated a better perceived health status, a high index of well-being and greater life satisfaction than in-centre HD patients.

In the United Kingdom a combined Manchester/ Oxford study undertook to review these questions in 159 dialysis patients (78 HD, 81 CAPD) [83]. This study again reported a marked deterioration in mobility on treatment as compared to that prior to commencement of therapy, and the same was also true for items of everyday life (shopping, cooking, travel, social life) [84]. However, subjective measures of quality of life as perceived by the patient showed no significant difference from a normal population [85]. On various psychological scales (Cantrill's life satisfaction, semantic differential, life stress, happiness and satisfaction scale), these patients perceived life to be satisfactory and comparable to a normal population. However, one group (males less than 60 years of age with risk factors such as diabetes and ischaemic heart disease) was consistently less satisfied with life than older groups.

Another cross-sectional study evaluated the relationships between various clinical variables and quality of life of 147 CAPD patients, using objective indicators of quality of life (Karnofsky's functional score and Parfrey's symptom score) and subjective indicators (index of psychological affect, indices of overall satisfaction, of well-being, and Cantril's life satisfaction ladder). It concluded that age, nutrition and technique-related complications (catheter related, peritonitis rates) were associated with lower quality of life scores while use of EPO and long-term CAPD treatment was associated with higher scores on factor analysis. The dose of dialysis had no influence on quality of life scores (P. Gokal and K. Fortunas, unpublished data).

More recent comparative studies

Health profile measurements. A review of the literature showed 14 different comparative studies (Table 6). These were selected for the comparative analysis of the HRQOL of patients on different dialysis modalities. Most studies were carried out in the USA (64%). However, the studies were done before 1992 and all the studies adopted a cross-sectional design. CAPD (13 studies), home HD (nine studies), in-centre HD (nine studies), and transplantation (seven studies) were the treatments most frequently evaluated. Most of the studies over-represented one treatment group.

Studies collected various patients' characteristics, which could affect the quality of life results. A varying number of quality of life instruments were used in the study. Eight studies used one to three instruments to measure quality of life; three studies three to six instruments and three studies more than six instruments. The majority of the studies used a generic and specific instrument of quality of life simultaneously. Patients on different modalities were not comparable in 11 out of the 14 studies due to differences in their sociodemographic and health characteristics.

The HRQOL results obtained from the studies reviewed suggest that patients on home dialysis (HD and CAPD) showed better quality of life than patients on in-centre HD. Only a few studies found statistically significant differences between groups and only in seven studies were results adjusted for patient differences. All these results should be treated with some caution. Studies were cross-sectional in design. This means that comparison was made at one point in time so that the quality of life refers to a particular moment and does not permit comparisons of outcomes over time. Longitudinal studies could show how quality of life is subject to variation over time, due to ageing, development of complications or changes in comorbidity, or due to the patient's adjustment to his/her situation. Longitudinal studies will provide more accurate information on effects of treatment on HRQOL. In addition patients were not randomly allocated to a treatment modality (an argument that also applies to survival statistics). The other problem relates to the use of multiple instruments in each study, because no gold standard, all-encompassing instrument has yet been developed to measure HRQOL. Few studies used specific instruments for ERSD patients.

A well-conducted large study done by Simmons *et al.* [86], assessed 766 patients who experienced one of the renal replacement therapies for at least

Table 6. Details of comparative studies on quality of life in HD and CAPD patients, giving the instruments used to assess health outcomes. HHD = home HD, CHD = centre HD, N = number of patients [95]

Study	Quality of Life instrument	Dimensions of Quality of Life assessed	Group	N
Rozembaum *et al.* 1985 [189]	Karnofsky (modified)	Work, physical activity, sleep, sexual activity, Self-assessment of Quality of Life	HHD CHD IPD CAPD	8 208 24 46
Evans *et al.* 1985 [6]	Karnofsky Index of psychological affect (1) Index of overall life satisfaction (2) Index of Well-Being (1 + 2)	Physical functioning ability to work Emotional well being, life satisfaction CAPD	HHD CHD 81	287 347
Hart and Evans 1987 [190]	Sickness Impact Profile	Physical and psychosocial function, sleep and rest, eating, work, home management, recreation and pastimes	HHD CHD CAPD	287 347 81
Soskolne and DeNour 1987 [127]	Non-standardized items list Brief Symptom Inventory Psychosocial Adjustment to Physical Illness Scale	Physical, Psychological, social functioning, general well-being, economic, situation, stressors satisfaction with health	HHD CAPD CHD	29 34 63
Bihl *et al.* 1988 [135]	Haemodialysis Stressors Scale, modified Quality of Life Index Rating Scale	Physical, psychological, social function, general well-being, economic situation, stressors, satisfaction with health	HD CAPD	18 18
Wolcott and Nissenson 1988 [87]	Karnofsky Global Adjustment to Illness Simmons self-esteem Scale Multidimensional Health Locus of Control Modality Specific Stress scale General Treatment Stress scale Global Illness Stress on Self and Others Illness Coping Patterns Dialysis Relations Quality scale Social Support Satisfaction scale Social/Leisure Activities Index Dialysis Relationship Quality Resources and Social Supports	Sociodemographic and medical status, Physical psychological, social cognitive function, General well-being	HD CAPD	33 33
Bremer 1989 [89]	Objective measures, not standardized Positive and Negative Affect Scales Affect Balance Scale Index of General Affect Index of Well-being Two seven-point adjective pairs Seven-point Scales of Satisfaction of Life Scale of Control and Scale of Sexual Satisfaction	Physical, psychological, social, cognitive functioning, General well-being, Economic self-control, sexual performance	HHD CHD CHD CAPD	47 105 41 79

Julius et al. 1989 [191]	Modified version of Katz's index of ADL Physical dysfunction dimension of SIP	Physical functioning	CHD CAPD	171 125
Morris and Jones 1989 [192]	Life Satisfaction Scored, not standardized General Health Questionnaire Locus of Control Scale (not standardized) Threatening Life Events	Psychological and social functioning, family support, self-control of life.	HHD CHD CAPD	24 24 21
Simmons and Abborress 1990 [119]	Index of Physical Well-Being, not standardized	Physical, social and emotional well-being	CHD	83
	Rosenberg Self-Esteem Scale Rosenberg Happiness Scale Bradburn Happiness Item Campbell's Index of Well-Being Index of General Affect Overall Life Satisfaction Measure Social measures 'previously used' not specified	CAPD	510	
Muthny and Koch 1991 [91]	A questionnaire not standardized	Medical status, Life satisfaction, Emotional well-being, work, social function (family situation, leisure activities)	HD CAPD	290 68
Tucker et al. 1991 [193]	Patient Life Situation Questionnaire Well-Being Scale Patient Control Index Ziller Self-Other Orientation Task Marital Happiness Index	Physical, psychological, cognitive and social functioning General well-being, Economic situation, Self-esteem and hope	HD CAPD	22 29
Griffin et al. 1994 [194]	ESRD Severity Index Karnofsky Beck Depression Inventory Spielberg Trait Anxiety Inventory Positive and Negative Affect Scales Illness Effects Questionnaire	Functional status, physical symptoms, psychological adjustment, social functioning and general well-being	HD PD	35 63
Gudex 1995 [93]	HMQ (Health Measurement Questionnaire) Rosser Classification of Illness States	Physical, psychological and social function and general well-being	HHD CHD PD	59 95 93

1 year, but who in addition were non-diabetic and aged between 19 and 56 years. The four groups that were studied were in-centre HD (83 patients from eight centres), CAPD (510 patients from 185 centres), current transplants (91 patients successfully transplanted between 1980 and 1984) and historical transplants (82 performed in the 1970s). Survey questionnaires were administered containing measures of physical, emotional and social well-being, vocational rehabilitation, and sexual adjustment. Case-mix differences were controlled, so far as possible, with an analysis of covariance; adjusted means were compared. Findings of the study again indicate that the quality of life for successful transplant recipients exceeded that of both dialysis groups for almost all variables; however, CAPD patients had significantly better life and therapy satisfactions as compared to in-centre HD patients.

In another comparative study by Wolcott and Nissenson [87] 33 matched pairs of CAPD and in-centre HD patients were assessed for various measures of quality of life. Here CAPD patients had a higher quality of life, lower illness, lower modality-related stress, lower mood disturbances, higher employment, higher community activities and better cognitive function. Similar results were found in the 'Battelle' series, which also demonstrated a better perceived health status, higher index of well-being and a good life satisfaction than in-centre HD patients. In addition Nissenson *et al.* [88] found that CAPD patients had superior psychosocial adaptation, and concluded that patients who had higher levels of stress on in-centre HD may benefit from CAPD therapy.

Additional studies of quality of life in ESRD have re-examined these issues. The first of these is by Bremmer *et al.* [89], which looked at a self-administered questionnaire assessing both objective and subjective quality of life in 489 ESRD patients. This study revealed that patients differed in both objective and subjective quality of life when examined as a function of treatment modality. They found that quality of life was similar for successful transplant and home HD patients; these patients appeared to fare better than other treatment groups on both objective and subjective measures. Patients receiving staff-assisted in-centre HD and CAPD reported markedly diminished quality of life; these differences remained after statistically controlling for non-treatment variables. One of the purposes of the study was to test how representative were the results from Evans *et al.* [6]. Indeed, Bremmer *et al.* [89] substantiated the results of Evans and colleagues. The

reproducibility supports the usefulness of these measures for evaluation of different treatment modalities for ESRD, and presumably for other chronic diseases.

Tucker *et al.* [90] again compared in-centre HD and CAPD patients on several quality of life variables: dietary adherence, self-esteem, hope, well-being, marital happiness, perceived control of life, marital status, number of emotional support persons and participation in social recreation and work activities. There were no statistically significant differences in the quality of life variables due to treatment modality or demographic variables. However, CAPD patients did engage in significantly more social and recreational activities, though not more work activity, than did in-centre HD patients. An interesting point was the skewed racial distribution in this US population in that 73% of the CAPD patients were Caucasian whilst 72% of the in-centre HD patients were of black origin. This skewed racial composition, also noted in previous research publications, suggests that a choice of treatment is occurring on the basis of some set of patient characteristics or perhaps systematic assignment is occurring on the basis of race, sex and/or education.

Another study by Muthny and Koch [91] also confirmed the favourable outcome of renal transplantation in terms of medical and vocational rehabilitation. This was also true for emotional well-being, complaints and satisfaction of different life areas (satisfaction with physical performance, intellectual functioning, partnership, family life, sex life and leisure time activities). This study also confirmed the findings of Evans *et al.* [6], but was in conflict with Kalman *et al.* [92], who did not find differences between treatment groups, especially in terms of psychiatric morbidity. For example, using the global anxiety score in this group of patients in Germany [91], there was no discrimination between the three groups of in-centre HD, CAPD, and renal transplantation patients.

A recent quality of life study in the UK in ESRD patients undergoing dialysis and transplant treatments shows interesting results. The objective of the study was to describe quality of life issues among these groups of patients to be used in a cost utility analysis of renal failure treatment in Britain. Patients comprised in-centre HD (95), home HD (59), CAPD (93) and transplant (367) groups. A patient questionnaire (the Health Measurement Questionnaire), a visual analogue scale to assess overall distress, as well as the degree of distress caused by a series of feelings, and a modified version of the Rosser Matrix, had been developed to assess quality of life data [93, 94]. Thus the questionnaire and data analysis took into account comorbidity, severity, an overall disability level and an overall distress level. Patients on dialysis were significantly more impaired in all disability domains than transplanted patients. Home HD patients showed less disability according to the Rosser categories than patients on other dialysis modalities. With respect to comparability of comorbidity, the response in this study differed from those involved in Bremer et al. [89] and Evans et al. [6]. This may simply reflect national difference in experience of illness, but may also be due to age differences (CAPD and transplant patients in this study were older than their counterparts in the other two studies). In this UK study [93], 35% of the dialysis respondents needed a walking aid or help to get outdoors, or were bedridden. One-third had a problem with some aspect of self-care, and 30% reported that their usual activity was either severely affected or unable to be carried out; 84% had a problem with some aspect of personal and social relationships. Social life, hobbies, leisure and sex life were affected in up to 75% of dialysis respondents (Table 7). However, there were few differences between dialysis groups and, in addition, those with a functioning transplant had a much better quality of life than those on dialysis [95].

Two additional comments of concern relating to the design of the research come to mind from this study. First, age was clearly an important factor, and in this study there were several areas where significant differences were due to age differences rather than the treatment modes themselves. Indeed, after adjusting for age and comorbidity, statistically significant differences between all groups disappeared. The second point that one should take into account relates to the questionnaires: quality of life questionnaires can vary considerably depending on the aim and emphasis of the authors. The questionnaire used in the study was designed so that it could be sent out to respondents by mail; whilst questionnaires were fairly short, they still aimed to be comprehensive. A

disadvantage of this method is a potential loss of data, either through non-completion or through misunderstandings arising from ambiguous or difficult questions. An alternative design is an interview-based questionnaire such as that developed by Parfry and colleagues [49, 96].

In a Spanish multicentre study [97], involving 1013 randomly selected stable patients who were undergoing in-centre HD (88%), CAPD (4%), haemodiafiltration (7%) and home HD (0.7%) treatments, evaluation of quality of life was made using the Karnofsky and Sickness Impact Profile instruments. There were no significant differences between these patients, relating to dialysis technique, dialysis solution or dialyser membrane, while better haemoglobin levels were related to better quality of life. Again advanced age and comorbidity index were related to worse quality of life scores. In another multicentre study Merkus et al. [98] assessed the impact of demographic, clinical, renal function, and dialysis characteristics on the quality of life of Dutch dialysis patients, 3 months after the start of chronic dialysis treatment and comparing it with the quality of life of the general population. The authors studied 120 HD patients and 106 CAPD patients using the patient's self-assessment of quality of life instrument SF-36. They found that in both modes of treatment, quality of life was significantly impaired in comparison to the general population sample, particularly with respect to role-functioning, and physical and general health perceptions. Overall, HD patients showed lower levels of quality of life than PD patients on physical functioning, role functioning, emotional, mental health, and pain, but on multivariate analysis they only demonstrated an impact of dialysis modality on mental health. Comorbid conditions, haemoglobin, and residual renal function could explain the poorer quality of life to a limited extent in both groups.

Finally, in recent studies on quality of life evaluation, Carmichael et al. [99] in the UK, using the Kidney Disease Questionnaire (Quality of Life–Short Form) on CAPD [96], and HD [49] found that dialysis patients did differ from the normal population but there was no difference between CAPD and HD patients, except better social functioning in PD patients. Walters et al. [100], in Finland, used the general instrument SF-36 in a total of 2779 (2483 HD, 199 CAPD, 83 CCPD and 14 home HD in 1995) and in 3039 (2830 HD, 121 CAPD, 36 CCPD and 52 home HD in 1997) patients, found similar results between the groups, while there were only small changes of quality of life issues between these two periods of study (1995–97).

Table 7. The UK quality of life study [93]. This shows the percentages of patients in whom the domains of social life, leisure life and sex were seriously and adversely affected

	In-centre HD	Home HD	CAPD	Transplant	General population
Social life	74.2	63.2	65.2	21.6	11.9
Leisure life	71.9	58.9	68.5	25.5	12.1
Sex life	67.9	67.9	68.7	30.8	7.8

Time trade-off, sickness impact profile, SF-36, uraemic index and disease-specific questionnaires

Preference-based measurements

These measures of quality of life in ESRD patients were utilized in a total of eight published studies (Table 8). These studies were difficult to compare, because their objectives differed and consequently their methodologies varied considerably. The specific preference values in these studies were variable. A time trade-off (TTO) instrument was used in three studies; the ESRD patients were the judges in all of them and only they assessed the desirability (or preference) of their own health state.

Time trade-off (TTO) score looks at the ratio between years of full health, which the patient would consider equivalent to a lifetime with ESRD [26]. TTO is the ratio of the two where zero equals death and one equals full health. These workers, studying four groups of patients in various renal replacement treatment modalities, found that scores in these groups were: in-centre HD, 0.43; home HD, 0.49; CAPD, 0.56; transplantation, 0.84. Again, transplantation had the highest score, while patients on home dialysis had a satisfactory score with peritoneal dialysis being second to transplantation. This instrument has also been used to assess the impact of change of dialysis to transplantation [101].

Sickness impact profile (SIP) [21] is still recognized as a strong instrument for quality of life assessments. One hundred and thirty-six questions are put into 12 categories and scores are expressed on a scale of 1–100 with higher scores denoting worse states. Normal individuals have scores between 2 and 3 and terminally ill patients around 35. Hart

Table 8. Preference-based instruments (PBI) for quality of life (QoL) studies

Main author	Reference	Year	Main objective
Churchill	[107]	1984	To describe the characteristics of a PBI
Churchill	[26]	1987	To describe the characteristics of a PBI
Revicki	[108]	1992	To compare the values obtained using different QoL instruments
Hornberger	[109]	1992	To compare the values obtained using different QoL instruments
Busschbach	[110]	1993	To investigate the influence of age on preference based measures
Gudex	[93]	1995	To compare HRQoL for different forms of dialysis

and Evans [39] looked at this index in 859 renal replacement therapy patients. Scores for the transplant groups were 5.5, home HD 10, CAPD 12.2, and in-centre HD 13.9. The 'Battelle' series reported by Evans [7] relates these SIP scores by treatment modality, breaking down the scores into physical and psychosocial dimensions. Again the superiority of transplantation is obvious, while there is little to choose between in-centre HD and CAPD.

The *Medical Outcome Studies (MOS) short-form health survey – SF-36* has been used in assessing the health and functional status of chronic dialysis patients and to compare their health to well subjects and patients with other chronic diseases. Quality of life studies have also been reported in children [102, 103] and in the elderly [38, 84, 104–106].

Parfrey and colleagues [49] have assessed a health questionnaire, The *Quality of Life Assessment*, specific for ESRD in 107 dialysis and 119 transplant recipients. They looked at the prevalence of 24 physical symptoms and a questionnaire was devised using two new indices (a symptom scale using 12 symptoms and an affect scale comprising 12 emotions) and six indices previously used in other chronic illnesses. Constructive validity for the questionnaire was shown by interviewing 97 dialysis and 82 transplant patients in whom the authors hypothesized that physical well-being would be better in transplant patients. After each initial matching the transplant group were more active, with a higher objective quality of life and free of physical symptoms, than the dialysis group. Subsequently, 63 stable dialysis and 67 stable transplant patients, 15 dialysis patients successfully transplanted in the intervening year and five failed transplant patients were interviewed 1 year later to assess the responsiveness of the questionnaire. In the group who had recently been successfully transplanted both physical affect and quality of life scores showed a major improvement following transplant. The authors conclude that this questionnaire is specific for ESRD patients, and examines physical, psychological and social well-being. The instrument is brief, easily administered and reproducible. It also has construct validity and is responsive to changes in therapy.

A new instrument, the *Renal-dependent Quality of Life instrument (RDQoL)*, based on that of the Audit of Diabetes Dependent Quality of Life (ADDQoL) diabetes-specific individualized Quality of Life questionnaire, has been developed recently [51]. This instrument is an individualized questionnaire measure of the impact of renal disease and its treatment on the quality of life of dialysis patients. The questionnaires specify life domains (19 domain-specific items) and the respondents rate personally applicable domains for importance and impact of the renal condition. Face and content validity is established for adult renal patients and is being further evaluated for research and clinical use (Manchester, unpublished data).

Another promising renal-specific instrument, the *Renal Quality of Life Questionnaire (RQLP)*, developed by Salek [52, 53] is based on constructs representing a renal patient's own quality of life determinants. It is a condition-specific and modality-independent quality of life instrument which measures individual perceptions and expectations of renal patients; it is self-administered, easy to complete and with no need of training. It is a brief and comprehensive instrument, suitable for research and routine use, reliable, with face validity. It contains 43 items describing health-related dysfunctional behaviours that are specific to ESRD patients, grouped into five categories (eating and drinking, physical activity, leisure, psychosocial aspects and treatment effects). It is currently in use for evaluation in research and clinical use.

Rehabilitation and employment

The number of patients who have ESRD is increasing world-wide and approximately half of these patients belong to the working age of 18–55 years [111, 112]. Nevertheless, only about 25% of them are employed, in contrast to the initial optimistic projection that 60% of dialysis patients of this age would have maintained employment [111–113]. However, discussions on rehabilitation cannot be limited to the employment issue alone. The goal of any renal replacement therapy is to achieve a level of rehabilitation equal to that of the predialysis and premorbid state. Rehabilitation encompasses restoration of the patient's physical condition, psychological well-being and vocational rehabilitation. Successful renal transplantation provides the best rehabilitation for ESRD patients, whilst chronic dialysis patients have a dismal rehabilitation irrespective of the mode of dialysis [114]. Many factors, such as old age, diabetes, and comorbidity, account for this. To improve rehabilitation programmes a Life Options Rehabilitation Advisory Council was formed in 1993, with financial support from Amgen Inc. The council identified several common characteristics underlying successful renal rehabilitation programmes [115]. A report entitled Renal Rehab-

Table 9. The five 'Es' of total rehabilitation

Rehabilitation comprises:
  Employment
  Exercise
  Education
  Encouragement
  Evaluation

ilitation: Bringing the Barriers (Life Option 1994) brought about the five key areas that must be targeted to achieve rehabilitation success. These are outlined in Table 9, and referred to as the 'five Es'.

While employment is an objective parameter of quality of life, it is a more difficult parameter to assess because it is related to social circumstances, reimbursement for employment, 'employability' in view of employer-related bias against dialysis and transplant patients, and placement of housewives in an unemployed category [86, 112, 113]. Nevertheless, available data seem to support better employability of successfully transplanted patients (Table 10).

For CAPD patients Fragola *et al.* [116] found a similar percentage employed after commencement of CAPD; this study was undertaken when the therapy was still in its infancy, in the early 1980s. Simmons *et al.* [86], found sharp differences in vocational rehabilitation in the four groups (male patients: historic transplants, 75%; current transplant, 64%; CAPD, 35%; in-centre HD, 19%. Female patients: 36%, 31%, 15%, 11%, respectively). Julius *et al.* [117] evaluated 742 patients from Michigan and reported that CAPD patients were 2.6 times more likely to work than in-centre HD patients.

Employment prospects are known to be related to the functional ability of patients. From the 'Battelle' series it is apparent that diabetics were less able initially than non-diabetics to work, although the outlook for all patients improved with time. Even 15 months after transplantation, 50% of the

Table 10. Percentages of patients who are actually working or able to work on various treatment modalities. Modified from Evans [7]

Modality	Working	Able to work
Home HD	36.2	59.2
In-centre HD	20.5	37.2
CAPD	16.2	24.7
EPO–HD	22.9	38.7
Transplant	45.9	74.1
Diabetic transplant	21.5	37

non-diabetics had returned to work compared to 25% of diabetics. Seedat *et al.* [118] also reported a decline in employment in both CAPD and in-centre HD groups, but none in the transplant groups. Thirty-two per cent of the CAPD and 42% of the in-centre HD patients were employed in this series from South Africa. Simmons *et al.* [119] noted that vocational rehabilitation is a particular area of concern. Overall transplant patients are the most likely to be working full-time, but they pointed out that regulations concerning disability payments under the ESRD programme operate as disincentives for employment. In this study 51% of CAPD patients agreed that they did not work because they were worried losing social security disability payments. Walcott and Nissenson [87] found that 88% of the in-centre HD subjects reported no current participation in school work or household activities as compared with 55% of CAPD subjects who reported absence of these vocational activities. These workers felt, therefore, that CAPD is independently associated with a higher frequency of maintained vocational function in chronic dialysis patients. Whether this differential level of vocational activity resulted from the relatively small differences in educational history in this population, physician bias to selectively encourage more active patients to begin CAPD, or from true modality effects on vocational function is uncertain, and needs further assessment. In the study of Ifudu *et al.* [114] in which 430 patients treated by HD alone were studied using the Karnofsky scale, they concluded that a significant proportion of these patients were functionally debilitated, and these comprised diabetics (36.5% of the patients), women, Hispanics, and the elderly. In a study by Julius *et al.* [117] the subsample of known diabetic patients aged 20–64 years from the Michigan ESRD population was analysed. Seven hundred and forty-two patients entered into this study and interviews were conducted from 1984 to 1986. A significantly higher percentage of the patients undergoing stable CAPD were in the labour force than those undergoing in-centre HD (27.4% vs 9.6%). Using logistic regression adjusted for sex, race, age, education, marital status, primary diagnosis and duration of the ESRD, this stable CAPD group was 2.6 times more likely to be employed than in-centre HD groups. Similar data were reported by Bremmer *et al.* [89] (28% employed full-time on CAPD vs 9% on in-centre HD). This group showed that in-centre HD patients were more likely to be employed part-time than CAPD (23% vs 10%). In Europe the situation is not any different.

In the Oxford/Manchester study [81] there was a dramatic decline in the percentage of patients that were employed while on dialysis as compared to those before dialysis therapy (CAPD 44% from 73%; in-centre HD 42% from 83%).

Muthny and Koch [91] in Germany found that the transplant group had the highest vocational rehabilitation. Excluding those above the age of 60 years from the analysis, 31% of the transplant patients, 16% of in-centre HD and 19% of CAPD patients were working full-time. These are lower rates than in other reported studies but relate to about 50% or so of these patients reporting their vocational status as 'retired'.

Several reports suggest that physical training and exercise have some beneficial effects in terms of rehabilitation [120, 121]. Restoration of physical condition adds to the psychological well-being of these patients [122]. Education, evaluation, and encouragement to recreational activities (hobbies, travel, reconstruction of a new role, volunteer work, learning experiences, etc.) will provide a positive meaning to their existence and will give strength to continue to try to live a life as close as possible to the normal [123].

Sexual functioning and psychosexual problems

This is an area that has been neglected through ignorance and embarrassment on the part of the renal care team. Nevertheless, studies in this area have shown a dramatic decline in sexual activity for patients on both treatments (PD and HD). Relatively few studies exist in this field and they are summarized in a review [124]. Auer *et al.* [83] showed a dramatic decline of sexual activity on dialysis compared to 12 months prior to commencement of therapy. This applied equally to PD and HD patients; only 31% of patients had satisfactory sexual activity as compared to nearly 60% prior to dialysis, whilst the nonexistent sexual activity category increased from 22% predialysis to nearly 50% on treatment. Furthermore, when the same cohorts in the study were asked about an affectionate relationship, 87% of married couples were satisfied with marriage but only 24% had satisfactory sexual relationships [125]. Simmons and Abress [119] reviewed satisfaction with sexual activity in male transplant, CAPD and in-centre HD patients. On a scale of 1 (complete dissatisfaction) to 7 (complete satisfaction), the three groups had scores of 4.87,

3.11, and 3.21. In the study by Gudex et al. [93] relating to patients in the UK, sex life became seriously affected on therapy in roughly 70% of all dialysis patients (home HD, in-centre HD and PD), but only 31% of transplant patients. For hobbies and leisure activities and social life being seriously affected, similar percentages of dissatisfaction were reported in the four treatment groups.

In the study by Muthny and Koch [91] relatively high contentedness was reported with respect to family life, partnership and role in the family; less than 10% in this German study showed mild dissatisfaction in these areas. In contrast, however, almost 30% reported marked dissatisfaction with sex life. The highest dissatisfied group, being 40% of the in-centre HD patients, 33% of the renal transplant, 43% of the HD and 56% of CAPD patients, reported that they had had no sexual intercourse in the previous 4 weeks. Bremmer et al. [89] found sexual activity quite markedly down in in-centre HD patients compared to CAPD, which in turn was worse than in transplanted patients. Days since last orgasm, with intercourse, was around 180 days in in-centre HD patients as opposed to around 28 days in the CAPD patients and 4 in the transplant patients. Steele et al. [126], in a CAPD population of 68 randomly selected patients, studied the actual and desired frequency of intercourse, and the results were correlated with standard measures of depression, anxiety, physical symptoms, adequacy of dialysis, nutrition and assessment of quality of life using a 1–10 analogue scale. Sixty-three per cent reported never having intercourse, 19% reported having intercourse less than twice per month, and 18% having intercourse more than twice per month. The first group had significantly higher depression and anxiety scores, more physical symptoms, less satisfaction with their sexual activity and a poorer overall quality of life in comparison with the last group; these results were independent of nutritional status, adequacy and duration of dialysis. It is apparent from the above that in chronic dialysis patients there is a diminished participation in social and leisure activities with increased marital and sexual problems, as is well highlighted in the study of Soskolne and DeNour [127].

Thus the ability to function sexually remains an important human need even in the face of a chronic illness. The nephrology team should have a working knowledge of sexual dysfunction of these patients, not hesitating to refer them to a specialist who could try to offer them a successful treatment to improve the quality of their lives [128]. It remains to be seen whether the recent availability of the drug Viagra will improve male impotence, a multifactorial and common problem in dialysis patients.

Psychosocial adjustment and dialysis-related stress

Depression and denial are the main responses to the stress of a life on renal replacement therapy [129]. Depression is associated with limitations in social and role functioning, and is an important prognostic factor in dialysis patients [130].

Ever since the beginning of the era of dialysis treatment, remarkable therapeutic advances have allowed depression and denial to be seen as normal steps on the path to adaptation to the new mode of living. At the same time health stabilization on dialysis permitted a better acceptance of the new life. However, non-compliance to dialysis still remains a problem for many patients [130]. Probably the most important causes of non-compliance are personal traits and sociocultural factors unrelated to dialysis. De-Nour and Czaczkes [65, 131] found that low frustration, tolerance and primary and secondary gains from assuming a sick role were the most frequent causes of non-compliance. Inability to resolve depression, anger and hostility, whether due to personal reasons or imposed conditions, will lead to denial and non-compliance.

Serial studies have looked at the effect of chronic disease and therapy modality on subjective indicators of quality of life such as physical well-being, emotional well-being and social well-being [132, 133]. Simmons et al. [86] found that physical, emotional and social well-being and satisfaction with therapy as clusters all correlated significantly with therapy type. These findings clearly indicate the existence of differences between the various modalities for all dimensions of quality of life. In the same study the effect of therapy type on each specific variable within the clusters was also compared. On most variables transplant cohorts scored more favourably than either the CAPD or the HD group. For most of the 23 variables, differences among the four therapy groups were statistically significant. Comparison of the HD and CAPD groups showed significant differences favouring the CAPD group on nine variables (healthier than before therapy, self esteem, happiness, index of well-being, overall life satisfaction, social life satisfaction, happiness with therapy and would still be happy to choose the same therapy). The CAPD patients showed significantly higher health satisfaction, therapy satisfaction, and higher self-esteem than the HD patients and rated at least higher on the other seven variables. When a differentiation in the groups with regard to the years spent on therapy was taken into account, the results showed that CAPD patients no longer demonstrated an advantage over HD patients. Thus, when background characteristics and disease history variables are controlled, the advantages of transplantation persist but the advantages of CAPD over HD do not. Juergensen *et al.* [134], studying 103 CAPD patients using a variety of instruments (Patient Related Anxiety Scale, Beck's Depression Inventory, Patient Self-assessed Quality of life, Kupfer-Detre System II Somatic Symptom Scale) came to the conclusion that higher depression and anxiety scores and a poorer quality of life rating were associated with higher complication rates in terms of hospitalization, peritonitis and exit-site infection rates. They suggested that screening of patients with objective measures of psychosocial functioning may enable caregivers to predict the patients at greater risk for developing medical complications.

Undoubtedly, dialysis does impart stress, and several factors have been identified as stressors. Simmons and Abress [119] looked at satisfaction as an indicator of stress and found that in-centre HD patients faired worse. Walcott and Nissenson [87] found that CAPD had a lower modality-related stress score; this group also found that, in males over 51 years of age, lower vocational activity was associated with poor adaptation to dialysis and increased stress. Bihl *et al.* [135] found that the severity of stressors in CAPD groups was related to uncertainty of the future, limits on vacations and frequent hospitalization; in the in-centre HD group stresses were found to be fatigue and boredom, limitation of fluid intake and length of treatment. Similar findings are reported by Eichel [136] and Fuchs and Schreiber [137].

These studies suggest that there is some difference between the treatments in relationship to stress. The stresses are different and there are differing anxieties on the various modalities. However, others found that patients with good family support, adequate premorbid stress defences, and agreeable personalities with presence of control over health, cope better with dialysis independent of the modality treatment [61, 138]; Sensky [129] concludes that, in terms of adjustment to dialysis, or rehabilitation or quality of life, some patients simply do better than others, regardless of the method of renal replacement therapy. Thus, adapting to ESRD and to dialysis has to do not only with the treatment modality that is offered, and to the differences that may exist between these treatments, but also with the psychosocial background of the patient present at the time of commencement of dialysis. This can be developed with adequate education and support of the caregivers and the family.

Withdrawal of dialysis

Withdrawal of dialysis is now the second most frequent single cause of death in dialysis patients in the USA [139], accounting for 17% of all deaths, with a higher percentage in patients over 65 years of age. The main reason for the increasing incidence of dialysis withdrawal is the greater acceptance of 'high-risk' patients on to dialysis. Advanced age and comorbidity factors are no longer contraindications to initiating renal replacement therapy, and this usually leads with time to a poor quality of survival where 'life is worse than death' [140]. This leads to the consideration of withdrawing dialysis treatment. Thus elective cessation of life support is predicated on the belief that prolonged, futile suffering can be avoided, and one may undergo a dignified, 'appropriate and good death' [141, 142]. One needs to preserve dignity in dying. Weisman [142] defined a good death as being the type of death that one would choose if there were a choice.

Attitudes of dialysis unit medical directors and personnel vary on withholding and withdrawing treatment. Most would favour a patient's wish (92%). However, in patients with dementia, 32% would stop dialysis but 68% would continue [143]. In a study of 125 anonymously surveyed nephrologists from various states of the US, 98% of them reported omissions in terminal care with the patient's knowledge and 80% without the patient's knowledge [144]. In contrast, 43% responded that they would never initiate measures in order to hasten death, even if it had to become legal. The ethical framework utilized for withdrawal of dialysis comprised: medical benefit (cancer as criterion, 48%; multisystem complications 84%, dementia 79%) and quality of life criteria. It is obvious that ethical and legal questions connected with aspects of withdrawing life-sustaining treatments and reactions among patients, relatives and nursing personnel will increase in the near future, given that the number of disabled patients taken on for chronic dialysis increases progressively [145–148]. It is clear that dealing with severely ill patients with poor quality of life, intolerable pain and loss of human dignity is not something that doctors or even the patients themselves wish to face. 'Letting die is better than helping to live' [149], especially 'when dialysis becomes worse than death' [140]. However, there are still controversies regarding euthanasia, and very few would openly carry this out. Differences exist, regarding withdrawal of dialysis between US and Europe. In the USA the decision of a mentally competent patient to discontinue dialysis is now accepted, and the right of a patient to refuse treatment has clearly been established. The American Medical Association has defined specific guidelines for physicians, who are obliged to promote the dignity and autonomy of dying patients [150]. In Europe there is not yet legal acceptance of euthanasia or withdrawing from life-sustaining measures, although in countries such as the Netherlands, current medical practice is to accept 'assisted suicide' from the physicians, an act that is protected by a body of case law and strong public support [151]. In the UK, in a meeting in Edinburgh in 1997 of the British Medical Association, members voted against any change in the laws for accepting euthanasia ('others rightly see us saving life, not embracing death. Do not do anything to betray that trust'), and a few months later the Doctor Assisted Dying Bill, to permit assisted suicide for the incurably ill, was heavily defeated in the UK parliament.

Simple answers to this difficult matter are not available today. The dilemma is not as simple as 'to be or not to be'. Nephrologists have to face up to the rights of a human to live a life with dignity and meaning, and to let death be peaceful. Dialysis is a life-prolonging treatment for an incurable disease. The decision when to continue and when to discontinue treatment gives rise to a plethora of medical, legal, moral, religious and ethical issues that clinical nephrologists have to resolve together with their patients and their families, and with the rest of the multidisciplinary team.

Nursing-home dialysis

It is estimated that US dialysis population will have increased to 300 000 patients by the year 2000 [152]. It is projected that 60% of the patients will be 65 or older and will live longer after the initiation of dialysis [153]. Diabetes, a disease accompanied by many complications and comorbid factors, is now the most common attributed cause of ESRD [152]. Hospitalization rates of these ESRD patients and economical pressure which accompany the overall treatment of these usually sicker and unstable patients, are very high [153]. The transfer of these high-risk patients from a high-level acute-care facility to a chronic-care facility makes economic and practical sense. It may allow better long-term health care planning and more stability for the family or care-givers [154]. An estimated 2000–3000 ESRD patients are admitted to nursing-homes each year in the USA [155]. Usually there is reluctance on the part of most nursing homes to accept dialysis patients, mainly because of the need for more intensive nursing, medical care and training of the personnel in dialysis procedures. Data on how successfully dialysis is applied in nursing homes are sparse. Haemodialysis is the preferred mode in these settings but still a significant percentage (13–15% of ESRD patients) are treated with PD. Anderson [156] reported a 10-year experience with CAPD in a nursing-home setting. A group of 109 patients with a mean age of 62.7 years (62.4% of them being diabetics), with a large number of comorbid factors, were studied. The overall 6- and 12-month survival rates were 51.7% and 37.2%, respectively. Age greater than 75 years, poor functional status, coronary artery disease and decubitus ulcers were significant mortality risk factors. Diabetics and patients older than 75 were less likely to be discharged. Despite the dismal outcome of these patients, the authors believe that PD in nursing homes is still a reasonable option for these patients. This is supported when comparison is made with the expected life-span for the general population, outcomes of in-centre HD patients in the same age group, and the life expectancy of diabetics with the burdens of several complications (amputations, infections, malnutrition). Jassal et al. [157], in a retrospective observational study over 5 years in 185 elderly patients (mean age 67 years; HD, 80%; CAPD, 20%) managed in a programme of rehabilitation and care for disabled patients, found that 35% of the patients died, 34% were discharged home and 13% were still resident at the completion of the study. These results may not be very persuasive, but are encouraging enough for development of such programmes throughout dialysis communities.

Further research and study are needed in this area to confirm if PD in nursing homes will provide improved hospitalization, advantages over HD, overall a better quality of life and a lower economic burden for health providers.

Quality of life of family caregivers

A major contributory factor for many individuals, for good quality of life, is the ability to enjoy family interactions [158]. Family caregivers of patients with ESRD often experience varying degrees of discomfort, stresses and burdens due to the chronic illness management and long-term assistance that these patients need [158, 159]. Thus the importance of recognizing that family caregivers are an integral part of the ESRD treatment, and incorporating them in the plan of optimal care, cannot be minimized.

The burden for the caregiver is a multidimensional phenomenon reflecting the physical, psychological, social and economical consequences of caring for an impaired or handicapped family member [160]. This burden can be differentiated into objective and subjective categories [161]. Subjective burden refers to the perceived strain or stress associated with providing care, and objective burden refers to the disruptions in family life and activities related to providing care [158]. Objective burden is clear and definite (i.e. dialysis therapy) while subjective burden is related to the caregiver's personality and feelings about the tangible changes that occur as a result of assuming the caregiving role [158, 161]. There are only a few longitudinal studies referring to changes of the quality of life of caregivers managing ESRD patients at home. These show that social and recreation activities appear most affected in the carers [162], while depression, psychological overload, role captivity, behavioural problems, and stress are also common between family caregivers [159, 163], and especially with mothers and spouses of severely ill patients [164]. These changes in quality of life threaten the meaningfulness of life of caregivers and diminishes their compliance and care of the patient leading to dismal outcomes. Support provided by a multidisciplinary team (home sisters, social workers, dieticians, babysitters), has shown that the burden can be ameliorated and 'burnout' prevented. It also provides valuable feedback on quality of life issues [165]. Growth of children was better in families with low burden of care [165]. A structured parents' group, with several meetings with social workers and psychologists, enabled caregivers to interchange their experiences and thus be supportive to each other and bring to the notice of medical staff the impact on their quality of life and ways to improve the situation [159, 165].

ESRD and home/self-care dialysis impose a variety of long-term stressors to which both patients and their family members struggle to adapt. Today's society is changing, as is the structure of families. Modern families are non-traditional in composition, smaller in size, and more culturally, ethically and socioeconomically diverse than in the past [159]. There is concern as to how long families can continue to provide the types of caregiving expected. The population is ageing and patients live longer lives as a variety of alternative treatments are offered to ESRD patients. Families are now expected to handle more difficult caregiving roles and for a longer period of time. Society and health providers have a great number of challenges ahead as the twenty-first century nears. A multidisciplinary approach to the dialysis patient and the family caregivers will allow both groups a better quality of life, and can possibly prevent any non-compliance and withdrawal of care, which could lead to institutionalized care, with all the consequences that this carries.

Quality of life in patients on automated peritoneal dialysis (APD)

APD, a peritoneal dialysis technique which uses a machine to perform the dialysis exchanges at night, was first used in the early 1960s by Boen [166] and Lasker [167] in the US to treat limited numbers of patients by intermittent peritoneal dialysis. This mode of treatment leaves the patient free from the need to perform manual CAPD exchanges. Diaz-Buxo and Suki [168] introduced the technique of continuous cyclic peritoneal dialysis (CCPD) in the late 1970s, a few years after the introduction of CAPD. Despite the attractions of this method, limitations due to the size of the machines and the cost did not allow its spread. Today, the percentage of peritoneal patients performing APD at home is increasing, APD ranks as the fastest-growing home dialysis modality, and it is estimated that 20% of the PD population is treated with APD, related to its advantages [169–171]. This mode of dialysis has the potential to ameliorate the quality of life of PD patients, offering them more free time, less discomfort and a better dialysis dose. Studies on quality of life of patients treated with this method are still in progress. McComb *et al.* [172] assessed the impact of the introduction of a portable APD system on

HRQOL of 26 CAPD patients, using the RAND 36 item Health Survey instrument. They found an increased Kt/V, unchanged serum albumin, but an insignificant improvement in pain scores ($p = 0.079$). They concluded that the portable APD systems did not bring about predicted improvements in HRQOL. This was probably because of insensitiveness of the HRQOL instrument or because of undefined biases.

Wrenger et al. [173], however, indirectly showed that quality of life of their patients improved. Some of their patients continued to be treated with PD, despite having abdominal hernias and dialysate leakage. APD offered free time and rehabilitation to 69% of their patients who were under 60 years of age and were employed or in school. They had less back pain and young patients felt better regarding their body image, which is a significant psychosocial problem, especially in young female patients.

With the rapid technical developments and the wider spread of this method, we will need good randomized studies using sensitive and valid instruments to prove that the advantages of this method will bring the necessary improvements in terms of adequacy, rehabilitation and quality of life.

Impact of erythropoietin on quality of life

The introduction of recombinant human erythropoietin (EPO) for the treatment of anaemia of ESRD patients has indeed been a significant advance in the last decade. The impact of EPO has been quite dramatic, and several studies have been published which have shown a significant improvement in quality of life in dialysis patients [70–77], including considerable improvement in energy, physical activity, employment, rehabilitation and sleep. The specific improvements in a patient's functional health status and well-being demonstrated by clinical trials include increased exercise capacity [73], decreased fatigue, improvement on tests of visual, conceptual and auditory–verbal learning and improved sexual function [77, 174]. The National Cooperative Recombinant Human Erythropoietin Study, designed to evaluate the medical and social impact of EPO therapy on the dialysis population in the US, was initiated in 1990 [76, 175]. This is an open-label, multicentre study of a non-random sample of dialysis patients (HD and CAPD) of approximately 2100 adult dialysis patients with a history of anaemia from 203 US dialysis facilities.

The instrument used for HRQOL assessment was based on the self-administered SF-36 with role activities items adapted from the Nottingham Health Profile. To better understand the health burden of chronic renal patients, quality of life results were also compared with those of the general US population and with those of patients with congestive heart failure and clinical depression. As a component of this study, 448 dialysis patients who had not previously been treated with EPO (new-to-EPO) were compared with 520 dialysis patients who were already receiving EPO (old-to-EPO).

At baseline, scores for both groups were below those observed in the general population, reflecting substantial impairments in functional status and well-being among patients with chronic renal failure. Significant improvements from baseline to follow-up were observed among new-to-EPO patients in vitality, physical and social functioning, mental heath, looking after home, social life, hobbies and satisfaction with sexual activity. Scores from old-to-EPO patients did not change significantly but were comparable with new-to-EPO patients at the time of follow-up. Analysis of the results showed that some of the beneficial quality of life effects of EPO were mediated through a change in haematocrit levels.

The optimal haematocrit required to provide an enhanced quality of life, and yet avoid some of the potential risk of EPO, still remains to be defined. Although there are references that show an improvement in the quality of life, morbidity and mortality, associated with increasing the haematocrit, a recent study shows the adverse effects of normal as compared with low haematocrit values in HD patients with cardiac disease treated with EPO [176]. The authors studied 1233 patients with clinical evidence of congestive heart failure or ischaemic heart disease treated with HD. A group of patients (618) were assigned to receive doses of EPO to achieve and maintain a haematocrit of 42%, and 615 were assigned to receive doses of EPO sufficient to maintain a haematocrit of 30% throughout the study. Researchers had to halt the study because among the group with normal haematocrit levels more deaths and episodes of first non-fatal myocardial infarctions were noticed (risk ratio 1.3 versus the low-haematocrit group) and the authors suggested that, in patients with clinically evident congestive heart failure or ischaemic heart disease on HD, administration of EPO to raise their haematocrit to 42% is not recommended.

However, the study itself provides some interesting points of disagreement with their statements

[177, 178]. Although there were more primary events in the normal haematocrit group, mortality actually decreased with increasing haematocrit values in both groups. Furthermore, 32 patients in the same group died 16–318 days after stopping the study therapy, when their haematocrit values would have been lower. In addition the deaths did not correlate with the haematocrit or the dose of EPO [176]. A prospective well-designed large study is probably needed to address the issue of the optimal haematocrit levels and the optimal dose of EPO for ESRD patients. However, there are numerous studies showing the beneficial effect of EPO in the improvement of many aspects of the quality of life of ESRD patients [75, 179–181]. These studies clearly establish an improvement in health-related quality of life in dialysis patients after the administration of EPO.

Summary of studies on quality of life and future trends

Many factors seem to play a role in assigning a particular modality of therapy to a patient. These reasons have been reviewed in an excellent article by Nissenson *et al.* [182]. This situation is further complicated since patients frequently change their modality of treatment for both medical and nonmedical reasons [183]. Therefore the timing of the study comparing modalities becomes a critical variable in itself [86, 184]. Because PD patients have a higher drop-out rate compared to in-centre HD patients [185, 186] studies later in the course of therapy can be biased in favour of PD in that 'survivors' of the technique are studied [187]. Very few longitudinal studies of quality of life of dialysis patients have been done, and none has adequately addressed the critical issue of selection bias. Modality selection is important as it has an impact on outcome and quality of life, and an analysis of medical decisions making such a modality selection must include an understanding of the potential costs and benefits of the decision. In addition to this, few if any studies on patients have been evaluated predialysis, to determine if quality of life patterns truly represent the effect of dialysis, or rather are more representative of the predialysis status of the patient [188]. Only a very few studies have evaluated patients early in the course of treatment to determine what if any effect dialysis of any type might have on the patient. Finally, the impact of recombinant

human erythropoietin has been such that one must question the validity of studies prior to the EPO era.

What we need to know and how to achieve it

Dialysis care can be divided into three major component parts: structure, process and outcome. The outcome of most interest is, currently, mortality. However, other outcomes of therapy, critical to assessing the quality of care, will be added to the ongoing evaluation of ESRD programmes. It is important therefore when making assessments of the outcomes of care that specific areas of structure and process of dialysis care must be examined. Patient-specific data and case-mix are important variables that have an impact on outcome. Information that describes the relative importance and effects of various comorbid conditions, weighted by severity, is essential. These data are needed to adjust and evaluate outcome such as mortality, hospitalization rates, cost of care, intensity of resource utilization, quality of life, rehabilitation and patient satisfaction. In addition more information is needed regarding the influence of psychosocial and demographic characteristics on outcomes. The effects of income, job status, family status, education and various psychological factors (such as depression or coping mechanism) need to be examined. Other specific areas that need to be built into the equation related to treatment that the patient receives, are the effect of dose of dialysis prescribed and delivered, time of treatment versus solute clearances, dialyser uses, and changes of modality of dialysis. Finally, how the choice of modality is made and how this decision is controlled by the physician or by other factors is also going to be important.

When all these factors are corrected for, one then has to decide on what instruments are available to assess this quality of life and outcome. Many instruments are available (Table 4) and have been used for assessing the quality of life of dialysis patients. The central theme has always been to arrive at an instrument which is comprehensive enough to include many dimensions of quality of life, short enough to minimize respondent burden, reliable and valid, easily scored and interpreted, and inexpensive. Such comprehensive overall instruments are limited and have their drawbacks but the SF-36, Sickness Impact Profile, Nottingham Health Profile and Karnofsky Performance Index (functional ability) are good instruments. It would be important to supplement these with disease-specific information which is incorporated in the Kidney Disease Questionnaire; the new ones, the Renal Disease Quality of Life Questionnaire (RDQOL) and the Renal Quality of Life Profile (RQLP) seem to provide nephrology researchers of quality of life issues with further useful and valid instruments. In terms of assessing patients' mental or emotional condition and social well-being, various instruments also exist, but those that are easy to utilize include POMS and PAIS. The overall scales of well-being, life satisfaction and psychological affect are also useful. One cannot stress enough the urgent need for a core battery to assess quality of life in ESRD patients. Amongst hundreds of published papers one can barely find half a dozen that are studied by the same methods to ascertain aspects of quality of life. This lack of agreement about methods of measurement is at least a partial explanation for the contradictory information that is presented above. There is no general agreement about the quality of life of patients in renal replacement therapy. Some results are very hard to accept (e.g. in the study by Evans [7], American home dialysis and transplant patients were found to be happier than the general American public). The lack of consensus about patients' quality of life is not only an academic problem but also a highly practical one. If we do not know a patient's adjustment how can we study and elucidate the factors that influence adjustment, how can we improve adjustment or how can we suggest to patients which of the available renal replacement therapies is better for them. In this respect it is of interest that the US Renal Data System case-mix-adequacy of dialysis study has commenced and, because of the size and complexity, is likely to provide useful data, relating to risk stratification based upon patient case-mix and the impact this has on quality of care provided and the outcome of this care.

Summary

Rehabilitation can be achieved by renal replacement therapy. Data to date would indicate that most successfully transplanted patients achieve rehabilitation both on objective and subjective criteria in a cost-effective manner; however, unsuccessful transplantation has a poor quality of life outcome. Home dialysis patients achieve this same goal to a certain extent. For in-centre HD and PD patients the objective evidence of rehabilitation is lacking; however, perceived quality of life on subjective measures shows results comparable to a normal population. Comparisons between in-centre HD and CAPD populations are difficult but different modality-related stressors impart different stresses to the patient. CAPD has marginal advantages over in-centre dialysis. What is needed in the future, in unravelling the many questions facing the end-stage renal dialysis community with respect to outcome, appears to be the development of a model of risk stratification based upon patient case-mix. Patients can then be characterized in sufficient detail to draw practical conclusions. Whilst the effect on patient survival is important, of much greater relevance is the effect of the treatment of renal failure on patient quality of life and that of the family. Improving this outcome should be the primary goal of end-stage renal failure care whether or not life is substantially prolonged. Future studies in this area, addressing the shortcomings of the available ones as outlined in this review, should be given high priority for research funding.

References

1. Spilker B, Molinek F, Jhnston K, Simpson RL, Tilson HH. Quality of life bibliography and indexes. Med Care 1990; 28 (suppl.): D51–77.
2. Wilkin D, Hallam L, Doggett M. Measure of Need and Outcome for Primary Care. Oxford: Oxford University Press, 1992.
3. Gokal R. Quality of life in patients undergoing renal replacement therapy. Kidney Int 1993; 43 (suppl. 40): S23–7.
4. Editorial. Quality of life and clinical trials. Lancet 1995; 346 (8966): 1–2
5. Medical Research Council. Advice to applicants of clinical trial proposal, July 1993.
6. Evans RW, Manninen DL, Garrison LP et al. The quality of life of patients with end-stage renal failure. N Engl J Med 1985; 312: 553–9.
7. Evans RW. Quality of life assessment and the treatment of end-stage renal disease. Transplant Rev 1990; 4: 28–51.
8. Mathers DF. Beyond survival. Dial Transplant 1980; 9: 657–61.
9. Hopkins A. How might measures of quality of life be useful to me as a Clinician? In: Hopkins A, ed. Measures of the Quality of Life. London: Royal College of Physicians of London Publications, 1992, pp. 1–13.
10. Guyatt GH, Feeny DH, Patrick DL. Measuring health related quality of life. Ann Intern Med 1993; 118: 622–9.
11. Fitzpatrik R, Fletcher A, Gore S, Jones D, Spiegelhalter D, Cox D. Quality of life measures in healthcare. I: Applications and issues in assessment. Br Med J 1992; 305: 1074–7.
12. Alexander JL, Willems EP. Quality of life: some measurement requirements. Arch Phys Med Rehabil 1981; 62: 261–5.
13. Stout J, Auer J. Rehabilitation and quality of life on CAPD. In: Gokal R, ed. Continuous Ambulatory Peritoneal Dialysis. Edinburgh: Churchill Livingstone, 1986, pp. 327–48.
14. Churchill DN. The effect of treatment modality on the quality of life for patients with end stage renal disease. Adv Perit Dial 1988; 8: 63–5.
15. Patrick DL, Erickson P. Health Status and Health Policy. Allocating Resources to Health Care. Oxford: Oxford University Press, 1993.

16. Hopkins A. Measuring the Quality of Medical Care. London: Royal College of Physicians of London Publications, 1990.

17. Black D. Ethical issues arising from measures of the Quality of Life. In: Hopkins A, ed. Measures of the Quality of Life. London: Royal College of Physicians of London Publications, 1992, pp. 121–9.

18. Black D. Paying for health. J Med Ethics 1991; 17: 117–23.

19. Dew MA, Simmons EG. The advantages of multiple measures of the Quality of Life. Scand J Urol Nephrol 1990; (suppl. 131): 23–30.

20. Meenan R, Gertman P, Mason J, Dunaif R. The arthritis impact measurement scales: further investigations of a Health Status instrument. Arch Rheum 1982; 19: 1048–53.

21. Fletcher A, Gore S, Jones D, Fitzpatrick R, Spiegelhalter D, Cox D. Quality of life measures in health care. II: Design, analysis, and interpretation. Br Med J 1992; 305: 1145–48.

22. Bergner M, Bobbert R, Carter W, Gibson B. The sickness impact profile: development and final revision of a health status measure. Med Care 1981; 19: 787–805.

23. Hunt S, McEwen J, McKenna S. Measuring Health Status. London: Croom Helm, 1986.

24. Ware JE, Sherbourne CD. The MOS 36-Item Short-Form Health Survey (SF-36): 1. Conceptual framework and item selection. Med Care 1992; 30: 473–83.

25. Spitzer W, Dobson A, Hall J *et al.* Measuring the Quality of Life of cancer patients: a concise QL-index for use by physicians. J Chron Dis 1981; 34: 585–97.

26. Churchill DN, Torrance GW, Taylor DE *et al.* Measurements of Quality of Life in end-stage renal failure. The time trade-off approach. Clin Invest Med 1987; 10: 14–27.

27. Cox D, Fitzpatrick R, Fletcher A *et al.* Quality of Life assessment: can we keep it simple? J R Stat Soc, Series A 1992; 155: 353–92.

28. Lomas J, Pickard L, Mohide A. Patients versus clinician item generation for Quality of Life measures. Med Care 1987; 25: 764–9.

29. Anderson R, Bury M. Living with Chronic Illness: the experience of patients and their families. London: Unwin, Hyman, 1988.

30. Guyatt G, Bernan L, Townsend M, Pingsey SO, Chambers LW. A measure of Quality of Life for clinical trials in chronic lung disease. Thorax 1987; 42: 773–8.

31. Stewart A, Greenfield S, Hays R *et al.* Functional status and well-being of patients with chronic conditions. JAMA 1989; 262: 907–13.

32. Jenkinson C, Fitzpatrick R. Measurements of health status in patients with chronic illness: comparison of the Nottingham Health Profile and the general health questionnaire. Fam Pract 1990; 7: 121–4.

33. Patrick D, Deyo R. Generic and disease specific measures in assessing health status and quality of life. Med Care 1989; 27: S217–32.

34. Guyatt G, Walter S, Norman G. Measuring changes over time: assessing the usefulness of evaluation instruments. J Chron Dis 1987; 40: 171–8.

35. Tugwell P, Bombardier C, Buchanan W *et al.* Methotrexate in rheumatoid arthritis: impact on Quality of Life assessed by traditional standard item and individual patient preference health status questionnaire. Arch Intern Med 1990; 150: 59–62.

36. Deniston OL, Carpenter-Alting P, Kneisly J, Hawthorne M, Port FK. Assessment of Quality of Life in end-stage renal disease. Health Serv Res 1989; 24: 555–78.

37. Evans RW. Recombinant human erythropoietin and the Quality of Life of end-stage renal disease patients: a comparative analysis. Am J Kidney Dis 1991; 18 (suppl. 1): 62–70.

38. McClennan WM, Anson C, Birkeli K, Tuttle E. Functional status and Quality of Life. Predictors of early mortality among patients entering treatment for end-stage renal disease. J Clin Epidemiol 1991; 44: 83–9.

39. Hart LG, Evans RW. The functional status of ESRD patients as measured by the sickness impact profile. J Chron Dis 1987; 40 (suppl. 1): S117–30.

40. Meyer KB, Espindle DM, DeGiacomo JM *et al.* Monitoring dialysis patients' health status. Am J Kidney Dis 1994; 24: 267–79.

41. Jenkinson C, Lawrence K, McWhinnie D, Gordon J. Sensitivity to changes of health status measures in a randomozed controlled trial: comparison of the COOP charts and the SF-36. Qual Lif Res 1995; 4; 47–52.

42. Hemingway H, Stafford M, Stansfeld S, Shipley M, Marmot M. Is the SF-36 a valid measure of change in population health? Results from the Whitehall II study. Br Med J 1997; 315: 1273–9.

43. Devins GM, Binik YM, Mandin H *et al.* The Kidney Diease Questionnaire: a test for measuring patient knowledge about end-stage renal disease. J Clin Epidemiol 1990; 43: 297–307.

44. Laupacis A, Muirhead N, Keown P, Wong C. A disease specific questionnaire for assessing quality of life in patients on haemodialysis. Nephron 1992; 60: 302–6.

45. Laupacis A, Wong C, Churchill D and the Canadian Erythropoitin Study Group. The use of generic and specific quality of life measures in haemodialysis patients treated with erythropoietinn. Control Clin Trials 1991; 12: 168–79S.

46. Hays RD, Kallich JD, Mapes DL, Coons SJ, Carter WB. Development of the Kidney Disease Quality of Life (KDQOL) Instrument. Qual Life Res 1994; 3: 329–38.

47. Hays RD, Kallich JD, Mapes DL, Coons SJ, Amin N, Carter WB. Kidney Disease Quality of Life Short Form (KDQOL-SF), Version 1.2: a manual for use and scoring. P-7928, Santa Monica, CA: Rand, 1995.

48. KDQOL Newsletter 1997; 3: 1–8.

49. Parfrey PS, Vavasour HM, Bullock M *et al.* Development of a health questionnaire specific for ESRD. Nephron 1989; 52: 20–9.

50. Churchill DN, Wallace JE, Ludwin D *et al.* A comparison of evaluative indices of quality of life and cognitive function in haemodialysis patients. Control Clin Trials 1991; 12: 159–67.

51. Bradley C. Design of a renal-dependent individualised quality of life questionnaire. Adv Perit Dial 1997; 13: 116–20.

52. Salek MS, Reakes AM. Quality of life assessment in end-stage renal disease using a renal-specific quality of life profile (RQLP): a practicality and validation study. Report I 1994, University of Wales, Cardiff.

53. Salek MS. Quality of life assessment in patients on peritoneal dialysis; a review of the state of the art. Perit Dial Int 1996; 16 (suppl.): S398–401.

54. McKevitt P 1980. Support and support systems in dialysis. Dial Transplant 1980; 9: 980–1.

55. Perras SP, Zappacosta. AR. Identifying candidates for CAPD. Dial Transplant 1981; 10: 108–12.

56. DeNour AK. Medical staff's attitude and patient rehabilitation. Proc EDTA 1980; 17: 520–3.

57. McKevitt P. Support in home and self-care. Dial Transplant 1980; 9: 1097–100.

58. Burton H, DeNour DK, Cowley JA, Wells CA, Wai L. Comparison of psychological adjustment to CAPD and home haemodialysis. Perit Dial Bull 1982; 2: 72–86.

59. Auer J. Quality of Life in CAPD related to sex and age: a comparison with haemodialysis. Proc EDTNA 1981; 9: 204–10.

60. Rasgon SA, Chemleski BL, Ho S *et al.* Benefits of a multidisciplinary predialysis program in maintaining employment among patients on home dialysis. Adv Perit Dial 1996; 12: 132–5.

61. Sesso R, Yoshihiro MM. Time of diagnosis of chronic renal failure and assessment of quality of life in haemodialysis patients. Nephrol Dial Transplant 1997; 12: 2111–16.

62. deWardener HE. Some ethical and economic problems associated with intermittent haemodialysis. In: Wolstenholme GEW, O'Conner M, eds. Ethics in Medicine. Boston: Luth Brown, 1966, pp. 104–26.

63. Evans RW, Blagg CR, Bryan FA. Implications for healthcare policy. A social and demographic profile of haemodialysis patients in the United States. JAMA 1981; 245: 487–92.

64. Hagberg B, Malnquist AA. A prospective study of patients on chronic haemodialysis. Pretreatment of psychiatric and psychological variables predicting outcome. J Psychosom Res 1974; 18: 315–22.

65. DeNour AK, Czaczkes JW. Adjustment to chronic haemodialysis. Israel J Med Sci 1974; 10: 498–505.

66. Gutman RA, Stead WW, Robinson RR *et al.* Physical activity and employment status of patients on maintenance haemodialysis. N Engl J Med 1981; 304: 309–13.

67. Rennie D. Renal rehabilitation – where are the data? N Engl J Med 1981; 304: 351–3.

68. Evans RW, Manninen DL, Garrison LP *et al.* Special reports: Fundings from the National Kidney Dialysis and Kidney Transplantation Study. HCFA Publ No. 3230, Baltimore, MD: Health Care Financing Administration, 1987.

69. National ESRD Patient Rehabilitation Task Force: Final report of the National ESRD Patient Rehabilitation Task Force. Transmitted by RA Guttman, June 1980.

70. Auer J, Simon G, Oliver DO, Anastassiades E, Stephens J, Gokal R. Improvements in quality of life on CAPD patients treated with subcutaneously administered erythropoietin for anaemia. Perit Dial Int 1992; 12: 40–2.

71. Deniiston QL, Luscombe FA, Buesching DP, Richer RE, Spinowitz BS. Effect of long term erythropoietin beta therapy on the quality of life of haemodialysis patients. Am Soc Artif Organs Transplant 1990; 36: M157–60.

72. Wolcott DL, Marsh JT, LaRue A, Carr C, Nissenson AR. Recombinant human erythropoietin treatment may improve quality of life and cognitive function in chronic haemodialysis patients. Am J Kidney Dis 1989; 14 (suppl. 1): 14–18.

73. Canadian Erythropoietin Study Group. Association between recombinant human erythropoietin and quality of life and exercise capacity of patients receiving haemodialysis. Br Med J 1990; 300: 573–8.

74. Evans RW. Recombinant human erythropoietin and the quality of life of endstage renal disease patients: a comparative analysis. Am J Kidney Dis 1991; 18 (suppl. 1): 62–70.

75. Evans RW, Rader B, Manninen DL. The quality of life of haemodialysis recipients treated with recombinant human erythropoietin. Cooperative multicentre EPO clinical trial group. JAMA 1990; 263: 825–30.

76. Nissenson AR. National cooperative rHuEPO study in patients with CRF. A phase IV multicentre study. Am J Kidney Dis 1991; 18 (suppl. 1): 24–33.

77. Beusterien KM, Nissenson AR, Port K, Kelly M, Steinwald B, Ware JE, Jr. The effects of recombinant human erythropoietin on functional health and well-being in chronic dialysis patients. J Am Soc Nephrol 1996; 7: 763–73.

78. Klahr S. Rationing of health care and the endstage renal disease programme. Am J Kidney Dis 1990; 16: 392–5.

79. Ari D, Held PJ, Pauly MV. The Medicare cost of renal dialysis. Med Care 1992; 30: 879–91.

80. Friedman EA. Nephrology and the rationing of healthcare. Contrib Nephrol 1993; 102: 200–36.

81. Maiorca R, Cancarini GC, Oreopoulos DG. PD or not PD? That is the question. Am J Kidney Dis 1997; 30: 445–7.

82. Morris PLP, Jones B. Transplantation versus dialysis: a study of Quality of Life. Transplant Proc 1988; 20: 23–6.

83. Auer J, Gokal R, Stout JP *et al.* The Oxford/Manchester study of dialysis patients. Scand J Urol Nephrol 1990; (suppl.) 131: 31–7.

84. Stout J. How does dialysis affect the lifestyle of renal patients? A comparative study between CAPD and HD. EDTNA J 1988; 9; 11–2.

85. Stout J, Gokal R, Hillier V *et al.* Quality of Life of high risk and elderly dialysis patients in the UK. Dial Transplant 1987; 16: 674–7.

86. Simmons RG, Anderson CR, Abress LK. Quality of Life and rehabilitation differences among four ESRD therapy groups. Scand J Urol Nephrol 1990; (suppl.) 131: 7–22.

87. Wolcott DL, Nissenson AR. Quality of Life in chronic dialysis patients: a critical comparison of CAPD and HD. Am J Kidney Dis 1988; 11: 402–12.

88. Nissenson AR, Maida CA, Katz AH *et al.* Psychological adaptation of CAPD and centre haemodialysis patients. Adv Perit Dial 1986; 4: 47–56.

89. Bremmer BA, McCauley CR, Wrona RM, Johnston JP. Quality of life in endstage renal disease: a re-examination. Am J Kidney Dis 1989; 13; 200–9.

90. Tucker CM, Ziller RC, Smith WR, Mars DR, Coone MP. Quality of Life of patients on incentre haemodialysis versus CAPD. Perit Dial Int 1991; 11: 341–6.

91. Muthny FA, Koch K. Quality of Life of patients with endstage renal failure. In: La Graca G, Olivares J, Feriani M, Passlick-Deitjen J, eds. CAPD – A Decade of Experience. Basel: Karger 1991, Vol. 89, pp. 265–73.

92. Kalman TP, Wilson PG, Kilman CM. Psychiatric morbidity in longterm renal transplant recipients and patients undergoing haemodialysis. JAMA 1983; 250: 55–8.

93. Gudex CM. Health-related quality of life in endstage renal failure. Qual Life Res 1995; 4; 359–66.

94. Rosser R, Kind P. A scale of valuations of State of Illness: is there a social consensus? Int J Epidemiol 1978; 7: 347–58.

95. Gokal R, Figueras M, Olle A, Rovira J, Badia X. Outcomes in peritoneal dialysis and haemodialysis – a comparative assessment of survival and quality of life. Nephrol Dial Transplant 1999; 14 (suppl. 6): 24–30.

96. Parfrey PS, Vavasour HM, Henry S *et al.* Clinical features and severity of non specific symptoms in dialysis patients. Nephron 1988; 50: 121–8.

97. Moreno F, Lopez-Gomez JM, Sanz-Guajardo D, Jofre R, Valderrabano F (on behalf of the Spanish Cooperative Renal Patients Quality of Life Study Group). Quality of life in dialysis patients. A Spanish multicentre study. Nephrol Dial Transplant 1996; 11 (suppl. 2): 125–9.

98. Merkus MP, Jager KJ, Dekker FW, Boeschoten EW, Stevens P, Krediet RT. Quality of life in patients on chronic dialysis; self-assessment 3 months after the start of treatment. The Necosad Study Group. Am J Kidney Dis 1997; 29: 584–92.

99. Carmichael P, Popola J, Carmichael AR, Prosser DI, Stevens PE. Assessment of quality of life in a single centre dialysis population using the KDQOL-SF questionnaire. J Am Soc Nephrol 1998; 9: 142A (abstract).

100. Walters BAJ, Bander SJ, Lin S, DiDominic V. Quality of life comparison between HD, HomeHD, CAPD and CCPD using the SF-36 quality of life instrument. J Am Soc Nephrol 1998; 9: 240A (abstract).

101. Russell JD, Beecroft ML, Ludwen D, Churchill DN. The quality of life measures in renal transplantation – a prospective study. Transplantation 1992; 54: 656–60.

102. Doyle CL, Flannigan J, Mabe C. Tidal peritoneal dialysis vs CAPD Children's preference. ANNA J 1992; 19: 249–54.

103. Roscoe JM, Smith CF, Wiliams EA *et al.* Medical and social outcome in adolescents with endstage renal failure. Kidney Int 1991; 40: 948–53.

104. Sandroni S, Arona N, Vidrene L, Moles K. Feasibility of incentre staff assisted cycler dialysis. Adv Perit Dial 1990; 6: 76–8.

105. Kutner NG, Brogan DJ. Assisted survival, ageing and rehabilitation needs: comparison in older diallysis patients and age matched peers. Arch Phys Med Rehabil 1992; 73: 309–15.

106. Avram MR, Pena C, Burrel D, Antignani A, Avram MM. Haemodialysis and the elderly patients: potential advantages as to quality of life. Urea generation, serum creatinine and less interdialysate weight gain. Am J Kidney Dis 1990; 16: 342–8.

107. Churchill D, Morgan J, Torrance G. Quality of life in endstage renal disease. Perit Dial Bull 1984; 4: 20–3.

108. Revicki D. Relationship between Health Utility and psychometric health status measures. Med Care 1992; 30: MS274–82.

109. Hornberger JC, Redelmeier DA, Petersen J. Variability among methods to assess patient's well-being and consequent effects on a cost-effectiveness analysis. J Clin Epidemiol 1992; 5: 505–12.

110. Busschbach JJ, Hessing DJ, de Charro FT. The utility of health at different stages in life: a quantitative approach. Soc Sci Med 1993; 37: 153–8.

111. Evans RW, Blagg C, Bryan FA. Implications for health care policy: a social and demographic profile of haemodialysis patients in the United States. JAMA 1981; 245: 487–91.

112. Gutman RA, Stead WW, Robinson RR. Physical activity and employment status of patients on maintenance dialysis. N Engl J Med 1981; 304: 309–13.

113. Peters VJ, Hazel LA, Finkel P, Colls J. Rehabilitation experience of patients receiving dialysis. ANNA 1994; 21: 419–26.

114. Ifudu O, Paul H, Mayers J et al. Pervasive failed rehabilitation in center-based maintenance haemodialysis patients. Am J Kidney Dis 1994; 23: 394–400.

115. Life Option Rehabilitation Advisory Council. Renal Rehabilitation: Bridging the Barriers. Madison, WI: Medical Education Institute, Inc., 1994.

116. Fragola JA, Grube S, VanBlock L, Bourke E. Multicentre study of physical activity and employment status of CAPD patients in the United States. Proc EDTA 1983; 20: 243–9.

117. Julius M, Kneisley J, Carpentier-Alting P, Hawthorne V, Wolfe R, Port K. A comparison of employment rates of patients treated with CAPD vs incentre haemodialysis. Arch Intern Med 1989; 149: 839–42.

118. Seedat YK, McIntosh CG, Subban JV. Quality of life for patients in an endstage renal disease programme. S Afr Med J 1987; 71: 500–4.

119. Simmons RG, Abress L. Quality of Life issues for endstage renal disease patients. Am J Kidney Dis 1990; 15: 201–8.

120. Goldberg AP, Geldman EM, Hagberg JM et al. Therapeutic benefits of exercise training for haemodialysis patients. Kidney Int 1983; 24 (suppl.): 303–9.

121. Ross DL, Grabeau GM, Smith S, Seymour M, Knierim N, Pitetti KH. Efficacy of exercise for endstage renal disease patients immediately following high efficiency haemodialysis: a pilot study. Am J Nephrol 1989; 9: 376–83.

122. Kouidi E, Iacovides A, Iordanidis P et al. Exercise renal rehabilitation program: psychosocial effects. Nephron 1997; 77: 152–8.

123. Oberley ET, Compton A. Nursing interventions for rehabilitating renal patients. ANNA J 1994; 21: 407–11.

124. Gokal R, Uttley L. A collection of problems in CAPD. Adv Perit Dial 1989; 5: 76–80.

125. Stout JP, Auer J, Kincey J et al. Sexual and marital relationships and dialysis patients' viewpoint. Perit Dial Bull 1987; 7: 97–101.

126. Steele TE, Wuerth D, Finkelstein S et al. Sexual experience of the CAPD patient. J Am Soc Nephrol 1996; 7: 1165–8.

127. Soskolne V, DeNour AK. Psychosocial adjustment of home HD, CAPD and hospital diaysis patients and their spouses. Nephron 1987; 47: 266–73.

128. Uttley L. Treatment of sexual dysfunction. Perit Dial Int 1996; 16 (suppl. 1): S402–5.

129. Sensky T. Psychosomatic aspects of endstage renal failure. Psychother Psychosom 1993; 59: 56–68.

130. Kimmel PL, Peterson RA, Simmens SJ et al. Psychosocial factors, behavioral compliance and survival in urban haemodialysis patients. Kidney Int 1998; 54: 245–54.

131. DeNour AK, Czaczkes JW. Personality factors in chronic haemodialysis patients causing non-compliance with medical regime. Psychosom Med 1972; 34: 333–44.

132. Wells KB, Stewart A, Hays RD et al. The functioning and well-being of depressed patients. Results from the Medical Outcomes Study. JAMA 1989; 262: 914–19.

133. Shidler NR, Peterson RA, Kimmel PL. Quality of life and psychosocial relationships in patients with chronic renal insufficiency. Am J Kidney Dis 1998; 32: 557–66.

134. Juergensen PH, Wuerth DB, Juergensen DM et al. Psychosocial factors and clinical outcome on CAPD. Adv Perit Dial 1997; 13: 121–4.

135. Bihl MA, Ferrans CE, Powers MJ. Comparing stressors and quality of llife of dialysis patients. ANNA J 1988; 15: 27–36.

136. Eichel CJ. Stress and coping in patients on CAPD compared to haemodialysis patients. ANNA J 1986; 13: 9–73.

137. Fuchs J, Schreiber M. Patients perceptive of CAPD and haemodialysis stressors. ANNA J; 1988; 15: 282–300.

138. Hoothay F, Leary EM. Life satisfaction and coping of diabetic haemodialysis patients. ANNA J 1990; 17: 361–5.

139. Agodoa LY, Eggers PW. Renal replacement therapy in the United States: data from the United States Renal Data System. Am J Kidney Dis 1995; 25: 119–33.

140. Sessa A. When dialysis becomes worse than death. Nephrol Dial Transplant 1995; 10: 1128–30.

141. Cohen LM, McCue JD, Germain M, Kjellstrand CM. Dialysis discontinuation. A 'good' death? Arch Intern Med 1995; 155: 42–7.

142. Weisman AD. On Dying and Denying: a psychiatric study of terminality. New York: Behavioral Publications Inc., 1972, pp. 32–41.

143. Moss AH, Stocking CB, Sachs GA, Siegler M. Variation in the attitudes of dialysis unit medical directors towards decisions to withhold and withdraw dialysis. J Am Soc Nephrol 1993; 4: 229–34.

144. Rutecki GW, Cugino A, Jarloura D, Kilner JF, Whittier FC. Nephrologists' subjective attitudes towards end-of-life issues and the conduct of terminal care. Clin Nephrol 1997; 48: 173–80.

145. Carlson RW. Editorial. Quality of death after discontinuation of dialysis. Arch Intern Med 1995; 155: 13.

146. Auer J. Dialysis withdrawal. Br J Renal Med 1997; 1: 18–20.

147. Sekkarie MA, Moss AH. Withholding and withdrawing dialysis: the role of physician specialty and education and patient functional status. Am J Kidney Dis 1998; 31: 464–72.

148. Moss AH. Managing conflict with families over dialysis discontinuation. Am J Kidney Dis 1998; 31: 868–83.

149. Oreopoulos DG. Withdrawal from dialysis: when letting die is better than helping to live. Lancet 1995; 346: 3–4.

150. Council on Ethical and Judicial Affairs, American Medical Association: decisions near the end of life. JAMA 1992; 267: 2229–33.

151. Angel M. Editorial, Euthanasia in Netherlands. Bad news or good news? N Engl J Med, 1996; 335: 22.

152. Annual data report of US Renal Data System. Incidence and prevalence of ESRD, 1998, pp. 23–35.

153. Annual data report of US Renal Data System. Incidence and prevalence of ESRD, 1998, pp. 121–32.

154. Schleifer CR. Nursing home dialysis: can we meet the challenge? Perit Dial Int 1997; 17: 234–5.

155. Anderson J, Kraus J, Sturgeon D. Incidence, prevalence, and outcomes of endstage renal disease patients placed in nursing homes. Am J Kidney Dis 1993; 21: 619–27.

156. Anderson JE. Ten years' experience with CAPD in a nursing home setting. Perit Dial Int 1997; 17: 255–61.

157. Jassal SV, Brissenden JE, Roscoe JM. Specialized chronic care for dialysis patients – a five year study. Clin Nephrol 1998; 50: 84–9.

158. Wicks MN, Milstead EJ, Hathaway DK, Cetingok M. Subjective burden and quality of life in family caregivers of patients with endstage renal disease. ANNA J 1997; 24: 527–38.

159. Campbell AR. Family caregivers: caring for ageing endstage renal disease partners. Adv Renal Replace Ther 1998; 5: 98–108.

160. Brunier GM, McKeever PT. The impact of home dialysis on the family: Literature review. ANNA J 1993; 20: 653–9.

161. Thompson JEH, Doll W. The burden of families coping with the mentally ill: an invisible family crisis. Fam Rel 1982; 31: 379–88.

162. LoGiudice D, Kerse N, Brown K *et al.* The psychosocial health status of carers of persons with dementia: a comparison with the chronically ill. Qual Life Res 1998; 7: 345–51.

163. Watson AR. Stress and burden of care in families with children commencing renal replacement therapy. Adv Perit Dial 1997; 13: 300–4.

164. Dunn SA, Bonner PN, Lewis SL, Meize-Grochowski A. Quality of life for spouses of CAPD patients. ANNA J 1994; 21: 237–47.

165. Watson AR. Home health and respite care. Perit Dial Int 1996; 16 (suppl. 1): S551–3.

166. Boen ST, Molinari AS, Dillar DH, Scribner BH. Periodic peritoneal dialysis in the management of chronic uraemia. Trans Am Soc Artif Intern Organs 1962; 8: 256–62.

167. Lasker N, McCauley EP, Passeroti CT. Chronic peritoneal dialysis. Trans Am Soc Artif Intern Organs 1966; 12: 94–7.

168. Diaz-Buxo JA, Suki WN. Automated Peritoneal Dialysis. In: Gokal R, Nolph KD, eds. Textbook of Peritoneal Dialysis. Dordrecht, Kluwer Academic Publishers, 1994, pp. 399–418.

169. KL, Cox P. Continuous cyclic peritoneal dialysis: a viable option in the treatment of chronic renal failure. Trans Am Soc Artif Intern Organs 1981; 27: 51–3.

170. Misra M, Nolph KD, Khanna R. Will automated peritoneal dialysis be the answer? Perit Dial Int 1997; 17: 435–9.

171. Williams P, Cartmel L, Holis J. The role of automated peritoneal dialysis (APD) in an integrated dialysis programme. Br Med J 1997; 53: 697–705.

172. Wrenger E, Krautzig S, Brunkhorst R. Adequacy and quality of life with automated peritoneal dialysis Perit Dial Int 1996; 16 (suppl. 1): S153–7.

173. McComb J, Morton R, Singer MA, Hopman WM, MacKenzie T. Impact of portable APD on patient perception of health related quality of life. Adv Perit Dial 1997; 13: 137–40.

174. Wrenger E, Krautzig S, Brunkhorst R. Adequacy and quality of life with automated peritoneal dialysis. Perit Dial Int 1996; 16 (suppl. 1): S153–7.

175. Nissenson AR. Recombinant human erythropoietin: impact on brain and cognitive function, exercise tolerance, sexual potency, and quality of life. Semin Nephrol 1989; 9 (suppl. 2): 25–31.

176. Levin NW, Lazarus M, Nissenson AR, for the National Cooperative rHu Erythropoietin Study Group: National Cooperative Hu Erythropoietin Study in patients with chronic renal failure – an interim report. Am J Kidney Dis 1993; 22 (suppl. 1): 3–12.

177. Besarab A, Bolton WK, Browne JK *et al.* The effects of normal as compared with low haematocrit values in patients with cardiac disease who are receiving haemodialysis and erythropoietin. N Engl J Med 1998; 339: 584–90.

178. Adamson JW, Eschbach JW. Editorial. Erythropoietin for endstage renal disease. N Engl J Med 1998; 339: 625–7.

179. Macdougal IC, Ritz E. The normal haematocrit trial in dialysis patients with cardiac disease: are we any the less confused about target haemoglobin? Nephrol Dial Transplant 1998; 13: 3030–3.

180. Eschbach HW, Abdulhadi MH, Brown JK *et al.* Recombinant human erythropoietin in anaemic patients with endstage renal disease: results of a phase III multicenter clinical trial. Ann Intern Med 1989; 111: 992–1000.

181. Beusterien KM, Nissenson AR, Port FK, Kely M, Steinwald B, Ware JE Jr. The effects of recombinant human erythropoietin on functional health and well-being in chronic dialysis patients. J Am Soc Nephrol 1996; 7 : 763–73.

182. Marsh JT, Brown WS, Wolcott D *et al.* RHuEPO treatment improves brain and cognitive function of anaemic dialysis patients. Kidney Int 1991; 39: 155–63.

183. Nissenson AR, Prichard SS, Cheng IKP *et al.* Non medical factors that impact on ESRD modality selection. Kidney Int 1993; 43 (suppl. 40): S120–7.

184. Porter GA, Lowson L, Buss J. Bias in selecting treatment for endstage renal disease. Kidney Int 1985; 28 (suppl. 17): S34–7.

185. Parfrey PS, Vavasour HM, Gault MH. A prospective study of health status in dialysis and transplant patients. Transplant Proc 1988; 20: 1231–2.

186. Gokal R, Jakubowksi C, King J *et al.* Outcome in patients in CAPD and haemodialysis: 4 year analysis of a prospective multicentre study. Lancet 1987; 2: 1105–9.

187. Serles KD, Blagg CR, Nolph KD, Vonesh EF, Shapiro F. Comparison of patient and technique survival in CAPD and haemodialysis: a multicentre study. Perit Dial Int 1990; 10: 15–19.

188. Kutner NG, Brogan D, Kutner MH. Endstage renal disease treatment modality and patients Quality of Life. Am J Nephrol 1986; 6: 396–402.

189. Oldenburg B, MacDonald GS, Perkins RJ. Prediction of quality of life in a cohort of endstage renal disease patients. J Clin Epidemiol 1988; 41: 555–64.

190. Rozembaum EA, Pliskin JS, Barnoon S, Chaimovitz C. Comparative study of costs and quality of life of CAPD and hemodialysis patients in Israel. Israel J Med Sc 1985; 21: 335–9.

191. Hart LG, Evans RW. The functional status of ESRD patients as measured by the sickness impact profile. J Chron Dis 1987; 40 (suppl. 1): S117–30.

192. Julius M, Hawthorne VM, Carpentier-Alting P, Kneisley J, Wolfe RA, Port FK. Independence in activities of daily living for end-stage renal disease patients: biomedical and demographic correlates. Am J Kidney Dis 1989; 13: 61–9.

193. Morris PLB, Jones B. Life satisfaction across treatment methods for patients with end-stage renal failure. Med J Aust 1989; 150: 428–32.

194. Tucker CM, Ziller RC, Smith WR, Mars DR, Coons MP. Quality of life in patients on in-centre hemodialysis versus CAPD. Perit Dial Int 1991; 11: 341–6.

195. Griffin KW, Wadwa NK, Friend R *et al.* Comparison of quality of life in hemodialysis and peritoneal dialysis patients. Adv Perit Dial 1994; 10: 104–8.

24 | The use of peritoneal dialysis in special situations

S. S. Prichard and J. M. Bargman

Introduction

Peritoneal dialysis (PD) is now widely and successfully used to treat end-stage renal disease (ESRD) patients. The continuous nature of the therapy and its home-based, self-care nature make it particularly advantageous for certain subgroups of patients. Using the peritoneal cavity as access provides additional uses of the therapy in both uraemic and non-uraemic states. This chapter focuses on the use of PD in special groups of ESRD patients and in a variety of non-uraemic conditions.

Renal failure: special situations

Pregnancy in ESRD

In 1978 a report from the European Dialysis and Transplantation Association (EDTA) reported on 115 pregnancies among 13 000 women of childbearing age followed by the registry [1]. Of the pregnancies that were not terminated, 16 livebirths occurred, representing a 23% success rate. Prematurity and low birth weight almost always occurred. Between 1980 and 1992, there were various reports of successful pregnancy [2–11]. More recent surveys have indicated a significantly higher incidence of pregnancy in women aged 14–44 years on dialysis [12–19]. In Belgium, 15 pregnancies were reported in 1472 women, giving an incidence of 0.3 per 100 patient-years [16]. The National Registry for Pregnancy in Dialysis Patients (NRPD) indicated an overall incidence between 1992 and 1995 in the US of 2.2%, with the frequency on haemodialysis being significantly higher (2.4%) compared to peritoneal dialysis (1.1%) [17]. Thus, pregnancy should no longer be considered a rarity among menstruating women on dialysis, and advice regarding contraceptives should be part of the care of these patients.

The rate of successful outcomes from pregnancy has also improved for dialysis patients. Hou reported that 21% of infants survived prior to 1990, and 52% after 1990 [18]. Most recently from the NRPD, 42% of infants survived [17]. However, there is a significant difference in the success of those pregnancies initiated prior to requiring dialysis compared to those in whom conception occurred in a patient already on dialysis, with infant survival being 73.8% and 40.2% respectively. With regard to dialysis modality and outcomes there appears to be no advantage of haemodialysis or PD, with infant survival being 39.5% and 37% respectively. Thus, there appears to be no reason to change treatment modality at the time of a pregnancy being diagnosed. Similarly, modality selection of patients initiating dialysis after becoming pregnant should be based on the medical and social determinants that are used for all patients.

General guidelines to optimize pregnancy outcome in pregnant dialysis patients have been published [15]. These include maintaining a dietary intake of 1 g/kg/day plus 20 g/day for fetal growth requirements; adequate antihypertensive treatment; maintenance of a haemoglobin between 100 and 110 g/L with the necessary increase in erythropoietin dosages; prevention of metabolic acidosis, hypocalcaemia and hypercalcaemia; and water-soluble vitamin supplementation. Targets of adequacy in PD remain empirical but should probably exceed a weekly Kt/V of 2.4. Since small volume exchanges are necessary as the pregnancy progresses, frequent exchanges and automated PD are usually required. With regard to antihypertensive treatment, alpha-methyldopa and hydralazine remain the drugs of first choice. Labetolol appears to be safe, whereas other beta-blockers have been reported to cause some fetal complications. However, beta-blockers and calcium channel blockers can be used in more difficult cases. ACE inhibitors and ATI blockers remain contraindicated.

PD offers several theoretical advantages to the pregnant patient: the continuous nature of the therapy avoids the fluid shifts and blood pressure varia-

R. Gokal, R. Khanna, R.Th. Krediet and K.D. Nolph (eds.), Textbook of Peritoneal Dialysis, 2nd Edition, 737–754.
© 2000 Kluwer Academic Publishers. Printed in Great Britain.

tions seen in haemodialysis, and no heparin is required, which should reduce bleeding complications, especially abruptio placentae. However, problems peculiar to continuous ambulatory peritoneal dialysis (CAPD) do occur. Peritonitis has been reported in three instances and in one episode at 24 weeks gestation, this was associated with the onset of premature labour and a stillbirth [5]. As the pregnancy advances, the intraperitoneal volume of fluid tolerated may be reduced, requiring more frequent small volume exchanges in order to achieve the usual targeted plasma urea level of less than 18 mmol/L [7]. Catheter placement can generally be achieved without complication at any stage of pregnancy [6]. One patient was reported to have developed a leak and one had several catheters fail, requiring a change to haemodialysis.

The present use of erythropoietin (EPO) has alleviated the high transfusion requirements reported in the ESRD pregnancies prior to 1988. However, hypertension, which often complicates pregnancy in dialysis, might be aggravated [8, 11]. Hou *et al.* reported on five cases treated with EPO, and in none was hypertension a difficult management issue. The CAPD patient in that series required no additional antihypertensive medication [8]. Most patients require a significant increase in their EPO dosage to maintain the target haemoglobin of 100–110 g/L.

Spontaneous haemoperitoneum in the non-pregnant young women on CAPD is rarely a cause for concern. In pregnancy, however, it may represent the onset of an abruptio or the rupture of a uterine vessel and should be treated seriously, including observation in hospital and urgent ultrasound assessment.

A potential therapeutic manoeuvre for CAPD patients with premature labour is the addition of magnesium to the bath. Careful attention must be paid to serum magnesium levels, particularly when intravenous boluses of magnesium are also used.

In summary, a successful outcome of pregnancy can be achieved in many patients on PD. The reason for the apparent lower rate of conception on PD compared to haemodialysis is unclear. Throughout the course of a pregnancy for a PD patient, attention to recommended practices and potential complications is essential.

HIV-infected patients

Renal disease, including ESRD, is a frequent complication of HIV-infected patients [20–24]. The prognosis for ESRD patients who are HIV-positive is poor, particularly for those with AIDS at the time of starting dialysis. However, as overall prognosis for HIV patients has improved in the 1990s with the introduction of antiviral therapies, so too has the prognosis for HIV-positive ESRD patients [23, 25, 26]. Currently, survival in HIV-positive ESRD patients is related mostly to their CD4 counts [23, 27], as is true for all HIV patients.

Both haemodialysis and PD have been used to manage these patients. There are some reasons to advocate the use of PD preferentially, including caloric supplementation provided by the dialysate glucose, the maintenance of a home environment, and reduced risk exposure for the health-care providers. There can also be disadvantages. Dialysate protein losses in these patients, who are often otherwise nutritionally compromised and/or nephrotic, may worsen their nutritional status. Neurologic involvement causing physical and intellectual impairment sometimes contraindicates home PD as an initial form of therapy, or may require a modality change to haemodialysis after some period of time on home-based PD. Finally, the immunocompromised state common to all HIV-positive patients could predispose to an increased incidence of peritonitis or exit-site infections with unusual and difficult-to-treat infecting organisms.

There are somewhat conflicting data in the literature on the incidence and type of peritonitis in HIV-infected patients. Cruz *et al.* reported on their experience with five patients in 1989 [28]. Their peritonitis rate was extremely high (1 in every 2.7 patient-months). The predominant organism was *Staphylococcus*. Their overall survival after starting CAPD was 7.8 ± 2.4 months. In 1990 Graham *et al.* reported on a multicentre trial in which data were collected from 32 CAPD units [29]. Fifty-eight per cent of the population were intravenous drug abusers. In this study population 53% were asymptomatic, 37% had AIDS and 10% had AIDS-related complex. Twenty-five of the 32 centres reported that home PD was the preferred modality for HIV patients. There were 226 episodes of peritonitis in the 79 patients. Over half (55%) of these were Gram-positive, with *Staphylococcus* being the predominant organism. Gram-negative infections comprised 20% of the reported peritonitis episodes, of which almost 30% were *Pseudomonas*. Fungal organisms were isolated in 6% of the episodes and there was no growth in 18%. There was a substantial rate (29%) of modality change to haemodialysis reported. This high incidence of pseudomonal and fungal peritonitis has also been reported by Dressler *et al.* [30] and Lewis *et al.* [31].

In 1991 Wasser *et al.* did not report an increased incidence of peritonitis in HIV patients, nor did they report a higher rate of Gram-negative or fungal peritonitis [32]. However, in 1992 Schloth *et al.* reported on their experience with HIV-positive patients [33]. There was a two-fold increase in peritonitis in this population compared to their HIV-negative population (1 in 4.6 vs. 1 in 9.9 patient-months). Although Gram-positive organisms were the most frequent infecting organisms, there was a tendency (though not statistically significant) for a higher rate of Gram-negative and fungal peritonitis. These authors could not correlate infection rates with serum albumin levels in the HIV-positive patients.

Tebben *et al.* [34] analysed their experience with 39 HIV-infected patients. The peritonitis rates were more than 2-fold higher in their HIV patients, with pseudomonal and fungal infections being notably more frequent. In contrast, Wasser *et al.* [35] reported on 16 HIV-positive patients and found no increase in peritonitis compared to their HIV-negative patients (1 in 13.15 vs. 1 in 11.04 patient-months). In both of the later studies the peritonitis rates are high for the non-HIV groups compared to the experience widely reported with disconnect flush-before-fill systems. Perhaps, once these baseline peritonitis rates are reduced, a more consistent difference between HIV-positive and HIV-negative patients will become apparent.

Retention rates at the end of 1 year for HIV patients are variably reported from 28% to 45% [28, 29, 33]. Drop-out occurs largely because of death. In addition, modality change is frequent, largely to haemodialysis, but also to automated PD because of an inability to cope with standard CAPD therapy. Frequent peritonitis may also require a modality change. Kemmel *et al.* report no difference in survival using PD or haemodialysis [36].

Management of the HIV population with ESRD requires an understanding of their primary disease, its clinical course, new and therapeutic options. In particular, appropriate adjustment for drug dosages must be made. Commonly administered drugs, including AZT, DDI, gancyclovir, acyclovir, intravenous pentamadine, and Foscarnet all require a decrease in dosage with advanced renal failure. The peritoneal clearance of these drugs is minimal. The use of amphotericin at any therapeutic dose may result in further loss of residual renal function.

The maintenance of adequate nutrition is essential and difficult because of frequent concurrent diarrhoea and oesophagitis. A careful record of dietary intake with appropriate supplementation will help maximize general well-being. Unlike other dialysis patients, a low serum albumin is not necessarily a good prognostic indicator for HIV patients, as its causes are multifactorial, including urinary protein loss, diarrhoea, poor dietary intake and chronic inflammation. CD4 counts give a better index of prognosis.

Peritoneal dialysate drainage contains the HIV antigen and as such is a potential source of contamination [37]. It is recommended that universal precautions, as proposed by the Center for Disease Control [38, 39], be followed for these patients. Disposal of the spent dialysate can be in the toilet after treatment with bleach (sodium hypochlorite). The empty dialysate bags should be double-bagged prior to disposal, and needles used at home should be taken back to the hospital centre for disposal. Adherence to these guidelines can minimize any risk of transmission of the virus. Some countries may have more stringent regulations with regard to HIV waste handling.

In summary, the prognosis for HIV ESRD patients is improving overall, and PD can be successfully used to manage them. There are reasons to favour this modality, but there are some circumstances in which PD may not be feasible. Peritonitis rates are high for this patient population, particularly for *Pseudomonas* and fungus, but this has not precluded the use of PD. Finally, retention rates are low due to a high mortality rate and a failure to cope with a self-care, home-based programme as the primary disease progresses.

A novel approach to HIV treatment has been reported by Chapman *et al.* [40]. Dextrin 2 sulphate, a sulphated polysaccharide with anti-HIV activity, is instilled into the peritoneal cavity three times a week. Although patients appear to tolerate this treatment well, its efficacy remains to be proven.

Chronic liver disease

PD offers several advantages over haemodialysis in the management of patients with advanced chronic liver disease, with or without ascites. The avoidance of anticoagulation and intradialytic hypotension, and the direct drainage of ascites, should facilitate patient care. However, there are surprisingly few reports on the use of PD in this population.

In 1977 Wilkinson *et al.* reported on a large series of patients using acute PD in 20 patients with chronic liver disease, and 50 patients with fulminant acute liver disease [41]. None of the cirrhotic groups survived to leave hospital. Perhaps these early poor results have discouraged the use of PD in cirrhotic patients. More recent reports have shown much better success using PD.

In 1992 Marcus *et al.* reported on a series of nine patients, all with ESRD and advanced cirrhoses with ascites, managed with PD [42]. These patients showed survivals of up to 8 years on CAPD, with three of the patients still being alive and well on PD after 18–24 months at the time of the report. Noted complications included: pleural effusions in two, with one of these patients developing an empyema; recurrence of repaired umbilical and other hernias; and a peritonitis rate similar to the overall centre experience. Interestingly, these patients' serum albumin levels remained unchanged while on PD.

Durand *et al.* have reported a series of four patients with chronic cirrhosis and tense ascites who have been successfully treated with PD for periods of 2–11 years [43]. They reported excellent peritoneal clearance and ultrafiltration, and nutritional deficiencies were not a problem. Horie *et al.* also reported on a single case treated successfully for 30 months with PD [44]. Macia and co-workers also reported a patient with ascites and cavernous transformation successfully treated with PD who had a D/P ratio of 4 h of 0.86 and a high rate of ultrafiltration [45].

Dadone *et al.* studied the transport characteristics of 10 patients on PD with chronic hepatic disease (CHD) compared to normals [46]. The duration of PD therapy at the time of study for the CHD group exceeded 12 months. This again underlines the usefulness of PD in managing these patients. With regard to water and solute transport, the CHD patients had higher rates of ultrafiltration and higher small solute transport, but no correlation between dialysate glucose absorption and ultrafiltration. These results are summarized in Table 1. On the basis of these observations one can presume that the ongoing production of ascites probably contributes to the excess ultrafiltration, and that a high rate of lymphatic absorption continues in CHD patients on peritoneal dialysis, just as is found in CHD patients not on dialysis. In spite of this, PD effectively maintained both fluid balance and adequate solute clearance.

Patients who have hepatitis B or C do shed viral particles into the peritoneal fluid. As such, handling of the patients' blood and spent dialysate should be similar to the procedure for HIV-contaminated fluids, and the guidelines recommended by the CDC should be followed [38, 39].

In summary, patients with ESRD and concurrent chronic liver disease can be successfully managed on PD. Since the peritoneal drainage also manages the ascites, PD may in fact be the modality of choice if the patient is able to carry out the therapy.

Acute renal failure

Acute renal failure (ARF) requiring a dialytic intervention can be treated with intermittent haemodialy-

Table 1. Peritoneal dialysis in special ESRD populations

Patient groups	Peritoneal dialysis potential advantages	Peritoneal dialysis potential disadvantages
Pregnancy	No anticoagulation. Stable blood pressure. Minimal blood loss. Stable chemistries. Home-based. May add magnesium to dialysate.	Requires frequent exchanges. Tolerance of only small intraperitoneal volumes. Peritonitis precipitating labour.
HIV infected patients	Reduced health care. Provider risk exposure. Caloric loading with glucose. Home-based. Minimal blood losses.	Additional protein losses in dialysate. Increased peritonitis especially pseudomonas and fungus. Inability to cope requiring modality change.
Chronic liver disease	No anticoagulation. Stable blood pressure. Direct ascites drainage. Caloric loading with glucose.	Recurrence of hernias. Pleural effusions (pleural–peritoneal communication). Large protein losses in dialysate.
Acute renal failure	No anticoagulation. No vascular access. Stable blood pressure. Continuous solute clearance. Caloric loading with glucose. Can be done in locations where haemodialysis expertise is unavailable.	Requires high-dose PD to achieve adequate clearance in catabolic patients. Requires an intact peritoneal cavity. Protein losses contribute to net nitrogen losses.

sis, continuous renal replacement (CVVHD or CAVHD) or PD [46–52]. PD offers the advantage of being a continuous therapy, which does not require anticoagulation or vascular access. Furthermore, it can be performed in hospitals or on wards where haemodialysis nursing expertise does not exist. However, it cannot be utilized in patients with open abdominal wounds or abdominal surgical drains. It can be used in patients with recent abdominal surgery provided the incision site is intact.

Acute renal failure patients are frequently severely catabolic. Therefore, a high-dose PD therapy is required to maintain adequate clearances for both small and larger molecular weight substances [47, 49, 50]. This may involve the use of up to 48 L of dialysate per 24-h period. The use of large doses of PD fluid also gives patients a substantial caloric load, which can help reduce the catabolic state.

Careful attention needs to be paid to the patients' net nitrogen loss in assessing the success of PD in ARF. Although azotaemia can be controlled, the patient may remain in net negative nitrogen balance [46]. Potentially, the addition of amino acids to the dialysate could improve nitrogen balance at the risk of worsening azotaemia [53]. If an appropriate balance between azotaemia and catabolism cannot be achieved, aggressive daily haemodialysis or continuous renal replacement therapy may be necessary.

Access for acute PD may be achieved either by a temporary stylet catheter or a chronic PD catheter. If the expertise is easily available for its insertion, the latter is generally preferable because of its longevity. In patients starting ESRD therapy it has been advocated to have the peritoneal catheter in place for several weeks prior to its use, because of the increased risk of leaks when it is used early. This delay is obviously not possible in ARF, but maintaining the patients in the recumbent position for the first few days after catheter insertion can reduce this risk.

In summary, patients with ARF can be managed with PD provided their peritoneal cavity is intact. In order to obtain adequate solute clearances, high-dose PD must be utilized, and additional nutritional support is often necessary even though the PD itself supplies a large caloric load. In reality, as the use of continuous renal replacement therapies becomes widespread, PD as a treatment modality in ARF is not usual.

A summary of the potential advantages and disadvantages of PD for ESRD patients with concurrent pregnancy, HIV infection and chronic liver disease, as well as patients with acute renal failure, is shown in Table 1.

Hypercalcaemia and hypocalcaemia

Hypercalcaemia in non-uraemic patients can virtually always be treated successfully with interventions using bisphosphonates, calcitonin, or mithramycin, in conjunction with rehydration. Prior to the development of these pharmacological agents there are scattered reports of using PD with low or zero calcium dialysate to treat hypercalcaemia [54].

Currently hypercalcaemia has become a frequent complication of patients with ESRD who are managed with calcium containing phosphate binders. The availability of a lower peritoneal calcium-dialysate has somewhat alleviated this problem, and this is discussed elsewhere in this book. However, there remain a small number of patients on PD who develop severe hypercalcaemia [55, 56]. These cases can be well managed by utilizing a calcium-free dialysate solution made up by the local hospital pharmacy using distilled water, 50% dextrose, NaCl, and $NaHCO_3$. Long-term use of 1.0 mmol/L Ca solution in CAPD puts patients in negative balance for calcium [57].

Similarly, non-uraemic hypocalcaemia patients can be managed medically with appropriate administration of calcium, vitamin D, and magnesium. There is, however, a subgroup of ESRD patients who have undergone parathyroidectomy who may benefit from intraperitoneal calcium supplementation. Both Thompson and Neale [58] and Benz et al. [59] have reported cases of hungry bone syndrome post-parathyroidectomy with prolonged hypocalcaemia in whom calcium gluconate was safely added to the peritoneal dialysate for periods of weeks to months. The continuous nature of CAPD gave all four of these cases excellent calcium control. Thus, prolonged post-parathyroidectomy hypocalcaemia in ESRD patients may be an additional indication for PD.

Non-uraemic indications for PD

Congestive heart failure

In the severest forms of cardiac failure the salt and water retention which accompanies this condition may become unresponsive to even the most potent diuretics. With pump failure, forward perfusion can become so compromised that renal blood flow is severely reduced and renal insufficiency supervenes. The decrease in peritubular blood flow and tubular fluid flow rate limits the delivery of diuretic to its target sites within the nephron. Furthermore, with limited renal blood flow even if the diuretic were to reach its effector site the resultant diuresis and natri-uresis is limited by counter-regulatory effects within the renal circulation. The end-result is the lack of response to diuretics in the face of severely limited renal blood flow.

In the 1960s intermittent PD (IPD) was reported to be useful in the treatment of volume overload in patients with cardiac disease. The dialysis effected rapid fluid removal (more than 7 L on average). Diuretic responsiveness was reported to be restored in the majority of patients, presumably by the subse-quent 'unloading' of the heart, increased inotropy and hence improved renal blood flow. Because the dialysis ultrafiltrate is hypotonic to plasma, the hyponatremia in these patients was corrected by the removal of water in excess of salt. It was postulated that PD could be used in the treatment of refractory congestive heart failure in patients with concomitant renal disease, severe hyponatraemia, or for the opti-mization of a patient prior to cardiac surgery [60]. This method was also successful in treating severe cardiac failure in babies and children with congenital heart disease. Although the improvement was tran-sient, it enabled the infants and children with cor-rectable lesions to undergo cardiac surgery [61]. Other reports of the use of IPD confirmed its useful-ness in severe heart failure. Dilution studies con-firmed that salt and water removal led to an increased cardiac index. The majority of patients treated in this manner entered remission and some were able to undergo corrective cardiac surgery such as valve replacement [62]. IPD was used in the setting of acute myocardial infarction with subse-quent severe cardiac failure and was again found to be effective in fluid removal and correction of electrolyte abnormalities. It was suggested that PD could be used to tide a patient over this period until the myocardium was able to repair itself from the ischaemic event [63].

In each of the above reports IPD was used tran-siently. The patients who had remediable disease were benefited by the ultrafiltration, and had an opportunity to recover or undergo corrective sur-gery. Those without potential for improvement in their cardiac disease succumbed at some point after the dialysis. It became clear that for this kind of patient the only option to extend life in any real way would be to provide repeated dialysis. Subsequently a patient with severe arteriosclerotic heart disease and normal renal function was described who received repeated sessions of IPD every few months and who survived for 21 months after his initial

presentation with anasarca and pulmonary oedema [64].

A larger cohort of patients with refractory conges-tive heart failure who received repeated IPD was reported more than a decade later by Shapira *et al.* Ten patients with severe cardiac disease and baseline serum creatinine concentrations ranging between 2.7 and 7.1 mg/dl received up to seven sessions of IPD. Between 4.5 and 15 L was ultrafiltrated with each dialysis. These patients experienced improvement in their quality of life with relief of pulmonary oedema or anasarca and a reduction in the frequency and length of hospitalizations. Interestingly, a dramatic increase in urine output was noted after the comple-tion of each dialysis, again presumably related to improved cardiac function and renal perfusion. Unfortunately, despite the implied improvement in overall quality of life (not formally examined), sur-vival remained short because of the severity of the heart disease [65]. Similar results were seen in the patients reported by Weinrauch *et al.*, who also noted that these patients did not tolerate ultrafiltra-tion by haemodialysis because of hypotension and angina, but were able to tolerate IPD somewhat better [66].

Continuous ambulatory PD (CAPD) was used in three patients with intractable congestive heart failure. Once again the dialysis effected an almost 10 kg weight loss with marked improvement in symptoms. However, recurrent peritonitis precluded continuation of CAPD, and all three patients died shortly after discontinuing dialysis [67].

Despite this disappointing initial report it was clear that CAPD, given its continuous nature, would be more suitable than IPD for the treatment of heart failure. With IPD there is the opportunity for reaccu-mulation of salt and water, and hence interdialytic weight gain. Furthermore, the rapid ultrafiltration which must occur during the IPD poses the risk of hypotension and unwanted electrolyte fluxes.

The optimism for CAPD was borne out by the report of a patient with severe ischaemic cardiomy-opathy, serum creatinine of 2.4 mg/dl and volume overload uncontrolled by diuretics, who was placed on CAPD, two or three exchanges daily, and was maintained successfully on this treatment for 2 years despite an ejection fraction of just 14% [68]. Subse-quent reports demonstrated that CAPD was success-ful in maintaining euvolaemia for months to years in patients with severe cardiac disease with or with-out renal impairment [69–72]. As a result of con-trolling hypervolaemia, long-term CAPD led to improvement in cardiac function in some patients [69, 70, 73].

Table 2. The effect of CAPD on patients with congestive heart failure

Parameter	Before CAPD	After 1.5–32 months CAPD
Systolic blood pressure	82	122
Diastolic blood pressure	55	72
Serum ANF (ng/L)	1253	295
Renin (pg/ ml)	12 730	3800
Aldosterone (ng/dl)	35	13
Na (mmol/L)	126	136

Other benefits noted included improved renal function; indeed, Shilo *et al.* noted an almost four-fold increase in renal plasma flow as measured by PAH clearance, and doubling of the creatinine and inulin clearance [71]. Presumably the improved renal perfusion was the result of increased left ventricular function. Coincident with correction of hypervolaemia there is an appropriate fall in plasma concentration of atrial natriuretic factor (ANF) and, in addition, the increased renal perfusion leads to a dramatic fall in plasma renin concentration and aldosterone levels [73]. Some results of this study are shown in Table 2.

The prognosis for these patients, however, must remain guarded. If the cardiac condition is not operable or self-limited, these patients are at risk for early cardiac death. Indeed, in one study 16 of 19 patients died a sudden death, probably the result of ventricular arrhythmias [72]. In Rubin and Ball's report overall median survival was less than 1 year, and the patients were hospitalized as often for dialysis-related problems as they had been before dialysis for cardiac-related problems [70].

Two more recent studies of larger numbers of patients further validate the use of PD in patients with intractable heart failure. Stegmayr *et al.* [74] reported in 1995 on 16 consecutive patients with NYHA Class III or IV treated successfully with PD, giving the patients improved functional status and reduced heart size.

Similarly in 1997, Ryckelynck and co-workers [75] reported another series of 16 patients, with intractable heart failure, 13 of whom did not have ESRD, all of whom demonstrated functional improvement and a better quality of life, including a reduction in hospitalization rates.

In summary, CAPD can be useful in the management of intractable congestive heart failure which has become unresponsive to drug therapy. PD is very effective in controlling salt and water overload and in correcting the hyponatraemia so frequently found in these patients. With the attendant ultra-filtration there have been reports of improved cardiac function, increased renal perfusion, and renewed responsiveness to diuretics. In the occasional patient there has been a remarkable prolongation of life, and in patients with transient cardiac dysfunction, intervention with ultrafiltration can be lifesaving. Overall, however, most patients are still left with very severe cardiac disease and so still have a poor prognosis.

Inborn errors of metabolism

The inborn errors of metabolism comprise a large and diverse group of diseases wherein there is often a missing intermediary step or enzyme abnormality leading to a block in the normal degradative pathways of metabolism. Such a block leads to the accumulation of precursors which can cause toxic manifestations, often in the neonatal period. Current therapy revolves around the recognition of the disorder, the rapid removal of the accumulated toxic metabolites, dietary modification, and vitamin supplementation [76].

Given the small molecular weight of the products to be cleared, dialysis has become important in the urgent removal of these toxic metabolites in the neonatal period.

Urea cycle defects and neonatal hyperammonaemia

In the hepatic urea cycle, several enzymes are involved in the metabolism of ammonia to urea. Deficiency of any of these enzymes can lead to a marked accumulation of ammonia in the blood, which manifests as neurological changes up to and including coma and death [76]. The mainstay of the treatment of this neonatal emergency is the rapid removal of ammonia.

The clearance of ammonia by haemodialysis and PD has been compared by several investigators, and in each case the clearance by haemodialysis was approximately 10-fold that achieved by PD [77–79]. Since the goal of treatment is to lower plasma ammonia levels as quickly as possible, it would seem prudent to use haemodialysis, if available, as the first line of therapy. As suggested by Wiegand *et al.*, PD may be useful adjunctive therapy once the ammonia levels have been lowered and dietary therapy is being introduced [78]. Indeed, in a baby with deficiency of the urea cycle enzyme ornithine transcarbamylase (OCT), treatment with rapid PD alone did not lower blood ammonia levels, and the baby died [80]. A recent report suggests that the combination of PD and venovenous haemofiltration can effectively reduce ammonia to safe levels [81].

Organic acidemias

Deficiency of a degradative enzyme leads to accumulation of organic acids with a number of deleterious consequences, including metabolic acidosis, elevated ammonia levels and, clinically, failure to thrive, poor feeding, vomiting, lethargy, and coma [76]. Absent proprionyl-CoA-carboxylase activity leads to proprionic acidaemia. Clinical outcome appears to be related to the plasma proprionic acid concentration. Russell *et al.* described acute PD to reduce plasma levels of proprionic acid; during the first 6 h of PD the blood levels decreased from 5.22 mmol/L to 0.66 mmol/L. Although the patient was being treated for sepsis simultaneously, the finding of proprionic acid in the dialysis fluid suggested that improvement was in large part due to the removal of the acid by dialysis [82]. Subsequent reports have confirmed the effectiveness of PD in the treatment of proprionic acidaemia, with [83] or without [84, 85] accompanying exchange transfusion.

Deficiency of the methylmalonyl-CoA mutase apoenzyme leads to methylmalonic acidaemia. The combination of acute PD and exchange transfusion proved lifesaving in a neonate with this condition, who unfortunately succumbed soon after to sepsis [86] Another $2\frac{1}{2}$-year-old child with methylmalonic acidaemia who was failing to thrive was placed on CAPD, six exchanges daily, to remove methylmalonate and control metabolic acidosis. The patient experienced a remarkable improvement, both clinically and biochemically, despite a number of dialysis-related complications [87].

Disorders of amino acid metabolism

Perhaps the most well known of these disorders is maple syrup urine disease (MSUD), so named because of the distinct odour of the urine. Infants with this condition present with feeding problems and neurological deterioration. The mechanism of the toxicity is unknown but an abnormality in myelin formation has been noted [88].

The biochemical defect is a block in the decarboxylation of the ketoacids of branched-chain amino acids (BCAA). Because of this block there is accumulation of the BCAA (leucine, isoleucine, valine) and their ketoacids. Again the goal of treatment has rested in part in removing the retained metabolites

and in inducing anabolism, but with foods deficient in BCAA.

Sallan and Cottom reported treating an infant with MSUD with 100 h of IPD, along with high-calorie feeding by the intravenous and nasogastric routes. There was a gratifying reduction in blood and cerebrospinal fluid BCAA levels, and the peritoneal clearance of leucine was similar to that of creatinine. The authors concluded that PD was more effective than repeated exchange transfusions for the urgent treatment of MSUD [89]. However, subsequent studies have revealed that haemodialysis results in a 7–10-fold increase in the clearance of BCAA and their ketoanalogues compared to PD [79].

However, as noted by McMahon and MacDonnell, haemodialysis and exchange transfusions are difficult, labour-intensive procedures carrying the risk of septicaemia and hypotension. Moreover, feeding, which is a crucial part of treatment, must often be suspended during these procedures. On the other hand, PD leads to a steady reduction of BCAA levels while allowing for the feeding of the infant [88]. This has been confirmed by reports of rapid reduction in plasma levels of BCAA with PD alone [85, 88]. Follow-up of patients with MSUD treated with PD in addition to parenteral and intestinal alimentation, has revealed normal somatic and intellectual development [90].

Disorders of carbohydrate metabolism

A 42-year-old woman with glucose-6-phosphatase deficiency (von Gierke disease) and renal failure was treated with CAPD. The use of hypertonic high-glucose solution overnight was able to prevent the nocturnal hypoglycaemia seen in this glycogen storage disease [91].

Type I hyperoxaluria

Liver transplantation is the treatment of choice for patients with type I hyperoxaluria. However, PD can remove a significant amount of oxalate and contribute to their management [92].

Acute pancreatitis

Acute inflammation of the pancreas leads to the elaboration of a number of potentially toxic substances from this organ into the peritoneal cavity. It is probable that these compounds are absorbed into the systemic circulation, where they contribute to the serious complications seen in severe pancreatitis, such as hypotension and non-cardiogenic pulmonary oedema. Suggested mediators produced by the inflamed pancreas include histamine, lipase, trypsin, kallikrein, kinins, and prostaglandins [93].

Lavage of the peritoneal cavity with dialysate or some other physiological fluid would seem to be an effective method to clear the potentially harmful mediators before they are absorbed. In 1965 Wall reported that the institution of PD for renal failure in three patients with acute pancreatitis led to rapid improvement in their overall status [94].

Subsequent animal studies suggested that peritoneal lavage conferred benefit in experimental acute pancreatitis. In dogs with pancreatitis induced by the injection of trypsin and taurocholate into the pancreatic duct, intervention with PD for 6 h led to a marked reduction of short-term mortality and, histologically, in decreased fat necrosis and pancreatic haemorrhage and necrosis [95]. More than two decades later similar results were obtained in dogs with pancreatitis induced by retrograde injection of bile and trypsin into the pancreatic duct. The survival rate was higher in dogs receiving peritoneal lavage and higher still in dogs lavaged with aprotinin, an inhibitor of trypsin, in the dialysis fluid. As in the first study, a marked reduction in necrotizing and haemorrhagic lesions was seen histologically [96]. Subsequent experimental work in rats also gave encouraging results [97–99].

In 1976 Ranson *et al.* randomized 10 patients with acute pancreatitis of mixed aetiology into two groups of equal severity. Five patients received PD with dialysate containing potassium, heparin and ampicillin for 48–96 h. Five patients received the usual supportive care. In the group receiving PD the duration of stay in the intensive-care unit was half that of those receiving conventional treatment. In addition, oral intake was resumed more quickly and the duration of hospitalization was shorter in the dialysed group [100]. However, after more experience with peritoneal lavage, these workers observed that, while PD led to a striking early improvement, there was no difference in overall mortality between the two groups. The later deaths in the dialysed patients were due to sepsis, particularly pancreatic abscesses [101]. To address the problem of late sepsis, Ranson and Berman randomized 29 patients presenting with acute pancreatitis to peritoneal lavage for 2 days or for 7 days. Once again ampicillin was added to the dialysate. The longer lavage reduced the frequency of sepsis and death from sepsis. In the subgroup of patients with many signs of poor prognosis, lavage for 7 days was associated with no deaths from sepsis compared to a 54% death rate in those receiving the 2-day lavage. These were small numbers, however, and it is interesting to note that the overall mortality in both groups was similar, with three deaths out of 15 patients receiving the short lavage, and two deaths (neither due to abscess) out of 14 in those receiving lavage for 7 days. The authors postulated that the longer dialysis is more effective because the inflamed pancreas continues to secrete enzymes and other harmful mediators for many days [102]. A trial of PD in acute alcoholic pancreatitis by Stone and Fabian noted a greater frequency of early improvement and lower mortality compared to those patients who received supportive care only [103].

Another important study led to a different conclusion. A large multicentre randomized study of 3 days of PD showed no difference in outcome in the 45 patients who received dialysis compared to the control group of 46 patients who received maximum supportive care. There were 13 deaths (28%) in the control group and 12 deaths (27%) in the lavage group. Furthermore, lavage did not change the length of survival or the incidence of pseudocyst or abscesses. (It is interesting to note that the lavage group lost a median of 44 g of protein daily in the dialysate.) Criticism of this study includes the fact that the median time to the start of dialysis was too long at 38 h, longer than the previous studies discussed above. The authors, however, suggest that the transperitoneal route of absorption of pancreatic toxins may not be as important as other routes, such as the lymphatics and pancreatic veins, so peritoneal lavage is not that crucial to treatment [104].

In summary, there is a good physiological and experimental basis to support using PD in severe acute pancreatitis. On the other hand, the human data have not convincingly demonstrated reduced overall mortality in those receiving peritoneal lavage. Probably this is related to the multisystem deterioration that acompanies severe acute pancreatitis; these patients are so ill that any one intervention may be unlikely to change overall outcome. Still, the treatment options are so limited in this devastating condition that a recent review on the management of acute pancreatitis still recommends PD for patients with severe pancreatitis who fail to improve with intensive supportive care during the first 24–48 h [105].

It should be noted that there are a number of cases reported in the literature in which PD is felt to have contributed to the aetiology of acute pancreatitis [106–108]. This remains an uncertain association [109].

Other surgical indications

A patient has been reported with chyloperitoneum associated with alcoholic pancreatitis. In addition to supportive measures the patient underwent PD with rapid improvement in abdominal pain and overall condition [109]. PD has also been successful in the management of traumatic haemoperitoneum [110] and to temporize in patients with perforated gastro-duodenal ulcers [111].

Psoriasis

The chance observations that psoriasis improved with both haemodialysis [112] and PD [113] led Twardowski and colleagues to try PD in non-urae-mic patients with severe forms of this skin disease [114]. Of the three patients, two experienced rapid improvement with almost complete resolution of the skin manifestations. Dialysis did not effect improvement in the third, who had pustular psoriasis. However, as the authors pointed out, the study was uncontrolled and spontaneous remissions are seen in this disease.

Since these original observations there have been numerous reports on the effect of PD on the natural history of psoriasis. Given the bias for reporting only positive results, it is perhaps not surprising that the majority of reports are of patients improving on dialysis [115–122]. Moreover, PD appeared to be more effective than haemodialysis in this respect [115, 121–123].

As emphasized by Kramer *et al.* [118], however, there are pitfalls in the interpretation of these studies. The ability of psychological factors to lead to improvement in psoriasis has been demonstrated [124]. Therefore the institution of dialysis may lead to remission by a 'placebo effect' rather than by removal of pro-psoriatic factors in the dialysate. In addition, if the treating physician truly believes the dialysis will be effective, the results could be misinterpreted. Finally, if the follow-up period is too short the relapse rate may be underestimated.

However, the study by Whittier *et al.* presented cogent evidence that PD led to real improvement in severe intractable plaque-type psoriasis [119]. In random order, patients received 48 h of sham or real PD weekly for 4 weeks. This was followed by a 2-month observation period after which the patient then received the alternative dialysis (sham or real PD) for 4 weeks, followed by another 2-month period of observation. Four of the five patients had a striking response to real PD, whereas none of the

patients showed improvement with the sham procedure. The results strongly suggested that PD is effective in altering the natural coure of psoriatic skin disease. The authors recommended trying PD in patients with severe plaque-type psoriasis (the pustular type appears more resistant to this treatment) [125] when other forms of treatment have failed.

If PD does indeed lead to improvement of psoriasis, the mechanism of the improvement is far from clear. How could the peritoneal cavity clear a factor(s) that the normally functioning kidney could not? Suggested explanations are that the factors are large molecular weight or extensively protein-bound, and therefore unable to pass through the glomerular capillary bed, but able to enter the peritoneal cavity. In a related fashion the factors may be rejected by electrostatic forces at the glomerular capillary wall. Finally, perhaps the factors are filtered, but completely reabsorbed by the renal tubules [126].

Glinski and colleagues suggest that the improvement seen with PD is the result of removing poly-morphonuclear leukocytes (PMNL) from the peritoneal cavity. These cells contain higher than normal amounts of proteases capable of inducing destructive changes in the stratum corneum of the skin. In a study of 16 patients with psoriasis there was a strong correlation between the number of PMNL removed by dialysis and the improvement in the skin disease. Content of the proteases in the PMNL was highest in the first few days of dialysis and fell thereafter. The authors speculated that the 'activated' PMNL are replaced over time by non-stimulated PMNL with normal or reduced content of proteolytic enzymes [127]. (Interestingly, Whittier *et al.* [119] could not find any correlation between the occurrence of peritonitis, with its high rate of neutrophilic exudation into the peritoneal cavity, and improvement of psoriasis.) These investigators also found that leukopheresis had a beneficial effect in psoriasis similar to that of PD, which is consonant with the hypothesis that the pro-psoriatic factor is contained within the PMNL [128].

Despite the flurry of favourable reports in the 1970s and 1980s, PD has not found widespread use in the treatment of severe, resistant psoriasis. It is expensive treatment and requires the involvement of nephrologists and nephrology nurses. There is the ever-present risk of peritonitis and other complications. Koebner's phenomenon may occur at the exit site [121], which could predispose to infection. Finally, the results do not appear, for the most part, to be long-lasting, and reactivation of disease may occur soon after discontinuation of dialysis [117, 121]. Therefore, this treatment should be reserved for the very exceptional cases of disabling plaque-type psoriasis where no improvement is effected by the current armamentarium of topical and systemic medications.

Acute hepatic failure

The liver possesses the capacity to regenerate. Because of this, the goal of treatment of fulminant hepatic failure has been to support the patient and optimize the status until the liver can begin to heal. Unfortunately, the advent of coma as a result of hyperammonaemia and other retained metabolites is a poor prognostic sign. Clinicians have attempted to remove the retained toxins by various methods to lessen the encephalopathy. PD has been said to be helpful in treating the coma resulting from liver failure.

In 1967 Krebs and Flynn reported on reversal of hepatic coma in a young man with viral hepatitis who received exchange transfusion and PD. The rationale for the concurrent use of dialysis was to aid in the removal of ammonia, not only that retained with liver failure but also that contained in the massive amount of old blood the patient received by transfusion. The authors were uncertain of the contribution of the dialysis to the patient's recovery [129]. Indeed, the use of dialysis in four patients (three PD, one haemodialysis) by Pirola *et al.* did not ameliorate hepatic coma [130].

A more optimistic report came from Mactier *et al.*, who used rapid-exchange IPD in five patients with fulminant hepatic failure of diverse aetiology. Four of the patients had concomitant renal failure. During the first period of IPD (up to 4 days) hepatic coma improved in four patients. Three of the patients recovered completely with normal hepatic and renal function on follow-up. The authors suggested that, because the overall prognosis of combined hepatic and renal function is poor, the recovery seen in three of the five patients suggests that PD indeed conferred a true benefit. The authors suggested that the results with IPD are comparable to those seen with haemoperfusion [131].

Perhaps the only real way to discern the effect of PD would be by means of a controlled clinical trial. This, of course, would be very difficult to carry out, particularly with the advent of successful liver transplantation for fulminant hepatic failure.

However, if the patient is not a transplant candidate, or there are no organs available, PD can prove helpful, particularly in the setting of associated renal failure. As suggested by Mactier [132], in contrast to charcoal haemoperfusion, PD can treat the extracellular fluid volume overload and hyponatraemia so often seen in this condition, remove uraemic and perhaps hepatic toxins, treat hypoglycaemia, and obviate the need for anticoagulation of an extracorporeal circuit.

Hypothermia and hyperthermia

In 1967 Lash *et al.* reported the use of PD as a method of core rewarming in patients with accidental hypothermia [133]. The use of external rewarming (blankets, etc.) in the absence of a method of core rewarming is felt to be dangerous. The peripheral vasodilation can lead to the shunting of cold peripheral blood to the core, producing further chilling of the heart and increasing the risk of serious arrhythmia. The vasodilation of peripheral vessels with external rewarming can also contribute to hypovolaemia by decreasing the circulating volume [134]. Dogs undergoing experimental hypothermia needed larger volumes of fluids and electrolytes when warmed externally compared to those who underwent core rewarming by cardiac bypass or PD [135]. The set-up for core rewarming by PD is not difficult, and should be available in most emergency units. As pointed out by Reuer and Parker [134], an added advantage to PD is the clearance of alcohol and some other drugs in those patients whose hypothermia is associated with an overdose of these substances.

There have been many reports of successful resuscitation from hypothermia with warmed PD [136–138] even when the original core temperature at presentation has been as low as 16°C [136].

Given the ease of access to the peritoneal cavity as a conduit for alteration of core temperature, it is not surprising that cold PD has been used in the hyperthermia associated with heat stroke [139] and meningococcal septicaemia [140].

Poisoning

The clearance of small molecular weight substances depends on blood and dialysate flow rates. For the majority of ingested poisons, which are of low molecular weight, clearance of toxins is consistently higher with haemodialysis than with PD [141].

The reports documenting the effectiveness of PD in the treatment of drug intoxication are generally from the time before haemodialysis gained wide-

Table 3. Intoxications treated by PD

Salicylates [142]
Barbiturates [143]
Isopropyl alcohol [148]
Potassium dichromate [149]
Bromates [150, 151]
Organophosphates [152, 153]
Carp gallbladder [154]
Lead [147]
Phenytoin [146]

spread use. PD proved beneficial in the treatment of salicylate poisoning [142] and barbiturate overdose [143], although the clearance of barbiturate is limited by its large volume of distribution [143]. Interestingly, the effectiveness of PD reported in Reye's syndrome [144] may have actually been the result of clearing salicylate by dialysis, before the association between salicylates and Reye's syndrome was appreciated [145].

Other intoxications in which PD has been used to increase clearance of the toxin are listed in Table 3.

There are perhaps some extraordinary circumstances where PD might be more effective than extracorporeal dialysis. For example, the anticonvulsant phenytoin is highly protein-bound and therefore poorly dialysable. However, a newborn with phenytoin poisoning was successfully treated by PD. The authors suggested that the permeability of the newborn's peritoneum is so great that the protein–phenytoin complexes were able to be cleared from the peritoneal cavity [146]. Intraperitoneal EDTA has been reported in the treatment of lead intoxication, but the patient had ESRD [147].

However, except in these unusual circumstances, or when haemodialysis is not available, PD should not be the treatment of choice for the management of poisoning. Haemodialysis affords higher small solute clearances which is important in the urgent treatment of intoxication.

Multiple myeloma

Although the causes of renal failure in multiple myeloma are diverse, the most frequent association is with 'myeloma kidney'. Histologically, there is deposition of immunoglobulin light chains in the tubules with surrounding inflammation. With progressive tubular damage renal failure supervenes.

Immunoglobulin light chains, present in high concentration in plasma cell disorders, are tubulotoxic. What is not clear is whether the removal of large amounts of light chains, by plasmapheresis or PD, is of benefit in reversing the renal failure of multiple myeloma. Although the total immunoglobulin has a molecular weight in the hundreds of thousands, depending on subtype, the light chain has a molecular weight of 22 000 and so may be partially transported across the peritoneum.

Yium *et al.* reported a 54-year-old man with IgG lambda myeloma who responded clinically to IPD. However, he was uraemic at presentation and improvement in his status could have resulted from the coincident treatment of sepsis and uraemia. Moreover, he remained in renal failure. However, the first IPD session removed 22 g of IgG, and the second removed 72 g of IgG. For this quantity to be removed by plasmapheresis instead would have entailed the removal of unacceptably large volumes of plasma [155]. On the other hand, when light chain rather than the whole immunoglobulin was measured, Russell and colleagues found that one 5 L plasma exchange removed 10 times as much Bence-Jones protein as 50 h worth of PD [156]. They concluded that plasma exchange was more efficient to remove light chains than PD. Moreover, Rosansky and Richards reported that PD removed just 104 mg of IgG per hour, which would extrapolate to about one-tenth as much IgG removed by this method than that reported by Yiu. Indeed, plasmapheresis removed over 100 times as much IgG per hour as did PD [157].

It remains controversial whether plasmapheresis has a role in the treatment of myeloma for reasons other than hyperviscosity, i.e. to remove light chains and so lessen the renal insult. Insofar as PD may be even less effective in removing significant amounts of Bence-Jones protein, it is doubtful that intervening with PD for reasons other than uraemia would benefit the patient with multiple myeloma.

Despite these concerns, however, there are some reports of patients with myeloma who improved after receiving PD. In one patient CAPD was commenced to increase the light chain clearance. The patient's renal function improved and repeat renal biopsy showed amelioration of the tubulopathy. However, chemotherapy was given concurrently and light chain clearance by PD was not documented, so the relationship of the PD to the improved kidney function remains tenuous [158]. Another patient with lambda light chain myeloma and renal failure was treated with CAPD. She refused chemotherapy but on dialysis alone experienced improvement in the haematological parameters [159]. Finally, a review by Cosio *et al.* of their myeloma patients and those in the literature gave perhaps the most intriguing results: if the patients were divided into those who recovered renal function and those who remained on chronic renal replacement therapy, the absence of light chain disease and the use of PD were both associated with increased recovery of renal function. In other words, patients treated with PD recovered renal function more often than patients undergoing haemodialysis. As the authors note, however, the number of patients treated by PD was small, and there may be a bias to reporting successful results [160].

While it is conceivable that PD could lessen the burden of immunoglobulin light chains presented to the kidney, there is insufficient evidence to recommend its use in non-uraemic patients. In the patient with renal failure, however, there may be an advantage to PD over haemodialysis because of the greater clearance of immunoglobulin light and heavy chains with PD. However, the role of light chain clearance, even by the more effective plasmapheresis, remains controversial, and it is well to remember that patients treated with haemodialysis have also shown improved renal function [161, 162].

Patients with myeloma, on CAPD, can do well with an acceptable rate of peritonitis. Their longevity is usually limited by the primary disease [163].

Aortic vascular prosthesis

Vascular disease is an increasingly common cause of ESRD as the population entering dialysis gets older. Concerns about the advisability of PD in patients with acute renal failure following abdominal vascular prosthesis placement have been raised in the light of possible leaks occurring and of peritonitis, which brings the site of infection and the graft into close proximity. However, a review of the use of PD in this setting would indicate that it is a safe alternative [164, 165].

Experimental uses for the peritoneal cavity: total peritoneal nutrition, paracorporeal membrane oxygenation, gene therapy

Total peritoneal nutrition

When the gut is unable to support enteral feedings, total parenteral nutrition has served as a useful alternative. However, the administration of large amounts of carbohydrates, lipids, and amino acids via the venous system has a number of drawbacks, both from a nutritional/metabolic standpoint and from a mechanical perspective. The latter includes exit-site infection, thrombosis, and septicaemia. Furthermore, these problems may be amplified in the paediatric population, where long-term venous access may be troublesome.

Given the transport capabilities of the peritoneal cavity, it became clear that not only intraperitoneal glucose but amino acids [166, 167] and lipids [168] were transported across the peritoneal membrane. Preliminary studies have documented the absorption of amino acids from dialysis fluid. A potentially useful role for the peritoneal cavity would be to absorb all the nutrients necessary for total nutritional support, in the event that oral feedings or intravenous alimentation were not feasible.

Sprague-Dawley rats were given nothing per os but were dialysed for 7 days with a solution containing 10% dextrose and 2% amino acids, electrolytes, vitamins, trace elements, carnitine, and choline [169]. They were compared to a cohort who underwent laparotomy and sham PD set-up but who were fed orally with the same amount of nutrients. The intraperitoneal feeding was found to support body weight and positive nitrogen balance. No hepatic steatosis developed in the animals fed intraperitoneally. The absorption of amino acid nitrogen and absorption of glucose from the peritoneal cavity averaged 95%.

The authors concluded that, even without data on lipid absorption, PD represents an alternative route for nutritional support. The peritoneal cavity might be especially useful in patients with problems with venous access, or in patients in whom large fluid loads directly into the vascular tree may pose difficulty, such as the patient with poor cardiac reserve. It remains to be seen if long-term nutritional support, with or without lipids, can be maintained in humans by the use of peritoneal nutrition.

Paracorporeal membrane oxygenation and removal of carbon dioxide

In acute lung disease, such as non-cardiogenic pulmonary oedema, the maintenance of tissue oxygenation is important for survival. There are a number of extracorporeal bypass-type membrane oxygenators that oxygenate the red cells and return them to the body. The peritoneal cavity has a large surface area with large splanchnic blood flow. If the peritoneal cavity could function as a paracorporeal membrane oxygenator it would obviate the need for the extracorporeal circuit or the attendant complex technology.

Table 4. The Peritoneum as membrane oxygenator (data from ref. 170)

Rabbit	Baseline PaO_2	12% FIO_2 (baseline)	12% FIO_2 + PD
1	86	39	87
2	128	34	111
3	61	29	62
4	139	78	150
5	85	46	74
6	111	43	82

New Zealand white rabbits were intubated and ventilated with a high nitrous oxide, low oxygen-containing gas to simulate severe hypoxia [170]. Two peritoneal catheters were inserted. Dialysate was bubbled with 100% O_2 and dialysis was carried out in this manner. The peritoneal oxygenation resulted in augmentation of p_{O_2} to very satisfactory levels. No gas trapping or surgical emphysema was noted. In addition, CO_2 was adequately removed by the dialysate Some results of this study are shown in Table 4. The authors concluded that peritoneal oxygenation is capable of augmenting oxygenation and carbon dioxide removal in the critically ill patient with acute respiratory failure [170].

In a different model the peritoneal cavity was simulated by a bubble oxygenator into which 10% CO_2 was added. The rate of CO_2 removal was a linear function of dialysate flow rate, gas flow rate, and concentration of bicarbonate. This model removed 60 ml/min of CO_2, which represents 30% of CO_2 production, a rate predicted to be able to treat hypercapnoea associated with acute respiratory failure [171]. It is hoped that further animal studies will be forthcoming on the potential of the peritoneal cavity as a gas exchange organ.

Gene therapy

Gene therapy is a technique in which genetic elements are inserted into the somatic cells of a patient, leading to *in-vivo* synthesis of a gene product or a change in endogenous expression of a gene. It has been used or proposed to be used in a variety of inherited or acquired diseases or to provide a new function for cells. The peritoneal mesothelial cells are an attractive target for gene therapy because they are a large cell population, easily accessible, stable, metabolically active, amenable to cell culture, and have proven to be genetically modifiable by viral and non-viral techniques [172–176].

The potential applications of gene therapy in the peritoneal cavity include:

1. Understanding peritoneal biology by adding or deleting a product thought to be important in normal peritoneal function such as transforming growth factor β or interleukin 1.
2. The prevention of surgical adhesion by inserting the production of tissue plasminogen activator.
3. The treatment of peritoneal malignancies using tumour suppressor genes or through the inactivation of functioning oncogenes, e.g. anti sense for K-ras.
4. The systemic delivery of therapeutic proteins such as human growth hormone or erythropoietin.

Although human clinical applications of gene therapy using the peritoneum remain to be proven, the potential of such therapeutic strategies is exciting.

References

1. Registration Committee of the European Dialysis and Tranplant Association. Successful pregnancies in women treated by dialysis and kidney transplantation. Br J Obstet Gynaecol 1980; 87: 839–5.
2. Hou S. Peritoneal dialysis and hemodialysis in pregnancy. Baillieres Clin Obstet Gynecol 1987; 1: 1009–25.
3. Hou S. Pregnancy in women requiring dialysis for renal failure. Am J Kidney Dis 1987; 9: 368–73.
4. Lavoie SD, Johnson-Whittaker L, Huard PJ et al. Two successful pregnancies on CAPD. Adv Perit Dial 1988; 4: 90–5.
5. Gadallah MF, Ahmad B, Karubian F et al. Pregnancy in patients on chronic ambulatory peritoneal dialysis. Am J Kidney Dis 1992; 20: 407–410.
6. Hou S. Pregnancy in continuous ambulatory peritoneal dialysis (CAPD) patients. Perit Dial Int 1990; 10: 201–4.
7. Redav M, Cherem L, Eliot J et al. Dialysis in the management of pregnant patients with renal insufficiency. Medicine 1988; 67: 199.
8. Hou S, Orlowski J, Pahl M et al. Pregnancy in women with end-stage renal disease: treatment of anemia and premature labor. Am J Kidney Dis 1993; 21: 16–22.
9. Nagiotte MP, Grundg HO. Pregnancy outcome in women requiring chronic hemodialysis. Obstet Gynecol 1988; 72: 456–9.
10. Barri YM, Al Furayh O, Quinibi WY et al. Pregnancy in women on regular hemodialysis. Dial Transplant 1991; 20: 652–6.
11. Fujimi S, Hori K, Mujemd C et al. Successful pregnancy and delivery in a patient following r Hu EPO therapy and on long-term dialysis. J Am Soc Nephrol 1990; 1: 397 (abstract).
12. Okundaye I, Hou S. Results of pregnancy in patients undergoing dialysis. J Am Soc Nephrol 1995; 6: 398 (abstract).
13. Hou S. Pregnancy in women treated with peritoneal dialysis: viewpoint 1996. Perit Dial Int 1996; 16: 442–3.
14. Okundaye I, Hou S. Management of pregnancy in women undergoing ambulatory peritoneal dialysis. Adv Perit Dial 1996; 12: 151–5.
15. Jungers P, Chauveau D. Pregnancy in renal disease. Kidney Int 1997; 52: 871–85.
16. Bagon JA, Vernaeve H, De Muylder X, Lafontaine JJ, Martens J, Van Roost G. Pregnancy and dialysis. Am J Kidney Dis 1998; 31: 756–65.
17. Okundaye I, Abrinko P, Hou S. Registry of pregnancy in dialysis patients. Am J Kidney Dis 1998; 31: 766–73.
18. Hou S. Pregnancy in chronic renal insufficiency and end-stage renal disease. Am J Kidney Dis 1999; 33: 235–52.

19. Buchler N, Schreiber M, Moodley SJ *et al.* Successful pregnancy with APD. Perit Dial Int 1997; 17: S57 (abstract).

20. Rao TK, Friedman EA, Nicastri AD. The types of renal disease in the acquired immunodeficiency syndrome. N Engl J Med 1987; 316: 1062–8.

21. Gardenswartz MH, Lerau CW, Seligson AR *et al.* Renal disease in patients with AIDS: a clinicopathological study. Clin Nephrol 1984; 21: 197–204.

22. Nochy D, Glotz D, Dosquet P *et al.* Renal disease associated with HIV infection: a multicentric study of 60 patients from Paris hospitals. Nephrol Dial Transplant 1993; 8: 11–19.

23. Laradi A, Mallet A, Beaufils H, Allouach M, Martinez F. HIV-associated nephropathy: outcome and prognosis factors. J Am Soc Nephrol 1998; 9: 2327–35.

24. Humphreys MH. Human immunodeficiency virus-associated glomerulosclerosis. Kidney Int 1995; 48: 311–20.

25. Ifudu O, Mayers JD, Matthew JJ *et al.* Uremia therapy in patients with end-stage renal disease and human immunodeficiency virus infection: has the outcome changed in the 1990s? Am J Kidney Dis 1997; 29: 549–52.

26. Breen C, Stein A, Hendry B. Outcome for patients with HIV-associated nephropathy on dialysis in the UK. J Am Soc Nephrol 1998; 9: 201A (abstract).

27. Perinbasekar S, Brod-Miller C, Pal S, Mattara J. Predictors of survival in HIV-infected patients on hemodialysis. Am J Nephrol 1996; 16: 280–6.

28. Cruz C, Kaul R, Markowitz N. Dialysis options for HIV infected patients. Perit Dial Int 1989; 9 (Suppl. 1): 89.

29. Graham MM, Bonini LA, Verdi MM. A multi-center study: clinical practices of HIV infected patients on CAPD/CCPD. Adv Perit Dial 1990; 3: 88–91.

30. Drissler R, Peters AT, Lynn RI. Pseudomonal and candidal peritonitis as a complication of continuous ambulatory peritoneal dialysis in human immunodeficiency virus-infected patients. Am J Med 1989; 86: 787–90.

31. Lewis M, Gorban-Brennan NL, Kliger A *et al.* Incidence and spectrum of organisms causing peritonitis in HIV positive patients on CAPD. Adv CAPD 1990; 6: 136–8.

32. Wasser WG, Beryl MJ, Brandons *et al.* HIV positivity does not predispose peritoneal dialysis patients to peritonitis. J Am Soc Nephrol 1991; 2: 369–73.

33. Schloth T, Genabe I, Pilgrim W *et al.* Peritonitis and the patient with human immunodeficiency virus (HIV). Adv Perit Dial 1992; 8: 250–2.

34. Tebben JA, Rigsby MO, Selwyn PA, Brennan N, Kliger A, Finkelstein FO. Outcome of HIV infected patients on continuous ambulatory peritoneal dialysis. Kidney Int 1993; 43: 191–8.

35. Wasser WG, Bajl MJ, Brandon S *et al.* HIV positivity does not predispose peritoneal dialysis patients to peritonitis. Perit Dial Int 1993; 13 (Suppl. 1): S88 (abstract).

36. Kimmel PL, Umana WO, Simmens SJ, Watson J, Bosch JP. Continuous ambulatory peritoneal dialysis and survival of HIV infected patients with end-stage renal disease. Kidney Int 1993; 44: 373–8.

37. Scheel, Jr. PJ, Farzadegan H, Ford D, Malan M, Watson A. Recovery of human immunodeficiency virus from peritoneal dialysis effluent. J Am Soc Nephrol 1995; 5: 1926–9.

38. Centre for Disease Control. Recommendations for providing dialysis treatment for patients infected with human-T-lymphotrophics virus type III/lymphadenopathy related virus. Ann Intern Med 1986; 106: 558–9.

39. MMWR. Recommendations for Prevention of HIV Transmission in Health Care Settings. 21 August 1987; 36: 25–185.

40. Chapman A, Wilkinson V, Peers EM, Brown CB. Intraperitoneal access for the treatment of peritonitis with AIDS. Perit Dial Int 1999; 19: S83 (abstract).

41. Wilkinson SP, Weston MJ, Parsons V *et al.* Dialysis in the treatment of renal failure in patients with liver disease. Clin Nephrol 1977; 8: 287–92.

42. Marcus RG, Messana J, Swartz R. Peritoneal dialysis in end-stage renal disease patients with preexisting chronic liver disease and ascites. Am J Med 1992; 93: 35–40.

43. Durand P-Y, Friedd P, Chanleau J *et al.* Long term follow up in cirrhotic patients with chronic renal failure undergoing CAPD. Perit Dial Int 1993; 13 (Suppl. 1): S47 (abstract).

44. Horie M, Kobayashi S. Nezassa S *et al.* A case report of hepatic cirrhosis with ascites and uremia treated by CAPD. Perit Dial Int 1993; 13 (Suppl. 1): S73 (abstract).

45. Macia M, del Castillo N, Pulido-Duque J, Garcia J. Successful maintenance CAPD in a diabetic patient with ascites and cavernous transformation of the portal vein. Perit Dial Int 1996; 16: 533–5.

46. Dadone C, Pincella G, Bonoldi G *et al.* Transport of water and solutes in uremic patients with chronic hepatic disease in CAPD. Adv Perit Dial 1990; 6: 23–5.

47. Steiner RW. Continuous equilibration peritoneal dialysis in acute renal failure. Perit Dial Int. 1989; 9: 5–7.

48. Cameron JS, Ogg CH, Trounce JR. Peritoneal dialysis in hypercatabolic acute renal failure. Lancet 1967; 1: 1188–91.

49. Posen GA, Luisello J. Continuous equilibration peritoneal dialysis in the treatment of acute renal failure. Perit Dial Bull 1981; 1: 6.

50. Katirtzoglous A, Kontesis P, Myopoulou-Symvoulidis D *et al.* Continuous equilibration peritoneal dialysis (CEPD) in hypercatabolic renal failure. Perit Dial Bull 1983; 3: 178–80.

51. Trevino-Becerra A, Munoz P, Avilez C *et al.* Equilibrium peritoneal dialysis (EPD) in acute renal failure (ARF) secondary to rhabdiomyolysis (sic). Perit Dial Bull 1987; 7: 244–6.

52. Siemons L, van den Heuvel P, Parizel G *et al.* Peritoneal dialysis in acute renal failure due to cholesterol embolization: two cases of recovery of renal function and extended survival. Clin Nephrol 1987; 28: 205–8.

53. Nolph KD. Peritoneal dialysis for acute renal failure. Trans Am Soc Artif Intern Organs 1988; 34: 54–5.

54. Hamilton JW, Lasrich M, Hergil P. Peritoneal dialysis in the treatment of severe hypercalcemia. J Dial 1980; 4: 129–35.

55. Heyburn PJ, Selby PL, Peacock M *et al.* Peritoneal dialysis in the management of severe hypercalcemia. Br Med J 1980; 280: 525–6.

56. Querfelf U, Salusky IB, Fine RN. Treatment of severe hypercalcemia with peritoneal dialysis in an infant with end-stage renal disease. Pediatr Nephrol 1988; 2: 323–5.

57. Weinreich T, Ritz E, Passlick-Deetjen J. Long-term dialysis with low-calcium solution (1.0 mmol/L) in CAPD: effects on bone mineral metabolism. Perit Dial Int 1996; 16: 260–8.

58. Thompson TJ, Neale TJ. Intraperitoneal calcium for resistant symptomatic hypocalcaemia after parathyroidectomy in chronic renal failure. Br Med J 1988; 296: 896–7.

59. Benz RL, Schleifer CR, Teehan BP *et al.* Successful treatment of postparathyroidectomy hypocalcemia using continuous ambulatory intraperitoneal calcium (CAIC) therapy. Perit Dial Int 1989; 9: 285–8.

60. Mailloux LU, Swartz CD, Onesti G *et al.* Peritoneal dialysis for refractory congestive heart failure. JAMA 1967; 199: 873–8.

61. Nora JJ, Trygstad CW, Mangos JA *et al.* Peritoneal dialysis in the treatment of intractable congestive heart failure of infancy and childhood. J Pediatr 1966; 68: 693–8.

62. Cairns KB, Porter GA, Kloster FE *et al.* Clinical and hemodynamic results of peritoneal dialysis for severe cardiac failure. Am Heart J 1968; 76: 227–34.

63. Malach M. Peritoneal dialysis for intractable heart failure in acute myocardial infarction. Am J Cardiol 1972; 29: 61–3.

64. Raja RM, Krasnoff SO, Moros JG *et al.* Repeated peritoneal dialysis in treatment of heart failure. JAMA 1970; 213: 2268–9.

65. Shapira J, Lang R, Jutrin I *et al.* Peritoneal dialysis in refractory congestive heart failure. Part I: Intermittent peritoneal dialysis (IPD). Perit Dial Bull 1983; July–Sept: 130–2.

66. Weinrauch LA, Kaldany A, Miller DG *et al.* Cardiorenal failure: treatment of refractory biventricular failure by peritoneal dialysis. Uremia Invest 1984; 8: 1–8.

67. Robson M, Biro A, Knobel B *et al.* Peritoneal dialysis in refractory congestive heart failure. Part II: Continuous ambulatory peritoneal dialysis (CAPD). Perit Dial Bull 1983; July–Sept: 133–4.

68. McKinnie JJ, Bourgeois RJ, Husserl FE. Long-term therapy for heart failure with continuous ambulatory peritoneal dialysis. Arch Intern Med 1985; 145: 1128–9.

69. Kim D, Khanna R, Wu G *et al.* Successful use of continuous ambulatory peritoneal dialysis in refractory heart failure. Perit Dial Bull 1985: 127–30.

70. Rubin J, Ball R. Continuous ambulatory peritoneal dialysis as treatment of severe congestive heart failure in the face of chronic renal failure. Arch Intern Med 1986; 146: 1533–5.

71. Shilo S, Slotki IN, Iaina A. Improved renal function following acute peritoneal dialysis in patients with intractable congestive heart failure. Isr J Med Sci 1987; 23: 821–4.

72. Mousson C, Tanter Y, Chalopin JM *et al.* Treatment of refractory congestive cardiac insufficiency by continuous ambulatory peritoneal dialysis. Long-term course. Presse Med 1988; 17: 1617–20.

73. Konig PS, Lhotta K, Kronenberg F *et al.* CAPD: a successful treatment in patients suffering from therapy_resistant congestive heart failure. In: Khanna R, Nolph KD, Prowant BF, Twardowski ZJ, Oreopoulos DG, eds. Advances in Peritoneal Dialysis. Toronto: Perit Dial Bull Inc., 1991; 7: 97–101.

74. Stegmayr BG, Banga R, Lundberg L, Wikdahl AN, Plum-Wirell M. PD treatment for severe congestive heart failure. Perit Dial Int 1996; 16: S231–5.

75. Ryckelynck J-P, Lobbedez T, Valette B, Le Goff C, Mazouz O, Levaltier B, Potier J–C, Hurault de Ligny B. Peritoneal ultrafiltration and refractory congestive heart failure. Adv Perit Dial 1997; 13: 93–7.

76. Burton BK. Inborn errors of metabolism: the clinical diagnosis in early infancy. Pediatrics 1987; 79: 359–69.

77. Donn SM, Swartz RD, Thoene JG. Comparison of exchange transfusion, peritoneal dialysis and hemodialysis for the treatment of hyperammonemia in an anuric newborn infant. J Pediatr 1979; 95: 67–70.

78. Wiegand C, Thompson T, Bock GH *et al.* The management of life-threatening hyperammonemia: a comparison of several therapeutic modalities. J Pediatr 1980; 96: 142–4.

79. Rutledge SL, Havens PL, Haymond MW *et al.* Neonatal hemodialysis: effective therapy for the encephalopathy of inborn errors of metabolism. J Pediatr 1990; 116: 125–8.

80. Siegel NJ, Brown RS. Peritoneal clearance of ammonia and creatinine in a neonate. J Pediatr 1973; 82: 1044–6.

81. Lettgen B, Bonzel KE, Colombo JP *et al.* Therapy of hyperammonemia in carbamyl phosphate synthase deficiency with peritoneal dialysis and venovenous hemofiltration. Monatsschr Kinderheilkd 1991; 139: 612–7.

82. Russell G, Thom H, Tarlow MJ *et al.* Reduction of plasma propionate by peritoneal dialysis. Pediatrics 1974; 53: 281–3.

83. Hsu WC, Lin SP, Huang FY *et al.* Propionic acidemia: report of a case that is successfully managed by peritoneal dialysis and sodium benzoate therapy. Chin Med J 1990; 46: 306–10.

84. Robert MF, Schultz DJ, Wolf B *et al.* Treatment of a neonate with propionic acidaemia and severe hyperammonemia by peritoneal dialysis. Arch Dis Child 1979; 54: 962–5.

85. Gortner L, Leupold D, Pohlandt F *et al.* Peritoneal dialysis in the treatment of metabolic crises caused by inherited disorders of organic and amino acid metabolism. Acta Paediats Scand 1989; 78: 706–11.

86. Sanjurjo P, Jaquotot C, Vallo A *et al.* Combined exchange transfusion and peritoneal dialysis treatment in a neonatal case of methylmalonic acidemia with severe hyperammonemia. An Esp Pediatr 1982; 17: 317–20.

87. Moreno-Vega A, Govantes JM. Methylmalonic acidemia treated by continuous ambulatory peritoneal dialysis (letter). N Engl J Med 1985; 312: 1641–2.

88. McMahon Y, MacDonnell RC Jr. Clearance of branched chain amino acids by peritoneal dialysis in maple syrup urine disease. In: Khanna R, Nolph KD, Prowant BF, Twardowski ZJ, Oreopoulos DG, eds. Advances in Peritoneal Dialysis. Toronto: Perit Dial Bull Inc., 1990; 6: 31–4.

89. Sallan SE, Cottom D. Peritoneal dialysis in maple syrup urine disease. Lancet 1969; 635: 1423–4.

90. Clow CL, Reade TM, Scriver CR. Outcome of early and long-term management of classical maple syrup urine disease. Pediatrics 1981; 68: 856–62.

91. Vandepitte K, Lins RL, Daelemans R *et al.* Continuous ambulatory peritoneal dialysis (CAPD) in a patient with glucose-6-phosphatase deficiency. Perit Dial Int 1989; 9: 111–14.

92. Bunchman TE, Swartz RD. Oxalate removal in type I hyperoxaluria or acquired oxalosis using HD and equilibration PD. Perit Dial Int 1994; 14: 81–4.

93. Lankisch PG, Koop H, Winckler K *et al.* Continuous peritoneal dialysis as treatment of acute experimental pancreatitis in the rat. II: analysis of its beneficial effect. Dig Dis Sci 1979; 24: 117–22.

94. Wall AJ. Peritoneal dialysis in the treatment of severe acute pancreatitis. Med J Aust 1965; 2: 281–3.

95. Rasmussen BL. Hypothermic peritoneal dialysis in the treatment of acute experimental hemorrhagic pancreatitis. Am J Surg 1967; 114: 716–21.

96. Bassi C, Briani G, Vesentini S *et al.* Continuous peritoneal dialysis in acute experimental pancreatitis in dogs. Effect of aprotinin in the dialysate medium. Int J Pancreatol 1989; 5: 69–75.

97. Lankisch PG, Koop H, Winckler K *et al.* Continuous peritoneal dialysis as treatment of acute experimental pancreatitis in the rat. I: Effect on length and rate of survival. Dig Dis Sci 1979; 24: 111–16.

98. Tilquin BM, O'Connor TC, Hancotte-LaHaye CM *et al.* The effect of peritoneal dialysis with and without aprotinin on acute experimental pancreatitis in rats. Int Surg 1990; 75: 174–8.

99. Fric P, Slaby J, Kosafirek E *et al.* Effective peritoneal therapy of acute pancreatitis in the rat with glutaryl-trialanin-ethylamide: a novel inhibitor of pancreatic elastase. Gut 1992; 33: 701–6.

100. Ranson JHC, Rifkind KM, Turner JW. Prognostic signs and nonoperative peritoneal lavage in acute pancreatitis. Surg Gynecol Obstet 1976; 143: 209–19.

101. Ranson JHC, Spencer FC. The role of peritoneal lavage in severe acute pancreatitis. Ann Surg 1978; 187: 565–75.

102. Ranson JHC, Berman RS. Long peritoneal lavage decreases pancreatic sepsis in acute pancreatitis. Ann Surg 1990; 211: 708–18.

103. Stone HH, Fabian TC. Peritoneal dialysis in the treatment of acute alcoholic pancreatitis. Surg Gynecol Obstet 1980; 150: 878–82.

104. Mayer AD, McMahon MJ, Corfield AP *et al.* Controlled clinical trial of peritoneal lavage for the treatment of severe acute pancreatitis. NEJM 1985; 312: 399–404.

105. Crist DW, Cameron JL. The current management of acute pancreatitis. Adv Surg 1987; 20: 69–123.

106. Joglar FM, Saadé M. Outcome and pancreatitis in CAPD and HD patients. Perit Dial Int 1995; 15: 264–73.

107. Ubara Y, Hara S, Katori H *et al.* Acute pancreatitis in a CAPD patient in association with hemolytic anemia. Perit Dial Int 1997; 17: 96–7.

108. Donnelly S, Levy M, Prichard S. Acute pancreatitis in continuous ambulatory peritoneal dialysis (CAPD). Perit Dial Int 1988; 8: 187–90.

109. Gupta A, Yi Yuan Z, Balaskas EV, Khanna R, Oreopoulos DG. CAPD and pancreatitis: no connection. Perit Dial Int 1992; 12: 309–16.

110. Moncade F, Fortier A, Guyon P *et al.* Peritoneal puncture dialysis in the monitoring and treatment of hemoperitoneum of traumatic origin? J Chir 1991; 128(6_7): 285–9.

111. Delaitre B, Attailia A, Chihaoui M. Perforated gastroduodenal ulcers. Treatment by peritoneal dialysis. 72 cases. Presse Med 1988; 17: 1297–300.

112. McEvoy J, Kelly AMT. Psoriatic clearance during hemodialysis. Ulster Med J 1976; 45: 76–8.

113. Twardowski ZJ. Abatement of psoriasis and repeated dialysis (letter). Ann Intern Med 1977; 86: 509–10.

114. Twardowski ZJ, Nolph KD, Rubin J et al. Peritoneal dialysis for psoriasis. An uncontrolled study. Ann Intern Med 1978; 88: 345–51.

115. Hanicki Z, Cichocki T, Klein A et al. Dialysis for psoriasis – preliminary remarks concerning mode of action. Arch Dermatol Res 1981; 271: 401–5.

116. Goring HD, Thieler H, Guldner G et al. Peritoneal dialysis therapy in psoriasis. Hautarzt 1981; 32: 173–8.

117. Halevy S, Halevy J, Boner G et al. Dialysis therapy for psoriasis. Report of three cases and review of the literature. Arch Dermatol 1981; 117: 69–72.

118. Kramer P, Brunner FP, Brynger H et al. Dialysis treatment and psoriasis in Europe. Clin Nephrol 1982; 18: 62–8.

119. Whittier FC, Evans DH, Anderson PC et al. Peritoneal dialysis for psoriasis: a controlled study. Ann Intern Med 1983; 99: 165–8.

120. Glinski W, Jablonska S, Imiela J et al. Peritoneal dialysis and leukopheresis in psoriasis: indications and contraindications. Hautarzt 1985; 36: 16–19.

121. Twardowski ZJ, Lempert KD, Lankhorst BJ et al. Continuous ambulatory peritoneal dialysis for psoriasis. A report of four cases. Arch Intern Med 1986; 146: 1177–9.

122. Sobh MA, Abdel Rasik MM, Moustafa FE et al. Dialysis therapy of severe psoriasis: a random study of forty cases. Nephrol Dial Transplant 1987; 2: 351–8.

123. Nissenson AR, Rapaport M, Gordon A et al. Hemodialysis in the treatment of psoriasis: a controlled trial. Ann Intern Med 1979; 91: 218–20.

124. Goldsmith LA, Fisher M, Wacks J. Psychological characteristics of psoriasis: implications for management. Arch Dermatol 1969; 100: 674.

125. Anderson PC. Dialysis treatment of psoriasis (editorial). Arch Dermatol 1981; 117: 67–8.

126. Chen WT, Hu CH, Schiltz JR et al. In search of 'psoriasis factor(s)': a new approach by extracorporeal treatment. Artif Organs 1978; 2: 203–5.

127. Glinski W, Zarebska Z, Jablonska S et al. The activity of polymorphonuclear leukocyte neutral proteinases and their inhibitors in patients with psoriasis treated with a continuous peritoneal dialysis. J Invest Dermatol 1980; 75: 481–7.

128. Glinski W, Jablonska S, Imiela J et al. Peritoneal dialysis and leukopheresis in psoriasis: indications and contraindications. Hautarzt 1985; 36: 16–19.

129. Krebs R, Flynn M. Treatment of hepatic coma with exchange transfusion and peritoneal dialysis. JAMA 1967; 199: 430–2.

130. Pirola RC, Ham JC, Elmslie RG. Management of hepatic coma complicating viral hepatitis. Gut 1969; 10: 898–903.

131. Mactier RA, Dobbie JW, Khanna R. Peritoneal dialysis in fulminant hepatic failure. Perit Dial Bull 1986; 6: 199–202.

132. Mactier R. Non-renal indications for peritoneal dialysis. In: Khanna R, Nolph KD, Prowant BF, Twardowski ZJ, Oreopoulos DG, eds. Advances in Peritoneal Dialysis. Toronto: Perit Dial Bull Inc 1992.

133. Lash RF, Burdette JA, Ozdil T. Accidental profound hypothermia and barbiturate intoxication: a report of rapid 'core' rewarming by peritoneal dialysis. JAMA 1967; 201: 269–70.

134. Reuler JB, Parker RA. Peritoneal dialysis in the management of hypothermia. JAMA 1978; 240: 2289–90.

135. Moss JF, Haklin M, Southwick HW et al. A model for the treatment of accidental severe hypothermia. J Trauma 1986; 26: 68–74.

136. DaVee TS, Reineberg EJ. Extreme hypothermia and ventricular fibrillation. Ann Emerg Med 1980; 9: 100–2.

137. Davis FM, Judson JA. Warm peritoneal dialysis in the management of accidental hypothermia: report of five cases. NZ Med J 1981; 94: 207–9.

138. Troelsen S, Rybro L, Knudsen F. Profound accidental hypothermia treated with peritoneal dialysis. Scand J Urol Nephrol 1986; 20: 221–4.

139. Horowitz BZ. The golden hour in heat stroke: use of iced peritoneal lavage. Am J Emerg Med 1989; 7: 616–19.

140. Khan IH, Henderson IS, Mactier RA. Hyperpyrexia due to meningococcal septicaemia treated with cold peritoneal lavage. Postgrad Med J 1992; 68: 129–31.

141. Blye E, Lorch J, Cortell S. Extracorporeal therapy in the treatment of intoxication. Am J Kidney Dis 1984; 3: 321–38.

142. Schlegel RJ, Altstatt LB, Canales L et al. Peritoneal dialysis for severe salicylism: an evaluation of indications and results. J Pediatr 1966; 69: 553–62.

143. Arieff AI, Friedman EA. Coma following nonnarcotic drug overdosage: management of 208 adult patients. Am J Med Sci 1973; 266: 405–26.

144. Pross DC, Bradford WD, Krueger RP. Reye's syndrome treated by peritoneal dialysis. Pediatrics 1970; 45: 845.

145. Shaw EB. Reye's syndrome and salicylate intoxication. Pediatrics 1970; 46: 976–7.

146. Narcy P, Zorza G, Taburet AM et al. Severe poisoning with intravenous phenytoin in the newborn. Value of peritoneal dialysis. Arch Fran Pediatr 1990; 47: 591–3.

147. Roger SD, Crimmins D, Yiannikas C et al. Lead intoxication in an anuric patient: management by intraperitoneal EDTA. Aust NZ J Med 1990; 20: 814–17.

148. Dua SL. Peritoneal dialysis for isopropyl alcohol poisoning (letter). JAMA 1974; 230: 35.

149. Kaufman DB, DiNicola W, McIntosh R. Acute potassium dichromate poisoning. Treated by peritoneal dialysis. Am J Dis Child 1970; 119: 374–6.

150. Lichtenberg R, Zeller WP, Gatson R et al. Bromate poisoning. J Pediatr 1989; 114: 891–4.

151. Warshaw BL. Treatment of bromate poisoning. J Pediatr 1989; 115: 660–1.

152. Duo LJ, Zhi ZG, Ji LY. Peritoneal dialysis in the treatment of severe poisoning with organophosphorus pesticides: experience with twenty-two patients. Perit Dial Int 1990; 10: 242–3.

153. Kassa J. Use of peritoneal dialysis as a therapeutic method in poisoning by Neguvon. Cesko Farm 1990; 39: 7–10.

154. Yamamoto Y, Wakisaka O, Fujimoto S et al. Acute renal failure caused by ingestion of the carp gall bladder – a report of 3 cases, with special reference to the reported cases in Japan. J Jap Soc Intern Med 1988; 77: 1268–73.

155. Yium J, Martinez-Maldonado M, Eknoyan G et al. Peritoneal dialysis in the treatment of renal failure in multiple myeloma. South Med J 1971; 64: 1403–5.

156. Russell JA, Fitzharris BM, Corringham R et al. Plasma exchange versus peritoneal dialysis for removing Bence Jones protein. Br Med J 1978; 2: 1397.

157. Rosansky SJ, Richards FW. Use of peritoneal dialysis in the treatment of patients with renal failure and paraproteinemia. Am J Nephrol 1985; 5: 361–5.

158. Rose PE, McGonigle R, Michael J et al. Renal failure and the histopathological features of myeloma kidney reversed by intensive chemotherapy and peritoneal dialysis. Br Med J 1987; 294: 411–12.

159. Boyce NW, Holdsworth SR, Thomson NM et al. 'Long-term' survival in light-chain myeloma with dialysis therapy alone. Aust NZ J Med 1984; 14: 676–7.

160. Cosio FG, Pence RV, Shapiro FL et al. Severe renal failure in multiple myeloma. Clin Nephrol 1981; 15: 206–10.

161. Brown WW, Herbert LA, Piering WF et al. Reversal of chronic end-stage renal failure due to myeloma kidney. Ann Intern Med 1979; 90: 793–4.

162. Johnson WJ, Kyle RA, Dahlberg PJ. Dialysis in the treatment of multiple myeloma. Mayo Clin Proc 1980; 55: 65–72.

163. Shetty A, Oreopoulos DG. Continuous ambulatory peritoneal dialysis in end-stage renal disease due to multiple myeloma. Perit Dial Int 1995; 15: 236–40.

164. Misra M, Goel S, Khanna R. Peritoneal dialyssi in patients with abdominal vascular prostheses. Adv Perit Dial 1998; 14: 95–7.

165. Vogt, J, Chlebowski H, Kniemeyer H-W, Grabensee B. Successful reinstitution of CAPD after retroperitoneal repair of an aortic aneurysm: a case report. Perit Dial Int 1995; 15: 71–2.

166. Goodship THJ, Lloyd S, McKenzie PW *et al.* Short-term studies on the use of amino acids as an osmotic agent in continuous ambulatory peritoneal dialysis. Clin Sci 1987; 73: 471–8.

167. Oreopoulos DG, Marliss EB, Anderson GH *et al.* Nutritional aspects of CAPD and the potential use of amino acid containing dialysis solutions. Perit Dial Bull 1983 (Suppl. 3): 510–12.

168. Mitwalli A, Rodella H, Brandes L *et al.* Is fat absorbed through the peritoneum? Perit Dial Bull 1985; 5: 165–8.

169. Pessa ME, Sitren HS, Copeland EM III *et al.* Nutritional support by intraperitoneal dialysis in the rat: maintenance of body weight with normal liver and plasma chemistries. J Parent Ent Nutr 1988; 12: 63–7.

170. Siriwardhana SA, Newfield AM, Lipton JM *et al.* Oxygen delivery by the peritoneal route. Can J Anesthes 1990; 37: S159.

171. Shah BS. An *in vitro* model for chemical extraction of carbon dioxide via modified peritoneal dialysis. ASAIO Trans 1988; 34: 112–15.

172. Hoff CM, Shockley TR. The potential of gene therapy in the peritoneal cavity. Perit Dial Int 1999; 19 (Suppl. 2): in press.

173. Hoff CM, Cusick JL, Masse EM, Jackman RW, Nagy JA, Shockley TR. Modulation of transgene expression in mesothelial cells by activation of an inducible promoter. Nephrol Dial Transplant 1998; 13: 1420–4.

174. Jackman RW, Stapleton TD, Masse EM *et al.* Enhancement of the functional repertoire of the rat parietal peritoneal mesothelium *In vivo*: directed expression of the anticoagulant and antiinflammatory molecule thrombomodulin. Human Gene Therapy 1998; 9: 1069–81.

175. Hoff CM, Shockley TR. Genetic modification of the peritoneal membrane: potential for improving peritoneal dialysis through gene therapy. Semin Dial 1998; 11: 218–27.

176. Nagy JA, Shockley TR, Masse EM, Harvey VS, Hoff CM, Jackman RW. Systemic delivery of a recombinant protein by genetically modified mesothelial cells reseeded on the parietal peritoneal surface. Gene Therapy 1995; 2: 402–10.

25 | Outcome with peritoneal dialysis compared to haemodialysis

R. Maiorca and G. C. Cancarini

Patient survival on CAPD and HD

Nephrologists are still questioning the ability of continuous ambulatory peritoneal dialysis (CAPD) to achieve the same results as haemodialysis (HD), although more than 20 years have passed from its introduction into clinical practice and many studies have been addressed to this topic.

Problems and limits of comparison

Clinical and ethical considerations, including the patients' right to choose the dialysis treatment they prefer, make it very difficult, if not impossible, to undertake prospective, randomized studies. Hence, comparisons are made on groups of patients arbitrarily put on CAPD or HD, thus with important pretreatment differences, only occasionally partially compensated for by sophisticated statistical analyses.

The first published survival studies were retrospective and in many of them no attempt was made to correct for case mix. Some studies looked at subgroups of patients (elderly, diabetics, etc.) or at the so-called 'standard population'. Some studies used statistical analysis to find the pretreatment factors affecting survival, in order to adjust for them. The search for risk factors has sometimes led to different results, or has been successful for one modality only. This is due to many reasons: different numbers of patients, different length of follow-up, number of fatalities too low for each cause to achieve statistical significance. It follows that risk factors emerged in higher numbers from the largest studies and, among them, in studies searching for more factors. Thus in many studies the statistical adjustment for case mix was only partial.

Another important point is the lack of gradation in comorbid conditions [1]: e.g. among patients with pretreatment 'ischaemic cardiopathy', patients with a single past episode of angina and others with a former extensive myocardial infarction can be included, and all of them are considered at the same risk from death.

The largest series (e.g. national registries, multicentre studies) actually give the best representation of the results obtained in the area, but present important drawbacks when modalities are compared: the participating centres may differ in their experience with CAPD, in the percentage of patients put on the two modalities, in the selection criteria, evaluation of comorbidity, incidence and treatment of complications, willingness to change modality when necessary. A large number of patients increases the statistical power of the analysis, with lower p-values, but not necessarily its reliability, as the consequences of methodological biases are also maximized. On the other hand, data coming from a single centre warrant uniformity in patient selection, in the evaluation of their comorbidity and in the quality of medical care on HD and PD. However results cannot be extrapolated to other centres, due to the centre effect. Probably data from a single centre or from a few homogeneous centres give a better comparison of the real ability of different modalities to preserve patient survival, whereas data from multicentre studies give a better analysis of what results the different modalities can obtain in routine medical practice.

One point that deserves much attention is how patients are selected for the study. Some studies analyse 'incident' patients (i.e. patients who start dialysis), others 'prevalent' patients (i.e. those on treatment at a certain date (e.g. 1 January of a particular year) or during a certain period of time, irrespective of when they started dialysis). The first method is able to analyse possible effects that become evident after some time on treatment; the second lacks this possibility.

As dialysis lifespan is long in some patients, they can start with a treatment and later switch to another treatment. Many studies do not take into account the first months on therapy, for financial reasons or in order to avoid the misleading effect of late patient referral. However, this practice can affect method com-

R. Gokal, R. Khanna, R.Th. Krediet and K.D. Nolph (eds.), Textbook of Peritoneal Dialysis, 2nd Edition, 755–783.
© 2000 *Kluwer Academic Publishers. Printed in Great Britain.*

parison as it excludes some early deaths related to the modality (i.e. for HD, adverse events related to venous catheterism, or gastrointestinal bleeding due to the uraemic syndrome but worsened by heparin, etc.).

Modality changes are also treated in different ways, depending on whether the 'history method' or 'intention-to-treat analysis' are selected. Studies using the 'history method' stop the observation when the patient changes modality and consider him/her as 'censored'. The risk with this method is to artifactually improve the results of the first modality and worsen those of the second, as those patients transferred because the method is performing badly can die a few days after the transfer. This bias can favour PD more than HD, because the drop-out is much more frequent for PD patients. This risk can be avoided or limited by ascribing to the first modality the deaths occurring during the first 2 months after shifting, and reasonably related to illnesses/problems that arise during the period on the first modality. A statistical comparison of demographic and other prognostic risk factors between patients withdrawing from and those continuing on the first modality could show if patients withdrawing from the modality are older and sicker than the others.

The studies using 'intention-to-treat analysis' do not take into account the method changes, and consider the patients as always on their first modality. With this kind of analysis the main risk is to attribute to the first modality deaths depending on the second. This bias might worsen PD results, as PD has more drop-outs than HD: all deaths occurring on HD in patients coming from PD would be attributed to this method, even if not causally or temporally related to it.

Some authors argue that a higher transplantation rate might worsen the results of dialysis methods, by leaving in the oldest and sickest patients. But the probability to be transplanted is, nowadays, similar for PD and HD patients. Moreover, if one modality has a higher transplantation rate, it is only because their patients had been positively selected: in this case the higher transplantation rate rebalances the two modalities.

In addition, results are greatly affected by differences in experience with the two methods, and this is particularly true for those countries where PD is used for a minority of uraemics. The CAPD technique is still insufficiently standardized, with important differences in connection systems, in the incidence of peritonitis and in catheter-related complications.

Finally, in the 'adequacy era', when the important effect on survival of the dialysis dose delivered is no longer questioned (see below), comparisons not taking this variable into account are at risk from wrong conclusions.

Mistrust can sometimes arise from the complicated statistical methods used to compare two populations, and sceptical people probably consider them too sophisticated and misleading. On the other hand, these methods need large numbers of patients and fatalities, and a long follow-up to identify those factors which affect survival. This can lead to an insufficient adjustment, or no adjustment at all, for those risk factors with low prevalence.

Patient survival in the 1980s

Table 1 shows patient survivals published in different studies throughout the 1980s. Studies not reporting survival percentages are not included. Results were similar for CAPD and HD [3–5, 8, 9, 12], or better for HD [2, 7, 11], and definitely better for home HD (HHD) [2, 6]. The presence of a higher percentage of diabetics worsened CAPD results. Patient survival was the same on CAPD and HD in 'standard' populations [4], in non-diabetics of similar ages [5], in subgroups of diabetics and non-diabetics [13], in patients without high risk of diabetes [12]. Cavalli *et al.* [10] observed better results with CAPD, in spite of a higher percentage of patients with diabetic nephropathy or aged 70 years or more, but the HD group included more patients with malignancy and hypertension. In a study by Capelli *et al.* [2], the differences in survival observed at 3 years (32% with CAPD versus 50% with in-centre HD (ICHD) disappeared after adjusting for age and diabetes only.

In the large series of Burton and Walls [14], life-expectancy was better with transplantation than with either form of dialysis ($p < 0.05$), and probably better with HD than with CAPD. In the Regional Piedmont Dialysis and Transplantation Registry there were no significant differences between CAPD, acetate-HD and bicarbonate-HD after 60 months. Patients on haemofiltration had significantly worse survival. The similarity of results for CAPD, bicarbonate-HD and acetate-HD was also confirmed for the subgroups of 'standard patients' and 'high-risk patients' [15]. Posen *et al.* [16] compared the non-diabetic patients of the Canadian Renal Failure Registry. The CAPD patients aged 15–44 had the same survival as comparable HD patients up to 30 months of follow-up. No differences were found for patients aged 45–64 after 42 months. For the age group 65 and older, survival on CAPD was

Table 1. Patients survival in some comparative studies throughout the 1980s

Reference	Years studied	Modality	Number of patients	Percentage of diabetics	Mean age	Percentage of survivors (years)						Comments
						1	2	3	4	5	6	
Capelli et al. [2]	1974–81	CAPD	88	35.2	55.7	86	50	32				
		IPD	26	42.3	53.2	70	20	10				
		ICHD	276	14.9	52.0	85	63	50				
		HHD	64	4.7	44.2	98	85	66				
Charytan et al. [3]	1980–81	CAPD	72	12.5	50.0		~80					
		ICHD	92	14.1	57.7		~80					
Mion et al. [4]	1978–82	CAPD; SP	20	0	42.8		90					
	1976–82	ICHD; SP	91	0	40.9		92					
	1976–82	HHD; SP	87	0	42.2		98					
	1976–82	HIPD; SP	30	0	39.8		100					
Kurtz et al. [5]	1979–83	CAPD; ND	21	0	49.6	91	91	78*				* = 32nd month
		HHD; ND	30	0	47.8	96	96	84*				* = 32nd month
Mailloux et al. [6]	1970–85	CAPD	46	n.a.	n.a.					43		
		ICHD	425	n.a.	n.a.					35		
		HHD	52	n.a.	n.a.					90		
Gokal et al. [7]	1983–86	CAPD	610	16	52				62			
		HD	329	4 (?)	48				74			
Maiorca et al. [8]	1981–86	CAPD	120	23	59	89	81	73	64	46		p = 0.2694 vs HD
		HD	139	9	48	92	88	80	72	66		
Maiorca et al. [9]	1981–87	CAPD	480	20.2	56.2	91	79	68	60	49	38	p = 0.0725 vs HD
		ICHD	373	7.2	50.0	92	84	79	67	62	54	
Cavalli et al. [10]	1981–88	CAPD	42	14.3	61.6			71				
		HD	48	7.1	57.8			58				
Gentil et al. [11]	1984–88	CAPD	272	28.7	n.a.	89	73	64				Mantel: p = 0.008
		ICHD	842	2.3	n.a.	91	85	80				Breslow: p = 0.17
Lupo et al. [12]	1985–89	CAPD	660	13	59.7					45		p = n.s. vs HD
		HD	968	8	53.6					54		
		CAPD; NHR	240	0	n.a.					65		p = n.s. vs HD
		HD; NHR	527	0	n.a.					66		
		CAPD; D	89	100	n.a.			45				p = n.s. vs HD
		HD; D	80	100	n.a.			50				

D = Diabetics, ND = non-diabetics, NHR = no high-risk patients, SP = standard population.

better than on HD at 6 and 12 months, but the difference narrowed after the 18th month and disappeared by the 36th month.

Patient survival in the 1990s

The increased experience with CAPD, and technical improvements occurring with both CAPD and HD during the 1980s have led to improved results during the 1990s. The main progress in HD has been: bicarbonate-based dialysis solutions, more compatible dialysers, technological advances in dialysis machines and the progressive adoption of the suggested targets of adequacy [17].

In the history of PD the improvements initially involved technical aspects (commercially available solutions, substitution of acetate base with lactate; closed, automated systems, etc.). Subsequently, increasing attention was paid to catheter-related infections and to patient nutritional status, to the unphysiology of dialysis, the study of peritoneal permeability and the search for an adequate dialysis dose.

However, the effects of such improvements have often been masked by the patients' increasing age at the beginning of dialysis, with a consequent increase in the number of comorbidities.

We will discuss, below, a few more recent studies comparing PD and HD [18–24], some of them obtained from large national registries, that have had a larger impact on the scientific community.

In 1995 Bloembergen et al. published a study on 170 700 Medicare patients, on treatment throughout 1987–89 [18]. Results showed that PD patients had a 1-year significantly higher risk of death than HD patients (1.19 versus 1.00 in HD; p < 0.001). Patients aged 55 or less had a similar risk of death with CAPD and HD. Patients aged 55 or more had a higher RR of death with PD and this increased with age ($p < 0.05$ at 55 years and $p < 0.01$ at about 67). The RR of death with PD was significantly higher in females (RR = 1.30; $p < 0.001$) and in diabetics (RR = 1.38; $p < 0.001$) but also in non-diabetics (RR = 1.11; $p < 0.001$) [18].

This study had considerable impact on the scientific community in the United States for its results, questioning the validity of CAPD in comparison with HD. However, when analysed in depth the study shows some methodological problems, acknowledged by the authors, which weaken its conclusions. The analysis of these problems is also useful to better understand other papers on the same topic.

The relative risk of death in PD patients was significantly higher than that of HD patients only after the age of 55 years, and became highly significant at 65 years and over. However, the study adjusted survival curves for comorbidity by taking into account only diabetes, and excluded all the other risk factors (e.g. ischaemic cardiopathy, malignancy, systemic disease, etc.) known for having significant effects on survival. Although adjustments for these factors were lacking in both CAPD and HD patients, one cannot exclude differences in case mix penalizing CAPD and becoming more and more evident, as happens with comorbidity, with patient age. Consequently one cannot exclude that the worst results of CAPD in the oldest age group are due to differences in case mix, with comorbidity being more frequent in the elderly. The worst case mix with PD compared to HD has been reported for those years in the USA [12].

It is generally agreed that results of a given therapy are affected by the physician/nurse's experience. The percentage of patients on PD in that study was low, about 13%, i.e. the 'HD patients/PD patients' ratio was 6.7. Such a ratio clearly indicates a selection of CAPD patients that cannot be defined, as information on pretreatment comorbidity, except diabetes, is lacking.

Bloembergen *et al.* examined all the patients prevalent on 1 January of three consecutive years, from 1987 to 1989, pooling the three cohorts in one and evaluating its 1-year survival. Such an approach can bias the results. Fenton *et al.* [20] have shown, in incident patients, that survival is better with PD than with HD for the first 2 years, PD being probably favoured, initially, by the better preservation of residual renal function (RRF). This advantage disappeared when the analysis was made on prevalent patients. Vonesh, re-examining incident plus prevalent patients of the USRDS database over the period

1987–93, obtained different results than Bloembergen *et al.*: less than 1% difference in the adjusted 1-year survival between PD and HD in non-diabetics; a statistically significant lower risk of death on PD for diabetics under the age of 50 and a significantly higher one for diabetics over the age of 50; no or little difference in RR of death for male diabetics in PD versus those on HD; significant worse survival for female diabetics on PD (personal communication). Furthermore, the Bloembergen *et al.* analysis puts together patients with different lengths of dialysis, who can be counted twice or thrice if their survival is sufficiently long. It also excludes the survival time before the beginning of observation.

The 'intention-to-treat' analysis used in the study does not consider changes of treatment, and one patient is always considered on the first modality. It can be that a patient spending only 1 month on PD and dying on HD 11 months later is registered as dying on PD.

Finally, the study compares patient survival throughout the years 1987–89 when Kt/V was already used in HD, and not in PD. Since later studies demonstrated [22, 25, 26] that adequate dialysis dose impacts on survival, PD was biased, in the study, by the inadequate dose delivered, in those years, in PD. Keshaviah *et al.* [27] found that the RR of death was similar on CAPD and HD when patients with equivalent (according to the peak concentration hypothesis) dose of dialysis were compared.

The results of the previous study on United States patients differ from the more recent results of the Canadian Register, first reported in 1993 [28] and then confirmed in 1996 [19].

At the end of 1994 this nationwide register had 9075 incident dialysis patients on file, 5725 (63%) on HD and 3350 (37%) on PD. The main data of the register can be summarized as follows: CAPD/CCPD patients aged 0–64 years have a reduced RR of death compared to HD patients: 0.90 (95% confidence interval 0.85–0.96; $p < 0.05$); patients diabetic or with vasculopathy as their primary renal disease have an increased RR (2.17; $p < 0.05$ and 1.36, $p < 0.05$, respectively) when compared to patients with glomerulonephritis; patients dialysed in 1990–94 have a lower RR than those treated in 1981–85 (RR = 1.57; $p < 0.05$) and 1986–89 (RR = 1.49; $p < 0.05$); there was a significant difference in the risk of death among the different Canadian provinces, with RRs ranging from 0.94 to 1.51 ($p < 0.05$).

Fenton *et al.* [20] compared mortality rates with HD and CAPD/CCPD in patients of the Canadian

Register, using only incident patients for whom data were available on predialysis conditions. This study, probably having the best statistical approach published so far, includes 11,633 ESRD patients starting treatment between 1990 and 1994, followed up for a maximum of 5 years. The ratio between HD ($n = 7792$) and PD patients ($n = 2841$) was 2.7; more balanced that in the Bloembergen *et al.* study. The survival analyses also took into account the first months on dialysis (usually lacking in the US studies, as the Medicare registration starts from the third month of dialysis) and were adjusted for known prognostic factors and predialysis comorbid conditions, and used Poisson regression, which accounts for treatment modality switches. A series of additional models were also used, based on Poisson regression but also on Cox regression model, to best analyse the results.

Twenty-six per cent of PD patients and 31% of HD patients died during follow-up. The RR associated with CAPD/CCPD was 0.74 (95% confidence interval 0.68–0.79) relative to HD = 1.00. The reduced mortality with PD was concentrated in the first 2 years after starting dialysis, maybe due to longer maintenance of the residual renal function, a finding lost when a prevalent analysis was made. Similar findings have been reported by Foley *et al.* [29], who used an intention-to-treat analysis and, in a cohort of 433 dialysis patients, found that the adjusted RR of death in PD compared to HD was 0.76 (95% confidence interval 0.45–1.27; $p = 0.28$, n.s.) in the first 2 years of treatment and 1.57 (95% confidence interval 0.97–2.53; $p = 0.06$, marginally not significant) in the following years. A recent observation that residual renal function is associated with a better lipid profile in CAPD patients [30] could be an additional cause of the better patient survival with CAPD during the first years of treatment.

The CAPD/CCPD advantage was lower among diabetics and patients aged 65 or more, and a statistically significant difference disappeared in diabetics aged 65 or more.

When an 'intention-to-treat' Cox regression model was used, like that used by Blombergen *et al.* [18], that does not account for change of modality and hence partially mixes the two modalities, the differences seen with the Poisson regression model disappeared [20].

Maiorca *et al.* [21] have recently extended their previous studies [8,9] comparing patient survival in PD and HD to the longest follow-up time published so far, more than 10 years. The analysis involved 578 new end-stage renal disease (ESRD) patients who started dialysis from January 1981 to December 1993 and survived for at least 2 months. Fifty-one per cent of them started on CAPD and 49% on HD. Survival analysis was based on the 'history method' that considers patients as 'censored' when they change from their first modality. All deaths occurring in the first 2 months after changing the dialysis modality, and reasonably referable to the previous modality, were attributed to it.

Patients on CAPD had the same mean follow-up as HD patients, but were 6 years older ($p = 0.0001$). Percentages of primary renal disease were different among CAPD and HD for glomerulonephritis, more frequent in HD patients, and diabetes and uncertain aetiologies more frequent in CAPD patients. Among the pretreatment risk factors assessed at the start of dialysis, the following were significantly more frequent with CAPD than with HD: arrhythmias, diabetes, and age more than 70. The number of risk factors increased with the patients' age (r: 0.5; $p < 0.001$) and in diabetics (4.2 ± 1.5 vs 2.4 ± 1.4, $p = 0.0001$).

At the end of follow-up, 42% of CAPD patients had died, 18% had changed modality, 7% had been given transplants, 2% had recovered renal function and 1% had been transferred to another centre. Among the 281 HD patients these figures were 28%, 3%, 18%, 1%, and 12%. The 10-year patient survival observed was 34.6% with HD and 14.4% with CAPD ($p = 0.004$). The Cox hazards regression model showed that the factors significantly impairing survival were: age, cerebrovascular disease, peripheral vascular disease, ischaemic cardiopathy, malignancy, chronic liver disease, tuberculosis and malignant hypertension. Interstitial nephropathy and the start of treatment after 1987 significantly improved survival. The adjusted survival on CAPD was not significantly different from that on HD.

For the old elderly the probability to survive was better with CAPD in the first years (unadjusted: 70% vs 47%, $p = 0.04$; adjusted for comorbidity: 78% vs 51%, $p < 0.02$), but the curves later became similar.

The same group has recently reviewed the data of its PD and HD programme; the observed patient survival with PD and HD is shown in Fig. 1. In the more recent 5-year experience, 155 HD and the 139 PD patients starting dialysis throughout 1991–96 were less affected by the limitations of the initial experience [31]. During recent years, the mean age of the incident HD patients has progressively increased, so approaching that of PD patients. Con-

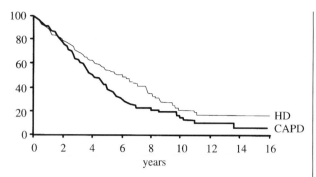

Figure 1. Observed patient survival throughout the period 1981–96 (HD = 371 patients, PD = 373 patients) at the Chair and Division of Nephrology, University and Spedali Civili of Brescia.

sequently, the prevalence of risk factors has also become very similar. This makes a statistical adjustment of data, always questionable, unnecessary. The adjusted survival curves were only marginally different from those unadjusted, that did not differ with PD and HD (log rank test: $p = 0.78$; Breslow: $p = 0.91$; Tarone-Ware: $p = 0.95$) (Fig. 2). These data strongly support the theory that PD can assure the same survival as HD when the two groups of patients are comparable.

The contrasting results obtained in the USA and in the Canada Registries are made even more evident by the Canusa study [22], which showed, on 680 PD patients, a mortality rate 1.93 times (95% confidence interval: 1.14–3.28) higher in the United States than in Canada. The 2-year probability to survive

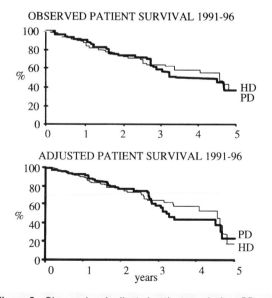

Figure 2. Observed and adjusted patient survival on PD and HD throughout the period 1991-96 at the Chair and Division of Nephrology, University and Spedali Civili of Brescia.

on CAPD in Canada was 79.7% versus 63.2% in the United States.

This difference was not explained by statistical analyses taking into account race, age, gender, functional status, diabetes, cardiovascular disease, nutritional status or adequacy of dialysis [23]. After taking into account the effects of the above variables on survival, the RR was still high: 1.80 (95% confidence interval 1.21–2.67). The analysis of further variables did not define factors able to significantly explain the difference. The only differences found were the following: higher RR of a non-fatal cardiovascular event in the United States compared with Canada (1.80; 95% confidence interval 1.21–2.67), higher acceptance rate in United States (211 per million population versus 100 in Canada) and lower prevalence of peritoneal dialysis in the United States (22% versus 48% in Canada). The high acceptance rate might explain the increased risk of cardiovascular event and the lower percentage of PD patients might indicate a lower experience with PD. It is interesting to note that the 18-month survival probability for patients aged less than 65 was similar in the two countries (89.2% in Canada and 88.6% in the United States), while a greater difference, but not statistically significant, was observed in patients aged 65 or more (82.0% versus 61.1%). Finally, one cannot exclude the fact that the four United States centres were not representative of the other centres in the country. For a more detailed analysis of such a comparison see the chapter 'Implications of the Canadian-USA (CANUSA) Multicentre Trial' in this book.

Another interesting comparison between two countries has been reported by Marcelli *et al.* [24]. That study groups together patients coming from the Case Mix Severity Special Study of the USRDS with those from the Lombardy Registry who started treatment from 1986 to 1987. In the overall population (USA + Lombardy), PD showed a RR of death of 1.34 (95% confidence interval 1.205–1.499; $p = 0.0001$) compared to 1.0 on HD and the Lombardy patients had a RR of 0.71 (95% confidence interval 0.628–0.806; $p = 0.0001$) compared to 1.0 in the United States patients. When the patients were stratified according to modality and country, and by considering the RR = 1 for United States HD patients, the RRs were: 0.64 for Lombardy HD patients ($p < 0.01$) and 1.17 ($p = 0.03$) for United States PD patients. No significant difference in RR was observed between Lombardy and United States PD patients.

Factors affecting patient survival

Modality

Many studies have been performed in an attempt to measure the differences in RR associated to either CAPD or HD, and their results are summarized in Table 2. Only four studies have shown statistically significant differences. In two of them [24, 33] the effect was in favour of HD and in the other two in favour of PD.

After adjusting data for pretreatment risk factors, Burton and Walls [14] estimated that the proportions of patients predicted to survive 10 years were 53% for CAPD, 45% for HD and 50% for transplantation. However, these figures were projections, calculated on the basis of clinical data with a follow-up of 5.5 years for transplantation and less than 2 years for CAPD. In the studies by Maiorca et al. [8, 9], the risk of death on each modality increased with age, but the RR increased more in old HD patients. In another study [36] patients aged 60 or older had similar patient survival on CAPD and HD but worse on IPD.

The higher drop-out on the CAPD technique might positively influence patient survival figures by dropping the worst patients and leaving the best patients on the treatment. If that be true, patients dropping out from CAPD should be at higher risk of death, e.g. should be older or have more risk factors. This was excluded in one study [37]: the only statistically significant differences between patients leaving the method and the others were incidence of systemic diseases (higher) and mean age (lower) in patients leaving CAPD.

Age

In any kind of disease, and in normal individuals, age heavily influences mortality. Shapiro and Umen [38] showed that age had a non-linear effect on patient survival in HD patients, the relative risk of death being 0.21 for patients 1–45 years old, 0.53 for 46–60 and 1.0 over 61. In one of the first studies on patient survival with CAPD [39], age was a powerful negative factor. For the patients of the EDTA-ERA Registry there were important differences between age groups in primary renal disease, but no differences between CAPD and HD for any of them, with survivals on CAPD no worse, and possibly better, than on other modes of treatment [40]. The relative risks of death due to age in different studies are shown in Table 3.

Table 2. Relative risk of death with PD and HD in different studies

| | | Relative risk of death for | | | |
| | | HD versus CAPD | | CAPD versus HD | |
		RR	p	RR	p
Gentil et al. [11]		0.82	n.s.		
Burton and Walls [32]		1.30	n.s.		
Maiorca et al. [8]				1.34	n.s.
Rubin et al. [33]	HHD			1.30	=0.02
	LCD			1.03	n.s.
Wolfe et al. [34]				0.98	n.s.
Maiorca et al. [9]				1.30	n.s.
Serkes et al. [13]	ND			0.62	n.s.
Lunde et al. [35]				1.025*	n.s.
Lupo et al. [12]		1.571	n.s.		
Canadian register [19]	ND (age: 0–64)			0.91	<0.05
	ND (age: 65+)			0.84	<0.05
	D (age: 0–64)			0.86	<0.05
	D (age: 65+)			0.97	n.s.
Fenton et al. [20]				0.74	0.68–0.79†
Maiorca et al. [21]				1.346	n.s.
Bloembergen et al. [18]				1.19	<0.001
Marcelli et al. [24]				1.344	<0.0001

* Patients ⩾ 65 years old.
† Significance level not available; 95% confidence interval is reported.
D = Diabetics, ND = non-diabetics.

Table 3. Effect of age on patient survival in different studies

Study	Age groups (years) increments	Relative risk	p	Notes
Capelli *et al.* [2]	10-year increment	1.20		
Burton and Walls [14]	10-year increment	1.68	< 0.0001	
Gokal *et al.* [7]	Age = 60	3.28	< 0.001	In CAPD patients
	Age = 60	2.3	< 0.05	HD patients
Maiorca *et al.* [8]	Age − 53.2	1.14	= 0.0003	CAPD + HD patients
Walker and Grove [41]	(Age − 51)/10	1.45	= 0.0003	CAPD + HD patients
Rubin *et al.* [33]	By 20 year difference	1.17	= 0.001	CAPD + HD patients
Wolfe *et al.* [34]	10-year increment	1.2	< 0.001	CAPD + ICHD patients 20–60 years old
Serkes *et al.* [13]	Age < 46	0.34	< 0.05	ND (age 46–60 = 1.00)
	Age > 60	2.77	< 0.003	ND (age 46–60 = 1.00)
Gentil *et al.* [11]	Age > 60	4.10	= 0.000	CAPD + ICHD
	Age > 60	4.10	< 0.001	ICHD
	Age > 60	3.69	< 0.001	CAPD
Maiorca *et al.* [9]	Age − 53.5	1.07	= 0.0001	CAPD + HD
Lupo *et al.* [12]	Age	1.047	= 0.000	CAPD + HD
	Age	1.040	= 0.025	CAPD
	Age	1.055	= 0.000	HD
Fenton *et al.* [20]	Age 0–14	0.93	–	CAPD/CCPD + HD
	Age 15–44	1.00	–	CAPD/CCPD + HD
	Age 45–64	2.14	= 1.85–2.47*	CAPD/CCPD + HD
	Age 65 +	3.69	= 3.21–4.25*	CAPD/CCPD + HD
Marcelli *et al.* [24]	One-year increment	1.043	< 0.0001	
Canadian Register [19]	ND, age 0–14 vs ND, 15–44	1.85	< 0.05	CAPD + HD
	ND, age 45–64 vs ND, 15–44	1.74	< 0.05	CAPD + HD
	D, age 45–4 vs D, 15–44	1.20	< 0.05	CAPD + HD
Maiorca *et al.* [21]	Age − 59	1.079	< 0.001	CAPD + HD

* Significance level not available; 95% confidence interval is reported.
D = Diabetics; ND = non-diabetics.

Only a few studies have compared the effect of age on CAPD and HD patients. In the USRDS Annual Data Report 1991 [42], survival with CAPD was lower than on HD for the elderly, and higher for younger patients. In the elderly, Gokal *et al.* found a greater risk of death with CAPD than with HD [7] whereas Gentil *et al.* [11] found that patients on ICHD had a higher risk than those on CAPD. Maiorca *et al.* [8] found that the rates of increase in mortality associated with increasing age were different for the two methods. After adjusting for the risk of death linked to pretreatment risk factors, survival was the same on CAPD and HD for patients aged 30–66, but not for patients 67 and over, who had a significantly lower mortality rate on CAPD than on HD [8]. When the study was extended to five other centres the statistically significant difference of survival in the elderly disappeared [9], but the risk of death associated with age increased at a greater rate with HD than with CAPD [43]. In a larger study [12] Lupo *et al.* also found that the impact of age on survival was greater with HD than with CAPD: 4-year patient survival was 85% on HD and 70% on CAPD for patients 21–50 years old, 63% and 54% for 51–65 years old and 30% and 40% for patients over 65.

Lunde *et al.* [35] compared mortality in 1552 elderly patients divided according to the treatment in use on the 120th day. Diabetes, hypertension, white race and age significantly increased the risk of death. They concluded that CAPD and HD had similar outcomes in geriatric non-diabetic patients. These data are questionable since they consider the events that occurred after the 120th day, even if patients changed treatment subsequently. Moreover, comorbid conditions other than primary renal disease were not considered.

The more recent studies have also confirmed the significant negative effect of age on survival. No further studies have been carried out on the effect of age in the different modalities, after adjustment for the other prognostic factors.

Table 4. Effect of gender on patient survival in different studies

Study	Gender	Relative risk	p
Maiorca *et al.* [8]	Female	0.65	n.s.
Serkes *et al.* [13]	Female diabetic	0.55	<0.03
	Female non-diabetic	0.70	n.s.
Maiorca *et al.* [9]	Female	1.13	n.s.
Burton and Walls [32]	Male	0.48	<0.001
Wolfe *et al.* [34]	Male (all)	1.09	n.s.
	Male (diabetics)	1.27	<0.01
Lunde *et al.* [35]	Male	1.05	n.s.
Marcelli *et al.* [24]	Male	1.116	=0.0157
Maiorca *et al.* [21]	Male	0.823	n.s.

Gender

In 672 non-diabetics on HD from 1976 to 1982, Shapiro and Umen found a negative effect of male gender on survival [38]. However, when other risk factors were simultaneously taken into account the gender influence disappeared. Presumably the higher mortality in males, not confirmed elsewhere, was to be attributed to the higher prevalence of cardiovascular disease in men. Table 4 shows how controversial is the topic of whether or not male or female sex has any influence on survival of uraemic patients. Marcelli *et al.* [24] found a significant negative effect of male gender in their patients, whereas Serkes *et al.* and Wolfe *et al.* [13, 34] found a similar significant higher risk of death in males, but only among diabetics.

An analysis on the possibility that the RR of death between PD and HD was different according to gender was carried out by Bloemergen *et al.* [18]. They found that females had a significantly higher risk of death with PD (RR = 1.30; $p < 0.001$) than with HD; a lower but significant RR was found for males (RR = 1.11; $p < 0.001$).

Race

The white race has also been attributed a negative effect on survival. This was true in the study by Wolfe *et al.* [34], who also found greater risk for patients with primary diagnoses of hypertension or diabetes, and the study by Lunde *et al.* for white patients aged 65 years and more [35]. However, this was not seen in other studies evaluating this variable [13, 18, 33].

Cardiac and vascular disease

Cardiovascular disease is the most frequent cause of death in dialysis patients, accounting for about 50% of all causes.

In many studies with long [9, 44], and others with shorter follow-ups, cardiovascular deaths were similar for CAPD and HD, but in the USRDS 1995 Report [45], there were more deaths with CAPD, at 1 year, for myocardial infarction and 'other cardiac' causes, except sudden death. These findings are surprising, because CAPD should be tolerated better than HD by cardiovascular patients, as noted below. It is quite possible that the metabolic derangements found in CAPD patients, especially more marked dyslipidaemia (see below), expose CAPD patients to more severe atherosclerosis and increased vascular mortality.

Cardiovascular, cerebrovascular and other vascular diseases were the main causes of death in HD patients, accounting for 48% in a study by Shapiro and Umen [38]. The relative risk of death due to this pathology was high, but decreased when age was simultaneously taken into account. The negative effect of pretreatment heart disease was confirmed by Khanna *et al.* for CAPD patients [39]: 2-year survival was 95% for patients without cardiac abnormalities before dialysis, 51% for patients with myocardial infarction and 62% for patients with angina. After 42 months the survival was 46% for patients with cardiomegaly compared to 88% for those without cardiac abnormalities. On the other hand, dialysis increases the risk of developing cardiovascular disease. Khanna *et al.* [39] showed that 40–59-year-old CAPD patients had cumulative incidences of *de-novo* ischaemic heart disease of 8.8% and 15% after 1 and 2 years. These percentages were not very different from the 12% and 18% found in HD patients [46] but greater than the 12.7% at 6 years found in the matched non-uraemic population of Framingham [47].

A strong negative effect of cardiovascular disease on patient survival has been assessed in analyses carried out using the Cox hazard regression model (Table 5).

Among the risk factors for cardiovascular disease are uraemic cardiomyopathy, with myocardial hypertrophy and intermyocardiocytic fibrosis, coronary artery disease, hypertension and dislipidaemia. Theoretically, CAPD has some haemodynamic advantages over HD: no need for an arteriovenous fistula, constant electrolyte and acid–base balance, constant removal of uraemic waste products (some of them possible aetiological factors in uraemic cardiopathy) and the lack of intradialytic or interdialytic changes in cardiac filling, inotropism and oxygen request, all detrimental to long-term performance of the heart. Another favourable effect of

Table 5. Effect of cardiovascular diseases on patients survival in some studies

Study	Definition	Relative risk	p
Burton and Walls [32]	Ischaemic heart disease	1.65	<0.025
Maiorca *et al.* [21]	Ischaemic cardiopathy	1.63	=0.002
Maiorca *et al.* [9]	Ischaemic cardiopathy	2.02	=0.0001
Walker and Grove [41]	Previous myocardial infaction	1.21	
Panarello *et al.* [36]	Heart failure	2.00	=0.002
Serkes *et al.* [13]	Arteriosclerotic heart disease; ND	1.14	n.s.
Serkes *et al.* [13]	Arteriosclerotic heart disease; D	1.93	<0.02
Gentil *et al.* [11]	Cardiovascular (CAPD + ICHD)	1.53	=0.038
Gentil *et al.* [11]	Cardiovascular (CAPD)	0.77	n.s.
Gentil *et al.* [11]	Cardiovascular (ICHD)	2.06	=0.003
Marcelli *et al.* [24]	Heart disease	1.40	<0.0001
Fenton *et al.* [20]	Cardiovascular (CAPD/CCPD + HD)	1.65	1.53–1.78*
Gokal *et al.* [7]	Cerebrovascular and cardiovascular disease	3.36	<0.001
Maiorca *et al.* [9]	Cerebrovascular disease	1.60	=0.0184
Maiorca *et al.* [21]	Cerebrovascular disease	1.80	<0.001
Fenton *et al.* [20]	Vascular disease (CAPD/CCPD + HD)	1.32	1.16–1.50*
Serkes *et al.* [13]	Peripheral vascular disease; ND	1.01	n.s.
Serkes *et al.* [13]	Peripheral vascular disease; D	1.84	<0.03
Panarello *et al.* [36]	Peripheral vascular disease	2.10	=0.002
Maiorca *et al.* [8]	Peripheral vascular disease	2.21	=0.0227
Maiorca *et al.* [9]	Peripheral vascular disease	1.61	=0.0103
Marcelli *et al.* [24]	Vascular disease	1.34	<0.0001
Maiorca *et al.* [21]	Peripheral vascular disease	1.95	<0.001

* Significance level not available; 95% confidence interval is reported.
D = Diabetics; ND = non-diabetics.

CAPD was, in the past, less anaemia, but this advantage is now minimized by the use of human recombinant erythropoietin.

Cardiac systolic function is usually normal in CAPD and HD patients but can be reduced in the elderly or in patients with ischaemic cardiopathy, and can become hyperdynamic on HD, in patients with high-output arteriovenous fistulas [48]. Diastolic function is, on the contrary, often altered in both methods, due to uraemic cardiomyopathy including left ventricular hypertrophy (LVH) and intermyocardiocytic fibrosis [49–53]. In the uraemics the left ventricle (LV) becomes progressively stiffer and in the early phase of diastole its dilation becomes progressively difficult and less efficient. LV end-systolic and end-diastolic pressures increase. Ventricular filling will depend more and more on atrial contraction, with consequent atrial hypertrophy and enlargement. During fluid retention, e.g. in the interhaemodialytic interval, such patients are at risk from atrial arrhythmias and pulmonary and peripheral congestion. Increased LV pressure and fibrosis are responsible for subendocardial ischaemia and for altered propagation of action potentials, with facilitated arrythmia of the re-entry type [54].

Alpert *et al.* [55] carried out a cross-sectional study of 54 patients on HD and 39 on CAPD, and found with the latter a lower incidence of end-diastolic and end-systolic left ventricular dilation, higher cardiac output, and lower mean velocity of circumferential fibre shortening. The same group obtained concordant results for patients switching from HD to CAPD and vice-versa. Septal and posterior wall thickness were increased by similar percentages in patients on the two methods. Canziani *et al.* [56] found that LVH is significantly more frequent in HD than in CAPD. Some studies have evaluated the echocardiographic changes in LVH during CAPD and HD. For 18 patients on CAPD for 6–12 months, Leenen and co-workers [57] observed decreases in left ventricular mass, wall thickness, end-diastolic and end-systolic dimensions. In a longitudinal study Timio and co-workers [58] observed, after 6 months of treatment, decreases in thickness of the myocardial interventricular septum, posterior wall mass and left ventricular mass index with CAPD, but not with HD. A decreased in left ventricular mass and end-diastolic volume with CAPD and an increase with HD were observed by Deligiannis *et al.* [59]. These data are in contrast with those published by Eisenberg *et al.* [50], who observed worsening of myocardial hypertrophy with CAPD, from normal/mild to moderate in five of 10 cases, and from moderate to severe in two of six cases. These differences may result from different case mixes, duration of diet and dialysis treatments, control of hypertension and extracellular volume (ECV).

LVH has many possible causes in uraemia, among them high blood pressure over 24 h rather than occasionally, anaemia, hyperparathyroidism, (local) renin system, endothelin, sympathetic overactivity, salt/ouabain-like factor, pulsatile vs steady LV workload [60]. Reduction of LVH with CAPD and not with HD has been related to the nocturnal blood pressure lessening, seen only on CAPD, although this is less than in physiological conditions, and to norepinephrine levels, lower on CAPD than on HD [58]. We saw no differences in nocturnal blood pressure between 15 elderly CAPD and 15 elderly HD randomly selected, mean ages 72 ± 5 and 71 ± 5 years, on dialysis for 31 ± 18 months and 31 ± 19 months. The 24 h blood pressure readings were taken with an automatic apparatus, choosing the short interval day for HD patients [43].

Intermyocardiocytic fibrosis is an early complication of uraemia. In parathyroidectomized and subtotally nephrectomized rats given parathyroid hormone (PTH) there is three times more myocardial interstitium and lesser capillary density [61]. There are no comparative studies of changes in intermyocardiocytic fibrosis with HD and CAPD; there is evidence that it progresses in patients on maintenance HD [62, 63]. Weiss et al. [64] showed a trend towards a more impaired diastolic function in HD patients when compared to PD patients.

On the basis of the data of the USRDS, Bloembergen et al. [18] found that patients on PD had a 20% higher probability of dying from stroke than their HD counterparts. This is even more impressive if one considers that in the USRDS study HD patients had a 50% higher underlying cerebrovascular disease prevalence than PD patients. More recently Mattana et al. [65] reported, in the dialysis patients of the USRDS, a cerebrovascular death rate of 11.6/1000 patient-years. When the effect of modality was considered, PD had a greater odds ratio in diabetics aged 45 or more and in non-diabetics aged 65 or more; in the other age groups the odds ratio was higher in HD patients. Maiorca et al. also noted a higher percentage of deaths due to stroke in CAPD than in HD patients [21]. In their series 21 out of 297 CAPD patients (23/1000 patient-years) and six out of 281 HD patients (7/1000 patient-years) died of stroke, but there were more diabetics, on CAPD. The increased prevalence of stroke in CAPD patients might be due to the higher preva-

lence of hyperlipidaemia in PD patients due to both the continuous glucose load from the peritoneal cavity and the lower plasma protein concentration (see chapter 'Nutritional Aspects of Peritoneal Dialysis' in this book).

Clinical data demonstrate that CAPD is effective in controlling hypertension. The continuous removal of sodium and excess water limits ECV fluctuation, avoiding those hypertensive peaks connected with fluid overfilling that can be seen with HD. Since the large majority of hypertensive states in uraemics can be corrected by ultrafiltration, blood pressure control with CAPD depends mostly on the accurate maintenance of the dry weight. This can be achieved through correct dosage of hypertonic dialysis fluid. In the 1987 Report of the NIH-CAPD Registry, 30% of 400 medicated patients were converted to normal within 1 year and others tended to take less medication [66]. In two other studies [67, 68], CAPD appeared to be as effective as HD, whereas in another one [55] there was better control of blood pressure with CAPD than with HD. A decreased vascular response to exogenous angiotensin infusion, possibly related to the peritoneal clearance of some still-unknown substance(s), enhancing the vascular effect of circulating vasopressive agents, has been observed [69]. In a study with continuous 24 h monitoring of blood pressure, CAPD, more than HD, decreased the nocturnal blood pressure, close to physiological values. It has been suggested that this effect contributes to the lessening of LVH on this method [70]. In contrast to these authors, Maiorca et al. [43] were not able, in randomly selected elderly patients, to find differences between the two methods. In their elderly population, treated for at least 6 months and up to 4 years, there were no differences in the percentages becoming normotensive or in the number of antihypertensive agents needed by the others [13].

Velasquez et al. [71] studied 21 patients, 10 of them transferred from CAPD to HD and 11 from HD to CAPD, and found a higher prevalence of hypertension with PD (71%) than with HD (43%). According to the authors the difference might depend on greater body fluid expansion with PD.

Arrhythmias, due to cardiovascular disease, but also to intercompartmental water and electrolyte shifts during dialysis, are frequent in HD patients. Moreover, as documented in patients with essential hypertension, LVH is a strong predictor of premature ventricular beats, cardiac arrhythmias and sudden death. In patients on HD or haemofiltration the incidence of premature beats was frequent, 25%, especially in the last 2 h of treatment [72]. In a multicentre, cross-sectional study, ventricular arrhythmias were seen in 79% of patients from the third hour of HD up to 5 h or more after dialysis; 21% of these arrhythmias were Lown class 4A or B. On the contrary, in a Holter study of 21 patients on CAPD [73] the incidence of arrhythmias was no different, even in elderly or cardiac patients, during treatment and on a day in which the treatment was deliberately withheld. In a comparative study with continuous 48 h Holter monitoring, supraventricular, isolated ventricular and bigeminal arrhythmias were seen, more frequently with HD than with CAPD, and in both treatments ventricular extrasystole rates correlated with blood norepinephrine levels. Only HD patients had ventricular tachycardic episodes, whereas with CAPD hypokinetic arrhythmias prevailed [70].

Occurrence of myocardial ischaemic episodes is frequent with HD, whereas there are no data for CAPD. Zuber *et al.* [72] observed ST depression, indicative of ischaemic episodes, prevalently in the last 2 h of HD or haemofiltration, in 25% of patients studied with continuous Holter registration. ECG changes lasted for 40–90 min and half of them were asymptomatic. None of these patients had objective signs of coronaropathy.

The appearance rates of *de-novo* coronary disease on CAPD and HD was, in separate studies, 8.8% at 1 year and 15% at 2 years, on CAPD [74], and 12% and 18% on HD [75]. Foley *et al.* [29] found that there is no difference between PD and HD for *de-novo* ischaemic heart disease (RR 1.37, $p = 0.33$), while PD had a lower RR for *de-novo* cardiac failure, statistically not significant (RR 0.70, $p = 0.18$).

A good performance of PD on cardiac diseases is reported by Elhalel-Dranitzki *et al.* [76] who, in CAPD patients with congestive heart failure class IV NYHA (New York Heart Association), observed improved functional capacity and significant reduction of hospitalization.

Hypotensive episodes and other intra- or peridialytic symptoms are common on HD and rare on CAPD. Hypotension, multifactorial in origin, can be ultimately referred to an imbalance between ultrafiltration rate and vascular refilling [77], which is frequent on HD and uncommon on CAPD. If the HD ECV rapid changes are the trigger for hypotension, uraemic, and elderly, when present, cardiomyopathies are the underlying cause: frequent hypotensive episodes are seen much more often in patients with LVH than in those without LVH [48].

In 92 patients on HD and 72 on CAPD undergoing treatment for up to 26 months, there were 15.6 episodes per patient per year with HD versus only 0.46 with CAPD, of hypotension or hypertension, significant arrhythmias, chest pain, seizures, muscle cramps, headaches, twitching, gastrointestinal troubles, symptoms all related to the treatment. Together, they occurred in 20% of HD treatments [78]. High hypotension rates, from 20% to 50% of dialyses, had been reported in the past [79–81] but better tolerance has probably been achieved since the introduction of convective or mixed techniques, bicarbonate buffer and automated ultrafiltration [82–84]. Maiorca *et al.* evaluated the incidence of hypotensive episodes (i.e. a drop of systolic blood pressure (SBP) to 90 mmHg or less, or a 20 mmHg drop if the initial SBP was 100 mmHg or less) in 1 year, in 63 patients (34 male, 29 female) mean age 62 ± 15 years, on dialysis for 87 ± 63 months, treated with bicarbonate-HD (59 patients) or acetate-HD (4 patients), all on automated ultrafiltration. In a total of 1034 treatments, hypotensive episodes occurred in 10.8%. Seventy-four per cent of the hypotensive episodes occurred in 30% of patients, not differing from the others for age (62 ± 16 versus 62 ± 15 years; $p = 0.95$) or time on dialysis (92 ± 62 versus 84 ± 63 months; $p = 0.68$) [37].

Dislipidaemia is also a risk factor for cardiovascular disease and CAPD treatment is associated with a more atherogenic lipoprotein profile than HD. Dialysis patients are hyperlipidaemic as a result of an increased production and a decreased removal of triglycerides with both CAPD and HD, positively correlated to plasma immunoreactive insulin levels [85]. Serum cholesterol is generally normal in HD patients, while it has been found increased [85, 86] or unchanged [87] in CAPD patients. In these patients plasma lipid concentrations before dialysis are relevant to their final concentrations during treatment. Patients having low plasma levels of triglyceride at the beginning of CAPD will have the lowest triglyceride [88, 89], and the highest HDL cholesterol levels, and no increase in VLDL [89]. This suggests that lipoprotein response to continuous glucose supply differs from patient to patient according to the efficiency of their lipoprotein metabolism [90].

In a longitudinal assessment the risk of atherogenesis did not differ with CAPD and HD over 24 months of follow-up; however, when on longer time, in a cross-sectional study, the risk appeared to be greater in patients on CAPD up to 70 months [91]. This probably indicates that a long time is necessary to develop significant lipid changes. Lipoprotein(a), an atherogenic serum component, is significantly higher in CAPD than in HD [92]. In a comparative study Avram et al. [93] found CAPD treatment to be associated with a more atherogenic lipoprotein profile than is HD, but the potential risk associated with hyperlipidaemia was far outweighed by the increased overall mortality of patients with hypolipidaemia due to malnutrition, malnutrition being a more important prognostic factor for patient survival.

In conclusion, it seems reasonable to consider CAPD as the method that preserves cardiovascular function better. Myocardial hypertrophy seems to progress with HD, whereas more reports indicate a regression with CAPD, provided that good control of ECV is obtained. On HD the progressively increasing impairment of early left ventricular filling can have devastating effects during the sessions, due to the rapid blood ultrafiltration that can dramatically worsen cardiovascular refilling and can bring on collapse, arrhythmia, or even sudden death [63]. Between the sessions HD patients are at increased risk from atrial, pulmonary and peripheral congestion and atrial arrhythmias. On CAPD all these effects are avoided by the continuous ultrafiltration. Moreover, the absence of the arteriovenous fistula; the constant acid–base balance; the constant concentrations of sodium, potassium and calcium; and the constant removal of uraemic waste products are all favourable factors in the control of uraemic cardiomyopathy.

On the other hand, CAPD has a more atherogenic lipid profile, the negative effects of which are hard to predict. However, the substantial lack of differences in the cardiovascular death rate seems to indicate that advantages and disadvantages of the two methods have equivalent weights.

Diabetes

Diabetes worsens patient survival, and this has been shown in many studies [7, 8, 11, 15, 18, 34, 35, 40], but survival has not been found different with CAPD or with HD in many studies [28, 94, 95]. The relative risk of death for dialysed diabetics versus non-diabetics ranges from 1.71 to 5.71 in different studies [7, 9, 11, 34–36, 41]. Bloembergen et al. found that in diabetic end-stage renal disease (ESRD) Medicare patients prevalent in the years 1987–89, the 1-year death rate was higher with CAPD than with HD [18]. Held et al., in a large sample of the ESRD Medicare patients incident in the years 1986–87 found that survival of diabetics, adjusted for comorbidity, was similar on CAPD and HD at 1 year

(83.3% and 85.4%) [96], but lower with CAPD at 2 years (54.0% compared to 64.6% for HD) and through the remainder of the follow-up period [96]. However, in this study the patients treated with CAPD were sicker, having more underlying peripheral vascular disease. These data are in contrast to those reported in the 1996 Canadian Registry Report [19] showing by Cox analysis a lower risk of death in diabetics on CAPD than on HD (relative risk significantly lower, 0.86, for patients 0–64 years of age, and 0.97, p = n.s., for patients 65 and over).

In a study by Maiorca et al. survival of diabetics after 4 years was about 60% versus about 90% for non-diabetics, after adjusting for the negative effects of other factors [8]. Survival was 60% versus 84% after 2 years in the CAPD patients of Khanna et al. [39]. This is contradicted by the data of Chandran et al. [97], who in CAPD patients found the same life-expectancy in diabetics as in non-diabetics, but the two groups had different ages. The risk of death for diabetics increased with age in the study of Capelli et al. [2], but not in that of Serkes et al. [13], where the RR increased with age only for non-diabetics.

According to Walker and Grove [41], the greater risk of death with dialysis for diabetics than for non-diabetics has lessened with time: from 5.71 in 1977 to 3.92 in 1980 and to 2.69 in 1983.

Different result for diabetic survivals on PD and HD have been reported. For diabetics 20–60 years old Wolfe found a significantly higher relative risk of death with CAPD than with ICHD [34]. In the USRDS Annual Data Report 1991 [42], 1-year survival was lower with CAPD than with HD (65.7% vs 69.6%), but the results were not adjusted for race or for diagnosis other than diabetes. The mean age was 53 for CAPD and 55 years for HD patients [42]. White patients with diabetic or hypertensive ESRD tended to survive better with CAPD up to approximately age 40, and to survive better with HD above that age. According to the investigators these data must be taken only as general trends, because of the small sample size and the substantial random variability in the individual estimates. In a study by Zimmerman et al. CAPD was the best primary modality for patients not to be given transplants [98]. Mejia and Zimmerman [94] analysed the results for diabetics obtained at the University of Wisconsin. Survival was no different with HD and CAPD for up to 12 months, after which it became higher with CAPD, and after 3 years it was 81%, versus 40% with HD [94]. In 298 diabetics of the Piedmont Dialysis and Transplantation Registry, Triolo *et al.* [95] found that 1-year survival was 85% for patients younger than 50 years versus 63% for patients older than 60. Survival was better with CAPD, haemofiltration and bicarbonate-HD (82%, 81% and 80%) than with acetate-HD (66%).

Survival was no different for diabetics on CAPD and HD in some studies [8, 9, 13] after adjusting for pretreatment differences.

The most frequent cause of death in diabetics on dialysis is cardiovascular disease, 55.8% of deaths versus 51.1% for non-diabetics in the EDTA report [99]. Infections caused 13.6% and 14.3% of deaths. For other causes only malignancy differed, causing 1% of deaths in diabetics and 4.6% in non-diabetics. In the study of Legrain *et al.* [100], the causes of death for HD and CAPD patients expressed as percentages of patients at risk, were: cerebrovascular + cardiac 12% versus 15%, arteritis + sepsis 10% in both, sepsis 9% versus 2%, treatment withdrawal 6% versus 2%, other causes 6% versus 2%. Peritonitis was the cause of death in 10% of CAPD patients, and hyperkalaemia and malnutrition each caused 4% of deaths in the HD group only.

The worst results obtained for diabetics are due to several factors, the principal one being the presence of complications of diabetes at the start of dialysis. Peripheral vascular disease, hypertension and retinopathy are present in a large majority of diabetics and 10–20% of them are blind at the start of dialysis [94, 101, 102].

Some of these complications seem to have progressed differently in patients on CAPD or on HD, in some studies. For example, diabetic retinopathy appeared to improve more frequently in patients on CAPD than in those on HD in the studies of Legrain *et al.* and Khauli *et al.* [100, 103], while its progression was the same on CAPD and HD in other studies [102, 104]. In spite of the different results these studies agree that control of hypertension is important for slowing the rate of progression of retinopathy [100, 104]. Legrain *et al.* reported data supporting better control of hypertension in CAPD than in HD patients, and this might explain the better results on the progression of retinopathy obtained with CAPD [100]. On the other hand, a major problem in diabetics, on both HD and CAPD, is hypotension [100], consequent to autonomic nervous system dysfunction due to both diabetes and uraemia. The results also do not fully agree regarding the control of neuropathy, some studies having found greater improvement with CAPD than with HD [103], and others no different results in the two methods [100].

Peripheral vascular disease is one of the most frequent complications in diabetes and 4–5% of diabetics on dialysis have amputations [98, 102]. Concerns have been raised about the possibility that CAPD worsens the course of peripheral vascular disease in diabetics as well as in non-diabetics [105]. However, the data for diabetics show similar incidences of amputation in both CAPD and HD patients [100, 103]. In HD patients the diabetic vascular disease negatively affects the duration of vascular access [100, 106]. On the other hand, the presence of arteriovenous fistula was significantly associated with hand gangrene in the same limb [106]. Mejia and Zimmerman showed that CAPD and HD diabetics had about the same incidence of complications (4.6 ± 1.2 episodes/patient-year versus 3.6 ± 0.7), but vascular access required interventions more often than peritoneal access (1.3 ± 0.5 episodes/patient-year versus 0.2 ± 0.1) [94].

In the more recent studies Fenton *et al.* [20] found that diabetic nephropathy increases the risk of death by about 70% (RR = 1.69; 95% confidence interval 1.49–1.91) and Marcelli *et al.* [24] found that the RR of death associated with diabetes was 1.499 ($p < 0.0001$). The effect of diabetes in the Canadian Organ Replacement Register has been analysed earlier, in the section on survival, being the data of that Register stratified by diabetic status.

In a study by Maiorca *et al.* [21] diabetes significantly affected survival when peripheral vascular disease was removed from the statistical model. When both the diseases were present in the model, diabetes lost the statistical significance, but peripheral vascular disease did not (RR = 1.95; $p < 0.001$).

Peritonitis

CAPD patients with higher incidence of peritonitis have the worst survival [107]. In 288 CAPD patients we found significantly different death rates in patients with less than 0.5 and more than one peritonitis episode per year [107]. The peritonitis rate was not related to time on CAPD or to the age of the patient at the start of treatment. In eight of nine patients who died of peritonitis there was a fungal aetiology. In patients with high peritonitis rates death was due, other than to peritonitis, to cardiovascular disease, liver disease, and other causes. It is difficult to say whether peritoneal infections are more likely in some diseases, such as liver and cardiac disease, or whether peritonitis becomes more severe or life-threatening in these conditions. Probably both of these hypotheses are true.

Uraemia impairs the immunological status, as demonstrated by lymphopenia, delayed rejection of allografts and leukocyte recruitment at the site of infections, cutaneous anergy, reduced chemotaxis and phagocytosis, attenuated humoral responses to vaccine administration and reduced interferon production [108–110]. These changes might be the cause of the increased susceptibility to infections and neoplasms in uraemics [111].

Many experimental studies have evaluated the capability of dialysis methods to improve the immunological status in uraemics, and results are often controversial. Dialysis *per se* may further impair the immunological status through depletion of useful proteins, trace metals and vitamins, or can stimulate an immune response through bioincompatibility of dialysis membranes and dialysis fluid or entry into the blood of microorganisms or endotoxins. Entry of microorganisms is frequent with HD, and accounts for approximately half of the life-threatening infections in dialysis patients [112]. Endotoxins can enter the blood stream more easily in uraemic patients, and important increases in plasma levels have been found in patients on conservative treatment (17.0 ± 2.0 ng/L), on HD (40.0 ± 4.7 ng/L) and on haemofiltration (19.0 ± 7.5 ng/L). On the contrary, levels were similar to those of healthy controls (7 ± 0.6 ng/L) in transplanted and PD patients [113].

Serum antibacterial activity is depressed in uraemics and further depressed by HD or CAPD [114]. Sera from HD patients and from non-dialysed uraemics showed non-complement-related antibacterial activity that did not appear in normal controls or in CAPD patients; this residual activity might be due to middle molecules more easily removed by peritoneal dialysis (PD) than by HD [114]. Neutrophils from CAPD patients had chemotactic and bactericidal activities similar to those from HD patients, but better phagocytic function [115]. There was significantly less chemiluminescence of stimulated polymorphonuclear neutrophil leukocyte (PMN) cells from HD patients, while PMN cells from CAPD patients did not differ from those of controls [110].

CAPD patients showed improvement in cellular immunity (tested by E-rosette count) and in delayed hypersensitivity reactions (tested by dinitrochlorobenzene and paraphenylenediamine skin test) in contrast to HD patients in whom no changes were found [116, 117]. Collart *et al.* [118] found increased OKT4+/OKT8+ ratios with both HD and CAPD due to reduced percentages of OKT8+ cells with normal values of OKT4+. OKT3+ were normal. In contrast, others [119] observed significant increases in percentages of OKT3+ and OKT4+ cells and a higher OKTA+/OKT8+ ratio only in CAPD patients. The lymphoblastic response in autologous serum was better in CAPD than in HD patients, perhaps because of the removal of some inhibitory factor(s) [110, 120, 121]. T-cell function appeared to be impaired in HD patients, as demonstrated by a complete loss of inducibility of the interleukin-2 gene and decreased inducibility of gamma-interferon mRNA, which appears to be normal in PD patients [122]. The proliferative response to mitogens is also similar or better with CAPD than with HD [118, 123, 124].

Sensitization to membrane or tubing or to sterilizing agents has been observed with HD. Similar percentages of patients (12%) with IgE antibodies against ethylene oxide have been found with HD, haemofiltration and intermittent peritoneal dialysis [125]. This was not confirmed by another study [126] in which positive skin tests were found in 9% of HD patients and not in patients on PD and positive radioallergosorbent tests in 12% of HD patients in contrast to only one in 41 of PD patients (and this single patient had previously been on HD for 2 years).

In conclusion, in the majority of the studies CAPD appears to preserve immune function better than HD. However, have the differences in laboratory tests any clinical importance? In a retrospective clinical study, HD patients required more admissions per patient-year than CAPD patients for infectious diseases other than those related to technique (infection of the access, peritonitis): 0.158 versus 0.096, but days of hospitalization were the same (1.55/patient-year) [37]. Respiratory tract infections comprised more than 45% of all causes. There was no statistically significant difference in the incidence of any other infectious disease. The incidence of malignancy did not significantly differ, 4.2% with HD and 5.9% with CAPD. The follow-up was comparable, but the mean age of patients on CAPD was 7 years older than on HD ($p < 0.001$), and this might have influenced the results. There were no significant differences in the localization of malignancies. Thus, clinical results do not seem to support the suggested better ability of CAPD to improve uraemic immunity.

Malignancy

Malignancy is obviously one of the illnesses with the highest relative risk, from 1.32 to 6.09, for survival of uraemics (p from 0.004 to less than 0.0001) [8, 9, 20, 21, 24, 36, 41]. It follows that correction for this factor is of paramount importance when comparing different methods, provided that the frequency of events is sufficiently high as to allow correct adjustment.

Other patient-related factors

Other factors have been shown, in single studies, to affect patient survival, sometimes adversely, sometimes favourably. Burton and Walls [14] found a negative effect of amyloidosis ($RR = 8.26$), acute presentation or 'acute on chronic' presentation ($RR = 2.73$) and convulsions ($RR = 3.17$). Parenthood ($RR = 0.45$), pyelonephritis ($RR = 0.48$) and residence in the Leicestershire area ($RR = 0.64$) had positive effects. Walker and Grove [41] and Wolfe *et al.* [34] found a significant positive effect of glomerulonephritis, and Maiorca *et al.* [21] reported a RR of 1.80 ($p = 0.03$) for tuberculosis, of 1.80 ($p = 0.014$) for chronic liver disease and a positive effect ($RR = 0.54; p = 0.025$) for interstitial nephropathy. In the Canadian Organ Replacement Register, in patients aged 0–64, renovascular disease as primary cause of ESRD had a RR of death of 1.32 ($p < 0.05$) when compared to glomerulonephritis. In non-diabetics aged 65 or more, polycystic kidney disease played a protective role ($RR = 0.79; p < 0.05$), while vascular disease and kidney diseases other than glomerulonephritis had an increased RR ($1.28; p < 0.05$, and 1.23, $p < 0.05$, respectively). In the study by Fenton *et al.* [20] chronic obstructive lung disease had a RR of 1.17 (95% confidence interval 1.05–1.29), and polycystic kidneys 0.66 (95% confidence interval 0.52–0.83), when compared to glomerulonephritis.

Interestingly, interstitial nephropathy was the only prognostic risk factor having a positive effect on survival [14, 21, 42], which might be greater with CAPD.

Early or late referral of ESRD patients

Survival on dialysis can be heavily affected by predialysis care and, above all, by when the patient is referred to the nephrologist, late referral being associated with higher mortality and hospitalization [129–132]. Since late referral can depend on the health-care organization, this might be one major factor explaining the differences in survival among countries.

Experience and technical improvement

Walker and Grove [41] found that for dialysis patients the RR of death decreases over time, irrespective of the modality. The risk of death related to modality, which was not different for CAPD and HD in 1980, dropped more for CAPD than for HD.

On the contrary, Wolfe *et al.* found an increase in the risk of death on dialysis by a factor of 1.04 per year after 1980 [34], but there were important differences between modalities, since the risk decreased by 1% per year in the CAPD patients ($p < $ n.s.) and increased significantly, by 6% per year ($p < 0.001$), in ICHD patients. This might be due to the increased experience with CAPD and a change in case mix.

Gentil *et al.* [11] found that, for CAPD and ICHD considered together, the relative risk of death declined by 0.84 per year after 1984. Separately the two modalities did not show any significant improvement with time. Maiorca *et al.* [21] showed, in patients from their centre, a reduction in the risk of death with time: patients starting dialysis after 1987 had a significantly better survival ($RR = 0.688; p = 0.021$) than those starting before.

The better survival, referable to technique and clinical improvements, is clearly shown by the data of the Canadian Organ Replacement Register [19]. For HD and PD patients kept together, putting the RR of death to 1.0 in 1990–94, it was 1.47 ($p < 0.05$) in 1981–85 and 1.45 ($p < 0.05$) in 1986–89 in non-diabetics and 1.77 ($p < 0.05$) and 1.50 ($p < 0.05$), respectively, in diabetics. Thus, the risk of death remained relatively stable in the first two periods, characterized by important improvements in the connection system, and dropped in the period 1990–94, characterized by the increasing perception of the need for an adequate dialysis dose.

Fenton *et al.* [20] found that patients treated in centres with less than 400 patients had a RR of death of 1.18 (95% confidence interval 1.10–1.28) when compared to those in centres with more than 400 patients.

Adequacy of dialysis

The problem of the adequacy of dialysis dose arose in PD in the first years of the 1990s, several years later than in HD (for a review in depth, see the chapter 'Adequacy of Peritoneal Dialysis' in this book). Many theoretical and clinical studies had been performed during the 1980s to define methods and targets for the dose of dialysis [133–142]. Clinical studies were few, retrospective, cross-sectional and on a limited number of patients, with consequently weak statistical analyses. Only two studies have prospectively analysed the effect of adequacy on survival. Maiorca *et al.* [25] looked for the adequate dialysis dose of CAPD, on the basis of Kt/V per week and on RRF (mean of urea and creatinine clearances). The study, starting with a cross-sectional analysis, followed by a prospective 3-year follow-up, was interventional, since the dialysis dose was adjusted for the loss of RRF. The analysis was adjusted for other confounding factors. In summary it showed that a weekly Kt/V of 1.96–2.03 and a renal + peritoneal creatinine clearance of > 70 L/week were the CAPD doses associated with the best survival (Fig. 3). The study also looked for the adequate Kt/V in HD patients, and found that Kt/V more or less than 1.7/week on CAPD and more or less than 1.0 on HD, respectively, gave similar survival rates. Furthermore, when based on the peak concentration hypothesis by Keshaviah *et al.* [143], and on the model suggested by Gotch [144] to compare Kt/V in the two methods, the CAPD adequate dose ($wKt/V = 2$) corresponded, for HD, to a Kt/V of 1.0 per treatment after the short interval, and 1.3 after the long interval.

The CANUSA study [22] separately analysed the effects of both Kt/V and weekly creatinine clearance (C_{Cr}) and of other nutritional parameters in incident patients maintained on a stable dialysis schedule. Kt/V and C_{Cr}, and also the nutritional parameters, significantly influenced survival, and creatinine clearance was also effective in predicting technique survival and hospitalization. Based on a large population of patients this study has strong statistical power. Nevertheless its design, and the lack of

adjustment for the declining RRF, made it unable to define the optimal Kt/V dose. A projection of its data over time has led to the hypothesis that there is an endless linear relationship between Kt/V and survival, which is questionable. This hypothesis is also in contrast with the old National Cooperative Dialysis Study which, for HD, demonstrated that above a certain Kt/V, further increase in the dialysis dose is of little or no clinical advantage.

Keshaviah *et al.* [145], comparing the patients of the CANUSA study and those of the Minnesota Regional Kidney Disease Program, found that survival for CAPD patients with weekly $Kt/V = 2$ was similar to that for HD patients with $Kt/V = 1.3$ per treatment; this result is consistent with the ones reported above by Maiorca *et al.*

Reviewing the available data the DOQI (Dialysis Outcome Quality Initiative, promoted by the National Kidney Foundation) [146] has recently suggested the adoption of $Kt/V = 2$/week as the adequate dialysis dose in CAPD. Unfortunately, according to the 1995 Report from the Core Indicators for Peritoneal Dialysis Study Group, in 1994 only 65% of the 1328 PD patients of the Regional ESRD Network in United States had at least one adequacy measurement during a 6-month observation [147].

Nutrition

Serum albumin has been considered a reliable index of nutritional status, although not by everybody [140–142, 148–157] and a strong relationship has been found between serum albumin level and survival [140, 158–161]. On the contrary, dementia/cachexia did not cause greater mortality with CAPD than with HD, even during extended follow-up [21], in spite of the larger number of patients older than 70 on CAPD and this supports former observations [43, 61]. This finding is a little surprising, because malnutrition, whether mild or severe, seems to be more frequent with CAPD than with HD [127, 128].

Hypoalbuminaemia is one of the most reliable signs of malnutrition in non-proteinuric and non-enteropathic patients, and has often been used to define the nutritional status of dialysed patients. CAPD may not completely correct the hypoalbuminaemia present before dialysis, whereas HD usually does [162]. An inverse relationship between albuminaemia and mortality in HD patients was also found in CAPD patients [142, 163]. On the other hand, one report showed that stable low serum levels of albumin in CAPD patients were not correlated with a worse patient outcome [164].

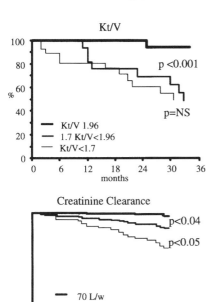

Figure 3. Effect of adequacy on survival.

In an international study of 224 CAPD patients using the 'subjective nutritional assessment', based on 21 variables derived from history and clinical examination, anthropometry and biochemistry, 8% of the patients were severely malnourished and 32.6% were mildly or moderately malnourished [162]. In an Italian multicentre study [128] the same method, applied to 256 HD and 204 CAPD patients, showed severe malnutrition in 3% of the HD and 7.8% of the CAPD patients, moderate/mild malnutrition in 27% and 33.8%, and good nutritional status in 70% and 58.3%, with differences between treatments statistically not significant. There was no relationship between mortality and subjective global assessment of nutritional status or serum albumin levels. When all the malnourished were combined, percentages of malnourished patients increased with age, with both HD and CAPD, and the increases were higher with HD than with CAPD in patients older than 65, suggesting that CAPD better preserves the nutritional status in the elderly. Other studies based on anthropometric measurements found no differences in nutritional status between CAPD and HD [165, 166]. In addition, the percentages of deaths due to cachexia were similar for HD and CAPD in a multicentre study [9].

Another approach to the problem is a longitudinal study of nutritional parameters in patients on each treatment. CAPD patients have lower serum protein levels than HD patients [162]. However, long-term CAPD patients, up to 8 years of treatment, maintain unchanged plasma levels of albumin and transferrin [167], indicating that long-term CAPD treatment is not necessarily associated with malnutrition. These data are in agreement with our other results that show stability of the protein catabolic rate and the creatinine appearance rate in patients on long-term CAPD treatment [167]. CAPD patients usually have lower protein intake than that recommended (1.1–1.3 g/kg body weight per day) for nitrogen balance [168, 169] and this should expose them to a greater risk of malnutrition [164, 167]. However, this protein need was assessed in patients 44–48 years old, a range quite different from the older range of CAPD patients. Studies also including elderly patients have shown that on CAPD as well as on HD there is an inverse relationship between normalized protein catabolic rate and age [167, 170]. According to these studies it seems reasonable to suggest that CAPD patients, the majority of whom are elderly, can have an average lower protein requirement than that usually suggested to maintain nitrogen balance.

The studies on adequacy have found that, besides the dose of dialysis, the nutritional parameters have important effects on survival. In the study by Maiorca *et al.* [25] serum albumin concentration less than 3.5 g/dl ($p < 0.001$) significantly affected survival. In the CANUSA study [22] the increase in serum albumin by 1 g/L decreases the RR of death to 0.94 (95% confidence interval 0.90–0.97) and the increase by 1 unit in the Subjective Global Assessment to 0.75 (95% confidence interval 0.66–0.85).

A relationship between dose of dialysis and nutritional status has been hypothesized, but the relationship seen by many authors, between Kt/V and normalized protein catabolic rate (NPCR), has been questioned, as it can be a mathematical artifact. Nevertheless, adequate dialysis is only one of the factors that can affect nutrition in dialysis. Diet should supply a correct amount of calories and amino acids. Acidosis, which stimulates protein breakdown and inhibits protein synthesis [171–174], should be corrected by using bags with higher buffer concentration or by giving sodium bicarbonate orally. Masticatory and gastrointestinal problems should be analysed and, when possible, resolved. If protein malnutrition is still present after these therapeutic attempts, the addition of amino acid supplements, in the bags or orally, or the transfer to HD, should be taken into consideration.

Residual renal function

After the first reports [175–177], suggesting a better capacity of CAPD over HD in preserving residual renal function, many papers confirmed this trend in non-diabetics [178–180] and in diabetics [176–178]. Moreover, in patients with acute worsening of chronic renal function, CAPD proved to allow a more frequent recovery of renal function enough to stop dialysis. In different studies [177, 179–181] this was seen in 1.0–8.0% of patients on CAPD, compared to 0.86%–1.20% of patients on HD. The recovery of renal function is more frequent in patients with nephroangiosclerosis, interstitial nephropathy and systemic disease [179–181]. This is in agreement with data by Cancarini *et al.* [177], who showed that the mean annual reduction of renal creatinine clearance was, with CAPD, much smaller in patients with nephrangiosclerosis and interstitial nephropathy than in patients with primary glomerulonephropathy. The preservation of renal function in dialysis patients has indisputable advantages as it allows the reduction of the administered dose of dialysis. In the study by Maiorca et al. [25], the Cox multivariate analysis showed a 17.5% reduction in RR of death for each 5 L/week of residual glomerular filtration rate (GFR). In the data of the Canusa study, Bargman et al. [185], analysing the residual GFR as a co-variable in a time-dependent model, found a 10% reduction in RR for each 5 L/week R-GFR. RRF is, thus, an important contributor to the dialysis adequacy, and its value probably goes beyond that measurable as Kt/V [134].

Causes of death

The causes of death varied in different series, but were often alike for CAPD and HD. Cardiovascular pathology is the main cause, being responsible for 27–54% of deaths with CAPD and for 29–50% with HD [7–9, 32, 98, 186]. According to the 1991 EDTA Registry [187], in 1990 on overall dialysis patients, cardiovascular deaths accounted for 51% with HD, for 55% with CAPD and for 36% in transplanted patients. These data do not take into account differences in age or other pretreatment risk factors. Among cardiovascular causes, deaths due to myocardial infarction were 14% with HD, 20% with PD and 17% in transplanted patients, cardiac arrests were 13%, 12% and 6%, cardiac failures 13%, 12% and 6%, cerebrovascular deaths 11%, 11% and 7%. Total and cardiovascular mortality in dialysis was, in the EDTA Registry, higher in northern than in southern Europe.

Other causes have different incidences in each method and in each study, and the only unequivocal but obvious difference between the two methods is in the deaths from peritonitis. Peritonitis is directly responsible for 7–10% of deaths with CAPD, i.e. for the death of 1.3–1.9% of all patients on this treatment [7–9, 32]. However, as peritonitis can have a serious impact on the nutritional status and the general condition of patients, it might be responsible for more deaths. Among the causes of death with CAPD, sclerosing encapsulating peritonitis seems to be less frequent after chlorhexidine and acetate buffer were identified as their major causes. Dementia and cachexia had similar incidences in CAPD and HD patients [9].

Hospitalization

The causes for hospitalization are partially different for PD and HD, and this must be considered when evaluating comparative results.

Several investigators have evaluated the need for hospitalization with CAPD and with HD, but their results are not really comparable, because there are important differences in centre policy towards hospitalization or ambulatory care. Case mix is another variable, since age and diabetes, at least, influence hospitalization rate [13, 32]. When comparing home treatment to in-centre treatment, it is important, for better comprehension, to separate the first hospitalization from later ones, as the training period, if done on a hospitalization regimen, can prolong the first hospitalization length considerably.

The incidence of hospitalization is greater with CAPD than with HD in some studies [5, 32, 37, 188] and similar in others [3, 13, 188]. In the study by Serkes et al. the difference was small but statistically significant [13]. In the study by Kurtz and Johnson [5], 43% of CAPD patients did not need to be hospitalized during the time of the study versus 23% of HHD patients but, once hospitalized, patients on CAPD had longer hospitalization. Diabetics on CAPD are admitted more often than non-diabetics [3, 13, 32]. Days of hospitalization for diabetics on CAPD have been reported to be more [13] or less [3, 34, 100] than those for diabetics on HD. Unfortunately, not all the studies give the percentage of diabetics, and this can influence the results. It is noteworthy that studies that report the incidence of hospitalization due to peritonitis [5, 189] or that divide the days of hospitalization according to their causes [7, 37] show that the difference between CAPD and HD disappears or becomes negative when admissions due to peritonitis are excluded.

Burton and Walls analysed the hospitalization of dialysis patients in greater depth [32]. They applied a generalized linear model to 227 patients on either CAPD or HD to identify confounding factors, estimate the magnitude of their effects and make adjustments for their biasing influence on hospitalization. Six of the 86 variables studied influenced hospitalization, some adversely, others beneficially. Diabetes and atherosclerotic disease significantly increased the hospitalization rate, while having a living spouse and the initial presentation via outpatient department reduced it. After correction for the above biases the investigators found a quadratic relationship between patient age and hospitalization rate: the ratio between the estimated rate at a specific age and the rate at 50 years of age increased below the age of 20, and much more above the age of 60 years. When hospitalization was examined according to the date of commencement of dialysis, it remained stable with HD over the course of the study, whereas it markedly diminished with CAPD, so that the annual hospitalization ratio between CAPD and HD fell, with time, from the initial 7.8 to 1.33 days/patient-month. The conclusion of the investigators is that, with growing experience, hospitalization levels with CAPD can become very close to those with HD. The same conclusion was reached by Khanna *et al.* [39], who observed a progressive reduction in the incidence of hospitalitazion of CAPD patients from 26.1 days/patient-year (13.1 due to peritonitis) in the period 1977–78 to 16 (5.1 due to peritonitis) in 1982. A similar positive trend was found by Nolph for all patients and the for 'standard patient' of the US CAPD Registry [190].

In another study, 254 CAPD and 240 HD patients treated in a single centre between January 1981 and December 1991were evaluated [37]. The two groups had comparable follow-ups (32 ± 29 months on HD vs. 34 ± 26 on CAPD). Hospitalizations were classified into: first hospitalization (diagnosis period, preparation of dialytic access, CAPD training); hospitalization due to technique-related problems (peritonitis, exit-site and tunnel infection, hernias, problems related to vascular access, etc.); hospitalizations in some way connected to pathology already present at the beginning of treatment (cardiovascular disease, diabetes, etc.); all other reasons for hospitalization (diagnostic needs, haemorrhages, infectious diseases, metabolic problems, surgical problems, etc.). First hospitalization, which included training as inpatients, was longer with CAPD than with HD, 32.5 days versus 22.1. The duration of hospitalization for all other admissions combined was longer with CAPD than with HD: 20.0 days/patient-year on CAPD, 12.4 on bicarbonate-HD, 9.1 on acetate-HD and 9.5 on HF/HDF. The incidence of days spent in hospital because of complications of the technique was almost twice as great for CAPD as for HD patients, the difference being due to peritonitis. There were no differences in hospitalizations due to pathologies already present at the start of treatment, whereas the length of hospitalization due to other causes was longer with CAPD and with bicarbonate-HD than with other methods.

In the 221 301 dialysis patients of the 1993 US RDS registry, Habach *et al.* [191] found that patients on PD had 1.9 admissions/year versus 1.7 on HD, and 21.9 hospital days/year vs 17.3. This higher incidence was also confirmed in the subgroups obtained according to age, gender, race, presence or absence of diabetes.

Another study [192] found that hospitalization rates among CAPD patients were slightly higher than for haemodialysis in each age group, with the exception of patients aged 65 years or more, for whom hospitalization was similar in PD and HD.

The effect of adequacy and nutrition on the number of days of hospitalization has been examined in the CANUSA study [22]. Any increase in serum albumin (multiplicative factor = 0.95 for 1 g/L), in subjective global assessment (0.82 for 1 unit) and in creatinine clearance (0.99 for 5 L/week per 1.73 m^2 of body surface area), was associated with a statistically significant reduction in hospital days. In the study by Maiorca *et al.* [21] patients with weekly $Kt/V < 1.7$ had a significantly higher hospitalization rate than those with weekly $Kt/V > 1.7$.

Technique failure

PD technique survival is one of the most widely discussed topics in the evaluation of method performance. Some investigators also include the death of patients among the causes of technique failures, since patient death can be considered as a failure of the method. However, it is well known that about 50% of deaths are due to cardiovascular disease and many other causes, and some of them, such as malignancy, cannot be related to method failure. This is why, in the evaluation of method survival, we, like many others, prefer to treat the patients who are dead as lost to follow-up. On the other hand, to include death among the final events of technique survival can be useful to evaluate the probability for one patient to live on the method. This approach, often called 'technique success analysis', can be important to predict the workload of the centre and the number of patients who will remain on the method within a certain period of time.

In the following analysis of the published studies we will discuss the two different approaches in different sections, the first called 'technique survival', the second 'technique success', to avoid confusion.

Technique survival

For intermittent peritoneal dialysis, technique survival is worse than for HD. In one prospective, randomized study [193], 49.2% of patients were switched from home intermittent peritoneal dialysis (HIPD) to HD versus only 9.1% from HHD to IPD.

More studies have compared technique survivals for CAPD and HD, some reporting worse results with CAPD [7–9, 11, 21], others with comparable results [10, 12]. In one study [16], reporting data from the Canadian Renal Failure Registry for non-diabetic patients, technique survival was worse for CAPD in youth, with differences progressively decreasing with age. For the age group 15–44 years, CAPD patients had the same technique survival as HD patients in the first 6 months, but afterwards the CAPD curve continued to decrease while the HD curve was stable, and after 30 months technique survival was 45% for CAPD and 85% for HD. A similar trend was observed in the age group 45–64, but the final differences were less than for younger patients (55% on CAPD versus 70% on HD). Finally, in the older age group (65 years or more), technique survival was better for CAPD in the first 24 months, but at 30 months any difference had disappeared. The conclusions of this study are supported by other observations, of better CAPD technique survival in the elderly [16], with the risk of changing method decreasing for CAPD, and increasing for ICHD, after 60 years of age [11].

Another paper [15] cites data from the Dialysis and Transplantation Registry of the Italian Piedmont Region in the period 1981–87. Technique survivals after 42 months were about 55% for CAPD (359 patients), 65% for bicarbonate-HD (431 patients), and 30% for acetate-HD (1231 patients). Comparison of the CAPD patients with 53 haemofiltration patients showed similar results after 24 months of treatment.

Several studies have attempted to identify causes of CAPD failure. Peritonitis frequency still stands as the most important cause and its frequency significantly affects technique survival (Fig. 4) [107]. Better technique survivals were obtained [10] after the introduction of flush-before-fill systems in the 1980s [194, 195]. The influence of peritonitis on technique survival was assessed in a cause-specific analysis [9]. When considering 'changes of modality due to peritonitis' as 'lost to follow-up' the relative

risk for CAPD versus HD dropped from 1.81 to 1.06, very close to that of HD, placed at 1.

Other studies have examined the role of diabetes in CAPD technique survival. Diabetics on CAPD have a higher risk of changing modality than non-diabetics or diabetics on HD [13]. However, another study has reported, for diabetics, a higher probability of remaining in CAPD and of shifting from HD to CAPD [11]. The presence of cerebro-cardiovascular disease was also associated with increased risk to change modality, from HD to CAPD [7] in one study, but not in another [11]. In an Italian study [9] no factor related to the patient was found to significantly affect technique survival, with a marginal non-significant adverse effect for female sex. Firanek et al. found a higher relative risk of changing, from CAPD to HD, in black than in white patients [196]. Italian Cooperative showed that diabetics have the same probability of technique failure as non-diabetics, and that the incidence of peritonitis was similar.

Other factors which are not patient-related influence technique survival. In a multicentre study, differences were seen among centres [9], probably due to different centre policies in patient selection, treatment, training and inclination to change method because of peritonitis or other technique-related complications. The Canusa study showed that both adequacy and nutrition play a role in technique failure. The increase by 1 g/L in serum albumin decreases the RR of failure to 0.95 (95% confidence interval 0.92–0.98); a similar degree of reduction in RR was associated with an increase by 5 L/week in creatinine clearance.

Maiorca et al. have pointed out that, in their experience, the shift from PD to HD did not artefactually improve patient survival in PD. Patients switching to HD or remaining on PD had the same survival rate [45]. In a recent paper, Van Biesen et al. [197] reported that the reasons for patient transfer from HD to PD are mainly PD-related complications, whereas transfer from HD to PD involves mostly severe cardiovascular problems. Patient survival is improved when patients are transferred from PD to HD, but not vice-versa. This was not due to worse survival on PD, because the survival curves were the same until the time of transfer.

Canaud and Mion suggest there should be no delay in the change from PD modality when indicated [198]. They found a greater risk of death during the first year due to a bad performance of PD in the last months before transfer.

All studies agree that PD modality has a lower technique survival than HD. The Canadian Register,

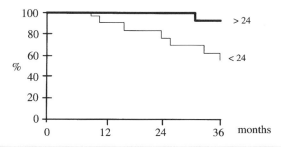

Figure 4. Technique survival (1991–96) according to the mean interval between episodes of peritonitis longer or shorter than 24 months.

which notes better patient survival with CAPD than with HD, also confirms that the incidence of method failure is higher on CAPD, 186 failures per 1000 patient-years, than with HD, 165 failures per 1000 patient-years [20].

Technique success

In one of the first studies, Rubin *et al.* [33] found a lower technique success rate (mortality and technique failure) with CAPD than with HD, 16% versus 43%. However, the two groups were not comparable because with CAPD there were more diabetics (25% versus 5%), more cardiovascular disease (37% versus 8%) and more patients with lower income. The mean age was 5 years greater for CAPD, but this difference was not statistically significant. In a study published in 1983 [4], the percentages of 'standard patients' continuing on their first treatment modality were 90% for HHD, 80% for CHD, 42% for IPD and 50% for CAPD. Interestingly, the main reason for transferring CAPD patients to another modality was loss of ultrafiltration, and peritonitis was the second reason. At that time acetate buffer was used, which has a proven negative effect on ultrafiltration.

In other studies the percentages of success were similar with CAPD and HD [3, 199] or worse with CAPD [11], even after adjustment for pretreatment differences [9].

Causes of technique failure

Among patients 3–7% per year change type of dialysis, as compared with 11–15% of CAPD patients [7–9, 13]. Peritonitis is the main reason for changing CAPD method (40–47%), loss of peritoneal function accounting for 15–19% and catheter-related problems for 9–15%. A very small percentage of drop-outs is due to malnutrition, 4–15% to patient preference. On the other hand, HD is discontinued for cardiovascular instability, loss of the vascular access and other medical reasons. In the most important Registries [200], peritonitis accounts for 27–52% of drop-outs, and loss of peritoneal function for 8–14%. The loss of peritoneal function was higher (30% after 2 years) in France [201]. In absolute figures 1.7–2.5% of patients at risk leave the treatment for loss of peritoneal function and 5–7.2% for peritonitis [7–9].

In Canada [19], 14% of PD patients changed modality in 1994, versus 12% in 1990. The more frequent reasons for changing were: peritonitis 29%, other abdominal complications 17%, inadequate dialysis 22%. Improvements in both connection system and therapy of peritonitis have reduced the risk of leaving PD: in the same Canadian Register, in 1990, these figures were 44%, 16% and 9%, respectively. On the other hand, the greater attention paid in the 1990s to the adequacy of dialysis leading to higher Kt/V targets, with increased prescription of bags and of dialysate volumes, are leading to a dramatic increase in drop-outs due to patient and partner burnout. In one paper these drop-outs rose to 9.1% during the period 1987–92, from 2.5% in 1981–86 [21].

An interesting observation regarding factors which can influence the outcome of CAPD has been made by Juergensen *et al.* [202], who found that patients with higher depression and anxiety scores have a higher incidence of medical complications (peritonitis, exit-site infection, days of admission).

Transplantation

Many groups have compared the transplantation outcomes in HD and CAPD patients and have shown no differences in patient and graft survival [203–216]. These results have also been confirmed for children [217, 218].

Transplanted patients coming from peritoneal dialysis are at risk of developing catheter-related infections. Post-tranplant prevalence of peritonitis varies from 0% to 40% [203, 204, 206, 209–212, 214–218]. Peritonitis developed very rarely in patients not using CAPD after surgery [198, 214]. In any case, post-transplant peritonitis is not a major problem if it is managed aggressively with antibiotic therapy and early catheter removal [196]. Diaz-Buxo *et al.* [203] suggest removing the catheter 1 day before transplantation of kidneys from living-related donors and 1–2 weeks after surgery for kidneys from cadaveric donors. Wood *et al.* [214] and Ogawa *et al.* [218] removed the catheter perioperatively, others 1–26 weeks after transplantation [203, 207, 212, 214, 215].

The percentages of transplanted patients with infections of the wound were similar in HD and CAPD [214], or greater in CAPD patients: 9% versus 9% [209], 26% versus 11% [215]. In the last study the percentage increased to 56%, only when patients needing CAPD post-transplantation were taken into account [215]. On the other hand, no wound infection was observed by Ogawa *et al.* [218] in 20 children, 16 of whom had the catheter removed at the time of transplant.

Exit-site infections occurred, in the post-transplant course, in 2–8% of patients [207, 211, 212, 214, 215] and leakage from the transplant wound in 1.8–5% [193, 211, 220]. Ascites developed in 2–20% of patients [204, 209, 220]. Incidence of infections other than peritonitis, wound infection and catheter exit-site infection were similar in CAPD and HD patients [220].

Fontan et al. [221] analysed the results of 92 PD and 587 HD patients who had received a cadaveric renal graft. PD patients had a higher prevalence of diabetes, 12% versus 4%; $p < 0.05$, and a shorter time on dialysis, 24 ± 29 months versus 45 ± 27; $p < 0.01$. Immediate graft function occurred in 68.5% of PD patients (46.5% in HD patients), delayed graft function in 22.5% (39% in HD patients), no function in 9% (14% in HD patients; $p < 0.001$). No difference was seen between the two groups in recipient-related, donor-related or graft related factors, with the exception of HD, performed immediately before transplantation in only 15% of PD patients but in 74% of HD patients; however, HD immediately before transplantation did not significantly affect the outcome of renal transplantation.

Long-term maintenance of residual renal function with CAPD allows these patients to have a higher bladder capacity at the time of transplantation [222], which allows a better ureteral–bladder anastomosis and could reduce the risk of ureteral reflux, urinomas and urinary tract infection [223]. Even if residual renal function is maintained with CAPD [180, 181], the patients on this modality have some degree of extracellular over-hydration. Patients who come from PD have a greater body weight loss (2.8 ± 2.9 kg) than patients coming from HD (0.9 ± 2.4 kg; $p = 0.009$) during the 10 days after renal transplantation.

Hepatitis B virus infection is associated, after transplantation, with a high incidence of liver disease, and this is a negative prognostic factor for patient survival [224]; its prevalence in patients on the waiting list has been reported as 13% on HD versus 2% on PD, $p < 0.05$ [222]. This was probably dependent on contamination during the in-centre HD treatment, a finding similar to that reported in the literature [225]. In the same study no significant difference was found in the prevalence of antibodies to anti-hepatitis C virus (Ab-HCV) (HD 14% versus PD 12%) and cytomegalovirus (96% versus 86%) between PD and HD patients. The short time spent on dialysis before renal transplantation could explain the low and similar prevalence on HD and PD.

Finally, PD does not negatively affect patient survival in the waiting period; survival has been reported as 93.0% with PD versus 95.4% with HD after 3 years, in agreement with former studies [21, 222]; this could also depend on the short time spent by both PD and HD patients on dialysis before transplantation, and on the positive patient selection for both modalities.

Technique survival in patients on the waiting list is better with HD; however, PD technique survival in these patients is better than that in the overall population [21], also considering the age class of the patients examined here.

Conclusions

All the collected evidence points to a longer maintenance of residual renal function on PD and a better survival during the first 2 years. PD patients also have the same chance as their HD counterparts of having a successful kidney transplantation. On the other hand, drop-out is definitely higher with PD than with HD, which precludes long-term PD therapy in about one-half of patients. However, it is reassuring that life-expectancy is not jeopardized when patients withdraw from the method in a timely fashion.

All these facts considered, PD can be suggested as the first dialysis modality in all patients with no clinical contraindication. Those transplanted in a reasonable period of time can, in this way, be dialysed at home, with their preferred PD modality, CAPD or APD, at reduced social costs. When PD no longer appears beneficial, or clearly becomes no longer accepted by the patient or his/her partner, a switch to HD must be decided, avoiding any delay that may have consequences later.

Other PD benefits may be considered. The first months on dialysis are quite stressing for the psychological impact of dialysis, and the need to go to the dialysis centre for HD three times a week worsens the stress. A start with home treatment can be accepted more easily. The money saved by using CAPD can permit other, more expensive treatments to be performed, e.g. in-line haemofiltration, haemodiafiltration, acetate-free biofiltration, etc., to satisfy the therapeutic need of those patients burdened by major cardiovascular complications. A period on PD can preserve vascular access sites longer. Finally, the risk of hepatitis B and C is reduced with CAPD [226] and this has a very favourable impact on transplantation outcome.

References

1. Nolph KD. Why are reported relative mortality risks for CAPD and HD so variable? (Inadequacy of the Cox proportional hazard model). Perit Dial Int 1996; 16: 15–18.

2. Capelli JP, Camiscioli TC, Vallorani RD. Comparative analysis of survival on home dialysis, in-center hemodialysis and chronic peritoneal dialysis (CAPD-IPD) therapies. Dial Transplant 1985; 14: 38–52.

3. Charytan C, Spinowitz BS, Galler M. A comparative study of continuous ambulatory peritoneal dialysis and center hemodialysis. Arch Intern Med 1986; 146: 1138–43.

4. Mion C, Mourad G, Canaud B et al. Maintenance dialysis: a survey of 17 years' experience in Languedoc-Roussillon with a comparison of methods in a 'standard populations'. ASAIO J 1983; 6: 205–13.

5. Kurtz SB, Johnson WJ. A four-year comparison of continuous ambulatory peritoneal dialysis and home hemodialysis: a preliminary report. Mayo Clin Proc 1984; 59: 659–62.

6. Mailloux LU, Bellucci AG, Mossey RT et al. Predictors of survival in patients undergoing dialysis. Am J Med 1988; 84: 855–62.

7. Gokal R, Jakubowski C, King J et al. Outcome in patients on continuous ambulatory peritoneal dialysis and haemodialysis: 4-year analysis of a prospective multicentre study. Lancet 1987; 14: 1105–9.

8. Maiorca R, Vonesh E, Cancarini GC et al. A six-year comparison of patient and technique survivals in CAPD and HD. Kidney Int 1988; 34: 518–24.

9. Maiorca R, Vonesh EF, Cavalli PL et al. A multicenter selection-adjusted comparison of patient and technique survivals on CAPD and hemodialysis. Perit Dial Int 1991; 11: 118–27.

10. Cavalli PL, Viglino G, Goia F, Cottino R, Mariano F, Gandolfo C. CAPD versus hemodialysis: 7 years of experience. Adv Perit Dial 1989; 5: 52–5.

11. Gentil MA, Cariazzo A, Pavon MI et al. Comparison of survival in continuous ambulatory peritoneal dialysis: a multicenter study. Nephrol Dial Transplant 1991; 6: 444–51.

12. Lupo A, Cancarini G, Catizone L et al. Comparison of survival in CAPD and hemodialysis: a multicenter study. Adv Perit Dial 1992; 8: 136–40.

13. Serkes KD, Blagg CR, Nolph KD, Vonesh EF, Shapiro F. Comparison of patient and technique survival in continuous ambulatory peritoneal dialysis and hemodialysis: a multicenter study. Perit Dial Int 1990; 10: 15–9.

14. Burton PR, Walls J. Selection-adjusted comparison of life-expectancy of patients on continuous ambulatory peritoneal dialysis, haemodialysis, and renal transplantation. Lancet 1987; 1: 1115–19.

15. Quarello F, Bonello F, Boero R et al. CAPD in a large population: a 7-year experience. Adv Perit Dial 1989; 5: 56–62.

16. Posen G, Arbus G, Hutchinson T, Jeffery A. Survival comparison of adult non-diabetic patients treated with either hemodialysis or CAPD for end-stage renal failure. Perit Dial Bull 1987; 7: 78–9.

17. Gotch FA, Sargent JA. A mechanistic analysis of the National Cooperative Dialysis Study (NCDS). Kidney Int 1985; 28: 526–34.

18. Bloembergen WE, Port KF, Mauger A, Wolfe RA. A comparison of mortality between patients treated with hemodialysis and peritoneal dialysis. J Am Soc Nephrol 1995; 6: 177–83.

19. Annual Report 1996, Vol. 1: Dialysis and Renal Transplantation, Canadian Organ Replacement Register. Ottawa, Ontario: Canadian Institute for Health Information, March 1996.

20. Fenton SSA, Schaubel DE, Desmeules M et al. Hemodialysis versus peritoneal dialysis: a comparison of adjusted mortality rates. Am J Kidney Dis 1997; 30: 334–42.

21. Maiorca R, Cancarini GC, Zubani R et al. CAPD viability: a long-term comparison with hemodialysis. Perit Dial Int 1996; 16: 276–87.

22. Canada–USA (CANUSA) Peritoneal Dialysis Study Group: Adequacy of dialysis and nutrition in continuous ambulatory peritoneal dialysis: association with clinical outcomes. J Am Soc Nephrol 1996; 7: 198–207.

23. Churchill DN, Thorpe KE, Vonesh E, Keshaviah PR, for the Canada–USA (CANUSA) Peritoneal Dialysis Study Group. Lower probability of patients survival with continuous ambulatory peritoneal dialysis in the United States compared with Canada. J Am Soc Nephrol 1997; 8: 965–71.

24. Marcelli D, Stannard D, Conte F, Held PJ, Locatelli F, Port FK. ESRD patient mortality with adjustment for comorbid conditions in Lombardy (Italy) versus the United States. Kidney Int 1996; 50: 1013–18.

25. Maiorca R, Brunori G, Zubani R et al. Predictive value of dialysis adequacy and nutritional indices for mortality and morbidity in CAPD and HD patients. A longitudinal study. Nephrol Dial Transplant 1995; 10: 2295–305.

26. Bloembergen WE, Stannard DC, Port FK et al. Relationship of dose of hemodialysis and cause-specific mortality. Kidney Int 1996; 50: 557–65.

27. Keshaviah PR, Ma J, Thorpe K, Churchill D, Collins A. Comparison of 2-year survival on hemodialysis and peritoneal dialysis with dose of dialysis matched using the peak concentration hypothesis. J Am Soc Nephrol 1995; 6: 540.

28. Canadian Organ Replacement Register, 1993 Annual Report. Don Mills, Ontario: Canadian Institute for Health Information, 1995.

29. Foley RN, Parfrey PS, Harnett JD et al. Mode of dialysis therapy and mortality in end-stage renal disease. J Am Soc Nephrol 1998; 9: 267–76.

30. Kagan A, Elimalech E, Lerner Z, Fink A, Bar-Khayim Y. Residual renal function affects lipid profile in patients undergoing continuous ambulatory peritoneal dialysis. Perit Dial Int 1997; 17: 243–9.

31. Cancarini GC, Brunori G, Zani R et al. Long-term outcomes of peritoneal dialysis. Perit Dial Int 1997; 17 (suppl. 2): S115–18.

32. Burton PR, Walls J. A selection adjusted comparison of hospitalization on continuous ambulatory peritoneal dialysis and haemodialysis. J Clin Epidemiol 1989; 42: 531–9.

33. Rubin J, Barnes T, Burns P et al. Comparison of home hemodialysis to continuous ambulatory peritoneal dialysis. Kidney Int 1983; 23: 51–6.

34. Wolfe RA, Port FK, Hawthorne VM, Guire KE. A comparison of survival among dialytic therapies of choice: in-center hemodialysis versus continuous ambulatory peritoneal dialysis at home. Am J Kidney Dis 1990; 15: 433–40.

35. Lunde NM, Port FK, Wolfe RA, Guire KE. Comparison of mortality risk by choice of CAPD versus hemodialysis among elderly patients. Adv Perit Dial 1991; 7: 68–72.

36. Panarello G, De Baz H, Cecchin E, Tesio F. Dialysis for the elderly: survival and risk factors. Adv Perit Dial 1989; 5: 49–51.

37. Maiorca R, Cancarini GC, Brunori G, Camerini C, Manili L. Morbidity and mortality of CAPD and hemodialysis. Kidney Int 1993; 43 (suppl. 40): S4–15.

38. Shapiro FL, Umen A. Risk factors in hemodialysis patient survival. ASAIO J 1983; 6: 176–84.

39. Khanna R, Wu G, Vas S, Oreopoulos DG. Mortality and morbidity on continuous ambulatory peritoneal dialysis. ASAIO J 1983; 6: 197–204.

40. Brunner FP, Brynger H, Challah S et al. Renal replacement therapy in patients with diabetic nephropathy, 1980–85. Report from the European Dialysis and Transplantation Association Registry. Nephrol Dial Transplant 1988; 3: 585–95.

41. Walker JV, Grove MA. Survival in a community hospital dialysis center. Am J Nephrol 1988; 8: 40–8.

42. Excerpts from United States Renal Data System. 1991 Annual Data Report. V. Survival probabilities and cause of death. Am J Kidney Dis 1991; 18 (suppl. 2): 49–60.

43. Maiorca R, Cancarini G, Brunori G *et al.* CAPD in the elderly. Perit Dial Int 1993; 13 (suppl. 2): S165–71.
44. Youmbissi J, Sellars L, Shore AC, Poon T, Wilkinson R. Blood pressure on CAPD: relationship to sodium status, renin, and aldosterone, compared to hemodialysis. In: Maher JF, Winchester JF, eds. Frontiers in Peritoneal Dialysis, Proceedings of the Congress of the International Society for Peritoneal Dialysis. New York: Field, Rich & Assoc., 1986, pp. 450–6.
45. US Renal Data System. 1993 Annual data report: patient survival. Am J Kidney Dis 1995; 25: 1–10.
46. Rostand SG, Gretes JC, Kirk KA, Rutsky EA, Andreoli TE. Ischemic heart disease in patients with uremia undergoing maintenance hemodialysis. Kidney Int 1979; 16: 600–11.
47. Kannel WB, Dawber TRE, Kagan A, Revotskie N, Stokes J. Factors of risk in the development of coronary heart disease: six-year follow-up experience. The Framingham study. Ann Intern Med 1961; 55: 33–50.
48. Wizemann V, Timio M, Alpert M Kramer W. Options in dialysis therapy: significance of cardiovascular findings. Kidney Int 1993; 43 (supp. 40): S85–91.
49. Levy D, Anderson K, Savage D, Balkus S, Kannel W, Castelli W. Echocardiographically detected left ventricular hypertrophy: prevalence and risk factors. The Framingham Hearth Study. Ann Intern Med 1988; 108: 7–13.
50. Eisenberg M, Prichard S, Barre P, Patton R, Hutchinson T, Sniderman A. Left ventricular hypertrophy in end-stage renal disease on peritoneal dialysis. Am J Cardiol 1987; 60: 418–19.
51. Silberberg DS, Barre P, Prichard S, Sniderman AD. Left ventricular hypertrophy: an independent determinant of survival in end-stage renal failure. Kidney Int 1989; 36: 286–90.
52. Harnett JD, Parfrey PS, Griffiths SM, Gault MH, Barre P, Bultmann RD. Left ventricular hypertrophy in end-stage renal disease. Nephron 1988; 48: 107–15.
53. Kramer W, Hüting J, Wizemann V. Left ventricular hypertrophy in end-stage renal failure: functional findings and therapeutical implications. In: Timio M, Wizemann V, eds. Cardionephrology. Milan: Wichtig Editore, 1991, pp. 97–100.
54. Levy D, Anderson KM, Savage DD, Balkus SA, Kannel WB, Castelli WP. Risk of ventricular arrhythmias in left ventricular hypertrophy. The Framingham Heart Study. Am J Cardiol 1987; 60: 560–5.
55. Alpert MA, Van Stone J, Twardwoski ZJ *et al.* Comparative cardiac effects of hemodialysis and continuous ambulatory peritoneal dialysis. Clin Cardiol 1986; 9: 52–60.
56. Canziani ME, Cendoroglio NM, Saragoca MA *et al.* Hemodialysis versus continuous ambulatory peritoneal dialysis: effects on the heart. Artif Organs 1995; 19: 241–4.
57. Leenen FHH, Smith DL, Khanna R, Oreopoulos DG. Changes in left ventricular hypertrophy and function in hypertensive patients started on continuous ambulatory peritoneal dialysis. Am Heart J 1985; 10: 102–5.
58. Timio M, Ronconi M, Lori G, Venanzi S, Pede S. Effetto differenziato dell'emodialisi e della dialisi peritoneale ambulatoriale continua (CAPD) sull'ipertrofia asimmetrica settale dei pazienti uremici. G Ital Nefrol 1985; 4: 157–60.
59. Deligiannis A, Paschalidou E, Sakellariou G *et al.* Changes in left ventricular anatomy during haemodialysis, continuous ambulatory peritoneal dialysis and after renal transplantation. Proc Eur Dial Transplant Assoc 1984; 21: 185–9.
60. Rambausek M, Amann K, Mall G, Ritz E. Structural causes of cardiac dysfunction in uremia. Ren Fail 1993; 15: 421–8.
61. Malle G, Rambausek M, Neumeister A, Kollmar S, Vetterlein F, Ritz E. Myocardial interstitial fibrosis in experimental uremia. Implications for cardiac compliance. Kidney Int 1988; 33: 804–11.
62. Malle G, Huther W, Schneider J, Lundin P, Ritz E. Diffuse intermyocardiocytic fibrosis in uremic patients. Nephrol Dial Transplant 1990; 5: 39–44.
63. Ritz E, Rambausek M, Mall G, Ruffmann K, Mandelbaum A. Cardiac changes in uremia and their possible relationship to cardiovascular instability on dialysis. Nephrol Dial Transplant 1990 (suppl. 1): 93–7.
64. Weiss G, Lhotta K, Reibnegger G, König P, Knapp E. Divergent effects of hemodialysis and continuous ambulatory peritoneal dialysis on cardiac diastolic function. Perit Dial Int 1997; 17: 353–9.
65. Mattana J, Effiong C, Gooneratne R, Singhal PC. Risk of fatal cerebrovascular accident in patients on peritoneal dialysis versus hemodialysis. J Am Soc Nephrol 1996; 8: 1342–7.
66. Report of the National CAPD Registry of the National Institutes of Health, 1987.
67. Ramos J, Gokal R, Siampoulos K, Ward MK, Wilkinson R, Kerr DNS. CAPD: three year experience. Q J Med 1983; 52: 165–86.
68. Young MA, Nolph KD, Dulton S, Prowant B. Anti-hypertensive drug requirements in continuous ambulatory peritoneal dialysis. Perit Dial Bull 1984; 4: 85–8.
69. Glasson PH, Favre H, Vallotton MB. Response of blood pressure and the renin–angiotensin–aldosterone system to chronic ambulatory peritoneal dialysis in hypertensive end-stage renal failure. Clin Sci 1982; 63: 207s.
70. Timio M. Clinica cardiologica nell'uremia. Ruolo terapeutico della dialisi peritoneale. Milan: Wichtig Editore, 1990, pp. 73–8.
71. Velasquez MT, Lew SQ, Von Albertini B, Mishkin GJ, Bosch JP. Control of hypertension is better during hemodialysis than during continuous ambulatory peritoneal dialysis in ESRD patients. Clin Nephrol 1997; 48: 341–5.
72. Zuber M, Steinmann E, Huser B, Ritz R, Thiel G, Brunner F. Incidence of arrhythmias and myocardial ischaemia during haemodialysis and haemofiltration Nephrol Dial Transplant 1989; 4: 632–4.
73. Peer G, Korzets A, Hochhauzer E, Eschchar Y, Blum M, Aviram A. Cardiac arrhythmia during continuous ambulatory peritoneal dialysis. Nephron 1987; 45: 192–5.
74. Wu G and the University of Toronto Collaborative Dialysis Group. Cardiovascular deaths among CAPD patients. Perit Dial Bull 1983; 3 (suppl): S23–6.
75. Rostand SG, Gretes JC, Kirk KA, Rutsky EA, Andreoli TE. Ischemic heart disease in patients with uremia undergoing maintenance hemodialysis. Kidney Int 1979; 16: 600–11.
76. Elhalel-Dranitzki M, Rubinger D, Moscovici A *et al.* CAPD to improve quality of life in patients with refractory heart failure. Nephrol Dial Transplant 1998; 13: 3041–2.
77. Maiorca R. Cardiovascular problems in the choice of dialysis therapy for the elderly. Cardionephrological Meeting, Assisi, 1993. Contrib Nephrol 1994; 106: 74–83.
78. Charytan C, Spinowitz BS, Galler M. A comparative study of continuous ambulatory peritoneal dialysis and center hemodialysis. Arch Intern Med 1986; 146: 1138–43.
79. Henderson LW. Symptomatic hypotension during hemodialysis. Kidney Int 1980; 17: 571–6.
80. Rosa AA, Fryd DS, Kyellstrand CM. Dialysis symptoms and stabilization in long-term dialysis. Arch Intern Med 1980; 140: 804–7.
81. Degoulet P, Reach I, Di Giulio S *et al.* Epidemiology of dialysis-induced hypotension. Proc Eur Dial Transplant Assoc 1981; 18: 133–8.
82. Ronco C, Fabris A, Chiaramonte S *et al.* Comparison of four different short dialysis techniques. Int J Artif Organs 1988; 11: 169–74.
83. De Vries PMJM, Olthof CG, Solf A *et al.* Fluid balance during haemodialysis and haemofiltration: the effect of dialysate sodium and a variable ultrafiltration rate. Nephrol Dial Transplant 1991; 6: 257–63.
84. Zucchelli P, Santoro A, Ferrari G, Spongano M. Acetate-free biofiltration: hemodiafiltration with base-free dialysate. Blood Purif 1990; 8: 14–22.
85. Chanz MK, Varghese Z, Persaud JW, Baillod RA, Moorhead JF. Hyperlipidemia in patients on maintenance hemo- and peritoneal dialysis: the relative pathogenetic role of tri-

glycerides production and triglyceride removal. Clin Nephrol 1982; 17: 183–90.

86. Von Baeyer H, Gahl GM, Riedinger H *et al*. Adaptation of CAPD patients to the continuous peritoneal energy uptake. Kidney Int 1983; 23: 29–34.

87. Lameire N, Matthys D, Matthys E, Beheydt. Effects of long-term CAPD on carbohydrate and lipid metabolism. Clin Nephrol 1988; 30 (suppl. 1): S53–8.

88. Cancarini GC, Brasa S, Camerini C, Maiorca R. I problemi della CAPD: quali progressi dopo 4 anni di esperienze. In: Giordano C, De Santo NG, eds. Dialisi peritoneale, Atti del II Convegno Nazionale. Milan: Wichtig Editore, 1984, pp. 77–82.

89. Breckenridge WC, Roncari DAK, Khanna R, Oreopoulos DG. The influence of continuous ambulatory peritoneal dialysis on plasma lipoproteins. Atherosclerosis 1982; 45: 249–58.

90. Lindholm B, Bergstrom J, Norbeck HE. Lipoprotein metabolism in patients on continuous ambulatory peritoneal dialysis. In: Gahl GM, Kessel M, Nolph KD, eds. Advances in Peritoneal Dialysis. Amsterdam: Excerpta Medica, 1981, pp. 434–6.

91. Tane D, Fein PA, Antignani A, Mittman N, Avram MM. The impact of CAPD treatment on lipid metabolism and cardiovascular risk. Adv Perit Dial 1990; 6: 234–7.

92. Kronenberg F, Konig P, Neyer U *et al*. Multicenter study of lipoprotein(a) and apolipoprotein(a) phenotypes in patients with end-stage renal disease treated by hemodialysis or continuous ambulatory peritoneal dialysis. J Am Soc Nephrol 1995; 6: 110–20.

93. Avram MM, Goldwasser P, Burrel DE, Antignani A, Fein PA, Mittman N. The uremic dislipidemia: a cross-sectional study. Am J Kidney Dis 1992; 20: 324–35.

94. Mejia G, Zimmerman SW. Comparison of continuous ambulatory peritoneal dialysis and hemodialysis for diabetics. Perit Dial Bull 1985; 5: 7–11.

95. Triolo G, Segoloni GP, Pacitti A *et al*. The treatment of uremic diabetic patient (UDP) in Piemonte (Dialysis and Transplantation Registry – RPDT): survival analysis. In: Andreucci VE, Dal Canton A, eds. New Therapeutic Strategies in Nephrology. Boston: Kluwer, 1991, pp. 440–2.

96. Held PJ, Port FK, Turenne MN, Gaylin DS, Harmburger RJ, Wolfe RA. Continuous ambulatory peritoneal dialysis and hemodialysis: comparison of patient mortality with adjustment for comorbid conditions. Kidney Int 1994; 45: 1163–9.

97. Chandran PK, Lane T, Flynn CT. Patient and technique survival for blind and sighted diabetics on continuous ambulatory peritoneal dialysis: a ten-year analysis. Int J Artif Organs 1991; 14: 262–8.

98. Zimmerman SW, Glass N, Sollinger H, Miller D, Belzer F. Treatment of end-stage diabetic nephropathy: over a decade of experience at one institution. Medicine 1984; 63: 311–7.

99. Brunner FP, Broyer M, Brynger H *et al*. Survival on renal replacement therapy: data from the EDTA Registry. Nephrol Dial Transplant 1988; 2: 109–22.

100. Legrain M, Rottembourg J, Bentchikou A *et al*. Dialysis treatment of insulin dependent diabetic patients: ten years experience. Clin Nephrol 1984; 21: 72–81.

101. Rottembourg J, Bellio P, Maiga K, Remaoun M, Rousselie F, Legrain M. Visual function, blood pressure and blood glucose in diabetic patients undergoing continuous ambulatory peritoneal dialysis. Proc Eur Dial Transplant Assoc 1985; 21: 330–4.

102. Catalano C, Postorino M, Kelly PJ, Fabrizi F, Enia G, Maggior Q. Diabetes and renal replacement therapy in Italy: mode of treatment and major complications. In: Andreucci VE, Dal Canton A, eds. New Therapeutic Strategies in Nephrology. Boston: Kluwer, 1991: 443–5.

103. Khauli RB, Novick AC, Steinmuller DR *et al*. Comparison of renal transplantation and dialysis in rehabilitation of dia-

104. Diaz-Buxo JA, Burgess WP, Greenman M, Chandler JT, Farme CD, Walker J. Visual function in diabetic patients undergoing dialysis: comparison of peritoneal and hemodialysis. Int J Artif Organs 1984; 7: 257–62.

105. Mion C. Practical use of peritoneal dialysis. In: Maher JF, ed. Replacement of Renal Function by Dialysis. Dordrecht: Kluwer, 1989, pp. 537–89.

106. Tzamaloukas AH, Murata GH, Harford AM *et al*. Hand gangrene in diabetic patients on chronic dialysis. ASAIO Trans 1991; 37: 638–43.

107. Maiorca R, Cancarini GC, Camerini C, Manili L, Brunori G. The impact of the Y-system and low peritonitis rate on CAPD results. In: Hatano M, ed. Nephrology. Tokyo: Springer-Verlag, 1991, pp. 1592–601.

108. Keane WF, Raij LR. Host defenses and infectious complications in maintenance hemodialysis patients. In: Drukker W, Parsons FM, Maher JF, ed. Replacement of Kidney Function by Dialysis, 2nd rev edn. Boston: Martinus Nijhoff, 1983, pp. 646–58.

109. Van der Meer JWM. Defects in host-defense mechanism. In: Rubin RH, Young LS, eds. Clinical Approach to Infection in the Compromised Host, 2nd edn. New York: Plenum, 1988, pp. 41–73.

110. Zucchelli P, Ferrari G, Catizone L, Beltrandi E. Clinical importance of immunological disturbances in hemodialysis and CAPD patients. In: La Greca G, Chiaramonte S, Fabris A, Feriani M, Ronco C, eds. Peritoneal Dialysis. Milan: Wichtig Editore, 1988, pp. 101–6.

111. Schollemeyer P, Bozkurt F. The immune status of the uremic patients: hemodialysis versus CAPD. Clin Nephrol 1988; 30 (suppl. 1): S37–40.

112. Tolkoff-Rubin NE, Rubin RH. Uremia and host defenses. N Engl J Med 1990; 322: 770–2.

113. Nisbeth U, Hällgren R, Eriksson Ö, Danielson BG. Endotoxemia in chronic renal failure. Nephron 1987; 45: 93–7.

114. Bertazzoni EM, Panzetta G. Effects of different forms of dialytic treatment on serum antibacterial activity in patients with chronic renal failure. Nephron 1984; 36: 224–9.

115. Huttenen K, Lampainen E, Silvennoinen-Kassinen S, Tiilikanen A. The neutrophil function of uremic patients treated by hemodialysis or CAPD. Scand J Urol Nephrol 1984; 18: 167–72.

116. Giacchino F, Quarello F, Pellerey M, Piccoli G. Continuous ambulatory peritoneal dialysis improves immunodeficiency in uremic patients. Nephron 1983; 35: 209–10.

117. Giacchino F, Pozzato M, Piccoli G. Evaluation of the influence of peritoneal dialysis on cellular immunity by the E-rosette inhibition test. Artif Organs 1984; 8: 156–60.

118. Collart F, Tielemans C, Dratwa M, Schandene L, Wybran J, Dupont E. Hemodialysis, continuous ambulatory peritoneal dialysis and cellular immunity. Proc Eur Dial Transplant Assoc 1983; 20: 190–4.

119. Guillou PJ, Will EJ, Davison AM, Giles GR. CAPD – a risk factor in renal transplantation? Br J Surg 1984; 71: 878–80.

120. Giacchino F, Alloatti S, Quarello F, Coppo R, Pellerey M, Piccoli G. The influence of peritoneal dialysis on cellular immunity. Perit Dial Bull 1982; 2: 165–8.

121. Giangrande A, Cantù; P, Limido A, de Francesco D, Malacrida V. Continuous ambulatory peritoneal dialysis and cellular immunity. Proc Eur Dial Transplant Assoc 1982; 19: 372–9.

122. Gerez L, Madar L, Shkolnik T *et al*. Regulation of interleukin-2 and interferon-gamma gene expression in rela failure. Kidney Int 1991; 40: 266–72.

123. Langhof E, Ladefoged J. Improved lymphocyte transformation *in vitro* of patients on continuous ambulatory peritoneal dialysis. Proc Eur Dial Transplant Assoc 1983; 20: 230–5.

124. Donnelly PK, Shenton BK, Lennard TWJ, Proud G, Taylor RMR. CAPD and renal transplantation. Br J Surg 1985; 72: 819–21.

125. Rumpf KW, Seubert S, Seubert A et al. Association of ethylene-oxide-induced IgE antibodies with symptoms in dialysis patients. Lancet 1985; 2: 1385–7.

126. Marshall C, Shimizu A, Smith EKM, Dolovich J. Ethylene oxide allergy in a dialysis center: prevalence in hemodialysis and peritoneal dialysis populations. Clin Nephrol 1984; 21: 346–9.

127. Marckmann P. Nutritional status of patients on hemodialysis and peritoneal dialysis. Clin Nephrol 1988; 29: 75–8.

128. Cianciaruso B, Brunori G, Kopple JD et al. Cross-sectional comparison of malnutrition in continuous ambulatory peritoneal dialysis and hemodialysis patients. Am J Kidney Dis 1995; 26: 475–86.

129. Jungers P, Zingraff J, Albouze P et al. Late referral to maintenance dialysis: detrimental consequence. Nephrol Dial Transplant 1993; 8: 1089–93.

130. Campbell JD, Ewingman B, Hosokawa M, Van Stone JC. The timing of referral of patients with end stage renal disease. Dial Transplant 1989; 18: 660–86.

131. Sesso R, Belasco AG. Late diagnosis of chronic renal failure and mortality in maintenance dialysis. Nephrol Dial Transplant 1996; 11: 2417–20.

132. Obrador GT, Pereira JG. Early referral to nephrologists and timely initiation of renal replacement therapy: a paradigm shift in the management of patients with chronic renal failure. Am J Kidney Dis 1998; 31: 398–417.

133. Teehan BP, Schleifer CR, Brown J. Urea kinetic modelling is an appropriate assessment of adequacy. Semin Dial 1992; 5: 189–92.

134. Lameire NH, Vanholder R, Veyt D, Lambert MC, Ringoir S. A longitudinal, five year survey of urea kinetic parameters in CAPD patients. Kidney Int 1992; 42: 426–32.

135. Acchiardo SR, Kraus AP Jr, LaHatte G et al. Urea kinetic evaluation of hemodialysis and CAPD Patients. In: Khanna R, Nolph KD, Prowant BF, Twardowski ZJ, Oreopoulos DG, eds. Advances in Peritoneal Dialysis. Toronto: Peritoneal Dialysis Bulletin Inc., 1992, pp. 55–8.

136. Mooraki A, Kliger AS, Gorban-Brennan NL, Juergensen P, Brown E, Finkelstein FO. Weekly KT/V urea and selected outcome criteria in 56 randomly selected CAPD patients. In: Khanna R, Nolph KD, Prowant BF, Twardowski ZJ, Oreopoulos DG, edd. Advances in Peritoneal Dialysis. Toronto: Peritoneal Dialysis Bulletin Inc., 1993, pp. 92–6.

137. Spinowitz BS, Gupta BK, Kulogowski J et al. Dialysis adequacy versus metabolic factors in the clinical assessment of CAPD. In: Khanna R, Nolph KD, Prowant BF, Twardowsky ZJ, Oreopoulos DG, eds. Advances in Continuous Ambulatory Peritoneal Dialysis. Toronto: Peritoneal Dialysis Bulletin Inc., 1992, pp. 295–8.

138. Goodship THJ, Pablick-Deetjen J, Ward MK, Wilkinson R. Adequacy and nutritional status in CAPD. Nephrol Dial Transplant 1993; 8: 1366–71.

139. Selgas R, Bajo MA, Fernandez-Reyes MJ et al. An analysis of dialysis in a selected population on CAPD for over 3 years: the influence of urea and creatinine kinetics. Nephrol Dial Transplant 1993; 8: 1244–53.

140. Nolph KD, Moore HL, Prowant B et al. Cross sectional assessment of weekly urea and creatinine clearance and indices of nutrition in continuous ambulatory peritoneal dialysis patients. Perit Dial Int 1993; 13: 178–183.

141. Blake PG, Sombolos K, Abraham G et al. Lack of correlation between urea kinetic indices and clinical outcome in CAPD patients. Kidney Int 1991; 39: 700–6.

142. Teehan BP, Schleifer CR, Brown JM, Sigler MH, Raimondo J. Urea kinetic analysis and clinical outcome on CAPD. A five-year longitudinal study. In: Khanna R, Nolph KD, Prowant BF, Twardowski ZJ, Oreopoulos DG, eds. Advances in Continuous Ambulatory Peritoneal Dialysis. Toronto: Peritoneal Dialysis Bulletin Inc., 1990, pp. 181–5.

143. Keshaviah P, Nolph K, Van Stone J. The peak concentration hypothesis: a urea kynetic approach to comparing the adequacy of continuous ambulatory peritoneal dialysis (CAPD) and hemodialysis. Perit Dial Int 1989; 9: 257–60.

144. Gotch FA. Prescription criteria in peritoneal dialysis. Perit Dial Intern 1994; 14 (suppl. 3): S83–7.

145. Keshaviah P, Ma J, Thorpe K, Churchill D, Collins A. Comparison of 2 year survival on hemodialysis and peritoneal dialysis with dose of dialysis matched using the peak concentration hypothesis. J Am Soc Nephrol 1995; 6: 540.

146. NFK-DOQI Clinical Practice Guidelines for the Treatment of Anemia of Chronic Renal Failure. New York: National Kidney Foundation, 1997.

147. Rocco MV, Flanigan MJ, Beaver S et al. Report from the 1995 core indicators for the Peritoneal Dialysis Study Group. Am J Kidney Dis 1997; 30: 165–73.

148. Heimbürger O, Bergström J, Lindholm B. Is serum albumin an index of nutritional status in continuous ambulatory peritoneal dialysis patients? Perit Dial Int 1994; 14: 108–14.

149. Kaysen GA, Schoenfeld PY. Albumin homeostasis in patients undergoing continuous ambulatory peritoneal dialysis. Kidney Int 1984; 25: 107–14.

150. Germain M, Harlow P, Mulhern J, Lipkowitz G, Braden G. Low protein catabolic rate and serum albumin correlate with increased mortality and abdominal complications in peritoneal dialysis patients. In: Khanna R, Nolph KD, Prowant BF, Twardowsky ZJ, Oreopoulos DG, eds. Advances in Continuous Ambulatory Peritoneal Dialysis. Toronto: Peritoneal Dialysis Bulletin Inc., 1992, pp. 113–15.

151. Spinowitz BS, Gupta BK, Kulogowski J, Charytan C. Dialysis adequacy in hypoalbuminemic continuous ambulatory peritoneal dialysis patients. Perit Dial Int 1993; 13 (suppl. 2): S221–3.

152. Lindsay RM, Spanner E. The lower serum albumin does reflect nutritional status. Semin Dial 1992; 5: 215–8.

153. Kawanishi H, Namba S, Morishi M, Takahashi N, Tanji H, Tsuchiya T. Adequate dialysis and morbidity in CAPD is greatly affected by peritoneal permeability. J Am Soc Nephrol 1993; 4: 410 (abstract).

154. Cancarini G, Costantino E, Brunori G et al. Nutritional status in long-term CAPD patients. In: Khanna R, Nolph KD, Prowant BF, Twardowsky ZJ, Oreopoulos DG, eds. Advances in Continuous Ambulatory Peritoneal Dialysis. Toronto: Peritoneal Dialysis Bulletin Inc., 1992, pp. 84–7.

155. Kumano K, Takagi Y, Yokota S, Shimura S, Sakai T. Urea kinetics and clinical features of long-term continuous ambulatory peritoneal dialysis patients. Perit Dial Int 1993; 13 (suppl. 2): S180–2.

156. Heimbürger O, Barany P, Tranaeus A, Bergstrom J, Lindholm B. KT/V and protein catabolic rate (PCR) in CAPD and CCPD patients. Perit Dial Int 1992; 12 (suppl. 1): 125 (abstract).

157. Abdo F, Clemente L, Davy J, Grant J, Laduocer D, Morton AR. Nutritional status and efficiency of dialysis in CAPD and CCPD patients. In: Khanna R, Nolph KD, Prowant BF, Twardowski ZJ, Oreopoulos DG, eds. Advances in Peritoneal Dialysis. Toronto: Peritoneal Dialysis Bulletin Inc., 1993, pp. 76–9.

158. Blake PG, Flowerdew G, Blake RM, Oreopoulos DG. Serum albumin in patients on continuous ambulatory peritoneal dialysis – predictors and correlations with outcomes. J Am Soc Nephrol 1993; 3: 1501–7.

159. Pollock CA, Ibels LS, Caterson RJ, Mahony JF, Waugh DA, Cocksedge B. Continuous ambulatory peritoneal dialysis, eight years of experience at a single center. Medicine 1989; 68: 293–308.

160. Gamba G, Mejia JL, Saldivar S, Pena JC, Correa-Rotter R. Death risk in CAPD patients. The predictive value of the initial clinical and laboratory variables. Nephron 1993; 65: 23–7.

161. Acchiardo SR, Kraus AP, Kaufman PA, Lahatte G, Atkins D. Serum albumin a marker for morbidity and mortality in CAPD patients. J Am Soc Nephrol 1993; 4: 412 (abstract).

162. Maiorca R, Cancarini G, Manili L *et al.* CAPD is a first class treatment: results of an eight-year experience with a comparison of patient and method survival in CAPD and hemodialysis. Clin Nephrol 1988; 30 (suppl. 1): S3–7.

163. Lowrie EG, Lew NL. Death risk in hemodialysis patients: the predictive value of commonly measured variables and an evaluation of death rate differences between facilities. Am J Kidney Dis 1990; 15: 458–82.

164. Fine A, Cox D. Modest reduction of serum albumin in continuous ambulatory peritoneal dialysis is common and of no apparent clinical consequence. Am J Kidney Dis 1992; 20: 50–4.

165. Nelson EE, Hong CD, Pesce AL *et al.* Anthropometric norms in the dialysis population. Am J Kidney Dis 1990; 16: 32–7.

166. Marckmann P. Nutritional status of patients on hemodialysis and peritoneal dialysis. Clin. Nephrol 1988; 29: 75–8.

167. Cancarini GC, Costantino E, Manili L *et al.* Nutritional status in long-term CAPD patients. Adv Perit Dial 1992; 8: 84–7.

168. Kopple JD, Blumenkrantz MJ. Nutritional requirements for patients undergoing continuous ambulatory peritoneal dialysis. Kidney Int 1983; 24 (suppl.): S295–302.

169. Blumenkrantz MJ, Kopple JD, Moran JK, Coburn JW. Metabolic balance studies and dietary protein requirements in patients undergoing continuous ambulatory peritoneal dialysis. Kidney Int 1982; 21: 849–61.

170. Movilli E, Mombelloni S, Gaggiotti M, Maiorca R. Effect of age on protein catabolic rate (PCRn), morbidity and mortality in uremic patients with adequate normalized dose of dialysis (Kt/V urea). Nephrol Dial Transplant (In press).

171. Reaich D, Channon SM, Scrimgeour CM *et al.* Ammonium chloride induced acidosis increases protein breakdown and amino acid oxidation in humans. Am J Physiol 1992; 263: E735–9.

172. Lindholm B, Bergström J. Nutritional requirements of peritoneal dialysis patients. In: Gokal R, Nolph KD, eds. The Textbook of Peritoneal Dialysis. Dordrecht: Kluwer, 1994, pp. 443–72.

173. Stein A, Baker F, Larrat C *et al.* Correction of metabolic acidosis and the protein catabolic rate in PD patients. Perit Dial Int 1994; 14: 187–96.

174. Stein A, Bennett S, Feehally J *et al.* Does low-calcium dialysate improve the nutritional status of CAPD patients? Perit Dial Int 1993; 13: 69.

175. Rottembourg J, Issad B, Gallego JL *et al.* Evolution of residual renal function in patients undergoing maintenance hemodialysis or continuous ambulatory peritoneal dialysis. Proc Eur Dial Tranplant Assoc 1982; 19: 397–409.

176. Rottembourg J, Issad B, Poignet JL *et al.* Residual renal function and control of blood glucose levels in insulin-dependent diabetic patients treated by CAPD. In: Keen H, Legrain M, eds. Prevention and Treatment of Diabetic Nephropathy. Lancaster: MTP, 1983, pp. 339–52.

177. Cancarini GC, Brunori G, Camerini C, Brasa S, Manili L, Maiorca R. Renal function recovery and maintenance of residual diuresis in CAPD and hemodialysis. Perit Dial Bull 1986; 6: 77–9.

178. Lysaght MJ, Vonesh EF, Gotch F *et al.* The influence of dialysis treatment modality on the decline of remaining renal function. Trans Am Soc Artif Internal Organs 1991; 37: 598–604.

179. Hallet M, Owen J, Becker G, Stewart J, Farrel PC. Maintenance of residual renal function: CAPD versus HD. Perit Dial Int 1992; 12 (suppl. 1): 124 (abstract).

180. Nolph KD. Is residual renal function preserved better with CAPD than with hemodialysis? Am Kidney Fund Lett 1990; 7: 1–7.

181. Coronel F, Hortal L, Naranjo P *et al.* Analysis of factors in the prognosis of diabetics on continuous ambulatory peritoneal dialysis: long-term experience. Perit Dial Int 1989; 3: 12–17.

182. Lindblad AS, Nolph KD. Recovery of renal function in continuous ambulatory peritoneal dialysis. A study of National CAPD Registry data. Perit Dial Int 1992; 12: 43–7.

183. Michel C, Haddoum F, Viron B, Mignon F. Reprise de la fonction rénale après traitement par dialyse péritonéale continue ambulatoire? Nephrologie 1989; 10 (suppl. 2): 53–5.

184. Rottembourg J, Issad B, Allouache M, Jacobs C. Recovery of renal function in patients treated by CAPD. Adv Perit Dial 1989; 5: 63–6.

185. Bargman JM, Thorpe KE, Churchill DN. The importance of residual renal function for survival in patients on peritoneal dialysis. 30th Annual Meeting of the American Society of Nephrology, San Antonio, Texas, 2 November 1997.

186. Heaton A, Rodger RSC, Sellars L *et al.* Continuous ambulatory peritoneal dialysis after the honeymoon: review of experience in Newcastle 1979–84. Br Med J 1986; 293: 938–41.

187. Brunner FP, Ehrich JHH, Fassbinder W *et al.* Combined report on regular dialysis and transplantation in Europe, XXI, 1990. Nephrol Dial Transplant 1991; 6 (suppl. 4): 5–29.

188. Blagg CR, Wahl PW, Lamers JY. Treatment of chronic renal failure at the Northwest Kidney Center, Seattle, from 1960 to 1982. ASAIO J 1983; 6: 170–5.

189. Frascino J. A comparison of self-care dialysis modalities. Home hemodialysis, continuous ambulatory peritoneal dialysis, in-center self-care hemodialysis. Dial Transplant 1985; 14: 13–6.

190. Nolph KD, Pyle WK, Hiatt M. Mortality and morbidity in continuous ambulatory peritoneal dialysis: full and selected Registry populations. ASAIO J 1983; 6: 220–6.

191. Habach G, Bloemebregren WE, Mauger EA, Wolfe RA, Port FK. Hospitalization among United States Dialysis patients: hemodialysis versus peritoneal dialysis. J Am Soc Nephrol 1995; 5: 1940–8.

192. Hospitalization. United States Renal Data System. Am J Kidney Dis 1997; 30 (suppl. 1): S145–59.

193. Gutman RA, Blumenkrantz MJ, Chan YK *et al.* Controlled comparison of hemodialysis and peritoneal dialysis: Veterans Administration multicenter study. Kidney Int 1984; 26: 459–70.

194. Buoncristiani U, Bianchi P, Cozzari M *et al.* A new safe simple connection system for CAPD. Int J Nephrol Urol Androl 1980; 1: 50–3.

195. Maiorca R, Cantaluppi A, Cancarini GC *et al.* Prospective controlled trial of a Y-connector and disinfectant to prevent peritonitis in continuous ambulatory peritoneal dialysis. Lancet 1983; 2: 642–4.

196. Firanek CA, Vonesh EF, Korbet SM. Patient and technique survival among an urban population of peritoneal dialysis patients: an 8-year experience. Am J Kidney Dis 1991; 18: 91–6.

197. Van Biesen W, Dequidt C, Vijt D, Vanholder R, Lameire N. Analysis of the reasons for transfers between hemodialysis and peritoneal dialysis and their effect on survival. Adv Perit Dial 1998; 14: 90–4.

198. Canaud B, Mion C. Place de la dialyse pèritonèale continue ambulatoire au sein d'un program de traitemen de l'insuffisance rènale chronique. Problèmes posèes par les transferts de DPCA en transplantation ou en hèmodialyse. Nèphrologie 1995; 16: 129–35.

199. Marichal JF, Cordier B, Faller B, Brignon P. Continuous ambulatory peritoneal dialysis (CAPD) or center hemodialysis? Retrospective evaluation of the success of both methods. Perit Dial Int 1990; 10: 205–8.

200. Nolph KD. Clinical results with peritoneal dialysis. Registry experiences. In: Twardowski Z, Nolph KD, Khanna R, Stein JH, eds. Peritoneal Dialysis. Contemporary Issues in Nephrology, vol. 22. New York: Churchill Livingstone, 1991, pp. 127–44.

201. Slingeneyer A, Canaud B, Mion C. Permanent loss of ultrafiltration capacity of the peritoneum in long-term peritoneal dialysis: an epidemiological study. Nephron 1983; 33: 133–8.

202. Juergensen PH, Wuerth DB, Juergensen DM *et al.* Psycho-social factors and clinical outcome on CAPD. Adv Perit Dial 1997; 13: 121–4.

203. Diaz-Buxo JA, Walker PJ, Burgess WP *et al.* The influence of peritoneal dialysis on the outcome of transplantation. Int J Artif Organs 1986; 9: 359–62.

204. Odor-Morales A, Casterona G, Jimeno C *et al.* Hemodialysis or continuous ambulatory peritoneal dialysis before transplantation: prospective comparison of clinical and hemodynamic outcome. Transplantation Proc 1987; 19: 2197–99.

205. Triolo G, Segoloni GP, Salomone M *et al.* Comparison between two dialytic populations undergoing renal transplantation. Adv Perit Dial 1990; 6: 72–5.

206. Kyllönen L, Helanterä A, Salmela K, Ahonen J. Dialysis method and kidney graft survival. Transplant Proc 1992; 24: 354.

207. O'Donoghue D, Manos J, Pearson R *et al.* Continuous ambulatory peritoneal dialysis and renal transplantation: a ten-year experience in a single center. Perit Dial Int 1992; 12: 242–9.

208. Taylor RMR, Proud G, Donnelly PK. Continuous ambulatory peritoneal dialysis. Br J Surg 1985; 72: 250.

209. Evangelista JB, Bennett-Jones D, Cameron JS *et al.* Renal transplantation in patients treated with haemodialysis and short term and long term continuous ambulatory peritoneal dialysis. Br Med J 1985; 291: 1004–7.

210. Shapira Z, Shmueli D, Yussim A, Boner G, Haimovitz C, Servadio C. Kidney transplantation in patients on continuous ambulatory peritoneal dialysis. Proc Eur Dial Transplant Assoc 1984; 21: 932–5.

211. Rubin J, Kirchner KA, Raju S, Krueger RP, Bower JD. CAPD patients as renal transplant patients. Am J Med Sci 1987; 294: 175–80.

212. Gokal R. Renal transplantation in patients on CAPD. In: La Greca G, Chiaramonte S, Fabris A, Feriani M, Ronco C, eds. Peritoneal Dialysis. Proc. 2nd International Course. Milan: Wichtig Editore, 1985, pp. 283–8.

213. Poole-Warren LA, Disney APS, Schindhelm K, Farrel PC. Australian renal, transplant experience in CAPD patients. In: La Greca, Chiaramonte S, Fabris A, Feriani M, Ronco C, eds. Peritoneal Dialysis. Proc. 2nd International Course. Milan: Wichtig Editore 1985, pp. 289–90.

214. Wood CJ, Thomson NM, Scott DF, Holdsworth SR, Boyce N, Atkins RC. Renal transplantation in patients on CAPD. In: Maher JF, Winchester JF, eds. Frontiers in Peritoneal Dialysis, New York: Field and Rich, 1986, pp. 353–6.

215. Tsakiris D, Brawell SP, Briggs JD, Junor BJR. Transplantation in patients undergoing CAPD. Perit Dial Bull 1985; 5: 161–4.

216. Cosio FG, Alamir A, Yim S *et al.* Patient survival after renal transplantation: I. The impact of dialysis pre-transplant. Kidney Int 1998; 53: 767–72.

217. Hymes LC, Warshaw BL. Renal transplantation in children undergoing peritoneal dialysis. Perit Dial Bull 1986; 6: 74–6.

218. Ogawa O, Hoshinaga K, Hasegawa A *et al.* Successful renal transplantation in children treated with CAPD. Transplant Proc 1989; 21: 1997–2000.

219. Robinson RJ, Leapman SB, Wetherington GM, Hamburger RJ, Fineberg NS, Filo RS. Surgical considerations of continuous ambulatory peritoneal dialysis. Surgery 1984; 96: 723–9.

220. Glass NR, Miller DT, Sollinger HW, Zimmerman SW, Simpson D, Belzer FO. Renal transplantation in patients on peritoneal dialysis. Perit Dial Bull 1985; 5: 157–60.

221. Fontan MP, Rodriguez-Carmona A, Bouza P *et al.* Delayed graft function after renal transplantation in patients undergoing peritoneal dialysis and hemodialysis. Adv Perit Dial 1996; 12: 101–4.

222. Maiorca R, Sandrini S, Cancarini GC *et al.* Integration of peritoneal dialysis and transplantation programs. Perit Dial Int 1997; 17 (suppl. 2): S170–4.

223. Pearson JC, Amend WJ Jr, Vincenti FG *et al.* Post-transplantation pyelonephritis: factors producing low patient and transplant morbidity. J Urol 1980; 123: 153–6.

224. Debure A, Degos F, Pol S *et al.* Liver disease and hepatic complications in renal transplant patients. Adv Nephrol 1988; 17: 375–400.

225. Mioli VA, Balestra E, Bibiano L *et al.* Epidemiology of viral hepatitis in dialysis centers: a national survey. Nephron 1992; 61: 278–83.

226. Cendorogio Neto M, Draube S, Silva A *et al.* Incidence of and risk for hepatitis B virus and hepatitis C virus infection among hemodialysis and CAPD patients: evidence for environmental transmission. Nephrol Dial Transplant 1995; 10: 240–6.

26 | Peritoneal dialysis registry data

P. G. Blake

Mortality comparisons between haemodialysis and peritoneal dialysis

The dramatic growth in popularity of CAPD in the decade after its first description in 1976 inevitably led to comparisons being made between the new modality and haemodialysis (HD) in terms of their relative effectiveness as renal replacement therapy. Even after initial improvements in PD technology led to a marked decrease in peritonitis rates, it remained clear that technique failure (TF) was more likely in CAPD. However, it also became apparent that, in most developed countries, CAPD was significantly less expensive and so, in spite of the excess TF, its widespread use would be justifiable if overall mortality rates were similar to, or lower than, those on HD. Given that studies looking for mortality differences between HD and PD patients will only have sufficient statistical power if they include large numbers of patients, and also, given the difficulty of addressing this issue with a prospective trial, it is not surprising that data from national renal registries have been the main resource used to address this issue. While registries have the advantage of including information from large numbers of patients, there is typically a limit to both the detail and quantity of these data and, even with the most exhaustive statistical techniques, the methodology will inevitably fall short compared to well-conducted randomized clinical trials [1]. In the absence of the latter, however, much attention has been focused on registry-based modality comparisons in recent years.

Early comparisons between the two modalities, based on European Registry data, suggested some advantage for HD [2]. However, between 1985 and 1992 a number of studies from various countries, including the US, Canada, the UK, Italy and Spain, suggested no consistent difference in mortality rates [3–8]. These studies used a variety of methodologies and encompassed the full range from single-centre to national registry-based analyses. They led to a general consensus that, despite higher TF rates on CAPD, the modalities were broadly equivalent in terms of patient survival. A reasonable clinical conclusion, therefore, was that in most cases modality selection was not primarily a medical issue and that the choice could thus be left to the patient to make. Furthermore, the combination of lower cost and equivalent mortality could be used to justify large-scale promotion of CAPD in countries with publicly provided renal replacement therapy (RRT) where cost considerations were paramount.

This consensus was strikingly disrupted in the mid-1990s with the publication of a large and widely quoted US Registry study by Bloembergen *et al.* which appeared to show significantly higher mortality in PD patients, as compared to those on HD, with the difference being most marked in females, diabetics and the elderly [9]. This study was published at the same time as the CANUSA study which questioned the adequacy of PD as long-term RRT, and these two landmark papers caused a degree of concern in the North American PD community [10]. In combination they may have contributed to the decrease in PD usage that has since occurred in North America, although other factors may have been more important [11].

This chapter will focus on the key registry studies from the 1990s addressing mortality comparisons between HD and PD, and will in particular examine the controversial US Registry data. It will also review in detail more recent studies from Canada and the US which have tended to redress the balance in favour of PD and, in the process, emphasized potential pitfalls of various comparative methodologies. Contemporary mortality comparisons from outside North America have been fewer and have perhaps had even greater methodological limitations, but will also be briefly reviewed.

Before addressing these individual studies, how-

R. Gokal, R. Khanna, R.Th. Krediet and K.D. Nolph (eds.), Textbook of Peritoneal Dialysis, 2nd Edition, 785–797.
© 2000 Kluwer Academic Publishers. Printed in Great Britain.

ever, it is very important to give attention to the wide array of methodological problems that arise when registry-based intermodality mortality comparisons are being made.

Methodological problems

Methodological issues in comparing outcomes on PD and HD can be roughly divided into those that are primarily statistical and those that pertain mainly to clinical practice (Table 1)

Statistical issues

The initial decision to be made when studying comparative outcomes is whether the analysis is to be an incident or prevalent one. An incident analysis looks at new patients starting PD or HD, whereas a prevalent one typically takes a cross-section of patients already on dialysis at a given time and studies their subsequent outcomes. This is a critical issue in intermodality comparisons as PD patients tend in most studies to do relatively better in their first 2 years on dialysis, whereas HD patients tend to do better in subsequent years (Fig. 1). Because of this apparent disproportionality in relative outcomes on the two modalities, the results of a comparison will differ substantially if a prevalent, rather than the more usual incident, methodology is used. Thus, a prevalent analysis such as that of Bloembergen *et al.* will give less weight to the early time on dialysis and so will favour HD, while the opposite will be the case with an incident analysis, such as that of Fenton *et al.* [9, 12]. In general, incident analyses are preferred as they will detect important early events more reliably than a prevalent analysis.

A question that arises in an incident study is when exactly to commence the analysis. It might seem obvious to suggest the day of the initial dialysis, but

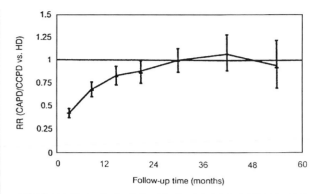

Figure 1. Mortality rate ratios for PD relative to HD, by follow-up interval adjusted for age, diabetic status and comorbid conditions, and estimated using Poisson regression. Follow-up time on each modality was calculated for each patient within each follow-up interval with deaths being allocated to the modality the patient was receiving at the time death occurred. Data come from over 14 000 patients initiating dialysis in Canada between 1990 and 1996. Figure reproduced with permission from Schaubel *et al.* [29].

this would result in the inclusion of patients who are truly cases of acute or acute-on-chronic renal failure. Also, it can be convincingly argued that deaths occurring in the initial months on dialysis are more appropriately attributed to pre-existing comorbidity than to either dialysis modality *per se*. Furthermore, many patients who intend to use PD as their initial definitive modality actually start on HD and may not be transferred to PD for some weeks, or even months, due to waiting lists or acute medical complications. In some centres, where HD spots are scarce, the converse may be the case; also, patients who require dialysis immediately or shortly after first presenting with renal failure may not have an opportunity to make a definitive modality selection until some weeks or months have passed. It is thus customary to use 60 days or 90 days post-initiation as 'time zero' for the purposes of the analysis. In many centres, such a waiting period may be too short, for the reasons already mentioned, and may lead to patients who plan eventually to do PD being included in the HD group, or vice versa.

Equally important is that it is also likely that the sickest, frailest, most medically complicated patients who present late will be, by their nature, treated with HD and, as this group inevitably has a higher early mortality, too short a waiting period may bias the analysis against HD. However, if the waiting period is too long a significant amount of patient time will be lost to the analysis. This may also lead to an inherent bias against the modality which is most effective early on. As there are substantial data

Table 1. Problem issues in intermodality comparative studies

Statistical	Clinical
Incident or prevalent?	Non-random allocation of patients to the two
'Intention to treat' or 'treatment received'?	patients to the two modalities
Correction for demographics, comorbidity, functional status, laboratory measures?	Changing clinical practices
Period of grace post-modality switch?	Non-contemporary studies
Period between initiation of dialysis and entry into dialysis?	A modality or a practice issue
Disproportionate risks	

suggesting PD is relatively more successful in the first 1–2 years, long waiting periods may particularly bias the analysis against PD [9, 12].

A second key issue is whether the analysis is to be an 'intention-to-treat' (ITT) one or based on 'treatment received' (TR). An ITT analysis has the advantage of being clinically very relevant in terms of the advice a patient should receive as end-stage renal disease (ESRD) approaches. In that context the key question to be answered is whether initial modality selection impacts in any way on eventual patient survival. If there is no effect, then, regardless of the possible inherent superiority of either modality, the matter can reasonably be left to patient choice.

The disadvantage of an ITT analysis is that the comparison may be very poor at detecting true differences in modality efficacy. Switches between the modalities, especially from PD to HD, are common and, of course, many patients on both modalities will receive renal transplants. Consequently, a true ITT analysis will tend to mask any differences between the modalities. An approach that is frequently used to get around this problem is to censor patients both at the time of transplantation and at the time of any modality switch. This, however, leads to the omission of a large proportion of patient-years from the analysis, especially in PD patients as they generally have a higher rate of switching. It also leads to concern that true differences in modality efficacy will be masked because patients who are doing poorly on one modality, and who may be at high risk of dying, may be switched to the other modality so that the resulting adverse outcome will be lost to the analysis. A further refinement, to get around this problem, is to introduce a 'period of grace' post-switch, during which time any mortality or other outcome being monitored is still attributed to the initial modality. This approach intuitively appears reasonable, but the approximate duration of the period of grace is problematic. If it is too short, mortality related to the initial modality may be understated but, if it is too long, mortality related to the second modality may be unfairly attributed to the first. Periods of grace typically vary from 30 to 120 days and, in practice, usually have only a modest influence on the results of comparative analyses, so this problem, while important to appreciate, may not always be critical. Obviously, when these refinements are introduced, the analysis is no longer a 'pure' ITT one.

With all these analytical dilemmas there is no single correct method, and it is ideal that the analysis be done in a variety of ways, comparing results with different periods of grace, waiting periods, and censoring policies.

The advantages of a TR type analysis are, first, that it is more likely to detect any true differences that exist between the modalities and, second, that it is more relevant to prevalent dialysis patients who might be considering switching from one modality to the other. If such an analysis is being done, all of the same issues concerning waiting periods and periods of grace arise. The latter is particularly important in a TR analysis because patients who switch modalities will now not leave the analysis completely, but will rather switch to the opposite group once the designated period of grace is complete. Thus, any bias from having too short or too long a period of grace will be compounded with the potential for deaths related to one modality being misleadingly attributed to the other. Again, the best compromise is to repeat the analysis with a variety of periods of grace and compare the results.

Of course, allocation of patients to HD and PD is not a random event, and the demographic, comorbid, and other characteristics of populations being compared cannot be presumed to be equivalent. For example, recent US Registry data suggest a significant age and comorbidity gap between the two modalities, with PD being used to treat a younger, and perhaps somewhat healthier, population [13]. Thus, any comparison requires some correction for these other variables which may themselves independently influence patient outcomes. This is typically done using the Cox proportional hazards statistical technique [14]. Most registry-based comparison studies routinely correct for age, gender, race and diabetic status. However, correction for other comorbidity is not always possible because registry data are often limited in scope. The Canadian Registry, for example, corrects for the number of comorbid conditions each patient has from a list comprising cardiac disease, peripheral vascular disease, cerebrovascular accidents, and cancer [12]. Such corrections are helpful but may be far from perfect, depending on the potentially variable enthusiasm with which forms are completed at participating centres, and a recent US study has pointed out how unreliable these can be [15]. More importantly, the number of comorbid conditions tells nothing about their severity, which may be much more important. Attempts to estimate this using standardized comorbidity scores may be feasible in smaller studies, but would be difficult to achieve in a nationwide registry.

Registries are also almost never able to correct for more subtle measures of patient well-being.

Examples would be functional status, ability to ambulate independently, and psychological well-being, all of which may be powerful predictors of patient outcome [16, 17]. It is thus doubtful if any registry-based, or even non-registry-based study can ever truly correct for all the relevant factors. Only a randomized controlled trial could completely get around this problem, and this is widely believed not to be a feasible option because of the probable unwillingness of most informed patients to be randomized between two such different modalities.

A further issue is correction for laboratory variables that have been shown to predict survival. These would include serum levels of albumin, urea, creatinine, C-reactive protein, and a variety of other indices. Equally, or more important, may be derived indices which assess adequacy of dialysis and nutrition, such as the fractional urea clearance (Kt/V) or the normalized protein equivalent of nitrogen appearance, which is a surrogate for protein intake.

Some interesting questions arise when correction for these indices is attempted. First, it is very difficult to compare serum and clearance values between the two modalities because one is intermittent and the other continuous. It is widely accepted that the same amount of clearance delivered continuously is more effective than when delivered intermittently, but the exact model on which any correction could be based is controversial and there is no consensus as to which is best [18–20]. This leads to a second concern, which is whether correction for issues inherent to the individual modalities being compared is valid. In other words, is it legitimate in a comparative intermodality study to correct for serum albumin when we know that it is inherent in PD that it be lower because of the inevitable dialysate protein losses? Similarly, is it reasonable to correct for residual renal function when it may be inherent to PD that it is better preserved than on HD? Furthermore, is it appropriate to correct for Kt/V, even if a model could be agreed upon, when the differences in Kt/V may, to some extent, be inherent to the therapies being compared? An analogy might be whether it would be legitimate in a comparison of survival rates in males and females to correct for serum testosterone levels! Most would agree that such a correction would be absurd.

One further point that needs to be made relates to the use of the Cox proportional hazards model to correct for patient characteristics and intermodality comparisons. This statistical model presumes hazards to be proportional – that is, the relative risks associated with various factors remain constant with time. We have increasingly learned that this is not the case. Not only are the influences on outcomes of factors such as diabetic status, comorbidity and hypoalbuminaemia variable with time, but so, it appears, are the relative risks between the modalities themselves [21]. As already pointed out, a consistent feature of recent studies is that PD does relatively better compared to HD in the initial years of dialysis as compared to the subsequent years [9, 12]. This may relate to better preservation of residual renal function, or to unmeasured comorbidity differences, or to other unclear factors, but it is a well-recognized finding. It is this disproportionality, in particular, that accounts for the perceived differences in results of incident and prevalent analyses, and it underlies much of the apparently contradictory findings in the recent literature [9, 12]. The simplest approach to this problem is to repeat the Cox analysis every 6–12 months using the beginning of each such period as a new 'time zero' to see how results vary. One study using this sort of methodology showed very different results in the first 2 years of dialysis compared to subsequently, and the authors who detected this have emphasized this issue strongly in their subsequent work [21, 22].

A conclusion from all this is that there is no single correct way to perform an intermodality comparative analysis. Variations in statistical methods have a large influence on the results achieved, and conclusions based on one methodology alone should be considered suspect, as a basis for clinical decision-making. If a finding is really robust it should persist even with variation of the method of analysis. Conversely, any comparison being made should be repeated with a variety of methods to see if the result holds constant.

Clinical issues

A number of clinical points arise when registries are used to make intermodality comparisons. First, allocation of patients to the two modalities in any region is never random but depends on a variety of factors. These include physician and provider biases, which may lead to healthier patients being preferentially put on one modality in one region and the other in another. It is thus likely that equivalent groups of patients are not being compared and, as already mentioned, adjustment for age, comorbidity and other factors may not be sufficient to correct for these discrepancies. This is one of the greatest potential weaknesses of registry-based comparisons.

Similarly, the proportion of patients managed on PD varies greatly within and between countries. Comparative studies for regions where both modalities are used by a relatively high percentage of patients may have broader relevance than those from regions where one or other modality is used only by a small minority.

Most important of all these clinical considerations, however, is the issue of constantly changing clinical practice in each modality. For example, over the past decade HD has altered significantly with more widespread use of volumetric machines, bicarbonate dialysate, and medium and high-flux dialysers. The application of urea kinetic modelling has improved clearances, and the introduction of recombinant erythropoietin has had a major impact. In the near future new trends such as blood volume monitoring and access surveillance programmes may further improve the practice of HD. PD has also altered within the same time-scale. Newer transfer systems have led to lower rates of peritonitis. Automated PD has proliferated, and there has been the introduction, more recently than in HD, of clearance targets and more heterogeneous prescription. Eythropoietin has also made an impact and, in the future, new dialysis solutions will further alter the modality. Thus comparative studies based on patient observations from even a few years ago can be considered to be out of date. It might even be argued that, by the time any registry review is analysed and published, the respective modalities may have changed sufficiently to raise the issue of whether the comparison is of anything more than historical interest. Furthermore, comparative practices in the two modalities may have evolved relatively more in one country than in another, and this may explain apparently contrasting results. For example, new superior double-bag systems were used in PD in Europe for many years prior to being introduced in Canada and subsequently in the US.

Following on from this, it is important to distinguish between a particular modality such as HD and PD and how it is practised in a given place at a given time. In other words, if a regional registry reports inferior survival on PD, it may be that the modality is inherently inferior or it may be that the practice of PD is not as good, relative to HD, as in other regions or, as already discussed, it may be that the data are incomplete or biased. Separating out these possibilities is exceedingly difficult. This dilemma has been well reviewed by Nolph and by Port *et al.* in recent publications [23, 24].

US Registry studies

The best-known of the US Registry-based studies published in the past decade is the 1995 analysis by Bloembergen *et al.* [9]. This study looked at over 170 000 patient-years of experience between January 1987 and January 1990. The analysis was rather unusual in that it attempted to deal with the issue of modality switches by attributing all patient events in a given calendar year to whichever modality the patients were receiving on 1 January of the year concerned. Thus, in a sense, each patient was treated as a new data subject every 1 January and, during the course of the 3-year study, a single patient could provide three distinct patient calendar years of follow-up, and if patients had switched modality, could be included in the analysis successively in both the PD and HD groups. This methodology resulted in no patient time after modality switches being excluded from the analysis.

The study overall showed that the relative risk of dying associated with being on PD was 1.19, and this was highly significant. The risk was particularly concentrated in subgroups of patients, particularly those who were older, females, diabetic or black (Table 2). It was also found to be more pronounced in patients who had been on PD for longer periods of time. The excess risk of death associated with PD was attributed to a variety of causes, most notably cardiovascular and infectious diseases [25].

It is interesting, however, to analyse this study, keeping in mind some of the various statistical and clinical points mentioned in the earlier part of this chapter. First, the study is a mix of incident and prevalent patients. Thus, it includes patients who were on dialysis for some time prior to 1987 as well as patients who started subsequent to that time. It also was an unusual mix of an ITT- and TR-based

Table 2. Relative risk of mortality associated with PD versus HD (where risk for HD is taken as 1.00), Bloembergen study

	Relative risk on PD
All patients	1.19*
Male	1.11*
Females	1.30*
Diabetics	1.30*
Non-diabetics	1.11*
<1 year on dialysis	1.14†
>1 year on dialysis	1.21*
Age < 55	1.00
Age > 55	Increasingly large*

$^* p < 0.001;$ $^† p < 0.05.$

analysis. It is ITT in the sense that events occurring in a given year are attributed to whatever modality the patient was on at the beginning of that year. However, it is a TR-type analysis in the sense that patients who eventually switched modality have subsequent events attributed to the second modality, provided that they were on it on 1 January of the year concerned. Obviously there are potential problems with this methodology. If a patient is on PD on 1 January but switches to HD on 5 January it seems inappropriate that a death occurring in December of the same year is attributed to PD.

Because of the methodology used, there was no consistent period of grace post-modality switch in the analysis. With regard to a waiting period after initiation of dialysis, the standard 90 days used routinely in USRDS studies was applied. Potentially more controversial, however, was the stipulation that no patient could enter the study until the 1 January following the end of the first 90 days after initiation of dialysis. It was thus conceivable for a patient to be on dialysis for almost 15 months before the data would be included in the study. For example, a patient who initiated dialysis on 2 October, 1987 would not complete the 90-day waiting period until 2 January, 1988 and so would not enter the analysis until 1 January 1989. The crucial point here is that a large proportion of the early period on dialysis for many patients is omitted. As has already been explained, this methodology tends to favour HD over PD as the latter modality performs relatively best in the first 1–2 years [9, 12, 22]. Conversely, mortality rates in HD tend to be relatively high in the first year, probably due to unmeasured comorbidity, and omission of this period will favour HD in any comparison.

Other criticisms of the Bloembergen study have been made. One is that, with the exception of correction for diabetes, no other adjustment for comorbidity was made. The study authors have argued that previous US Registry-based analyses have not shown excess comorbidity in PD patients relative to those on HD, and that it is therefore unlikely that any more sophisticated adjustment for comorbidity would alter the results [26]. Nevertheless, the study would have been strengthened by more detailed correction for comorbidity.

From a clinical perspective an additional criticism of the study is that by the time it was published it dealt with a time period that was 5–7 years earlier. As already outlined, both modalities have changed significantly since the 1980s, so the relevance of findings for present practice may be limited.

A recent follow-up analysis, using the same methodology, has been carried out by Vonesh and Moran [27]. Deriving data from US Registry Annual Data Reports, the authors repeated the analysis not only for the 3-year period beginning 1987 but also for subsequent 3-year periods up to the one beginning 1992. Furthermore, they did separate analyses for both diabetic and non-diabetic patients. The most notable finding of their study was that the relative risks of mortality on PD relative to HD declined in the 3-year periods subsequent to that beginning in 1987, and in three of the most recent four 3-year periods there was no significant difference between mortality rates on the two modalities (Fig. 2). At first sight this interesting finding might suggest that the gap between the two modalities is narrowing due to disproportionately greater improvements in PD. This explanation may be partly correct, but there is an additional factor. In the three-year period beginning 1989, the US Registry changed its methodology and started including in the analysis for each year all patients who were incident during that year. Under the old methodology these patients would not have been included until the beginning of the following year. This alteration brings a lot of early patient dialysis time into the analysis that would not previously have been included and, as explained previously, this tends to favour PD relative to HD. Hence, a significant part of the decrease in the relative risks of mortality on PD may have resulted from this. However, given that the omission of early patient dialysis time in the previous methodology was somewhat arbitrary, and varied with the time of the year the patient started dialysis, it would seem that the newer methodology is more appropriate and the results potentially more valid.

Although Vonesh's reanalysis of US Registry data found the excess mortality on PD was no longer statistically significant, there did remain a significant difference for particular subgroups. These included diabetics, females and older patients. On further analysis Vonesh determined that the excess mortality on PD was concentrated in older female diabetics and that, if this group was extracted from the analysis, there was almost no statistically or clinically significant difference in patient outcomes. One other group that continued to show an excess mortality in PD, however, was black patients [27].

It is worth noting at this point that the Bloembergen analysis was not the only major intermodality comparison study produced by the US Registry in recent years. In 1992 Held *et al.* did a detailed ITT analysis, with and without censoring 30 days after

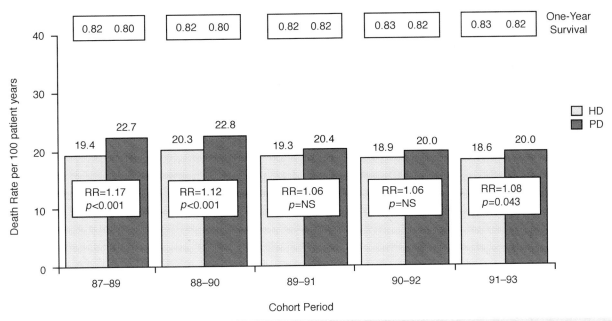

Figure 2. Trends in death rates for patients treated with HD and PD in prevalent cohorts of US patients analysed over 3-year periods between 1987 and 1993. Death rates are adjusted for age, sex, race and diabetic status. Relative risks (RR) are expressed as the risk of death on PD as compared to HD where HD is taken to be 1.00. One-year survival estimates are adjusted for age, sex, race, and diabetic status. Data come from USRDS Annual Data Reports and are reproduced with permission from Vonesh *et al.* [27].

modality switch [26]. Although this study was relatively small, comprising just over 4000 patients, it had the advantage of having detailed information on baseline comorbidity and functional status. The study covered an apparently representative cohort of incident patients from the years 1986 and 1987 who had survived 90 days on dialysis. Patients were attributed to whatever modality they were using after 30 days of dialysis, with the result that 17% were PD and 83% HD. The mean age was 58 years and 42% were diabetic. Follow-up was between 2.25 and 4.25 years with censoring at transplantation. Correction was made for five co-morbidities, three estimates of functional status, standard demographics, systolic blood pressure and three biochemical indices, all measured at baseline. Non-diabetics and diabetics were analysed separately and relative mortality risk was 16% lower for PD in non-diabetics and 20% lower for HD in diabetics, although only the latter observation was statistically significant (Table 3). On further analysis the excess risk on PD in diabetics was concentrated in those aged more than 58 years at onset of ESRD. While this excess risk was most notable after 1 year on dialysis, no significant disproportionality of the hazard function for modality by time could be identified. Interestingly, the relative risks were no different when a

Table 3. Relative risks of mortality associated with PD versus HD, where HD = 1.00 in Held study [28]

	Relative risk on PD
Diabetics	1.26*
Non-diabetics	0.86
Diabetic aged 68.7 years	1.45
Non-diabetic aged 68.7 years	0.95

* $p < 0.05$.

pure ITT analysis was done as opposed to one with censoring [26]. Overall, when compared to the subsequent Bloembergen analysis, this study is more favourable to PD but it shows a similar trend for older diabetics to be at extra risk on PD. Although it is a smaller study, it is more rigorous in that correction for baseline comorbidity is much more complete, and in that a variety of methodologies were successfully applied to confirm the sensitivity of the results. However, the major difference between the two studies is that the Held one is an incident, ITT-type analysis while the Bloembergen one is mainly prevalent and is a mix of ITT and TR analyses. As already explained, incident analyses tend to be more favourable to PD.

Table 4. Relative risks of mortality by modality, sex and diabetic status, in Collins study [28] where risk in males aged >55 years and on HD is taken as 1.0

Modality/diabetic status	Males		Females	
	<55 years	>55 years	<55 years	>55 years
HD/diabetic	0.51	1.00	0.50	0.93
PD/diabetic	0.47	1.05	0.46	1.16†
HD/non-diabetic	0.40	1.00	0.38	0.99
PD/non-diabetic	0.31*	0.91*	0.26*	0.89*

*Lower mortality on PD relative to HD at $p < 0.05$.
†Lower mortality on HD relative to PD at $p < 0.05$.

In 1998 Collins *et al.* presented a more up-to-date analysis, similar to that of Held, using Health Care Financing Authority data for over 106,000 incident dialysis patients between 1994 and 1998 [28]. The methodology was ITT, based on modality at 90 days but with censoring 60 days after any modality switch. Again, diabetics and non-diabetics were analysed separately. Correction was for age and race only. The relative risk of all-cause mortality was significantly lower in non-diabetics on PD than on HD, but the reverse was the case for older diabetics and, just as in the Bloembergen and Vonesh studies, the excess risk in older diabetics was greater in females (Table 4). Again this is an incident study dealing with the early years on dialysis and so is favourable for PD. The absence of a correction for comorbidity is a concern, given the recognition that PD patients tend to be healthier than those on HD. However, like the Vonesh and Held papers, it redresses somewhat the impression from the Bloembergen study that PD is associated with substantially inferior survival compared to HD.

A consensus from these US Registry-based data is that PD and HD are broadly equivalent in terms of patient survival, at least in the early years on dialysis, and that apparently discrepant findings are mainly a consequence of using prevalent rather than incident patient-based methodology. If there is a concern about PD, it is concentrated in the older female diabetic subgroup of patients. The reason for this is not obvious and merits further explanation. Possibilities include body-size issues, peritoneal transport differences and vascular access problems leading to the sickest of these patients being directed to PD. A second concern about PD is the tendency for relative mortality rates to rise in the later years on dialysis, perhaps due to loss of residual renal function which, if prescriptions are not altered, will lead to lower clearance and less effective fluid removal.

Canadian Registry data

Data published from the Canadian Registry in 1997 and again in 1998 have also helped to allay some of the concern in the PD community that followed the publication of the Bloembergen Study [12, 29]. The Canadian Registry is particularly suitable for comparative intermodality studies because of its very complete collection of patient information and also because of the relatively more equal distribution of patients between the two modalities in Canada, compared to the US. The recent publications have been based on almost 15 000 ESRD patients who initiated treatment in Canada between 1990 and 1996. Baseline data were available for these patients with regard to the presence or absence of a variety of common comorbid conditions. The comparative analysis was done using both ITT and TR methodologies, and based on incident patients in each case. With the TR methodology, patients were monitored from the date of initiation of dialysis and were not censored at transplantation. No period of grace was allowed after modality switches. In the ITT model, patients were attributed to the modality they were using 90 days post-initiation of dialysis and were censored only at transplantation. In each case correction was done for age, race, primary disease, centre size, and the number of predialysis comorbid conditions.

The result of the TR analysis showed that the relative risk of mortality was 27% less for all patients treated with PD, as compared to HD (Table 5). The advantage for PD was substantial and significant in non-diabetics above and below the age of 65 and

Table 5. Mortality rate ratios for PD relative to HD (where HD is 1.00) in Fenton study [29] of Canadian patients initiating dialysis 1990 to 1995 using 'treatment received' and 'intention to treat' analysis

	Treatment received: relative risk (95% CI)	Intention-to-treat: hazard risks (95% CI)
All	0.73 (0.69–0.77)*	0.93 (0.87–0.99)*
Non-diabetic <65 years	0.53 (0.46–0.60)*	0.84 (0.87–0.99)*
Non-diabetic >65 years	0.75 (0.65–0.86)*	0.95 (0.86–1.05)
Diabetic <65 years	0.76 (0.65–0.83)*	0.90 (0.82–1.10)
Diabetic >65 years	0.88 (0.75–1.04)	1.04 (0.87–1.24)

CI = Confidence interval.
*Confidence interval does not cross 1.0 so $p < 0.05$.

also in diabetics below the age of 65. For diabetics over the age of 65 there was a trend towards an advantage for PD, but it did not reach significance [12, 29]. In the ITT analysis there was also a significant advantage for PD with a 7% lower risk for the patient population as a whole. On subgroup analysis this risk was significantly lower only in non-diabetics aged less than 65 (Table 4) [29].

A number of other features were apparent on closer review of this study. First, the advantage of PD in the TR analysis was apparent only during the first 2 years of treatment [12]. Indeed, mortality on the two modalities followed different patterns (Fig. 1). Mortality on PD started low, but gradually increased with time. Mortality on HD started much higher than that on PD, but fell over the first 9 months before rising gradually over the ensuing 3 years. Prior to 18 months, mortality was always lower on PD, but after that time the rates converged.

With both the TR and the ITT analysis the authors varied different aspects of the methodology in order to see how robust the results were [12]. If, for example, periods of grace varying from 30 to 90 days after modality switches were introduced into the TR analysis, there was no real change in the results. If, however, the first 90 days post-initiation of dialysis were included in the ITT analysis, then the advantage for PD was more apparent. It will be recalled that these first 90 days were included in the TR analysis and so may be central to the advantage seen for PD in this study. As has already been pointed out, the inclusion of more of the early time on dialysis tends to give an advantage to PD over HD in modality comparisons.

There are two possible interpretations for the apparent superiority of PD over HD in these Canadian Registry studies. One is that PD is an inherently superior modality in the early years of dialysis, perhaps related to better retention of residual renal function [30]. The other is that there are unmeasured differences in comorbidity between HD and PD patients that are not satisfactorily corrected for in the analysis. It is a frequent observation that patients who present for dialysis late are in a generally unstable medical condition and are much more likely to be treated with HD than PD. These patients, by their nature, have a high early mortality rate and their inclusion in the analysis may make PD look particularly good, relative to HD. Despite the efforts made to correct for demographics and comorbidity between the two modalities, there may still have been an unmeasured residual excess baseline risk in the HD patients. This may be the real cause of the difference in outcomes and may, in particular, explain the high early mortality rate on HD and why the inclusion of the initial 3-month period in either the TR or ITT analysis makes HD look worse. Thus, while the Canadian Registry study appears to show PD to be a superior therapy, a certain amount of scepticism may be justified, and a safer conclusion might be to say that the therapies are broadly equivalent, with perhaps a suggestion that PD may be particularly advantageous in the early years on dialysis, especially when used in relatively stable patients.

This conclusion is supported by a more recent Canadian multicentre study from Murphy *et al.* [31]. This analysis is based on 822 incident Canadian patients at 11 centres in 1993 and 1994, and has the advantage of including extensive correction for the severity and number of comorbidity conditions as well as for functional status. The study showed that baseline comorbidity was significantly higher in HD and that, in an ITT analysis, hazard ratios were, indeed, lower on PD before adjustment is made for comorbidity, but were not significantly different, once full adjustment was carried out. Again, this important study suggests that insufficiently adjusted registry data can be misleading.

US/Canada comparisons

In the aftermath of the publication of the US Registry data from Bloembergen *et al.* and the Canadian Registry data from Fenton *et al.*, there was some degree of consternation in the dialysis community as to how such apparently conflicting results could come from two studies, addressing essentially the same subject, in adjacent countries. This, in particular, led to speculation that there were serious problems in the practice of PD in the US. This argument appeared to have been reinforced when Churchill *et al.*, in an analysis from the Canada/USA PD Adequacy Study, reported that the relative risk of mortality was over 90% higher in the US as compared to Canadian PD patients, even after comprehensive correction had been done for demographics, comorbidity, nutritional and adequacy indices (Fig. 3) [32].

However, a number of points should be made before these results are interpreted as showing a particular deficiency in the practice of PD in the US. First, it is hoped that the review of the registry studies carried out above has pointed out that the methodology used in the Bloembergen study may

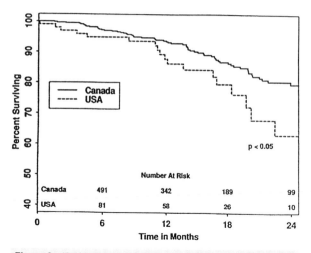

Figure 3. Kaplan–Meier patient survival curves for CANUSA study patients in Canada and the United States. Two-year survival probabilities are 79.7% in Canada and 63.2% in the United States ($p > 0.05$). The survival curves are adjusted for the effects of demographic and baseline clinical variables, for nutritional status, adequacy of dialysis and for interaction between these variables. Data are reproduced with permission from Churchill *et al.* [32].

have exaggerated the superiority of HD in the US, and the Fenton study may have similarly exaggerated the superiority of PD in Canada [9, 12]. Comparison of the more recent analyses by Vonesh *et al.*, Collins *et al.* and Murphy *et al.* would suggest that this may be so [27, 28, 31]. The second point that must be kept in mind is that acceptance rates for dialysis are more than twice as high in the US as compared to Canada [33]. Even when correction for the different ethnic mix of the population is made, acceptance rates are still about 50% higher in the US. This would suggest that the frailer, sicker patients are being treated in the US and this, rather than any difference in the actual practice of dialysis, may explain a large part of the discrepancy in mortality rates. It is likely that a similar discrepancy in mortality rates to that seen in the Canada/USA PD Adequacy Study would be seen if mortality rates in HD were compared in the same fashion. Of course, there may be other differences between the dialysis population in the two countries. One possibility is that rates of non-compliance with PD exchanges are greater in the US than in Canada. This has been suggested in a number of studies using assessments of patients' dialysis solution inventory, and it recently appears to have been confirmed by a questionnaire-based study which suggests that non-compliance is almost three times as common in US CAPD patients [34–36]. This and other areas per-

taining to the characteristics of the dialysis population of the two countries merit further attention.

Other international registry studies

There have been a number of single-centre and multicentre studies from Europe comparing outcome on HD and PD [2, 3, 7]. However, these have tended to be relatively small and statistically underpowered, and there is a disappointing lack of large-scale registry-based comparisons analogous to those done in North America. In 1995 the Australia/New Zealand Registry published an ITT analysis with censoring at modality switch on over 6600 dialysis patients treated between 1983 and 1992 [37]. Correction was done for age, sex, race, year of initiation and primary renal disease and PD was associated with a relative risk of mortality of 1.31, relative to HD. In 1996, however, investigators from the same registry found no difference in death rates between the two modalities using a prevalent-type TR analysis in over 5000 patients. This still-unpublished study had two advantages. It was based on a more contemporary period, 1991–1995 and, unlike its predecessor, it also corrected for baseline comorbidity [38].

More recently the European Renal Association Registry reported comparative survival data from the period 1975–1992 (R. Gokal, personal communication). As multiple countries are involved the completeness of this database may be questioned. However, data on 243 000 patients aged between 20 and 75 years who started dialysis between 1975 and 1992 were reviewed. Approximately 84% of these patients were treated with HD and 16% with PD. The analysis was done using an ITT methodology and there was correction for age, gender, diabetic status and year of initiating dialysis. As expected, the results showed that diabetic and older patients did worse, but there was also a 25% higher mortality rate in those initially treated with PD. Mortality on both HD and PD decreased over the 17-year period and this decrease was more pronounced in PD patients so that the excess risk associated with PD seems to be lessening with time. Thus, the adjusted relative risk was 1.3 between 1975 and 1983, but less than 1.2 between 1984 and 1992. This excess risk associated with PD, just as in the US studies, became most apparent after the first 2 years of dialysis treatment. This study has not yet been published, but there are apparent weaknesses. One is that it lacks correction for comorbidity and it is likely that in individual European countries there will be biases that determine modality allocation. A second concern relates to the almost inevitable incompleteness of data in such a large multinational registry. The greatest concern, however, is that the study covers a 17-year period and, as mentioned earlier, HD and PD have changed markedly during this time. For example, PD patients in 1975 would have been treated with intermittent rather than continuous PD. The relevance of such observations to contemporary practice may be limited. Nevertheless, it is interesting to see that some of the patterns noted in North American studies are also apparent in Europe. In particular, the tendency of PD patients to do relatively less well, compared to those on HD, as the years pass, is a consistent finding reflecting perhaps loss of residual renal function, inadequate clearances, the cumulative effects of peritonitis or some variety of 'treatment burnout'.

The most complete comparative registry-based study outside North America comes from the Lombardy Registry in northern Italy [39]. This comprehensive registry covers 44 renal units and in 1995 it reported 10 years of experience with almost 7000 patients. The average age on initiation of dialysis was 56.6 years, and 68% started on HD as compared to 32% on PD. In this study an ITT methodology was used with censoring 2 months after any modality switch. Patients had to survive 30 days on dialysis to become eligible for the analysis. Correction was carried out for age, sex, primary renal disease and for some basic baseline comorbidity. A Cox model was used and a total of over 17000 patient-years was analysed. An excess mortality was noted in patients initiated on PD with a relative risk of 1.42, after correction for the above-mentioned factors. In contrast to the US studies, the excess risk associated with PD was apparent within 12 months of initiation of dialysis. It did not appear to differ with the age of the patient and was found in diabetics and non-diabetics alike. The main concern in this study is that there was an excess of comorbidity in PD patients. This pattern, the opposite to what is seen in North America, involved the patients being, on average, more than 7 years older on PD and being substantially more likely to have excess comorbidity. While these factors were adjusted for in the analysis, just as in the Canadian Study, one is concerned that corrections may be less than complete in a setting where there appears to be a systematic bias towards putting healthier patients on one modality relative to the other. Nevertheless, the Lombardy Study, to some extent, supports the findings of the preliminary European Renal Association analysis. There clearly needs to be further investigation into the relative risks of the two modalities in Europe. It is worth noting, in this context, that studies from Maiorca in northeastern Italy have tended to show that patients on PD do at least as well as those on HD, and that patient survival is significantly better on PD in the subgroup of patients aged more than 53.5 years [5]. This latter study is not registry-based and is relatively small, but shows that, even within one country, there can be quite striking differences in comparative mortality rates.

Conclusion

As is apparent from this review, comparison of mortality rates on HD and PD is fraught with problems. The data from the US in particular, but also from Canada, indicate that the method of analysis used has the potential to alter greatly the ultimate result of the study. While this will be apparent to those familiar with the vagaries of epidemiology and biostatistics, there is clearly a concern that the casual observer may over-interpret the implications of findings that have more to do with the methodology used than with clinically meaningful differences [1, 28]. Thus, studies that use a variety of methodologies and still find consistent results are potentially more meaningful [12].

It is suggested that the most appropriate methodology for intermodality comparisons is an incident one, using both ITT and TR, and with censoring after a 60–90-day period of grace post-modality switch. In general, analyses that include a large proportion of early time on dialysis will tend to favour PD, whereas those that do not will tend to favour HD. Underlying this is the likelihood that a substantial subset of patients initiating HD are a high-risk, particularly ill group who are on HD precisely for this reason. Leading on from this, a recurrent concern about all these studies is that the corrections for comorbidity and functional status are inevitably inadequate. Clearly there are systematic biases in modality selection that vary from country to country so that, for example, PD patients in the US and Canada tend to be healthier than their HD counterparts, whereas the opposite is the case in northern Italy [11, 26, 39].

The ultimate answer to the question of which modality is superior would require a randomized controlled clinical trial, but this may not be feasible. The differences between the two modalities are so great in terms of lifestyle implications that most informed patients will be unlikely to agree to randomization. A reasonable conclusion from the available evidence would seem to be that neither modality has been proven to be superior to the other. In general, PD seems to perform well in the first 1–3 years, particularly in non-diabetic patients and in those who are relatively younger. As time on dialysis passes, HD outcomes relative to PD tend to improve. This probably relates to the loss of the residual renal function which is such an advantage in the early years in PD patients. It may reflect not just decreased clearances, but also better regulation of volume and consequent protection against cardiovascular complications. A crucial question is whether, with the recent greater attention to clearances in PD, good early results with the modality can be extended to later years. However, all the problems associated with long-term PD may not pertain to clearance and fluid removal. Even with the relatively low contemporary rates of peritonitis the cumulative effect of recurrent episodes can lead to peritoneal cavity damage or patient 'burnout'. Nevertheless, even if long-term PD technique survival continues to be limited for most patients, the modality should still have a major role to play in patients who are expecting early transplantation, in those who have limited life-expectancy because of comorbidity, and in those who simply wish to have more independence in their early years on dialysis.

A question that inevitably arises from reviewing all these studies is whether there is any purpose, given their obvious limitations, in continuing to do these analyses. In favour of this argument is the fact that these studies can be misleading and that, in general, PD and HD should be seen as complementary rather than competitive modalities. Many patients will need to do both and also, perhaps, receive a renal transplant at some stage in their course. The two modalities should be seen as continuously evolving treatments and attention should be focused on continuing to improve them both. In contrast, it can be argued that these comparative studies have been helpful in focusing attention on areas where there may be a problem, and have led practitioners of both modalities to re-examine and attempt to improve their practices. For example, the relatively high early mortality on HD and the relatively high late mortality on PD are important observations that require a response from the nephrology community. A fair conclusion is that these studies should continue to be done and that, provided the results are examined critically, they can be a spur to future improvements in practice.

References

1. Ward RA, Brier ME. Retrospective analyses of large medical data bases: what do they tell us? J Am Soc Nephrol 1999; 10: 429–32.
2. Jacobs C, Broyer M, Brunner FP *et al.* Combined report on regular dialysis and transplantation in Europe, 1980. Proc Eur Dial Transplant Assoc 1981; 15: 2–58.
3. Burton PR, Walls J. Selection-adjusted comparison of life-expectancy of patients on continuous ambulatory peritoneal dialysis, haemodialysis and renal transplantation. Lancet 1987; 1: 1115–19.
4. Serkes KD, Blagg CR, Nolph KD, Vonesh EF, Shapiro F. Comparison of patient and technique survival in continuous ambulatory peritoneal dialysis and hemodialysis, a multi-center study. Perit Dial Int 1990; 10: 15–19.
5. Maiorca R, Vonesh EF, Cavalli P *et al.* A multi-center selection-adjusted comparison of patient and technique study survivals on CAPD and hemodialysis. Perit Dial Int 1991; 11: 118–27.
6. Posen GA, Jeffery JR, Fenton SSA, Arbus GS. Results from the Canadian Renal Failure Registry. Am J Kidney Dis 1990; 15: 397–401.
7. Gentil MA, Carriazo A, Pavon MI *et al.* Comparison of survival in continuous ambulatory peritoneal dialysis in hospital, haemodialysis: a multi centric study. Nephrol Dial Transplant 1991; 6: 444–51.
8. Nelson CB, Port FK, Wolfe RA, Guire KE. Comparison of continuous ambulatory peritoneal dialysis in hemodialysis patient survival with evaluation of trends during the 1980s. J Am Soc Nephrol 1992; 3: 1147–55.
9. Bloembergen WE, Port FK, Mauger EA, Wolfe RA. Comparison in mortality between patients treated with hemodialysis and peritoneal dialysis. J Am Soc Nephrol 1995; 6: 177–83.
10. Canada–USA (CANUSA) Peritoneal Dialysis Study Group. Adequacy of dialysis and nutrition in continuous peritoneal dialysis; association with clinical outcome. J Am Soc Nephrol 1996; 7: 198–207.
11. Blake PG, Bloembergen WE, Fenton SSA. Changes in the demographics and prescription of peritoneal dialysis during the last decade. Am J Kidney Dis 1998; 32: (suppl. 4): S44–51.
12. Fenton SS, Schaubel DE, Desmeules M *et al.* Hemodialysis versus peritoneal dialysis: a comparison of adjusted mortality rates. Am J Kidney Dis 1997; 30: 334–42.
13. Held PJ, Bloembergen WE, Young EW *et al.* A comparison of patients initiating hemodialysis and peritoneal dialysis in the US. J Am Soc Nephrol 1997; 8: 219A.
14. Cox DR. Regression models and life tables (with discussion). J R Stat Soc B 1972; 34: 187–220.
15. Longnecker JC, Klag MJ, Koresh J *et al.* Validation of comorbid conditions on the ESRD medical evidence report by medical record review: the choices for healthy outcomes in caring for ESRD (CHOICE) study. J Am Soc Nephrol 1998; 9: 218A.
16. McClellan W, Anson C, Birkeli K, Tuttle E. Functional status and quality of life: predictors of early mortality among patients entering treatment for end stage renal disease. J Clin Epidemiol 1991 44: 83.
17. Wai L, Burton H, Richmond J, Lindsay R. Influence of psychosocial factors on survival of home-dialysis patients. Lancet 1981; 2: 155–7.
18. Keshaviah PR, Nolph KD, Van Stone JC. The peak concentration hypothesis: a urea kinetic approach to comparing the adequacy of continuous ambulatory peritoneal dialysis and hemodialysis. Perit Dial Int 1989; 9: 257–60.
19. Depner TA. Quantifying hemodialysis and peritoneal dialysis: examination of the peak concentration hypothesis. Semin Dial 1994; 7: 315–17.
20. Casino FG, Lopez T. The equivalent renal urea clearance: a new parameter to assess dialysis dose. Nephrol Dial Transplant 1996; 11: 1574–81.

21. Foley RN, Parfrey PS, Kent GM. Early and late mortality in ESRD: hazards of the Cox model. J Am Soc Nephrol 1997; 8: 284A.

22. Foley RN, Parfrey PS, Harnett JD et al. Mode of dialysis therapy and mortality in end-stage renal disease. J Am Soc Nephrol 1998; 9: 267–76.

23. Nolph KD. Why are reported relative mortality risks for CAPD and HD so variable? Perit Dial Int 1996; 16: 15–18.

24. Port FK, Wolfe RA, Bloembergen WE, Held PJ, Young EW. The study of outcomes for CAPD versus hemodialysis patients. Perit Dial Int 1996; 16: 628–33.

25. Bloembergen WE, Port FK, Mauger EA, Wolfe RA. A comparison of cause of death between patients treated with hemodialysis and peritoneal dialysis. J Am Soc Nephrol 1995, 6: 184–91.

26. Held PJ, Port FK, Turenne MN et al. Continuous ambulatory peritoneal dialysis and hemodialysis: comparison of patient mortality with adjustment for comorbid conditions. Kidney Int 1994, 45: 1163–9.

27. Vonesh EF, Moran J. Mortality in ESRD: a reassessment of differences between patients treated with hemodialysis and peritoneal dialysis. J Am Soc Nephrol 1999, 10: 354–65.

28. Collins A, Ma J, Xia H, Ebben J. CAPD/CCPD in incident patients is equal to or better than hemodialysis, except in females aged ⩾ 55 years. J Am Soc Nephrol 1998, 9: 204A.

29. Schaubel DE, Morrison HI, Fenton SS. Comparing mortality rates in CAPD/CCPD and hemodialysis. The Canadian experience: fact or fiction? Perit Dial Int 1998 18: 478–84.

30. Lysaght MJ, Vonesh EF, Gotch F et al. The influence of dialysis treatment modality on the decline of remaining renal function. ASAIO Trans 1991; 37: 598–604.

31. Murphy SE, Foley RN, Barrett BJ et al. Comparative mortality of HD and PD in Canada. J Am Soc Nephrol 1998, 9: 1208A.

32. CANUSA, Churchill DN, Thorpe KE, Vonesh EF, Keshaviah PR, For the Canada–USA Peritoneal Dialysis Study Group. Lower probability of patient survival with continuous peritoneal dialysis in the United States compared with Canada. J Am Soc Nephrol 1997; 8: 965–71.

33. Mendelssohn DC, Kriger F, Winchester J. A comparison of dialysis in the US and Canada. Can Dial Nephrol 1993; 14: 27–31.

34. Fine A. Compliance with CAPD prescription is good. Perit Dial Int 1997; 17: 343–6.

35. Bernardini J, Pirano B. Measuring compliance with prescribed exchanges in CAPD and CCPD patients. Perit Dial Int 1997; 17: 338–42.

36. Blake P, Korbet S, Blake R et al. Admitted non-compliance with CAPD exchanges is more common in US than Canadian patients. J Am Soc Nephrol 1997; 8: A1277 (abstract).

37. Disney AP. Demography and survival of patients receiving treatment for chronic renal failure in Australia and New Zealand: report on dialysis and renal transplantation treatment from the Australia and New Zealand Dialysis and Transplant Registry. Am J Kidney Dis 1995; 25: 165–75.

38. Murphy BG, Carlin JB, Livingston B, Disney A, Becker G. An analysis of factors predicting mortality in patients on renal replacement therapy. J Am Soc Nephrol 1996; 7: 748A.

39. Locatelli F, Marcelli D, Conte F et al. 1983–1992: Report on regular dialysis and transplantation in Lombardy. Am J Kidney Dis 1995; 25: 196–205.

27 | Implications of the Canada–USA (CANUSA) multicentre trial

D. N. CHURCHILL

Introduction

The Canada–USA study of peritoneal dialysis was published in July 1996 [1] and has become the focus of considerable discussion related to the methodology and clinical implications of the results [2–4]. There have been five publications based on the data collected by the CANUSA study group [1, 5–8] as well as two abstracts addressing the clinical impact of peritonitis [9] and the role of residual renal function [10] in this population (Table 1). The clinical implications of the published studies include the association of adequacy of dialysis and nutritional status with clinical outcomes [1], the relationship between residual renal function at initiation of dialysis and clinical outcomes, the clearances of urea and creatinine required to maintain good nutrition [5], outcomes in patients with type I and type II diabetes mellitus [6], reasons for poorer outcomes in patients from the USA compared to Canada [7] and the poorer outcomes in patients with higher peritoneal membrane transport [8].

The objective of this chapter is to review the data in the published studies and to discuss the clinical implications of these data.

Association of adequacy of dialysis and nutritional status with clinical outcomes [1]

Objective

The objective of this study was to evaluate the association of adequacy of dialysis and nutritional status with clinical outcomes.

Methodology

The CANUSA study group included 14 centres in North America; 10 in Canada and four in the USA.

Table 1. CANUSA bibliography

Publications
J Am Soc Nephrol 1996; 7: 198–207 [1]
Kidney Int 1996; 50 (suppl. 56): S56–61 [5]
Semin Dial 1997; 10: 215–18 [6]
J Am Soc Nephrol 1997; 8: 965–71 [7]
J Am Soc Nephrol 1998; 9: 1285–92 [8]

Abstracts
Perit Dial Int 1996; 16 (suppl. 2): 541 [9]
J Am Soc Nephrol 1997; 8: 185A [10]

There were 680 consecutive new continuous peritoneal dialysis patients enrolled between 1 September 1990 and 31 December 1992 with follow-up censored on 31 December 1993. Exclusion criteria were unlikely to survive for 6 months, living-related renal allograft scheduled within 6 months, HIV or hepatitis B-positive or active systemic inflammatory disease. The majority were treated with CAPD (98%); changes in dialysis prescription were made by the nephrologists within each clinical centre without data from the coordinating centre.

Adequacy of dialysis was estimated by measurement of total (renal plus peritoneal) weekly Kt/V for urea and total weekly creatinine clearance (C_{Cr}). Total body water (V) was estimated from the formula of Watson et al. [11]. The renal contribution to total C_{Cr} was estimated from the average of renal urea and creatinine clearances. This is an accurate estimate of glomerular filtration rate (GFR) [12]. The total weekly C_{Cr} was expressed per 1.73 m^2 body surface area (BSA) from the formula of Dubois and Dubois [13]. Adequacy of dialysis was estimated at the conclusion of training for peritoneal dialysis and every 6 months thereafter.

Estimates of nutritional status were obtained at the same intervals as for adequacy. These included the serum albumin concentration, the subjective global assessment (SGA) of nutrition [14], protein catabolic rate (PCR) according to Randerson et al.

R. Gokal, R. Khanna, R.Th. KPediet and K.D. Nolph (eds.), Textbook of Peritoneal Dialysis, 2nd Edition, 799–807.
© 2000 Kluwer Academic Publishers. Printed in Great Britain.

[15] normalized to standard body weight $(0.58/V)$ and percentage lean body mass (%LBM) from creatinine kinetics [16].

The statistical analysis used the Cox proportional hazards model with estimates of adequacy and nutritional status as time-dependent covariates [17, 18].

Results

The patients had a mean age of 54 years, mean weight 67.8 kg and a mean body mass index of 24.6 kg/m². The racial groups included 82.1% Caucasian; 8.4% African-American and 5.6% Asian. Diabetes was the cause for ESRD for 29.7% of the study population; 58.9% were male.

The relative risk (RR) of death was increased with increased age, dialysis in the USA compared to Canada, those with diabetes and prescribed insulin, history of cardiovascular disease (CVD), lower serum albumin concentration and worse nutritional status according to SGA and %LBM (Table 2). The RR of death was decreased by 6% for a 0.1 unit increase in the weekly Kt/V and decreased by 7% for a 5 L/1.73m² per week increase in C_{Cr}.

Data from the multivariate analysis were used to create a mathematical model to predict survival at different levels of weekly Kt/V and C_{Cr}. This model assumes that peritoneal and renal clearances are equivalent, and predicts the probability of survival, in this population, if total weekly clearances could be maintained at stable levels by increasing peritoneal clearance as renal clearance is lost. The predicted 2-year survival probabilities are shown in Table 3. Over the range of adequacy studied, there was a progressive increase in the probability of survival with increased Kt/V and C_{Cr}.

Clinical implications

These results, using a multivariate statistical analysis which controlled for other important independent

Table 2. Cox proportional hazards model

Variables	Relative mortality risk	95% confidence interval
Age (per year)	1.03	1.01–1.05
IDDM	1.45	0.89–2.36
CVD	2.09	1.33–3.28
Country (USA)	1.93	1.14–3.28
Serum albumin (↑1 g/L)	0.94	0.90–0.97
Kt/V (↑0.1 units/week)	0.94	0.90–0.99
SGA (↑1 unit)	0.75	0.66–0.85

Citation: Table 4 from J Am Soc Nephrol 1996; 7: 198–207.

Table 3. Expected 2-year patient survival according to sustained weekly Kt/V and C_{Cr} (L/1.73 m²)

Kt/V	Survival (%)	C_{Cr}	Survival (%)
2.3	81	95	86
2.1	78	80	81
1.9	74	70	78
1.7	71	55	72
1.5	66	40	65

Citation: Table 6 from J Am Soc Nephrol 1996; 7: 198–207.

variables and recognized changes in adequacy and nutritional status, showed a clinically important and statistically significant decrease in the RR of death with increased Kt/V and C_{Cr}. Previous smaller studies [19–22], using univariate analysis, had, with one exception [19], suggested this relationship. In a study of prevalent continuous peritoneal dialysis patients, Maiorca and colleagues have reported similar findings [23].

Selection of a target Kt/V or C_{Cr} for adequate dialysis was based on theoretical constructs. As originally conceived by Moncreif and Popovich [24, 25], the target weekly Kt/V for an anephric 70 kg male would have been 2.0 [26]. Others, using kinetic modelling approaches, suggest weekly Kt/V values of 2.0–2.2 [27, 28]. Accordingly, we selected a weekly Kt/V of 2.1 as the adequacy target. This is, in the mathematical model derived from the CANUSA data, associated with a predicted 2-year patient survival of 78%. There are no corresponding theoretical constructs on which to select an adequacy target expressed as C_{Cr}. However, the predicted 2-year survival of 78% was associated with a modelled weekly C_{Cr} of 70 L/1.73 m² and this value was selected. The Dialysis Outcome Quality Initiative (DOQI) recommends a target weekly Kt/V of 2.0 and a weekly C_{Cr} of 60 L/1.73 m² [29], values close to those recommended by CANUSA [1]. The slightly lower C_{Cr} target recognizes the relationship between C_{Cr} and Kt/V among prevalent peritoneal dialysis patients [23].

These data have focused attention on the importance of delivering adequate dialysis, in terms of clearance of urea and creatinine, for patients treated with continuous peritoneal dialysis. These data are observational rather than the result of a randomized clinical trial and should be considered as hypothesis-generating rather than hypothesis-testing. Gotch and colleagues have completed a randomized clinical trial in which patients were randomized to a total weekly Kt/V of either 1.7 or 2.1 with monthly estimates of total Kt/V. The peritoneal urea clearance

Table 4. Clinical and research questions

Equivalence of peritoneal and renal clearances?
Which estimate of adequacy, Kt/V or C_{Cr}
Adequate or optimum?

(Kt_p/V) was adjusted to maintain the total weekly Kt/V within the target ranges. This study was terminated early due to excess mortality in the group randomized to a weekly Kt/V of 1.7 [30]. The observational data from the CANUSA study are supported by this latter study.

Other questions have evolved from the CANUSA study [1]. These questions are listed in Table 4 and address the equivalence of peritoneal and renal clearances, whether Kt/V or C_{Cr} is the better estimate of adequacy and whether adequate or optimum dialysis is the objective of treatment.

Studies of adequacy of peritoneal dialysis have traditionally assumed that peritoneal and renal clearances of urea (Kt/V) and creatinine (C_{Cr}) are equivalent and have used total weekly values in the statistical analyses. In the CANUSA study [1], the initial weekly Kt/V value was 2.38 (1.67 peritoneal and 0.71 renal). The mean weekly peritoneal Kt/V value, for those who remained on CAPD, did not change. The value at 24 months was 1.70. On the other hand, the mean weekly renal Kt/V decreased to 0.28 at 24 months. When, using CANUSA study data [1], the renal and peritoneal clearances were entered separately into the Cox proportional hazards model and treated as time-dependent covariates [17, 18], the renal Kt/V has a much stronger association with patient survival than does peritoneal Kt/V [10]. This does not appear to be related to lack of variability in peritoneal clearances among these patients. The first and third quartile values for weekly renal Kt/V, at initiation of dialysis, were 0.30 and 0.99 respectively. For incident patients there are two other potential explanations for the stronger association with renal than with peritoneal Kt/V. Patients with higher renal Kt/V at initiation of dialysis may have started dialysis earlier as a result of either earlier referral or earlier scheduled initiation of dialysis. The former, and possibly the latter, are associated with better clinical outcomes on dialysis [31]. If this were the case, higher renal Kt/V is associated with better outcomes due to the relationship with referral and initiation, and represents a confounder in the analysis. Another explanation is obvious. Residual renal function provides more than clearance of low molecular weight solutes. More residual renal function is associated with increased

urine output and better-preserved endocrine function. The better outcomes associated with greater residual renal function are more likely associated with renal functions other than with clearance of urea or creatinine.

Peritoneal and renal clearances of urea or creatinine should be equivalent with respect to associations with clinical outcomes and the current convention of adding clearances appears reasonable. Residual renal function almost certainly provides benefit beyond that estimated by simply measuring clearance of small molecular weight solutes. Residual renal function should be estimated by a technique other than urea and creatinine clearance, and entered as a separate independent variable in statistical analyses addressing adequacy of dialysis.

C_{Cr} is associated with more clinical outcomes than is Kt/V in the CANUSA study [1]. While both were associated with the probability of patient survival, C_{Cr} but not Kt/V was associated with the relative risk of technique failure and hospitalization. This may be an artifact related to the greater contribution of renal, as compared to peritoneal, clearance, to total weekly C_{Cr} and to total weekly Kt/V. For C_{Cr}, renal clearance accounted for 47% of total weekly C_{Cr} at initiation of dialysis, while renal clearance contributed 30% of the total Kt/V. The association of C_{Cr} with more clinical outcomes than Kt/V may be due to residual renal function contributing more to total C_{Cr} than to total Kt/V. Residual renal function, either as a surrogate for earlier referral or initiation or as a reflection of renal function other than clearance of small molecular weight solutes, may explain these associations. The DOQI recommendation is that Kt/V be used as the preferred estimate of adequacy of small molecular weight solute clearance due to the relationship with protein metabolism and being less affected by variation in residual renal function [29].

There has been considerable debate about adequate as opposed to optimum dialysis for peritoneal dialysis patients. Gotch has used a kinetic model, based on thrice-weekly haemodialysis in the United States, to suggest that Kt/V greater than 2.0 would not be associated with improved patient survival [4]. The model developed by the CANUSA study [1] predicts increasing survival probabilities as weekly Kt/V increases from 1.5 to 2.3. The statistical criticism of the CANUSA model is that measurement of adequacy every 6 months did not provide sufficient precision to justify the prediction [4]. The Gotch model, based on comparison with thrice-weekly haemodialysis, may not be directly applicable to a continuous therapy. For outcomes other than patient survival there are data from nocturnal haemodialysis programmes which deliver much higher weekly Kt/V than thrice-weekly haemodialysis, indicating much-improved biochemistry and quality of life among patients with greater removal of uraemic solutes [32]. Although these data suggest added benefit with increased Kt/V, the controversy remains unresolved. One approach is to provide incremental doses of dialysis to achieve the target Kt/V while another is to provide as much clearance as is possible without decreasing patient quality of life or imposing unacceptable costs on the individual or the state.

How much peritoneal dialysis is required for the maintenance of a good nutritional state? [5]

Objective

The primary objective of this study was to evaluate the association of changes in adequacy of dialysis with changes in nutritional status. A secondary objective was to evaluate the relationship of residual renal function at initiation of dialysis with nutritional status at initiation, and to evaluate the relationship between initial nutritional status and clinical outcome.

Methodology

The patient population and measurement techniques were identical to those described for the study of adequacy of peritoneal dialysis [1]. In order to evaluate the association between adequacy of dialysis and nutritional status, the hypotheses were that the increased clearance associated with initiation of peritoneal dialysis would be associated with improvement in nutritional status and that loss of residual renal function (without a compensatory increase in peritoneal clearance) would be associated with a decrease in nutritional status. The first 6 months were chosen to evaluate the effect of increased peritoneal clearance and the next 12 months were chosen to evaluate the effect of loss of residual renal function. The relationship between residual renal function at initiation of peritoneal dialysis and nutritional status at that time was evaluated by dividing the patients into tertiles representing those with the highest, middle and lowest third with respect to residual renal function. Both renal Kt/V

and C_{Cr} were used to create these tertiles. For each of the nutritional markers, patient survival was determined for three levels of that nutritional marker.

Results

The mean increment in weekly Kt/V during the first 6 months of peritoneal dialysis was a peritoneal Kt/V of 1.67 (first and third quartiles 1.37 and 1.89 respectively). This was associated with an increase in PCR, %LBM and SGA score, but not in the serum albumin. The mean decrement in residual renal function, expressed as weekly Kt/V, between the 6th and 18th month of follow-up was 0.19 while the GFR decreased by 9.7 L/1.73 m². There were decreases in PCR, %LBM and SGA over this time period.

Whether estimated from weekly renal Kt/V or GFR, there was progressively worse nutritional status with less residual function at the initiation of peritoneal dialysis (Tables 5 and 6). For serum albumin, %LBM and PCR, the 2-year patient survival was better for those with better initial residual renal function (Table 7).

Table 5. Mean values of nutritional status at initiation of dialysis according to residual renal function estimated by weekly Kt/V tertiles ($n = 680$)

Kt/V	Albumin (g/L)	SGA (units)	LBM (%)	PCR (g/kg)
>0.89	35.4	5.4	71.6	1.12
0.44–0.89	35.0	5.1	68.0	1.03
<0.44	34.2	5.1	64.8	0.98
ANOVA p	<0.05	<0.05	<0.001	<0.001

Citation: Table 3 from Nephrol Dial Transplant 1998; 13 (suppl. 6): 158–63.

Table 6. Mean values of nutritional status at initiation of dialysis according to residual renal function estimated by weekly GFR/1.73 m² tertiles ($n = 680$)

GFR	Albumin (g/L)	SGA (units)	LBM (%)	PCR (g/kg)
>50	35.8	5.4	73.8	1.10
25–50	34.8	5.2	68.1	1.04
<25	34.1	5.0	58.0	0.99
ANOVA p	<0.01	<0.05	<0.001	<0.001

Citation: Table 4 from Nephrol Dial Transplant 1998; 13 (suppl. 6): 158–63.

Table 7. Two-year survival probabilities according to nutritional status at initiation of dialysis

Albumin (g/L)		LBM (%)		nPCR (g/kg)	
<30	(64%)	<63	(65%)	<0.09	(71%)
30–35	(75%)	63–73	(81%)	0.09–1.02	(80%)
>35	(85%)	>73	(88%)	>1.02	(83%)
Log-rank *p*					
<0.001		<0.001		<0.001	

Citation: Table 5 from Nephrol Dial Transplant 1998; 13 (suppl. 6): 158–63.

Clinical implications

The improvement in nutritional status during the first 6 months of dialysis provides evidence that peritoneal clearance is valuable in this regard. The decline with loss of residual renal function indicates that replacement of that clearance by increased peritoneal clearance is necessary to maintain that nutritional status. The decline in nutritional status occurred despite total weekly Kt/V falling only to 2.02, a value considered adequate by DOQI [29]. The inference is that the weekly Kt/V should be maintained at the mean 6-month level of 2.25 in the CANUSA study [1]. However, while perhaps necessary, maintaining total weekly Kt/V at 2.25 may not be sufficient if factors associated with residual renal function, other than clearance of small molecular weight solutes, are responsible for the development of malnutrition.

The worse nutritional status associated with less residual renal function at initiation is consistent with the observations of Ikizler *et al.* [33] for patients in usual clinical practice. This may be due to late referral, late initiation and minimal dietary instruction [31]. In a research setting such as the Modification of Diet in Renal Disease (MDRD) study, with skilled dietary intervention, there was evidence for mild malnutrition, but these patients were started on dialysis much earlier than the patients in the CANUSA study [1]. The mean GFR was 9.1 ml/min/1.73 m² [34] compared to 3.8 ml/min/1.73 m² in the CANUSA study.

These data strongly support the need for early referral of patients with chronic renal failure and close clinical follow-up with frequent skilled dietary intervention. Initiation of dialysis, based on a renal weekly Kt/V of <2.0 (C_{Cr} 9–14 ml/min/1.73 m²) with evidence for malnutrition, as recommended by DOQI, is consistent with these data [29].

Treatment of diabetics with end-stage renal disease: lessons from the Canada–USA (CANUSA) study of peritoneal dialysis [6]

Objective

The objective of this study was to re-evaluate the CANUSA study results with respect to patients with diabetes mellitus. In the original analysis diabetes was identified as a cause for renal disease as a baseline demographic variable. Patients with diabetes for whom insulin was prescribed represented those with diabetic comorbidity. In this report [6], diabetes mellitus was defined more precisely and the data were reanalysed.

Methodology

All clinical investigators were asked to review original patient records and to redefine diabetic patients according to the algorithm described by Cowie and colleagues [35]. A patient was considered to have type I diabetes mellitus if the diagnosis had been made before age 25 and if insulin had been prescribed within 3 months of diagnosis. Type I and type II diabetes mellitus were entered as separate independent variables in the Cox proportional hazards model as described in the CANUSA study [1].

Results

There were 203 patients with diabetes mellitus, 29.6% of the CANUSA study population. There were 99 with type I and 104 with type II diabetes mellitus. The type I diabetics were younger at initiation of dialysis, age 44 vs 61 years; were more likely male, 70% vs 51%; and were more likely to be Caucasian, 89% vs 72%. They were more likely to function independently, 55% vs 38%; were less likely to have a history of cardiovascular disease, 36% vs 47%. They were not different with respect to serum albumin concentration, SGA or residual renal function at initiation of dialysis. The 2-year patient survival probabilities were 79% for non-diabetics, 83% for type I diabetes mellitus and 66% for those with type II diabetes mellitus. The relative risk of death, compared to the referent of non-diabetic patients, was calculated with age and country as the other independent variables. For those with type I diabetes mellitus the relative risk was 1.76; for those with type II it was 1.46. With the addition of cardiovascular disease history, serum albumin, SGA and esti-mates of adequacy of dialysis, the relative risk of death was 1.08 and 1.18 for type I and type II diabetes mellitus respectively. Non-diabetic patients were hospitalized 14.6 days per year compared to 25.7 days for those with type I and 33.5 days for those with type II diabetes mellitus, respectively.

Clinical implications

These data show the importance of accurate defini-tion of diabetes mellitus as either type I or type II for epidemiological studies, and for accurate attribu-tion of the risks associated with diabetes and the associated comorbid conditions. The patients with type II diabetes mellitus are older, have a higher proportion of non-Caucasians, are less likely to be independent and have cardiac disease at the initia-tion of dialysis. Predialysis management should be directed at prevention of the development of cardiac disease in these patients.

Lower probability of patient survival with continuous peritoneal dialysis in the United States compared with Canada [7]

Objective

The objective of this report was to evaluate the reasons for the difference in survival probabilities for patients treated in Canada and the USA in the CANUSA study. The relative risk of death was 1.93 for patients in the USA centres compared to Canada [1].

Methodology

The factors evaluated were baseline demographic and clinical factors, residual renal function at initia-tion of dialysis, initial nutritional status, total weekly Kt/V and C_{Cr}. Cardiovascular disease was reclassi-fied according to severity of disease.

Results

There was no difference between patients from the USA and Canada with respect to age, gender, proportion with diabetes mellitus or history of cardiovascular disease. Neither was there a differ-ence in the severity of the cardiovascular disease. Patients from the USA were more likely to be Afri-

can-American (30% vs 4%) and had an average BSA of 1.80 m^2 compared to 1.74 m^2 for Canadian patients. Analysis excluding African-American patients increased the difference between the coun-tries with respect to survival. There was an increased relative risk of a non-fatal cardiovascular event among patients in the USA compared to Canada; RR 1.80 (95% CI 1.21–2.67).

In the absence of an explanation, from the data in the CANUSA study, for the worse patient survival among patients in the USA, several speculative explanations were advanced. The first is that patients were negatively selected for peritoneal dialysis in the USA; the second was that the much higher rate of acceptance for dialysis in the USA than in Canada resulted in acceptance of patients with more comor-bidity than in Canada; the third was that patients in the USA were less compliant than those in Canada.

There is no direct method available to evaluate the contention that there is negative patient selection in the USA. The rate acceptance of new dialysis patients in the USA during the study period was 211 per million per year compared to 100 per million population per year in Canada. If one restricts this to Caucasians, the rate in the USA was 162 per million population per year. The suggestion that there is more non-compliance in the USA is sup-ported by two small studies, one from Pittsburgh [36] and one from Winnipeg [37]. Using compara-ble methodology involving comparison of prescribed compared to consumed inventory at the patient's home, the rate of non-compliance, defined as use of <90% of prescribed exchanges, was 40% in the American centre compared to 12% in the Canadian centre. A multicentre study used a questionnaire to compare admitted non-compliance and found a smaller, as expected, rate of non-compliance, but the relative difference between countries was similar to that in the studies with an objective estimate of non-compliance [38].

Clinical relevance

The difference in patient survival between Canada and the USA does not appear explained by overt comorbidity or systematic differences in prescribed therapy. Higher rates of acceptance for dialysis are associated with increased numbers of comorbid con-ditions [39]. These are not captured in the comorbid factors recorded in the CANUSA study [1]. Future studies should use validated comorbidity indices, an example of which has been published by Barrett and colleagues [40]. The success of home therapies, such as continuous peritoneal dialysis, is very sensitive to compliance. A systematic approach to enhance and monitor compliance in these programmes is essential.

Increased peritoneal membrane transport is associated with decreased patient and technique survival for continuous peritoneal dialysis patients [8]

Objective

The objective of this study was to evaluate the association between peritoneal membrane transport, determined 1 month following initiation of dialysis, and clinical outcomes among patients treated with continuous peritoneal dialysis.

Methodology

Among the 680 patients reported in the CANUSA study, 606 had a peritoneal equilibrium test (PET) performed, according to the method described by Twardowski and colleagues [41], at the initiation of dialysis. Peritoneal membrane transport was classified as low, low average, high average and high (L, LA, HA, H) [41].

Results

Higher transport was associated with increased age, male gender and diabetes mellitus, both type I and type II. The 2-year technique survival probabilities were 94%, 76%, 72% and 68% for L, LA, HA and H respectively. The 2-year patient survival probabilities were 91%, 80%, 72% and 71% for L, LA, HA and H respectively. The 2-year probabilities of both technique and patient survival were 86%, 61%, 52% and 48% for L, LA, HA and H respectively. The Cox proportional hazards analysis showed that the relative risk of either technique failure of death, compared to L, was 2.54 for LA, 3.39 for HA and 4.00 for H (Table 8). The mean drain volumes (litres) in the PET were 2.53, 2,45, 2.33 and 2.16 for L, LA, HA and H respectively while the 24 h drain volumes were 9.38, 8.93, 8.59 and 8.22 L for L, LA, HA and H respectively. The mean serum albumin values, about 1 month after initiation of dialysis, were 37.8, 36.2, 33.8 and 32.8 g/L for L, LA, HA, H respectively.

Table 8. Relative risk of death, technique failure, or either according to peritoneal transport

Group	death	Transfer to HD or IPD	Either death or transfer
L	1.00	1.00	1.00
LA	1.60	3.26	2.54
HA	2.30	4.04	3.39
H	1.94	5.82	4.00

Citation: Table 4 from J Am Soc Nephrol 1998; 9: 1285–92.

There was no difference among the peritoneal transport groups with respect to SGA, %LBM or NPCR. Neither was there any difference among groups with respect to residual renal function, whether estimated from Kt/V or C_{cr}. The trend was to more residual renal function with higher peritoneal transport. The weekly peritoneal Kt/V was slightly, but not statistically significant, lower in the H group. The weekly peritoneal C_{Cr} was higher, as expected, with increased peritoneal transport. The 24 h losses of both albumin and protein increased with higher peritoneal transport (Table 9). When followed over 18 months there were no further changes in any of the estimates of nutritional status or serum albumin, within each transport category.

Clinical implications

The finding of worse technique and patient survival among patients with higher peritoneal membrane transport is counter-intuitive. One would expect higher clearances of urea and creatinine with higher transport and this was the case with the exception of Kt/V for high peritoneal transport where decreased drain volumes may have been responsible. In the multivariate analysis, higher Kt/V and C_{Cr} are still associated with a decreased relative risk of death, but there is a significant increase in the relative risk of technique failure or death with increased peritoneal membrane transport.

Table 9. Dialysate protein and albumin losses at baseline by transport group

Group	n	Protein* (g/24 h) (SD)	n	Albumin* (g/24 h) (SD)
L	40	5.29 (2.22)	29	3.09 (1.40)
LA	191	6.19 (2.11)	134	3.86 (1.57)
HA	280	7.10 (2.56)	177	4.27 (1.81)
H	93	8.77 (4.05)	54	5.61 (3.17)

Citation: Table 7 from J Am Soc Nephrol 1998; 9: 1285–92.
* $p < 0.001$ by ANCOVA.

These associations were first suggested by Nolph *et al.* [42], Heaf [43] and Wu *et al.* [44], and have been confirmed by others [45–47]. The mechanism is speculative. Nolph had reported evidence of malnutrition after about 18 months treatment and attributed this to loss of protein in peritoneal dialysate [42]. However, we have shown the decreased serum albumin to be present about 1 month after the initiation of dialysis. It is not progressive and other estimates of nutritional status are not impaired with increased peritoneal membrane transport. Ultrafiltration failure may contribute to fluid overload with the low serum albumin due to dilution and death due to cardiac disease. High transport may be associated with increased inflammation with low albumin representing a negative acute-phase reactant. Increased glucose absorption may mediate adverse cardiovascular events.

The clinical reactions to higher peritoneal membrane transport with hypoalbuminaemia and/or fluid overload include a transfer to nocturnal cycling peritoneal dialysis or haemodialysis. The former has been associated with more ultrafiltration per gram of glucose absorbed but no decrease in the loss of protein in the dialysate [48]. The impact of nocturnal cycling peritoneal dialysis and haemodialysis on outcomes for patients with high peritoneal transport is unknown. The suggestion that exposure to glucose increases peritoneal membrane transport indicates a need to continue research into alternative osmotic agents for peritoneal dialysis.

Canada–USA Peritoneal Dialysis Study Group: AFFILIATIONS

D. N. Churchill, D. W. Taylor, K. E. Thorpe, M. L. Beecroft, St Joseph's Hospital, McMaster University, Hamilton, Ontario; P. R. Keshaviah, G. deVeber, L. W. Henderson, Baxter Healthcare; K. K. Jindal, Victoria General Hospital, Halifax, Nova Scotia; S. S. A. Fenton, J. M. Bargman, D. G. Oreopoulos, The Toronto Hospital, Toronto, Ontario; G. G. Wu, Credit Valley Hospital, Mississauga, Ontario; S. D. Lavoie, Ottawa Civic Hospital, Ottawa, Ontario; A. Fine, St Boniface Hospital, Winnipeg, Mannitoba; E. Burgess, Foothills Hospital, Calgary, Alberta; J. C. Brandes, Medical College of Wisconsin, Milwaukee, Wisconsin; K. D. Nolph, B. F. Prowant, University of Missouri Medical Center, Columbia, Missouri; D. Pagé, Ottawa General Hospital, Ottawa, Ontario; F. X. McCusker, B. P. Teehan, Lankenau Hospital, Thomas Jefferson Medical College, Philadelphia, Pennsylvania; M. K. Dasgupta, University of Alberta Hospital, Edmonton, Alberta; R. Caruana, Medical College of Georgia, Augusta, Georgia

References

1. Churchill DN, Taylor DW, Keshaviah PR for the CANUSA Peritoneal Dialysis Study Group. Adequacy of dialysis and nutrition in continuous peritoneal dialysis: association with clinical outcomes. J Am Soc Nephrol 1996; 7: 198–207.
2. Blake PG. A critique of the Canada–USA (CANUSA) peritoneal dialysis study. Perit Dial Int 1996; 16: 243–5.
3. Jindal KK. Commentary on the findings of the CANUSA study. Perit Dial Int 1996; 16: 246–7.
4. Gotch FA. The CANUSA study. Perit Dial Int 1997; 17 (suppl. 2): S111–14.
5. McKusker FX, Teehan BP, Thorpe KE, Keshaviah PR, Churchill DN for the CANUSA Peritoneal Dialysis Study Group. How much peritoneal dialysis is required for the maintenance of a good nutritional state? Kidney Int 1996; 50 (suppl. 56): S56–61.
6. Churchill DN, Thorpe KE, Teehan BP for the CANUSA Peritoneal Dialysis Study Group. Treatment of diabetics with end-stage renal disease: lessons from the Canada–USA (CANUSA) study of peritoneal dialysis. Semin Dial 1997; 10: 215–18.
7. Churchill DN, Thorpe KE, Vonesh EF, Keshaviah PR for the CANUSA Peritoneal Dialysis Study Group. Lower probability of patient survival with continuous peritoneal dialysis in the United States compared with Canada. J Am Soc Nephrol 1997; 8: 965–71.
8. Churchill DN, Thorpe KE, Nolph KD, Keshaviah PR, Oreopoulos DG, Page D for the CANUSA Peritoneal Dialysis Study Group. Increased peritoneal membrane transport is associated with decreased patient and technique survival for continuous peritoneal dialysis patients. J Am Soc Nephrol 1998; 9: 1285–92.
9. Jindal K, Thorpe KE, Lavoie S, Bargman J, Dasgupta M, Churchill DN for the CANUSA Peritoneal Dialysis Study Group. Multivariate analysis of peritonitis in peritoneal dialysis; the CANUSA experience. Perit Dial Int 1996; 16 (suppl. 2): S41.
10. Bargman JM, Thorpe KE, Churchill DN. The importance of residual renal function for survival in patients on peritoneal dialysis. J Am Soc Nephrol 1997; 8: 185A.
11. Watson PE, Watson ID, Batt RD. Total body water volumes for adult males and females estimated from simple anthropometric measurements. Am J Clin Nutr 1980; 33: 27–39.
12. Van Olden RW, Krediet RT, Struijk DG, Arisz L. Measurement of residual renal function in patients treated with continuous peritoneal dialysis. J Am Soc Nephrol 1996; 7: 745–50.
13. Du Bois D, Du Bois EF. A formula to estimate the approximate surface area if height and weight are known. Arch Int Med 1916; 17: 863–71.
14. Baker JP, Detsky AS, Wesson DE *et al.* Nutritional assessment: a comparison of clinical judgement and objective measurements. N Engl J Med 1982; 306: 969–72.
15. Randerson DH, Chapman GV, Farrell PC. Amino acid and dietary status in CAPD patients. In: Atkins RC, Farrell PC, Thompson N, eds. Peritoneal Dialysis. Edinburgh: Churchill-Livingstone, 1981, pp. 180–91.
16. Keshaviah PR, Nolph KD, Moore HL *et al.* Lean body mass estimation by creatinine kinetics. J Am Soc Nephrol 1994; 4: 1475–85.
17. Cox D. Regression models and life-tables. J R Stat Soc 1972; 34: 187–201.
18. Cox DR, Oakes D. Analysis of Survival Data. London: Chapman & Hall, 1984.

19. Blake PG, Sombolos K, Abraham G *et al.* Lack of correlation between urea kinetic indices and clinical outcomes in CAPD patients. Kidney Int 1991; 39: 700–6.

20. Teehan BP, Scheifler CR, Brown J. Urea kinetic modelling is an appropriate assessment of adequacy. Semin Dial 1992; 5: 189–92.

21. DeAlvarro F, Bajo MA, Alvarez-Ude F *et al.* Does *Kt/V* have the same predictive value as in HD? A multicentre study. Adv Perit Dial 1992; 8: 93–7.

22. Lameire NH, Vanholder R, Veyt D, Lambert MC, Ringoir S. A longitudinal 5 year survey of kinetic parameters in CAPD patients. Kidney Int 1992; 42: 426–32.

23. Maiorca R, Brunori G, Zubani R *et al.* Predictive value of adequacy of dialysis and nutritional indices for mortality and morbidity in CAPD and HD patients. A longitudinal study. Nephrol Dial Transplant 1995; 10: 2295–305.

24. Popovich RP, Moncrief JW, Dechard JB, Bomar JB, Pyle WK. The definition of a novel portable/wearable equilibrium peritoneal dialysis technique. ASAIO Trans 1976; 5: 64.

25. Popovich RP, Moncrief JW. Kinetic modelling of peritoneal transport. Contrib Nephol 1979; 17: 59–72.

26. Churchill DN: Adequacy of peritoneal dialysis: how much dialysis do we need? Kidney Int 1994; 46 (suppl. 48): S2–6.

27. Teehan BP, Scheifler CR, Sigler MH, Gilgore GS. A quantitative approach to the CAPD prescription. Perit Dial Bull 1985; 5: 152–6.

28. Keshaviah PR. Adequacy of CAPD: a quantitative approach. Kidney Int 1992; 42 (suppl. 38): S160–4.

29. NKF-DOQI Clinical Practice Guidelines for Peritoneal Dialysis Adequacy. New York: National Kidney Foundation, 1997.

30. Gotch F. Update on the randomized multicentre trial on CAPD prescription. Presented at Symposium on Dialysis Schedule in Hemodialysis and Peritoneal Dialysis. Perugia, Italy, 24–26 November 1996.

31. Churchill DN. An evidence-based approach to earlier initiation of dialysis. Am J Kidney Dis 1997; 30: 899–906.

32. Pierratos A, Ouwendyk M, Francoeur R *et al.* Nocturnal hemodialysis: three year experience. J Am Soc Nephrol 1998; 9: 859–68.

33. Ikizler TA, Greene JH, Wingard RL, Parker RA, Hakim RM. Spontaneous dietary protein intake during progression of chronic renal failure. J Am Soc Nephrol 1995; 6: 1386–91.

34. Levey AS, Greene T, Burkart J for the MDRD Study Group. Comprehensive assessment of the level of renal function at the initiation of dialysis in the MDRD study. J Am Soc Nephrol 1998; 9: 153A.

35. Cowie CC, Port Fk, Wolfe RA, Savage PJ, Moll PP, Hawthorne VM. Disparities in incidence of diabetic end-stage renal disease according to race and type of diabetes. N Engl J Med 1989; 321: 1074–9.

36. Bernardini J, Piraino B. Measuring compliance with prescribed exchanges in CAPD and CCPD patients. Perit Dial Int 1997; 17: 338–42.

37. Fine A. Compliance with the CAPD prescription is good. Perit Dial Int 1997; 17: 343–6.

38. Blake P, Korbet S, Blake R *et al.* Admitted non-compliance with CAPD exchanges is more common in US than Canadian patients. J Am Soc Nephrol 1997; 8: 278A.

39. Keane WF, Collins AJ. Influence of co-morbidity on mortality and morbidity in patients treated with hemodialysis. Am J Kidney Dis 1994; 24: 1010–18.

40. Barrett BJ, Parfrey PS, Morgan J *et al.* Prediction of early death in end-stage renal disease patients starting dialysis. Am J Kidney Dis 1997; 29: 214–22.

41. Twardowski ZJ, Nolph KD, Khanna R. Peritoneal equilibrium test. Perit Dial Bull 1987; 7: 138–47.

42. Nolph KD, Moore HL, Prowant B. Continuous peritoneal dialysis with a high flux membrane. ASAIO J 1993; 39: 904–9.

43. Heaf J. CAPD adequacy and dialysis morbidity: detrimental effect of a high peritoneal equilibration rate. Renal Fail 1995; 17: 575–87.

44. Wu C, Huang C, Huang J, Wu M, Leu M. High flux peritoneal membrane is a risk factor in survival of CAPD treatment. Adv Perit Dial 1996; 12: 105–9.

45. Fried L. Higher membrane permeability predicts poorer patient survival. Perit Dial Int 1997; 17: 387–89.

46. Wang T, Heimburger O, Waniewski J, Bergstrom J, Lindholm B. Increased peritoneal permeability is associated with decreased fluid and small solute removal and higher mortality in CAPD patients. Nephrol Dial Transplant 1998; 13: 1242–9.

47. Davies SJ, Phillips L, Russell GI. Peritoneal solute transport predicts survival independently of residual renal function. Nephrol Dial Transplant 1998; 13: 962–8.

48. Twardowski ZJ, Nolph KD, Khanna R, Gluck Z, Prowant BF, Ryan LP. Daily clearances with CAPD and NIPD. ASAIO Trans 1986; 23: 575–9.

28 | Intraperitoneal chemotherapy

M. F. FLESSNER AND R. L. DEDRICK

Introduction

A wide variety of therapeutic drugs are administered into the peritoneal cavity as a portal of entry to the body and as a localized treatment. Because of intravenous access problems in neonates, transfusion of packed red blood cells was one of the earliest uses of intraperitoneal (i.p.) therapy [1, 2]. Insulin is often placed in the dialysate in order to treat glucose intolerance during peritoneal dialysis [3], and i.p. insulin delivery is currently undergoing investigation as a means of long-term therapy in diabetes [4]. Erythropoietin, prescribed as replacement therapy for the anaemia related to end-stage renal disease (ESRD), has recently been administered intraperitoneally [5, 6]. In contrast to these forms of i.p. therapy which are designed to treat systemic illnesses, antibacterial agents are injected intraperitoneally in order to treat peritonitis [7, 8]. In the past 20 years i.p. chemotherapy has increasingly been evaluated for treatment of malignancies localized to the peritoneal cavity [9–22].

Prior to prescribing i.p. therapy, the critical point which the clinician must determine is the usefulness of such an approach. Is there a pharmacokinetic advantage of administering the drug regionally (i.p.) versus systemically (intravenously or i.v.)? In other words: does the drug achieve therapeutic concentration in the region of interest, while maintaining an acceptably low level in the general circulation?

On the other hand, the i.p. administration of a drug such as erythropoietin, which has a site of action in the bone marrow and not the peritoneal cavity, may not be an appropriate use of this route. Because of a slow rate of systemic absorption, very large concentrations of erythropoietin must be injected with the peritoneal dialysate to attain levels in the blood which are equivalent to those attained with i.v. or subcutaneous (s.c.) dosing. Much of this expensive agent must be wasted, since the solution must be drained from the patient before the drug is fully absorbed [5].

What follows is an analytical approach to the evaluation of the i.p. route of administration with respect to the i.v. route. The approach assumes that the target of the therapy is either a cellular component in the peritoneal cavity (bacteria or tumour ascites cells) or the tissues surrounding the peritoneal cavity.

At steady state the quantitative formula for pharmacokinetic advantage (R_d) in its simplest form is [23]:

$$R_d = \frac{\left(\dfrac{C_P}{C_B}\right)_{i.p.}}{\left(\dfrac{C_P}{C_B}\right)_{i.v.}} \qquad (1)$$

where: C_P = concentration in the peritoneal cavity, C_B = concentration in the systemic circulation, and the subscripts indicate the route of administration. In planning a therapeutic strategy the physician would like to predict R_d prior to administration of the drug in humans. The pharmacokinetics of a particular drug are based on the transport physiology of the region in which it is administered, as well as pharmacokinetic processes in the rest of the body.

Physiological characteristics of the peritoneal cavity which cause it to be advantageous for removal of waste metabolites and poisons from the body also provide an excellent portal of entry into the body for many drugs. The tissue space surrounding the cavity is capable of absorbing almost any agent, including cell-sized materials, placed in the cavity. As illustrated in Fig. 1, blood and lymphatic capillary networks are contained within the tissue space. The density of these networks depends on the specific organ tissue. As drugs transport into the tissue from the cavity, they will be taken up by these networks and returned to the general circulation. The rate of a drug's transfer to the blood is governed by its effective diffusivity and convection (solvent drag) within the tissue space, the permeability–

R. Gokal, R. Khanna, R.Th. Krediet and K.D. Nolph (eds.), *Textbook of Peritoneal Dialysis, 2nd Edition*, 809–827.
© 2000 *Kluwer Academic Publishers. Printed in Great Britain.*

TRANSPORT BETWEEN THE
BLOOD AND PERITONEAL CAVITY

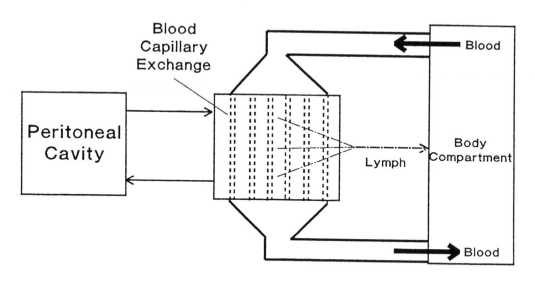

Figure 1. Distributed model concept in which blood flows through exchange capillaries which are distributed uniformly in the tissue surrounding the peritoneal cavity. Drugs introduced into the peritoneal cavity transport into the surrounding tissue interstitium. From the tissue interstitium the solutes transfer into either blood capillaries (small molecules) or lymphatic capillaries (the pathway for macromolecules)

surface area of the blood and lymphatic capillaries for a given volume of tissue, and the blood perfusion. The process of drug uptake from the peritoneal cavity includes the same physiological mechanisms responsible for transport during dialysis, except that the direction of transfer is reversed.

Our goal in this chapter is to illustrate how the physician can implement the above equation to estimate the pharmacokinetic advantage in a proposed therapy which utilizes the peritoneal cavity as a drug-delivery system. We will first present a detailed conceptual model of peritoneal transport, followed by a brief explanation of the mathematical consequences of this conceptual model over a range of molecular weights. Then we will give a number of examples in which the theory is applied.

Model concept

Although the simplicity of the concept presented in Fig. 1 is appealing, the anatomy and physiology of

the peritoneal cavity are far more complex. Figure 2 illustrates a conceptual model which attempts to include some of the diversity of organ physiology which exists in the tissue surrounding the peritoneal cavity [24].

The body is shown as a single compartment in Fig. 2, but it could be represented by multiple compartments, if the pharmacokinetic characteristics of the drug demand it. For example, a drug which has its major effect or chief site of metabolism in the liver would be a candidate for such a model, in which the relative rates of absorption into each tissue would determine the overall effectiveness of the medication. The volume of the body compartment equals the volume of distribution of the drug in the total body excluding the tissues surrounding the peritoneal cavity. Its concentration is assumed to equal the arterial concentration. The drug is cleared at some rate CL_{BC} and there may exist some rate of input into the compartment (I_{BC}). Blood flows from the body compartment through each peritoneal

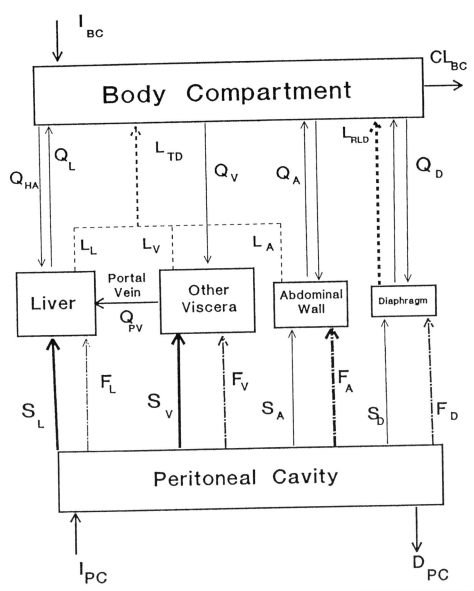

Figure 2. Compartmental model concept of intraperitoneal drug delivery in which transport occurs between the cavity and specific tissues surrounding the cavity. *Symbols:* I = infusion; CL = clearance; D = drainage from the cavity; Q = blood flow through organ or vessel; L = lymph flow from tissue to body compartment; F = rate of convection from the cavity to tissue; S = rate of solute transfer from the cavity to tissue. *Subscripts:* A = abdominal wall and psoas; BC = body compartment; D = diaphragm; HA = hepatic artery; L = liver, PC = peritoneal cavity; PV = portal vein; RLD = right lymph duct; TD = thoracic duct; V = other viscera including the intestines, stomach, pancreas, and spleen. See text for a full desription.

compartment with rate Q_i. Lymph flows from each organ system (L_i) through two major systems into the body compartment: the thoracic duct (L_{TD}) and the right lymph duct (L_{RLD}).

The single 'peritoneal tissue' compartment has been divided into four major compartments. Each of these compartments receives blood originating in the body compartment. The blood flows through capillary exchange vessels distributed throughout the tissue (as illustrated in Fig. 1 but left out of Fig. 2 for clarity) and returns to the body compartment. Lymph flows from each tissue space to the body compartment as illustrated in Figs 1 and 2. Each tissue compartment receives solutes from the peritoneal cavity with a solute mass transfer rate of S and fluid at rate F (S and F are illustrated as positive from the cavity into the tissue).

The diaphragm is included as a separate compartment because of the specialized subdiaphragmatic lymphatic system [25, 26] which accepts cell sizes to 25 μm in diameter [27] and which accounts for 70–80% of the total lymph flow from the cavity [28–30]. The diaphragm also experiences relatively large but variable hydrostatic pressure gradients during respiration, because of its position between the thoracic and abdominal cavities. Expiration facilitates direct fluid movement into the diaphragmatic interstitium and into the lacuna of the subdiaphragmatic lymphatic apparatus [25, 26].

The abdominal wall is shown as a separate compartment because it is the single largest recipient of fluid transfer from the cavity. In animal experiments this amounts to 40–50% of the total fluid movement out of the cavity [28–31]. The reason for this fluid movement has been attributed to the hydrostatic pressure gradient across the abdominal wall. In addition, the lymphatics are not well developed in this tissue and therefore do not provide the safety valve that they do in intestinal tissue [32]. Proteins or other macromolecular drugs which are carried into the tissue as a result of the hydrostatic pressure-driven convection will circulate to the body compartment very slowly [31, 33].

The liver is separated from the other visceral tissues because of its unique portal circulation coupled with its role in drug metabolism. The liver may be primarily responsible for protein losses into the cavity. The 'other viscera' include the spleen, stomach, intestines, and the pancreas, which are lumped together in a single tissue compartment.

The peritoneal cavity compartment is assumed to be well mixed; i.e. the concentration is the same throughout the cavity. The cavity may have a solute input rate of I_{PC} and a drainage rate of D_{PC}. The cavity does not exchange directly with the body compartment; transport occurs only with the tissue compartments.

Model implementation

In order to use equation (1), C_P must be estimated. In order to do this, the mathematical model corresponding to the conceptual model of Fig. 2 must be solved. This consists of: (a) a series of mass and volume balances of each compartment; (b) rate equations (defining each S and CL); and (c) boundary conditions (defining initial concentrations, volumes, and inputs (I) and outputs (D)). Critical to the solution of these equations are a large number of parameters which describe the system.

Estimation of solute-independent parameters

A necessary step in the solution is the determination of the parameters in Fig. 2: Q_i, L_i, and F_i. Each of these numbers depends not on solute characteristics but upon the underlying physiology of the tissue. Table 1 is a listing of these parameters. Because many of these numbers had to be estimated from incomplete information or scaled from animal experiments, they should be considered order-of-magnitude.

The first two columns concern peritoneal surface area. The first column specifies the percentage of the total peritoneal surface area, while the second tabulates the total surface area in cm². We chose Rubin *et al.* [34] because the measurements were more conservative than those of Esperanca and Collins [35], since the mesentery was not included. The areas have been scaled to a 70 kg body weight by the factor (body weight)$^{0.7}$ [23]. It should be noted that these are total surface areas which have resulted from the dissection of each tissue and its surface area measured by planimetry; these area values may not represent the true area of contact between the peritoneal fluid and the tissue.

Table 1. Adult human parameters which are independent of solute size (scaled to 70 kg body weight)

Tissue	Percentage total surface area	A_i (cm²)	Weight (g)	q_i (ml/min/g)	Q_{tot} (ml/min)	L (ml/min)	F (ml/min)	L/F
Liver	13.2	1056	1800	0.83	1500	0.46	0.07	6.83
Other viscera (intestines spleen, stomach)	67.9	5432	1700	0.65	1100	0.97	0.33	2.91
Abdominal wall	11	880	1960	0.06	118	0.04	0.67	0.05
Diaphragm	7.9	632	190	0.3	57	0.27	0.27	1.01

The tissue weights were estimated as follows. The liver weight was taken directly from a table in Ludwig [36]. The 'other viscera' weight was computed from the sum of the spleen (0.14 kg) and intestines. The latter were estimated from the product of the total surface area [34], the average thickness of 2.5 mm [37], and the specific gravity of these tissues, which was assumed to equal 1 g/cm³. The thicknesses of the abdominal wall and diaphragm were estimated to be 2 cm and 0.3 cm [38, 39], respectively, and the tissue weight was calculated in the same fashion as in the case of the hollow viscera.

There have been a number of estimates of the rate of perfusion (q_i) of the abdominal tissues. We used Rubin *et al.*'s [40] measurement in the control animals for the parietal wall (0.06 ml/min/g tissue) and diaphragm (0.31). Other estimates [41] for the parietal wall tended to be much higher, because of the specific preparation and use of vasodilators. The perfusion rates in the 'other viscera' and the liver (includes both hepatic artery and portal flow) were estimated from total organ blood flows [42, 43] and divided by the weight of each system. The estimates for the gastrointestinal tract agree with several other measurements made in a variety of tissues from other species [44–46]. The total blood flows for the diaphragm and abdominal wall (Q_i) can be calculated from the product of the organ weight and q_i.

Thoracic duct lymph flow has been measured in humans and typically has a flow rate of 1–1.6 ml/h/kg body weight [47, 48]. Non-ruminant animals have flow rates on the order of 2–3 ml/h/kg body weight [29, 49–51]. Morris [51] estimates that the contributions of the liver and gastrointestinal tract amount to 30% and 64%, respectively, of the thoracic duct flow. The remaining 6% of the total flow is from all the skeletal muscle below the diaphragm, including the psoas, the abdominal wall, and the lower limbs. In order to estimate the lymph flow for humans, the mean value for the thoracic duct (1.3 ml/h/kg body weight) was multiplied by the percentages obtained by Morris for each organ system: 30% for liver and 64% for other viscera. One-third of the remaining 6% was arbitrarily assumed to be the contribution of the abdominal wall. Total lymph flows were then calculated by multiplying each tissue-specific lymph flow rate by the body weight (70 kg) and converting to ml/min.

Of the lymph which exclusively leaves the peritoneal cavity 70–80% occurs through the subdiaphragmatic system [52]. This is a major site for transport of fluids, macromolecules, and cellular materials from the cavity to the blood. Values for

flow range from 0.6–1.8 ml/h/kg body weight in the anaesthetized rat [29] to 0.1 ml/h/kg in anaesthetized sheep and 0.50 ml/h/kg in awake sheep [53]. Flow rates in awake, healthy continuous ambulatory peritoneal dialysis (CAPD) patients vary from 0.14 to 0.28 ml/h/kg body weight [54, 55]. The rates appear to increase in cirrhosis to 0.43 ml/h/kg [56]. We have chosen the mean rate of 0.23 ml/h/kg and multiplied it by 70 kg to find the diaphragmatic lymph flow rate of 16.1 ml/h.

The next to last column in Table 1 lists estimated total flow rates of fluid in ml/min to each organ system. The total flow from the cavity has been estimated from the average of three studies in healthy CAPD patients [53–55, 57] to be 1.33 ml/min. This flow is driven by the hydrostatic pressure in the cavity [29, 58, 59] and occurs in the face of hyperosmolar solutions which draw fluid into the cavity [31, 33, 59–61]. These studies have shown that protein acts as a marker for fluid movement. The total hourly flow rate has been partitioned to each set of tissues on the basis of the fraction of protein deposition from the cavity of the rat [31] with corrections for the rates of lymph flow from each tissue.

Peritoneal transport of small molecules: theory

The next step in the implementation of our model concept is the definition of the appropriate rate equations. This has been rigorously performed only for small molecules.

Transfer of small molecules from the peritoneal cavity can be viewed as a process of diffusion from the fluid in the cavity into the adjacent tissues followed by absorption from the tissue extracellular space into blood in the exchange vessels (Fig. 1). Convection generally does not play a quantitatively significant role for small solutes, and lymphatic uptake is negligible compared with removal from the tissue by the flowing blood. The result is that a concentration profile is established within the tissue. At steady state the rate of diffusion down the profile at any location is exactly balanced by the combination of irreversible chemical reaction in the tissue and removal by flowing blood. For a non-reactive solute and a uniformly distributed capillary network, it is easily shown that the rate of uptake into blood perfusing the viscera may be calculated from the equation [62]:

$$S_V = \sqrt{D_V(p_V a_V)} A_V(C_P - C_B) \qquad (2)$$

where S_V = net rate of uptake of the solute (μg/min), D_V = the effective diffusivity of the solute in the viscera (cm²/min), p_V = the intrinsic permeability of the blood capillaries in the viscera (cm/min), a_V = the capillary surface area per unit tissue volume (cm²/cm³), A_V = the superficial surface area of the viscera exposed to peritoneal fluid (cm²), C = the free solute concentration (μg/cm³), and the subscripts P and B refer to peritoneal fluid and blood, respectively. The effective diffusivity is equal to the diffusivity in the tissue interstitial space multiplied by the tissue fractional interstitial space, which is available to the solute.

A number of observations may be made about equation (2). First, the effective diffusivity, capillary permeability and capillary surface area enter as their square root so that doubling of the capillary permeability, for example, would be expected to be associated with only a 41% increase in mass transfer ($2^{1/2} = 1.41$); second, the net transport rate is proportional to the superficial area of the tissue; and, third, the rate of transport is proportional to the difference in the free concentration of solute between the peritoneal fluid and blood.

Equation (2) serves as the basis for the definition of an equivalent 'permeability' P_V of the tissue. If there were a thin membrane separating the peritoneal fluid from the blood, the rate of uptake would be given by

$$S_V = P_V A_V (C_P - C_B) \tag{3}$$

Comparison of equations (2) and (3) shows that the equivalent tissue permeability can be calculated from

$$P_V = \sqrt{D_V (p_V a_V)} \tag{4}$$

Either equation (2) or (3) can be used to calculate the rate of absorption of a drug from the peritoneal cavity into the blood as they are exactly equivalent. The spatially distributed view of the tissue offers certain advantages because it provides some insight into the underlying transport mechanisms and how these might be altered by pathological processes or pharmacological manipulations. It also serves as a natural link to the very large body of literature on capillary physiology, and provides a natural framework to incorporate this into descriptions and predictions of peritoneal transport rates. Further, it explicitly predicts that a concentration profile extends a finite depth into the tissue, and tissue penetration is an important consideration if the goal of i.p. therapy is to treat disease in the tissue or disease of finite thickness such as peritoneal carcino-

matosis on serosal surfaces. Explicitly, the concentration profile is given by:

$$\frac{C - C_B}{C_P - C_B} = \exp - \sqrt{\frac{p_V a_V}{D_V}} \, x \tag{5}$$

where x is the distance from the serosal surface.

Equations similar to (2) and (3) can be written for as many types of peritoneal tissue as desirable. Since uptake rates into the various tissue types are parallel processes, they may be summed to provide:

$$S = [(PA_L) + (P_V A_V) + (P_A A_A) \\ + (P_D A_D)](C_P - C_B) \tag{6}$$

with the subscripts defined in Fig. 2.

Equation (6) is usually given simply as:

$$S = (PA)(C_P - C_B) \tag{7}$$

where PA is the mass transfer coefficient which incorporates all absorbing structures in contact with peritoneal fluid. The PA product is a single parameter defined as the sum of the individual tissue PA values as indicated by comparison of equations (6) and (7).

The 'A' should not, in general, be equated to the topological surface area of the peritoneum but to the area in contact with the dialysis fluid contained in the cavity. Chagnac and colleagues recently developed a new technique which utilizes stereological methods combined with computerized tomography scanning of the peritoneal cavity filled with dialysate containing contrast fluid [63], and their determinations in three patients produced a mean value for A of 0.58 m². This is less than the conservative estimate of 0.8 m² in Table 1 or the determinations of dissected tissue area which approach the total body area [64].

Estimation of parameters dependent on molecular weight

It is instructive to examine the magnitudes of some of the parameters that have been discussed above in order to place them in quantitative perspective.

Variation of PA with molecular weight

The value of PA has been studied extensively because of its importance to peritoneal dialysis. Therefore, our best data exist for the common indicators of azotaemia and physiological markers that have been measured in this context. Figure 3 shows some values of PA plotted against molecular weight [65].

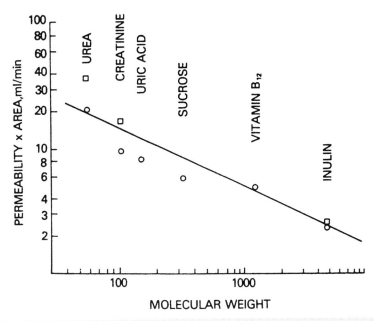

Figure 3. Peritoneal permeability times area (or mass-transfer-area coefficient) versus molecular weight. See text for a complete discussion. From ref. 65.

The data vary approximately as the inverse of the square root of molecular weight. This would be expected from the penetration model if the capillary permeability varies with the -0.63 power of molecular weight (Fig. 4) and the diffusivity in tissue varies with the -0.45 power of molecular weight observed for diffusion in water [62]. From this correlation, PA for sucrose would equal 8.5 ml/min; the PA for inulin would be 2.8 ml/min. Rubin [3] measured a mass-transfer-area coefficient (MTAC, a parameter equivalent to PA) for inulin to be 3.3 ml/min in humans. However, the convective component of blood-to-peritoneal cavity transport has probably been included in Rubin's calculation [3], and this would produce a higher estimate than that due to diffusion alone. Values for the IgG PA have been estimated by Rippe [66] to be 0.05 ml/min, and by Krediet *et al.* [67] to be on the order of 0.04 ml/min.

Variation of PA with body size

Figure 5 shows the PA product for urea and inulin for the rat, rabbit, dog and human; these species cover a body-weight range from 200 g to 70 kg [23]. The parameter increases as the 0.62–0.74 power of body weight for inulin and urea, respectively. The average of these two values is very close to the 2/3 expected for body-surface-area scaling. We note that Keshaviah and colleagues [68] demonstrated a linear correlation between the volume at which PA was maximum and the body surface area in a study

of 10 patients with body surface areas ranging from 1.4 to 2.3 m^2. Since the characteristic time for absorption from the peritoneal cavity is equal to V_p/ PA, similar time scales can be achieved in humans and experimental animals if the volume is scaled as the 2/3 power of the body weight. For example, 2 L in the peritoneal cavity of the 70 kg human patient (29 ml/kg) would be equivalent to 40 ml in a 200 g rat (200 ml/kg) because $(200/70\,000)^{2/3}(2000) = 40$. These scaling criteria permit the design of experiments which more accurately reflect in small animals dialysis which is carried out in humans.

Areas for transport

The peritoneal surface area of the adult human has been estimated to be of the order of 8000 to 10 000 cm^2 [34, 35]. Of this value, the surface of the liver constitutes about 6–13% (range of averages from the two references), the diaphragm 4–8%, the peritoneal walls 11% (anterior abdominal wall 7%). Corresponding percentages for the 595 cm^2 surface area of the adult rat were: liver, 16%; diaphragm, 3%; peritoneal walls, 19% [34]. From equation (2) the rate of transfer is directly dependent on the actual area in contact with the dialysis fluid. In studies with chambers which isolated specific areas on the rat peritoneum [69], the P-values for different surfaces were determined as well as the dissected areas (presumed to equal the maximum area available to the dialysis fluid) of the entire

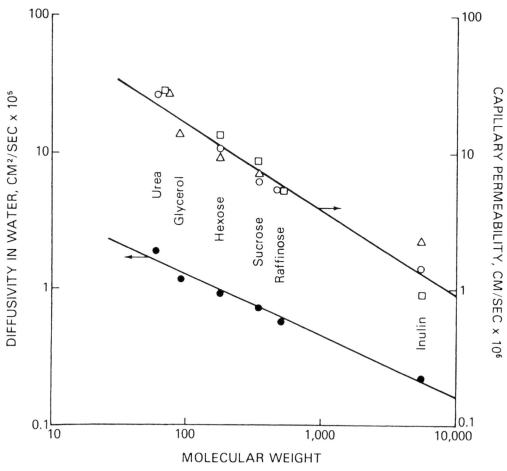

Figure 4. Capillary permeability versus molecular weight (right axis) and diffusivity in water versus molecular weight (left axis). Adapted from ref. 62.

peritoneum. When the values for P were multiplied times the corresponding dissected areas and summed, the resulting number was three to four times the PA obtained with a volume corresponding to 2000 ml in a human (40–50 ml in 200 to 300 g rats, see previous subsection). Separate animals were dialysed with solution containing an intensely staining dye in order to detect which surfaces were in contact with the fluid. Significant parts of the peritoneum had no staining, including one side of the caecum, one side of the stomach, and large parts of the abdominal wall and diaphragm. Levitt and colleagues [70] measured the rate of transport of urea, creatinine, and glucose in rats at rest or agitated with an orbital shaker and found a fourfold increase in PA. Others [71] found similar results to Levitt in analogous studies. With the assumption that the experimental manoeuvres to increase the PA do not change P, these studies all imply that only 25–30% of the anatomical peritoneum is available to the

dialysis solution during quiescent conditions. The single study in humans [63], from which the wetted area in three patients was estimated to be 0.6 m², would appear to agree with the principle that the wetted area is significantly less than that of the dissected area.

The wetted area is also dependent on the volume in the cavity and the body size (see above). Keshaviah and colleagues [68] carried out a study in 10 patients in which the PA values for urea, creatinine, and glucose were determined for different dwell volumes varying from 500 to 3000 ml. They found a nearly linear relationship between MTAC and dialysate volume until a peak at 2500–3000 ml of 'true dialysate volume'. While there was no way to separate P from A, the authors attributed the correlation to an increase in A with increasing peritoneal volume.

As reviewed recently [72] studies adequate to define the difference between the functional surface

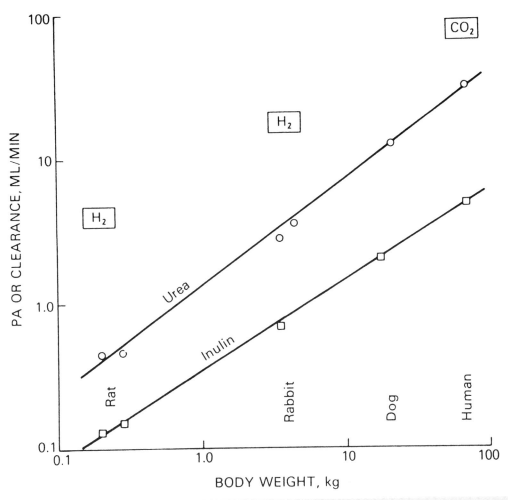

Figure 5. Peritoneal permeability times area (or mass-transfer-area coefficient) for the indicated gases, urea, and inulin versus body weight. From ref. 62.

area and the anatomical surface area in human subjects have not been conducted. Further, clinically applicable techniques to substantially increase the functional surface area and better expose targeted disease on serosal surfaces have not been persuasive. A recent trial was conducted of continuous hyperthermic peritoneal perfusion (CHPP) with carboplatin (CBDCA) in six patients with small-volume residual ovarian cancer [73]. Pharmacokinetic data adequate to calculate PA were obtained from five of these. Even if we exclude one patient who probably had an artifactually high PA because of extensive fluid absorption, the average value of PA was 42 ml/min. This is approximately four times the value expected from published studies of conventional intraperitoneal CBDCA administration, consistent with the laboratory studies described above. The CHPP involved rapid recirculation (1.5 L/min) of drug-containing solution through the peritoneal

cavity by means of a two-catheter system combined with vigorous manual shaking of the abdomen. Temperature uniformity was documented with three probes. While an important effect of the elevated temperature on transport was not definitively excluded, the authors argued that elevated temperature alone was unlikely to be the cause of the large increase in PA.

Role of capillary permeability

Figure 3 shows that the PA product for a 250-dalton hydrophilic drug in a human would be expected to be about 10 ml/min. If the peritoneal surface area is approximately 6000 cm^2, as discussed above, then the average equivalent peritoneal permeability would be 1.7×10^{-3} cm/min. Figure 4 shows that the intrinsic permeability, p, of mammalian muscle capillaries is 10^{-5} cm/s or 0.6×10^{-3} cm/min. This remarkable similarity is probably fortuitous. Peritoneal transport appears to derive its selectivity partly from the properties of the capillaries shown in equation (4).

Regional permeabilities

Experiments to determine values for P for specific tissues require isolation of the transport process to a specific area of the tissue. To do this, experiments were carried out in anaesthetized rats, whose peritoneum was exposed surgically by laparotomy. Plastic chambers were glued to portions of the peritoneum overlying the liver, caecum, stomach, and abdominal wall.

The chamber was filled with an isotonic solution, which could be sampled during the experiment, and the volume of which could be determined. Labelled mannitol was infused continuously i.v. or was mixed with the solution in the chamber. By measuring the volume in the chamber and the mannitol concentration versus time, the rate of appearance of mannitol into the chamber, or the rate of disappearance from the chamber, could be calculated. By determining the mannitol concentration in the plasma, and after substituting the chamber concentration and area of the base of the chamber for C_P and A_V in equation (3), P could be calculated. The results demonstrated that there was no significant difference among the four tissues and no dependence on the direction of transport (overall average = $2.14 \pm 0.37 \times 10^{-3}$ cm/min) [69]. Similar results have been found for urea [74]. While the equivalence of transport directions (peritoneal cavity to blood and blood to peritoneal cavity) was expected, the equivalence of transport across the surface of diverse tissues was not. Subsequent studies of the tissue concentration profiles of these substances have demonstrated very similar results in each tissue (unpublished observations). If it is assumed that the human peritoneum is similar in its physiological properties to the rat, then these data justify the lumping of the surfaces together into one PA. They also imply that the critical variable in determination of PA is the area which is in contact with the solution in the cavity.

The transport of large proteins, such as IgG, is dominated chiefly by convection or solvent drag from the cavity [31, 33]. Once in the tissue they are removed by lymphatic flow. Table 1, therefore, lists values for L/F for each tissue. These suggest that the transport of protein from the cavity to the blood may be limited by its transport from the cavity to

the tissue space in the diaphragm, viscera, and the liver, which contain extensive lymphatic systems. On the other hand, transport of protein from the cavity via the abdominal wall interstitium is limited by the lymphatic flow.

Lipid solubility

Increasing lipid solubility increases the rate of transfer of a drug from the cavity into the surrounding tissue and the blood. Torres *et al.* [75] measured the absorption of model compounds dissolved in 50 ml of saline in the rat. They found that as the heptane–water partition coefficient (K_{hep}) increased above 0.001, the rate of absorption increased significantly. Barbital with a K_{hep} of 0.001 was found to have an absorption of 57% at the end of 1 h. On the other hand, thiopental, with a K_{hep} of 3.3, had an absorption of 96% at the end of 1 h. Subsequent studies with the lipid-soluble drugs hexamethylmelamine in the mouse [76] and thioTEPA in human subjects [77] have shown peritoneal clearances about an order of magnitude greater than would be expected for hydrophilic drugs. Unfortunately, capillary permeabilities and tissue diffusivities are not available for these compounds.

Blood flow

Estimates of the effective blood flow surrounding the peritoneal cavity suggest that transport between the blood and the cavity is not limited by the supply of blood. Physiologists have attempted to estimate the 'effective' blood flow by measuring the clearances of various gases from the peritoneal cavity, assuming that these were limited by blood flow only. Gas clearances of hydrogen [78, 79] and CO_2 [80] have been determined in small mammals and found to be equal to 4–7% of the cardiac output. However, this method of determining the effective peritoneal blood flow may actually underestimate the true blood flow. Collins [81], who studied absorption of several inert gases from peritoneal gas pockets in pigs, found almost a three-fold range in clearance which correlated with the gas diffusivity in water. If the transport of these gases was limited by blood flow, the clearance of each gas would have been the same. The results imply that the transport of these gases is not limited by blood flow but by resistance to diffusion in the tissue. Gas clearance data therefore underestimate the true peritoneal blood flow, and the conclusion, based on lumped clearance data, would be that blood flow limitation in the peritoneal cavity is unlikely.

The lumped clearance argument, however, does not rule out specific limitations in a portion of the peritoneal cavity, which may be offset by another set of tissues. To investigate the possibility of blood flow limitation of transport across specific surfaces of the peritoneum, the chamber technique (discussed in the section entitled 'Regional permeabilities') was utilized to answer the question of 'local' limitations of blood flow on urea (which should diffuse rapidly due to its small molecular weight and which would be more likely to demonstrate blood flow limitations) transport across the liver, stomach, caecum, and abdominal wall. The mass transfer rates of urea were determined under conditions of: control blood flow, blood flow reduced by 50–80%, and no blood flow (postmortem); the blood flow was monitored simultaneously with laser Doppler flowmetry. While all four tissues showed marked decreases in urea transport after cessation of blood flow, only the liver displayed a decrease in the rate of transfer during periods of reduced blood flow. Further studies with the chamber technique tested the effects of blood flow on osmotically induced water flow from the same four tissues; results demonstrated statistically non-significant decreases in water flow in the caecum, stomach, and abdominal wall [82]. Analogous to the solute data, the liver demonstrated a significant drop in water transfer with reduced blood flow. Thus transport of both solute and water across the surface of the liver is limited by blood flow. Zakaria and co-workers [83] have shown in rats that the liver is responsible for only a very small amount of the actual area of transfer; this implies that a drop in blood flow to the liver would have minimal effects on overall transperitoneal transport. These data support and extend earlier studies of peritoneal dialysis in dogs during conditions of shock [84] and support the use of the technique for solute or fluid removal during periods of low systemic blood pressure and the probable low blood perfusion of the organs surrounding the peritoneal cavity.

Pharmacokinetic advantage: theory

If a drug is infused at a constant rate into a fixed volume of fluid in the peritoneal cavity until steady state is achieved, then a regional advantage will be observed:

$$R_{i.p.} = (C_P/C_B)_{i.p.} \qquad (8)$$

Similarly, if the drug is infused at a constant rate intravenously with the same fixed i.p. volume of fluid, then the corresponding concentration ratio may be defined

$$R_{i.v.} = (C_P/C_B)_{i.v.} \qquad (9)$$

The pharmacokinetic advantage R_d is defined as the ratio:

$$R_d = R_{i.p.}/R_{i.v.} \qquad (10)$$

Conceptually, R_d expresses the relative advantage that may be achieved by administration of a drug directly into the peritoneal cavity compared with i.v. administration. It has been shown [23] that the pharmacokinetic advantage may be expressed as a remarkably simple equation if there is no elimination of the drug from the peritoneal region:

$$R_d = 1 + CL_{TB}/PA \qquad (11)$$

where CL_{TB} = total body clearance (cm^3/min). The same equation may be used for drug that is not administered by continuous infusion to steady state if the exposure terms are defined as the areas under the peritoneal and plasma concentration curves (AUC$_P$ and AUC$_B$) following any schedule of administration if the system is linear in the sense that none of the relevant parameters change with drug concentration or time.

Equation (11) indicates a large pharmacokinetic advantage for most hydrophilic drugs administered to the peritoneal cavity. For example, a typical antibiotic would be expected to have a PA of the order of 10 ml/min (Fig. 3). If the drug is cleared from the body by glomerular filtration at the rate of inulin, 125 ml/min [85], then the expected value of R_d is approximately 14.

Many drugs are eliminated by tissues within the peritoneal cavity, particularly the liver. This provides a first-pass effect which has the effect of increasing the natural pharmacokinetic advantage given by equation (11). The regional advantage expected in the presence of some extraction of the drug by liver may be obtained from Dedrick [23]:

$$R_{i.p.} = \frac{1 + \dfrac{CL_{TB}}{PA}}{1 - fE} \qquad (12)$$

where f = the fraction of the absorbed drug that enters the liver through the portal system or by direct absorption into its surface, and E = the fraction of that drug which is removed by the liver on a single pass. The quantity $(1 - fE)$ is the fraction of the absorbed drug that reaches the systemic circulation. If this fraction is small, then the natural advantage to regional administration can be considerably enhanced.

We do not have adequate information on the value of f. It is generally thought that small molecular weight compounds are absorbed primarily through the portal system [86]; however, there is evidence that some significant fraction of the absorbed drug can bypass the liver [11]. In the Speyer study, concentrations of 5-fluorouracil were observed to be higher in a peripheral artery than in the hepatic vein in three of four patients. Calculation of f was not reliable because analysis of the data depended upon knowledge of the blood flows in the portal vein and drug metabolism by gastrointestinal tissues, and these were not measured. The fact that about 15–20% of the peritoneal surface area covers tissues which are not portal to the liver is consistent with the transport observations.

Application of model to evaluation of the pharmacokinetic advantage

Antineoplastic agents

The pharmacokinetic rationale for the i.p. administration of drugs in the treatment of microscopic residual ovarian cancer was described in 1978 [65]. The procedure has been the subject of numerous preclinical and clinical studies during subsequent years, and these have been reviewed periodically [87–89]. The pharmacokinetic theory has been consistently validated, and there is clear evidence of response in terms of surgically staged complete remissions in a number of studies. Markman *et al.* [17] reviewed several of these and concluded that there may be an advantage to regional drug delivery of cisplatin-based therapy for small-volume refractory residual ovarian cancer. Subsequently, Markman *et al.* [90] concluded that attainment of a surgically staged complete remission may have a favourable impact on survival. Recently, Muggia *et al.* [21] demonstrated substantial activity with i.p. floxuridine (FUDR). However, the role of i.p. drug therapy in the management of abdominal cancer remains controversial [91].

One randomized prospective clinical trial established increased activity by i.p. drug administration [92]. This was the cooperative Southwest Oncology Group (SWOG) and Gynecologic Oncology Group (GOG) trial of cyclophosphamide and cisplatin for the treatment of patients with optimal stage III ovarian cancer. In this trial the only difference was the route of administration of the cisplatin: i.v. compared with i.p. The cyclophosphamide was administered intravenously in both groups. The i.p. group showed a clear survival advantage (hazard ratio 0.76). Remarkably, the i.p. group also experienced less tinnitus, clinical hearing loss, neutropenia and neuromuscular toxicity. There is a need for additional properly designed trials to define the activity of new agents, other combinations and the characteristics of the patient populations which would be most likely to benefit from regional therapy.

While the place of i.p. drug administration in cancer chemotherapy has not been adequately defined, some important pharmacological principles have been explored during the investigation of antineoplastic agents. Some of these principles are illustrated by a discussion of two specific drugs: *cis*-diamminedichloroplatinum(II) (cisplatin) and 5-fluorouracil (5-FU). At issue are both the pharmacology of intracavitary administration and the depth of penetration of drug into both normal and neoplastic tissues.

Cisplatin

Cisplatin is among the most active agents used in the treatment of ovarian cancer. Its pharmacokinetics have been studied extensively, and a physiological model has been developed and applied to several species [93–95]. Briefly, the drug reacts with both small and large molecular weight nucleophiles in plasma and tissue compartments. The tissue-specific rate constants vary among the tissues but are relatively constant across species. Release of (presumably inactive) platinum from macromolecules is dominated by their catabolism.

Goel *et al.* [96] studied the i.p. administration of cisplatin in combination with etoposide, and examined the effect of concurrent administration of sodium thiosulphate to protect the kidney against platinum toxicity. They administered the drug combination in 2 L of normal saline and observed a cisplatin clearance from the peritoneal cavity of 15 ml/min and a clearance from the plasma of 329 ml/min. These clearances resulted in a regional advantage (AUC_P/AUC_B) of 26 in those patients who did not receive sodium thiosulphate. This advantage is similar to the value of 16 obtained by Piccart *et al.* [97] for cisplatin administered in combination with melphalan.

Los *et al.* [98] conducted pharmacokinetic studies of cisplatin in rats bearing CC531 colonic adenocarcinoma on serosal surfaces of the peritoneal cavity in order to determine the effect of route of administration on tumour and normal tissue levels of platinum. The AUC_B was approximately the same following both i.v. and i.p. administration, while the regional advantage was 7.6 based on ultrafiltered plasma and peritoneal fluid. Clearance from the peritoneal cavity may be calculated from their data to be 0.42 ml/min for a 200 g rat. The rat clearance is thus predictive of the human values on the basis of body weight to the 2/3 power in general agreement with the allometric variation in Fig. 5.

Average tumour levels of platinum in the i.p. group were twice those in the i.v. group; however, the excess platinum was confined to the periphery of the tumour. Measurements of platinum concentrations by proton-induced X-ray emission (PIXE) showed substantially higher levels in the outer 1.0 mm of the tumour; concentrations at 1.5 and 2.2 mm from the surface were independent of route of administration of the drug. This limited penetration is consistent with theoretical calculations for hexose [62] and experimental data for [^{14}C]EDTA [99] in normal tissues. It is instructive to apply a penetration model to cisplatin. As a rough approximation, let us assume that the diffusivity in tissue, D, is 1.9×10^{-6} cm^2/s based on transport in brain [100]; that the capillary pa product is of the order of 1.4×10^{-3} s^{-1} based on hexose in jejunum; and that the tissue-specific reaction rate, k, is 8×10^{-5} s^{-1} based on muscle [94]. Then the nominal diffusion distance $[D/(pa+k)]^{1/2}$ is 0.4 mm, which would imply that 9/10 of the gradient would be confined to the first millimetre from the surface of the tissue. While these calculations are provided for illustrative purposes, and are very approximate, they are almost certainly much better that order-of-magnitude. They support the idea that direct diffusion of cisplatin into tissue is very limited in extent.

The above reaction ($k = 8 \times 10^{-5}$ s^{-1}) and permeability (1.4×10^{-3} s^{-1}) parameters predict that $[1.4 \times 10^{-5}/(1.4 \times 10^{-3} + 8 \times 10^{-5})](100) = 95\%$ of the drug would be expected to be absorbed into the systemic circulation. This large bioavailability is consistent with the observations of Los *et al.* [98] in the tumour-bearing rat and of Pretorius *et al.* [101] in the dog, as well as with considerable human experience.

5-Fluorouracil

As discussed by Chabner [102], phosphorylation of 5-FU to nucleotide analogues appears necessary for its subsequent biological effects. Elimination from the body is primarily by metabolism believed to require reduction of the pyrimidine ring by dihydrouracil dehydrogenase. This enzyme is present in both the liver and other tissues such as the gastrointestinal mucosa. 5-FU exhibits strongly non-linear elimination in human subjects with a half-saturating concentration of 15 µM as reviewed and discussed in the development of a physiological pharmacokinetic model [103]. Further, the observation of total-body clearances at low infusion rates that considerably exceed expected hepatic blood flow suggests the presence of extensive extrahepatic metabolism.

5-FU has pharmacological properties which commended it to i.p. trials in the treatment of intraabdominal cancer. It is a hydrophilic drug with a molecular weight of 130 daltons which would be expected to have a relatively slow clearance from the peritoneal cavity (Fig. 3) and a total-body clearance ranging from 0.94 L/min at an infusion rate of 134 mg/kg/day to as high as 4–7 L/min at infusion rates of 10–30 mg/kg/day [103]. In addition to the high ratio of CL_{TB} to predicted PA, significant removal of the drug by peritoneal tissues would be expected to further limit systemic exposure.

The prediction of a high regional advantage has been shown in a number of clinical trials. Values of the AUC ratio between peritoneal cavity and plasma have been reported to be strongly dose-dependent, ranging from 124 at a dose of 3.5 mmol/L to 461 at a dose of 2.0 mM [15]. These are in general agreement with the observations of Speyer *et al.* [10], who observed peritoneal-to-plasma concentration ratios of 298 at 4 h and of Sugarbaker *et al.* [104] who reported a mean AUC ratio of 200 in patients administered 5-FU in the immediate postoperative period. Clearance from the peritoneal cavity has been in good agreement with the predictions from Fig. 3: 14 ml/min [10] and 24 ml/min [15]. Non-linearity in systemic exposure deriving from the saturable metabolism (and possible saturable first-pass effect) of the agent was associated with an extraordinarily steep dose–response curve [10].

There has been considerable interest in the detailed mechanism of absorption of 5-FU from the peritoneal cavity because of the possibility of using this route as a way to perfuse the liver through the portal vein. Speyer *et al.* [11] placed catheters in the portal vein, hepatic vein, peripheral artery and peripheral vein of human patients. The hepatic extraction was calculated to decrease slightly from about 0.7 to 0.6 from the first to the seventh exchange. The estimated value of the fraction, f, of the absorbed drug entering the portal system was strongly dependent on assumptions relating to the blood flow rate in the portal vein and metabolism by tissues draining into the portal system, neither of which was directly assessed. Estimated values of f ranged from 0.3 to 1 depending on the assumptions made. There was direct evidence of drug bypassing the portal system in three of the four patients in whom the AUC in the peripheral artery actually exceeded the AUC in the hepatic vein. In studies in rats, Archer *et al.* [105] observed that systemic 5-FU levels were significantly lower during mesenteric vein infusion ($0.9 \pm 0.2 \, \mu M$) compared with i.p. infusion at the same rate ($2.1 \pm 0.3 \, \mu M$).

Indirect evidence of a pharmacological first-pass effect is provided by the observations of Gianola *et al.* [106], who were able to administer a mean of 1.5 g per treatment cycle intraperitoneally but only 1.0 g intravenously; the i.p. route was actually accompanied by less haematological toxicity.

Penetration of 5-FU into tissues surrounding the peritoneal cavity has not been studied experimentally. Collins *et al.* [107] observed a strongly concentration-dependent rate of 5-FU disappearance from the peritoneal cavity of the rat. The peritoneal clearance increased from 0.20 ml/min, consistent with its molecular weight, to 10 times that value as the peritoneal concentration was decreased from 10 mM to 20 μM. This was explained by assuming that the drug is metabolized in tissues adjacent to the peritoneal cavity. A one-dimensional diffusion model with saturable intratissue metabolism ($V_{max} = 36 \, nmol/min/g$, $K_M = 5 \, \mu M$) simulated the peritoneal concentrations reasonably well. The model predicted that the concentration in the tissue would be 10% of its value at the tissue surface at a depth of 0.6 mm following a 12 mM dose; the corresponding 10% level would be reached at only 0.13 mm following a 24 μM dose. Observations that the toxicity profile associated with i.p. administration is similar to that observed following i.v. administration [10, 106] seem to confirm limited tissue penetration. If the drug reached the gastrointestinal crypt cells in high concentration, one would expect substantial toxicity there.

Antibiotics: vancomycin

Intraperitoneal antibiotic therapy is used to treat localized peritonitis. The goal of such therapy is the same as that of antineoplastic agents: to maximize the concentration in the cavity in order to target the superficial tissues in the peritoneal cavity. Since the subject of i.p. antibiotic therapy has been covered thoroughly in another chapter of this text, we will illustrate the general approach to calculation of the regional pharmacokinetic advantage by application of the theory to vancomycin, a drug which is currently one of the recommended therapies for i.p. infections due to Gram-positive organisms which are resistant to cephalosporins and penicillins [8].

Vancomycin has a molecular weight of 1500; 55% of the drug is bound to serum protein [108–110]. Its volume of distribution is variable and is cited over a range of 0.64 L/kg in normal young humans [108] to 0.93 L/kg in the elderly [108, 109]. Patients with renal failure (creatinine clearance less than 10 ml/min) have volumes of distribution averaging 0.9 L/kg [103]. The serum half-life of vancomycin is typically 6 h. However, since 90% of the injected dose is excreted by the kidney [111, 112], the normal half-life of 6 h becomes markedly prolonged in renal failure. Clearance of the drug in a normal (70 kg) patient is 100–140 ml/min. In the patient with renal failure the clearance is correlated with iothalamate, a marker for glomerular filtration rate [111]. Typical clearance rates for patients with creatinine clearance less than 10 ml/min average approximately 5 ml/min [110, 113].

The overall PA estimated from Fig. 3 is 4.0 ml/min. For the purpose of illustration let us assume that the overall clearance from the body of our patient on peritoneal dialysis is 5 ml/min and that the drug is given by continuous infusion. Under these circumstances the relative advantage of i.p. administration relative to i.v. administration is calculated from equation (11) modified to account for protein binding: $R_d = 1 + 5/(4.0 \times 0.45) = 3.8$.

Because of the long half-life and the toxicity of high serum levels which might result if continuous infusion were performed [109], the drug is usually given in either a single i.p. dialysate dwell every 24 h or as an i.v. infusion approximately once a week. Bunke *et al.* [114] studied vancomycin pharmacokinetics by dosing patients with either 10 mg/kg i.v. in a saline solution over 30 min or 10 mg/kg diluted in 2 L of 1.5% dextrose dialysate, which was allowed to dwell over 4 h. By computing the AUC_P/AUC_B for i.p. delivery during the first 24 h, the regional advantage ($R_{i.p.}$) is $429/109 = 3.9$. Repeating the same for i.v. delivery, the AUC_P/AUC_B ($R_{i.v.}$) is $78.4/297 = 0.26$. The pharmacokinetic advantage would then be $R_{i.p.}/R_{i.v.} = 3.9/0.26 = 15$. This provides a strong theoretical and experimental argument for i.p. vancomycin in appropriate cases of peritonitis.

Intraperitoneal insulin

Human insulin is a small protein with a molecular weight of 5808, which is secreted by the beta cells of the pancreatic islets of Langerhans in response to a glucose load in the plasma [115]. The secretion occurs directly into blood which circulates via the portal vein to the liver. The bulk of the hormone in the blood is in the unbound form [116]. Extraction of the hormone by the liver is receptor-mediated, saturable, and typically amounts to 40–60% of the drug delivered in the portal system [117]. After entering the general circulation, insulin distributes to the entire extracellular space [118]. In particular insulin circulates to the kidney and muscle, which, aside from the liver, are its other major targets. Under normal conditions there is a portal-to-peripheral insulin concentration gradient, with the highest concentrations in the liver [116]. In an effort to control diabetic hyperglycaemia in a more physiological way, replacement insulin is increasingly being administered intraperitoneally in order to mimic the normal physiology [117, 118].

Insulin is often administered dissolved in the dialysate to diabetic patients who suffer from ESRD and are treated with CAPD [119]. This results in the simultaneous transfer of insulin and dextrose from the cavity into the body and generally results in stable levels of blood glucose and insulin, which are below the corresponding levels with subcutaneous insulin [120]. Because of the extensive extraction by the liver, equation (12) must be used in order to predict the regional advantage of i.p. insulin therapy. Rubin [3] has shown that the transport properties of insulin (mass-transfer-area coefficient or MTAC = 2.9 ml/min) are nearly identical to those of inulin (MTAC = 3.3 ml/min). Because of similar molecular size, parameters for inulin are typically substituted for those of insulin. Transport is probably highest across the surfaces of the liver and of other viscera because their combined surface area makes up 60–65% of the total peritoneal area. In equation (12), assume that $f = 0.9$ and $E = 0.5$ and the PA_{tot} from Fig. 3 is 2.3 ml/min. While the normal total body clearance of insulin is typically 650–750 ml/min (referenced to 1.73 m^2), the clearance of [125I]insulin is approximately half or 350 ml/min in chronic renal failure [121, 122]. The regional advantage can be calculated from equation (12): $R_R = [1 + 350/2.3]/(1 - 0.9(0.5)) = 278$. The

measured ratio of intraperitoneally administered [125I]insulin (AUC_P/AUC_B) was approximately 500 in dogs [119] and the value was 200–300 in humans [123].

Recent efforts in insulin replacement therapy for patients who suffer from diabetes mellitus, but who are not on dialysis, have tested i.p. administration as a more physiological method of drug delivery [118]. In a study which compared free insulin peaks after i.m., s.c., and i.p. injections, i.p. insulin produced serum insulin peaks at 15 min, while i.m. and s.c. insulin resulted in a much slower increase with peaks at 60 and 90 min, respectively [124]. The rapid rise in serum insulin, produced by i.p. administration, followed by a gradual fall in concentration, more closely mimics the true pancreas. The same study demonstrated that insulin delivered to the upper part of the peritoneal cavity was more quickly absorbed than insulin introduced into the lower part of the cavity. This is probably due to the rapid transfer into tissues of the gastrointestinal tract and direct diffusion into the liver. Delivery into the cavity by a pump has also led to more consistent serum levels than with administration into s.c. tissue, which produces variability in absorption rates [125].

In contrast to the relatively steady delivery of i.p. insulin in CAPD, this i.p. delivery therapy is typically given episodically in small volumes in the upper part of the cavity. The ratio of portal to systemic venous levels of insulin (AUC_{portal}/AUC_B) can give us a rough estimate of the utility of the delivery technique. It should be pointed out that the concentration in the portal vein probably reflects only a portion of the insulin delivered to the liver, since direct absorption across the surface of the liver is known to occur [126]. Selam et al. [127] have demonstrated in dogs that the ratio of i.p. insulin delivery to the portal vein over the amount appearing in the plasma is 17. This supports the concept of i.p. delivery of insulin in order to re-establish a more normal portal-to-peripheral insulin concentration gradient.

Intraperitoneal antibody therapy

An alternative to the typical antineoplastic agent in cancer therapy is the use of i.p.-administered monoclonal antibodies (Mab) in the treatment of intra-abdominal cancers. These antibodies, which are typically linked to some toxic agent, react specifically with antigens on the tumour cell and bind strongly, with subsequent killing of the cell [128].

As outlined in Dedrick and Flessner [129] the general equation for the calculation of the pharmacokinetic advantage is the same as that for small substances (see equation (11)). The PA for immunoglobulin has been estimated from pore theory to be 0.05 ml/min [67]. The total-body clearance of IgG has been estimated to be 0.5–1.0 ml/min [129]. Inserting this into equation (11), one may calculate a R_d of 17–33. This suggests a considerable pharmacokinetic advantage in i.p. administration of monoclonal antibody.

The usefulness of this therapy must also be assessed in terms of the ultimate goal. Free ascites cells are readily accessible to MAbs [130]; in this case the R_d would be the number calculated by equation (11). Unlike smaller molecules, however, large proteins do not penetrate tissues readily. Because of their large size (molecular radius = 52 Å), the effective diffusivity in tissue is on the order of 10^{-7}–10^{-9} cm^2/s [131–133]. Since this is two orders of magnitude less than the diffusivity of small molecules, the diffusive transport of macromolecules such as IgG within normal or neoplastic tissue is very slow. Recent mathematical analyses have also shown that MAbs with high affinity to their antigens are even more severely retarded by the 'binding-site barrier' [131, 134–136]. The transport of these molecules is typically dominated by convection, both within the interstitial space [137, 138] and across capillary endothelium [139]. Tissue penetration studies of antibodies administered i.p. in animals [33, 133] have shown that most of the IgG is contained in the initial 300–400 μm of tissue during the first 3 h. These studies also demonstrated that diffusion probably plays only a minor role in the transport of the protein. Studies in tumour-bearing animals confirm these findings, and have not demonstrated large advantages of i.p. MAb administration over i.v. administration [130, 140]. This means that there may be limitations in the treatment of solid tumours and metastases with MAbs or other macromolecules.

Summary

Intraperitoneal chemotherapy should be considered as an alternative to i.v. therapy when the target is contained within the peritoneal cavity or within the adjacent tissue. The distributed model concept has been used to formulate a mathematical scheme in order to evaluate the solute transport to specific tissue groups surrounding the cavity. With parameters derived from the literature, the model can be used to solve for the steady-state concentrations in the peritoneal cavity and the plasma. The ratio of these two concentrations defines the regional advantage of i.p. therapy. Several applications of the theory are presented in order to illustrate the method in which a new i.p. therapy may be evaluated prior to use in patients.

References

1. Cole WCC, Montgomery JC. Intraperitoneal blood transfusion. Amer J Dis Child 1929; 37: 497–510.
2. Clausen J. Studies on the effects of intraperitoneal blood transfusion. Acta Paediatr, Stockholm 1940; 27: 24–31.
3. Rubin JA, Reed V, Adair C, Bower J, Klein E. Effect of intraperitoneal insulin on solute kinetics in CAPD: insulin kinetics in CAPD. Am J Med Sci 1986; 291: 81–7.
4. Pitt HA, Saudek CD, Zacur HA. Long-term intraperitoneal insulin delivery. Ann Surg 1992; 216: 483–92.
5. Bargman JM, Jones JE, Petro JM. The pharmacokinetics of intraperitoneal erythropoietin administered undiluted and diluted in dilaysate. Perit Dial Int 1992; 12: 369–72.
6. Reddingius RE, de Boer AW, Scroder CH, Willems JL, Monnens LAH. Increase of the bioavailability of intraperitoneal erythropoietin in children on peritoneal dialysis by administration in small dialysis bags. Perit Dial Int 1997; 17: 467–70.
7. Hirszel P, Lameire N, Bogaert M. Pharmacologic alterations of peritoneal transport rates and pharmacokinetics of the peritoneum. In: Gokal R, Nolph KD, eds. The Textbook of Peritoneal Dialysis. Dordrecht: Kluwer, 1994, pp. 161–232.
8. Keane WF, Alexander SR, Bailie GR et al. Peritoneal dialysis-related peritonitis treatment recommendations: 1996 update. Perit Dial Int 1996; 16: 557–73.
9. Jones RB, Myers CE, Guarino AM, Dedrick RL, Hubbard SM, DeVita VT. High volume intraperitoneal chemotherapy ('Belly Bath') for ovarian cancer. Cancer Chemother Pharm 1978; 1: 161–6.
10. Speyer JL, Collins JM, Dedrick RL et al. Phase I and pharmacological studies of 5-fluorouracil administered intraperitoneally. Canc Res 1980; 40: 567–72.
11. Speyer JL, Sugarbaker PH, Collins JM, Dedrick RL, Klecker RW, Jr, Myers CE. Portal levels and hepatic clearance of 5-fluorouracil after intraperitoneal administration in humans. Cancer Res 1981; 41: 1916–22.
12. Markman M. Intraperitoneal therapy for ovarian cancer. Semin Oncol 1998; 25: 356–60.
13. Ozols RF, Young RC, Speyer JL et al. Phase I and pharmacological studies of adriamycin administered intraperitoneally to patients with ovarian cancer. Cancer Res 1982; 42: 4265–9.
14. Gianni L, Jenkins JF, Greene RF, Lichter AS, Myers CE, Collins JM. Pharmacokinetics of the hypoxic radiosensitizers misonidazole and demethylmisonidazole after intraperitoneal administration in humans. Cancer Res 1983; 43: 913–16.
15. Arbuck SG, Trave F, Douglas Jr HO, Nava H, Zakrzewski S, Rustum YM. Phase I and pharmacologic studies of intraperitoneal leucovorin and 5-fluorouracil in patients with advanced cancer. J Clin Oncol 1986; 4: 1510–17.
16. Urba WJ, Clark JW, Steis RG et al. Intraperitoneal lymphokine-activated killer cell/interleukin-2 therapy in patients with intra-abdominal cancer: immunologic considerations. J Nat Cancer Inst 1989; 81: 602–11.
17. Markman M, Hakes T, Reichmann B, Hoskins W, Rubin S, Lewis Jr JL. Intraperitoneal versus intravenous cisplatin-based therapy in small-volume residual refractory ovarian cancer: evidence supporting an advantage for local drug delivery. Reg Cancer Treat 1990; 3: 10–12.

18. Alberts DS, Liu PY, Hannigan EV *et al.* Intraperitoneal cisplatin plus intravenous cyclophosphamide versus intravenous cisplatin plus intravenous cyclophosphamide for stage III ovarian cancer. N Engl J Med 1996; 335: 1950–5.

19. Markman M, Rowinsky E, Hakes T *et al.* Phase I trial of intraperitoneal taxol: a Gynecologic Oncology Group Study. J Clin Oncol 1992; 10: 1485–1491.

20. Markman M, Brady MF, Spirtos NM, Hanjani P, Rubin SC. Phase II trial of intraperitoneal paclitaxel in carcinoma of the ovary, tube, and peritoneum: a Gynecologic Oncology Group study. J Clin Oncol 1998; 16: 2620–4.

21. Muggia FM, Liu PY, Alberts DS *et al.* Intraperitoneal mitoxantrone or floxuridine: effects on time-to-failure and survival in patients with minimal residual ovarian cancer after second-look laparotomy – a randomized phase II study by the Southwest Oncology Group. Gynecol Oncol 1996; 61: 395–402.

22. Howell SB, Pfeifle CE, Wung WE, Olshen RA. Intraperitoneal *cis*-diamminedichloroplatinum with systemic thiosulfate protection. Cancer Res 1983; 43: 1426–31.

23. Dedrick RL. Interspecies scaling of regional drug delivery. J Pharm Sci 1986; 75: 1047–52.

24. Crafts RC. A Textbook of Human Anatomy, 2nd edn. New York: John Wiley, 1979, pp. 213–345.

25. Leak LB, Rahil K. Permeability of the diaphragmatic mesothelium: the ultrastructural basis for 'stomata'. Am J Anat 1978; 151: 557–94.

26. Bettendorf U. Lymph flow mechanism of the subperitoneal diaphragmatic lymphatics. Lymphology 1978; 11: 111–16.

27. Allen L. On the penetrability of the lymphatics of the diaphragm. Anat Rec 1956; 124: 639–58.

28. Yoffey JM, Courtice FC. Lymphatics, Lymph, and the Lymphomyeloid Complex. New York: Academic Press, 1970.

29. Flessner MF, Parker RJ, Sieber SM. Peritoneal lymphatic uptake of fibrinogen and erythrocytes in the rat. Am J Physiol 1983; 244: H89–96.

30. Abernathy NJ, Chin W, Hay JB, Rodela H, Oreopoulos D, Johnston MG. Lymphatic drainage of the peritoneal cavity in sheep. Am J Physiol 1991; 260: F353–8.

31. Flessner MF, Dedrick RL, Reynolds JC. Bidirectional peritoneal transport of immunoglobulin in rats: compartmental kinetics. Am J Physiol 1992; 262: F275–87.

32. Pearson CM. Circulation in skeletal muscle. In: Abramson DI, ed. Blood Vessels and Lymphatics. New York: Academic Press, 1962, pp. 520–1.

33. Flessner MF, Dedrick RL, Reynolds JC. Bidirectional peritoneal transport of immunoglobulin in rats: tissue concentration profiles. Am J Physiol 1992; 263: F15–23.

34. Rubin J, Clawson M, Planch A, Jones Q. Measurements of peritoneal surface area in man and rat. Am J Med Sci 1988; 295: 453–8.

35. Esperanca MJ, Collins DL. Peritoneal dialysis efficiency in relation to body weight. J Pediatr Surg 1966; 1: 162–9.

36. Ludwig J. Current Methods of Autopsy Practice. Philadelphia: WB Saunders, 1972.

37. Rhodin JAG. Histology: A Text and Atlas. New York: Oxford University Press, 1974.

38. Richardson KC. Illustrations of Light Microscopical Preparations from Various Tissues and Organs. Baltimore: University of Maryland School of Medicine, 1976.

39. diFiore MSH. Atlas of Human Histology. Philadelphia: Lea & Febiger, 1981.

40. Rubin J, Jones Q, Planch A, Stanek K. Systems of membranes involved in peritoneal dialysis. J Lab Clin Med 1987; 110: 448–53.

41. Vetterlein F, Schmidt G. Functional capillary density in skeletal muscle during vasodilation induced by isoprenaline and muscular exercise. Microvasc Res 1980; 20: 156–64.

42. Guyton AC. Textbook of Medical Physiology, 6th edn. Philadelphia: WB Saunders, 1981, p. 349.

43. Mapleson WW. An electric analogue for uptake and exchange of inert gases and other agents. J Appl Physiol 1963; 18: 197–204.

44. Bonaccorsi A, Dejana E, Quintana A. Organ blood flow measured with microspheres in the unanesthetized rat: effects of three room temperatures. J Pharmacol Meth 1978; 1: 321–8.

45. Grim E. The flow of blood in the mesenteric vessels. In: Hamilton WF, Dow P, eds. Handbook of Physiology. vol. II, sect 2, Washington: American Physiological Society, 1963, pp. 1443–56.

46. Chow CC, Grassmick B. Motility and blood flow distribution within the wall of the gastrointestinal tract. Am J Physiol 1978; 235: H34–9.

47. Crandall LA Jr, Barker SB, Graham DG. A study of the lymph flow from a patient with thoracic duct fistula. Gastroenterology 1943; 1: 1040.

48. Courtice FC, Simonds WJ, Steinbeck AW. Some investigations on lymph from a thoracic duct fistula in man. Austral J Exp Biol Med Sci 1951; 29: 201.

49. O'Morchoe CCC, O'Morchoe DJ, Holmes MJ, Jarosz HM. Flow of renal hilar lymph from volume expansion and saline diuresis. Lymphology 1978; 11: 27–31.

50. Shad H, Brechtelsbauer H. Thoracic duct lymph in conscious dog at rest and during changes of physical activity. Pfluegers Arch 1978; 367: 235–40.

51. Morris B. The exchange of protein between the plasma and the liver and intestinal lymph. Q J Exp Physiol 1956; 41: 326.

52. Yoffey JM, Courtice FC. Lymphatics, Lymph, and Lymphoid Tissue. Cambridge, MA: Harvard University Press, 1956: pp. 121–35.

53. Tran L, Rodela H, Abernethy NJ *et al.* Lymphatic drainage of hypertonic solution from peritoneal cavity of anesthetized and conscious sheep. J Appl Physiol 1993; 74: 859–67.

54. Daugirdas JT, Ing TS, Gandhi VC, Hano JE, Chen WT, Yuan L. Kinetics of peritoneal fluid absorption in patients with chronic renal failure. J Lab Clin Med 1980; 85: 351–61.

55. Rippe B, Stelin G, Ahlmen J. Lymph flow from the peritoneal cavity in CAPD patients. In: Maher JF, Winchester JF, eds. Frontiers in Peritoneal Dialysis. New York: Field, Rich, 1986, pp. 24–30.

56. Dykes PW, Jones JH. Albumin exchange between plasma and ascites fluid. Clin Sci 1964; 34: 185–97.

57. Mactier RA, Khanna R, Twardowski Z, Nolph KD. Role of peritoneal cavity lymphatic absorption in peritoneal dialysis. Kidney Int 1987; 32: 165–74.

58. Zink J, Greenway CV. Control of ascites absorption in anesthetized cats: effects of intraperitoneal pressure, protein, and furosemide diuresis. Gastroenterology 1974; 73: 1119–24.

59. Flessner MF, Schwab A. Pressure threshold for fluid loss from the peritoneal cavity. Am J Physiol 1992; 270: F377–90.

60. Nolph KD, Mactier R, Khanna R, Twardowski ZJ, Moore H, McGary T. The kinetics of ultrafiltration during peritoneal dialysis: the role of lymphatics. Kidney Int 1987; 32: 219–26.

61. Flessner MF. Net ultrafiltration in peritoneal dialysis: role of direct fluid absorption into peritoneal tissue. Blood Purif 1992; 10: 136–47.

62. Dedrick RL, Flessner MF, Collins JM, Schultz JS. Is the peritoneum a membrane? ASAIO J 1982; 5: 1–8.

63. Chagnac A, Herskovitz P, Weinstein T *et al.* The peritoneal membrane in peritoneal dialysis patients: estimation of its functional surface area by applying stereological methods to CT scans. J Am Soc Nephrol 1999; 10: 342–6.

64. Putiloff PV. Materials for the study of the laws of growth of the human body in relation to the surface areas of different systems; the trial on Russian subjects of planigraphic anatomy as a means for exact anthropometry – one of the problems of anthropology. Report of Dr P. V. Putiloff at the meeting of the Siberian Branch of the Russian Geographic Society, 29 October 1884, Omsk, 1886.

65. Dedrick RL, Myers CE, Bungay PM, DeVita VT. Pharmacokinetic rationale for peritoneal drug administration in the treatment of ovarian cancer. Cancer Treat Rep 1978; 61: 1–11.

66. Rippe B, Stelin G, Ahlmen J. Basal permeability of the peritoneal membrane during continuous ambulatory peritoneal

dialysis (CAPD). In: Maher J, ed. Advances in Peritoneal Dialysis, 1981. Amsterdam: Excerpta Medica, 1981, pp. 5–9.

67. Krediet RT, Struijk DG, Koomen GCM *et al.* Peritoneal transport of macromolecules in patients on CAPD. Contrib Nephrol 1991; 89: 161–74.

68. Keshaviah P, Emerson PF, Vonesh EF, Brandes JC. Relationship between body size, fill volume, and mass transfer area coefficient in peritoneal dialysis. J Am Soc Nephrol 1994; 4: 1820–6.

69. Flessner MF. Small solute transport across specific peritoneal tissue surfaces in the rat. J Am Soc Nephrol 1996; 7: 225–33.

70. Levitt MD, Kneip JM, Overdahl MC. Influence of shaking on peritoneal transfer in rats. Kidney Int 1989; 35: 1145–50.

71. Zakaria ER, Carlsson O, Rippe B. Limitation of small-solute exchange across the visceral peritoneum: effects of vibration. Perit Dial Int 1996; 17: 72–9.

72. Dedrick RL, Flessner MF. Pharmacokinetic problems in peritoneal drug administration: tissue penetration and surface exposure. J Natl Cancer Inst 1997; 89: 480–7.

73. Steller MA, Egorin MJ, Trimble EL *et al.* A pilot phase I trial of continuous hyperthermic peritoneal perfusion (CHPP) with high-dose carboplatin (CBDCA) as primary treatment of patients with small volume residual ovarian cancer. Cancer Chemother Pharmacol 1999; 43: 106–14.

74. Kim M, Lofthouse J, Flessner MF. Blood flow limitations of solute transport across the visceral peritoneum. J Am Soc Nephrol 1997; 8: 1946–50.

75. Torres IJ, Litterst CL, Guarino AM. Transport of model compounds across the peritoneal membrane in the rat. Pharmacology 1978; 17: 330–40.

76. Wikes AD, Howell SB. Pharmacokinetics of hexamethylmelamine administered via the ip route in an oil emulsion vehicle. Cancer Treat Rep 1985; 69: 657–62.

77. Lewis C, Lawson N, Rankin EM *et al.* Phase I and pharmacokinetic study of intraperitoneal thioTEPA in patients with ovarian cancer. Cancer Chemother Pharmacol 1990; 26: 283–7.

78. Aune S. Transperitoneal exchange. II. Peritoneal blood flow estimated by hydrogen gas clearance. Scand J Gastroenterol 1970; 5: 99–104.

79. Flessner MF. Transport of water soluble solutes between the peritoneal cavity and the plasma in the rat. (Dissertation.) Ann Arbor, MI: Department of Chemical Engineering, University of Michigan, 1981.

80. Grzegorzewska AE, Moore HL, Nolph KD, Chen TW. Ultrafiltration and effective peritoneal blood flow during peritoneal dialysis in the rat. Kidney Int 1991; 39: 608–17.

81. Collins JM. Inert gas exchange of subcutaneous and intraperitoneal gas pockets in piglets. Resp Phys 1981; 46: 391–404.

82. Demissachew H, Lofthouse J, Flessner MF. Tissue sources and blood flow limitations of osmotic water flow across the peritoneum. J Am Soc Nephrol 1999; 10: 347–53.

83. Zakaria ER, Carlsson O, Rippe B. Liver is not essential for solute transport during peritoneal dialysis. Kidney Int 1996; 50: 298–303.

84. Erb RW, Greene JA Jr, Weller JM. Peritoneal dialysis during hemorrhagic shock. J Appl Physiol 1967; 22: 131–5.

85. Pitts RF. Physiology of the Kidney and Body Fluids. Chicago: Year Book Medical Publishers, 1963, p. 63.

86. Lukas G, Brindle SD, Greengard P. The route of absorption of intraperitonelly administered compounds. J Pharmacol Exp Ther 1971; 178: 562–6.

87. Myers CE, Collins JM. Pharmacology of intraperitoneal chemotherapy. Cancer Invest 1983; 1: 395–407.

88. Brenner DE. Intraperitoneal chemotherapy: a review. J Clin Oncol 1986; 4: 1135–47.

89. Los G, McVie JG. Experimental and clinical status of intraperitoneal chemotherapy. Eur J Cancer 1990; 26: 755–62.

90. Markman M, Reichman B, Hakes T *et al.* Impact on survival of surgically defined favorable responses to salvage intraperitoneal chemotherapy in small-volume residual ovaian cancer. J Clin Oncol 1992; 10: 1479–84.

91. Ozols RF. Intraperitoneal chemotherapy. Current Prob Cancer 1992; 16: 99–101.

92. Alberts DS, Liu PY, Hannigan EV *et al.* Intraperitoneal cisplatin plus intravenous cyclophosphamide versus intravenous cisplatin plus intravenous cyclophosphamide for stage III ovarian cancer. N Engl J Med 1996; 335: 1950–5.

93. Farris FF, King FG, Dedrick RL, Litterst CL. Physiological model for the pharmacokinetics of *cis*-dichlorodiammineplatinum(II) (DDP) in the tumored rat. J Pharmacokin Biopharmacol 1985; 13: 13–39.

94. King FG, Dedrick RL, Farris FF. Physiological pharmacokinetic modeling of *cis*-dichlorodiammineplatinum(II) (DDP) in several species. J Pharmacokin Biopharm 1986; 14: 131–55.

95. King FG, Dedrick RL. Physiological pharmacokinetic parameters for *cis*-dichlorodiammineplatinum(II) (DDP) in the mouse. J Pharmacokin Biopharmacol 1992; 20: 95–9.

96. Goel R, Cleary SM, Horton C *et al.* Effect of sodium thiosulfate on the pharmacokinetics and toxicity of cisplatin. J Nat Cancer Inst 1989; 81: 1552–60.

97. Piccart MJ, Abrams J, Dodian PF *et al.* Intraperitoneal chemotherapy with cisplatin and melphalan. J Natl Cancer Inst 1988; 80: 1118–24.

98. Los G, Mutsaers PHA, van der Vigh WJF, Baldew GS, de Graaf PW, McVie JG. Direct diffusion of *cis*-diamminedichloroplatinum(II) in intraperitoneal rat tumors after intraperitoneal chemotherapy: a comparison with systemic chemotherapy. Cancer Res 1989; 49: 3380–4.

99. Flessner MF, Fenstermacher JD, Dedrick RL, Blasberg RG. A distributed model of peritoneal–plasma transport: tissue concentration gradients. Am J Physiol 1985; 248: F425–35.

100. Morrison PF, Dedrick RL. Transport of cisplatin in rat brain following microinfusion: an analysis. J Pharm Sci 1986; 75: 120–8.

101. Pretorius RG, Petrilli ES, Kean C, Ford LC, Hoeschele JD, Lagasse LD. Comparison of the iv and ip routes of cisplatin in dogs. Cancer Treat Rep 1981; 65: 1055–62.

102. Chabner BA. Fluorinated pyrimidines. In: Chabner B, ed. Pharmacologic Principles of Cancer Treatment. Philadelphia: WB Saunders, 1982, pp. 183–212.

103. Collins JM, Dedrick RL, King FG, Speyer JL, Myers CE. Nonlinear pharmacokinetic models for 5-fluorouracil in man: intravenous and intraperitoneal routes. Clin Pharmacol Ther 1980; 28: 235–46.

104. Sugarbaker PH, Graves T, DeBruijn EA *et al.* Early postoperative intraperitoneal chemotherapy as an adjuvant therapy to surgery for peritoneal carcinomatosis from gastrointestinal cancer: pharmacological studies. Cancer Res 1990; 50: 5790–4.

105. Archer SG, McCulloch RK, Gray BN. A comparative study of the pharmacokinetics of continuous portal vein infusion versus intraperitoneal infusion of 5-fluorouracil. Reg Cancer Treat 1989; 2: 105–11.

106. Gianola FJ, Sugarbaker PH, Barofsky I, White DE, Meyers CE. Toxicity studies of adjuvant intravenous versus intraperitoneal 5-FU in patients with advanced primary colon or rectal cancer. Am J Clin Oncol 1986; 9: 403–10.

107. Collins JM, Dedrick RL, Flessner MF, Guarino AM. Concentration-dependent disappearance of fluorouracil from peritoneal fluid in the rat: experimental observations and distributed modeling. J Pharm Sci 1982; 71: 735–8.

108. Cutler NR, Narang PK, Lesko LJ, Ninos M, Power M. Vancomycin disposition: the importance of age. Clin Pharmacol Ther 1984; 36: 803–10.

109. Moellering RC. Pharmacokinetics of vancomycin. J Antimicrob Chemother 1984; 14 (suppl.): D43–52.

110. Matzke GR, McGory RW, Halstenson CE, Keane WF. Pharmacokinetics of vancomycin in patients with various degrees of renal function. Antimicrob Agents Chemother 1984; 25: 433–7.

111. Rotschafer JC, Crossley K, Zaske DE, Mead K, Sawcuk RJ, Solem LD. Pharmacokinetics of vancomycin: observations

in 28 patients and dosage recommendations. Antimicrob Agents Chemother 1982; 22: 391–4.

112. Nielsen HE, Hansen HE, Korsager B, Skov PE. Renal excretion of vancomycin in kidney disease. Acta Med Scand 1975; 197: 261–4.

113. Cunha BA, Ristuccia AM. Clinical usefulness of vancomycin. Clin Pharmacol 1983; 2: 417–24.

114. Bunke CM, Aronoff GR, Brier ME, Sloan RS, Luft FC. Vancomycin kinetics during continuous ambulatory peritoneal dialysis. Clin Pharmacol Ther 1983; 34: 621–37.

115. Guyton AC. Textbook of Medical Physiology, 6th edn. Philadelphia: WB Saunders, 1981, p. 959.

116. Larner J. Insulin and oral hypoglycemic drugs and glucagon. In: Gilman AG, Goodman LS, Rall TW, Murad F, eds. Goodman and Gilman's The Pharmacological Basis of Therapeutics, 7th edn. New York: Macmillan, 1985, pp. 1490–503.

117. Duckworth WC. Insulin degradation: mechanisms, products, and significance. Endocrine Rev 1988; 9: 319–45.

118. Duckworth WC, Saudek CD, Henry RR. Why intraperitoneal delivery of insulin with implantable pumps in NIDDM? Diabetes 1992; 41: 657–61.

119. Shapiro DJ, Blumenkrantz MJ, Levin SR, Coburn JW. Absorption and action of insulin added to peritoneal dialysate in dogs. Nephron 1979; 23: 174–80.

120. Scarpioni L, Ballocchi S. Castelli A. Scarpioni R. Insulin therapy in uremic diabetic patients on continuous ambulatory peritoneal dialysis; comparison of intraperitoneal and subcutaneous administration. Perit Dial Int 1994; 14: 127–31.

121. Fuss M, Bergans A, Brauman H et al. ^{125}I-insulin metabolism in chronic renal failure treated by renal transplantation. Kidney Int 1974; 5: 372–7.

122. Navalesi R, Pilo A, Lenzi S, Donato L. Insulin metabolism in chronic uremia and in the anephric state: effect of the dialytic treatment. J Clin Endocrinol Metab 1975; 40: 70–85.

123. Wideroe T-E, Smeby LC, Berg KJ, Jorstad S, Svart TM. Intraperitoneal (^{125}I) insulin absorption during intermittent and continous peritoneal dialysis. Kidney Int 1983; 23: 22–8.

124. Micossi P, Cristallo M, Librenti MC et al. Free-insulin profiles after intraperitoneal, intramuscular, and subcutaneous insulin administration. Diabet Care 1986; 9: 575–8.

125. Williams G, Pickup J, Clark A, Bowcock S, Cooke E, Keen H. Changes in blood flow close to subcutaneous insulin injection site in stable and brittle diabetics. Diabetes 1983; 32: 466–73.

126. Zingg W, Rappaport AM, Leibel BS. Studies on transhepatic absorption. Can J Physiol Pharmacol 1986; 64: 231–4.

127. Selam J-L, Bergman RN, Raccah D, Jean-Didier N, Lozano J, Charles MA. Determination of portal insulin absorption from peritoneum via novel nonisotopic method. Diabetes 1990; 39: 1361–5.

128. Ward BG, Mather SJ, Hawkins LR et al. Localization of radioiodine conjugated to the monoclonal antibody HMFG2 in human ovarian carcinoma: assessment of intravenous and intraperitoneal routes of administration. Cancer Res 1987; 47: 4719–23.

129. Dedrick RL, Flessner MF. Pharmacokinetic Considerations on Monoclonal Antibodies. Immunity to Cancer. II. New York: Alan R. Liss, 1989, pp. 429–38.

130. Griffin TW, Collins J, Bokhari F et al. Intraperitoneal immunoconjugates. Cancer Res 1990; 50: 1031–8s.

131. Clauss MA, Jain RK. Interstitial transport of rabbit and sheep antibodies in normal and neoplastic tissues. Cancer Res 1990; 50: 3487–92.

132. Flessner MF, Lofthouse J, Zakaria ER. *In vivo* diffusion of immunoglobulin G in muscle: effects of binding, solute exclusion, and lymphatic removal. Am J Physiol 1997; 273: H2783–93.

133. Berk DA, Yuan F, Leunig M, Jain RK. Direct *in vivo* measurement of targeted binding in a human tumor xenograft. Biophysisics 1997; 94: 1785–90.

134. Fujimori K, Covell DG, Fletcher JE, Weinstein JN. Modeling analysis of the global and microscopic distribution of immunoglobulin G, F(ab')$_2$, and Fab in tumors. Cancer Res 1989; 49: 5656–63.

135. Fujimori K, Covell DB, Fletcher JE, Weinstein JN. A modeling analysis of monoclonal antibody percolation through tumors: a binding-site barrier. J Nucl Med 1990; 31: 1191–8.

136. van Osdol W, Fujimori K, Weinstein JN. An analysis of monoclonal antibody distribution in microscopic tumor nodules: consequences of a 'binding site barrier'. Cancer Res 1991; 51: 4776–84.

137. Flessner MF. Peritoneal transport physiology: insights from basic research. J Am Soc Nephrol 1991; 2: 122–35.

138. Flessner MF, Dedrick RL. Tissue-level transport mechanisms of intraperitoneally-administered monoclonal antibodies. J Controlled Rel 1998; 53: 69–75.

139. Rippe B, Haraldsson B. Fluid and protein fluxes across small and large pores in the microvasculature. Application of two-pore equations. Acta Physiol Scand 1987; 131: 411–28.

140. Flessner MF, Dedrick RL. Monoclonal antibody delivery to intraperitoneal tumors in rats: effects of route of administration and intraperitoneal solution osmolality. Cancer Res. 1994; 54: 4376–84.

29 | Peritoneal dialysis in developing countries

G. ABRAHAM AND A. GUPTA

Introduction

The incidence of new end-stage renal disease (ESRD) is gradually increasing because of increasing awareness about renal problems and greater availability of treatment facilities for this condition. In India itself it is reported that the incidence of new ESRD patients varies between 80 and 100/1 million population every year. However, the choice of treatment of ESRD depends on various non-medical factors such as the financial situation of the family, availability of a family donor for transplant, social and cultural habits, availability of facilities for dialysis and last but not least on the preference of the treating nephrologist. In most developing countries facilities for maintenance haemodialysis are limited and a cadaveric transplantation programme is yet to become a reality. There are only 0.3 haemodialysis centred/million population in India for maintenance haemodialysis [1]. The socioeconomic statuses of the various regions of the world are diverse and the gross domestic product (GDP) and per-capita income is low in the developing countries. In India the average per-capita income is US$500 per year. Even today 75% of the dialysis resources are reserved for only 15% of the world's poulation, and in many countries the sole alternative to dialysis or transplantation is death [2]. In large areas of Africa, Latin America, the Indian subcontinent and Southeast Asia, renal replacement therapy for renal failure is poorly developed and is affordable for only a small minority. The policies for treatment of patients with ESRD vary greatly from the developed to the developing world. This is largely based on government and medical insurance reimbursement policies, type of renal replacement therapy (RRT) done, and physician incentive to introduce peritoneal dialysis as an equal or better alternative form to haemodialysis.

Manual intermittent peritoneal dialysis (IPD) as a short-term modality for treatment of acute and chronic renal failure is being used in many developing countries because it is simple and does not require expensive and specialized equipment. Even today in many renal units in the developing countries stylet catheters are being inserted at the bedside to perform acute intermittent peritoneal dialysis using 1–2 L of fluid in glass bottles or non-collapsible plastic bags. However, repeated punctures have to be made for access into the peritoneal cavity twice a week for the IPD, which leads to a number of technical complications. These complications include peritonitis, from infection along the tunnel and from manually changing the bottles, and in the long run lead to the development of adhesions and obliteration of the peritoneal cavity [3–5].

Continuous ambulatory peritoneal dialysis (CAPD) as a modality of treatment in some Asian and South American countries started in the early 1980s. However, its use in most developing countries, including India, began only in the 1990s, and it is gratifying to note that during the past decade the maximum annual growth of CAPD in the world has been reported from these countries.

There are several problems in starting a CAPD programme in the developing world. There is still considerable lack of awareness and information about the benefits of CAPD both amongst the lay public and the medical community. Even many nephrologists consider CAPD to be inferior to haemodialysis and do not accept the potential advantages of CAPD. They are under the impression that the tropical climate would lead to a greater incidence of peritonitis. Patients in developing countries usually report for renal replacement therapy when they have advanced renal failure and significant malnutrition. As a result they are physically incapable of performing self-dialysis and are dependent on other family members. Further, because of prevailing cultural habits, relatives of patients would themselves not agree to patients participating in their own treatment. However since doing three or four exchanges every day is physically demanding,

R. Gokal, R. Khanna, R.Th. Krediet and K.D. Nolph (eds.), Textbook of Peritoneal Dialysis, 2nd Edition, 829–847.
© 2000 *Kluwer Academic Publishers. Printed in Great Britain.*

family support tends to wane after a certain period of time because of exhaustion on the part of the caregiver. There is also a certain inherent fear amongst people about doing CAPD at home, and they are not very confident about performing the procedure by themselves without supervision. Most developing countries lack good support systems, which are important if patients develop problems in the course of their treatment. Lack of reliable microbiology laboratories in smaller towns, and communication and transport problems, are some of these problems. Although these problems appear as minor constraints they limit the selection of patients to be put on CAPD.

The most important problem is, however, financial. Most developing countries have no health insurance system. In some of the countries partial to complete medical reimbursement is available only to government employees. The majority of patients are thus financing their own treatment. Presently the cost of consumables used in CAPD, such as fluid bags and delivery sets, is very high. In India the monthly expenditure for doing three exchanges/day by the cheapest system (straight-line system) is around US$300, while average per-capita income is around US$500/year. The cost of haemodialysis three times a week in India is around US$200/month. As a result patients who are put on CAPD after a certain period either drop out or do fewer exchanges than prescribed. The effects of under-dialysis have been seen by many nephrologists who have initiated CAPD programmes at their centres.

There is a mix of various systems being used in developing countries. While people from the more affluent sections of society have opted for the disconnect systems (such as Y-set, double-bag, etc.) patients coming to government hospitals have opted for the cheaper straight-line systems. This choice would also have an impact on infection rates of the patients.

In the following section of the chapter we have tried to focus on the penetration of CAPD and associated problems, some of which are unique to the developing countries.

PD growth in developing countries

There has been a general increase in the number of ESRD patients on PD in Asia in 1997 as compared to 1996 (Fig. 1). However, this trend was not seen in a large number of countries from South America. The exact reason for this negative growth is not clear; however, in Mexico over 90% of patients on renal replacement therapy are being treated on some form of PD.

There is also a great deal of variability in growth rate among different countries in the same continent. In Asia, countries such as Pakistan, India, Bangladesh, and Sri Lanka have shown the maximum growth. There are several reasons for this; one of them is that in many of these countries unrelated renal transplants are becoming illegal unless approved by specific committees. As a result many patients who could have had an unrelated renal transplant are now not able to get it done, and are having to opt for long-term dialysis. Since haemodialysis is not very readily available, because of shortage of dialysis machines, CAPD is gaining more popularity. Further there is now perhaps a greater awareness about this form of treatment in these countries, and some of the local industrial companies have started manufacturing the consumables locally, thereby making these products more easily available. Companies marketing CAPD products have also appointed clinical nurse coordinators who are able to visit these patients at their homes and to solve problems. This has led to a reduction in the drop-out rate and greater confidence of patients and their relatives in this form of therapy.

PD in Asia

PD utilization varies in different Asian countries [6]. In the 1980s chronic PD was initiated in Taiwan, China, Hong Kong, Singapore, Korea and Brunei [6]. It the 1990s the CAPD programme was started in India, Sri Lanka, Bangladesh, and Pakistan [7, 8]. The socioeconomic status of the Asian countries is diverse, and the cost of PD, government funding, insurance policies, and patient's choice influences the decision to put the patient on CAPD. Among various modalities of PD, CAPD is the commonest therapy being used in most Asian countries. The rate of utilization of PD systems varies greatly among different Asian countries. Automated PD is expensive as compared to conventional CAPD and is therefore not very frequently used. The cheaper systems such as conventional straight-line and the disconnect 'O' system, remain the dominant PD systems used in many Asian countries. However, there has been a progressive shift from the straight-line systems to disconnect systems during the past few years in these countries. PD utiliza-

PD PATIENTS

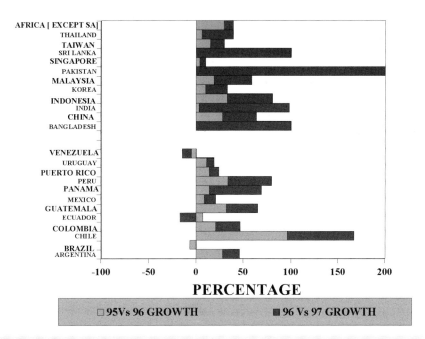

Figure 1. Patients on PD in Asia in 1997, compared with 1996.

tion rate appears to have a biphasic relationship with GDP per-capita income [6]. Countries with the highest (i.e. Japan and Taiwan) and lowest treatment rates (i.e. India, Indonesia, Pakistan, Bangladesh, Sri Lanka) tend to have lower PD utilization rates, whereas countries with modest treatment rates have higher PD utilization rates [6]. In countries with low treatment rates the complete lack of government reimbursement, and the fact that PD is almost twice as expensive as haemodialysis (HD), prevents the growth of the CAPD programme. The highest utilization rate in Asia has been reported in Hong Kong (74.3%) and this has been as a result of a deliberate policy to use CAPD as a first-line treatment for all ESRD patients because CAPD is considered to be more cost-effective than in-centre HD [6]. The lowest utilization rate in Asia has been reported from Pakistan [9].

The average number of daily CAPD exchanges varies among Asian countries. In most of the poorer countries the number of daily exchanges performed is usually three. The use of a lower number of exchanges was introduced initially as a cost-saving measure. The justification for the use of a low number of exchanges has been supported by a study from Hong Kong which showed

that patients routinely given 6 L daily exchanges have survival rates comparable to that of Caucasian patients routinely given 8 L daily exchanges or more exchanges [6]. This may be because Asian patients have a smaller body size.

PD in South America

There is variable penetration of PD as a modality of treatment for ESRD in the South American continent. While in Mexico over 90% of all ESRD patients are on PD, CAPD was introduced in Chile only in 1994, prior to which all ESRD patients were treated with HD. The prevalence of PD in Mexico is around 199.6 per million population [10]. About half of these patients are on IPD and the remainder are on CAPD. The rates of peritonitis in Mexico are about 1/24 patient-months on IPD and 1/15 patient-months on CAPD [10]. The annual mortality rates have been reported as 34% on IPD and 17% on CAPD [10]. In another centre from Mexico the survival of patients on CAPD is 67% and 48% at 1 and 3 years respectively [11]. Gamba *et al.* [11] reported that at their centre, after a follow-up of 12 ± 11 months, 32% of their patients were dead, 6% had discontinued treatment and 18% had received a kidney transplantation. Malnutrition is often present on CAPD, and contributes to morbidity and mortality. Espinoso *et al.* [12] studied 90 patients on CAPD for evidence of malnutrition. Ninety-one per cent of diabetics on CAPD and 76% of non-diabetics on CAPD showed some form of malnutrition. The authors concluded that diabetes mellitus and female sex were strong predictors for moderate and severe malnutrition [12]. It has been reported that peritonitis is an independent predictor of death in CAPD. Leanos-Miranda [13] has reported that IPD, peritonitis rates and level of basal serum albumin were associated with decreased survival in a univariate analysis. In a multivariate analysis the author reported that only high rate of peritonitis was associated with an increase in mortality rate, independent from other variables [13]. The cumulative survival in this Mexican centre has been reported as 64%, 29% and 13% at 12, 24 and 33 months [13]. Gamba *et al.* [11] from Mexico in their study showed that multivariate survival analysis according to the Cox proportional hazard model revealed that the most powerful predictor associated with a high risk of death was low serum albumin levels. Other independent variables associated with high risk of death on CAPD were advancing age, low serum creatinine concentration and elevated serum cholesterol levels [11].

In Brazil, while there was rapid initial growth, of late the number of patients on CAPD has levelled off [14]. The reason for this is not very clear. Patient survival was 78.6% and 40.7% at 1 and 5 years. Technique survival was 57.4% and 10.1% at 1 and 5 years [14]. Cost analysis of various treatment modalities for ESRD in Brazil has shown that CAPD is the most expensive. After 2 years of starting treatment the cost per year of survival was: CAPD $12 134, HD $10 065, cadaver transplant $6978 and live-related transplant $3022 [15]. However, this study also reported that although CAPD was less cost-effective, it yielded more years of survival after the initial 2 years of treatment [15]. In Mexico, however, the cost of treatment is covered by the treating institution.

CAPD has been used for treating children with ESRD both in Brazil and Argentina [14, 16]. In Argentina the incidence of peritonitis in children on CAPD was 1/15 patient-months [16]. Gram-positive organisms were present on culture in 60% of these episodes. Children with frequent episodes of peritonitis or with nephrotic syndrome had a poorer growth index for height [10]. The average duration of treatment with CAPD was around 4 years [16].

Catheter-related infections have become a prominent morbidity factor in CAPD. A study from Brazil by Alves *et al.* [17] has demonstrated that catheter-related infection occurred at a rate of 1/8 patient-months. Twenty-six per cent of all the episodes of peritonitis occurred secondary to catheter-related infection and almost half of catheter losses were due to this problem. Catheter-related infections were similar with both swan-neck or Tenckhoff catheters, or with 'O' set and disposable 'Y' set [17]. Catheter-related infections were found to be higher in the hotter months ($>32°C$) compared to months when the temperature was $<28°C$ (1/9 vs 1/19 patient-months, $p < 0.05$) [17]. It has been suggested that hot climate can adversely affect the rates of catheter-related infections.

The prevalence of hepatitis B and C infections in CAPD patients in South America is lower than in HD. Cendoroglo Neto *et al.* [18] from Brazil reported that HD treatment was the only risk factor significantly associated with HBV and HCV infections. The seroconversion for HbsAg on HD was 0.19/patient-year and for CAPD it was 0.01/patient-year. Seroconversion for anti-HCV on HD was 0.15/patient-year and for CAPD it was 0.03/patient-year [18]. The prevalence of hepatitis C among CAPD patients from another unit in Brazil has been reported as 17% [19] and there is great concern about the high prevalence of hepatitis C in the dialysis population in Brazil.

In Chile initial experience with CAPD has been encouraging. Fierro *et al.* [20] reported a peritonitis rate of 1/23.3 patient-months in CAPD patients and 1/36.7 patient-months in CCPD patients. The cumulative survival was 93.8% at 3 years. Amair *et al.* [21] from Venezuela reported that, although technique survival in CAPD patients at 5 years is inferior to HD (15% vs 39%), the crude mortality rate figures both at 1 and 5 years are better than for HD (HD 1 and 5 years 14.5% and 20.5%, CAPD 1 and 5 years 12.5% and 18.8%). The patient and technique survival in CAPD patients in Venezuela has been reported as 90% and 80% respectively at 1 year, and 35% and 20% respectively at 8 years on CAPD [21].

PD in central and eastern Europe

There has been a tremendous growth of PD in these countries. Over a 7-year period there has been an increment of 368% (400 patients in 1990 compared with 1873 patients in 1997) [22]. The majority of patients are on CAPD (94.5%). Reimbursement of PD treatment was from the government in the majority of the countries. In the Baltic countries, compared to a previous report [23] much progress has occurred. While in Estonia 25% of the ESRD patients are on CAPD, the figures are 8% in Latvia and 2% in Lithuania [24].

Peritonitis

Peritonitis and exit-site infections have been the major cause of morbidity and catheter loss in CAPD patients. With the development of newer catheters, better techniques of catheter placement, disconnect PD systems and better training the incidence of peritonitis and exit-site infections has been greatly reduced. Peritonitis rates have improved from one episode/4.5 patient-months as reported by al-Hilali et al. from Kuwait [25] in 1988 to one episode in 39.6 patient-months reported by Nitedvoravit et al. [31] from Thailand in 1998. Table 1 gives a comparison of peritonitis rates from various countries.

Gram-positive organisms lead to peritonitis more often than do Gram-negative organisms. Of the Gram-positive, coagulase-negative Staphylococcus is the most common offending organism [29]. Gram-negative peritonitis accounts for about one-third of all episodes of peritonitis. Lye et al. [45] reported an incidence of 28.6% of Gram-negative peritonitis

with E. coli (31.5%), P. aeruginosa (20%), Acinetobacter (15%) and Klebsiella (10%). Gram-negative infections can be successfully treated with aminoglycosides. Of the Gram-negative organisms, Pseudomonas is a difficult one to treat. Chan et al. [46] reported that Pseudomonas peritonitis accounted for 4.8% of all peritonitis. Pseudomonas infections recur very often, and prolonged treatment with two antibiotics (ceftazidime plus aminoglycoside) needs to be given for at least 3 weeks. Occasionally removal of the catheter may be necessary. Xanthomonas multiphalia (Gram-negative) has also been reported to cause peritonitis in CAPD patients. Szeto et al. [47] had six cases of peritonitis caused by this bacterium, accounting for 1.5% of all episodes of peritonitis. Recent bacterial peritonitis and treatment with broad-spectrum antibiotics are the major risk factors. In most instances the catheter would need to be replaced for complete eradication of this organism.

In the past it has been shown that the incidence of peritonitis is generally lower in patients on CCPD as compared to patients maintained on CAPD. However, with more advanced systems being introduced there has been a marked decrease in peritonitis rates. A study by Gahrmani et al. [28] has shown that both peritonitis and exit-site infections were significantly less in patients using ultra-bag systems for CAPD as

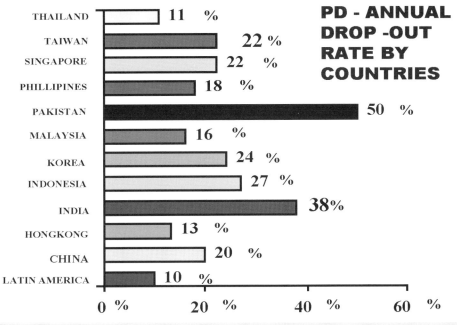

Figure 2. PD annual drop-out rates by country (data provided by Baxter, India, 1998).

Table 1. Peritonitis rates in various countries

Country and authors	Peritonitis (patient-months)	Organisms	Remarks
Kuwait			
al-Hilali *et al.* [25]	1/4.5	Gram + ve 34 Gram − ve 17	
Israel			
Benjamin *et al.* [26]	High risk 1/5.7 Low risk 1/13.2	Gram + ve 62.2% central nervous system (CNS) 55%	
Taiwan			
Chiou *et al.* [27]	1/15.2	CNS 32.4% *S. aureus* 14.7%	Manual spikes 1/4.6 'O' st 1/22.2
Iran			
Gahrmani *et al.* [28]	CAPD 1/23 CCPD 1/14.4		Ultra bag $p < 0.05$
Singapore			
Lee and Woo [29]	1/20.4	Gram + ve 54% CNS 24%	Catheter removal 14%
India			
Annigeri *et al.* [30]		Gram + ve 20% Gram − ve 10% Sterile 40%	'O' set
Abraham *et al.* [7]	1/20		
Thailand			
Nitedvoravit *et al.* [31]	1/31.6	CNS 53.19% methicillin resistant *Staphylococcus aureus* 10.6% Gram − ve 10.6%	
Mexico			
Su-Hernandez *et al.* [10]	IPD 1/24 CAPD 1/15		
Argentina			
Ramirez *et al.* [15]	1/15		Children on CAPD
Chile			
Fierro *et al.* [20]	CAPD 1/23.3 continuous cyclic peritoneal dialysis 1/36.7		
China			
Dai *et al.* [32]	1/28		
Han and Fan [33]	1/22.3		
Greece			
Konomopoulos *et al.* [34]	1/15		
Poland			
Rutkowski *et al.* [22]	1/19		
South Korea			
Kim *et al.* [35]	1/23		

There is some variation in the incidence of peritonitis reported from various developing countries. This may probably relate to the geographical, socioeconomic and educational background of the patients. Figure 4 gives the rates of incidence of peritonitis and exit-site infections in various countries [7, 10, 16, 20, 22, 25–44].

compared to CCPD (peritonitis, CAPD 1/23 patient-months vs CCPD 1/14.4 patient-months; exit-site infections, CAPD 1/35 patient-months vs CCPD 1/11.5 patient-months).

Patients with preexisting exit-site infections generally have more episodes of peritonitis. Exit-site infections are most often caused by *S. aureus* infection [29]. Persistent exit-site infections would require removal and replacement of the catheter. The duration of CAPD has not been found to influence the frequency of exit-site infections or peritonitis.

Patients with diabetes mellitus may have a higher incidence of peritonitis. Lye *et al.* [48] reported that diabetic patients on ESRD had a significantly higher incidence of peritonitis as compared to non-diabetics (1/10 episodes/patient-month vs 1/15 episodes/patient-month; $p < 0.005$).

The incidence of peritonitis in children being treated with CAPD is no different from that of adults. Chiou *et al.* [27] reported an incidence of peritonitis of one episode every 15.2 patient-months. Coagulase-negative *Staphylococcus* was responsible in 32.4% and *S. aureus* in 14.7. They also reported that children on manual spike straight-line systems had a higher incidence of peritonitis as compared to disconnect systems such as 'O' set (1/4.6 patient-months vs 1/12.2 patient-months).

Recurrent or resistant peritonitis in CAPD is often treated by removal of the catheter and putting the patient temporarily on HD. Locatelli *et al.* [49], however, reported their success in treating recurrent peritonitis in three patients by stopping CAPD for 2–4 weeks, leaving the catheter *in situ* and continuing antibiotic treatment.

The new Moncrief technique of burying the entire length of the catheter for at least 6 weeks prior to the start of CAPD has given good results in reducing the incidence of periluminal infections leading to peritonitis [50]. In a study by Han *et al.* [51] it was demonstrated that the incidence of peritonitis was significantly reduced using the Moncrief technique as compared to the conventional technique (1/14 patient-months vs 1/10.7 patient-months). It was also reported that there were fewer episodes of simultaneous peritonitis and exit-site infections using the Moncrief technique, thus suggesting that this technique eliminates infection by the periluminal route for establishing the diagnosis of peritonitis. In the lesser-developed countries, lack of well-established microbiological facilities at remote places is a major constraint for obtaining proper peritoneal fluid cultures. For this reason many CAPD centres

in India and other countries have a high incidence of culture-negative peritonitis (30–40%). It has been suggested that large volumes of the dialysate need to be centrifuged, and that the precipitate be used for inoculating the media for better yield. Superior methods of culture such as Bactac may provide better results [52]. Ishizakio *et al.* [53] have suggested that the endotoxin test, if used in CAPD patients, is 100% sensitive and specific for diagnosing Gram-negative peritonitis. The test takes about $1–1\frac{1}{2}$ h to perform; however this test cannot replace culture but may be a quick technique helpful in identifying Gram-negative infections. Peritoneal nitric oxide can be used as a marker for assessing treatment efficacy in CAPD patients with peritonitis. Yang *et al.* [54] reported a 5.1-fold increase in peak nitrite levels during bacterial peritonitis, and levels returned to normal after effective antibiotic treatment.

The conventional antibiotic regime of cefazolin and aminoglycoside is used for initiating treatment for peritonitis, as recommended by the International Society for Peritoneal Dialysis. However, for purposes of convenience, and reducing cost, some centres use different regimes with varying success. Dutta and Choudhary [55] reported that a 2-week course of oral ciprofloxacin (500 mg b.i.d.) and intraperitoneal gentamicin (single bag daily) was as effective as cefazolin and gentamicin or vancomycin and ceftazidime. This regime reduced the cost of treatment by 75% [55]; however a study by Cheng *et al.* [56] found oral ciprofloxacin to be ineffective, and these workers recommended using intraperitoneal ciprofloxacin at a dose of 50 mg/L to maintain adequate peritoneal trough levels.

Choice of catheters, break-in period, exit-site care and infections

Both straight Tenckhoff catheters and swan-neck catheters are being used. Straight catheters are cheaper and more widely available; however, certain centres have demonstrated that patients receiving swan-neck catheters have had a lower incidence of cuff extrusion, pericatheter leakage and catheter migration [57]. The incidence of exit-site/tunnel infections and catheter migration has been reported to be less with a swan-neck coiled catheter as compared to a straight Tenckhoff catheter. Lye *et al.* [58] reported exit-site infections of 0.29 episode per patient-year with swan-neck coiled versus 0.60 episode per patient-year with straight catheters. The coiled component of the catheter led to fewer episodes of catheter-tip migration [58]. It has also been recommended by some workers that fixing the catheter at two places can prevent its migration [59].

The use of prophylactic antibiotics at the time of insertion of the catheter is followed by many units, although a study by Lee *et al.* [60] revealed that preoperative administration of antibiotic as a prophylaxis (cefazolin and gentamicin) did not reduce the number of exit-site infections or peritonitis after insertion of the catheter.

Breaking in after catheter implantation is an important factor in the development of early catheter-related infections in CAPD patients. Lye *et al.* [61] studied two groups of patients who either had the catheter rested until the 14th day (group 1) after insertion or immediate use of the catheter for IPD (group 2). The authors reported no significant difference in the number of exit-site infections between groups 1 and 2. Many units routinely put patients on supine IPD with small volumes and short dwell times during the break-in period.

The technique of exit-site care is variable, ranging from daily cleansing to once a week, or using occlusive or non-occlusive dressings. However, most centres use povidone-iodine for cleansing, and hydrogen peroxide in addition in case of infection at the exit site. Tanaka [62] demonstrated that cleaning the exit site once a week and sealing it completely with an occlusive dressing leads to many fewer episodes of exit-site infection compared to daily care. However, this observation would not be readily acceptable in tropical countries where, because of humidity and warm climate, daily dressing would be required. Whether povidone-iodine is a good disinfectant is controversial, and Shino *et al.* [63] demonstrated that 46.8% of patients had a positive exit-site culture 1 h after cleaning with povidone-iodine.

The organisms causing exit-site infections are *S. aureus* (45%), *S. epidermidis* (15%), *E. coli* (15%), *P. aeruginosa* (5%) and *K. pneumoniae* (5%) [64]. Extrusion of the external cuff may be associated with recurrent exit-site infection. It has been shown that an external cuff reduces the episodes of exit-site infection from 0.79 episode/patient-year to 0.06 episode/patient-year [64]. Cuff shaving may be made easier if the external cuff is soaked in alcohol [65]. Catheter survival after cuff shaving may be as high as 50% [65]. The incidence of exit-site infections ranges from one episode in 27.3 patient-months [29], 1/35 patient-months [28] to 1/41.9 patient-

months [58]. These figures compare favourably with the incidence of exit-site infection in advanced countries.

Fungal peritonitis

The prevalence of fungal peritonitis is about the same as in the developed countries of the world. Chan *et al.* [66] and Wang *et al.* [67] from Hong Kong reported that 6.3–6.5% of all peritonitis episodes are due to fungal infections. From India Manjari *et al.* [68] reported an incidence of 6.73% of fungal peritonitis. Patients with more frequent bacterial peritonitis are at a higher risk of developing fungal peritonitis, and 28.6% of the cases in the study by Chan *et al.* [66] occurred after antimicrobial therapy. It has been reported that patients recently suffering from bacterial peritonitis (and if the infections are resistant to antibiotics) are at a greater risk of suffering from fungal peritonitis [69]. The majority of fungal peritonitis infections are caused by *Candida* (69–85%) [67, 70] but non-*Candida* fungal peritonitis episodes have been reported from India, Brazil, and Hong Kong [52, 71, 72]. *Candida albicans* peritonitis is associated with a worse outcome than non-*C. albicans* peritonitis. In one series 22% of patients with *C. albicans* infection could resume CAPD as compared to 42% of patients with non-*C. albicans* infection [67]. Patients who develop *de-novo* fungal peritonitis show lower mortality compared to patients developing fungal peritonitis after bacterial peritonitis [67]. The treatment of fungal peritonitis would include combination treatment with fluconazole, amphotericin B and removal of the catheter. Chan *et al.* [66] reported that giving treatment with fluconazole therapy alone, without catheter removal, the cure rate was only 9.5%, whereas with fluconazole plus catheter removal the cure rate improved to 66.7%. Addition of intravenous amphotericin B can be performed in patients not responding to fluconazole and catheter removal. Lee *et al.* [73] successfully used intracatheter amphotericin B and oral flucytosine for a period of 5 weeks for treating fungal peritonitis without catheter removal.

Mortality due to fungal peritonitis has ranged from 14.3% to 46% [66, 67]. CAPD can be successfully reinstituted after a waiting period of 4–6 weeks. There is a low prevalence of peritoneal adhesions and subsequent CAPD failure. Lo *et al.* [74] recommended that oral nystatin prophylaxis (500 000 units four times a day) may be given with each antibiotic prescription, since they found that this significantly reduced the rate of *Candida* peritonitis in CAPD patients.

Tuberculous peritonitis

The true incidence of tuberculosis (TB) in CAPD patients is unknown. Although TB peritonitis is a relatively rare entity, and accounts for 1–2% of peritonitis in developed countries, with the rapid expansion of PD in developing regions the incidence of TB peritonitis may be higher [75–78]. Occasionally patients may have concurrent fungal and tuberculous peritonitis [79]. Tuberculosis leading to peritonitis or reactivation of the disease with pulmonary and extrapulmonary involvement can manifest as prolonged fever, weight loss, anorexia, cough with haemoptysis or peritonitis. It can also present as non-specific symptoms in patients undergoing PD. TB peritonitis can result due to the spread of infection from an adjacent TB focus such as a mesenteric or para-aortic lymph node, intestine, Fallopian tube in women or during the course of miliary TB [80]. It is never due to primary infection through the catheter. In TB peritonitis a positive tuberculin test is seen in 30–100% of cases, and evidence of pleuropulmonary involvement is present in 25–83% of patients [80]. The clinical presentation is with abdominal pain, fever, and cloudy fluid. Although peritoneal lymphocytosis is reported, this is not a consistent finding, as predominant neutrophilia had been observed [79]. The peritoneal effluent is a poor specimen for demonstration of acid-fast bacillus (AFB) since only low numbers are present and the AFB cultures had been positive in only 25% of patients [81]. Occasionally a diagnostic laparoscopy, laparotomy and histological and microbiological examination of peritoneal biopsy specimens may be necessary for establishing the diagnosis [82]. The consequences of TB peritonitis, as it is a chronic disease, are malnutrition and loss of ultrafiltration capacity due to peritoneal sclerosis. Catheter removal appears not to be mandatory in all cases, provided prompt diagnosis and chemotherapy are carried out [83, 84]. Late ultrafiltration failure may develop after TB peritonitis if the PD is continued during chemotherapy. This is seen most frequently in patients in whom anti-tuberculous therapy has been delayed for more than 5 weeks after the onset of peritonitis [79, 85]. Therefore early diagnosis and chemotherapy for this unusual infection is crucial [86]. The chemotherapy consists of a combination of at least three drugs including rifampicin 600 mg, isoniazid 300 mg/day and pyrazinamide 1.5 g/day for 12 months [86]. Since streptomycin, even in reduced doses, may cause ototoxicity after prolonged use, it should not be administered in the ESRD patient. Similarly, ethambutal, because of the high risk of optic neuritis, is not recommended. Ciprofloxacin 750 mg/day, or ofloxacin 600–800 mg/day, or levofloxacin 750 mg/day may be used if four-drug therapy is required. Peritonitis that is culture, negative, unresponsive to treatment with conventional antibiotics, and that tends to relapse, with predominance of lymphocyte response in the dialysis effluent the diagnosis of TB, has to be considered. Appropriate therapy should be instituted as the disease carries a high degree of morbidity and mortality, especially in areas of developing countries where TB is endemic and in HIV-positive patients. Non-tubercular mycobacterial infection can occur during CAPD, and the presentation is similar to typical bacterial peritonitis. Along with appropriate therapy catheter removal may be required for management [87].

In developing countries where TB is endemic and a high proportion of patients on CAPD are diabetics, appropriate screening for TB, including Mantoux test and chest radiography, must be done before initiating patients on CAPD/CCPD. Appropriate chemotherapy should be given to prevent activation of the disease if patients have not been adequately treated previously.

Hepatitis B infection

Huang *et al.* [88] have demonstrated that 75% of CAPD patients were anti-HBsAg-positive as compared to 91.8% of normal controls (no significant difference). This probably reflects acquisition of HBV infection by CAPD patients before initiation of chronic dialysis therapy in a region hyperendemic for HBV. Patients on HD are more prone to become hepatitis B-positive as compared to patients on CAPD. In a study from Brazil [18] seroconversion on HD was found to be 0.19/patient-year, while on CAPD it was 0.01/patient-year. A Cox proportional hazards model showed that HD treatment was the only risk factor significantly associated with HBV infection, thus suggesting transmission through the environment [18]. The HBV attack rate in HD patients in Brazil has been found to be around 4.5% per year (range 0–6%) and an average 9.4% of HD patients are chronic carriers of hepatitis B virus

[19]. Pruritus is another common manifestation of viral hepatitis due to HBV in CAPD patients [89]. HBV infection, unlike HCV infection, did not cause significant serum aminotransferase elevation in CAPD patients; in fact CAPD patients in general were found to have significantly lower alanine amino transferase and aspartate amino transferase levels compared to adult controls who were HBV-positive [90].

Hepatitis C infection

HCV is an important agent of hepatitis in CAPD patients [91]. The prevalence of hepatitis C infection among patients on CAPD is significantly less than in patients on HD. There have been varying reports concerning the prevalence of HCV positivity from different countries (Table 2).

The prevalence of HCV infection is related to the duration and requirement of transfusion during HD [92, 93]. The risk of HCV infection is significantly increased in those who had received more than 5 units of blood transfusion [92]. However, a study from Japan [97] found no difference in the prevalence of HCV positivity in patients with a history of blood transfusion (32%) and those without this history (21%, $p > 0.05$). This study revealed that the frequency of becoming HCV-positive increased with

time on dialysis, the frequency being 50% with a dialysis period of more than 10 years.

The prevalence of anti-HCV has not been found to increase with the duration of CAPD. It has been suggested that CAPD offers better control of HCV infection [91]. A study from Brazil [18] showed that seroconversion from HCV-negative to HCV-positive was 0.15/patient-year for HD patients and 0.03/patient-year for CAPD patients. The hazard ratio for HCV infection in HD patients was 5.7 compared to CAPD patients. The prevalence of coexisting HBV and HCV infection in CAPD patients depends on the HCV status of the individual [88]. The detection of HCV can be improved by using the second-generation assays in uraemic patients [98]. Patients having severe pruritus are more prone to have infection with HCV, and screening for HCV infection should be done in uraemic patients on CAPD with unexplained itching. HCV is an important cause of chronic liver disease in CAPD patients and 31% of patients positive for anti-HCV were found to develop liver disease [97]. Hung *et al.* [90] suggested that serum aminotransferase cut-off values should be modified for screening viral hepatitis in CAPD patients. In their study they demonstrated that the conventional cut-off values of AST (40 IU/L) and ALT (40 IU/L) for detecting viral hepatitis yielded a sensitivity of 27.3% and 18.2% respectively. On the contrary, if the cut-off values were lowered, AST (24 IU/L) and ALT (17 IU/L), the sensitivity improved to 72.7% and 63.6%. For serial aminotransferase values the sensitivities of AST and ALT for detecting HCV were 36.4% and 27.3% by conventional criteria but 81.8% by their revised criteria [90].

Table 2. Prevalence of HCV positivity in various countries

Country	CAPD (%)	HD (%)	General population (%)
Hong Kong			
Chan *et al.* [92]	1.8	13.2	
South Korea			
Lee *et al.* [93]	5.3	27.8	
Taiwan			
Ng *et al.* [94]	29.7		4.2
Huang *et al.* [91]	15.4		
Hung *et al.* [88]	17.2		
Singapore			
Lee *et al.* [95]	6.5		
Saudi Arabia			1.4
al-Mugeiren *et al.* [96]	4.8	11.2	
Japan			
Nakashima *et al.* [97]	28		
Brazil			
Vanderborght *et al.* [19]	17	65	

Hepatitis G virus infection

Huang *et al.* [99] have demonstrated that the prevalence of GBV-C/HGV viraemia in CAPD patients was 23.3% compared with 1% in healthy adults ($p < 0.05$). Patients with GBV-C/HGV infection alone had received more blood transfusions. There are no significant differences between viraemic and non-viraemic groups with respect to age, gender, duration of previous HD, previous history of surgery and coinfection with HBV or HCV. It is known that GB virus C or hepatitis G virus can be transmitted parenterally, very probably sharing common routes of transmission with HCV. Mean ALT levels have been found to be significantly higher in the group with GBV-C/HGV infection compared to those without HBV, HCV infections [99].

Noh et al. [100] from South Korea reported a similar prevalence of HBV infection in patients on HD and CAPD (9.8% vs 12.7%). In both HD and CAPD patients HGV RNA was not related to age, sex, duration of dialysis, history of transfusion, history of hepatitis or to the presence of HBV or HCV markers [100]. It has been suggested that HGB infection does not seem to be associated with clinically significant hepatitis. The routes of HGV transmission other than transfusion or contamination during the HD procedure should be suspected [100, 101].

PD in CAPD patients with HIV infection

CAPD has been used as a renal replacement therapy for HIV-positive patients in developing countries [102, 103]. In Kenya, where there is a high prevalence of HIV infection, McLigeyo [102] reported the use of CAPD with a standard spike connection system. He reported a peritonitis rate of 1/1.5 patient-months in HIV-positive patients as compared to 1/5.7 patient-months in HIV-negative patients.

CAPD in children with ESRD

It is often difficult to dialyse children with ESRD or acute renal failure (ARF) with HD and PD (IPD or CAPD) has been found to be useful in dialysing these patients. The Japanese National Registry data on paediatric CAPD patients [104] provide interesting information. Over a period of 10 years, 434 children were on CAPD (8.5% of them being less than 1 year of age, 37.8% under 6 years of age). Half of these children were less than 20 kg in weight. The duration of CAPD was 2 years in 54% of the children and 11% of the children had been on CAPD for 5 years or more. About 10.5% of the children died, and 18% received a renal transplant. The patient survival rate was 85.6% at 3 years and 81.7% at 5 years. The technique survival was 74.9% at 3 years and 63.5% at 5 years. The rate of peritonitis was 1/28.6 patient-months. The peritonitis rates, catheter removal rate and rates of tunnel infection were worse in children less than 6 years of age. These data suggest that CAPD is an effective treatment for children with ESRD.

Chiou et al. [105] performed CAPD in 10 children (age 4–16 years) over a 3-year period. They found no evidence of malnutrition, and physical development improved. The most common compli-

cation in their series was peritonitis. In a larger series reported by the same group [27] the incidence of peritonitis was reported as 1/15.2 patient-months among 24 children on CAPD (mean age 2–17 years). Gram-positive organisms were responsible for peritonitis in 76.4% (coagulase-negative Staphylococcus 32.4% and S. aureus 14.7%). The manual spike straight-lime system was associated with a much higher incidence of peritonitis (1/4.6 patient-months) as compared to the disconnect systems such as 'O' set (1/22.2 patient-months). The authors felt that the main cause of peritonitis arose from contamination by the technical aspect of the procedure.

Munoz-Arizpe et al. [106] reported a peritonitis rate of 1/22 patient-months in uraemic children of low socioeconomic class on chronic PD. Many of their children developed malnutrition hypovolaemia and sepsis. Bahat et al. [107] from Turkey reported that the incidence of peritonitis is reduced as the time on CAPD increases. In their centre the incidence of peritonitis in children was 1/2.3 patient-months in the first 6 months of starting CAPD but it improved to 1/19 patient-months during the third year of PD. They did not find any correlation between the nutritional status and peritonitis rates. From India Abraham et al. [108] reported a peritonitis rate of 1/14 patient-months using disconnect systems in children. As has been reported in adults, the prevalence of anti-HCV in children on HD is significantly higher than in children on CAPD. al-Mugeiren et al. [96] reported a prevalence of 11.2% in Saudi children on HD, 4.8% in children on CAPD and 1.4% in normal children. According to those workers the high prevalence of anti-HCV in the HD group was possibly because of environmental contamination, and CAPD therapy might be helpful in reducing transmission of the HCV infection in children with ESRD. The incidence of peritonitis in Saudi children on CAPD has been reported as 1/9 patient-months [109]. This series reported that the majority of episodes were due to Gram-negative organisms (42%) followed by Gram-positive (20%), C. albicans (6%) and culture-negative in 32%. Peritoneal membrane loss was reported in 7/64 children and the morbidity rate was 4.6%, although none of the deaths was related to peritonitis or dialysis [109]. Araki et al. [110] reported that in long-term PD in children there is a high rate of development of sclerosing encapsulating peritonitis characterized by partial or intermittent bowel obstruction and marked sclerotic thickening of the peritoneal membrane.

PD has also been used to treat ARF in children. Kohli et al. [111] reported their experience in treating 31 infants and children with PD using a surgically placed Tenckhoff catheter. After an initial 24–48 h of continuous PD children were given 10 exchanges daily at 1 h intervals. The infection rate was less when a cycler was used as compared to the manual technique. In the opinion of Kohli *et al.* [111] this form of dialysis can be performed in remote places and is an effective and safe mode of treatment for children with ARF either using a Tenckhoff catheter or with a stylet PD catheter. The organisms causing peritonitis in children on acute PD are same as those in children treated by CAPD (*S. aureus* and coagulase-negative *Staphylococcus*) [112].

CAPD in diabetics with ESRD

Diabetic nephropathy is the leading cause of ESRD in the world, and a large number of diabetic ESRD patients are being accepted for renal replacement programmes. In India diabetes is the leading cause of ESRD among CAPD patients in most centres. This is because many of these patients are either elderly or have various comorbid conditions, particularly coronary artery disease, and therefore are not suitable for renal transplantation. Chan *et al.* [113] in 1987 reported that although diabetics on CAPD were significantly older than non-diabetics at their centre, they had a comparable biochemistry. The incidence of exit-site infection was 1/9.7 patient-months and the frequency of peritonitis was 1/94 patient-months [113]. Most of the diabetics in CAPD in their unit returned to work. They found good glycaemic control irrespective of the route of administration of insulin. There was no progressive increase in cholesterol or triglyceride. The cumulative patient survival at 2 years was 86% and technique survival was 100%.

Wei *et al.* [114] from Singapore reported their experience in 42 type II diabetics with ESRD on CAPD for a period of 18 months. Blood glucose was controlled either by diet and hypoglycaemic agents or insulin. The glucose control was similar in the three groups. These workers found no peritoneal membrane failure.

Lye *et al.* [48] reported peritonitis rates to be higher in diabetics on CAPD as compared to non-diabetics on CAPD (1/10 in diabetics vs 1/15 patient-months in non-diabetics; *p* < 0.05). However, they found no difference in the incidence of exit-site or tunnel infection, catheter loss or patient drop-out rates [48].

Diabetics on CAPD have been reported to have a greater prevalence of malnutrition than non-diabetics. Espinosa *et al.* [12] reported that, while 91% of diabetics on CAPD had evidence of malnutrition, only 76% of non-diabetics had a similar problem (*p* = 0.02). According to these authors [12] moderate to severe malnutrition was more frequent in diabetics.

Lee *et al.* [115] analysed their diabetic ESRD patients on CAPD and HD. Diabetic CAPD patients had more hospital admissions, more days of stay in hospital and higher withdrawal rates from dialysis compared to HD patients. The technique survival was, however, similar in both CAPD and HD. The mortality was lower in CAPD than HD in patients younger than 50 years of age, while it was higher in CAPD than HD in patients more than 50 years of age. An interesting observation by Wu *et al.* [116] was that diabetic patients on CAPD with poor glycaemic control predialysis had increased morbidity and shortened survival.

Nutrition

The incidence of malnutrition is high in the PD population, with approximately 50% of patients showing signs of malnutrition [117, 118]. The nutritional status may influence dialysis efficacy, the long-term survival rate and the quality of life of CAPD patients [118]. The factors contributing to malnutrition in dialysis patients include catabolic illness, poor dietary intake, and large losses of protein through the peritoneum, often exacerbated by bouts of peritonitis. It has been estimated that 0.5–2.0 g of protein is lost per litre of dialysate [119]. Pinlac and Danguclan [120] reported malnutrition with serum albumin of less than 4.0 g/dl in 80% of patients while starting CAPD in the Philippines, which increased mortality and morbidity. In most developing countries, ESRD patients wait until they are very ill before they start renal replacement therapy, and strict dietary protein restrictions imposed as part of conservative treatment during the predialysis phase further worsen the malnutrition. Malnutrition is a major factor affecting patient survival on PD therapy, as this predisposes to peritonitis, worsening of anaemia and other complications. In India and certain neighbouring countries a large percentage of CAPD patients are pure vegetarian, and significant malnutrition as assessed by anthropometric and biochemical markers has been encountered in these patients [121]. Jayanthi *et al.* [121] reported that vegetarians on

CAPD showed protein–calorie malnutrition, muscle wasting, low serum albumin, and low haemoglobin and transferrin levels, leading to an increased incidence of peritonitis. Malnutrition is more marked in CAPD patients who are diabetic as compared to non-diabetics [12, 122]. Espinoso et al. [12] reported that diabetes mellitus and female sex were strong predictors for moderate and severe malnutrition. Gamba [11] reported that a low serum albumin was the most powerful predictor of death. CAPD patients are advised to consume a protein intake of 1.2–1.5 g/kg/day. Yuan et al. [123] and Chen et al. [124] have shown that good nutritional management can improve the nutritional status in CAPD patients. The benefit of Chinese traditional medicine in improving the nutritional condition of CAPD patients has recently been reported [125].

Peritoneal membrane characteristics

The permeability of the peritoneal membrane varies considerably in patients from the developing countries [126–130], as demonstrated by the peritoneal equilibration test (PET). This is depicted in Fig. 4. There are no long-term data on the survival of CAPD patients according to peritoneal membrane characteristics from the developing countries. While in India it has been observed that the majority of patients are high transporters, other countries have not reported this. Korean patients show slightly lower peritoneal solute transfer rates than previously reported results in North American patients. The solute transfer rates of Korean patients decreases with time on peritoneal dialysis [131]. However, Cueto-Manzano et al. [132] reported that transport type as evaluated by PET was consistent over time in Mexican patients. Kumar et al. [126] found no statistically significant difference between diabetics and non-diabetics, vegetarians and non-vegetarians, or between females and males. The CANUSA study has shown a higher 2-year mortality in high transporters as compared to low transporters. This has also been reported by others from Asia [133, 134]. These high transporters may develop symptomatic fluid retention on CAPD. Thus it could be argued that the higher mortality seen in high transporters may reflect the adverse effect of fluid retention on underlying cardiovascular disease. This volume expansion would also explain some of the association on hypoalbuminaemia with high transport status and adverse outcomes. Whether transferring these patients to daytime short-dwell ambulatory peritoneal dialysis (DAPD) or switching the patients to cycler PD (CCPD) at night would favourably influence the outcome should be looked into in the future. In developing countries such as India, where the cost of CCPD is much higher, it would be advisable to transfer these patients to HD. An alternative approach might be to use a new osmotic agent such as icodextrin in the high transporter group [135].

PET RESULTS IN VARIOUS COUNTRIES

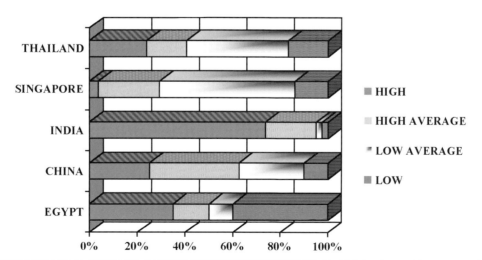

Figure 3. PET results in various countries.

PERITONITIS & EXIT SITE INFECTION RATE

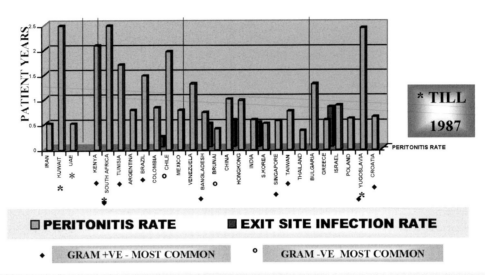

Figure 4. Peritonitis and exit-site infection rates.

PD annual drop-out rate

The annual drop-out rate from PD varies from 10% to 50% in various developing countries (Fig. 3). The major causes of drop-out are deaths (majority due to cardiovascular disease and malnutrition); transferred to HD (because of recurrent peritonitis/exit-site infection, fungal infections); transplant or stoppage of treatment for economic reasons.

Adequacy and long-term outcome of CAPD

The optimal dialysis level for the Asian population and its clinical impact have not been defined. The CANUSA study found an association of lower mortality and higher urea and creatinine clearances in CAPD patients. It is, however, uncertain if guidelines with regard to dialysis adequacy can be applied uniformly to Asians and Caucasians. The usual dialysis prescription in many Asian countries is three 2 L exchanges/day because of financial constraints; this dialysis prescription would be considered suboptimal by Western standards. Szeto et al. [136] reported that 78% of their patients were on three exchanges/day while the remainder were on four exchanges/day. Patients who were performing four exchanges/day had a higher Kt/V ($\geqslant 1.7$), higher

haemoglobin and higher nPCR. However, patients on three exchanges/day ($Kt/V < 1.7$) had a 5-year survival of 79% and their rehabilitation status was the same as those for four exchanges/day [136]. The authors felt that small-volume dialysis may be possible in the Asian population because of smaller body size and the dietary difference compared to the Western population. This has been the impression of other workers who feel that, because of the smaller surface area, it may be easier to maintain the patient with fewer exchanges [137]. Kim et al. [138] observed that patients with lower body surface area had better serum albumin levels when given three exchanges/day. It appears that small body size is the key for adequate dialysis and nutrition.

However, recently Noh et al. [139] compared patients whose $Kt/V > 2.1$ with those whose $Kt/V < 2.1$. While the 2-year survival was same in the two groups (97.9% vs 95.6%), the 5-year survival was significantly better in patients with higher Kt/V (97.9% vs 66.8%). These authors [139] felt that, even in Asian patients who have a smaller body surface area, the dose of dialysis (Kt/V) would determine long-term patient survival.

There is considerable debate about the long-term outcome of CAPD. Okada et al. [140] suggested that the time limit for CAPD can be expected to be approximately 6–8 years in a stable CAPD patient because of problems induced by CAPD on the peritoneal membrane. In their study [140] they observed the dose relationship between mean dialysate osmolality and duration of CAPD. As the duration of CAPD increased there was an increase in serum creatinine and osmolality which resulted in problems in clearances and ultrafiltration. Kawaguchi *et al.* [141] reported their 16-year experience with 224 patients. They observed that ultrafiltration loss was the most prominent cause of withdrawal from CAPD in patients who were on CAPD for more than 6 years.

Gamba *et al.* [11] from Mexico reported survival rates of 67% and 48% at 1 and 3 years. Multivariate analysis according to the Cox proportional hazards model showed that the most powerful predictor associated with high risk of death was low serum albumin. Other independent variables were advancing age, low serum creatinine concentration and elevated serum cholesterol levels. Zent *et al.* [142] from South Africa reported an overall mean survival time on CAPD of 17.3 months. Multivariate analysis demonstrated increased peritonitis rates associated with age, black race, diabetes, psychosocial factors and socioeconomic variables.

Ye *et al.* [143] reported that long-term survival of Chinese patients was less than that of patients from Western countries. Patients with age > 55 years, weight < 50 kg, poor socioeconomic state, residual urine output < 550 ml/day, haemoglobin < 6 g/dl, serum albumin < 33 g/L, serum creatinine < 800 µmol/L can all lead to lower survival probabilities. The survival reported by Ye *et al.* [143] at 1, 2, 3 and 4 years was 85.6%, 67.1%, 56.9% and 44.4%.

From India Palanirajan *et al.* [144] and Aparajitha *et al.* [145] reported drop-out rates of around 50%. Most of the drops-outs were related to deaths secondary to associated comorbid conditions. Peritonitis contributed to 20% of the drop-outs in one of the series [144].

The survival of patients on CAPD has been found to be related to residual renal function. Lo *et al.* [146] reported that survival in patients who had higher initial residual renal function was much better, and thus recommend an early start of CAPD. Kobayashi *et al.* [147] suggested that CAPD should be started before the patient loses residual renal function because four bag exchanges as the standard CAPD prescription might not be adequate once the patient becomes progressively anuric.

It has also been reported that high transporters have significantly higher mortality, and this may be related to low serum albumin concentration and fluid retention. Chu *et al.* [133] reported a significant difference in the survival of high and low transporters at both 1 and 3 years. Lee *et al.* [134] observed a significant decrease of serum albumin levels in high transporters, and this decrease was seen after 31–36 months CAPD.

What then are the important issues that need to be addressed so that survival on CAPD may be prolonged. Kawaguchi *et al.* [148] from Japan state that although there is a reduction in peritonitis rates (1/40–1/60 patient-months in Japan) the incidence of exit-site/tunnel infection is still around 1/30 patient-months. New techniques need to be devised to prevent this infection. The peritoneal membrane gradually deteriorates as the duration of CAPD is increased, and there are reports of excapsulating peritonitis. An ideal PD solution needs to be developed. Further, Kawaguchi *et al.* [148] observed that 26% of the CAPD patients at their centre were malnourished; this problem also needs urgent attention. Further research needs to be done on the nutritional status of the patient, peritoneal membrane characteristics, clearances and patient outcome. In developing countries the caregivers should understand their patients' complex needs and recognize the importance of professional development. It is also important to develop a manual in local languages with graphic descriptions and simple protocols which are easy to follow, with a step-by-step guide for the management of the patient. This would provide consistent and routine emergency medical care to patients living in remote areas where there is no prior experience with CAPD. The most important thing, however, is to make CAPD cheaper and economically viable for ESRD patients from the poorer countries of the world. The majority of patients from the developing countries are financing their own treatment since there is no health insurance available. The use of fewer exchanges has been introduced as a cost-saving measure in poorer countries [6]. Studies performed to compare the quality of life of CAPD and HD patients found no significant difference [149]. If CAPD becomes cheaper and more affordable, it will become as popular as HD because of its inherent advantages.

Acknowledgements

The authors gratefully acknowledge help in preparation of this chapter from Dr Revathi Suppiah, Miss Jyothi Mutreja and Mr Santosh Kumar Verma. The authors also thank Baxter, India, for providing the relevant data.

References

1. Sakhuja V, Jha V, Ghosh AK *et al.* Chronic renal failure in India. Nephrol Dial Transplant 1994; 9: 871–2.

2. Maiorca R, Maggiore R, Mordacci E *et al.* Ethical problems in dialysis and transplantation. Nephrol Dial Transplant 1996; 11 (suppl. 9): 100–12.

3. Rashid HU, Azhar MA, Rahman A. Management of end stage renal disease with intermittent peritoneal dialysis. Perit Dial Bull 1986; 6: 214.

4. Trevino-Becerra A. Intermittent peritoneal dialysis with a cycler may be the answer. Perit Dial Bull 1984; 4: 112.

5. Tripathi K, Jai Prakash. Peritoneal dialysis in post-abdominal surgery in elderly patients developing acute renal failure. Perit Dial Bull 1987; 7: S78.

6. Cheng IK. Peritoneal dialysis in Asia. Perit Dial Int 1996; 16 (suppl. 1): S381–5.

7. Abraham G, Bhaskaran S, Soundarajan P *et al.* Continuous ambulatory peritoneal dialysis. J Assoc Phys India 1996; 44: 599–601.

8. Samad MA. CAPD: experience in Bangladesh. Perit Dial Int 1998; 18 (suppl. 2): S24.

9. Rizvi SAH. Present state of dialysis and transplantation in Pakistan. Am J Kidney Dis 1998; 31: x/v–x/viii.

10. Su-Hernandez L, Abascal Macias A, Mendez Bueno FJ *et al.* Epidemiologic and demographic aspects of peritoneal dialysis in Mexico. Perit Dial Int 1996; 16: 362–5.

11. Gamba G, Mejia JL, Saldivav S *et al.* Death risk in CAPD patients. The predictive values of the initial clinical and laboratory variables. Nephron 1993; 65: 23–7.

12. Espinoso A, Cueto Manzano AM, Velazquez Alva C *et al.* Prevalence of malnutrition in Mexican CAPD diabetic and nondiabetic patients. Adv Perit Dial 1996; 12: 302–6.

13. Leanos Miranda A. Factors predicting survival in patients on peritoneal dialysis. Rev Invest Clin 1997; 49: 355–60.

14. Thome FS, Rodrigues AT, Bruno R *et al.* CAPD in southern Brazil: an epidemiological study. Adv Perit Dial 1997; 13: 141–5.

15. Sesso R, Eisenberg JM, Stabile C *et al.* Cost effectiveness analysis of the treatment of end stage renal disease in Brazil. Int J Technol Assess Health Care 1990; S6: 107–14.

16. Ramirez JA, Ruiz S, Ferraris T *et al.* Continuous ambulatory peritoneal dialysis (CAPD): an alternative for the treatment of children with terminal chronic renal insufficiency in Argentina. Bol Med Hosp Infant Mex 1991; 48: 140–3.

17. Alves FR, Dantas RC, Lugon JR. Higher incidence of catheter related infections in a tropical climate. Adv Perit Dial 1993; 9: 244–7.

18. Cendoroglo Neto M, Draibe SA, Silva AE *et al.* Incidence of and risk factors for hepatitis B virus and hepatitis C virus infection among haemodialysis and CAPD patients: evidence for environmental transmission. Nephrol Dial Transplant, 1995; 10: 240–6.

19. Vanderborght BO, Rouzere C, Ginuino CF *et al.* High prevalence of hepatitis C infection among Brazilian haemodialysis patients in Rio de Janeiro: a one year follow up study. Rev Inst Med Trop Sao Paulo, 1995; 37: 75–9.

20. Fierro JA, Gomez E, Labbe E *et al.* Peritoneal dialysis new ESRD treatment in Chile. Perit Dial Int 1998; 18 (suppl. 2): S19.

21. Amair P, Betancor J, Weisenger JR. Comparison between CAPD and haemodialysis (HD) mortality rates. Perit Dial Int 1998; 18 (suppl. 2): S17.

22. Rutkowski B, Lichodziejewska-Niemeierko M, Reneke M *et al.* Current status of peritoneal dialysis (PD) in Poland. Perit Dial Int 1998; 18 (suppl. 2): S14.

23. Lazovkis I. Nephrology, dialysis and renal transplantation in Latvia: problems of our speciality in a country of the former Soviet block. Nephrol Dial Transplant 1994; 9: 214–16.

24. Petersons A, Ritz E. Nephrology in the Baltic countries. Nephrol Dial Transplant 1998; 13: 2779–80.

25. al-Hilali N, Cozma G, Abu Romesh S *et al.* Incidence of peritonitis on CAPD in Kuwait APMIS Suppl. 1988; 3: 101–3.

26. Benjamin J, Ben Ezer Gradus D, Mostoslavski M *et al.* Peritonitis in continuous ambulatory peritoneal dialysis patients in Southern Israel. Isr J Med Sci 1989; 25: 699–702.

27. Chiou YY, Chen WP, Yang LY, Lin CY. Peritonitis in children being treated with continuous ambulatory peritoneal dialysis. CAPD Team Chung Hua Min Kuo Hsiao Erh Ko L Hsueh Hui Tsa Chth 1995; 36: 176–83.

28. Gahrmani N, Gorban Brennan N, Kliger AS, Finkelstein FO. Infection rates in end stage renal disease patients treated with CCPD and CAPD using the ultra bag system. Adv Perit Dial. 1995; 11: 164–7.

29. Lee GS, Woo KT. Infection in continuous ambulatory peritoneal dialysis (CAPD): etiology, complications and risk factors. Ann Acad Med Singapore 1992; 21: 354–60.

30. Annigeri RA, Prakash GK, Balasubramaniyam R *et al.* 'O' set connector system in CAPD. J Assoc Phys India 1996; 44: 602–5.

31. Nitedvoravit S, Sivivongs D, Chunleritrith D. Outcome of peritonitis in CAPD in a Thai Medical centre. Perit Dial Int 1998; 18 (suppl. 2): S78.

32. Dai J, Hu Y, Zheng ZH. Nursing care can improve quality of dialysis in CAPD patients Perit Dial Int 1998; 18 (suppl. 2): S46.

33. Han QF, Fan MH. Five years' peritoneal dialysis experience in China. Perit Dial Int 1998; 18 (suppl. 2): S19.

34. Konomopoulos D, Dombros N, Balaskas E *et al.* Survival and complications of 103 catheters used in CAPD and intraperitoneal chemotherapy. Perit Dial Int 1998; 8: 75.

35. Kim JK, Shin YH, Park YK *et al.* Clinical observation of CAPD and HD patients. Perit Dial Int 1998; 18 (suppl. 2): S19.

36. Alwi K, Dwarkanathan R, Chin S, Chin LS, Krishnan Aung. CAPD: is it an adequate therapy for end stage renal patients in developing countries? Perit Dial Int 1988; 18: S28.

37. el-Matri A, Ben Abdallah T, Kechrid C *et al.* Continuous ambulatory peritoneal dialysis in Tunisia. Nephrologie 1990; 11: 153–6.

38. Salahudeen AK, D'Costa K, Pingle A. Successful experience with CAPD in UAE. Perit Dial Bull 1987; 7: S66.

39. Agastini L, Leon L, Rojas M. Treatment with CAPD for 54 months of a patient with end stage renal disease due to multiple myeloma. Perit Dial Bull 1986; 6: 46.

40. Drinovec J, Bren A, Gucek A *et al.* 42 months overview of CAPD peritonitis in one center. Perit Dial Bull 1987; 7: S26.

41. Laradi A, Krowri A, Drif M. Management of a CAPD program in developing country – an Algerian perspective. Perit Dial Int 1988; 8: 84.

42. Balista AV, Dangilan RA. The prevalence of peritonitis in renal patients on CAPD. Perit Dial Int 1998; 18 (suppl. 2): S78.

43. Henao JE, Meija G, Arbelaez M *et al.* Six and a half years of experience with three two liter daily exchanges in CAPD. Perit Dial Int 1988; 8: 207–10.

44. Jankroic N, Varlaj V, Pavloic D. The morbidity and mortality rate in CAPD patients. Perit Dial Int 1998; 18: S82.

45. Lye WC, Van der Straaten JC, Leong SO *et al.* Once daily intraperitoneal gentamycin is effective therapy for Gram negative CAPD peritonitis. Perit Dial Int 1998; 18 (suppl. 2): S74.

46. Chan MK, Chan PC, Cheng IP *et al.* Pseudomonas peritonitis in CAPD patients: characteristics and outcome of treatment. Nephrol Dial Transplant 1989; 4: 814–7.

47. Szeto CC, Li PK, Leung CB *et al. Xanthomonas maltophilia* in uremic patients receiving ambulatory peritoneal dialysis. Am J Kidney Dis 1997; 29: 91–5.

48. Lye WC, Leong SO, vander Straaten JC, Lee EJ. A prospective study of peritoneal dialysis related infections in CAPD patients with diabetes mellitus. Adv Perit Dial 1993; 9: 195–7.

49. Locatlli A, Quiroga MA, De Benedetti L *et al.* Treatment of recurrent and resistant CAPD peritonitis by temporary with-

drawal of peritoneal dialysis without removal of the catheter. Adv Perit Dial 1995; 11: 176–8.

50. Park MS, Yim AS, Chung SH *et al.* Effect of prolonged subcutaneous implantation of peritoneal catheter on peritonitis rate during CAPD: a prospective randomized study. Blood Purif 1998; 16: 171–8.

51. Han DC, Cha HK, So IN *et al.* Subcutaneously implanted catheters reduce the incidence of peritonitis during CAPD by eliminating infection by periluminal route. Adv Perit Dial 1992; 8: 298–301.

52. Gupta A. Fungal and bacterial infection in peritoneal dialysis. Personal communication.

53. Ishizaki M, Oikawa K, Miyashita E. Usefulness of the endotoxin test for assessing CAPD peritonitis by gram negative organisms. Adv Perit Dial 1996; 12: 199–202.

54. Yang CW, Hwang TL, Wu CH *et al.* Peritoneal nitric oxide is a marker of peritonitis in patients on continuous ambulatory peritoneal dialysis. Nephrol Dial Transplant 1996; 11: 2466–71.

55. Dutta AR, Choudhary S. Oral ciprofloxacin and intraperitoneal gentamycin: effective and cheap therapy for peritonitis. Perit Dial Int 1998; 18 (suppl. 2): S75.

56. Cheng IK, Chan CY, Wong WT *et al.* A randomized prospective comparison of oral versus intraperitoneal ciprofloxacin as the primary treatment of peritonitis complicating continuous ambulatory peritoneal dialysis. Perit Dial Int 1993; 13 (suppl. 2): S351–4.

57. Hwang TL, Huang CC. Comparison of swan-neck catheter with Tenckhoff catheter for CAPD. Adv Perit Dial 1994; 10: 203–5.

58. Lye WC, Kour NW, Van der Straten JC *et al.* A prospective randomized comparison of the Swan neck, coiled and straight Tenckhoff catheters in patients on CAPD. Perit Dial Int 1996; 16 (suppl. 1): S333–5.

59. Yeh TJ, Wei CF, Chiu TW. Catheter related complications of continuous ambulatory peritoneal dialysis. Eur J Surg 1992; 158: 277–9.

60. Lee WC, Lee EJ, Tan CC. Prophylactic antibiotics in the insertion of Tenckhoff catheters. Scand J Urol Nephrol 1992; 26: 177–80.

61. Lye WE, Giang MM, Vander Straaten JC, Lee EJ. Breaking in after insertion of Tenckhoff catheters: a comparison of two techniques. Adv Perit Dial 1993; 9: 236–9.

62. Tanaka S. Sealing the catheter exit site with dressing film and its effectiveness in preventing exit site infection: bacterial culture. Adv Perit Dial 1996; 12: 214–17.

63. Shino T, Okade T, Matsumoto H, Nakao T. Ineffectiveness of disinfectant treatment using povidone iodine in the prevention of exit site infection in peritoneal dialysis. Perit Dial Int 1998; 18 (suppl. 2): S37.

64. Kim JH, Park SH, Kim JC *et al.* Outcome of external cuff shaving for persistent exit site infection in CAPD. Perit Dial Int 1998; 18 (suppl. 2): S15.

65. Thiruventhiran T, Fitzgerald GH, Tan SY. Catheter cuff shaving procedure: description of a novel technique using the common catheter. Perit Dial Int 1998; 18 (suppl. 2): S16.

66. Chan TM, Chan CY, Cheng SW *et al.* Treatment of fungal peritonitis complicating ambulatory peritoneal dialysis with fluconazole: a series of 21 patients. Nephrol Dial Transplant 1994; 9: 539–42.

67. Wang AYM, Yu AWY, Li PKT *et al.* An analysis of a nine-year trend of fungal peritonitis in CAPD patients. Perit Dial Int 1998; 18 (suppl. 2): S75.

68. Manjari M, Abraham G, Sekhar U *et al.* Outcome of patients on CAPD with fungal peritonitis. Ind J Perit Dial 1998; 1: 37–9.

69. Zhu Z, Zhang W, Yang X *et al.* The factors related to fungal peritonitis in patients on peritoneal dialysis. J Tongji Med Univ 1997; 17: 123–5.

70. Cheng IK, Fang GX, Chan TM, Chan PC, Chan MK. Fungal peritonitis complicating peritoneal dialysis: a report of 25 cases and review of treatment. Q J Med 1989; 71: 407–16.

71. Lopes JO, Alves SH, Benevenga JP, Rosa AL. The second case of peritonitis due to *Histoplasma capsulatum*. Mycoses 1994; 37: 161–3.

72. Chan TH, Koehler A, Li PK. *Paecilomyces varioti* peritonitis in patients on continuous ambulatory peritoneal dialysis. Am J Kidney Dis 1996; 27: 138–42.

73. Lee SH, Chiang SS, Hseih SJ, Shen HM. Intra catheter amphotericin B retention for fungal peritonitis in continuous ambulatory peritoneal dialysis. J Formos Med Assoc 1995; 94: 132–4.

74. Lo WK, Chan CY, Cheng SW, Poon JF. A prospective randomized control study of oral nystatin prophylaxis for Candida peritonitis complicating continuous ambulatory peritoneal dialysis. Am J Kidney Dis 1996; 28: 549–52.

75. Lui SL, Lo CY, Choy BY *et al.* Optimal treatment and long term outcome of tuberculous peritonitis complicating continuous ambulatory peritoneal dialysis. Am J Kidney Dis 1996; 28: 747–51.

76. Vathsala A, Thomas A, Ng BL, Lim CH. An unusual case of peritonitis. An Acad Med Singapore 1987; 16: 666–70.

77. Tsai TC, Hsu JC, Chou LH, Lee ML. Tuberculous peritonitis in a child undergoing continuous ambulatory peritoneal dialysis. Chung Hua Min Kuo Hsiao Erh Ko L Hseuh Hui Tsa Chih. 1994; 35: 455–9.

78. Aparajitha C, Abraham G, Sekhar U *et al.* Tuberculosis in a cohort of CAPD population. Perit Dial Int 1998; 18 (suppl. 2): S37.

79. Zimmerman S, Abraham G. Was CAPD the answer to the patient's complex problems? Perit Dial Int 1997; 17: 630–6.

80. Bastani B, Shariatzadeh MR, Dehdasthi F. Tuberculous peritonitis: report of 30 cases and review of literature. Q J Med 1985; 56: 549–57.

81. Fernandez-Rodriguez CM, Perez-Arguelles BS, Ledo L *et al.* Ascitic adenosine deaminase activity is decreased in tuberculous ascites with low protein content. Am J Gastroenterol 1991; 86: 1500–3.

82. Singh MM, Bhargava AN, Jain KP. Tuberculous peritonitis: an evaluation of pathogenic mechanism, diagnostic procedures and therapeutic measures. N Engl J Med 1969; 281: 1091–4.

83. Mallet SG, Brensitner JM. Tuberculous peritonitis in a CAPD patient cured without catheter removal – case report, review of the literature and guidelines for treatment and diagnosis. Am J Kidney Dis 1989; 13: 57.

84. Tan D, Fein PA, Jorden A, Avram MM. Successful treatment of tuberculous peritonitis while maintaining patient on CAPD. Adv Perit Dial 1991; 7: 102–4.

85. Vas SI. Renaissance of tuberculosis in the 1990's. Lessons for the nephrologist. Perit Dial Int 1994; 14: 209–14.

86. Keane WF, Alexander SR, Baile GR *et al.* Peritoneal dialysis related peritonitis, treatment recommendations 1996 update. Perit Dial Int 1996; 16: 557–73.

87. Dunmire RB, Breyer JA. Nontuberculous mycobacterial peritonitis during continuous ambulatory peritoneal dialysis: case report and review of diagnostic and therapeutic strategies. Am J Kidney Dis 1991; 18: 126–30.

88. Hung KY, Shyu RS, Huang CH, Tsai TJ, Chen WY. Viral hepatitis in continuous ambulatory peritoneal dialysis patients in an endemic area for hepatitis B and C infection: the Taiwan experience. Blood Purif 1997; 15: 195–9.

89. Hung KY, Shyu RS, Tsai TJ, Chen WY. Viral hepatitis infection should be considered for evaluating uremic pruritus in continuous ambulatory peritoneal dialysis patients. Blod Purif 1998; 16: 147–53.

90. Hung KY, Lee KC, Yen CJ *et al.* Revised cutoff values of serum aminotransferase in detecting viral hepatitis among CAPD patients: experience from Taiwan, an endemic area for hepatitis B. Nephrol Dial Transplant 1997; 12: 180–3.

91. Huang CC, Wu MS, Lin DY, Liaw YF. The prevalence of hepatitis C virus antibodies in patients treated with continuous ambulatory peritoneal dialysis. Perit Dial Int 1992; 12: 31–3.

92. Chan TM, Lok AS, Cheng IK. Hepatitis C infection among dialysis patients: a comparison between patents on maintenance haemodialysis and continuous ambulatory peritoneal dialysis. Nephrol Dial Transplant 1991; 6: 944–7.

93. Lee HY, Kang DH, Park CS et al. Comparative study of hepatitis C virus antibody between haemodialysis and continuous ambulatory peritoneal dialysis patients. Yon sei Med J 1993; 34: 371–80.

94. Ng YY, Lee SD, Wu SC et al. Antibodies to hepatitis C virus in uremic patients on continuous ambulatory peritoneal dialysis. J Med Virol 1991; 35: 263–6.

95. Lee GS, Roy DK, Fan FY et al. Hepatitis C antibodies in patients on peritoneal dialysis: prevalence and risk factors. Perit Dial Int 1996; 16 (suppl. 1): S424–8.

96. al-Mugeiren M, al-Rasheed S, al-Sallum A et al. Hepatitis C virus infection in two groups of pediatric patients: one maintained on hemodialysis and the other on continuous ambulatory peritoneal dialysis. Ann Trop Pediatr 1996; 16: 335–9.

97. Nakashima F, Sate M, Takeshi S et al. Incidence of antibodies to hepatitis C virus in patients undergoing chronic dialysis or CAPD. Murume Med J 1993; 40: 249–53.

98. Ng YY, Lee SD, Wu SC et al. The need for second generation anti-hepatitis C virus testing in uremic patients on continuous ambulatory peritoneal dialysis. Perit Dial Int 193; 13: 132–5.

99. Huang CH, Kao JH, Kuo YM et al. GB virus C/hepatitis G virus infection in patients on continuous ambulatory peritoneal dialysis. Nephrol Dial Transplant 1988; 13: 2914–19.

100. Noh H, Kang SW, Choi SH et al. Hepatitis G virus infection in hemodialysis and continuous ambulatory peritoneal dialysis patients. Yonsei Med J 1998; 39: 116–21.

101. Kim BS, Park JH, Shin YS et al. The incidence and clinical impact of hepatitis G virus infection in peritoneal dialysis and haemodialysis patients. Perit Dial Int 1998; 18 (suppl. 2): S12.

102. McLigeyo SO. Initial experience with CAPD in patients with HIV infection in a developing country. Perit Dial Int 1992; 12: 267–8.

103. Abraham G, Ravi R, Venkat R et al. Successful use of CAPD as ESRD treatment in a HIV patient. JAPI 1994; 42: 828–9.

104. Honda M, Iitika K, Kawaguchi H et al. The Japanese National Registry data on pediatric CAPD patients: a ten year experience. A report of the study group of Pediatric PD conference. Perit Dial Int 1996; 16: 269–75.

105. Chiou YH, Chen WP, Lin CY. Continuous ambulatory peritoneal dialysis for children with end stage renal disease. Chung Hua Min Kuo Hsiao Erh Ko I Hsueh Hui Tsa Chih 1990; 31: 280–7.

106. Munoz-Arizpe R, Salazar-Gutierrez ML, Gordillo-Paniagua G. Adequacy of chronic peritoneal dialysis in low socio economic class uremic children. Int J Pediatr Nephrol 1986; 7: 81–4.

107. Bahat E, Akman S, Ozcan S et al. CAPD adaptation period and the relationship with the peritonitis rate in children. Perit Dial Int 1998; 18 (suppl. 2): S57.

108. Abraham G, Padma G, Mattew M, Shroff S. Ambulatory peritoneal dialysis in children: our experience. Ind J Perit Dial 1998; 1: 57.

109. Mirza K, Elzonki AY. Peritonitis in continuous ambulatory peritoneal dialysis in children living in Saudi Arabia. Pediatr Nephrol 1997; 11: 325–7.

110. Araki Y, Hataya H, Tanaka Y et al. High incidence of peritoneal dialysis sclerosis in children in long term PD. Perit Dial Int 1998; 18 (suppl. 2): S54.

111. Kohli HS, Arora P, Kher V et al. Daily peritoneal dialysis using a surgically placed Tenckhoff catheter for acute renal failure in children. Renal Failure 1995; 17: 51–56.

112. Kim JH, Kim PK. Clinical study of continuous ambulatory peritoneal dialysis (CAPD) and acute peritoneal dialysis in children. Perit Dial Int 1998; 18 (suppl. 2): S57.

113. Chan MK, Lam SS, Chin KW. Continuous ambulatory peritoneal dialysis (CAPD) in diabetic patients with end stage renal failure in Hong Kong. J Diabet Compli 1987; 1: 11–15.

114. Wei SS, Lee GS, Woo KT, LiM CH. Continuous ambulatory peritoneal dialysis in Type II diabetics Ann Acad Med Singapore 1993; 22: 629–33.

115. Lee HB. Dialysis in patients with diabetic nephropathy: CAPD vs HD. Perit Dial Int 1996; 16 (suppl. 1): S269–74.

116. Wu MS, Yu CC, Wu CH et al. Predialysis glycemic control is an independent predictor of mortality in type II diabetic patient on CAPD. Perit Dial Int 1998; 18 (suppl. 2): S10.

117. Young GA, Kopple JB, Lindholm B et al. Nutritional assessment of CAPD patients: an interpersonal study. Am J Kidney Dis 1991; 17: 462–71.

118. Guo D, Wang G, Jiang Y. Assessment of the nutritional status in 52 cases of CAPD patients. Perit Dial Int 1998; 18 (suppl. 2): S53.

119. Harty J, Gokal R. Nutritional status in PD. J Renal Nutr 1995; 5: 2–10.

120. Pinlac G, Danguclan RA. Nutritional parameters in new CAPD gpatients. Perit Dial Int 1998; 18 (suppl. 2): S52.

121. Jayanthi V, Ravichandran P, Abraham G. Nutritional problems in patients on CAPD. Perit Dial Int 1998; 18 (suppl. 2): S49.

122. Hong D: Nutritional status in CAPD patients. Perit Dial Int 1998; 18 (suppl. 2): S52.

123. Yuan B, Zhang Y, Chen X et al. The influence of dietary management on nutritional status in continuous ambulatory peritoneal dialysis patients. Perit Dial Int 1998; 18 (suppl. 2): S51.

124. Chen TP, Lee HP. Oral nutritional supplement improves nutritional status of CAPD patients. Perit Dial Int 1998; 18 (suppl. 2): S50.

125. Kong W. Clinical observation of CAPD patients nutritional condition in the use of Chinese traditional medicine. Perit Dial Int 1998; 18 (suppl. 2): S52.

126. Kumar R, Abraham G, Padma G et al. Peritoneal equilibration test in a CAPD population. Ind J Perit Dial 1998; 1: 34–6.

127. Naga SS, El-Belbessi A. Peritoneal equilibration test (PET) in acute peritoneal dilaysis (APD). Perit Dial Int 1998; 18 (suppl. 2): S3.

128. Sirivongs D, Chunlertrith D, Seetaso K. A modified PET for small size CAPD patients. Perit Dial Int 1998; 18 (suppl. 2): S3.

129. Wang NS, Tong LQ, Gao XP et al. Clinical use of PET. Kt/V and PCR in peritoneal dialysis patients. Perit Dial Int 1998; 18 (suppl. 2): S6.

130. Lye WC, vander Straaten JC, Leong SO et al. A cross sectional study on adequacy of dialysis, peritoneal equilibration test and nutrition in Asian CAPD patients. Perit Dial Int 1998; 18 (suppl. 2): S3.

131. Park JH, Koh SH, Kim BS et al. Reference range of values of peritoneal equilibration test and changes in peritoneal kinetics in long term Korean patients. Perit Dial Int 1998; 18 (suppl. 2): S61.

132. Cueto-Manzano AM, Gamba G, Abasta-Jimenez M, Correa-Rotter R. Consistency of the peritoneal equilibration test in a cohort of non selected Mexican CAPD patients. Adv Perit Dial 1995; 11: 114–18.

133. Chu WS, Yi HA, Kim YH et al. Peritoneal membrane hyperpermeability is a risk factor for CAPD mortality. Perit Dial Int 1998; 18 (suppl. 2): S10.

134. Lee IH, Kim BS, Hwang JH et al. Serial changes of serum albumin according to the peritoneal membrane transport characteristics in long term CAPD patients. Perit Dial Int 1998; 18 (suppl. 2): S11.

135. Peers E, Gokal R. Icodextrin: overview of clinical experience. Perit Dial Int 1997; 17: 22–6.

136. Szeto CC, Lai KN, Yu AW et al. Dialysis adequacy of Asian patients receiving small volume continuous ambulatory peritoneal dialysis. Int J Artif Organs 1997; 20: 428–35.

137. Lye WC, vander Straaten JC, Leong SD *et al.* A cross sectional study on adequacy of dialysis, peritoneal equilibration test and nutrition in Asian CAPD patients. Perit Dial Int 1998; 18 (suppl. 2): S3.

138. Kim YL, Kim JH, Kim SJ *et al.* Nutrition and dialysis adequacy of Korean patients on long term continuous ambulatory peritoneal dialysis. Perit Dial Int 1998; 18 (suppl. 2): S3.

139. Noh HT, Shin SK, Kang SW *et al.* Impact of dialysis dose on clinical outcomes in Korean continuous ambulatory peritoneal dialysis (CAPD) patients. Perit Dial Int 1998; 18 (suppl. 2): S-1.

140. Okada K, Takahashi S, Higuchi T *et al.* How long can continuous ambulatory peritoneal dialysis be continued? Nippon Jinzo Gokkai Shi 1993; 35: 65–71.

141. Kawaguchi Y, Hasegava T, Kubo H *et al.* Current issues of continuous ambulatory peritoneal dialysis. Artif Organs 1995; 19: 1204–9.

142. Zent R, Myers JE, Donald D, Rayner BL. Continuous ambulatory peritoneal dialysis: an option in the developing world? Perit Dial Int 1994; 14: 48–51.

143. Ye RG, Lu CS, Li HQ. Survival probability and multivariate analysis of prognostic factors in CAPD patients. Perit Dial Int 1998; 18 (suppl. 2): S11.

144. Palanirajan S, Prakash KC. Dropouts in continuous ambulatory peritoneal dialysis in India since 1993: a single centre experience. Perit Dial Int 1998; 18 (suppl. 2): S22.

145. Aparajitha C, Chaitanya C, Abraham G *et al.* Causes of dropout from CAPD in a developing country. Perit dial Int 1998; 18 (suppl. 2): S24.

146. Lo WK, Lo LY, Cheng SW *et al.* Early commencement of dialysis is important for better CAPD patient survival. Perit Dial Int 1998; 18 (suppl. 2): S2.

147. Kobayashi H, Kasai K, Terawaki H *et al.* Significance of residual renal functions of patients with end stage renal failure undergoing continuous ambulatory peritoneal dialysis. Nippon Jinzo Gakki Shi 1997; 39: 783–9.

148. Kawaguchi Y, Hasegawa T, Nakayama M *et al.* Issues affecting the longevity of continuous ambulatory peritoneal dialysis therapy. Kidney Int 1997; 62: S105–7.

149. Wang T, Lin B, Ye RG. Comparison of quality of life in continuous ambulatory peritoneal dialysis and hemodialysis patients. Chung Hua Nei Ko Tsa Chi 1993; 32: 754–6.

Index